Physiology and Medicine of Hyperbaric Oxygen Therapy

Physiology and Medicine of Hyperbaric Oxygen Therapy

Tom S. Neuman, MD, FACP, FACPM

Emeritus Professor of Medicine
University of California, San Diego
San Diego, California

Stephen R. Thom, MD, PhD

Professor of Emergency Medicine
Chief, Hyperbaric Medicine
University of Pennsylvania
Philadelphia, Pennsylvania

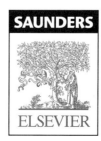

SAUNDERS

ELSEVIER

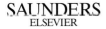

1600 John F. Kennedy Blvd.
Ste 1800
Philadelphia, PA 19103-2899

PHYSIOLOGY AND MEDICINE OF HYPERBARIC OXYGEN THERAPY   ISBN: 978-1-4160-3406-3

Notice

Knowledge and best practice in this field are constantly changing. As new research and experience broaden our knowledge, changes in practice, treatment, and drug therapy may become necessary or appropriate. Readers are advised to check the most current information provided (i) on procedures featured or (ii) by the manufacturer of each product to be administered, to verify the recommended dose or formula, the method and duration of administration, and contraindications. It is the responsibility of the practitioner, relying on their own experience and knowledge of the patient, to make diagnoses, to determine dosages and the best treatment for each individual patient, and to take all appropriate safety precautions. To the fullest extent of the law, neither the Publisher nor the Editors assume any liability for any injury and/or damage to persons or property arising out of or related to any use of the material contained in this book.

The Publisher

Library of Congress Cataloging-in-Publication Data

Physiology and medicine of hyperbaric oxygen therapy / [edited by] Tom S. Neuman, Stephen R. Thom. – 1st ed.
    p. ; cm.
Includes bibliographical references and index.
ISBN 978-1-4160-3406-3
1. Hyperbaric oxygenation. I. Neuman, Tom S. II. Thom, Stephen R.
[DNLM: 1. Hyperbaric Oxygenation. WB 342 P578 2008]
RM666.O83P49 2008
615.8'36–dc22

2007044397

Editor: Dolores Meloni
Developmental Editor: Kim DePaul
Project Manager: Mary Stermel
Design Direction: Louis Forgione
Marketing Manager: Paul Leese

Printed in the United States of America

Last digit is the print number: 9 8 7 6 5 4 3 2 1

Dedication

To all of our colleagues in the practice of hyperbaric medicine who have worked so tirelessly to bring our specialty into the mainstream of medicine.

And, most importantly, to our best friends and wives—Doris and Lynne.

Preface

If one is to be candid, the field of hyperbaric medicine is a relatively new one. The biological effects of pressure were sporadically investigated in the 18th and early 19th centuries, but the first cohesive, scientific analysis was carried out by Paul Bert, who published *La Pression Barometrique* in 1878. Hyperbaric chambers were used initially to treat a variety of "humors," but then interest began to focus on decompression sickness. It was not until the second half of the 20th century that hyperbaric chambers were used to treat conditions other than decompression illness on a more frequent basis. As such, early pioneers were clinically oriented and had their roots in either diving or aerospace medicine.

Thus hyperbaric medicine began as a clinical discipline. Early practitioners had a physiological rationale for hyperbaric oxygen therapy (HBOT), but clinical utilization was emphasized over basic science. It has been only recently that the basic science behind hyperbaric medicine has been explored, and this continues with ever-increasing sophistication. Of equal importance, it has been only recently that more rigor has been applied to the clinical situations in which HBOT might benefit patients. There is now a pool of knowledge concerning basic physiology and clinical outcomes that would benefit from being collected into one volume.

This was the purpose of this textbook. It was our goal to try to assemble all of the important physiological information, as well as the carefully conducted clinical investigations of HBOT. This text is meant to be a reference tool for researchers and clinicians to help them gain a better understanding of the fundamental mechanisms of HBOT; it also serves as a critical review of the indications for HBOT. It is not intended to be a simple recitation of the virtues of hyperbaric medicine but rather an academic approach to the subject. With this in mind the book is organized to deal with the practical issues of HBOT and the physiology behind the treatment. It addresses each of the generally accepted indications for HBOT with what the editors hope is fair academic vigor.

We feel that two chapters deserve special mention. The first of these is the chapter devoted to "Fitness to Dive." Because so many of the current clinicians practicing hyperbaric medicine no longer have their background in diving medicine, we felt this chapter was especially important. Practicing hyperbaric physicians are often called upon to examine commercial and sport divers to assess their fitness to dive, and at times to treat diving-related injuries. Our coverage of other diving medicine topics was limited, however, because there are several excellent texts in this area. The reader is referred to Bennett and Elliott's *Physiology of Medicine and Diving* as well as Bove and Davis's *Diving Medicine*. This text is not meant to replace those texts but rather to accompany them, and for all to be found side by side at any hyperbaric chamber installation. The second chapter that warrants special mention is devoted to the unconventional uses of hyperbaric medicine. In current times, with medicine being scrutinized carefully for its ever-increasing costs, this chapter turns a critical eye to conditions for which HBOT has been advocated without there being a firm rationale and/or data for its use. We make no apologies for the critical nature of this chapter. We believe such directness is overdue within the field of hyperbaric medicine.

With so many individuals as authors, the editors have tried to the best of their abilities to create a more or less uniform style for the chapters so that the reader may go from one chapter to another more easily. The symbols for respiratory abbreviations and concepts are those used by Elsevier throughout their publications. The units of pressure are those used most frequently in the field of hyperbaric medicine.

We hope this book meets the needs of our many colleagues.

Tom S. Neuman, MD, FACP, FACPM
Stephen R. Thom, MD, PhD

Contributors

Oskar Baenziger, MD
Professor
University of Zurich
Director, Department of Intensive Care
    and Neonatology
University Children's Hospital
Zurich, Switzerland

Richard C. Baynosa, MD
Plastic Surgery Resident
University of Nevada School of Medicine
Las Vegas, Nevada

**Michael H. Bennett, MBBS, MD,
MM(Clin Epi), FANZCA**
Associate Professor, Faculty of Medicine
The University of New South Wales
Senior Staff Specialist, Department of Diving
    and Hyperbaric Medicine
Division of Anaesthesia
Prince of Wales Hospital
Sydney, Australia

Alfred A. Bove, MD, PhD
Emeritus Professor of Medicine
Chief, Section of Cardiology
Temple University School of Medicine
Medical Staff
Temple University Hospital
Philadelphia, Pennsylvania

Jon A. Buras, MD, PhD
Research Associate Professor
Northeastern University
New England Inflammation and Tissue
    Protection Institute Consortium
Departments of Biology and Pharmaceutical
    Sciences
Boston, Massachusetts
Staff Physician in Emergency Medicine,
    Wound Care, and Hyperbaric Medicine
South Shore Hospital
Weymouth, Massachusetts
Consultant in Hyperbaric Medicine
Massachusetts Eye and Ear Infirmary
Boston, Massachusetts

Frank K. Butler, Jr., MD
Adjunct Associate Professor of Military
    and Emergency Medicine
F. Edward Hebert School of Medicine
Uniformed Services University of the Health
    Sciences
Medical College of Georgia
Augusta, Georgia
Staff Ophthalmologist
Naval Hospital
Pensacola, Florida

James M. Clark, MD, PhD
Clinical Associate Professor of Environmental
    Medicine in Pharmacology
Institute for Environmental Medicine
University of Pennsylvania School of Medicine
Philadelphia, Pennsylvania

Dick Clarke
Director, The Baromedical Research
    Foundation
Columbia, South Carolina

Dominic P. D'Agostino, PhD
Postdoctoral Fellow, Department of Molecular
  Pharmacology and Physiology
University of South Florida
School of Basic Biomedical Sciences, College
  of Medicine
Tampa, Florida

Jay B. Dean, PhD
Professor of Molecular Pharmacology
  and Physiology
Head of Hyperbaric Biomedical Research
  Laboratory
University of South Florida
Tampa, Florida

John J. Feldmeier, DO, FACRO
Professor and Chairman, Radiation Oncology
  Department
University of Toledo
Chairman and Clinical Director, Department
  of Radiation Oncology
University of Toledo Medical Center
Toledo, Ohio

Nachum Gall, MD
Director, Institute of Hyperbaric Medicine
  and Wound Care Center
Assaf Harofeh Medical Center
Zerifin, Israel

Lisardo Garcia-Covarrubias, MD
Cardiothoracic Surgery Fellow
University of Miami/Jackson Memorial Hospital
Miami, Florida

Anthony J. Gerbino, MD
Clinical Assistant Professor
University of Washington School of Medicine
Head, Section of Pulmonary/Critical Care
  Medicine
Virginia Mason Medical Center
Seattle, Washington

Peter Gilbey, MD
Head of Otolaryngology, Head and Neck Surgery
Sieff Medical Center
Zefat, Israel

Des F. Gorman, MBChB, MD, PhD
Head of the School of Medicine
The University of Auckland
Auckland, New Zealand

Catherine Hagan, MD
Senior Resident
Naval Medical Center
San Diego, California

Neil B. Hampson, MD
Clinical Professor of Medicine
University of Washington School of Medicine
Medical Director, Center for Hyperbaric
  Medicine
Virginia Mason Medical Center
Seattle, Washington

Kevin Hardy, MD
Assistant Professor, Department of Emergency
  Medicine
University of Pennsylvania
Attending Physician in Emergency Medicine
Attending Physician in Hyperbaric Medicine
Hospital of the University of Pennsylvania
Philadelphia, Pennsylvania

Harriet W. Hopf, MD
Professor, Director of Translational Research
University of Utah School of Medicine
Medical Director, Wound Care Services
LDS Hospital/Urban Central Region
Salt Lake City, Utah

Irving Jacoby, MD, FACP, FACEP, FAAEM
Clinical Professor of Medicine and Surgery
University of California, San Diego, School
  of Medicine
La Jolla, California
Attending Physician
Hyperbaric Medicine Center and Department
  of Emergency Medicine
University of California, San Diego, Medical
  Center
San Diego, California

Sarah H. Kagan, PhD, RN
Professor of Gerontological Nursing, School of
  Nursing and Secondary Faculty
Department of Otorhinolaryngology: Head and
  Neck Surgery
University of Pennsylvania School of Medicine
Clinical Nurse Specialist
Abramson Cancer Center
University of Pennsylvania
Philadelphia, Pennsylvania

Matthew Kelly, MD
Hyperbaric and Wound Care Physician
St. Francis Hospital
San Francisco, California

Jan P. Lehm, MD, FANZCA, DipDHM
Conjoint Senior Lecturer
The University of New South Wales
Sydney, Australia
Senior Staff Specialist, Department of Diving
    and Hyperbaric Medicine
Division of Anaesthesia
Prince of Wales Hospital
Senior Visiting Medical Officer, Department of
    Anaesthesia
Royal Hospital for Women
Randwick, Australia

D. Mathieu, MD, PhD
Professor of Critical Care Medicine
University of Lille
Head of the Critical Care and Hyperbaric
    Medicine Department
University Hospital
Lille, France

**Simon J. Mitchell, MBChB, PhD, DipDHM,
DipOccMed, FANZCA**
Senior Lecturer, Department of Anaesthesia
School of Medicine, Faculty of Medicine and
    Health Sciences
The University of Auckland
Consultant Anaesthetist
Auckland City Hospital
Auckland, New Zealand

Richard E. Moon, MD, FACP, FCCP, FRCPC
Professor of Anesthesiology, Professor of Medicine
Duke University
Medical Director, Center for Hyperbaric
    Medicine and Environmental Physiology
Duke University Medical Center
Durham, North Carolina

Tom S. Neuman, MD, FACP, FACPM
Emeritus Professor of Medicine
University of California, San Diego
San Diego, California

Herbert B. Newton, MD, FAAN
Professor of Neurology and Oncology,
    Department of Neurology and
    Hyperbaric Medicine Program
Ohio State University Medical Center and
    James Cancer Hospital
Ohio State University College of Medicine and
    Public Health
Columbus, Ohio

Juha Niinikoski, MD, PhD
Professor of Surgery and Chairman, Department
    of Surgery
University of Turku
Turku, Finland

Claude A. Piantadosi, MD
Professor of Medicine
Director, Center for Hyperbaric Medicine and
    Environmental Physiology
Duke University Medical Center
Durham, North Carolina

Dag Shapshak, MD
Assistant Professor, Department of
    Medicine
Division of Emergency Medicine
Medical University of South Carolina
Charleston, South Carolina

Avi Shupak, MD
Head, Unit of Otoneurology
Carmel Medical Center
Lin Medical Center
Haifa, Israel

Michael B. Strauss, MD, FACS, AAOS
Clinical Professor, Orthopaedic Surgery
University of Irvine College of Medicine
Irvine, California
Clinical Associate Professor, Orthopaedic
    Surgery
Harbor/UCLA Medical Center
Torrance, California
Active Staff, Departments of Orthopaedic
    Surgery and Hyperbaric Medicine
Long Beach Memorial Medical Center and
    Miller Children's Hospital
Attending Physician PACT (Preservation-
    Amputation, Care and Treatment) Clinic
Veterans Agency Medical Center
Long Beach, California

Stephen R. Thom, MD, PhD

Professor of Emergency Medicine
Chief, Hyperbaric Medicine
University of Pennsylvania
Philadelphia, Pennsylvania

Robert J. Turner, MBBS, FANZCA, DipDHM

Conjoint Lecturer
The University of New South Wales
Sydney, Australia
Senior Staff Specialist, Department of Diving
    and Hyperbaric Medicine
Division of Anaesthesia and Intensive Care
Prince of Wales Hospital
Randwick, Australia

Karen Van Hoesen, MD

Clinical Professor of Medicine, Department of
    Emergency Medicine
Director, Undersea and Hyperbaric Medicine
    Fellowship
Director, Diving Medicine Center
University of California, San Diego (UCSD)
San Diego, California

Dan Waisman, MD

Lecturer, Faculty of Medicine
Technion–Israel Institute of Technology
Director of the Newborn Unit, Department of
    Neonatology
Carmel Medical Center
Member, Reserve Medical Team
Israel Naval Medical Institute (INMI)
Haifa, Israel

Lindell Weaver, MD

Professor, Department of Medicine
University of Utah School of Medicine
Medical Director, Hyperbaric Medicine
LDS Hospital
Salt Lake City, Utah
Medical Director, Hyperbaric Medicine
Medical Co-director, Shock Trauma ICU
Intermountain Medical Center
Murray, Utah

William A. Zamboni, MD, FACS

Professor and Chairman, Department of Surgery
Chief, Division of Plastic Surgery
Program Director, Plastic Surgery Residency
    Program
University of Nevada School of Medicine
Las Vegas, Nevada

Contents

Section V

Side Effects and Complications 511

History **I**

Chapter 1 History of Hyperbaric Therapy

History 1
of Hyperbaric
Therapy

Dick Clarke

One of the earliest medical technologies still in use today, the history of hyperbaric medicine extends back almost 350 years. The first recorded attempt to use alterations in atmospheric pressure for therapeutic purposes is attributed to Henshaw, an English physician and clergyman, in 1662.[1] Apparently inspired by the salutary effects some investigators associated with changes in climate, and presumably secondary to differences in barometric pressure, Henshaw sought to artificially control climate. His "domicilium" was nothing more than a sealed room. Attached to it was a pair of large organ bellows. By manipulation of a series of valves and operation of the bellows, the atmosphere within the room could be "condensed" (compressed) or "rarified" (decompressed).

These changes were designed to simulate the effects of climate change experienced as one traveled to higher altitudes (the mountains) or lower altitudes (the coast). Henshaw chose the condensed atmosphere to treat certain acute conditions and the rarified atmosphere for several chronic diseases. There was even an opportunity for the unafflicted. Henshaw suggested,[1] "In times of good health this domicilium is proposed as a good expedient to help digestion, to promote insensible respiration, to facilitate breathing and expectoration, and consequently, of excellent use for the prevention of most affections at the lungs" (p. 10).

It is unlikely that patients experienced anything more than a temporary sense of improvement at best. The degree to which any alteration in the domicilium's pressure could be achieved certainly would have been modest, given the limitations of hand-operated bellows and the integrity of the room. This was probably fortuitous. Too low a pressure could have produced clinically significant hypoxia, or worse. Exposure to too high a pressure could have placed patients at risk for decompression sickness, a complication of compressed air exposure not to be identified for another 200 years. It was also unlikely that the domicilium's atmosphere was renewed during its occupancy. Consequently, Henshaw's "encouraging" reports of changes in respiration and insensible perspiration were possibly the result of an accumulation of metabolic waste products.

That Henshaw's domicilium produced any meaningful benefits is highly improbable, for it was almost 200 years before any further interest in hyperbaric therapy was recorded. Perhaps the most notable aspect of his work was that it preceded the discovery of oxygen by more than 100 years.

Oxygen was first discovered by Carl Wilhelm Scheele, a Swedish chemist, in 1772. However, he did not publish his observations until 1777.[2] In the meantime, Joseph Priestly, an English chemist, independently discovered oxygen in 1775 and published his findings that same year, 2 years before Scheele.[3] As a result, Priestly is commonly credited with the discovery of oxygen.

There were no other reports of attempts to improve illness or disease with simulated climate change until the 19th century, despite efforts to promote its scientific scrutiny. In 1782, the Royal Society of Sciences, in Haarlem, The Netherlands, introduced a prize for the design of an apparatus that would enable study of the effects of high pressures on animal and vegetable life.[4] There were no applicants, despite the prize being offered again on three other occasions through 1791.

COMPRESSED AIR BATHS

Emile Tabarie, a physician practicing in Montpellier, France, is credited with rekindling interest in hyperbaric medicine.[5] In 1832, he presented to the French Academy of Scientists a detailed description of the workings of a pneumatic laboratory. That same year he undertook a series of studies that investigated the effects of lowered air pressures, both locally and systemically.[5] By generating a reversal of this environment through an increase in ambient pressure, Tabarie hypothesized that healthful conditions would be further improved on and certain diseases might be successfully overcome. He suggested that the "indispensable nature" of atmospheric air would, by its modification, "represent an inexhaustible source of beneficial influence on man."[6] Tabarie claimed to have successfully treated 49 cases of mostly respiratory diseases.[6]

One final comment on Tabarie relates to the procedure he adopted to optimize hyperbaric comfort and safety. He advocated increasing air pressure gradually, maintaining it steadily at a predetermined maximum pressure, often in the order of two fifths of an additional atmosphere, then slowly lowering it. The entire process took approximately 2 hours and was somewhat similar to modern therapeutic dosing schedules, the exception being higher pressures in use today.

Junod, another French physician, is credited with the introduction of the first purpose-built hyperbaric chamber.[7] The chamber was commissioned in 1834, and it was based on a design by James Watt, of steam engine fame. The chamber was spherical, built of copper, and capable of compression to 4.0 atmospheres absolute (ATA). Junod exposed his patients to higher pressures and faster rates of compression and decompression than Tabarie. This apparently caused consistent difficulties sufficient to lead some to state that hyperbaric devices did not belong in the practice of medicine.[1]

Junod believed that a patient's perfusion was enhanced while in his chamber. That patients would report a greater sense of well-being during their occupancy he believed to be proof positive. A more modern analysis might conclude that the narcotic property of nitrogen in air at pressures of 4.0 ATA (reported 100 years later by another Frenchman, Jacques Cousteau, which he termed *rapture of the deep*) was the likely cause of what was certainly only a temporary sense of any such well-being.

The largest chamber complex of this period was built in 1837 by Pravaz and installed in the French city of Lyon.[8] It could accommodate 12 patients. Pravaz named this therapy *"le bain d'air comprime."* He was of the opinion that these "compressed air baths" served to dilate the bronchi, thereby proving beneficial in a wide range of pulmonary and related conditions, including tuberculosis.[9]

By the 1850s, great interest in compressed air therapy was apparent throughout much of

Western Europe. In 1855, Bertin constructed his own hyperbaric chamber and wrote the first textbook describing this medical technology.[10] His facility attracted patients from as far away as North America. In 1875, Forlanini, recognized as the pioneer of artificial pneumothorax in the treatment of tuberculosis, described his "pneumatic institute," which he had installed in Milan, Italy.[11]

As quickly as new diseases and illnesses were discovered, it seemed as if hyperbaric proponents suggested that the chamber represented its treatment or cure. Perhaps not surprisingly, a wave of enthusiasm spread rapidly, and chambers soon became operational in Scandinavia, England, Germany, The Netherlands, Belgium, and Austria.[12]

In 1879, Fontaine introduced a mobile hyperbaric operating room; it was capable of accommodating up to 12 people.[13] He suggested that this would allow surgery to extend from hospitals to sanatoriums, and even into private homes. A prominent surgeon of the day, Pean, used the chamber to perform some 27 different types of surgeries over a 3-month period. All surgeries were considered successful, and it was reported that his hyperbaric patients recovered more quickly from the crude anesthesia of the day, experienced little vomiting, and had no cyanosis. These observations led to the planning of a large hyperbaric surgical amphitheater, one that would hold up to 300 people. It was never completed. Sadly, Fontaine became the first known hyperbaric practitioner fatality after a construction accident while his hyperbaric amphitheater was under construction.

A series of seemingly unrelated events paralleled the introduction of "compressed air baths." These events were soon to converge and would eventually provide hyperbaric medicine with a firm mechanistic basis and its first clear treatment indication.

COMPRESSED AIR CAISSON TECHNOLOGY

During the late 18th century, major changes in European and North American economy and society took place. This period was sub-sequently termed the Industrial Revolution. These changes resulted from technologic advances in the use of iron and steel, the invention of new machines that would increase production and efficiency, and the introduction of the factory system. Coal replaced wood as the primary energy source.

As these changes became widely adopted, the search for new sources of coal took on the frenetic pace that characterizes today's search for oil and gas deposits. In northern France, sizable deposits of coal were discovered beneath the Loire River and below quicksand. Efforts to mine these deposits were hampered by the surrounding water table, which readily flooded mine shafts that penetrated the ground. Jean Triger, a French paleontologist and mining engineer, introduced a technology that was to overcome the flooding problem.[14] Triger's technique was based on an idea that Sir Thomas Cochrane patented in 1830, which detailed the use of compressed air in tunneling through water-bearing strata.[15]

Triger's design involved the connecting together of a series of 5-foot diameter circular steel rings to form a hollow shaft (Fig. 1.1). This shaft (or *caisson,* French meaning "box") was lowered through mud and quicksand, with additional rings added until the shaft came to rest on coal deposits beneath. The combined weight of the steel rings served to force the shaft down, as loose earth and sand was excavated away. The shaft was sealed with an "air lock." Connected to the shaft and air lock was an air compressor. Compressed air would be introduced until the pressure within the shaft reached the pressure at the bottom of the shaft, expelling whatever water and moist sand was present.

The purpose of the air lock was to allow men to enter and exit the shaft without its loss of pressure and resultant flooding. Once men were inside the air lock and its outer hatch sealed, compressed air would be introduced into the lock until its pressure equaled that of the previously pressurized mine shaft. The inner hatch of the air lock would then be opened and access to the shaft afforded. Excavated materials and coal were transferred out by reversing this sequence of hatch operation. In this manner, "dry" coal mining

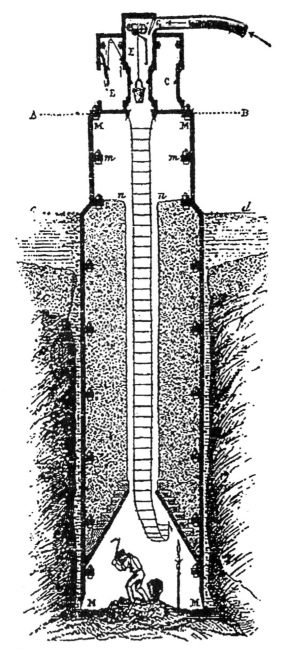

Figure 1.1 One of the first caissons used in France. *(Reprinted with permission of the Undersea and Hyperbaric Medical Society.)*

became possible, and it opened up access to the greater sources of coal needed to fuel the expanding Industrial Revolution.

Ultimately, some of these caissons were pressurized to as high as 4.25 ATA (107 feet of sea water equivalent). With a typical 4-hour work period, these caisson exposures placed the occupants at great risk for decom-

pression sickness.[16] At the time of Triger's pioneering efforts, however, the fact that caisson exposures might result in decompression sickness was not appreciated. After his own exposure on one particular occasion, Triger noted the next day, "[K]nee pains appeared in the left side, and we felt a rather severe painful discomfort for several days afterwards." He went on to note, "After we were quite free of these pains, we were anxious to try the experiment again. At the same hour, this is, 20 hours after our exit from compressed air, we felt in the right side pains just like the former ones, which kept us numb for four or five days."[17]

Today, we recognize these complaints as common clinical manifestations of decompression sickness, a condition unknown to Triger. Similar complaints in compressed-air workers received little sympathy and were frequently considered to have coincided with some nightly excesses by the workers between their caisson shifts![18] Triger was fortunate that his injuries were reversible and not any more severe. However, worse results were soon to follow.

Some 64 workers were eventually employed in the caissons operating in Douchy, northern France. Several of them subsequently complained of similar symptoms to those of Triger; one suffered complete paralysis of his arms and legs, lasting 12 hours, and two died. This newly introduced and valuable engineering technology was clearly outpacing medical science, and with fatal consequences.

By now, a relation between exposure to compressed air and these complaints was being suggested. At the request of Triger, two physicians, Pol and Watelle, went to the Douchy mines to study this phenomenon. Pol and Watelle would subsequently describe the medical problems encountered in these mines. They noted, among other things, "The danger does not lie in going into the compressed air. It is not a disadvantage to stop there a longer or shorter time." Their findings, published in 1854,[19] represented the earliest observations of decompression sickness in humans. Although they missed the significance of increasing exposure times, Pol and Watelle did acknowledge the veracity of the miners who observed that they "pay only when leaving the caisson."

Based on autopsy observations, Pol and Watelle considered the underlying problem as one of "superoxygenation and congestion."[19] They further noted that decompression was necessary to produce symptoms and recompression reduced symptom severity. This latter observation appeared to be based on statements by injured miners to the effect that their symptoms would improve on returning to the pressurized mine shaft for their next shift.

It was another 15 years before anyone drew attention to a similar presentation to those seen in compressed-air workers and those occurring in divers, who likewise breathed compression air.[20] Paul Bert, the dominant figure of this period, was the first to piece things together. Bert, another Frenchman, is considered by many to be the "father of pressure physiology," yet his early career left no clues as to his ultimate legacy. He was first an engineer, then a law student, before becoming one of Claude Bernard's (the celebrated 19th century physician and scientist) most brilliant pupils. On graduation as a doctor of medicine and a doctor of science, Bert was appointed to successive physiology positions at Bordeaux and the Sorbonne. His scientific activity was diverse, but his main achievements concerned the biological effects of barometric pressure. His classic work, *La Pression Barometrique,*[21] represented an enormously comprehensive investigation of the physiological effects of air under both increased and decreased atmospheric pressures. Applying Dalton's and Henry's gas laws,[16] Bert recognized that too rapid a decompression from the air pressures encountered in these caissons induced a pathophysiologic insult secondary to excess tissue nitrogen tensions.

Some 79% of atmospheric air is composed of nitrogen, which is largely inert. As environmental pressures are raised, increased amounts of nitrogen (and other gases present in air) are delivered to the lung (Dalton's Law). These gases are transferred to the blood and on to the tissues in their soluble state (Henry's Law). Here, nitrogen, being largely inert, accumulates as a function of pressure

and time. On return to normal atmospheric pressure (decompression), this accumulated nitrogen begins its return journey, along the same pathway, and still in its soluble state. If the rate of decompression becomes too great, tissues of the body and blood become supersaturated with nitrogen. Nitrogen may then evolve from its soluble form to a gaseous form, in a manner similar to the release of carbon dioxide when one opens a carbonated beverage container. Resulting bubbles may traumatize critical tissues, obstruct vascular flow, or coalesce. Resulting signs and symptoms will vary as a function of the amount of gas involved and its anatomic location. The extent of the injury will range from joint discomfort to death.

Bert noted, "All symptoms, from the slightest to those that bring on sudden death, are the consequences of the liberation of bubbles of nitrogen in the blood, and even in the tissues, when compression has lasted long enough." He added, "The great protection is slowness of decompression. ..."[21] He was of the opinion that slowing the rate of decompression would reduce the likelihood of this injury pattern, yet provided no guidance as to how best to do this. Specific measures would be introduced in the coming decades.

Bert's second significant contribution to the practice of hyperbaric medicine was his identification of the toxicity of oxygen on the central nervous system when applied at pressures in excess of approximately 1.75 ATA.[21] A range of premonitory signs and symptoms now identify such toxicity. Unless the partial pressure of oxygen is quickly reduced, a grand mal seizure may result. This complication of hyperbaric oxygenation is frequently referred to as the "Paul Bert effect." Central nervous system oxygen toxicity would not become clinically important for several decades, when sufficiently high partial pressures of oxygen were used clinically.

The compressed air caisson concept was quickly grasped by civil engineers as a tool that would allow them to undertake projects not otherwise possible. Bridges could now be designed to cross large bodies of water, with submerged caissons providing support for columns that held up the bridge spans. Underground mass transit systems would now be built within water table areas.

Unfortunately, news of the caisson concept traveled more quickly than news of the complications resulting from inadequate decompression from compressed-air environments. Paul Bert's suggestion that slowed decompression was of value in reducing the incidence of decompression injury was not published for several years, and then frequently not accepted or fully embraced. Not surprisingly, significant morbidity and mortality would plague subsequent compressed-air–based construction projects.

The building of the world's first steel arch bridge span, constructed in St. Louis, Missouri, and crossing the Mississippi River, was a case in point.[22] Construction on the bridge began in 1869. The caisson used for construction had its walls and roof reinforced; however, there was no floor. Once the caisson had been maneuvered into place, weight was added to its roof until it sank. Compressed air was introduced into each caisson to displace the water; then workers entered through an air lock to dig away the loose material beneath. The caisson's

weight continued to force it down until bedrock was reached. Once this occurred, the caisson was filled with concrete, which then formed the foundation for each bridge support column (Fig. 1.2). Manned exposures within the bridge support caissons reached 4.45 ATA (the equivalent of 114 feet of sea water.[23]

With exposure times of several hours, resultant nitrogen loading was frequently physiologically intolerable at the higher pressures. Of the 352 workers so exposed, 5% died and another 10% suffered serious forms of decompression sickness. Because construction had commenced before the publication of *La Pression Barometrique,* one might appreciate why morbidity and mortality would be as high as it was. There was simply no local knowledge of an association between decompression from compressed-air exposure and decompression sickness. Further complicating the issue was that this project involved significantly higher pressures (greater nitrogen loading) than its European counterparts. The bridge's designer, and head of its construction, James Eads, for whom the bridge was named, asked his physician friend to investigate these caisson-related mishaps. Dr. Alphonse Jaminet

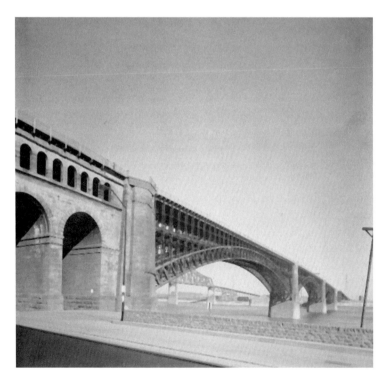

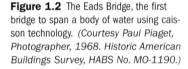

Figure 1.2 The Eads Bridge, the first bridge to span a body of water using caisson technology. *(Courtesy Paul Piaget, Photographer, 1968. Historic American Buildings Survey, HABS No. MO-1190.)*

subsequently made many descents into the Eads Bridge caissons.[23] On one such occasion he spent in excess of 2 hours at a pressure greater than 4.0 ATA. Subsequent decompression took only 4 minutes, which by today's standards would be quite rapid. On exiting the caisson's air lock, Jaminet became paralyzed and aphasic, implying decompression sickness involving the brain and spinal cord.[24] He was fortunate to eventually recover much of his premorbid function.

The second caisson project of note, from a decompression injury perspective, was in the building of the Brooklyn Bridge, which spans the East River.[25] Work began in 1870 and lasted 13 years. As with the construction of the Eads Bridge, the Brooklyn Bridge caissons were much larger than their European counterparts and involved higher ambient air pressures. The Brooklyn Bridge project was supervised by Washington Roebling, who assumed this responsibility on the death of his father John Roebling, one of the bridge's principal designers. The younger Roebling was aware of the serious medical complications associated with the Eads Bridge. He decided, therefore, that an on-site physician was necessary, and engaged Dr. Andrew Smith. Although Smith's tenure lasted only 5 months, he was faced with 110 cases of decompression injury, which he termed *caisson disease*. Smith first published his clinical experiences in 1870.[26] Smith's observations provided early and valuable insight into the various presentations of decompression sickness. Roebling himself suffered permanent paralysis as a result of his visits to the caissons, and ultimately succumbed to sepsis secondary to pressure ulcers.

Of the two Brooklyn Bridge caissons, the one on the Manhattan side ended up considerably deeper, eventually reaching 35 pounds per square inch gauge (psig; 3.38 ATA). Bedrock was first encountered at 33 psig (3.24 ATA). Just 1.0 psig deeper two fatalities occurred, with both men dying soon after exiting the caisson. At 35 psig (3.38 ATA), a third man died. Roebling decided, therefore, to halt any further evacuation even though bedrock was not uniformly exposed across the base of the caisson.

This turned out to be a reasonable compromise as both the bridge and Roebling's reputation remain intact today.

One lost opportunity was Smith's recommendation that a recompression chamber, fed by the caisson's air compressors, be made available. He was clearly of the opinion that improvement occurred in injured miners who returned to the pressurized caisson. Smith's position was that an on-site recompression chamber would allow treatment to be instituted immediately on presentation rather than the miner waiting for the next day's shift for possible and likely limited benefit while back in the caisson. Had Smith insisted on its availability, it is possible that one or more of the Brooklyn Bridge fatalities might have been avoided and many of the other serious injuries successfully treated. Had he gone one step further and argued that his chamber idea also be incorporated into the caisson itself, he would have better controlled decompression and been the first to actually prevent many cases of decompression sickness. He had, after all, observed that one clear cause was "the transition to normal atmospheric pressure, after prolonged sojourn in a highly condensed atmosphere."[27]

Controlled decompression via a medical lock built into the caisson first occurred several years after Smith's observations, and just a few miles away. New York's Hudson River tunnel was the first tunnel to be constructed using compressed-air technology.[28] In its latter stages, it was also the first caisson to incorporate a decompression chamber into the top of the caisson shaft. This project was likewise the scene of enormous decompression morbidity and mortality before the decompression chamber became operational. Work commenced in 1879, several years before the completion of the Brooklyn Bridge, and on the opposite side of Manhattan. In 1882, Moir[28] observed that "the men had been dying at a rate of one man per month, out of 45 or 50 men employed, a death rate of about 25% per annum" (p. 574). Work stopped this same year. It was not the result of any medical, legal, or employment issue. It was something more fundamental. The construction company had simply exhausted its funds.

Alternative financial support was acquired several years later, and work recommenced in 1889. At this point, a decompression chamber had been installed into the top of the caisson. It was used to carefully control the decompression rate from pressures now ranging from 30 to 35 psig (3.0–3.38 ATA). It was also used to treat cases of decompression sickness, by recompression. There were only two more deaths in the following 15 months,[29] and cures were affected in some cases of decompression sickness by using the chamber to recompress workers (the forerunner of the work-site recompression chamber). These cases of decompression sickness were successfully treated by using as its mechanistic basis the inverse relation of pressure and volume described by Boyle's Law.[16]

Between 1906 and 1908, construction of two more New York tunnels took place, both under the East River. Pressures reached 42 psig (3.86 ATA) and frequently involved twice-daily exposures. Despite the more gradual decompression process in use at this time, decompression sickness climbed in concert with the higher pressures and twice-daily exposures. Keays reported enormous morbidity and mortality, involving more than 3500 cases and 20 fatalities from some 500,000 manned caisson compressions.[30]

In the following two decades, decompression chambers became an integral part of caisson technology, and an increasing number of these chambers were constructed to function independent of the caisson. This would permit treatment of those who exited the caisson and became symptomatic without the need to return to it, thereby interfering with its routine operation. Although more gradual caisson decompression rates had by now become commonplace, the actual process was by no means uniform.

It was not until 1907 that some form of order was established. The British Admiralty, eager to capitalize on high-pressure environments for military diving, engaged J. Scott Haldane to investigate air decompression procedures. With colleagues Boycott and Damant, Haldane's work led to the first standardized set of decompression tables.[31,32]

From this point forward the navies of the world took a leading role in improving the safety of exposure to compressed-air environments and advancing depth and time exposures, to undertake a wide range of deep-sea diving operations. Civil engineers readily adopted navy decompression procedures and their variants. Testament to the effectiveness of Haldanian-based decompression tables was the subsequent and significant reduction in the incidence of decompression sickness. The construction of the Dartford Tunnel in southern England during the 1950s was characteristic of improved morbidity and mortality. The decompression sickness incidence rate was just 0.50% (689 cases in 122,000 compressions, of which only 35 were considered to be serious).[33]

HYPERBARIC MEDICINE

Several "firsts" are attributed to J. Leonard Corning, a New York neurologist. In the late 1880s, he was the first to introduce "compressed air baths" in the United States.[34] His 6-foot diameter hyperbaric chamber was the first to operate with an electrically powered air compressor, and he would eventually become more widely recognized as the first to use spinal anesthesia.

Corning's interest in hyperbaric medicine stemmed from his visits to the Hudson River Tunnel construction site. He observed numerous cases of paralytic decompression sickness, leading him to consider this condition as essentially an affliction of the spinal cord. Corning clearly saw promise in the ability of air recompression to resolve many of these cases, and he chose to use compressed-air therapy for a broader range of nondecompression-related brain and spinal cord illness and disease. This may have been based on his opinion that compressed-air workers exhibited "a striking exacerbation of mental and physical vigor."[34]

Corning's hyperbaric treatments would last from 1 to 2 hours, involving pressures of up to 3.0 ATA. Corning[34] certainly recognized the risk for decompression sickness and ensured "that fifteen to twenty minutes are consumed in the operation of reducing the pressure in the chamber" (p. 229). Corning appeared to use the chamber more as a facilitator of various medicinal solutions in the treatment of nervous and mental conditions than as stand-alone compressed-air therapy. Although he appeared to believe that some additive or synergistic benefit existed, his hyperbaric practices failed to impress the medical establishment. Within several years, use of hyperbaric air chambers for conditions other than decompression sickness was largely discontinued; however, chamber use for nondecompression-related conditions would soon return.

In the waning months of World War I an influenza pandemic swept the world. It has been estimated that between 25 and 50 million people died. In the United States alone, more than 500,000 people died of influenza. Orval Cunningham, chairman of the Department of Anesthesiology at Kansas University Medical School who was recognized as an "excellent teacher and practitioner of anesthesiology and remarkably keen clinical observer" (p. 40),[35] noted that the pandemic's morbidity and mortality rates were greater in areas of high elevation than they were in coastal regions. This observation intrigued Cunningham. He considered the only significant variable to be a change in barometric pressure. To determine whether this was a clinically significant event, he borrowed a hyperbaric chamber from a local bridge construction company. Beginning in 1918, he treated moribund influenza patients in the chamber with seemingly encouraging results: "Patients whose lips bore the blue-black livid stamp of the kiss of death and were deeply unconscious, but if not too far beyond the brink, in a matter of minutes were brought back to normal color and to a return of consciousness."[35]

These findings stimulated Cunningham. He eventually acquired a larger chamber and continued to report encouraging improvements in these cases. Cunningham's "validation" of hyperbaric treatments as essential in influenza may have stemmed from one unfortunate and tragic event. His patients would occasionally spend many days to several weeks at a time under the chamber's elevated air pressures. One night a mechanical failure brought the air compressors to a standstill. The chamber's

pressure decreased rapidly to normal atmospheric pressure. All its occupants died. Cunningham was now convinced that hyperbaric air alone had kept these patients alive, and they had died because they could not be supported on leaving it.[35] A modern analysis would deduce that death resulted from the overwhelming effects of decompression sickness secondary to high nitrogen tensions, as well as possible cases of pulmonary barotrauma of ascent.

As the pandemic ebbed and pulmonary cases decreased, Cunningham sought out other conditions to treat with hyperbaric air. It was unlikely that he was initially motivated by profit. As an anesthesiologist, he had rarely billed his patients, preferring to accept whatever was offered. He seemed to be of the opinion that inhalation of compressed air offered a meaningful therapeutic option.

Cunningham went on to treat arthritis, glaucoma, pernicious anemia, diabetes, syphilis, and certain cancers. His rationale was that arthritis was likewise influenced by alterations in barometric pressure and anaerobic bacteria were at the center of these other conditions.[35] Cunningham may have based his assumptions, in part, on Bert's observations that oxygen content varied throughout the body, and that lower oxygen tensions were evident in bone and connective tissue.[21]

One grateful patient, a close friend of a wealthy industrialist, who was "cured" by Cunningham, provided Cunningham the financial means to make his hyperbaric treatments more widely available. The result was the construction of the first in a planned series of huge chambers to be located across the country. The Timken-Cunningham Ball stood five stories high and 64 feet in diameter. Each floor had 12 bedrooms and the amenities of a good hotel.[36]

Cunningham's activities generated a great deal of interest within the lay community and an equal amount of concern within the medical establishment.[35,36] Cunningham did nothing to assuage his critiques by submitting clinical data requested of him for peer review. His only report related to hyperbaric medicine was published in 1927.[37] In this report, he argued the basis for his treatment approach but provided no supportive data and only a passing "outcomes" comment that "we have had encouraging results with five of twenty-seven cases of hopeless carcinoma."[37]

Cunningham was further challenged to produce more substantive data by the American Medical Association's Bureau of Investigation. Efforts by the American Medical Association continued without success, leading them to eventually censor Cunningham in 1928.[38] Cunningham subsequently closed his hyperbaric practice, and finally retired in 1935. Two subsequent owners attempted to keep this hyperbaric facility viable, but it was eventually abandoned in 1936. The chamber was subsequently used as a conventional hospital before closing permanently in 1940. Two years later, it was scrapped. This essentially marked the end of the compressed-air era of hyperbaric medicine for therapeutic purposes other than the treatment of decompression sickness.

EARLY HYPERBARIC OXYGEN THERAPY

The first practice of hyperbaric *oxygen* therapy is attributed to a South American whose contributions remain largely overlooked today. Although he is arguably deserving of the title "father of hyperbaric oxygen therapy," this accolade has been bestowed on the Dutch cardiovascular surgeon Ita Boerema, whose involvement in hyperbaric medicine, albeit considerable, did not begin until more than 20 years later. In 1934, the Brazilian Academy of Sciences held a special meeting in honor of the recently deceased Madam Curie. A Brazilian physician, Álvaro Osório de Almeida, who had trained under Curie (and several of Paul Bert's disciples) and had become her close friend, spoke at the meeting. His presentations were of particular interest to this audience in that they addressed hyperbaric oxygen–induced central nervous system toxicity, work he undertook as a prelude to treating cancer patients with hyperbaric oxygen.[39,40]

It was probably not high ambient air pressures that attracted de Almeida to hyperbaric medicine; rather, it was the ability of the chamber to deliver high amounts of oxygen. De Almeida hypothesized that malignant cells would be sensitive to high doses of oxygen. Initially, he sought to determine whether higher organisms could safely tolerate the levels of oxygen he considered necessary to injure malignant cells.[41,42] De Almeida reported that experimentally implanted tumors in rats invariably "softened" after repeated exposures to 6.0 ATA oxygen for 3 hours. Tumor breakup was perceptible after several days, with some resorption of tumor mass. Encouraged, de Almeida quickly moved on to human studies.[42] This proved more complicated, as 6.0 ATA oxygen was clearly too toxic an exposure level. Greatly increased sensitivity to oxygen was apparent, even when a strict dietary intake (200 daily calories) was enforced.

Not deterred, de Almeida attempted to combine radiation therapy and a hyperbaric dose of 3.0 ATA.[43] Madam Curie was able to make available radium for his studies, which was carried to Rio de Janeiro in the hand luggage of his friends, colleagues, and family members! His human work led him to conclude that the effects of combination hyperbaric oxygen and radium therapy are "greater than just the effects of one summed up with the effects of the other."[43]

De Almeida also studied the effects of hyperbaric oxygen on leprosy[44] and gas gangrene.[45] It was necessary to conduct all of this research in the basement of his home to avoid the stigma of being labeled a "dog doctor," which was commonly directed at academics during this period.

Despite publishing his work in three different languages, de Almeida's pioneering application of hyperbaric *oxygen* therapy goes largely unnoticed today.

DIVING MEDICINE

The U.S. Navy began experimenting with hyperbaric oxygen in the treatment of decompression sickness soon after de Almeida, reporting their early experience in 1937.[46] Behnke and Shaw were clearly cognizant of the ability of air recompression to resolve many, particularly less severe, cases of decompression sickness. They were dissatisfied, however, with the greatly extended decompressions necessary to safely return the patient and his attendants to the surface. Decompressions in excess of 24 hours were not uncommon.

Others, beginning with Bert,[21] had suggested that oxygen replace air during the treatment process. Behnke and Shaw became the first to attempt this. Their work resulted in treatment recommendations based on severity of injury, and included the first application of nitrogen-oxygen mixtures other than air.[46] An important aspect of this early work was the identification of safe time-dose oxygen exposure limits—that is, exposure to the highest oxygen pressure for the longest period with minimum possible risk for central nervous system oxygen toxicity.[47] Subsequent navy interest in oxygen extended to accelerating the decompression process to improve efficiency (time spent working vs time spent decompressing) and safety (getting the diver out of the water more quickly).[16]

Significant reductions in in-water decompression time resulted. Eventually, the practice of oxygen-enhanced decompression was extended to surface oxygen decompression procedures.[16] With these procedures, the diver exits the water well in advance of the time normally required for standard in-water air decompression to be completed. Once at the surface, the diver is immediately recompressed in a waiting hyperbaric chamber. Oxygen breathing is instituted, and subsequent decompression conducted. The stage used to recover the diver is now free to transport the next diver to the work site. Although this process appears hazardous—that is, exiting the water before elimination of what would normally be considered sufficient tissue nitrogen to surface safely—the incidence of decompression sickness is no greater than that associated with standard in-water air decompression.[47] One might argue that planned surfacing in such a manner would set the disease process in motion and is, therefore, dangerous. Others could counter that it is actually safer to do this, rather than undergo in-water decompression, in that the diver is no longer in a relatively hazardous environment, and his or her subsequent decompression can be more carefully controlled.

The next significant evolution in military diving and oxygen use occurred in 1960. Until that time, recompression of those suffering decompression sickness was commonly accomplished with patients breathing compressed air, with only limited oxygen exposures, despite Behnke and Shaw's[46] encouraging work with animals.

By the 1960s, a disturbing trend in U.S. Navy recompression treatment experience had become apparent. Treatment table failure rates were steadily climbing and were attributed, in part, to increasing intervals between symptom onset and therapeutic compression.[48] Delays were particularly common in recreational divers, whereas military and professional divers invariably work from a diving platform that incorporates recompression capability. The interval between symptom onset and therapeutic compression, therefore, is brief. Recreational divers rarely have such readily available support, frequently diving in medical and geographic isolation. Provision of treatment in these cases can be delayed from many hours to several days.

Goodman, Workman, and their colleagues[49] tackled the issue of lengthy decompressions from treatment pressure and treatment table failure rates. Their work culminated in the adoption by the U.S. Navy of the Minimal-Recompression Oxygen-Breathing treatment tables. These treatment tables remain in use today and are employed internationally.

RADIATION SENSITIZATION

During the early 1950s, several observations laid the groundwork for the introduction of hyperbaric oxygen as a radiation sensitizer. Gray and colleagues[50] observed that curability of small animal tumors with radiotherapy is limited by the radioresistance of the portion of cells that retain their reproductive integrity. Tumor cell sensitivity to irradiation was seen to increase when experimental mice breathed hyperbaric doses of oxygen.

Gray's group[51] further observed that radiobiological damage demonstrates dependence on the concentration of oxygen in the immediate vicinity of tumor cells at the time of radiation. It soon became evident that many solid tumor cell populations exist within a wide range of oxygen tensions.[52]

These findings were sufficiently encouraging to warrant an early clinical trial. This was undertaken at St. Thomas's Hospital in London, England, by Churchill-Davidson, Sanger, and Thomlinson.[53] Their protocol included placing patients into barbiturate coma to limit the likelihood of oxygen seizures and inserting tympanic membrane ventilation tubes to avoid ear barotrauma. Patients were then placed into a naval diving chamber modified to accommodate a recessed Perspex window, and its pressure was increased with oxygen to 3.0 ATA.[54]

It was through this window that X-rays were delivered in a single treatment to breast and lung cancers, the only tumor sites that would "match" the viewport. A unique method was used to assess any difference afforded by hyperbaric oxygen. Only patients with tumors large enough to be divided into two were recruited. Half of the tumor was irradiated conventionally, whereas the other half was shielded. Shielding was reversed and the second half of the tumor irradiated while the patient was exposed to hyperbaric oxygen.[53] Within 2 years, this group was able to report 35 patients successfully managed in this way.[55] Damage to the tumor areas irradiated in the chamber was more pronounced.

Great interest in this method of radiation delivery resulted,[56-59] but radiation oncologists were invariably frustrated by the lack of "anatomic visibility" afforded by the small and limited number of windows available in the largely steel hyperbaric chambers of the day. Such was the interest in hyperbaric oxygen radiosensitization that access to all tumors, regardless of where they were anatomically, was sought. Industry was challenged, and it responded by adding more windows into purpose-built chambers. By the early 1960s, a completely acrylic hyperbaric chamber had been produced.

Within a decade of the advent of hyperbaric oxygen radiation sensitization, doubts about its safety were being expressed. Some suggested that the incidence of new primary tumors and metastatic disease appeared to be greater in those patients irradiated in hyperbaric chambers.[60,61] Coupled with an apparent lack of consistent survival advantage, the introduction of alternative radiation sensitizers, and a lack of uniformity in radiation dosing (making comparisons difficult), interest in hyperbaric radiation sensitization waned, and had largely ceased by the mid-1970s.

CARDIAC SURGERY

The decade of the 1950s witnessed another significant hyperbaric event, one that resulted in the identification of a second therapeutic mechanism. Boerema's[62] introduction of controlled hypothermia had served to double the ischemic time from normothermic cardiac surgery. This doubling, however, still represented only a total of approximately 5 minutes. Boerema's search for more effective methods led him to consider hyperbaric oxygenation. He was aware of the practice of hyperbaric oxygen therapy as it related to the treatment of decompression sickness.

Using a small-animal chamber, he first demonstrated that dogs could tolerate much longer periods of cardiac arrest when both cooled and exposed to 3.0 ATA oxygen.[62] His foundation for hyperbaric dosing would be the work by Behnke and Shaw,[46] who had proposed 3.0 ATA for 3 hours as the upper safe threshold to avoid overt central nervous system oxygen toxicity. He next exposed pigs to this same pressure where they underwent exchange transfusion, first using plasma. He later switched to Macrodex, adding salts to produce a Ringer's-like solution. Although hemoglobin levels declined to essentially zero, there was clearly sufficient oxygen transport within plasma to support oxygen-dependent functions. This work was published in the first issue of *Journal of Cardiovascular Surgery,* under the title "Life Without Blood."[63]

By 1959, Boerema and colleagues[64] were performing cardiac surgery on infants and adults with a specially built hyperbaric operating room (Figs. 1.3 and 1.4). Successful cross-clamp ischemic times of between 13 and 14 minutes were achieved. Hyperbaric operating rooms were soon installed in many hospitals throughout the world.

Bernhard and colleagues[65] at Harvard Medical School were the first to perform hyperbaric cardiac surgery in the United States in 1963. They developed several complementary techniques, one a miniature extracorporeal circulation oxygenator that they used successfully with hyperbaric oxygenation and hypothermia. Soon thereafter, Bernhard's group[65] was routinely operating on infants with congenital cardiac abnormalities. Pressures between 3.0 and 3.6 ATA were used and titrated to overcome low arterial oxygen levels. The greater the degree of cyanosis, the higher the pressure. In accordance with Boerema's protocol, compression would begin once the chest was opened. Decompression commenced on repair of the defect and before closure of the thoracotomy, and took up to 150 minutes.

During this period of hyperbaric cardiac surgery enthusiasm, steady advances in the development of extracorporeal circulation devices were under way. By 1960, this technology was considered safe enough to support coronary artery bypass grafting, usually in conjunction with controlled hypothermia. Over the ensuing decade, the practice of hyperbaric surgery began to falter. Its disadvantages, namely, higher costs, risk for decompression sickness, ear barotrauma, and confinement anxiety issues (Boerema found that some 50% of those who would otherwise have been considered hyperbaric team members could not sufficiently tolerate its environment), became difficult to justify. Extracorporeal circulation technology eventually won the day.

What remained, however, was a second and important hyperbaric oxygen–induced therapeutic mechanism. Boerema had conclusively demonstrated that large volumes of oxygen could be transported in simple solution and in the absence of hemoglobin.[63] This effect would eventually become the treatment basis for acute carbon monoxide intoxication, crush injuries and other acute ischemias, inadequately perfused skin flaps, and exceptional blood loss anemia.

Although the ability of hyperbaric therapy to increase blood oxygen transport is intuitive today, only 20 years before Boerema's findings this concept had been ridiculed. According to the highly respected chairman of the University of Chicago Department of Medicine in a letter to the editor of *Journal of the American Medical Association*,[66] "[T]he claim that the method (hyperbaric therapy) has any effect on oxygen supply or oxygen tension in the tissues is

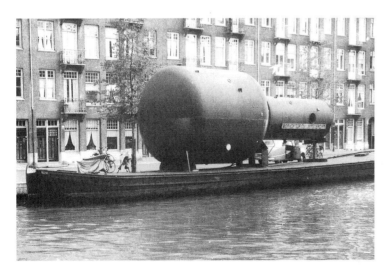

Figure 1.3 Boerema's hyperbaric operating room being delivered via an Amsterdam canal to Hospital Wilhelmina Gasthius. *(Permission granted by Best Publishing Company, Bakker DJ and Cramer FS: Hyperbaric Surgery, Perioperative Care, Flagstaff, Ariz, 2002.)*

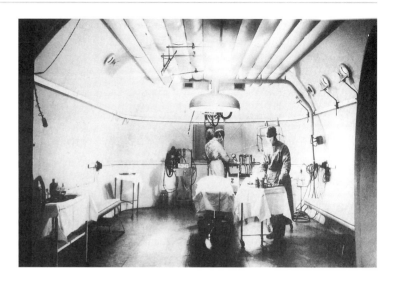

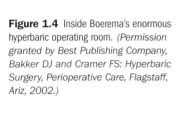

Figure 1.4 Inside Boerema's enormous hyperbaric operating room. *(Permission granted by Best Publishing Company, Bakker DJ and Cramer FS: Hyperbaric Surgery, Perioperative Care, Flagstaff, Ariz, 2002.)*

absurd. To claim that oxygen may be made to reach tissues at higher tensions is only to display ignorance of the mechanism by which oxygen is transported to and given off to the tissues"(p.1808). Even in the 1960s, some scientists remained convinced that the only way to increase oxygen delivery was to increase hemoglobin. They thought that dissolved oxygen was insignificant in oxygen transport.[67]

CLINICAL HYPERBARIC MEDICINE

Several members of Western Infirmary's Department of Surgery, Glasgow, Scotland, extended the investigation of hyperbaric oxygen therapy during this period, with an emphasis on acute ischemias.[68-72] Using a converted autoclave, Smith and Lawson studied the effects of hyperbaric oxygenation in a dog model of coronary artery occlusion.[71] After ligation of the circumflex coronary artery, dogs were randomized to receive 2.0 ATA oxygen or normal atmospheric air. They reported that 90% of the hyperbaric group was protected from the ventricular fibrillation that killed 60% of control animals. Similar findings were reported elsewhere.[73]

The first clinical experience of hyperbaric oxygen in the treatment of acute myocardial infarction was reported in 1962 by the Glasgow

group, initially involving a single patient.[70] Within 2 years they were able to report a randomized trial involving 36 cases, 18 treated at 2.0 ATA oxygen and 18 control subjects. No statistically significant difference was observed between the groups.[74]

Hyperbaric oxygen has, however, continued to be of research interest in myocardial infarction over the ensuing years. It has been found somewhat beneficial when used in concert with thrombolytic agents in both animals[75] and humans,[76,77] and as a method to reduce complications after stent placements.[78] The current role of hyperbaric oxygen therapy in acute coronary syndrome has recently been reviewed.[79]

It is somewhat surprising that it took until 1960 to treat the first human carbon monoxide poisoning with hyperbaric oxygen. Haldane[80] had demonstrated its value in animals some 50 years earlier. Subsequent animal studies determined that hyperbaric oxygen hastened the elimination of carbon monoxide from blood and provided sufficient plasma-borne oxygen to overcome failure of hemoglobin transport.[81-83] Pace and coworkers[84] confirmed these effects in healthy human volunteers.

The Glasgow group's first two carbon monoxide patients were particularly compromised. Their prompt recovery was attributed to treatment with 2.0 ATA oxygen therapy, and this dose of oxygen soon became a treatment standard at Western University. By 1962, their case experience had grown to 22 patients.[85]

ANTIMICROBIAL EFFECTS

Shortly after he introduced hyperbaric cardiac surgery, Boerema[86] used his chamber to treat a "hopeless" case of gas gangrene, that is, hopeless in that limb amputation was not an option. Boerema elected to use hyperbaric oxygen therapy at 3.0 ATA for 2 hours daily. A dramatic arrest of the advancing infection was observed, and systemic toxicity soon resolved. Boerema, Brummelkamp, and colleagues subsequently accumulated 40 cases[87] and then 80 cases.[88] In most patients, *Clostridial perfringens* was the primary organism. The use of oxygen to treat gas gangrene was, however, not new; it too had been injected directly into infected tissues of soldiers during World War I, used by Hinton in the same manner 30 years later,[89] and had already been delivered hyperbarically by de Almeida.[45]

The somewhat arbitrary selection of 3.0 ATA as the treatment pressure appeared fortuitous. Van Unnik[90] subsequently showed that alpha toxin production by *Clostridial perfringens* was inhibited, although not arrested, at 3.0 ATA, but not at lesser pressures.

A growing body of animal and clinical evidence followed. It became apparent that the action of hyperbaric oxygen was based on the formation of oxygen free radicals in the relative absence of free radical degrading enzymes such as superoxide dismutases, catalases, and peroxidases.[91-93] Although hyperbaric oxygen does not kill clostridia directly, it is bacteriostatic in vivo and in vitro.[94-96] In a dog model, the greatest reduction in morbidity was achieved when hyperbaric oxygen was combined with antibiotics and surgery.[97]

Hyperbaric oxygen was subsequently reported to be useful in the treatment of chronic osteomyelitis. Experimental work and clinical experience demonstrated enhanced osteogenesis,[98,99] improved bacterial cell wall antibiotic transport,[100] and heightened leukocyte-mediated killing of aerobic organisms.[101]

Application of the antimicrobial properties of hyperbaric oxygen was extended to the treatment of necrotizing soft-tissue infections caused by aerobic, anaerobic, and mixed bacterial flora.[102-104]

WOUND HEALING

In 1965, in Japan, Wada and colleagues[105] reported an observation that was to have a profound effect on the practice of hyperbaric medicine. Survivors of a coal mine fire with carbon monoxide poisoning were treated with hyperbaric oxygen. Some of these miners suffered concurrent burns. It was the impression of Wada's group that those patients treated with hyperbaric oxygen enjoyed improved burn wound healing compared with those burned miners who did not require hyperbaric oxygen therapy for carbon monoxide poisoning.

This observation prompted several investigators to study the potential of hyperbaric oxygen in animals, invariably involving a second-degree burn model. Hyperbaric oxygen was found to reduce burn wound edema,[106] improve healing time,[107] reduce infection rates,[107] produce an earlier return to capillary potency, and minimize inflammatory response.[108]

Published clinical experience was slow to accumulate. One small, randomized trial demonstrated reduced fluid requirements, faster healing rates, and reduced mortality rates.[109] Other reports, largely retrospective, suggested reduced skin grafting requirements,[110] lowered mortality and reduced hospital stays,[111] reduced infection rates,[112] and lower costs[113] when hyperbaric oxygen was incorporated into standard burn care management.

Despite these purported benefits, hyperbaric oxygen therapy has not been embraced by the burn wound community. It is possible that issues involving patient stabilization and management requirements, patient absence from the tightly controlled burn care environment, and concern about cross-contamination demand better scientific support before hyperbaric oxygen is accepted as treatment for burn victims.

Having initially concerned themselves with acute ischemias, the Glasgow group extended their interest in hyperbaric oxygen therapy to chronic obliterate vascular disorders. Some modest successes were reported in ischemic ulcers, but overall results were disappointing. It was hypothesized by others at Western University that a possible explanation for the lack of apparent benefit from hyperbaric oxygen was due to its vasoconstrictive effect. Blood vessels of the eye had been observed to constrict while volunteers breathed 100% oxygen under normal atmospheric conditions.[114] The same effect was observed within the cerebral vasculature and magnified at 3.5 ATA oxygen.[115] If blood flow to the limb was reduced in the same way, it was proposed that the benefit of hyperbaric oxygen to increase oxygen content might be lost.[116] Should this be the case, it might explain the failure of hyperbaric oxygen to produce improvement in patients with peripheral vascular disease.

Using young healthy volunteers, Bird and Telfer[116] measured forearm blood flow by occlusion plethysmography at 1.0 and 2.0 ATA oxygen. Mean blood flow decreased by 11.2% and 18.91%, respectively. The authors concluded that a homeostatic mechanism existed in ischemic limbs. As oxygen content is increased, blood flow correspondingly decreases, so that hyperbaric doses of oxygen never reach ischemic tissues.

Unfortunately, these researchers were unable to measure oxygen content. Had they been able to do so, they would have observed its profound increase as subsequent authors reported.[117,118] These tissue oxygen increases are largely dependent on adequate large-vessel patency.

Although unhelpful for chronic arterial occlusive disease, the vasoconstrictive effect of hyperbaric oxygen, occurring without concurrent hypoxia, has proved therapeutic elsewhere. Vasoconstriction occurs at the level of the arteriole. Venules are unaffected, so outflow is maintained. The net effect of hyperoxic-induced vasoconstriction, therefore, is to reduce edema. Indications include the impending stage of compartment syndrome,[119] acute thermal burns,[110] and edematous skin flaps.[120]

By the 1970s, the practice of hyperbaric medicine was based on several and frequently complementary effects. The inverse relation of absolute pressure to gas bubble volume (Boyle's Law) served as the mechanistic basis for the treatment of decompression sickness. This effect was enhanced with the provision of oxygen. Hyperoxygenation was used to support hypoxic tissues secondary to acute ischemic events, and to facilitate disassociation and hasten elimination of carbon monoxide. Antimicrobial activities were used in the treatment of both anaerobic and mixed anaerobic and aerobic infections, as well as to support leukocyte-mediated phagocytosis in infected and chronically infected bone. Vasoconstriction reduced compartment pressures and improved edematous states.

During this same period, treatment of conditions related to the above effects brought to light another potential hyperbaric application. It appeared as if some chronic wounds, related or otherwise to the primary hyperbaric indication, were healed as a consequence of hyperbaric oxygen treatments.[67]

This suggestion was counterintuitive to some scientists, who appreciated that the central environment of the healing wound was hypoxia, with resulting accumulations of lactate. Would not hyperbaric oxygen overwhelm the wound and eliminate this presumably normal healing environment?

This answer was no. It became evident that although lactate initiates wound repair, many of its subsequent reparative phases are oxygen dependent.[121-126] If a wound is compromised by local *tissue* hypoxia, it will stall or completely fail to heal. Hyperbaric oxygen, in the setting of adequate regional perfusion, will reestablish the necessary wound oxygen gradient. To determine whether a particular patient has sufficient physiologic capacity to respond locally (the wound) to centrally delivered hyperoxia, transcutaneous oxygen testing proved helpful.[127] The most precise indication for hyperbaric oxygen therapy in the management of a chronic wound is a low (<40 mm Hg) periwound transcutaneous oxygen value that briskly reverses on oxygen inhalation.[128]

Transcutaneous oximetry, applied algorithmically, will aid in patient selection, identify nonresponders, and suggest a therapeutic end point.[129] This screening process serves to enhance clinical outcome and the cost-effectiveness of hyperbaric oxygen therapy.

Hyperbaric wound referrals now extend to arterial insufficiency,[130] diabetic,[131,132] and soft-tissue radionecrosis[133,134] causative agents. Some of the stronger evidence relates to mandibular osteoradionecrosis. A clear understanding of its pathophysiology has emerged,[135] and so, too, has evidence that hyperbaric but not normobaric oxygen will stimulate angiogenesis.[136]

The sixth and most recently identified benefit of hyperbaric oxygen relates to ischemia-reperfusion injury. What was initially considered by some as a harmful effect of high levels of oxygen[137] is emerging as a potentially valuable therapeutic and preconditioning agent.

Prolonged periods of acute interruption in blood flow result in injury to the microcirculation and may lead to cell death. Paradoxically, subsequent reperfusion may actually accelerate these deleterious effects.[138] Reperfusion, by adjuvant therapy, decompression, or revascularization, has the potential to induce a complex interplay between adhesion molecules and neuropils with resulting microvascular plugging. This secondary ischemic state is frequently referred to as the "flow/no reflow phenomenon."

The well-documented deleterious effects of oxygen-derived free radicals might suggest that hyperbaric oxygen as a treatment or preventative measure is counterintuitive. One might expect an exacerbation of ischemia-reperfusion injury secondary to increased production of oxygen-derived free radicals associated with hyperbaric oxygenation. Animal studies have, however, failed to identify any harmful effect; in fact, the reverse has been demonstrated. In rats and rabbits, involving liver, brain, heart, skeletal muscle, small intestine, skin, and endothelial cell ischemia-reperfusion preparations, improved outcome was uniformly noted when hyperbaric oxygen was applied immediately before, during, or immediately after acute ischemia.[139] The effect of hyperbaric oxygen appears principally the result of a down-regulation of adhesion molecule function on leukocytes and vascular endothelium.[140]

These findings suggest a clinical foundation for the employment of hyperbaric oxygen therapy in several high-risk settings for ischemia-reperfusion injury. Examples include acute traumatic peripheral ischemias, compartment surgery, hypoxic birth, injury, and cardiac surgery. This latter example has already been the subject of a randomized clinical trial,[141] with encouraging results. Hyperbaric oxygen is already being advocated in all patients with revascularization or replanted extremities involving ischemia times greater than 6 hours.[142]

REFERENCES

1. Simpson A: Compressed Air, as a Therapeutic Agent in the Treatment of Consumption, Asthma, Chronic Bronchitis, and Other Diseases. Edinburgh, Scotland, Sutherland and Knox, 1857.
2. Lane N: Oxygen: The Molecule That Made the World, Oxford, United Kingdom, Oxford University Press, 2002.
3. Priestly J: Experiments and Observations on Different Kinds of Air. Birmingham, England, 1775.
4. Arntzenius AKW: De Pneumatische Therapie. Boekhandel, Amsterdam, Scheltema & Holkema's, 1887.
5. Tabarie E: Recherches sur les effets des variations dans la pression atmospherique a la surface du corps. Compt Rend 6:896, 1838.
6. Tabarie E: Sur l' action therapeutique de l'air comprime. Compt Rend 11:26, 1840.
7. Junod VT: Recherches physiologiques et therapeutiques sur les effets de la compression ed de la rarefaction de l'air, tant sur le corps que sur les members isoles. Rev Med Franc Etrange 3:350, 1834.
8. Pravaz C: Memoire sur l'application du bain in d'air comprime au traitement des affections tuberculenses, des hemorrhagies capillaries et des surdites catarrhales. Bull Acad Natl Med (Paris) 2:985, 1837-1838.
9. Pravaz C: Memoire sur l'emploi du bain d'air comprime au traitement des affections tuberculenses, des hemorrhagies capillaries et des surdites catarrhales. Bull Acad Natl Med (Paris) 5:177, 1840.
10. Bertin E: Etude clinique de l'emploi et des effets du bain d'air comprime dans le traitement des maladies de poitrine. Montpellier Med 1868.
11. Forlanini C: Brevissimi cenni sull' aeroterapia e sullo stabilimento medico-pneumatico di Milano. Gazz Med Lombarda Ser 7.2:371, 385, 397, 405, 1875.
12. Jacobson J, Morsch J, Rendell-Baker L: The historical perspective of hyperbaric therapy. Ann N Y Acad Sci 117:651–670, 1965.
13. Fontaine JA: Effets Physiologiques et Applications Therapeutiques de l' Air Comprime. Paris, France, Germer-Bailliere, 1877.

14. Triger: Memoir sur un appareil a air comprime par le placement des puit de mines at autres travaux, sous le eaux et dans les sables submerges. Comptes rendus de l'Academie des Sciences 13:884-896, 1841, as cited in Bert P: Barometric Pressure: Researchers in Experimental Physiology (originally published 1878). Hitchcock MA, Hitchcock FA (trans.). Columbus, Ohio, College Book Company, 1943.

15. Cochrane T: Apparatus for excavating, sinking, and mining. Patent Application 1830 No. 6018, London, 1831.

16. United States Navy Diving Manual. Rev. 4. Washington, DC, Superintendent of Documents U.S. Government Printing Office, 1999.

17. Triger AG: Lettre a M. Arago. Comptes Rendus de l'Academie des Sciences 20:445-449, 1845.

18. Blavier M: Rapport sur le procede suivi, a Douchy, pour traverser des nappes d'eau considerables. Ann des Mines, 4e ser 9:349-364, 1846.

19. Pol B, Watelle TJJ: Memoire sur les effets de la compression de l'air appliqué au creusement des puits a houille. Ann D'Hygiene Publique et de Medecine Legale 1(Ser 2):241-279, 1854, as cited in Bert P: Barometric Pressure: Researches in Experimental Physiology (originally published 1878). Hitchcock MA, Hitchcock FA (trans.). Columbus, Ohio, College Book Company, 1943. Republished: Bethesda, Md, Undersea and Hyperbaric Medical Society, 1978, pp 362-367, and Snell EH: Compressed Air Illness or So-called Caisson Disease. London, HK Lewis, 1896, pp 10-16.

20. De Mericourt L: Considerations sur l'Hygiene des Pecheurs d'Eponges. Ann Hyg Publ 31:274-286, 1869.

21. Bert P: La Pression Barometrique. 1879. Bert P: Barometric Pressure. Researches in Experimental Physiology. Hitchcock MA, Hitchcock FA (trans.). Columbus, Ohio, College Book Company, 1943.

22. Bauer: Pathological effects upon the brain and spinal cord of men exposed to the action of a largely increased atmospheric pressure. St. Louis Medical and Surgical Journal, New Series 7:234-245, May 1870.

23. Jaminet A: Physical Effects of Compressed Air and of the Causes of Pathological Symptoms Produced on Man, by Increased Atmospheric Pressure Employed for the Sinking of Piers, in the Construction of the Illinois and St. Louis Bridge over the Mississippi River at St. Louis, Missouri. St. Louis, Ennis, 1871.

24. Jarcho S: Alphonse Jaminet on caisson disease (1871). Wilderness Environ Med 10:112-114, 1999.

25. McCullough D: The Great Bridge. New York, Simon and Schuster, 1972.

26. Smith AH: St. Louis Medicine and Surgery Journal (3), 1870, quoted by Hill L: Caisson Sickness and the Physiology of Work in Compressed Air. London, Arnold, 1912.

27. Smith AH: The Effects of High Atmospheric Pressure Including Caisson Disease. Brooklyn, NY, Eagle Book and Job Printing Department, 1873.

28. Moir EW: Tunnelling by compressed air. Journal of the Society of Arts 567-585, 1896.

29. Boycott GWM: Caisson-disease at the new high-level bridge, Newcastle-on-Tyne, England, Trans Inst Civil Engineering CLXV, 1906, pp 231-237.

30. Keays FL: Compressed air illness, with a report of 3,692 cases. Dept Med Publ, Cornell University Medical College 2:1-55, 1909.

31. Haldane JS, Boycott AE, Damant GCC, et al: Report of a Committee Appointed by the Lord Commissioners of the Admiralty to Consider and Report upon the Condition of Deep Water Diving. London, His Majesty's Stationary Office, CN 1549/1907.

32. Boycott AE, Damant GCC, Haldane JS: The prevention of compressed air illness. J Hyg Camb 8:342-443, 1908.

33. Golding FC, Griffiths P, Hempleman HV, et al: Decompression sickness during construction of the Dartford Tunnel. Br J Ind Med 17:167-180, 1960.

34. Corning J: The use of compressed air in conjunction with medicinal solutions in the treatment of nervous and mental affections. Medical Reports, New York 40:225-232, 1891.

35. Sellers LM: The fallibility of the Forrestian principle. Anesth Analg 44:L40, 1965.

36. Brown IW, Fuson RL, Mauney FM, et al: Hyperbaric oxygenation (hybaroxia): current status, possibilities and limitations. Adv Surg 1:285-349, 1965.

37. Cunningham O: Oxygen therapy by means of compressed air. Anesth Analg 64-66, 1927.

38. Bureau of Investigation: The Cunningham 'tank treatment.' J Am Med Assoc 90:1494-1495, 1928.

39. Almeida AO: Recherches sur l'action toxique des hautes pressions d'oxygene. Societe de Biologie de Paris (Meeting Proceedings) 66:1225, 1934.

40. Almeida AO: Recherches sur laction toxique de l'oxygene sous haute pression sur l'homme. Archivos da Fundacao Gaffree-Guinle, Oxygenio e Cancer (supp):17-22, 1935.

41. Almeida AO: Do emprego do oxygenio em alta pressao no tratamento do cancer esperimental do rato e no cancer do homen. Separata dos Archivos da Fundacao Gaffree e Guinle 11-15, 1934-1935.

42. Almeida AO: Essais du traitement du cancer humain par l'oxygene sous pression. Annaes da Academia Brazileira de Sciencias 7:191-194, 1935.

43. Almeida AO: Research on the treatment of experimental and human cancer by oxygen under pressure. Archivos da Fundacao Gaffree-Guinle, Oxygenio e Cancer (suppl):29-36, 1938.

44. Almeida AO, Costa HM: Treatment of leprosy by oxygen under high pressure associated with methylene blue. Revista Brasileira de Leprologia 6(suppl):237-265, 1938.

45. Almeida AO, Pacheco G: Ensaios de tratamento das gangrenes gazozas experimentais pelo oxigenio em altas pressoes e pelo oxigenio em estado nascente. Revista Brasileira de Biologia 1:1-10, 1941.

46. Behnke AR, Shaw LA: The use of oxygen in the treatment of compressed-air illness. U.S. Navy Med Bull 35:61-73, 1937.

47. Clarke D: Diver medics: The first ten years. Proceedings International Diving Symposium. New Orleans, Association of Diving Contractors, 1984.

48. Rivera JC: Decompression sickness among divers: An analysis of 935 cases. Mil Med 129:314-334, 1964.

49. Goodman MW, Workman RD, Hedgepath CH, et al: Minimal-recompression, oxygen-breathing approach to

treatment of decompression sickness in divers and aviators. Research Report 5-65. Washington, DC, U.S. Navy Experimental Diving Unit, 1965.

50. Gray LH: Radiobiologic basis of oxygen as a modifying factor in radiation therapy. Am J Roentgenol 84:803-815, 1961.

51. Gray LH, Couger AD, Ebert M, et al: Concentration of oxygen dissolved in tissues at time of irradiation as a factor in radiation therapy. Br J Radiol 26:638, 1953.

52. Gray LH: Oxygen in radiotherapy. Br J Radiol 30:403, 1957.

53. Churchill-Davidson I, Sanger C, Thomlinson RH, et al: High-pressure oxygen and radiotherapy. Lancet 1091-1095, 1955.

54. Churchill-Davidson I, Sanger C, Thomlinson RH, et al: Oxygenation in radiotherapy. Br J Radiol 30:406, 1957.

55. Churchill-Davidson I, Sanger C, Thomlinson RH: Oxygenation in radiotherapy. II. Clinical application. Br J Radiol 30:406-422, 1957.

56. Emery EW, Lucas BG, Williams KG: Technique of irradiation of conscious patients under increased oxygen pressure. Lancet 1:248-250, 1960.

57. Sanger C: High pressure oxygen and radiation therapy. Am J Roentgenol 81:498-503, 1959.

58. Atkins HL, Seaman WB, Jacox HW, et al: Experience with hyperbaric oxygenation in clinical radiotherapy. Am J Roentgenol 93:651-663, 1965.

59. Cater DB, Schoeniger EL, Watkinson DA: Effect on oxygen tension of tumors of breathing oxygen at high pressures. Lancet 2:381-383, 1962.

60. Evans JC: Metastasis following radiotherapy in hyperbaric oxygen. Radiology 93:1155-1157, 1969.

61. Kagan AR, Bryant TL, Johnson RE: Hyperbaric oxygen effect on experimental tumor growth. Radiology 88:775-777, 1967.

62. Boerema I, Wildshut A, Schmidt WJH, et al: Experimental researches into hypothermia as an aid to surgery of the heart. Arch Chir Neerl 3:25, 1951.

63. Boerema I, Meyne NG, Brummelkamp WK, et al: Life without blood (a study of the influence of high atmospheric pressure and hypothermia on dilution of the blood). J Cardiovasc Surg 1:133-146, 1960.

64. Boerema I, Vermeulen-Cranch DMC, Meijne NG, et al: Observations during operation on deeply cyanotic young children breathing oxygen at three atmospheres absolute. Pediatr Surg 52:796-799, 1962.

65. Bernhard WF, Tank ES, Frittelli G: The feasibility of hypothermic perfusion under hyperbaric conditions in the surgical management of infants with cyanotic congenital heart disease. J Thorac Cardiovasc Surg 46:651-664, 1963.

66. McLean FC: J Am Med Assoc 90:1808, 1928.

67. Hunt TK, Gimbel ML: Hyperbaric oxygen and wound healing. Hyperbaric Surgery Perioperative Care. Flagstaff, Ariz, Best Publishing, 2002.

68. Illingworth CFW: Treatment of arterial occlusion under oxygen at two-atmospheres pressure. Br Med J 5315, November 1962.

69. Illingworth CFW, Smith G, Lawson DD, et al: Surgical and physiological observations in an experimental pressure chamber. Br J Surg 49:222-227, 1961.

70. Ledingham I: Some clinical and experimental applications of high pressure oxygen. Proc R Soc Med 56:31-34, 1963.

71. Smith G, Lawson DA: Experimental coronary arterial occlusion: effects of the administration of oxygen under pressure. Scot Med J 3:346-350, 1958.

72. Lawson DD, McCallister RA, Smith G: Treatment of acute experimental carbon-monoxide poisoning with oxygen under pressure. Lancet 800-802, April 1961.

73. Trapp WG, Creighton R: Experimental studies of increased atmospheric pressure on myocardial ischemia after coronary ligation. J Thorac Cardiovasc Surg 47:687-692, 1964.

74. Cameron AJV, Hutton I, Kenmure AC, et al: Controlled clinical trial of oxygen at 2 atmospheres in myocardial infarction. In: Boerema I (ed): Clinical Application of Hyperbaric Oxygen. Amsterdam, Elsevier Press, 1964, p 75.

75. Thomas MP, Brown LA, Sponseller DR, et al: Myocardial infarct size reduction by the synergistic effect of hyperbaric oxygen and recombinant tissue plasminogen activator. Am Heart J 120:791-800, 1990.

76. Shandling AH, Ellestad MH, Hart GB, et al: Hyperbaric oxygen and thrombolysis in myocardial infarction: The 'Hot MI' pilot study. Am Heart J 134:544-550, 1997.

77. Dekleva M, Neskovic A, Vlahovic A, et al: Adjunctive effect of hyperbaric oxygen treatment after thrombolysis on left ventricular function in patients with acute myocardial infarction. Am Heart J 148:E14, 2004.

78. Sharifi M, Fares W, Abdel-Karim I, et al: Inhibition of restenosis by hyperbaric oxygen: A novel indication for an old modality. Cardiovasc Radiat Med 3:124-126, 2003.

79. Bennett M, Jepson N, Lehm JP: Hyperbaric oxygen for acute coronary syndrome. Cochrane Database Syst Rev (2):CD004818.PUB2, 2005.

80. Haldane JBS: Reflection of action of carbonic acid to oxygen tension. J Physiol 18:201, 1895.

81. End E, Long CW: Oxygen under pressure in carbon monoxide poisoning. J Ind Hyg Technol 24:302-306, 1942.

82. Bronston PK, Corre KA, Decker SJ: Carbon monoxide poisoning: A review, topics in emergency medicine 8(4):50-59, 1987.

83. Douglas TA, Lawson DD, Ledingham I, et al: Carbon monoxide poisoning. Lancet 68, January 1962.

84. Pace N, Strajman E, Walker EL: Acceleration of carbon monoxide elimination in man by high pressure oxygen. Science 3:652-654, 1950.

85. Smith G: Treatment of coal-gas poisoning with oxygen at 2 atmospheres pressure. Lancet 816-818, April 1962.

86. Boerema I, Groeneveld PHA: Gas gangrene treated with hyperbaric oxygenation. Proceedings of the 4th International Congress on Hyperbaric Medicine, Sapporo, Japan. Baltimore, Williams & Wilkins, 1969, pp 255-262.

87. Brummelkamp WH, Hogendijk J, Boerema I: Treatment of anaerobic infections (clostridial myositis) by drenching the tissues with oxygen under high atmospheric pressure. Surgery 49:299-302, 1961.

88. Groeneveld PHA: Current therapy of gas gangrene. Advances and Perceives in the Management of Bacteriological Infections. San Francisco, University of California, San Francisco, 1967.

89. Hinton D: A method for the arrest of spreading gas gangrene by oxygen injection. Lancet 32:228-232, 1947.

90. Van Unnik AJM: Inhibition of toxin production in clostridium perfringens in vitro by hyperbaric oxygen. Antonie Van Leeuwenhoek 31:181-186, 1965.

91. Hirn M: Hyperbaric oxygen in the treatment of gas gangrene and perineal necrotizing fasciitis. Eur J Surg Suppl 570:1-36, 1993.

92. Hirn M, Niinikoski J, Lehtonen OP: Effect of hyperbaric oxygen and surgery on experimental multimicrobial gas gangrene. Eur Surg Res 25:265-269, 1993.

93. Bakker DJ, Van der Kleij AJ: Clostridial myonecrosis. Handbook on Hyperbaric Medicine. Springer, 1996, pp 362-385.

94. Kaye D: Effect of hyperbaric oxygen on clostridia in vitro and in vivo. Proc Soc Exp Biol Med 124:360-366, 1967.

95. Hill GB, Osterhout S: Effects of hyperbaric oxygen on clostridial species and experimental anaerobic infections. Proceedings of the 4th International Congress on Hyperbaric Medicine, Sapporo, Japan. Baltimore, Williams & Wilkins, 1969, pp 282-287.

96. Muhvich KH, Anderson LH, Mehm WJ: Evaluation of antimicrobials combined with hyperbaric oxygen in a mouse model of clostridial myonecrosis. J Trauma 36:7-10, 1994.

97. Demello FJ, Haglin JJ, Hitchcock CR: Comparative study of experimental clostridium perfringens infection in dogs treated with antibiotics, surgery, and HBO. Surgery 73:936-941, 1973.

98. Coulson DB, Ferguson AB, Diehl RC: Effect of hyperbaric oxygen on the healing femur of the rat. Surg Forum 17:449-450, 1966.

99. Stead DL: Enhancement of osteogenesis with hyperbaric oxygen therapy. A clinical study. J Dent Res 61A:288, 1982.

100. Mader JT, Adams KR, Couch LA, et al: Potentiation of tobramycin by hyperbaric oxygen in experimental *Pseudomonas aeruginosa* osteomyelitis. Paper presented at the 27th Interscience Conference on Antimicrobial Agents and Chemotherapy, 1987.

101. Mader JT, Brown GL, Guckian JC, et al: A mechanism for the amelioration by hyperbaric oxygen of experimental staphylococcal osteomyelitis in rabbits. J Infect Dis 142:915-922, 1980.

102. Hirn M: Hyperbaric oxygen in the treatment of gas gangrene and perineal necrotizing fasciitis. Eur J Surg Suppl 570:1-36, 1993.

103. Riseman JA, Zamboni WA, Curtis A, et al: Hyperbaric oxygen therapy for necrotizing fasciitis reduces mortality and the need for debridements. Surgery 108:847-850, 1990.

104. Hollabaugh RS, Dmochowski RR, Hickerson WL, et al: Fournier's gangrene: Therapeutic impact of hyperbaric oxygen. Plast Reconstr Surg 101:94-100, 1998.

105. Wada J, Ikeda T, Kamata K, et al: Oxygen hyperbaric treatment for carbon monoxide poisoning and severe burn in coal mine gas explosion. (hokutanyubari) Igakunoaymi (Japan) 5:53, 1965.

106. Ikeda K, Ajiki H, Nagao H, et al: Experimental and clinical use of hyperbaric oxygen in burns. Proceedings of the 4th International Congress on Hyperbaric Medicine, Sapporo, Japan. Baltimore, Williams & Wilkins 377-380, 1969.

107. Ketchum SA, Zubrin JR, Thomas AN, et al: Effect of hyperbaric oxygen on small first, second, and third degree burns. Surg Forum 18:65-67, 1967.

108. Korn H, Wheeler ES, Miller TA: Effect of hyperbaric oxygen on second-degree burn wound healing. Arch Surg 112:732-737, 1977.

109. Hart GB, Oreilly RR, Broussard ND, et al: Treatment of burns with hyperbaric oxygen. Surg Gynecol Obstet 139:693-696, 1974.

110. Cianci PE, Lueders HW, Lee H, et al: Adjunctive hyperbaric oxygen reduces the need for surgery in 40-80% burns. J Hyperb Med 3:97-101, 1988.

111. Cianci PE, Lueders HW, Lee H, et al: Adjunctive hyperbaric oxygen therapy reduces length of hospitalization in thermal burns. J Burn Care Rehabil 10:432-435, 1989.

112. Waisbren BA, Schutz D, Collentine G, et al: Hyperbaric oxygen in severe burns. Burns 8:176-179, 1982.

113. Cianci PE, Williams C, Lueders H, et al: Adjunctive hyperbaric oxygen in the treatment of thermal burns: An economic analysis. J Burn Care Rehabil 11:140-143, 1990.

114. Dollery CT, Hill DW, Mailer CM, et al: High oxygen pressure and the retinal blood-vessels. Lancet 291-292, August 1964.

115. Lambertsen CJ, Kough RH, Cooper DY, et al: Oxygen toxicity. Effects in man of oxygen inhalation at 1 and 3.5 atmospheres upon blood gas transport, cerebral circulation and cerebral metabolism. Appl Physiol 5:471-486, 1953.

116. Bird AD, Telfer AMB: Effect of hyperbaric oxygen on limb circulation. Lancet 355-356, February 1965.

117. Wells CH, Goodpasture JE, Horrigan D, et al: Tissue gas measurements during hyperbaric oxygen exposure. Proceedings of the 6th International Congress on Hyperbaric Medicine. Aberdeen, Scotland, Aberdeen University Press, 1977, pp 118-124.

118. Sheffield PJ: Tissue oxygen measurements with respect to soft-tissue wound healing with normobaric and hyperbaric oxygen. HBO Rev 6:18-46, 1985.

119. Strauss MB, Hart GB: Compartment syndromes: Update and role of hyperbaric oxygen. HBO Rev 5:163-182, 1985.

120. Zamboni WA: Applications of hyperbaric oxygen therapy in plastic-surgery. Handbook on Hyperbaric Medicine. Berlin, Springer, 1996, pp 443-483.

121. Lavan FB, Hunt TK: Oxygen and wound healing. Clin Plast Surg 17:463-472, 1990.

122. Johnson K, Hunt T, Mathes S: Oxygen as an isolated variable influences resistance to infection. Ann Surg 208:783-787, 1988.

123. Skover GR: Cellular and biochemical dynamics of wound repair. Wound environment in collagen regeneration. Clin Podiatr Med Surg 8:723-756, 1991.

124. Knighton DR, Silver IA, Hunt TK: Regulation of wound-healing angiogenesis effect of oxygen gradients and inspired oxygen concentration. Surgery 90:262-270, 1981.

125. Winter GD: Oxygen and epidermal wound healing. Adv Exp Med Biol 94:673-678, 1977.

126. Kivisaari J, Niinikioski J: Effects of hyperbaric oxygenation and prolonged hypoxia on the healing of open wounds. Acta Chir Scand 141:14-19, 1975.

127. Sheffield PJ: Tissue oxygen measurements. Problem Wounds: The Role of Oxygen. New York, Elsevier Publishing Company, 1988, pp 17-39.

128. Hunt TK, Gimbel ML: Hyperbaric oxygen in wound healing. Hyperbaric Surgery. Flagstaff, Ariz, Best Publishing Company, 2002, pp 429–459.

129. Clarke D: An evidence-based approach to hyperbaric wound healing. Blood Gas News 7:14–20, 1998.

130. Hammarlund C, Sundberg T: Hyperbaric oxygen reduced size of chronic leg ulcers: A randomized double-blind study. Plast Reconstr Surg 93:829–834, 1994.

131. Faglia E, Favales F, Aldehgi A, et al: Adjunctive systemic hyperbaric oxygen therapy in treatment of severe prevalently ischemic diabetic foot ulcer. Diabetes Care 19:1338–1343, 1996.

132. Kalani M, Jorneskog G, Naderi N, et al: Hyperbaric oxygen (HBO) therapy in treatment of diabetic foot ulcers. Long-term follow-up. J Diabetes Complicat 16:153–158, 2002.

133. Bevers RFM, Bakker DJ, Kurth KH: Hyperbaric oxygen treatment for haemorrhagic radiation cystitis. Lancet 346:803–805, 1995.

134. Feldmeier JJ, Heimbach RD, Davolt DA, et al: Hyperbaric oxygen as an adjunctive treatment for delayed radiation injury of the chest wall: A retrospective review of twenty-three cases. Undersea Hyperb Med 22:383–393, 1995.

135. Marx RE: Osteoradionecrosis: A new concept of its pathophysiology. J Oral Maxillofac Surg 41:283–288, 1983.

136. Marx RE, Ehler WJ, Tayapongsak P, et al: Relationship of oxygen dose to angiogenesis induction in irradiated tissue. Am J Surg 160:519–524, 1990.

137. Benke PJ: Jessica in the well: Ischemia and reperfusion injury. JAMA 259:1326, 1988.

138. Russell RC, Roth AC, Kucan JO, et al: Reperfusion injury and oxygen free radicals. A review. J Reconstr Microsurg 5:79, 1989.

139. Buras J: Basic mechanisms of hyperbaric oxygen in the treatment of ischemia-reperfusion injury. Int Anesthesiol Clin 38:91–108, 2000.

140. Buras JA, Stahl GL, Svoboda KKH, et al: Hyperbaric oxygen down regulates ICAM-1 expression induced by hypoxia and hypoglycemia: The role of Nos. Am J Physiol Cell Physiol 278:C292–C302, 2000.

141. Zamboni WA: Hyperbaric Medicine Practice. Kindwall EP (ed). Flagstaff, Ariz, Best Publishing Company, 1995.

142. Alex J, Laden G, Cale ARJ, et al: Pretreatment with hyperbaric oxygen and its effect on neuropsychometric dysfunction and systemic inflammatory response after cardiopulmonary bypass: A prospective randomized double-blind trial. J Thorac Cardiovasc Surg 130:1623–1630, 2005.

Technical **II** Aspects

Monoplace Hyperbaric Chambers

2

Lindell Weaver, MD

Monoplace hyperbaric chambers are designed to compress a single individual to greater than sea level pressure. Monoplace chambers have been used to treat patients for more than 50 years. For purposes of clinical hyperbaric oxygen delivery, the pressure must exceed 1.4 atmospheres absolute (ATA).[1] Topical oxygen is not hyperbaric oxygen and will not be reviewed in this chapter. Topical oxygen consists of placing a patient's wound within an oxygen-filled bag or chamber at pressures nom-inally greater than sea level pressure and should not be considered as "hyperbaric oxygen."[2] The Gamow bag is an inflatable hyperbaric chamber device used to alleviate symptoms and signs of high-altitude illness, and therapeutic pressures may be less than or equivalent to sea level (1 ATA); it is also not considered hyperbaric oxygen therapy (HBOT).[3]

Clinical monoplace hyperbaric chambers are cylindrical, range from 25 to 40 inches in diameter, and are customarily 8 feet in length. Monoplace chambers are generally made of acrylic, although some monoplace chambers have only 4 feet of acrylic with the lower part of the chamber made of steel to reduce costs. They usually are supported by four castors, one on each corner of their support platform (Fig. 2.1). The chamber room needs to be large enough to accommodate a fully opened chamber and connected gurney (more than 17 feet in length).

Pressurization of some monoplace chambers is now automated: The chamber operator specifies a specific chamber pressure, rate of chamber pressurization and chamber depressurization, and interval of time at pressure, and the chamber will automatically follow this pressure–time profile. Other chambers are manually operated and require a chamber operator to pressurize and depressurize the chamber. With this design, the

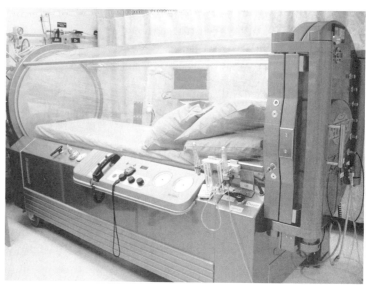

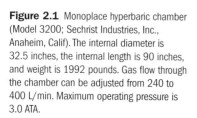

Figure 2.1 Monoplace hyperbaric chamber (Model 3200; Sechrist Industries, Inc., Anaheim, Calif). The internal diameter is 32.5 inches, the internal length is 90 inches, and weight is 1992 pounds. Gas flow through the chamber can be adjusted from 240 to 400 L/min. Maximum operating pressure is 3.0 ATA.

chamber operator must keep track of time at pressure to determine when the holding pressure or clinical treatment is to end and decompression should begin.

Most clinical monoplace chambers have a cam-operated hatch closure, which is a simple and efficient way to open and close the entry hatch. With larger diameter chambers, patients can sit up at 30 degrees, or even upright in the largest chambers.

Monoplace chambers are generally filled with 100% oxygen and require flow rates through the chamber ranging from 100 to 400 L/min. The gas supply to the chamber must be sufficiently robust to accommodate the pressurization of the chamber to 3 ATA, as well as 400 L/min flow through the chamber. Many hospital wall oxygen delivery systems cannot provide sufficient gas flow to operate two or more monoplace hyperbaric chambers simultaneously without installing an oxygen delivery system that provides additional gas flow. One chamber manufacturer, Sechrist Industries (Anaheim, Calif), has recently developed a monoplace chamber that uses less gas than others, and this design may be useful in facilities with limited gas delivery for their chambers.

It is important to flush the monoplace chamber with high oxygen flows, especially with larger diameter chambers that are now available. If chamber gas flows are low

(175 L/min), it may require more than 20 minutes before the concentration of oxygen in the chamber approaches 100%. With high chamber exhaust flows (350 L/min), the oxygen concentration approaches 100% in approximately 7 minutes.[4]

It is possible to fill and compress a monoplace chamber with air and have the patient breathe 100% oxygen through a hood or mask that provides oxygen from an external source. If the monoplace chamber is filled with air, even if hospital grade, it is important to properly filter the air coming to the chamber, with approved filters available from chamber manufacturers or chamber supply outlets.

Because of the inherent risk of oxygen-filled environments, a number of codes and standards regulate monoplace hyperbaric chamber manufacture and operation. The chamber itself should be designed and manufactured in accordance with *ANSI/ASME PVHO-1: Safety Standard for Pressure Vessels for Human Occupancy* (American Society of Mechanical Engineers, New York, NY). The hyperbaric department must follow all applicable rules from the National Fire Protection Association (NFPA), including *NFPA 99: Health Care Facilities* and *NFPA 53: Recommended Practice on Materials, Equipment, and Systems Used in Oxygen Enriched Environments* (National Fire Protection Association, Quincy, Mass).

Additional resources that discuss monoplace chambers include the Monoplace Hyperbaric Chamber Safety Guidelines[5] and the chapter Operational Use and Patient Care in the Monoplace Chamber, published in *Respiratory Care Clinics of North America.*[6]

TREATMENT PROTOCOLS

Hyperbaric oxygen treatments in monoplace chambers follow protocols similar to those provided in multiplace chambers. Common protocols include 2.0 ATA for 90 to 120 minutes, at pressure, or 2.4 ATA for 90 minutes with two 5-minute air periods (30 minutes oxygen, 5 minutes air, 30 minutes oxygen, 5 minutes air, then 30 minutes oxygen).[7] Air-breathing periods are used to reduce oxygen toxicity[8,9] and may be delivered with a mask[10] or a SCUBA mouthpiece fitted with a demand regulator.[11] It appears that patients can breathe more easily if the demand regulator is supplied with air at 85 pounds per square inch gauge (psig), rather than from the hospital source, which is 55 psig.[11] It is inefficient to provide air-breathing periods by switching the chamber gas supply from oxygen to air, because when the chamber gas supply is switched back from air to oxygen, the oxygen concentration recovery time is unacceptably long.[12]

One recommended protocol for acute carbon monoxide poisoning compresses the patient to 3.0 ATA and specifies air-breathing periods.[13] In addition, the U.S. Navy Treatment Tables 5 and 6 specify air-breathing periods.[14] Thus, if a monoplace chamber facility anticipates using such protocols, it should have the appropriate equipment (masks, mouthpieces, nose clips, a medical oxygen-approved demand regulator, and air delivered to the regulator at a pressure of at least 80 psig).

Research/Blinding

Clinical trials can be conducted with monoplace hyperbaric chambers. In a double-blind, randomized trial in acute carbon monoxide poisoning, patients were compressed randomly to either 3 or 1 ATA (2.2 psig at our altitude).[15] Blinding was accomplished by the chamber operator covering all chamber gauges and the clinicians leaving the immediate area of the chamber during therapy. A separate chamber treatment record maintained confidentiality during the course of the clinical trial.

PATIENT CARE

Electrocardiographic (ECG) monitoring is accomplished by passing out the necessary six monitoring leads onto a medical ECG monitor (Fig. 2.2). A connector for the ECG can be "hard-wired" within the chamber hatch, so the patient cable only has to be connected to the receptacle located in the hatch. The hospital's bioengineering department should be involved in this process.

Noninvasive blood pressure (NIBP) monitoring can be accomplished using an automated blood pressure machine made specifically for the monoplace chamber,[16] the Oscillomate Hyperbaric NIBP Monitor, Model 1630 (CAS Medical Systems, Branford, Conn). With this system, the monitor is located outside the chamber. Inflation of the blood pressure cuff and pressure monitoring are achieved with four tubes that pass through the chamber hatch using special attachments. We have found this instrument to operate well to 2 ATA, but at 3 ATA, it is less reproducible. In lieu of a dedicated NIBP monitor, a blood pressure cuff inflated and deflated from outside the chamber with a Doppler flow probe taped over a distal artery can be used.[17]

Invasive Pressure Monitoring

Arterial blood pressure, central venous pressure, intercompartmental pressures, and so forth can be measured in patients compressed within the monoplace chamber. Physiological transducers can be placed inside the chamber with their leads passing out of the chamber and onto a medical physiologic monitor. As with the ECG, it is convenient to have receptacles for invasive pressure transducers

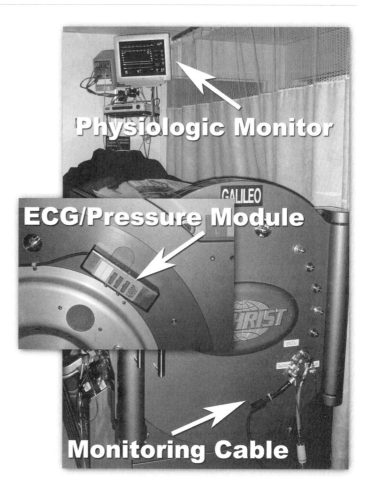

Figure 2.2 Physiologic monitoring of patients compressed in the monoplace hyperbaric chamber is accomplished by connecting the patient leads and cables to a module inside the chamber (depicted). Conductors pass outside the chamber through an electrical pass-through onto the physiologic monitor. ECG, electrocardiographic.

mounted inside the chamber (see Fig. 2.2). The transducers need to have a zero point established at the right atrial level before chamber pressurization. The fluid for the continuous flush device needs to be pressurized (hyperbaric pressure infuser, Catalog No. 4085; Ethox Corp. Medical Products, Buffalo, NY) to maintain continuous flushing of arterial catheters during HBOT. Hospital bioengineering services need to be involved with the installation and maintenance of these monitoring systems.

Pulmonary Arterial Pressure Monitoring

Pulmonary arterial or Swan-Ganz catheter monitoring can be done on research subjects[18] or patients compressed in the monoplace hyperbaric chamber.[19] This technique requires specially designed pass-through devices. This technique has been described previously and goes beyond the scope of this chapter.

Suction can be accomplished inside the monoplace chamber by using medically approved suction regulators located inside the chamber[20] (Fig. 2.3). The gradient of pressure from the pressurized chamber to outside the chamber drives the suction regulator. By regulating the flow of gas through the regulator, from inside to outside the chamber, the operator can adjust the degree of vacuum the regulator delivers from outside the chamber. This suction may be used for vacuum wound closures, nasogastric tubes, chest tubes, or drains. It is important that the vacuum regulator is adjusted properly to prevent excessive suction applied to the site.

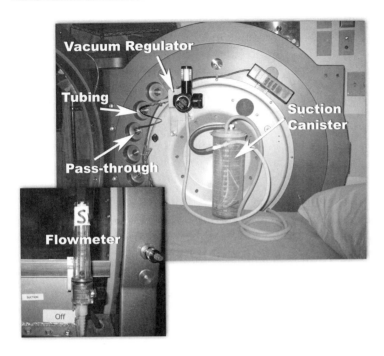

Figure 2.3 Suction of drains, vacuum closure devices, or nasogastric tubes is accomplished by placing a vacuum regulator inside the chamber.[20] The vacuum that drives the regulator derives from the pressure gradient from inside to outside the pressurized chamber. The degree of vacuum can be adjusted by use of a flowmeter outside the chamber, which is connected to the tubing passing outside the chamber.

Safety

As with multiplace chambers, fire safety with the operation of the monoplace chamber is paramount. Many organizations recommend that chamber operators and clinicians obtain formal training or at least rigorous familiarity with published references such as Workman's text, Hyperbaric Facility Safety[21]; the pertinent sections of the NFPA dealing with hyperbaric chambers (e.g., NFPA 99 and NFPA 53); and the Monoplace Hyperbaric Chamber Safety Guidelines[5] and the Operations Committee Report[22] (both available from the Undersea and Hyperbaric Medical Society).

Fires and explosions resulting in fatalities have occurred from improper operation of monoplace chambers.[21] In some of these catastrophes, operators failed to adhere to electrical safety standards, patients were wearing nonapproved garments while compressed in the chamber, or the patient introduced and activated an electrical or heating device while pressurized.[21]

Patients treated in the monoplace chamber need to wear antistatic, 100% cotton garments, and patients need to be grounded. Grounding is accomplished by affixing an ECG lead or grounding pad to the patient, which is connected to a solid earthen ground inside the chamber. Grounding adequacy should be verified by the hospital's biomedical engineering department. The patient needs to be questioned and inspected before each hyperbaric oxygen session regarding any electrical device on their person, such as watches, hearing aids, heated hand warmers, and so forth. Only approved devices may go inside the chamber, such as an approved implanted cardiac pacemaker. Currently, no readily available comprehensive list of monoplace-approved equipment exists. Monoplace chamber manufacturers can be a resource about certain equipment for monoplace chamber use. Also, the Safety Committee of the Undersea and Hyperbaric Medical Society (www.uhms.org) may be helpful to address questions pertinent to what equipment has been used or is considered safe in the monoplace chamber.

Children

Children can be treated inside the monoplace chamber. Older children may be treated similarly as adults, although they may feel more comfortable if their parent is near the chamber and visible to them. Young children are probably optimally managed inside a multiplace chamber because family or hyperbaric staff can attend them, but they can be treated in monoplace chambers (Fig. 2.4). Sometimes younger children may need to be treated with an adult accompanying them inside the chamber. When this is done, it is advisable to provide the adult with a nonrebreathing, reservoir face mask to deliver air or oxygen. In this way, the accompanying adult can be provided with interspersed periods of air and oxygen to reduce the risk for hyperoxic seizures (air breathing) and decompression sickness (oxygen breathing). Although this adult is not a patient, he or she needs to be evaluated and found suitable to be exposed to hyperbaric air and oxygen. Alternatively, oral or intravenous sedation can be provided to a child before exposure to hyperbaric oxygen. Providing sedation to children requires skill and experience The input of pediatricians, emergency physicians, or anesthesiologists can be helpful when sedating children. Intubated infants and children can also be treated with hyperbaric oxygen, given the appropriate equipment and staff. For these children, sedation can be continued during hyperbaric oxygen and titrated to the desired effect. Information is available in the literature about children treated with hyperbaric oxygen.[23-26]

Pacemakers, Internal Cardiac Defibrillators, and Nerve and Spinal Stimulators

Implanted pacemakers, internal cardiac defibrillators (ICDs), nerve and spinal stimulators, and implanted drug delivery devices have the same concerns in the monoplace chamber as in the multiplace chamber. Verification must be obtained that the specific device will function at the intended treatment pressure. Many pacemakers are acceptable, and the manufacturer should be able to provide their recommendations for exposure to hyperbaric pressurization.

ICDs warrant special discussion.[27] Manufacturers do not specifically state that their device may be safe in a hyperbaric chamber. Some of the leads from ICDs have failed,[28] and if discharge of the ICD were to occur in the setting of a damaged lead, high voltage could "spark" across the damaged lead (personal communication, Medtronics technical representative, February 2006). It is unlikely that

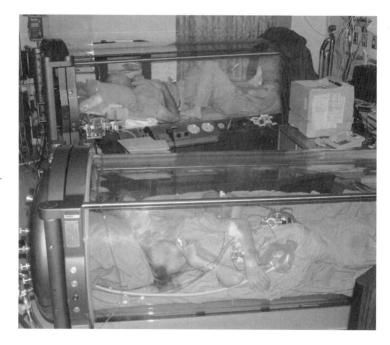

Figure 2.4 One parent and one child, in each of two monoplace chambers, are treated with hyperbaric oxygen for acute carbon monoxide poisoning.

ignition of tissue could occur; nevertheless, prudent practice is to deactivate ICDs just before each hyperbaric oxygen treatment and then reactivate them after decompression and discharge from the hyperbaric medicine department. Under such circumstances, a patient's ECG must be monitored during treatment and the facility must have the capability to defibrillate the patient, if necessary. Before treating patients with ICDs, it is imperative to consult with the patient's cardiologist.

Instances arise when it may not be prudent to treat patients with HBOT. For example, a device may have a pressure limit that is too close to the intended treatment pressure, or a drug delivery device may be influenced by chamber pressure, thus altering the rate of drug delivery.

Cleaning

After each patient compression, it is appropriate to clean the hyperbaric stretcher and the chamber acrylic. LpH se (#6466-08; Steris Corporation, St. Louis) can be used following the manufacturer's directions. For patients with methicillin-resistant, vancomycin-resistant, or other highly resistant infections with the possibility of nosocomial spread, we follow standard hospital policies for isolation.

Gurneys

Monoplace hyperbaric chambers require special gurneys. These gurneys mate to the chamber, permitting the patient portion of the gurney to slide inside the chamber. Some gurneys may be height-adjusted hydraulically, which is helpful when transferring nonambulatory patients to and from other beds.

Patient Comfort

All items used inside 100% oxygen-filled environments need to minimize static electric charge accumulation. Pillows should be made of 100% down fabric completely enclosed and sealed (approved pillows are sold by chamber manufacturers). Pillowcases need to be made of 100% antistatic cotton. All bedding linens and patient garments need to be made of 100% cotton or other hyperbaric chamber-approved material. Gel foam pads are available to reduce risk for decubitus ulceration from pressure and may be used during HBOT (Action Products, Hagerstown, Md).

STAFFING

In the United States, monoplace chambers are staffed in a variety of ways. A credentialed physician must be in attendance and supervising HBOT. Some hyperbaric facilities utilize nurse practitioners or physician assistants to supervise HBOT, but a hyperbaric physician should be available. Monoplace chambers can be operated by nurses, respiratory therapists, or technicians. Certified Hyperbaric Technologist (CHT and CHRN) credentialing through the National Board of Diving and Hyperbaric Medical Technology (www.nbdhmt.com) is not mandated, but this certification is recommended for chamber operators.[22]

Respiratory therapists, certified nurse assistants, and nurses can also manage the patients and deliver HBOT. For routine outpatients, two chamber patients can generally be managed by one chamber operator, with a certified nurse assistant to assist the chamber operator. For critically ill, intubated patients, the chamber is more appropriately operated by an individual capable of managing the hyperbaric ventilator such as a critical care respiratory therapist. It may be appropriate for a patient's critical care nurse to be present in the department, as well as a hyperbaric medicine credentialed nurse practitioner and credentialed physician.

MANAGEMENT OF COMPLICATIONS

Emergency decompression rarely is necessary in the setting of cardiac arrhythmia, hypotension, or equipment or ventilator problems in a critically ill patient. If a patient has a generalized seizure, emergency decompression should not be done, because cerebral gas embolism could occur if the patient has a closed glottis during decompression.[29]

Seizures during clinical HBOT are rare, with incidences ranging from 2 seizures in 80,679 patient treatments[30] to 6 in 20,238 (0.03%) patient treatments.[31] Patients with dysbarism have greater seizure rates (0.6%),[32] as do patients with acute carbon monoxide poisoning (0.3-2%, depending on the hyperbaric oxygen protocol).[33] If a patient has a history of seizure disorder, they may benefit from therapeutic levels of anticonvulsants and/or an appropriate benzodiazepine before treatment.

Seizures that occur during HBOT in the monoplace chamber may be managed by switching the chamber gas supply to air and increasing the rate of air flow through the chamber to reduce the fractional inspired concentration of oxygen to the patient, which often is sufficient to stop the seizure. Once the patient is removed from the chamber, the patient needs to be evaluated and managed as any patient who has just had a seizure. This may include ECG monitoring, providing a patent airway, and provision of supplemental oxygen. Oropharyngeal suction may be necessary and should be available in the chamber area at all times. The postictal patient will be confused and need to be supported until lucidity returns.

ACKNOWLEDGMENTS

I appreciate editorial and photographic assistance from Kayla Deru and also chapter critique by Susan Churchill, NP.

REFERENCES

1. Feldmeier JJ (ed): Hyperbaric oxygen therapy: 2003 committee report. Rev. ed. Kensington, Md, Undersea and Hyperbaric Medical Society, 2003.
2. Feldmeier JJ, Hopf HW, Warriner RA 3rd, et al: UHMS position statement: Topical oxygen for chronic wounds. Undersea Hyperb Med 32:157-168, 2005.
3. Freeman K, Shalit M, Stroh G: Use of the Gamow Bag by EMT-basic park rangers for treatment of high-altitude pulmonary edema and high-altitude cerebral edema. Wilderness Environ Med 15:198-201, 2004.
4. Worth ER, Cochran SLK, Dale HM: Oxygen concentration rise in a monoplace chamber [abstract]. Undersea Hyperb Med 32(4):280, 2005.
5. Weaver LK, Strauss MB (eds): Monoplace hyperbaric chamber safety guidelines. Bethesda, Md, Undersea and Hyperbaric Medical Society, September 1991.
6. Weaver LK: Operational use and patient care in the monoplace chamber. In Moon R, McIntyre N (eds): Respiratory Care Clinics of North America—Hyperbaric Medicine, Part I. Philadelphia, WB Saunders Company, 1999, pp 51-92.
7. Feldmeier JJ (ed): Hyperbaric Oxygen 2003. Indications and Results: The Hyperbaric Oxygen Therapy Committee Report. Kensington, Md, Undersea and Hyperbaric Medical Society, 2003.
8. Clark JM: Extension of oxygen tolerance by interrupted exposure. Undersea Hyperb Med 31:195-198, 2004.
9. Piantadosi CA: A mini-forum on air breaks and O2 toxicity in clinical HBO2 therapy. Undersea Hyperb Med 31:185, 2004.
10. Kindwall EP, Goldmann RW, Thombs PA: Use of the monoplace vs. multiplace chamber in the treatment of diving diseases. J Hyperb Med 3:5-10, 1988.
11. Weaver LK: Monoplace hyperbaric chamber use of US Navy Table 6—a 20-year experience. Undersea Hyperb Med 33:85-88, 2006.
12. Raleigh GW: Air breaks in the Sechrist model 2500-B monoplace hyperbaric chamber. J Hyperb Med 3:11-14, 1988.
13. Weaver LK, Hopkins RO, Chan KJ, et al: Hyperbaric oxygen for acute carbon monoxide poisoning. N Engl J Med 347:1057-1067, 2002.
14. U.S. Naval Sea Systems Command: Recompression therapy. In U.S. Navy Diving Manual, 4th rev. (Baton Rouge: Claitor's Publishing Division, 1999), Flagstaff, Ariz, Best Publishing, 5:1-49, 1999.
15. Weaver LK, Hopkins RO, Churchill S, Haberstock D: Double-blinding is possible in hyperbaric oxygen (HBO2) randomized clinical trials (RCT) using a minimal chamber pressurization as control. Undersea Hyperb Med 24(suppl):36, 1997.
16. Meyer GW, Hart GB, Strauss MB: Noninvasive blood pressure monitoring in the hyperbaric monoplace chamber. J Hyperb Med 4:211-216, 1990.
17. Weaver LK, Howe S: Non-invasive Doppler blood pressure monitoring in the monoplace hyperbaric chamber. J Clin Monit 7:304-308, 1991.
18. Weaver LK, Howe S: Normal human hemodynamic response to hyperbaric air and oxygen. Undersea Hyperb Med 21(suppl):77-78, 1994.
19. Weaver LK: Technique of Swan-Ganz catheter monitoring in patients treated in the monoplace hyperbaric chamber. J Hyperb Med 7:1-18, 1992.
20. Weaver LK. A functional suction apparatus within the monoplace hyperbaric chamber. J Hyperb Med 3:165-171, 1988.
21. Workman WT (ed): Hyperbaric Facility Safety: A Practical Guide. Flagstaff, Ariz, Best Publishing, 1999.
22. Kimbell PN (ed): Operations committee report. Kensington, Md, Undersea and Hyperbaric Medical Society, 2000.

23. Keenan HT, Bratton SL, Norkool DM, et al: Delivery of hyperbaric oxygen therapy to critically ill, mechanically ventilated children. J Crit Care 13:7-12, 1998.

24. Waisman D, Shupak A, Weisz G, Melamed Y: Hyperbaric oxygen therapy in the pediatric patient: The experience of the Israel Naval Medical Institute. Pediatrics 102:E53, 1998.

25. Chou KJ, Fisher JL, Silver EJ: Characteristics and outcome of children with carbon monoxide poisoning with and without smoke exposure referred for hyperbaric oxygen therapy. Pediatr Emerg Care 16:151-155, 2000.

26. Santamaria JP, Williams ET 3rd, Desautels DA: Hyperbaric oxygen therapy in pediatrics. Adv Pediatr 42:335-366, 1995.

27. Schmitz S, Churchill S, Weaver LK: Hyperbaric oxygen in patients with implanted cardiac defibrillators and pacemakers. Undersea Hyperb Med 33(5):349-350, 2006.

28. Schultz DG: FDA Preliminary Public Health Notification: Guidant VENTAK PRIZM® 2 DR and CONTAK RENEWAL® Implantable Cardioverter Defibrillators. Rockville, Md, U.S. Food and Drug Administration, July 14, 2005.

29. Bond GF: Arterial gas embolism. In Davis JC, Hunt TK (eds): Hyperbaric Oxygen Therapy. Bethesda, Md, Undersea Medical Society, 1977, pp 141-152.

30. Yildiz S, Aktas S, Cimsit M, et al: Seizure incidence in 80,000 patient treatments with hyperbaric oxygen. Aviat Space Environ Med 75:992-994, 2004.

31. Hampson N, Atik D: Central nervous system oxygen toxicity during routine hyperbaric oxygen therapy. Undersea Hyperb Med 30:147-153, 2003.

32. Smerz RW: Incidence of oxygen toxicity during the treatment of dysbarism. Undersea Hyperb Med 31:199-202, 2004.

33. Hampson NB, Simonson SG, Kramer CC, Piantadosi CA: Central nervous system oxygen toxicity during hyperbaric treatment of patients with carbon monoxide poisoning. Undersea Hyperb Med 23:215-219, 1996.

Multiplace Hyperbaric Chambers

3

Anthony J. Gerbino, MD,
and Neil B. Hampson, MD

Multiplace hyperbaric chambers are pressure vessels intended for occupancy by more than one person. They are defined by the National Fire Protection Association (NFPA) as Class A chambers. They range from "duo-place" chambers designed for 1 patient and an accompanying attendant to large chambers the size of a room capable of accommodating 20 or more seated patients with 1 or more inside attendants (Fig. 3.1).

Multiplace chambers are typically constructed from steel, although the U.S. Air Force built a prototype chamber made of prestressed concrete in Texas in the 1990s. The most common configuration for a steel chamber is a horizontal cylinder (see Fig. 3.1), although vertical cylinders (Fig. 3.2), rectangular rib-enforced chambers (Figs. 3.3 and 3.4), and spherical chambers are also in use.

Design, fabrication, and testing of multiplace chambers are governed by the American Society of Mechanical Engineers Pressure Vessels for Human Occupancy (ASME-PVHO-1) code. Hydrostatic pressure testing of the chamber to a pressure 1.5 times the maximum working pressure is required when the chamber is manufactured and if the pressure boundary is modified.

Most clinical multiplace hyperbaric chambers have more than one compartment or "lock." Single-lock multiplace chambers have a treatment compartment only. The most common configurations are either two or three locks (Fig. 3.5). Double-lock chambers typically have a treatment compartment and an entry compartment. Triple-lock chambers usually have two treatment compartments and an entry compartment. Although more than one lock can allow independent treatment of patients on different protocols, the most important advantage to a multilock system is the ability to move patients or staff into or out

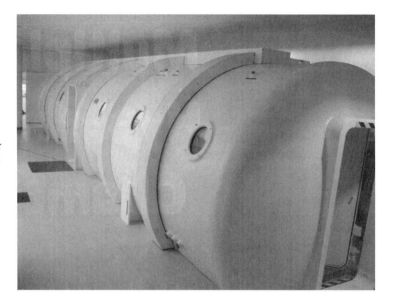

Figure 3.1 Triple-lock multiplace hyperbaric chamber with a horizontal cylinder configuration (installed 2005, Virginia Mason Medical Center, Seattle).

of the pressurized chamber. Most multiplace chambers also have smaller, wall-mounted pass-through locks through which items such as food, medication, and equipment can be locked into the pressurized chamber and items such as blood samples can be locked out.

Important components of a multiplace hyperbaric chamber include a compressor, a volume tank for storing compressed air, an oxygen supply, an emergency supply of commonly breathed gases such as oxygen and air, and a fire suppression system (Fig. 3.6). Typically, one or more compressors generate pressurized gas used to compress the hyperbaric chamber. In most countries, multiplace chambers are pressurized with air to decrease the fire risk associated with greater fractional concentrations of

oxygen. Because air heats when compressed, it cannot be directly used to pressurize an occupied chamber. Instead, air is sent from a compressor to high-pressure volume tanks for cooling and storage until needed. Cylinders of pressurized air can be used to pressurize small multiplace chambers that are used infrequently, or as an emergency backup source for chambers pressurized by compressors.

Patients within a multiplace hyperbaric chamber breathe 100% oxygen via one of several types of oxygen delivery systems. Most commonly these include soft plastic head hoods that are fitted tightly about the neck with a latex seal (Fig. 3.7), nonrebreather oronasal face masks, or endotracheal tubes. Head hoods are constant flow delivery systems that minimize

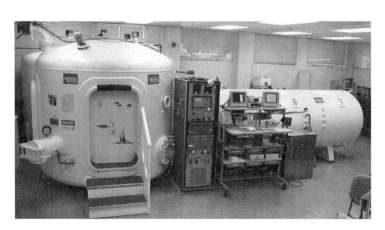

Figure 3.2 Dual-lock multiplace hyperbaric chamber, hybrid configuration with vertical and horizontal cylinders (in service 1970-2005, Virginia Mason Medical Center, Seattle).

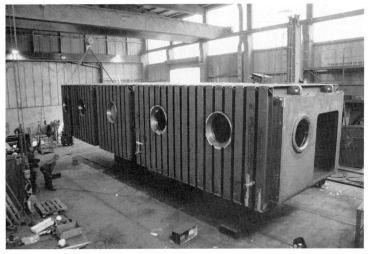

Figure 3.3 Rectangular multiplace hyperbaric chamber with external reinforcing ribs (installed 2006, Karolinska Institute, Stockholm, Sweden).

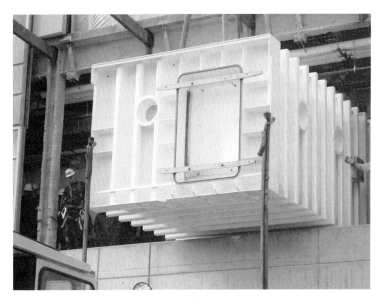

Figure 3.4 Rectangular multiplace hyperbaric chamber with external reinforcing ribs (installed 2006, Intermountain Medical Center, Murray, Utah).

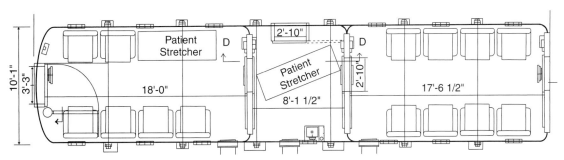

Figure 3.5 Schematic depiction of a triple-lock multiplace hyperbaric chamber (Virginia Mason Medical Center, Seattle). The system has two multipatient treatment locks and a central entry lock. Exit doors are located at each end of the chamber and from the central entry lock.

Configuration of a Double-Lock Multiplace Chamber

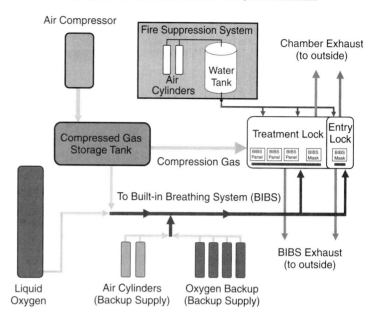

Figure 3.6 Schematic depicting typical components of a double-lock multiplace hyperbaric chamber. *(Adapted from Sheffield RB: Hyperbaric Chamber Systems, Hyperbaric Team Training Course Syllabus, San Antonio, Tex, International ATMO, Inc., 2006. Reprinted by permission of International ATMO, Inc.)*

resistance to breathing. The hood serves as a gas reservoir and must be ventilated at a rate sufficient to prevent carbon dioxide accumulation. With constant flow systems, the oxygen supply pressure must be higher only than the pressure of the chamber environment. In contrast, oronasal face masks are demand delivery systems that minimize gas consumption. The oxygen supply pressure must be a specific amount greater than the chamber environment to properly drive the demand valve. These systems must be tight fitting to minimize leaks of oxygen into the chamber or air into the breathing gas. Exhaled gas from either oxygen delivery system is predominantly oxygen and, therefore, must be routed out of the chamber to minimize accumulation in the chamber environment, which would increase fire risk.

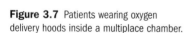

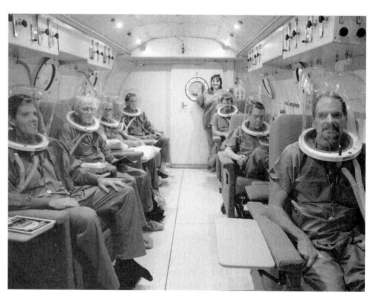

Figure 3.7 Patients wearing oxygen delivery hoods inside a multiplace chamber.

All clinical hyperbaric chambers have an oxygen supply. Liquid oxygen is the most efficient source when large volumes of oxygen are consumed. Cylinders of oxygen are used when smaller volumes are consumed or as an emergency backup source to liquid oxygen supply.

NFPA 99 also requires Class A hyperbaric chambers to have a fire suppression system. Testing has demonstrated that water is the agent of choice to extinguish a fire in the hyperbaric environment. Fire suppression systems are typically composed of both a handheld water hose operated by chamber occupants and an overhead sprinkler system that deluges the entire area of the chamber interior when activated. Either chamber occupants or the chamber operator can activate the deluge system.

Other components typically present in multiplace chambers are hull penetrators, pressure relief valves, and acrylic view ports. Penetrators are used to pass piping, wiring, and lighting through the pressure boundary. When a chamber is constructed, it is desirable to install excess penetrators so that future needs do not require modification of the pressure boundary and subsequent hydrostatic testing. Pressure relief or "pop-off" valves release pressure if it exceeds the design limit of the chamber or piping.

Acrylic ports have a finite lifetime of structural integrity. That lifetime is shortened by physical stress from chamber pressurization, exposure to ultraviolet light, and exposure to organic solvents. ASME/PVHO-1 requires regular inspection of acrylic ports to look for cracks and monitor crazing.

CHAMBER DISTRIBUTION IN THE UNITED STATES AND WORLDWIDE

Data are limited with regard to the number of hyperbaric chambers throughout the world. With regard to the United States, the Undersea and Hyperbaric Medical Society (UHMS) Chamber Directory lists 503 hyperbaric facili-

ties in 47 states and the District of Columbia (Table 3.1).[1] Of these, 396 have monoplace chambers, 85 have multiplace chambers, and 22 have both types. Forty-five states have monoplace chamber facilities, whereas only 32 have multiplace facilities. Multiplace chambers are more common in coastal locations. For example, multiplace chambers are present in 14 of 21 or 67% of U.S. states with saltwater coastline. These data likely underestimate the total number of chambers because facilities must report their information to the UHMS to be listed.

Outside of the United States, multiplace chambers are much more common than monoplace chambers. Informal listings of worldwide chamber numbers have been compiled by Tom Workman (UHMS, Director of Quality Assurance and Regulatory Affairs)[2] and Sunny Sonnenrein (Reimers Systems, Inc., Lorton, Va).[3] The number of chamber facilities varies widely among countries (Table 3.2), with estimates indicating a 100-fold difference in the number of chambers per capita (Fig. 3.8). As the number of chambers worldwide is ever-expanding, the reader is advised to consult the OXYNET Web site (www.oxynet.org) for updated information.

MULTIPLACE VERSUS MONOPLACE CHAMBERS

Multiplace and monoplace chambers each have distinct advantages and disadvantages. Issues that differentiate them include: (1) space requirements, (2) pressurization capabilities, (3) economics, (4) capacity issues, (5) patient comfort and acceptance, (6) patient management considerations, and (7) safety.

Multiplace chamber facilities require more space than monoplace chambers. Minimum space for a single monoplace chamber is 256 square feet of floor space (16 × 16 feet), whereas multiplace facilities typically occupy at least 2,000 to 2,500 square feet. The decision to install a multiplace chamber in a medical center should be viewed as a long-term institutional commitment to hyperbaric medicine because space needs are high and new construction may be necessary for installation. Because

Table 3.1 Hyperbaric Chamber Distribution by U.S. State

STATE	NUMBER OF FACILITIES	NUMBER OF FACILITIES WITH MONOPLACE CHAMBERS	NUMBER OF FACILITIES WITH MULTIPLACE CHAMBERS
Alaska	3	1	2
Alabama	6	4	3
Arkansas	9	9	0
Arizona	11	10	1
California	43	35	10
Colorado	7	5	2
Connecticut	4	2	2
District of Columbia	1	1	0
Florida	58	43	22
Georgia	16	14	3
Hawaii	2	0	2
Idaho	1	1	0
Illinois	18	14	4
Indiana	17	16	2
Iowa	6	5	1
Kansas	4	4	0
Kentucky	4	4	0
Louisiana	26	22	6
Maine	2	2	0
Maryland	4	3	1
Massachusetts	2	2	0
Michigan	10	8	2
Minnesota	1	0	1
Mississippi	11	11	0
Missouri	17	16	2
Montana	1	1	0
Nebraska	2	1	1
Nevada	5	3	3
New Hampshire	5	5	0
New Jersey	5	5	0
New York	21	16	6
North Carolina	9	7	2
Ohio	12	11	2
Oklahoma	5	5	1
Oregon	1	1	0
Pennsylvania	24	22	2
Rhode Island	2	2	0
South Carolina	6	5	1
South Dakota	2	2	0
Tennessee	14	13	1
Texas	70	59	13
Utah	5	4	1
Virginia	17	14	3
Washington	6	3	3
West Virginia	2	1	1
Wisconsin	5	5	1
Wyoming	1	1	0

Data from Undersea and Hyperbaric Medical Society Chamber Directory. Available at www.uhms.org/Chambers/CHAMBER DIRECTORY2.ASP. Accessed April 3, 2007.

Table 3.2 Estimated Number and Location of Hyperbaric Facilities Worldwide as of 2006

COUNTRY	NUMBER OF FACILITIES	COUNTRY	NUMBER OF FACILITIES
Argentina	15	Madagascar	1
Australia	12	Malaysia	4
Austria	2	Malta	1
Belgium	11	Mauritius	1
Brazil	71	Mexico	306
British West Indies	1	New Zealand	2
Canada	27	Norway	2
Chile	3	Panama	9
Columbia	60	P.R. China	3000
Cuba	9	Peru	35
Cyprus	1	Philippines	5
Denmark	3	Poland	1
Dominican Republic	5	Portugal	1
El Salvador	2	Russia	3000
England	16	Scotland	2
Estonia	5	Singapore	1
Finland	2	South Africa	14
France	21	South Korea	150
Germany	100	Spain	16
Greece	2	Sweden	11
Honduras	1	Switzerland	18
Hong Kong	3	Taiwan	10
India	4	Thailand	24
Indonesia	6	The Netherlands	2
Ireland	4	Turkey	1
Israel	3	United States	503
Italy	22	Venezuela	5
Japan	115	Serbia and Montenegro	2
Latvia	10		

Data courtesy of Workman WT: Director, Undersea and Hyperbaric Medical Society Quality Assurance and Regulatory Affairs. Personal communication, August 2006; and Sunny Sonnenrein: Reimers Systems, Inc. Personal communication, November 2006.

of their size and mobility, it is possible to install and operate one or more monoplace chambers on a temporary basis, removing them should a decision be made to discontinue the service.

Most multiplace chambers are designed and rated to treat patients up to a maximum pressure of 6 atmospheres absolute (ATA), whereas monoplace chambers typically have a maximum treatment pressure of 3 ATA. This becomes relevant when treating patients with arterial gas embolism if the decision is made to use a U.S. Navy Treatment Table 6A. This table includes an excursion to 165 feet sea water (fsw) pressure, equivalent to 6 ATA. This capability is not available in a monoplace chamber. Because most cases of gas embolism

treated in hyperbaric chambers are due to diving accidents, multiplace chambers have historically been favored in locations that treat large numbers of divers. However, the use of U.S. Navy Treatment Table 6A has been declining in recent years,[4] and pressure capability greater than 3 ATA may not confer a great advantage by itself.

With regard to economics, it is beyond the scope of this chapter to describe a complete economic analysis of multiplace versus monoplace facility operation. A large number of factors are involved, many specific to local or regional needs or economics. Two major considerations are the chamber acquisition cost and staffing. The following numbers are used

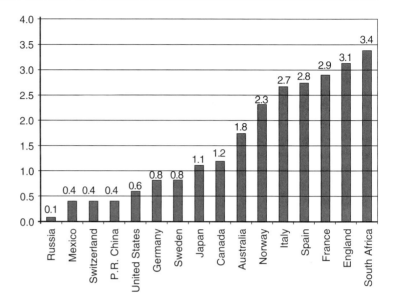

Figure 3.8 Population per hyperbaric facility in selected countries (in millions per facility).

as an example to illustrate the types of considerations involved. If a monoplace chamber costs $100,000 to acquire and is used for 10,000 compressions in its life, the hardware cost for each is $10. If a multiplace chamber costs $1,000,000 to acquire and is used for 25,000 compressions, each compression costs $40. This becomes economically advantageous for the multiplace chamber when occupancy per treatment averages more than four patients.

Similar calculations can be made for staffing. If one staff person is required to administer a monoplace chamber treatment, a facility has one monoplace chamber, and three routine 2-hour treatments can be administered in an 8-hour day, a simplified estimate is that each treatment will cost one third of a full-time staff position. If a facility has a multiplace chamber requiring two staff outside for operation and one inside to attend the patients, economic advantage is gained by the multiplace facility when the daily treatment volume averages more than nine patients. If the monoplace facility has two chambers and a single staff person can operate both simultaneously, the multiplace facility does not gain operational staff cost advantage until more than 18 patients are treated daily. However, these calculations are greatly simplified. For example, this analysis does not include the

additional cost of physician attendance and supervision, as is required for Medicare patients in the United States.

Patient comfort and acceptance may vary according to chamber type. Group socialization and support is possible when more than one patient is treated simultaneously in the multiplace chamber. In contrast, monoplace treatments isolate the patient from others during treatment. Confinement anxiety is a relatively small problem in multiplace chambers. In one series of 52,758 treatments performed at 2.4 ATA, only 28 patients (0.05%) required removal from the chamber for claustrophobia.[5] Claustrophobia may be a greater problem in monoplace chambers, especially when used to treat patients on long protocols. In a series of 90 divers with decompression illness treated using a U.S. Navy Treatment Table 6 profile in 25- or 32-inch monoplace chambers, 3 (3%) experienced claustrophobia sufficiently severe to require removal from the chamber and termination of the treatment.[6]

Multiplace chambers possess a safety advantage over monoplace chambers in several specific clinical emergencies because of the presence of an inside attendant who can provide earlier diagnosis and treatment. For example, an inside attendant may diagnose a pneumothorax while at depth or during ascent, and insert a vascular catheter or thoracostomy tube in the pleural space before chamber decompression. In the case of cardiac arrest, an inside attendant may provide earlier cardiopulmonary resuscitation and cardiac defibrillation. However, most advise rapid decompression of the multiplace chamber before defibrillation because this decreases fire risk and body tissues remain well oxygenated for a brief period after hyperbaric treatment. In a sedated or delirious patient, the inside attendant may physically intervene if the patient inadvertently attempts to remove vascular catheters or an endotracheal tube. In the case of central nervous system oxygen toxicity, an inside attendant may quickly remove the patient's oxygen hood before a seizure, or better position a seizing patient to prevent aspiration. Although each of these scenarios may be better managed by an inside attendant in a multiplace chamber, these events are rare, and safety considerations alone should not dictate one's choice of chamber.

The lower fractional concentration of oxygen in a multiplace versus monoplace chamber improves the chance of chamber occupants surviving a fire. Although the lower fractional concentration of oxygen decreases fire risk, hyperbaric chamber fires have occurred in both multiplace and monoplace chambers. Sheffield and Desautels[7] identified 11 monoplace and 8 multiplace chamber fires from 1980 to 1996. Of the multiplace fires, three occurred in chambers that were pressurized with oxygen rather than air. The only survivors of chamber fires have been those who occupied multiplace chambers pressurized with air, indicating that a lower percentage of oxygen within a chamber dictates the chance for survival rather than chamber size.

TYPICAL TREATMENT PROTOCOLS

Although diagnoses such as carbon monoxide poisoning, necrotizing fasciitis, and decompression illness may have distinct hyperbaric treatment profiles, most multiplace chambers treat problem wounds and chronic radiation tissue injury with a standard "wound healing" protocol. These protocols typically call for patients to breathe 100% oxygen for 90 to 120 minutes at pressures ranging from 2.0 to 2.4 ATA.

The "Jefferson Davis wound healing protocol" (Fig. 3.9A) is considered by some to be the standard wound healing protocol for multiplace chambers in North America.[8] This protocol was shaped by physiologic, experimental, and practical considerations during its development in the 1970s. The 90-minute period of oxygen breathing was based on Boerema's gas gangrene protocol in which patients were treated at 3.0 ATA.[9] However, the cumulative risk for central nervous system oxygen toxicity at a pressure of 3.0 ATA was considered too high to justify use of this pressure to treat conditions that were not immediately life-threatening and required a large number of treatments. Experience at that time indicated that 2.0 ATA was an effective pressure for treatment of chronic wounds.[8] Because of concerns that poorly fitting oxygen masks would entrain air and reduce the effective oxygen tension, Davis targeted the pressure at its current 45 fsw (2.36 ATA) to guarantee an actual inspired oxygen tension of 2.0 ATA. The oxygen-breathing interval was lengthened from 20 to 30 minutes in the 1970s because a rebreather hood system that had just been introduced required nearly 10 minutes to achieve 100% oxygen within the hood. Because the oxygen-breathing interval had been increased, the 5-minute air-breathing interval adopted from U.S. Navy treatment tables was also increased to 10 minutes to avoid central nervous system oxygen toxicity. Thus, the Jefferson Davis wound healing protocol commonly in use today includes three 30-minute oxygen-breathing sessions at 2.36 ATA with two intervening 10-minute air-breathing periods (air "breaks").[10] Variations have been introduced to the Davis protocol that include minor changes in oxygen-breathing or air-breathing intervals (e.g., see Figs. 3.9B and C). It is unclear whether minor variations in the length of oxygen-breathing or air-breathing intervals alter the frequency of seizures related to central nervous system oxygen toxicity.[11]

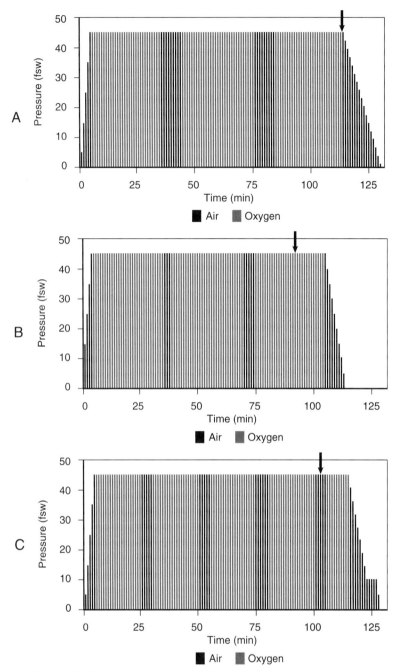

Figure 3.9 Typical treatment protocols used in a multiplace hyperbaric chamber. *Arrows* indicate when oxygen-breathing begins for the inside attendant. *A,* Jefferson Davis protocol: 30-minute O_2 breathing alternating with 10-minute air-breathing periods; attendant breathes O_2 during ascent. *B,* Virginia Mason protocol: 30-minute O_2 breathing alternating with 5-minute air-breathing periods; attendant breathes O_2 for 10 minutes at 45 feet sea water (fsw) and during ascent. *C,* Virginia Mason protocol modified to decrease central nervous system O_2 toxicity: 20-minute O_2 breathing alternating with 5-minute air-breathing periods, then a final 10-minute O_2 breathing period; attendant breathes O_2 for 10 minutes at 45 fsw, for 5 minutes at 10 fsw, and during ascent.

However, reported seizure rates are low regardless of which "wound healing" protocol is used.[11-13]

APPROACH TO SAFETY AND DAILY OPERATIONS

Leadership by a qualified medical and technical team is necessary for safe operation of a hyperbaric chamber. According to the UHMS Guidelines for Hyperbaric Facility Operation,[14] required leadership for a multiplace chamber includes a medical director, a safety director, a technical director, and a hyperbaric nurse/manager. The medical director is a physician who is ultimately responsible for all aspects of the hyperbaric practice. The safety director is responsible for assuring compliance with all safety-related standards. The technical director is responsible for safe operation and day-to-day maintenance of the hyperbaric chamber and related support systems. He or she must have more than 5 years' experience in hyperbaric facility operations.[14] The hyperbaric nurse manager is responsible for directing day-to-day clinical operations including patient care. These individuals are responsible for establishing a safety program, creating a culture of safety, and assuring adherence to established safety standards.

The European Code of Good Practice for Hyperbaric Oxygen Therapy[15] recommends that treatments in a multiplace facility be supervised by a team consisting at minimum of a hyperbaric physician, an inside attendant, and a chamber operator. The UHMS Guidelines for Hyperbaric Facility Operation[14] require the presence of a nurse or technician certified in hyperbaric medicine when a chamber is in operation. A hyperbaric-trained physician should be available to treat urgent and routine medical problems before, during, and after a treatment session. In the United States, Medicare requires the presence of a physician during treatment to bill for both the professional and technical aspects of hyperbaric treatments.

Because patient acuity and chamber size and configuration vary, more than one inside attendant may be necessary for each treatment. In general, one attendant can supervise up to 8 to 10 patients if these patients are of low acuity and are familiar with and comfortable in a hyperbaric environment.[16] If several patients are receiving hyperbaric treatments for the first time or require special attention (e.g., children), a lower patient-to-attendant ratio is advisable. Critically ill, mechanically ventilated patients are typically treated individually and are best served by two inside attendants, one of whom has critical care experience. Positioning the ventilator outside the chamber simplifies staffing because the inside attendants need not be trained in respiratory therapy. In this case, the respiratory therapist and a physician familiar with critically ill patients should be available in the hyperbaric facility.

Patients should be evaluated briefly before each hyperbaric treatment. This assessment includes vital signs and an updated history including ear complaints and stability of major medical problems. Commonly encountered problems that require intervention include otic barotrauma and poorly controlled hypertension or diabetes mellitus. Those whose history suggests otic barotrauma may require physician evaluation, pretreatment with nasal decongestants, or slower compression rates. Those with elevated systemic blood pressures may require treatment with a rapid-onset antihypertensive. Patients with diabetes with hypoglycemia are treated with an oral glucose source. In addition to the daily screening that is typically performed by a hyperbaric nurse, physicians should formally evaluate patients on a periodic basis to determine response to treatment and medical stability.

The UHMS provides safety and quality guidelines that assist the leadership team in delivering high-quality hyperbaric medicine. The UHMS has helped establish quality standards for hyperbaric personnel,[17,18] such as board certification for nurses, technicians, and physicians. The UHMS also provides opportunities for continuing medical education including courses devoted exclusively to safety. For physicians involved in the practice of hyperbaric medicine who are not board certified, a minimum of 40 to 60 hours of coursework in hyperbaric medicine is recommended.[14,15] The UHMS hyperbaric facility accreditation program increases the likelihood that hyperbaric centers are aware of and implement good safety practices.

Another important feature of safe hyperbaric chamber operation is design of a system that minimizes errors. Medical errors are commonplace in current health-care systems and cause considerable harm to patients.[19] Even when safety guidelines are in place, adherence may be compromised in a busy multiplace hyperbaric practice when patient volume is high or part-time staff is routinely used. Omission of a routine safety practice, such as checking patients for contraband that increases fire risk before chamber compression, can have devastating consequences.

Near-perfect safety records may be associated with unacceptable outcomes in some industries such as commercial aviation. To prevent errors in complex systems, these industries develop robust systems that emphasize safety.[20] Systems typically include standard operating procedures ("standard work") and successive safety checks to ensure errors are detected and corrected.

Incorporating these design principles into daily practice can enhance the safety of a busy multiplace hyperbaric practice. For example, standard work for hyperbaric patients could include changing into cotton-based surgical "scrubs" before treatment. Standard work for an inside attendant could include completion of a written checklist of pretreatment tasks (Table 3.3) and a verbal review of contraband items with patients before each treatment session (Table 3.4). Standard work for the chamber technician could include receiving the inside attendant's pretreatment checklist before pressurization of the chamber, and periodically verifying that routine maintenance checks have been performed and documented. Such

a system of successive safety checks should be built into many aspects of daily hyperbaric practice and will detect and correct inevitable human errors.

Each hyperbaric facility should develop its own operating manual.[15] This manual should include standard work for anticipated activities within the facility, as well as emergency procedures to cover unplanned events. The operating manual must be immediately available to staff. A proposed framework for an operating manual is provided in the European Code of Good Practice for Hyperbaric Oxygen Therapy.[15]

FIRE SAFETY

Fire is a rare but devastating complication of hyperbaric oxygen treatment. Because an oxygen-enriched environment causes fire to burn at hotter temperatures and spread more quickly, most hyperbaric chamber fires are fatal for chamber occupants. During the period from 1967 to 1996, there were 60 deaths in 21 of the 24 clinical hyperbaric chamber fires.[7] In this period, two clinical hyperbaric chamber fires occurred in North America (neither resulting in fatalities), and three fires resulting in two fatalities occurred in European clinical hyperbaric facilities. Nineteen of the 24 clinical hyperbaric chamber fires during this period occurred in Asia, resulting in 58 fatalities. Analysis of these fires reveals multiple errors including elevated fractional concentration of oxygen within a multiplace chamber, ignition sources inadvertently allowed in the chamber, the presence of unnecessary fuels within the chamber, faulty electrical equipment, and inadequate fire suppression systems.[7] Potential causes of fire in a multiplace hyperbaric chamber and safety measures taken to decrease fire risk due to these hazards are summarized in Table 3.5.

The primary focus of a hyperbaric fire safety program is prevention. Preventive measures focus on limiting the presence of fuel, an ignition source, and oxygen to the extent possible. When the oxygen fraction is

Table 3.3 Written Safety Checklist Completed by Inside Attendant and Reviewed by the Chamber Operator before Each Pressurization

INSIDE ATTENDANT PRETREATMENT CHECKLIST

Check contents of equipment cart	_____
Replace contents as needed	_____
List of patient names and risks	_____
Hood/Trach/Hose assembly for each patient	_____
Chair or stretcher for each patient	_____
Linen supplies as needed	_____
Water for all occupants	_____
Suction kit complete and assembled	_____
Fire Suppression System cabinets clear—must be able to open cabinet	_____
Pass-through lock door closed	_____
Mask/Hose assembly for each inside attendant	_____
Communication belt pack	_____
Your surface interval noted in logbook	_____
Glucose testing supplies available	_____
Compression log initialed when checklist complete	_____
Your Name: _____	Dive #: _____

sufficiently low, nitrogen impedes interaction between oxygen and fuel and fire cannot occur. Once the minimum fraction of oxygen is exceeded, burn rates increase exponentially with increasing oxygen fraction.[21] The NFPA forbids pressurization of the multiplace chamber with 100% oxygen, and requires that the oxygen concentration within the chamber not exceed 23.5%. This is accomplished by pressurizing the chamber with air, assuring adequate venting of patients' head hoods, continuously monitoring the fractional oxygen content within the chamber, and ventilating the chamber with air as needed to maintain the oxygen concentration at less than 23.5%.

Preventing fuel and ignition sources from entering the hyperbaric chamber is a major emphasis of fire prevention programs. The most common cause of hyperbaric fires since 1980 in North American and European clinical hyperbaric centers[7] has been contraband that was inadvertently brought into the chamber. Hand warmers, children's toys that create sparks, and cigarette lighters have all ignited hyperbaric chamber fires in recent years (Table 3.6). Patients are educated about potentially dangerous items to decrease the risk that contraband is brought into a hyperbaric chamber. Before each treatment, patients change into surgical "scrubs," are observed for the presence of prohibited items, and are read a list of prohibited items (see Table 3.4).

The multiplace chamber should be inspected routinely for the presence of potential fuel that may ignite easily. Flammable material such as garments, blankets, wound dressings, and salves

Table 3.4 Fire Safety Check Read Aloud by the Inside Attendant to Patients before Each Pressurization

"DOES ANYONE HAVE ANY OF THE FOLLOWING PROHIBITED ITEMS IN THE CHAMBER TODAY?"

· Cigarette lighters, matches, or hand warmers
· Flammable ointments, cosmetics, lip balms, or hairdressings
· ThermaCare (or similar) heat patches
· Wool, silk, synthetic clothing (including nylon stockings), or yarn
· Battery-powered devices, hearing aids, cellular phones, or pagers
· Newspapers or other loose papers
· Toys that create friction, static electricity, or sparks

Table 3.5 Potential Causes of Fire in the Hyperbaric Environment and Preventive Measures

FIRE HAZARD	PREVENTIVE MEASURES
Contraband that creates sparks, heat, or fire	· Educate patients regarding fire risks · Review fire safety checklist with patients before each treatment (see Table 3.4) · Limit personal belongings that each patient brings into the chamber
Faulty electrical equipment	· Eliminate all unnecessary equipment · Appropriate testing and maintenance of equipment to prevent overheating and electrical arcing
Static electricity	· Avoid high-static clothing (wear cotton) · Appropriate grounding of surfaces · Maintain high relative chamber humidity · Antistatic materials applied to fabrics
Easily ignited fuel	· Prohibit newspapers, loose papers · Avoid using or allowing hydrocarbon-based substances in the chamber · Avoid wearing street shoes in the chamber
Inadequate fire suppression system	· Handheld water hose and externally controlled deluge system in place · Routine testing of the fire suppression system every 6–12 months · All staff capable of operating the fire suppression system
Overheated items sent into the chamber	· Avoid overheating or uneven heating of preheated objects sent into the chamber

should not be stored in the hyperbaric chamber. Patients are instructed to avoid applying petroleum products to their skin or hair. Some centers treat garments with a fire retardant. Housekeeping procedures appropriate for other parts of the hospital need to be modified so that waxes and other hydrocarbon-based products are not used to clean chamber surfaces. Street shoes must be removed before entering the chamber so that oil or petroleum on shoe soles does not enter the chamber.

Electrical ignition was a common cause of hyperbaric fires before the 1990s (see Table 3.6). Improved fire safety codes, proper engineering, and diligent maintenance have virtually eliminated ignition from electrical arcing as a cause of chamber fires in most countries.[22] Modern electronic equipment such as cellular telephones represents a new potential source of electrical ignition that must be kept out of the hyperbaric environment.

The importance of static electricity in igniting hyperbaric chamber fires is controversial. Four clinical hyperbaric chamber fires in China that were reported to the UHMS Chamber Experience and Mishap Database[23] in the 1980s were attributed to static electricity, but additional detail is unavailable. Electrical charge is transferred between materials when dissimilar materials are rubbed together, and its release produces energy that may ignite a fire. Because release of static electricity produces only small

Table 3.6 Reported Causes of Fires in Clinical Hyperbaric Chambers from 1967 to 1998 (Includes Multiplace and Monoplace Chambers)

PROBABLE CAUSE	NUMBER OF EVENTS (YEAR)
Chemical hand warmer	5 (1997, 1996, 1993, 1989, 1967)
Spark from child's toy	3 (1997, 1987, 1987)
Static electricity	7 (1989, 1987, 1986, 1984, 1983, 1978, 1976)
Electrical spark	7 (1994, 1994, 1993, 1993, 1986, 1974, 1969)
Cigarette smoking/lighter use	6 (1998, 1996, 1993, 1993, 1979, 1967)
Microwave-heated blanket	1 (1989)

Data from Sheffield PJ: Hyperbaric chamber fires: To what extent is the problem? In: Workman WT (ed): Hyperbaric Facility Safety: A Practical Guide. Flagstaff, Ariz, Best Publishing, 1999, pp 487–493.

amounts of energy, the likelihood of ignition is low. However, fuel such as volatile vapors, if inadvertently present, ignites easily, suggesting it is prudent to prevent static electricity. Therefore, chamber occupants wear cotton because synthetic fabrics, yarn, and wool generate static electricity and are not permitted in the hyperbaric environment. Electronic equipment must be grounded appropriately. Humidification of oxygen and air sources also decreases static electricity.

Detailed fire safety codes and standards for multiplace chambers are described in the NFPA 99, *Standard for Health Care Facilities* (Chapter 19, Hyperbaric Facilities).[21] NFPA 99 was developed in response to fatal hyperbaric fires in the 1960s and has since been updated several times. At the time it was originally written, there were no fire safety standards for oxygen-enriched atmospheres in the United States. NFPA is a voluntary, nongovernment association that develops fire safety codes and standards. These recommendations may be adopted by regulatory agencies, but NFPA does not enforce these standards. NFPA 99 should be available at every clinical hyperbaric facility.

DECOMPRESSION ILLNESS IN INSIDE ATTENDANTS

Inside attendants breathe air during most or all of a hyperbaric treatment session and are therefore at risk for decompression illness. The frequency of decompression illness in attendants varies with the hyperbaric treatment protocol, the decompression profile, and the individual risks of the attendant. It has been demonstrated that chamber attendants can experience decompression stress with development of venous gas emboli, as detected by ultrasound Doppler.[24] Fortunately, treatment protocols currently in use rarely cause clinical decompression illness.[25,26] Baker[26] surveyed 33 multiplace hyperbaric chambers in North America and reported a 0.1% to 0.6% incidence rate of decompression illness following standard "wound healing" protocols. Similarly, possible or certain decompression illness occurred in 0.1% of inside attendants supervising a total of 19,000 hyperbaric treatments from 1992 to 2006 at Virginia Mason Medical Center in Seattle, Washington.

Appropriate decompression of inside attendants is based on decompression tables originally generated for underwater diving. However, the risk for decompression illness in inside attendants is unacceptably high when underwater decompression tables are used without modification.[25] For example, Thalmann[27] estimated a 6% to 11% risk for decompression illness when inside attendants breathe air while supervising a U.S. Navy Treatment Table 6. Consequently, decompression profiles suggested by standard dive tables are typically modified to provide an additional margin of safety for inside attendants.

Several factors decrease the risk for decompression illness. Decreasing treatment pressures from 2.4 to 2.0 ATA and increasing the interval between exposures have both been associated with lower rates of attendant decompression illness.[26] Rotating inside attendants so there is no decompression obligation is also effective, but may be impractical in the case of staff shortages in busy multiplace facilities.

The most effective practical measure to decrease the risk for decompression illness in inside attendants is to have the attendant breathe oxygen at pressure.[25-27] By preventing additional nitrogen loading and speeding unloading of tissue nitrogen, oxygen breathing effectively shortens time at depth and decreases decompression stress. The risk for decompression illness declines significantly as the duration of oxygen breathing increases. For example, the estimated risk for decompression illness following a U.S. Navy Treatment Table 6 is 6% to 11% when the inside attendant breathes air, 3% to 6% when oxygen is breathed for 30 minutes during ascent, and 0% when oxygen is breathed for 30 minutes at 2.8 ATA and then 30 minutes during ascent.[27]

In practice, inside attendants supervising routine wound healing protocols breathe oxygen during and sometimes before ascent.

For example, attendants typically breathe oxygen during ascent in the Davis wound healing protocol (see Fig. 3.9A). As decompression stress increases with increasing treatment duration or other factors, the period of oxygen breathing for the inside attendant is also typically extended. For example, in a commonly used variant of the Davis protocol (see Fig. 3.9B), attendants breathe oxygen for 10 minutes before and 9 minutes during ascent. When a patient is at risk for central nervous system oxygen toxicity, air-breathing intervals are more frequent, and total treatment length increases. Consequently, the attendant's oxygen-breathing period is also lengthened to decrease the risk for decompression illness (see Fig. 3.9C).

To further decrease the risk for decompression illness following a standard "wound healing" protocol, attendants are typically limited to supervision of one treatment per day, assuring a surface interval of nearly 24 hours. Similarly, they should avoid flying or driving to altitude for 24 hours after serving as inside attendant. Staff members should be educated about the increased risk for decompression illness created by dehydration, alcohol use, and heavy physical activity.[15]

Because early treatment of decompression illness improves outcome, attendants must be well informed about its signs and symptoms. Appropriate education should result in a low threshold to report possible decompression illness, even when dive profiles are benign, and prompt treatment of suspected cases.

Individuals who want to work as inside attendants should undergo a detailed medical examination by a physician who is trained in hyperbaric medicine. The evaluation should include a chest radiograph to evaluate for structural lung disease that might predispose to pulmonary barotrauma and a baseline audiogram given possible hearing loss associated with otic barotrauma. Spirometry is reserved for those with a history of asthma, chronic obstructive pulmonary disease, significant tobacco use, or wheezing on physical examination. Contraindications to serving as an inside attendant in a hyperbaric chamber are similar to those recommended for evaluation of underwater divers (Table 3.7).

ACCREDITATION OF MULTIPLACE HYPERBARIC FACILITIES

Beginning in 2002, the UHMS developed a voluntary clinical hyperbaric facility accreditation program. Because the installation, operation, and maintenance of a multiplace hyperbaric facility are more complex than for a monoplace chamber, this program is especially beneficial to those who operate multiplace hyperbaric chambers. The philosophy of the UHMS is that the accreditation process represents a quality improvement program rather than a bureaucratically mandated inspection. Areas

Table 3.7 Contraindications to Serving as an Inside Attendant in a Clinical Multiplace Hyperbaric Chamber

ABSOLUTE	RELATIVE
Seizure disorder	
History of spontaneous pneumothorax	
Significant hearing loss	Difficulty equalizing middle ear pressure
Active chronic obstructive pulmonary disease or asthma	
Residua of decompression illness	Previous unexplained decompression illness
Current or impending pregnancy	
Psychiatric disorder	Diabetes with frequent hypoglycemia
Congestive heart failure	
Lung bullae or cysts	

Table 3.8 Areas of Emphasis of the Undersea and Hyperbaric Medical Society Clinical Hyperbaric Facility Accreditation Program

GOVERNANCE	CHAMBER ELEC-TRICAL SYSTEMS	PROFESSIONAL IMPROVEMENT
Administration	Gas Handling	Leadership
Operations	Patient Rights	Human Resources
Maintenance	Patient Assessment	Information Management
Facility Construction	Patient Care	Infection Control
Chamber Fabrication	Environment of Care	Medical Staff
Chamber Ventilation	Patient Education	Teaching and Publication
Chamber Fire Protection	Quality Improvement	Clinical Research

of emphasis for the accreditation program are based on a number of regulatory guidelines[14,17,18,21,28-46] and are shown in Table 3.8. The UHMS believes its accreditation program is the most efficient method to ensure that:

1. Clinical hyperbaric facilities are staffed with proper specialists who are well trained
2. Clinical hyperbaric facilities are using quality equipment that has been properly installed and maintained, and is being operated with the highest level of safety
3. Clinical hyperbaric facilities are providing high-quality patient care
4. Clinical hyperbaric facilities are maintaining appropriate documentation of informed consent, patient treatment procedures, physician involvement, etc.

Each survey team consists of a hyperbaric physician, hyperbaric nurse, and a Certified Hyperbaric Technologist with special experience in the type of facility being surveyed. For example, a Certified Hyperbaric Technologist with extensive experience in multiplace hyperbaric chamber operations would be assigned to survey a multiplace hyperbaric facility. Of the concentration areas listed in Table 3.8, daily operations, maintenance, chamber ventilation, fire protection, electrical systems, gas handling, and human resources receive additional emphasis during an accreditation survey for a multiplace chamber facility. At the completion of each

2-day survey, the Certified Hyperbaric Technologist team member provides a list of recommendations and opportunities for technical improvement to the facility. If improvements are made in each facility surveyed, then over time, the collective quality of care will improve across the spectrum of hyperbaric facilities.

As of March 2007, 73 clinical hyperbaric facilities have been initially accredited by the UHMS. More than one fourth (21/73) of clinical hyperbaric facilities accredited by the UHMS operate multiplace hyperbaric chambers. Recent reaccreditation surveys indicate that notable improvements in each of the 24 concentration areas have been made. For organizations in the initial stages of planning a hyperbaric facility (regardless of the type of hyperbaric chamber planned), a copy of the UHMS Clinical Hyperbaric Facility Accreditation Program Manual can be obtained free of charge from the UHMS. This document is an excellent guide to developing the necessary policies and procedures required to operate a safe, high-quality, cost-effective clinical hyperbaric medicine program. By all indications, the UHMS Clinical Hyperbaric Facility Accreditation Program has established its relevance to the practice of hyperbaric medicine.

REFERENCES

1. Undersea and Hyperbaric Medical Society Chamber Directory. Available at www.uhms.org/Chambers/CHAMBER DIRECTORY2.ASP. Accessed April 3, 2007.
2. Workman WT: Director, Undersea and Hyperbaric Medical Society Quality Assurance and Regulatory Affairs. Personal communication, August 2006.

3. Sunny Sonnenrein: Reimers Systems, Inc. Personal communication, November 2006.

4. Dunford RG, Hampson NB: Use of USN Table 6A for the treatment of arterial gas embolism in divers in the United States. Undersea Hyperb Med 28(suppl):49, 2001.

5. Davis JC: Hyperbaric oxygen therapy. J Intensive Care Med 4:55-57, 1989.

6. Weaver LK: Monoplace hyperbaric chamber use of U.S. Navy Table 6: A 20-year experience. Undersea Hyperb Med 33:85-88, 2006.

7. Sheffield PJ, Desautels DA: Hyperbaric and hypobaric chamber fires: A 73-year analysis. Undersea Hyperb Med 24:153-164, 1997.

8. Sheffield PJ: How the Davis 2.36 ATA wound healing enhancement treatment table was established. Undersea Hyperb Med 31:193-194, 2004.

9. Brummelkamp WH, Hogendijk J, Boerema I: Treatment of anaerobic infections (clostridial myositis) by drenching the tissues with oxygen under high atmospheric pressure. Surgery 49:299-302, 1961.

10. Sheffield PJ, Workman WT: Transcutaneous oxygen monitoring in patients undergoing hyperbaric oxygen therapy. In: Huch R, Huch A (eds): Continuous Transcutaneous Blood Gas Monitoring. New York, Marcel Dekker, 1983, pp 667-672.

11. Piantadosi CA: A mini-forum on air breaks and O_2 toxicity in clinical HBO_2 therapy. Undersea Hyperb Med 31:185-191, 2004.

12. Hampson NB, Atik D: Central nervous system oxygen toxicity during routine hyperbaric oxygen therapy. Undersea Hyperb Med 30:147-153, 2003.

13. Davis JC: Hyperbaric oxygen therapy. J Intensive Care Med 4:55-57, 1989.

14. Workman WT (ed): UHMS Guidelines for Hyperbaric Facility Operation. Dunkirk, Md, Undersea and Hyperbaric Medical Society, 2004.

15. Kot J, Desola J, Simao AG, et al: A European Code of Good Practice for Hyperbaric Oxygen Therapy, COST Action B14, May 2004. Available at www.oxynet.org. Accessed April 30, 2007.

16. Kemmer A, Muth C, Mathieu D: Patient management. In: Mathieu D (ed): Handbook on Hyperbaric Medicine. Dordrecht, The Netherlands, Springer, 2006, pp 637-650.

17. Guidelines for Standards of Care for the Hyperbaric Patient Receiving Hyperbaric Oxygen Therapy. Columbia, SC, Baromedical Nurses Association.

18. Reiner A, Brown B: Manual of Patient Care Standards. Gaithersburg, Md, Aspen Publishers, 1991.

19. Kohn LT, Corrigan JM, Donaldson MS (eds): To Err Is Human: Building a Safer Health System. Institute of Medicine, Washington, DC, The National Academies Press, 2000.

20. Perrow C: Aircraft and airways. In: Perrow C (ed): Normal Accidents. Princeton, NJ, Princeton University Press, 1999, pp 123-169.

21. NFPA 99, Health Care Facilities (1999 edition). Quincy, Mass, National Fire Protection Association, 1999.

22. Sheffield PJ: Hyperbaric chamber fires: To what extent is the problem? In: Workman WT (ed): Hyperbaric Facility Safety: A Practical Guide. Flagstaff, Ariz, Best Publishing, 1999, pp 487-493.

23. Desautels DA: UHMS Chamber Experience and Mishap Database (1923-1998). Available at www.uhms.org/Safety/saf%20comm%20(articles).htm. Accessed April 3, 2007.

24. Risberg J, Englund M, Aanderud L, et al: Venous gas embolism in chamber attendants after hyperbaric exposure. Underse Hyperb Med 31:417-429, 2004.

25. Sheffield PJ, Pirone CJ: Decompression sickness in inside attendants. In: Workman WT (ed): Hyperbaric Facility Safety: A Practical Guide. Flagstaff, Ariz, Best Publishing, 1999, pp 643-664.

26. Baker PC: Decompression sickness incidence in inside attendants. Associates: BNA Pre-course on Chamber Safety, Undersea and Hyperbaric Medical Society Annual Scientific meeting, Cancun, Mexico, June 15-22, 1997.

27. Thalmann ED: Principles of U.S. Navy recompression treatments for decompression sickness. In: Moon RE, Sheffield PJ (ed s): Treatment of Decompression Illness, 45th UHMS Workshop. Kensington, Md, Undersea and Hyperbaric Medical Society, 1996, pp 75-95.

28. ASME Boiler and Pressure Vessel Code. New York, American Society of Mechanical Engineers, 2001.

29. ASME PVHO-1-2002, Safety Standard for Pressure Vessels for Human Occupancy. New York, American Society of Mechanical Engineers, 2003.

30. ASME PVHO-2-2003, Safety Standard for Pressure Vessels for Human Occupancy In-Service Guidelines for PVHO Acrylic Windows. New York, American Society of Mechanical Engineers, 2004.

31. CGA C-9-1988, Standard Color Marking of Compressed Gas Containers Intended for Medical Use. Arlington, Va, Compressed Gas Association, Inc., 1998.

32. CGA G-4-1996, Oxygen. Arlington, Va, Compressed Gas Association, Inc., 1996.

33. CGA G-4.3-2000, Commodity Specification for Oxygen. Arlington, Va, Compressed Gas Association, Inc., 2000.

34. CGA G-7-1990, Compressed Air for Human Respiration. Arlington, Va, Compressed Gas Association, Inc., 1990.

35. CGA G-7.1-1997, Commodity Specification for Air. Arlington, Va, Compressed Gas Association, Inc., 1997.

36. CGA P-2-1996, Characteristics and Safe Handling of Medical Gases. Arlington, Va, Compressed Gas Association, Inc., 1996.

37. CGA P-2.7-2000, Guide for the Safe Storage, Handling, and Use of Portable Liquid Oxygen Systems in Health Care Facilities, 2nd ed. Arlington, Va, Compressed Gas Association, Inc., 2000.

38. Comprehensive Accreditation Manual for Hospitals: The Official Handbook (2004). Oakbrook Terrace, Ill, Joint Commission on Accreditation of Healthcare Organizations, 2004.

39. Medical Device Amendments to the Federal Food, Drug, and Cosmetic Act, May 1976. 21 CFR 807.87.

40. Medical Device Amendments to the Federal Food, Drug, and Cosmetic Act, May 1976. 21 CFR 868.5470.

41. NFPA 13, Installation of Sprinkler Systems, 1999. Quincy, Mass, National Fire Protection Association, 1999.

42. NFPA 25, Standard for the Inspection, Testing, and Maintenance of Water-Based Fire Protection Systems, 1998. Quincy, Mass, National Fire Protection Association, 1998.
43. NFPA 50, Standard for Bulk Oxygen Systems at Consumer Sites, 2001. Quincy, Mass, National Fire Protection Association, 2001.
44. NFPA 70, National Electric Code. Quincy, Mass, National Fire Protection Association, 1999.
45. NFPA 99, Health Care Facilities (2005 edition). Quincy, Mass, National Fire Protection Association, 2005.
46. NFPA 101, Life Safety Code, 2000. Quincy, Mass, National Fire Protection Association, 2000.

The Physics **4** of Hyperbaric Oxygen Therapy

Kevin Hardy, MD

By definition, hyperbaric oxygen therapy (HBOT) is a treatment in which a patient breathes 100% oxygen while inside a pressure vessel or treatment chamber at a pressure that is higher than sea-level atmospheric pressure. Therefore, health-care professionals and providers of HBOT must be well versed in the basic physical principles that are applicable to the interactions of pressure, gases, and physiologic systems. It is not the intent of this chapter to provide a comprehensive review of elementary physics. (Any reader who requires a more thorough review is referred to any of the many excellent textbooks in physics.) On the contrary, this chapter focuses on the key physical principles required for a fundamental understanding of the HBOT environment. Furthermore, although physical principles that apply to HBOT and the diving environment are significantly interrelated, this chapter focuses on those aspects that apply specifically to HBOT. More in-depth discussions concerning diving medicine can be found in the literature.[1-5]

SYMBOLS

Any discussions that involve basic physics require the use of the symbols related to units of measurement, especially in this case those pertaining to pressure. For better or worse, HBOT has evolved over the years from various scientific and engineering developments. As a result, the field is saddled with a wide variety of symbols and the terminology they represent. The symbols and abbreviations used in this chapter are those generally utilized in the customary system of the United States (in most cases, avoirdupois) and the international metric system. In addition, because of the previously mentioned close association between diving and HBOT, some terminology and symbols are based on those used in the diving community. Table 4.1 lists symbols for common units of measurement.

Table 4.1 Symbols for Units of Measurement

SYMBOL	UNIT
atm	atmospheres
ATA	atmospheres absolute
cm	centimeter
cm^2	square centimeter
fsw	feet of sea water
kg	kilogram
kg/cm^2	kilograms per square centimeter
kPa	kilopascal
L	liter
m	meter
mm	millimeter
mm Hg	millimeters of mercury
Pa	Pascals
psi (lb/in^2)	pounds per square inch

Table 4.2 shows comparisons and conversions for commonly used units of pressure.

PRESSURE

Pressure is defined as the amount of force applied over unit of area. In the HBOT community, units commonly used to quantify pressure include atmospheres (atm) and atmospheres absolute (ATA), pounds per square inch (psi), kilograms per square centimeter (kg/cm^2), kilopascals (kPa), and feet of sea water (fsw). Given that the atmosphere is a unit that is independent of both the avoirdupois and metric systems, it is often considered to be the most useful international unit for pressure measurement in the hyperbaric community.

Atmospheric pressure is defined as the pressure exerted by Earth's atmosphere on all objects, whether animate or inanimate. At sea level, this atmospheric pressure is equal to 1 ATA, 1 atm, 14.7 psi, 1.03 kg/cm^2, 101.32 kPa, and 33 fsw. At higher elevations, the pressure exerted by Earth's atmosphere decreases and, therefore, atmospheric pressure is lower. In the hyperbaric therapy environment, pressure is, of course, increased and, therefore, will be greater than 1 ATA.

Gauge pressure is a term that refers directly to the pressure being measured. Generally speaking, it does not include atmospheric pressure, and most gauges are calibrated so that they read zero at normal atmospheric pressure.

Ambient pressure is defined as the total pressure surrounding or encompassing an object. This is equivalent to *absolute pressure* and is expressed in those terms and units of measurement. Whereas in the diving environment ambient pressure is equal to the sum of the atmospheric pressure and hydrostatic pressure (force resulting from the weight of the surrounding fluid on the submerged object), in the HBOT environment, ambient pressure and absolute pressure are synonymous. This absolute pressure can be calculated by adding the atmospheric pressure and the gauge pressure. Absolute pressure is expressed by the following equation:

$$P_{abs} = P_{atm} + P_{gauge}$$

As an example, let us consider a common hyperbaric treatment protocol calling for administration of 100% oxygen at 2.4 ATA. Let us further assume that this treatment is

Table 4.2 Conversions for Commonly Used Units of Pressure

	ATMOSPHERES (ATM)	PSI (LB/IN^2)	KG/CM^2	KPA	FEET OF SEA WATER (FSW)	MM HG (TORR)
1 atm	1	14.69	1.033	101.3	33	760.0
1 psi (lb/in^2)	0.068	1	0.070	6.895	2.246	51.72
1 kg/cm^2	0.968	14.22	1	98.07	32.04	735.6
1 kPa	0.010	0.145	0.010	1	0.326	7.501
1 fsw	0.030	0.445	0.031	3.070	1	23.04
1 mm Hg (torr)	0.0013	0.0193	0.0014	0.1333	0.0434	1

occurring at a coastal facility. Therefore, the local atmospheric pressure is 1.0 ATA. The chamber operator would then be instructed to compress the chamber to a gauge pressure of 1.4 ATA, which, added to the atmospheric pressure, gives the desired absolute pressure of 2.4 ATA. This value also represents the ambient pressure *inside* the chamber during the treatment.

$$P_{abs}\ (2.4\,\text{ATA}) = P_{atm}\ (1.0\,\text{ATA}) \\ + P_{gauge}\ (1.4\,\text{ATA})$$

The preceding example brings to mind another issue that can be of importance to the practitioner of hyperbaric medicine. It is the issue of treatment at altitude. As noted earlier, atmospheric pressure decreases as altitude increases. Thus, a chamber that provides HBOT for a hospital located in the mountains must use a higher-gauge pressure to achieve the same absolute treatment pressure as a similar chamber located in a sea-level facility.

The concept of *partial pressure* should also be considered. Any mixture of gases exerts pressure, such as the air in our atmosphere that is composed of multiple gases. The proportion of that pressure exerted by any single gas in the mixture is referred to as its partial pressure. It is in direct proportion to its percentage of the total volume of the gas mixture and also is a direct determinate of the amount of absorbed gas in tissues. The concept of absorbed gas in tissues is important and is more fully explained in the chapters that deal with air embolism, decompression sickness (DCS), and oxygen toxicity (see Chapters 13, 14, and 23).

GASES

As mentioned in the introduction, HBOT consists of the administration of oxygen in a pressurized chamber. These treatment chambers are typically pressurized by the use of compressed air but may utilize pure oxygen and, in unusual situations, various gas mixes. Therefore, any discussion of HBOT must include a review of the diverse constituent gases.

Atmospheric air is composed of nitrogen (79.1%), oxygen (20.9%), carbon dioxide (0.03%), water vapor, and a variety of trace gases. Despite the presence of miniscule amounts of suspended solids, air still has quite a low density and is, therefore, quite compressible, especially in comparison with liquids and solids. Its behavior is generally governed by and can be predicted by simple laws of physics that pertain to ideal gases. As noted earlier, nitrogen is the preponderant component of air. It is colorless, odorless, and tasteless in its free state. Although considered inert (which is true of the free state), it can be soluble in various fluids including body tissues under increased ambient pressure. It can be physiologically active on the central nervous system, causing intoxicant or anesthetic effects. Although these properties of nitrogen have little effect on the patient undergoing hyperbaric therapy, they are essential in understanding the pathophysiology of patients with DCS. Furthermore, facilities that utilize multiple patient chambers that use inside medical attendants must take into account the risks for DCS and nitrogen narcosis for the attendant when developing treatment protocols.

Oxygen, as any elementary school child can relate, is the essential component of air. It is the only gas capable of supporting human life. It is also colorless, odorless, and tasteless in its free state. The human organism generally has tolerance for only a narrow range of oxygen partial pressure. Below a partial pressure of 0.16 ATA, hypoxia and subsequent altered mental status and loss of consciousness may ensue. However, it should be noted that there have been reported instances of humans surviving for short periods at high altitude with less than 0.1 ATA oxygen in their inspired air. These issues do not significantly impact the HBOT environment unless a disastrous (and usually negligent) error is made with the oxygen supply lines. High partial pressures of oxygen are a more pertinent concern to the HBOT provider. Prolonged exposure to an oxygen partial pressure at or above 0.5 ATA can result in pulmonary oxygen toxicity. Shorter exposures to more than 1.8 ATA partial pressure oxygen can produce central nervous system effects. The most concerning, but fortunately most rare, of these neurologic events is a hyperoxia-induced seizure (see Chapter 23).

Oxygen is also readily soluble in body fluids and tissues. However, it is far from inert and is rather metabolically active. Consequently, no concomitant concern exists that patients treated with hyperbaric oxygen will be at risk for clinical DCS as when exposed to inert gases. In fact, this principle is used to reduce the risk of multiplace chamber tenders by including a period of oxygen breathing at the end of certain treatment tables to help "wash out" the inert gases breathed by the tender. These issues and other oxygen effects such as transient vasoconstriction are discussed in detail in Chapter 23. Before closing the subject of oxygen, however, it is important to emphasize its impact on the flammability of other substances. Although oxygen itself is inflammable, increasing partial pressure of oxygen in a hyperbaric chamber significantly increases the speed of the oxidation process known as fire. Subsequently, fire safety is of paramount importance in the HBOT environment.

Carbon dioxide, which is also colorless and tasteless in normal concentrations, is a waste product of human metabolism. Significantly elevated partial pressures are dangerous to humans, and untoward effects begin with respiratory acidosis and altered mental status potentially leading to loss of consciousness and death. Removal of carbon dioxide from the hyperbaric environment can be accomplished by the use of so-called carbon dioxide scrubbers that use chemical absorption (such as with lithium carbonate), or more typically by intermittent venting of the chamber.

Carbon monoxide is another odorless, colorless, and tasteless gas that is the product of incomplete combustion of a carbon-containing fuel. It is highly poisonous to humans, and its effects and treatment are discussed in Chapter 15. Notably, a number of hyperbaric chambers create compressed gases for therapy by the use of fuel-burning compressors. In these circumstances, care must be taken that the exhaust from compressor engines is safely separated from the air intake to avoid contamination.

Helium is another colorless, odorless, tasteless, and inert gas. It is furthermore nontoxic and nonexplosive, and it has virtually none of the central nervous system narcotic effects associated with nitrogen. Accordingly, some experts tout it as a superior replacement for the use of medical attendants treating patients who require recompression therapy at pressures greater than 3.0 ATA. These situations are rare, however, and the advantage of helium in breathing-gas mixtures must be balanced against its cost, supply logistics, and effect on the user's speech (Mickey Mouse effect), which can become unintelligible.

Other trace gases found in normal air such as *hydrogen* and *argon* may play certain roles in the breathing mixtures of commercial or other saturation divers but have no real impact or use in the HBOT community. A more in-depth understanding of the uses of these gases and their subsequent impact on saturation divers is the purview of the specialized commercial or scientific physician.

BREATHING-GAS MIXTURES

The definition of a breathing-gas mixture is a gas containing oxygen and one or more inert gases. Composition of these mixtures can be quite complex in the diving arena. Applicable considerations include the diver's metabolic and oxygen partial pressure needs, narcosis potential, cost, logistics, and safety including risks for fire or explosion. Although these issues also apply to the HBOT environment, the selection of mixtures is much simpler because treatment pressures are generally confined to a range of 1.4 to 3.0 ATA.

Atmospheric air (composition noted earlier in this chapter) is the most common mixture used in the compression of hyperbaric chambers because of its advantages of easier availability, lower cost, and improved safety profile. It is also almost universally used as the breathing gas for multiplace chamber attendants to prevent any untoward effects that repeat exposures to increased partial pressures of oxygen (much more numerous than any patient) would create. However, its nitrogen content with associated increased partial pressure and tissue solubility in hyperbaric conditions must be accounted for when planning treatment profiles and repetitive tender exposures or "dives."

Alterations in the proportions of nitrogen and oxygen are sometimes used in HBOT. These mixtures are often referred to by the somewhat misleading nomenclature of *nitrogen-oxygen* or *nitrox*. For all intents and purposes, atmospheric air is essentially *nitrox* 79:21—that is, a nitrogen-to-oxygen ratio of 79:21. That said, the term *nitrox* generally refers to mixtures that are enriched in oxygen. A number of such mixtures are used for diving, but less so for HBOT. However, one well-known example is in use for the venerable U.S. Navy Treatment Table 6A. This table is used at times for cases of air embolism and severe DCS. Because it involves compression to 6.0 ATA, the use of 100% oxygen is contraindicated because of an unacceptable oxygen toxicity profile. Therefore, a nitrogen-to-oxygen 50:50 breathing mixture is used for the patient with a subsequent reduction in total oxygen tension to 3.0 ATA to reduce the oxygen toxicity risk. Other breathing mixtures such as *helium-oxygen (heliox)*, *trimix*, and *argon-oxygen* are used to a significant extent in saturation diving, but a discussion of these mixtures is inapplicable to HBOT.

GAS LAWS

The solitary gases discussed earlier can be considered to be ideal gases for the purpose of understanding their physical behavior. This behavior of any one ideal gas is the same for all ideal gases or mixtures of these gases. The minute quantities of suspended solid impurities are so small that effects are minimal and air may also be considered an ideal gas by its physical behavior.

The behavior of ideal gases such as nitrogen and oxygen is governed by the intimately related factors of pressure, volume, and temperature. A change in any one of these three factors, such as an increase in pressure, results in a measurable and mathematically verifiable change in the other factors. These pressure, volume, and temperature relationships may be expressed by equations that mathematically describe the laws governing the behavior of any ideal gas or gas mixture as noted earlier. When discussing gas laws, pressures and temperatures are expressed in absolute terms with their corresponding units of measure. All other units of measure used in the equation must be in a single system of measure. The ideal gas laws that concern the hyperbaric practitioner are Boyle's Law, Guy–Lussac's Law, Charles' Law, Dalton's Law, and Henry's Law.

Boyle's Law

Boyle's Law states that if the temperature of a fixed mass of gas is kept constant, the volume of that given gas mass is inversely proportional to its absolute pressure. Mathematically, this means that the product of the pressure and volume will remain constant. This can be expressed by the following equation:

$$PV = k$$

where P is absolute pressure, V is volume, and K is a constant. Thus, when the pressure is doubled, the volume is reduced to half of the original volume. Another way of considering Boyle's Law is to use sequential subscripts to denote two different temporal states of a gas at the same temperature. It follows then that Boyle's Law may also be written as:

$$P_1 V_1 = P_2 V_2$$

As an example of Boyle's Law, let us assume that a closed flexible container of air, such as a pressure bag for intravenous fluids, with a volume of 1 L at sea level, is compressed to a pressure of 2.0 ATA. The volume at the new depth can be calculated using the above formula:

$$P_1 V_1 = P_2 V_2$$

$$1\ \text{ATA} \times 1\ \text{L} = 2\ \text{ATA} \times V_2$$

$$0.5\ \text{L} = V_2$$

where P_1 is atmospheric pressure expressed in absolute units, V_1 is the volume at P_1 of 1 L, P_2 is the chosen compression pressure, and V_2

is the new volume at the chosen pressure. Note that the volume decreases by 50%, although the chosen compression pressure is not at all extreme and is, in fact, a commonly used hyperbaric therapy pressure. Reversing the direction of the equation, one can see that during decompression, the decreasing ambient pressure would necessitate a doubling of the volume under pressure.

The implications for HBOT of the gas behavior described by Boyle's Law are varied and multiple. During the initial compression phase of the treatment, as pressure increases, the volume of gas in any air space in the body will decrease. This volume change, in turn, creates a pressure differential between the relatively lower pressure air space and the relatively higher pressure surrounding tissues. If additional (compressed) gas does not enter the space to equalize this pressure differential, tissue distortion with accompanying congestion, edema, and hemorrhage ensues. As a corollary, during the decompression phase of HBOT, the volume of gas in body air spaces increases or expands. If this air becomes trapped, for example, in the middle ear because of eustachian tube congestion or in the alveoli because of obstructive airways disease, the subsequent increased volume will create stretching and increased pressure in the surrounding tissues. These examples are various facets of treatment-related barotrauma and are discussed in further detail in Chapter 22.

Implications for other air-filled spaces in a hyperbaric treatment chamber must also be considered when contemplating Boyle's Law. Air in endotracheal tube cuffs, suction devices including Hemavac reservoirs and Jackson–Pratt bulbs, and therapy adjuncts such as pressure bags must be periodically observed and appropriately vented.

Gay–Lussac's Law

Gay-Lussac's Law states that, at a constant volume, the absolute pressure of a given mass of gas is directly proportional to the absolute temperature. This relationship is expressed by the following formula:

$$P_1/T_1 = P_2/T_2$$

where P and T are absolute measurements of pressure and temperature at times or conditions 1 and 2. The application of this law to the hyperbaric environment explains why in the rigid walled chamber (fixed volume) ambient temperature increases during compression and decreases during decompression, a fact most patients notice immediately and for which they should receive anticipatory counseling.

Charles' Law

Charles' Law states that, at a constant pressure, the volume of a given mass of gas is directly proportional to the absolute temperature. This relationship is expressed by the following formula:

$$V_1/T_1 = V_2/T_2$$

where V and T are absolute measurements of volume and temperature at times or conditions 1 and 2.

Guy–Lussac's and Charles' laws are sometimes combined mathematically to create the following algebraic expression:

$$PV = RT$$

where P is the absolute pressure, V is volume, T is absolute temperature, and R is a universal constant for all gases.

General Gas Law

The preceding discussion of Boyle's, Guy-Lussac's, and Charles' laws and the immediately preceding equation show that in considering the behavior of gases in the HBOT arena, the factors of temperature, volume, and pressure are so interrelated that a change in any one must result in a corresponding change in one or both of the others. The general gas law is a convenient expression of these relationships and can be used to predict the behavior of a given mass of gas when changes may be expected in any or all of the variables. The general gas law equation is typically noted to be:

$$PV/T = k$$

where P is the absolute pressure, V is volume, T is absolute temperature, and k is a constant. Because this is so, another perhaps more mathematically useful expression of the law denoting two conditions or states of the gas under consideration with subscripts is as follows:

$$P_1V_1/T_1 = P_2V_2/T_2$$

An example of the application of this formula's principle would be in the choice of location of either low- or high-pressure storage tanks used to store the compressed air and, in some cases, other gases used in hyperbaric therapy. If such tanks are subjected to extremes of temperature, significant changes in pressure of the fixed volume gases will result. The implications for gas reserves for proper treatment and patient and staff safety should be evident, and these are considerations that hyperbaric program directors and safety officers face daily.

Dalton's Law

Dalton's Law states that the total pressure exerted by a mixture of "n" gases is the sum of the pressure that would be exerted by each gas if each occupied the total volume. This deals with the concept of partial pressure. Algebraically, this relationship is expressed as:

$$P_t = P_a + P_b + P_c + \ldots + P_n$$

where P_t is the absolute pressure of the gas mixture; P is the partial pressure of the constituent gases including gases a, b, and c denoted by the subscripts; and n is the final constituent gas.

The partial pressure (P_a) of a given gas "a" in a mixture may be calculated by the following formula:

$$P_a = P_t \cdot F_a$$

where P_t is the absolute pressure of the gas mixture, and F_a is the percentage by volume of gas "a" in the mixture annotated as a decimal fraction. As an example, the partial pressure of oxygen (21% by volume, assuming no oxygen leaks from faulty or ill-fitting delivery systems) in the air of a chamber compressed to 2.8 ATA can be calculated as follows:

$$P_{O_2} = 2.8\,ATA \times 0.21 = 0.588\,ATA\,O_2$$

This calculation can be used to show that hyperbaric *air*, even at a relatively high treatment pressure, provides no more oxygen to a biologic system than a tight-fitting nonrebreather mask. The partial pressures of nitrogen and oxygen in air at various treatment pressures are noted in Table 4.3.

Henry's Law

Henry's Law states that the number of molecules or the mass of a gas that will dissolve in a liquid at a given temperature is directly proportional to the partial pressure of that gas. Henry's Law is related to Dalton's Law in that it deals with the relationship of the partial pressure of a gas to its absorption. The actual volume of a gas when it is in solution is negligible. Hence, there is no appreciable increase in the volume of the dissolving liquid. Gas solubility is also dependent on the temperature of the liquid. The lower the fluid temperature, the higher the solubility. Gas absorption is also dependant on the properties of the fluid. For example, the solubility of nitrogen in an oil such as fat is about five times its solubility in a mostly watery fluid such as plasma at the same pressure.

Henry's and Dalton's laws are useful when contemplating the diffusion of gases in the human body under pressure. The difference between the partial pressure (sometimes referred to as *tension*) of a gas dissolved in a liquid and its partial pressure in the ambient gas mixture will determine the direction and rate of diffusion into or out of solution. This pressure differential is often called the *gradient*. If a gas-free liquid is exposed to a gas, the inward gradient is high, and the rate at which gas molecules will migrate into the liquid is high. As the gas tension in the liquid increases, the rate of diffusion decreases.

Table 4.3 Partial Pressures of Nitrogen and Oxygen at Various Treatment Pressures

| | TREATMENT PRESSURE | | | PARTIAL PRESSURE | | | | | |
| | | | | NITROGEN | | | OXYGEN | | |
fsw (gauge)	ATA	kPa	psi	ATA	psi	kPa	ATA	psi	kPa
0	1.0	101	14.7	0.79	11.6	80	0.21	3.1	21
33	2.0	203	29.4	1.58	23.2	160	0.42	6.2	43
45	2.4	243	35.3	1.90	27.9	192	0.50	7.4	51
60	2.8	284	41.2	2.21	32.5	224	0.59	8.7	60
66	3.0	304	44.1	2.37	34.8	240	0.63	9.3	64
165	6.0	608	88.2	4.74	69.6	480	1.26	18.6	128

ATA, atmospheres absolute; fsw, feet of sea water; kPa, kilopascals; psi, pounds per square inch.

Equilibrium is achieved when the dissolved and ambient gas tensions are equal. The liquid is then considered saturated for those conditions. These concepts of gas solubility and diffusion are important in the study of nitrogen narcosis and DCS (see discussion in Chapters 10 and 14).

REFERENCES

1. Bove AA (ed): Bove and Davis' Diving Medicine, 4 ed. Philadelphia, Saunders, 2003.
2. Brubakk AO, Neuman TS (eds): Bennett and Elliott's Physiology and Medicine of Diving, 5 ed. Edinburgh, Saunders, 2003.
3. Edmonds C, Lowry C, Pennefather J, Walker R (eds): Diving and Subaquatic Medicine, 4 ed. London, Arnold, 2002.
4. Joiner JT (ed): NOAA Diving Manual, 4 ed. Flagstaff, Ariz, Best, 2001.
5. U.S. Navy Diving Manual [NAVSEA 0927-LP-001-9011]. Flagstaff, Ariz, Best, 1996.

Clearance to Dive and Fitness for Work

5

Simon J. Mitchell, MBChB, PhD,
DipDHM, DipOccMed, FANZCA,
and Michael H. Bennett, MBBS, MD,
MM(Clin Epi), FANZCA

Hyperbaric physicians may be consulted by prospective divers seeking clearance to dive and by occupational divers fulfilling statutory diving clearance and health surveillance requirements. Consultations are often sought when the candidate's medical history raises concerns about diving. Hyperbaric physicians should, therefore, expect to evaluate the most complex issues relating to clearance to dive. In addition, hyperbaric physicians supervising multiplace hyperbaric units are usually responsible for assessing and monitoring the fitness of their attendant staff for hyperbaric work.

This chapter reviews the medical evaluation of a prospective diver or hyperbaric worker. Ideally, the reader should already be familiar with environmental, medical, and practical issues of diving; comprehensive accounts of these issues can be found elsewhere.[1] This chapter begins with a discussion of diving activities and the functional capabilities necessary for safe participation. This is followed by a summary of modern trends in the philosophy of diving clearance assessments, typical models for administration of diving clearance issues, and a discussion of who should perform the assessments. An approach to a diving clearance consultation is described, and the implications of selected relevant medical issues or problems are discussed. We note that diving medicine is a field largely bereft of hard evidence to guide practice. Many "beliefs" are just that; they are supported by observational evidence at best. As Russi[2] succinctly states, "This unsatisfactory situation explains why numerous topics remain controversial even among experts in the field." It follows that in the subsequent discussion there are numerous conundrums that cannot be resolved by reference to definitive data.

DIVING APPLICATIONS AND ACTIVITIES

Diving may be divided into "recreational" or "occupational" categories. Recreational divers are a diverse group spanning a wide age range, some with significant medical problems. In contrast, occupational divers are a more homogeneous group, and less commonly are found to have diseases of relevance to diving safety. They are usually young men between the ages of 20 and 45 years who are fit and healthy.

Recreational diving is an unpaid, "for-pleasure" activity; however, the sobriquet "recreational" also embraces focused enthusiasts including photographers, cave divers, and wreck divers who may use gas mixtures, devices such as rebreathers, and advanced diving techniques. These divers often refer to themselves as "technical divers." Occupational diving is paid underwater work and includes those working on projects such as underwater building, drilling, dredging, and ship husbandry, as well as military, police, scientific, and public safety divers. Recreational diving instructors have long argued that they are not truly occupational divers, but there appears to be little basis in logic for such an argument. They are paid, and they assume responsibility for the safety of others during the course of their work. The hyperbaric physician performing diving medical examinations could expect to see members of all of these groups.

Whether occupational or recreational, diving is a physical activity that occurs in a potentially hostile environment, and that requires application of knowledge and skills for safe outcomes. It follows that awareness of the cognitive, psychological, physical, and physiologic requirements of diving activity is central to effective evaluation of candidates. For many hyperbaric physicians, this awareness comes from participation in diving themselves, but for guidance of the nondiving hyperbaric physician, we propose a generic suite of capabilities that reflects a "functional analysis" of diving.

Divers should be capable of performing the following actions:

- Acquiring and applying a relevant diving theory knowledge base
- Working as a team, and adhering to pre-agreed systems and a dive plan
- Tolerating the psychological stress of total submergence in water well beyond "standing depth"
- Lifting and carrying individual items of diving equipment on land
- Standing from sitting and walking 30 m (without fins) in standard scuba equipment

- Ascending a 1.5-m vertical ladder from the water wearing standard scuba equipment
- Swimming underwater at 0.5 knot for 30 minutes wearing standard scuba equipment adjusted for neutral buoyancy
- Swimming underwater at 1.2 knots (or making slow progress against a 1-knot current) for 5 minutes
- Insufflating the middle ears via the eustachian tubes
- Maintaining a protected airway with a scuba mouthpiece in place when totally immersed
- Seeing both near and far objects to allow reading of gauges and recognition of entry and exit points. Corrected visual acuity of at least 6/12 is recommended

These parameters are somewhat arbitrary, and no consensus has been published on a functional analysis for diving. The choice of a 0.5-knot swim relates to Bove's observation[3] that a "typical dive by an average recreational diver" results in energy expenditure around 3 mets, which represents an underwater swim of approximately 0.5 knot with scuba equipment.[4] Similarly, Bove[3] suggests that there is a realistic expectation of the need for a 12-met output for short periods under adverse conditions. This corresponds with an underwater swim at approximately 1.2 knots. A candidate who may fail to meet one or more of these performance requirements is not necessarily unsuitable for all diving. For example, candidates with disabilities who would be unable to meet a number of these performance requirements have learned to dive. However, their risk profile is different, and they cannot be "cleared" for unrestricted diving in the usual sense. The circumstances of their diving must be tailored to their disability.[5]

PHILOSOPHY OF MEDICAL CLEARANCE FOR DIVING

Diving medical assessments may be predicated on either a proscriptive model or a risk assessment model. In the former, the physician uses history, examination, and possibly laboratory investigations to identify potentially problematic diagnoses, consults a list of "contraindications to diving," and disallows diving by a candidate whose problem appears on such a list. A definitive statement is issued (usually expressed in terms such as "fit" or "unfit" for diving) that determines whether a candidate will be permitted to undertake dive training. One of the attractions of this approach is that the casting of the medical examiner as a "policeman" removes the need to communicate risk accurately, but this may result in unintended problems. For example, aggrieved candidates may seek alternative opinions and withhold health information without understanding the risk to which they are exposing themselves.[6] The adverse consequences of this phenomenon are also seen in other sports.[7]

A 2003 South Pacific Underwater Medicine Society workshop[8] identified several other problems with the proscriptive approach. These include the difficulty in providing sufficient numbers of appropriately trained physicians, the time-consuming and expensive nature of the compulsory consultations, and the potential for bias toward rendering a favorable decision when a candidate is required to pay for the assessment.[9] In addition, an accurate pronouncement of unequivocal "fitness" to dive requires a functional assessment that may exceed the capabilities of an office medical consultation.

The alternative to this rather unsatisfactory situation is a system with a discretionary approach based on risk assessment. In practice, such discretion usually extends to a judgment about who receives a formal dive medical consultation at all (see Administrative Models for Medical Clearance for Diving section later in this chapter) (Fig. 5.1). Where a medical consultation is required, usually because a screening questionnaire revealed a potential problem, the practitioner is expected to provide a detailed risk assessment for each individual. Medical conditions such as asthma no longer automatically exclude the candidate but do trigger an assessment of the potential risk they represent. The diver, in turn, assumes and acknowledges the role of an informed risk acceptor. Clearance determinations made under a discretionary system need no longer be couched in the form of dichotomous statements ("fit for diving" vs. "not fit for diving"). For example, whereas the South Pacific Underwater Medicine Society diving medical examination protocol required such a statement from the physician until 1999, the current declaration uses the more guarded *"I can find no conditions incompatible with SCUBA diving,"* accompanied, if necessary, by comments appended to the declaration.

The "risk assessment" approach is not without problems and limitations. These include difficulties in calculating and communicating risk, defining a level of risk that is acceptable, and protecting the interests of risk acceptors other than the candidate (such as spouses, dive instructors, and future dive partners). It is mainly for the latter reason that not all medical concerns can be set aside simply because the candidate is prepared to accept the risk. A small number of absolute contraindications to diving remain, and many potential scenarios exist where the medical examiner would consider the risk too great to allow the candidate to proceed. Risk perception is personal and variable.[10] Therefore, explanations should be objective and unambiguous. Where relevant, written guidelines should be provided, and the individual should accept responsibility for following these guidelines.

ADMINISTRATIVE MODELS FOR MEDICAL CLEARANCE FOR DIVING

Significant regional differences exist in the administrative approach to screening of prospective divers, particularly recreational divers. It is beyond the scope of this chapter to detail these differences, but a general description is provided and summarized in Figure 5.1.

Recreational Divers

The most prevalent model for medical clearance of recreational divers involves the candidate completing a questionnaire designed to screen for medical or psychological problems of potential significance in diving. If there are no positive responses, the candidate can proceed to training with no formal medical evaluation. If there are any positive responses, the candidate must complete a formal medical evaluation. The most widely used screening questionnaire (Fig. 5.2) was developed by the Recreational Scuba Training Council, a cooperative body of recreational diver training agencies, in conjunction with the Diving Committee of the Undersea and Hyperbaric Medicine Society.[11] In contrast, in the Commonwealth nations, there has been a tradition of requiring medical examinations of all recreational diving candidates.

Debate has raged for some years over which of the above systems is most appropriate; a debate that has been devoid of reference to relevant data until relatively recently. During the 1990s, the Scottish Sub-Aqua Club operated the traditional Commonwealth system. Glen and colleagues[12] evaluated 2962 medical forms completed by examining physicians and compared them with responses on questionnaires from the diver candidates. They report that no unexpected abnormalities were found, and that conditions preventing the subjects from diving were detected by the questionnaire. In response, the Scottish Sub-Aqua Club adopted the "American model" of requiring only candidates with a positive questionnaire to be examined, albeit by a doctor with diving medicine training. An audit of the consequent outcomes over 3 years[13] found that no incidents occurred because of undetected preexisting medical conditions, and concluded that the questionnaire system appeared effective. Traditionalists express concern that questionnaires might be answered dishonestly, and some unsuitable candidates might "pass" the questionnaire process. Although this is almost certainly correct, it does not automatically follow that compulsory medical consultations would be any more effective in identifying significant medical problems in an evasive candidate.

There has been a conspicuous absence of systems for ongoing health surveillance of

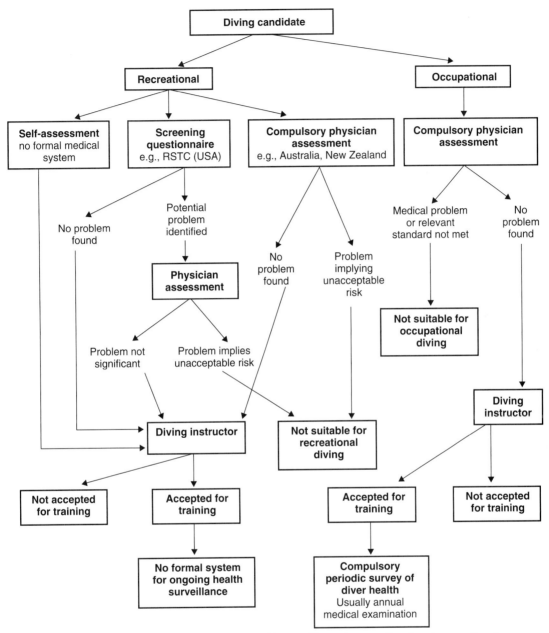

Figure 5.1 Systems for assessment and health surveillance in recreational and occupational divers. RSTC, Recreational Scuba Training Council.

recreational divers. Most training organizations require that diver health is resurveyed (usually by questionnaire) before participation in continuing education courses, and some of the more traditional recreational diving organizations do promote periodic review.[12] Formal requirements for periodic evaluations are rarely imposed.

Occupational Divers

Systems for evaluation and surveillance of occupational divers are driven largely by duty of care responsibilities that arise from health and safety in employment legislation.[6] Typically, the occupational diving candidate must have a consultation with a physician trained

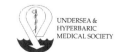

UNDERSEA &
HYPERBARIC
MEDICAL SOCIETY

MEDICAL STATEMENT
Participant Record (Confidential Information)

Please read carefully before signing.

This is a statement in which you are informed of some potential risks involved in scuba diving and of the conduct required of you during the scuba training program. Your signature on this statement is required for you to participate in the scuba training program offered

by_____and
　　　　　　　　　　　　　　Instructor

_____located in the
　　　　　　　　　　Facility

city of_____, state/province of _____.

　　　Read this statement prior to signing it. You must complete this Medical Statement, which includes the medical questionnaire section, to enroll in the scuba training program. If you are a minor, you must have this Statement signed by a parent or guardian.
　　　Diving is an exciting and demanding activity. When performed correctly, applying correct techniques, it is relatively safe. When

established safety procedures are not followed, however, there are increased risks.
　　　To scuba dive safely, you should not be extremely overweight or out of condition. Diving can be strenuous under certain conditions. Your respiratory and circulatory systems must be in good health. All body air spaces must be normal and healthy. A person with coronary disease, a current cold or congestion, epilepsy, a severe medical problem or who is under the influence of alcohol or drugs should not dive. If you have asthma, heart disease, other chronic medical conditions or you are taking medications on a regular basis, you should consult your doctor and the instructor before participating in this program, and on a regular basis thereafter upon completion. You will also learn from the instructor the important safety rules regarding breathing and equalization while scuba diving. Improper use of scuba equipment can result in serious injury. You must be thoroughly instructed in its use under direct supervision of a qualified instructor to use it safely.
　　　If you have any additional questions regarding this Medical Statement or the Medical Questionnaire section, review them with your instructor before signing.

Divers Medical Questionnaire
To the Participant:

The purpose of this Medical Questionnaire is to find out if you should be examined by your doctor before participating in recreational diver training. A positive response to a question does not necessarily disqualify you from diving. A positive response means that there is a preexisting condition that may affect your safety while diving and you must seek the advice of your physician prior to engaging in dive activities.

_____ Could you be pregnant, or are you attempting to become pregnant?

_____ Are you presently taking prescription medications? (with the exception of birth control or anti-malarial)

_____ Are you over 45 years of age and can answer YES to one or more of the following?
  * currently smoke a pipe, cigars or cigarettes
  * have a high cholesterol level
  * have a family history of heart attack or stroke
  * are currently receiving medical care
  * high blood pressure
  * diabetes mellitus, even if controlled by diet alone

Have you ever had or do you currently have...

_____ Asthma, or wheezing with breathing, or wheezing with exercise?

_____ Frequent or severe attacks of hayfever or allergy?

_____ Frequent colds, sinusitis or bronchitis?

_____ Any form of lung disease?

_____ Pneumothorax (collapsed lung)?

_____ Other chest disease or chest surgery?

_____ Behavioral health, mental or psychological problems (Panic attack, fear of closed or open spaces)?

_____ Epilepsy, seizures, convulsions or take medications to prevent them?

_____ Recurring complicated migraine headaches or take medications to prevent them?

_____ Blackouts or fainting (full/partial loss of consciousness)?

_____ Frequent or severe suffering from motion sickness (seasick, carsick, etc.)?

Please answer the following questions on your past or present medical history with a YES or NO. If you are not sure, answer YES. If any of these items apply to you, we must request that you consult with a physician prior to participating in scuba diving. Your instructor will supply you with an RSTC Medical Statement and Guidelines for Recreational Scuba Diver's Physical Examination to take to your physician.

_____ Dysentery or dehydration requiring medical intervention?

_____ Any dive accidents or decompression sickness?

_____ Inability to perform moderate exercise (example: walk 1.6 km/one mile within 12 mins.)?

_____ Head injury with loss of consciousness in the past five years?

_____ Recurrent back problems?

_____ Back or spinal surgery?

_____ Diabetes?

_____ Back, arm or leg problems following surgery, injury or fracture?

_____ High blood pressure or take medicine to control blood pressure?

_____ Heart disease?

_____ Heart attack?

_____ Angina, heart surgery or blood vessel surgery?

_____ Sinus surgery?

_____ Ear disease or surgery, hearing loss or problems with balance?

_____ Recurrent ear problems?

_____ Bleeding or other blood disorders?

_____ Hernia?

_____ Ulcers or ulcer surgery ?

_____ A colostomy or ileostomy?

_____ Recreational drug use or treatment for, or alcoholism in the past five years?

The information I have provided about my medical history is accurate to the best of my knowledge. *I agree to accept responsibility for omissions regarding my failure to disclose any existing or past health condition.*

_____ _____ _____ _____
　　　　Signature　　　　　　　　　　Date　　　　　Signature of Parent or Guardian　　　　　Date

PRODUCT NO. 10063 (Rev. 9/01) Ver. 2.0

© Recreational Scuba Training Council, Inc. 1989, 1990, 1998, 2001

Figure 5.2 Recreational Scuba Training Council (RSTC) screening questionnaire. *(Reprinted with the express permission of the Recreational Scuba Training Council [RSTC]. ©Recreational Scuba Training Council, all rights reserved.)*

in diving medical examination who will determine the candidate's suitability. Unilateral determinations by the examining physician may be flawed because doctors may not appreciate that their interaction is as a "commissioned agent of a third party" (usually the diver's employer) and does not constitute a "doctor–patient relationship."[6] Inappropriate advocacy behavior may result, especially because the diver is often paying a substantial fee for the service. The problem can be circumvented to some extent by a system of central review and arbitration, such as in New Zealand. Such systems have been advocated for similar reasons in professional sporting situations in the United States.[14]

The health of occupational divers is also surveyed annually, most commonly in the form of a repeat consultation and examination. As Gorman[6] has pointed out, there is little logic to either this frequency or the associated repetition of investigations such as spirometry that are unlikely to have changed in the course of a year. One alternative is currently undergoing trials in New Zealand, where comprehensive examinations take place on entry to the industry and then every 5 years, with annual completion of a health status questionnaire. The questionnaire responses are reviewed by a central arbitrator who either issues an ongoing clearance to dive or directs that a more comprehensive review take place.

WHO SHOULD PERFORM CLEARANCE TO DIVE ASSESSMENTS?

Pleas for the medical assessment of diving candidates by appropriately trained doctors have been made for decades.[15,16] Recreational training organizations attempt to circumvent the obvious difficulties that might be encountered by doctors with no diving medicine training by providing information and guidelines on the medical forms themselves,[11] but such guidelines are subject to variable interpretation.[17] There is no simple solution to this conundrum, but to summarize, we strongly endorse the view that diving clearance evaluations requiring medical input *should* be conducted by doctors with training in diving medicine. The diving instructor also has an important role in evaluating suitability for diving, particularly with regard to functional issues that cannot be easily assessed in a physician's office. Regardless of any prior opinion from a physician, he or she is entitled to refuse to train a seemingly unsuitable candidate.[18]

DIVING CLEARANCE CONSULTATION

History and Systems Review

The history should elicit known medical problems with emphasis on identifying conditions that may be exacerbated by diving, make a diving medical problem more likely, or compromise physical performance or safety underwater. This analytic approach contrasts with simply referring to lists of "contraindications" or "relative contraindications" to diving, which fails to allow for degrees of severity of a problem and other potentially mitigating issues.

It is usual practice to elicit information by administration of a questionnaire. The most common questionnaire in use is contained in the Recreational Scuba Training Council Medical Statement for recreational diving (see Fig. 5.2). The physician should supplement this information with his or her own questions because important issues are often overlooked. For example, although the Recreational Scuba Training Council questionnaire asks about "recurrent ear problems," it does not specifically address difficulty with insufflation of the middle ears via the eustachian tubes, which might be indicated by recurrent problems during flight. Also, an occupational history and a history of previous diving (and any associated problems) or other hobbies is often omitted from these questionnaires. Such issues may influence diving clearance determinations or the nature of any risk versus benefit discussion.

Examination

Examination of the diving candidate follows usual medical practice, but some important points are worthy of emphasis. It is important to ensure that the candidate is capable of insufflating both middle ears via the eustachian tubes. This may be achieved with standard techniques, typically otoscopic visualization of tympanic membrane movement during a Valsalva maneuver, or by obtaining objective evidence of middle-ear insufflation using "dynamic tympanometry" during Valsalva maneuver.[19] Indeed, both observation of the tympanic membrane during Valsalva and dynamic tympanometry were predictive of barotrauma in patients undergoing hyperbaric oxygen therapy.[19] Uzun and coworkers[20] found the "nine-step inflation/deflation test"[21] was a superior predictor of barotrauma than the less complicated iteration of dynamic tympanometry using Valsalva maneuver described by Lehm and Bennett.[19] This prompted Sim and Youngs[22] to suggest that "the Valsalva maneuver cannot be recommended for the evaluation of fitness to dive," but this is almost certainly an overinterpretation of the limited data that Uzun and coworkers[20] presented. Whatever method is adopted, it is notable that successful insufflation of the middle ear in the physician's office does not always predict a similar ability during a dive.[23]

The neurologic examination follows normal practice, and it is particularly important that any abnormalities are quantitatively documented should the candidate ever need treatment for neurologic decompression sickness (DCS). The sharpened Romberg test has been proposed as a sensitive marker of dysfunction in neurologic DCS,[24,25] and consideration should be given to performing four repetitions of this test and recording the best attempt as the baseline score. Lee[25] provides a detailed description of the test.

Investigations

The utility of routine investigations in diving clearance consultations is controversial. Edmonds[15] deems it "extraordinary" that more than half of a group of surveyed physicians performing recreational diving medicals did not routinely order a pure-tone audiogram, chest radiograph (CXR), or spirometry. Yet, in many countries, the regional experts accept that recreational diving candidates do not routinely require a medical consultation at all, let alone any investigations. A lack of hard data limits arguments.

The audiogram is arguably the most justifiable of investigations because there is a risk for otic barotrauma and inner-ear DCS during diving. In addition, gradual deterioration in hearing thresholds have been associated with long-term diving,[26] although this is most likely a result of noise exposure rather than diving per se.[27,28] A baseline audiogram would aid with evaluations of these problems and facilitate discussion of risks and benefits associated with diving in a candidate found to have pre-existing hearing loss.

The performance of spirometry is based on the notion that abnormal indices may predict risk for pulmonary barotrauma (PBT). It has proved difficult, however, to demonstrate that an obstructive spirometric picture (a low forced expiratory volume in 1 second/forced vital capacity [FEV_1/FVC] ratio) indicates a risk for air trapping and PBT. When Benton and colleagues[29] reviewed the preaccident spirometry from 10 cases of PBT arising from 115,090 submarine escape training ascents, they found that only an FVC less than the predicted value for age and height was significantly associated with increased risk, not the FEV_1/FVC ratio. This association was judged as insufficiently specific to be useful as an exclusion criterion for submarine escape training.

Similar concerns about specificity arose over work by Tetzlaff and colleagues,[30] who demonstrated that divers who had suffered PBT had similar FEV_1/FVC ratios but significantly lower flows at 50% and 25% of FVC (maximal expiratory flow at 50% [MEF_{50}] and MEF_{25}, respectively) when compared with divers who had suffered DCS without PBT. They recommended that an assessment of mid and late expiratory flow rates be included in screening of diving candidates, and that the MEF_{50} and MEF_{25} "should at least reach 80% of the predicted values." Neuman and Clausen[31] were critical of this proposal, however, because intersubject and intrasubject variability impose large standard deviations on the distribution of results, and those with measurements less than 80% of predicted will constitute 25% of candidates.

This discussion must take account of the infrequent occurrence of PBT and arterial gas embolism (AGE), which are estimated to occur in approximately 1 in 20,000 to 35,000 dives in military divers.[32] Therefore, it could be argued that spirometry is a nonspecific screen for risk for a rare event, and its routine use cannot be justified. Alternatively, a conservative approach based around a nonspecific test may be justified on the basis that an AGE is potentially catastrophic. Yildiz and coworkers[33] have articulated their support of a conservative policy for selection of Turkish submarine escape trainees. They screen all candidates using spirometry and exclude those whose FVC, FEV_1, or FEV_1/FVC ratio falls below 80% of predicted. In part, they attribute their record of 41,183 training ascents without PBT to this policy; though given the low prevalence of PBT in any diving population, the claim is difficult to evaluate. Denison[34] sensibly summed up the issue by suggesting that abnormalities in spirometric indices should trigger closer scrutiny of the candidate, especially with regard to exercise capacity, and not be interpreted by pass/fail thresholds.

The routine performance of a CXR in diving clearance consultations is based mainly around the notion that it can detect pulmonary abnormalities that predispose to PBT.[35] There can be little doubt that this is possible. For example, a case of PBT and AGE in a diver was presumed related to a preexisting emphysematous bulla detectable by plain CXR.[36] Similar unpublished cases are known from the authors' own practice. Despite this, much debate surrounds the imposition of routine CXRs. Concern exists over radiation exposure, the fact that PBT is rare, and the poor sensitivity and negative predictive value of CXR because adverse events can readily occur even when a CXR is normal.[37] Nevertheless, as with spirometry, some authors consider routine CXR justified[38] because the consequences of PBT are so serious. Computed tomography (CT) scanning is more sensitive. Indeed, CT scanning was used to detect small lung cysts that were undetectable using CXR in divers who had suffered PBT,[30,39] prompting the suggestion that a single CT scan may be appropriate on entry to occupational diving.[39] However, there is uncertainty over the relation between these lesions and PBT, and concern about the low specificity of the technique given that modern scanners detect such lesions in many "normal" subjects.[37]

Despite occasional case reports of diving deaths potentially linked to disorders such as long QT syndrome,[40,41] an electrocardiogram (ECG) is rarely advocated as routine for recreational diving evaluations. Although an ECG may reveal evidence of myocardial ischemia, structural abnormality, or an electrophysiologic or rhythm disturbance, it will not identify inducible ischemia or intermittent dysrhythmias. Moreover, the extent to which an ECG would increase the sensitivity of an accurate history in relation to most of these problems is debatable. Elliott[42] observes that there are no published data that demonstrate the ECG to be of value in the evaluation of diver fitness, and Wilmshurst[43] is also skeptical about its utility in the absence of relevant history. Despite these concerns, a routine ECG is still required by many occupational diving standards.

Routine measurement of hemoglobin (Hb), some other hematologic indices, cholesterol, and a screen for sickle cell trait are required for medical clearance of occupational divers in many countries but are rarely performed for recreational divers. A position article by Risberg[44] recommends measurement of Hb, erythrocyte sedimentation rate, sickle cell index, cholesterol, and blood type at the initial clearance consultation with repeated annual measures of Hb and erythrocyte sedimentation rate. Debate over the necessity and utility of these investigations resulted in consensus that blood typing and sickle cell index were unnecessary.[45] The latter was based on an assumption that patients with full sickle cell disease would be well aware of their diagnosis and unlikely to present for a diving clearance, and that there was no reason to prevent a candidate with sickle cell trait from diving. Controversy remains over Hb, erythrocyte sedimentation rate, and cholesterol screenings.

Radiographs of the shoulders, hips, and knees have been advocated for pre-employment and periodic follow-up of occupational divers because of the incidence of dysbaric osteonecrosis in these divers and in tunnel workers.[46] Detection of new juxta-articular lesions is considered to preclude further occupational diving to try to reduce the risk for subsequent joint collapse.[47] Occupational divers were originally singled out for actuarial reasons[48] and because the risk for dysbaric osteonecrosis appeared to be related to decompression diving exposures beyond 30 m that are typical of occupational activity. Radiographic screening is not required for recreational divers, and dysbaric osteonecrosis has proved to be rare in this group,[49] though this may change with the increase in deep recreational "technical" diving.

EVALUATION OF MEDICAL CONDITIONS IN RELATION TO DIVING

Many medical conditions may pose limitations and alter risk for diving. We limit this discussion to issues that arise commonly. Discussion of a wider range of medical conditions and diving can be found in dedicated books (e.g., Parker[50]).

A Generic Approach

The implications of many medical conditions in diving can be derived from a "first principles" approach. Concerns that might warrant further research or referral to a diving medicine specialist can be identified using a simple

template that addresses the following three questions[51]:

1. Could the condition predispose to a diving illness?
2. Could the condition be provoked by diving?
3. Could the condition compromise the diver's safety or performance underwater?

If the answer to any of these questions is "yes" or "don't know," then the issue deserves review in more depth; if definitively "yes," then a careful risk versus benefit analysis should be made in relation to diving.

Age Issues: Children and Diving

Children commonly participate in recreational diving; the Professional Association of Diving Instructors offers several programs for children as young as age 8. Progressive lowering of threshold ages for participation in diving activities has generated concerns about safety.[52] In this regard, there are some accident reports[53] and some reassuring anecdotes,[54] but no definitive data.[55] In one of the few relevant studies, Vandenhoven and others[56] followed 205 children involved in 2216 open-water dives over an 8-year period. Interestingly, four children (2%) suffered tympanic membrane perforations during pool training, but no accidents occurred during the open-water dives. Given the low accident rate in adult recreational dives, however, it is difficult to draw conclusions from these data. In the absence of data, the debate over the safety of diving by children usually defaults to the theoretical concerns that arise from the physical, physiologic, pathophysiologic, and psychological differences between adults and children, which are summarized by Mitchell.[54] With all issues considered, we can see no reason to prevent children from participating in the diving activities deemed appropriate for their age group by the diving training agencies. However, parents should clearly be made aware of the small risks involved.

Age Issues: Older Divers

Physiologic and pathologic changes associated with aging may alter risks of diving. A review of 877 diving fatalities attributed 130 (14%) to cardiovascular disease, with a sharply increased stratified risk for those older than 50 years.[57]

Evidence also is available that increased age may be associated with a greater risk for DCS. Older age was associated with greater venous bubble numbers after hypobaric decompression,[58] experimental open-water dives,[59] and uncontrolled open-water dives.[60] In addition, a retrospective review of data from altitude (flight) exposures showed a strong trend to increased risk for clinical DCS in participants older than 42 years.[61] Bradley[62] cites a number of references to historical data that suggest greater risk for DCS for older working divers and caisson workers. Despite this, establishing advanced age as a risk factor for clinical DCS in modern recreational divers has proved difficult. A recent retrospective cohort study failed to find an association between risk for DCS and age.[63] Some occupational groups such as the military impose conservative age limits on divers. However, in recreational diving, older age is best seen as a trigger for careful assessment with a high index of suspicion for ischemic heart disease, periodic review, and more detailed counseling of the candidate about risk. Older age is not in itself a reason to prescribe against recreational diving.

Cardiovascular Problems

Ischemic Heart Disease

Ischemic heart disease has consistently been the most common medical condition associated with diving fatalities.[64] The most troublesome problem is the approach to assessment of nonsymptomatic diving candidates with recognized risk factors[65] who may suffer "silent" myocardial ischemia. It has been suggested that candidates older than 45 years with risk factors undergo a cardiac stress test,[57] and Bove[66] recommends that any candidate older than 50 to 55 years should have a stress test regardless of the individual's risk factor history. Another problem is the diving candidate or established diver presenting for clearance to dive after intervention for coronary artery disease. Such candidates are directed to wait at least 6 months after their intervention and require a negative stress test before any consideration is given to diving.[66] The medication profile should also be reviewed. Potent antiplatelet agents, such as clopidogrel and ticlopidine, and anticoagulants are not recommended in diving. Beta-blockers have been anecdotally associated with immersion pulmonary edema[67] and may reduce exercise tolerance. However, they should not be stopped to ameliorate risk in diving if considered important for myocardial protection.

Valvular Heart Disease

Significant valvular heart disease may predispose to myocardial ischemia, pulmonary edema, arrhythmias, syncopal events, and limitation of exercise tolerance. On the rare occasions that candidates with symptomatic valvular heart disease present for diving clearance examinations, they should be strongly advised not to dive because there is potential for sudden death or incapacitation in the water and drowning.

Systolic murmurs that do not radiate in young candidates (teenage years and third decade of life) with an excellent history of exercise tolerance may be "innocent."[68] Nevertheless, because echocardiography provides a relatively cheap and noninvasive means of investigating cardiac structure and function, it is appropriate to investigate murmurs that have not been diagnosed previously. Most importantly, the murmur of hypertrophic cardiomyopathy may be easily misinterpreted as an innocent murmur because both are outflow tract systolic murmurs.

The two most common "innocent" murmurs are mitral valve prolapse and a bicuspid aortic valve, which affect 10% to 12% and 1% of the population, respectively.[66,68] Consensus among diving cardiologists is that the mild asymptomatic forms of both lesions do not contraindicate diving.[43,66] In contrast, any stenosis or regurgitation beyond trivial levels in either aortic or mitral valves justifies withholding of clearance to dive.

Prosthetic heart valves are not considered an absolute contraindication to diving[66] provided the functional history is good and the patient is healthy in all other respects. However, patients with mechanical valves take potent anticoagulants, and in theory, these may exacerbate bleeding in barotrauma and possibly some forms of spinal DCS in which white matter hemorrhage has been reported.[69]

Hypertension

Hypertension is a risk factor for coronary artery disease,[65] and it is possible that both hypertension[70] and its treatment with beta-blocker[67] may imply increased risk for immersion-induced pulmonary edema. Thus, we consider that the correct response to the discovery of undiagnosed or uncontrolled hypertension in a diving candidate is to refer them back to their primary care practitioner for review and initiation of antihypertensive treatment. Diving may be considered once the blood pressure is controlled. Bove[66] suggests a systolic pressure of greater than 150 mm Hg and a diastolic pressure of greater than 95 mm Hg as a suitable definition of hypertension in divers.

Patent Foramen Ovale

A patent foramen ovale (PFO) is present in 20% to 34% (depending on age) of "normal" humans at autopsy.[71] In life, these lesions are usually sought using transesophageal echocardiography (TEE) or transthoracic echocardiography during administration of bubble contrast through a peripheral vein. Shunting of bubbles from the right to left atrium is then provoked using strategies such as the Valsalva maneuver. TEE is frequently referred to as the more sensitive of the two echocardiographic techniques.[72] Not surprisingly, when these techniques were used in healthy divers (who had never suffered DCS), 31% were found to have a PFO.[73]

An association between PFO and nondiving disorders involving venous-to-arterial shunting of emboli has been known for some time. In theory, venous bubbles that are commonly formed after dives[60] and that are normally filtered by the pulmonary capillary bed[74] could also be introduced to the arterial circulation through a PFO. Using transthoracic echocardiography and bubble contrast, Moon and coworkers[75] found that 37% of 30 divers with a history of DCS had a PFO, a proportion not markedly greater than found in the general population. However, when they stratified their divers according to severity, they found that 61% of 18 divers with serious neurologic DCS had a PFO. Similarly, Wilmshurst and colleagues[76] found that 41% of 61 divers with a history of DCS had a PFO, compared with 66% of 29 divers with rapid-onset neurologic DCS. These data indicated that patients with a PFO were over-represented among victims of serious or rapid-onset neurologic DCS.

Subsequent studies have also linked PFO with neurologic and other forms of DCS. Using TEE and bubble contrast, Germonpre and coworkers[77] found a PFO that shunted right to left spontaneously or could be readily provoked into shunting in 51% of 37 divers who had suffered neurologic DCS and in 70% of a subgroup whose symptoms were mainly cerebral. This contrasted with 25% and 15%, respectively, of matched diver controls who had never suffered DCS. Using TEE and bubble contrast, Wilmshurst and Bryson[78] found medium-to-large PFOs (based on numbers of bubbles observed to shunt) in 52% of 100 divers with neurologic DCS and 12% of control divers who had not suffered DCS. Spinal DCS occurred in a significantly greater proportion of divers with a medium-to-large shunt than those without. In a subsequent study using similar methods, Wilmshurst and coworkers[79] showed that 49% of 61 divers with a history of cutaneous DCS had a spontaneous right-to-left shunt at rest compared with 5% of control divers without DCS. In another case–control study involving 101 divers with a history of DCS and 101 control divers with no such history, Cantais and others[80] showed that a major right-to-left shunt was present in 12% of control subjects versus 71% of vestibulocochlear cases, 62% of cerebral cases, 32% of spinal cases, and 15% of musculoskeletal cases. Shunting was detected using transcranial arterial Doppler imaging after injection of bubble contrast into a peripheral vein and, therefore, was not definitively linked to a PFO. A "major" shunt was indicated by detection of arterial bubbles above a threshold number in the absence of any provocation maneuvers. This over-representation of right-to-left shunt among divers with vestibulocochlear DCS was supported by a case series in which all nine victims were found to have a right-to-left shunt.[81] Finally, Torti and colleagues[82] surveyed the health history and performed TEE on 230 experienced divers. They reported an incidence of DCS symptoms clearly related to spinal or cerebral involvement of 5 per 10,000 dives in divers with a medium-to-large PFO versus 1 per 10,000 dives in divers with a small PFO or no PFO. The "size" of PFO was gauged from numbers of shunted bubbles.

Another line of research related to PFO and diving arose around the finding of hyperintense cerebral white matter lesions in divers who underwent magnetic resonance imaging (MRI) scans.[83] Subsequently, Knauth and co-workers[84] subjected 87 experienced divers to cerebral MRI scans and bubble contrast transcranial Doppler imaging to detect any right-to-left shunt. Eleven of the 87 subjects had hyperintense white matter lesions, and only subjects with a significant shunt exhibited multiple lesions. Schwerzmann and colleagues[85] performed a similar study that included experienced divers ($n = 52$) and a control group of nondivers ($n = 52$). All subjects underwent cerebral MRI scans and a TEE to detect a PFO. The authors found 1.23 and 0.64 cerebral white matter lesions per diver and 0.22 and 0.12 lesion per nondiver with and without PFO, respectively. This study suggests that both diving and a PFO are cumulative risk factors for these lesions, but it remains unestablished what these lesions represent and whether they have any functional significance.

In summary, a PFO is associated with cerebral, spinal, vestibulocochlear, and cutaneous DCS, and with the finding of hyperintense cerebral white matter lesions in both divers and nondivers on MRI scans. The size of the shunt facilitated by the PFO has consistently been found to be significant, with large and spontaneous shunts being important, and small shunts being unimportant. This latter point is consistent with the greater risk for paradoxical embolic events in other contexts as PFO size increases.[86] Taken at face value, these studies suggest a PFO is a significant risk factor for serious DCS, and by logical extension, they support a case for screening of prospective divers for PFO after an episode of neurologic or cutaneous DCS, or even before entry to the sport or vocation. Many divers have enthusiastically embraced this concept. When participants on Internet diving discussion forums report an episode of DCS, a chorus of advice to check for a PFO inevitably follows. At least one prominent "technical diving" group insists on all participants being screened before participation in diving. Prediving screening also has its medical advocates.[87] Not surprisingly, percutaneous transcatheter PFO repairs for the purposes of facilitating diving are becoming more common,[88] particularly in enthusiastic divers who have suffered DCS and subsequently had a PFO detected.

In the face of this trend toward screening and invasive PFO repair procedures, others have urged caution in interpreting the hazards associated with a PFO in diving. Moon and Bove[89] correctly point out that although PFO is common, serious DCS of the type associated with PFO remains rare. Arguably the best contemporary attempt at estimating the incidence of DCS across its entire range of severity in recreational divers found 1 case per 10,000 dives.[90] Less than half of these cases could be expected to exhibit objective neurologic signs[91] (and therefore be suffering from the DCS variants associated with PFO). It follows that the incidence of those forms of DCS made more likely by a PFO is less than 1 in 20,000 dives in recreational diving. As Moon and Bove[89] point out, this "disconnection" between a prevalent risk factor and a rare disease is amplified when it is considered that the formation of venous bubbles, the right-to-left shunting of which is the only plausible mechanism of risk from a PFO,[92] is common in recreational diving.[60] It appears clear that, although a PFO is a risk factor for neurological DCS, there are other factors, some of which are unclear, that must also combine to produce problems. Estimates of the relative risk of neurologic DCS implied by the presence of a PFO vary from 2.5[93] to 5.[82] Based on the incidence of neurologic DCS proposed earlier, this would increase the absolute risk in recreational diving to somewhere between 1 in 4000 and 1 in 8000 dives.

Although this risk remains small, population statistics and the concepts of relative and absolute risk often do not resonate deeply with the individual diver anxious about his or her own risk for DCS. Therefore, the diving physician will often be asked for referral for a TEE or other screening test. We consider such referrals to be justified after an episode of neurologic, vestibulocochlear, or cutaneous DCS occurring after relatively nonprovocative diving, and not unreasonable in the context of recurrent episodes of these DCS variants regardless of whether the diving was provocative. We do not consider referral appropriate after an episode of musculoskeletal DCS or for the purpose of routine screening before diver training. One possible exception to the latter is the technical diver who will be performing deep decompression dives. Anecdote among diving physicians supports the notion that these divers are at greater risk for neurologic DCS. Given the nature of the diving involved, it is also plausible that they are at greater risk for development of the large venous bubble loads that, in theory, become more significant in the presence of a PFO.

Any referral for investigation for PFO should be accompanied by thorough counseling about the implications. Our own practice is to make the following points that are designed to rectify prevalent omissions and misconceptions in our candidates' reasoning around the issue:

1. Although major harm is vanishingly rare during TEE, the procedure is uncomfortable, and probe insertion is abandoned in 1% to 2% of examinations because of poor patient compliance.[94] It is also expensive.
2. A positive test, which is likely in 25% to 30% of examinations, does not mean the diver will experience DCS if the lesion is not repaired. Indeed, those lesions that shunt small numbers of bubbles and only with significant provocation probably have little bearing on the risk for DCS.
3. Notwithstanding the previous point, if the diver elects to proceed with screening, there is a significant chance that a PFO of relevant size or shunting behavior will be discovered, and he or she will then be faced with a decision about what to do about it. Options include ceasing diving, modifying diving practice, or having the PFO repaired; but if there is no intent to follow one of these paths, there is little point in having the test.
4. A negative test does not mean the diver is "resistant" to DCS, as many seem to believe.
5. The discovery of a PFO after an episode of neurologic DCS does not prove that the PFO caused the problem.
6. As a corollary to the previous point, although the repair of a significant PFO after neurologic DCS may reduce future risk, it does not guarantee that a similar DCS event will not occur again.
7. Repair of a PFO is an invasive procedure and carries significant risks.

Once a PFO has been discovered in a diving candidate or diver, some potentially difficult decisions must be made. When consulted by an untrained diving candidate with a known PFO, our response depends on the nature of the lesion. If the PFO was considered "large" or could be readily provoked into shunting, we would discourage diving on the basis that the candidate has a recognized but poorly understood risk factor for serious DCS and little emotional or financial investment in diving to date. We would discourage repair of the lesion to facilitate diving under these circumstances. If the PFO was considered "small" with minimal shunting even on provocation, we would clear the candidate for diving after counseling the individual about the negligible relevance of the lesion to risk for DCS.

Dealing with the established diver who discovers a PFO is more difficult. Our approach is dependent once again on the nature of the lesion, but also on the circumstances under which it was discovered. A diver with no history of neurologic DCS who discovers a small lesion with minimal shunting despite provocation would be cleared to return to diving after counseling about the negligible relevance of the lesion to risk for DCS. At the opposite end of the spectrum, a diver with a moderate, large, or spontaneous shunt discovered after an episode of neurologic DCS would be counseled in detail about the options mentioned in point 3 of the above list. These options include ceasing diving, modifying diving practice, or having the lesion repaired. Modification of diving practice is aimed at reducing venous bubble formation by selecting conservative dive profiles and avoiding any postdive activities that might promote right-to-left shunting (such as lifting or straining).[95] Notably, if the DCS event was particularly serious, occurred early in the diver's career, or occurred after a nonprovocative dive, we might omit the option of continuing diving with just a modification of practice because the risk implied by the previous event might be too high. If repair of the PFO were contemplated, then there must be a clear understanding that although repair procedures are frequently described as safe, they still carry significant risks.[96] Whether the benefit of a PFO repair justifies these risks will depend significantly on individual circumstances and would be difficult to determine objectively. Under some circumstances it might be the only option that would make us comfortable with endorsing continuation of diving.

Other Intracardiac Shunts

No data define the diving risks associated with intracardiac and extracardiac shunts other than PFO, and the reader is referred to discussions by expert commentators on this subject.[66] In brief, diving is not recommended in virtually all patients with an atrial septal defect, but there is minimal extra risk implied by a small, hemodynamically insignificant ventricular septal defect or patent ductus arteriosis.

Rhythm Disturbances

Any history of a cardiac rhythm disturbance that causes syncope or incapacitation should result in withholding of clearance to dive, at least until the problem is resolved.[66] The use of modern permanent pacemakers in some of these conditions may allow individuals to successfully participate in moderately strenuous activity including diving.[7,66] If diving is contemplated, the interval pacemaker checks must be up to date, and the pressure tolerance of each individual device should be checked with its manufacturer. In contrast, the use of implantable defibrillators as a "backstop" in relevant disorders such as long QT syndrome disorders is not an acceptable solution for the purposes of facilitating diving because the subject may be transiently incapacitated despite successful operation of the device.

Respiratory Problems

Asthma

Asthma is a clinical syndrome characterized by wheezing, cough, shortness of breath, and chest tightness. Inflammatory changes cause the bronchial smooth muscle to be hyperresponsive to a variety of stimuli including exercise and dry air. During an asthma attack, there is both muscular constriction of the airways and inflammatory swelling of the respiratory endothelium. The narrowed airways combined with the production of thick, dry mucus may limit airflow.

Historically, recent or currently active asthma has been considered an absolute contraindication to compressed gas diving.[97] Since the mid-1990s, this position has come under increasing scrutiny, with both the Undersea and Hyperbaric Medicine Society and the South Pacific Underwater Medicine Society devoting recent workshops to the question: Should asthmatics dive?[98,99] Both workshops identify several reasons why divers with asthma may be at greater risk:

1. Bronchial hyper-responsiveness may lead to air trapping during ascent and overpressure within the lung units involved, therefore increasing the risk for PBT and cerebral arterial gas embolism (CAGE).
2. Even in an individual with well-controlled asthma, an exacerbation may be provoked

in response to exercise, saltwater aspiration, or breathing dry, cold air. Such an exacerbation is difficult to treat while submerged and may restrict the ability of a diver to safely complete or abort the dive.

3. A diving regulator may produce a fine mist of seawater (hypertonic saline with added biomass), which may provoke broncho-constriction. This assertion has yet to be clearly demonstrated in practice.

4. Added resistance in the regulator and increased gas density at depth will increase the work of breathing, further exhausting an individual with acute bronchospasm.

5. A possibility exists that bronchodilators may provoke the passage of venous bubbles across the pulmonary capillary bed and, therefore, predispose an individual with asthma to DCS. This has been demonstrated in dogs given aminophylline[74] but has not been investigated in humans.

Despite these concerns, some evidence has been reported that individuals with asthma are represented in the diving population in a proportion comparable with the general population,[100] and it has proved difficult to show with confidence that those divers are at significantly greater risk than divers without asthma. Table 5.1 summarizes the published data on the rate of diving-related injuries in divers with versus without asthma. Farrell and Glanvill[101] were the first to attempt to address whether individuals with asthma were over-represented in dive injury statistics. They and others concluded there was no good evidence of a significantly increased risk for DCS or PBT.[102-106] Exceptions to these general conclusions were reported by Edmonds[107] and Corson and coworkers.[108] Edmonds[107] retrospectively reviewed 100 diving fatality reports and concluded that 9% were associated with asthma. He assumed that the prevalence of asthma in active divers was less than 1% and concluded that asthmatics were over-represented in these fatalities. Corson and coworkers[108] compared an estimate of the incidence of DCS and CAGE in divers with asthma to group data from unselected British divers and concluded that the odds of DCS in divers with

asthma were significantly greater than in the control divers (odds ratio, 4.16). Despite this, most authorities seem to have accepted that individuals with asthma are not significantly over-represented in either diving fatalities or diving injury statistics.[98]

Asthma treatment guidelines are under constant evolution.[109] Current guidelines for treatment are published and updated annually by the National Heart, Lung and Blood Institute and can be found online through the National Guideline Clearinghouse (www.guideline.gov).[110] The general approach to pharmacologic therapy is to step up medication until control of symptoms is achieved, as summarized in Table 5.2. Assuming that patients have been assessed and treated according to this schema, and accepting that each decision will be highly individual, it appears likely that those who have moved beyond step 2 or 3 above would be advised not to dive by many diving physicians.

A proposed schema for dealing with a diving candidate with asthma is proposed in Figure 5.3. Most diving physicians accept that candidates with an asthma history and abnormal lung function (FVC or FEV_1 ≥20% less than predicted, or FEV_1/FVC ratio <75% of predicted) on simple spirometry should be advised not to undertake compressed gas diving. It is possible that such candidates may improve their results after optimization of medication, and that retesting could then be undertaken (see Fig. 5.3). The most contentious problem is how to advise asymptomatic "active" asthmatics (wheeze or medication within 5 years) who have normal spirometry. Normal spirometry implies "normal" lung function, but the airways may remain hyper-reactive, and resistance in peripheral airways may be increased despite a normal FEV_1.[111] One logical approach to this conundrum is to further evaluate the candidate's current tendency to bronchial hyper-reactivity using a bronchial provocation test chosen to have some relevance to diving.

The role of bronchial provocation testing in the setting of the diving medical examination has been reviewed by the Thoracic Society of Australia and New Zealand,[112] and a summary of some of the available tests is given in Table 5.3.

Table 5.1 Summary of Studies Investigating the Association between Asthma and Diving Mishaps

PUBLISHED DATA	SUBJECTS	OUTCOME	CONCLUSIONS
Farrell and Glanvill, 1990[101]	104 divers with asthma (survey responders)	12,864 dives; 2 episodes of DCS; 21% dived within 12 hours of wheezing	Low incidence of DCS—BSAC policy of waiting 48 hours after wheezing is safe
Edmonds, 1991[107]	Retrospective review of 100 diving fatalities	9% associated with asthma compared with an assumed <1% prevalence rate of asthma among divers	If history of asthma in last 5 years or evidence of hyper-responsiveness, should not dive
Corson and colleagues, 1991[102]	Retrospective review of DAN accident data 1987 to 1990 (1213 cases vs. 696 control divers)	Overall prevalence rate of 4.5% for cases vs. 5.3% for control subjects OR for AGE: 1.58 (95% CI, 0.80–2.99) OR for DCS: 0.74 (95% CI, 0.43–1.24)	No statistically significant increase in risk overall Perhaps as much as double risk for AGE in current individuals with asthma—possible small increased risk for AGE
Corson and colleagues, 1992[108]	279 divers with asthma (survey responders)	56,334 dives; 11 episodes of DCS in 8 individuals; this rate was compared with an estimated risk for unselected divers	OR for DCS in asthmatics: 4.16; $P = 0.00001$
Neuman and colleagues, 1994[103]		5% prevalence of asthma among U.S. divers; 1 asthmatic fatality in 2132 deaths	Risks in individuals with inactive asthma are probably similar to individuals without asthma
Dovenbarger, 1996[104]	Retrospective review of DAN accident data 1988 to 1994	6.2% prevalence rate of asthma among divers with AGE; 4.5% prevalence rate of asthma among divers with DCS	No good evidence of overrepresentation for individuals with asthma, but denominator unknown
Koehle and colleagues, 2003[105]	Systematic review including Farrell and Glanvill, 1990[101]; Corson, 1991[102]; Corson, 1992[108]	Critical analysis of published data to 2003 to gain an overall estimate of any increased risk	Some weak evidence of an increased risk for DCS in individuals with asthma—decision to dive should be made through informed, shared assessment
Glanvill and colleagues, 2005[106]	Cohort of 100 divers with asthma and studied over 5 years (12,697 dives)	One case of DCS; unrelated to wheezing and found to have a large PFO, 12 divers reported wheezing underwater	Individuals with well-controlled asthma have low risk

AGE, arterial gas embolism; BSAC, British Sub-Aqua Club; CI, confidence interval; DAN, Divers Alert Network; DCS, decompression sickness; OR, odds ratio; PFO, patent foramen ovale.
    Data from Walker R: Are asthmatics fit to dive? Diving Hyperb Med 36:213-219, 2006.

These tests may be classified as "direct" or "indirect." Direct methods involve spirometry before and after exposure to a nebulized pharmacologic agent (typically methacholine or histamine) that directly stimulates bronchial smooth muscle receptors. These tests actually assess hyper-reactivity and are not specific for asthma.[113] Given a high enough dose, nearly all individuals will react with bronchial constric-

tion, and it is not clear there is any case for excluding an individual from diving based on these tests in isolation. We favor indirect tests that involve the performance of spirometry before and after dry-air hyperpnea, exercise, or exposure to nebulized hypertonic saline. Most authorities accept a reduction in FEV_1 of greater than 15% as a "positive response" to indirect challenges, and the same implication is derived

Table 5.2 Therapeutic Steps in Achieving Asthma Control

STEP AND THE MOST RECOMMENDED THERAPY	PATIENT TYPE	EVIDENCE LEVEL OF TREATMENT RECOMMENDATION
One: As needed reliever medication *Rapid-acting β_2 agonist*	1. Untreated patients with occasional daytime symptoms, occasional nocturnal symptoms; normal lung function between episodes 2. Exercise-induced asthma as only manifestation	(B) Some randomized evidence, but not definitive (A) Good randomized evidence
Two: Reliever plus single controller *Rapid-acting β_2 agonist plus low-dose inhaled glucocorticoid*	Symptoms more frequent than above, or not controlled with step one	(A) Good randomized evidence
Three: Reliever plus two controllers *Rapid-acting β_2 agonist plus inhaled glucocorticoid*	If symptoms not controlled at step two, consider adding LABA *or* increasing to medium-dose ICS	(A) Good randomized evidence
Four: Reliever plus two or more controllers *Rapid-acting β_2 agonist plus inhaled glucocorticoid plus third agent*	If not controlled at step three, should be referred to specialist Use medium- or high-dose ICS with LABA; may need to add a leukotriene inhibitor or long-acting theophylline	(B) Some randomized evidence, but not definitive
Five: Reliever plus additional controller options	Consider oral glucocorticoids or Anti-IgE	(D) Expert panel opinion (A) Randomized evidence

ICS, inhaled corticosteroid; LABA, long-acting β_2 agonist.
From Global Initiative for Asthma (GINA): Global strategy for asthma management and prevention. Bethesda, Md, National Heart, Lung and Blood Institute (NHLBI), 2006.

from demonstrating more than a 15% improvement with the administration of a bronchodilator. The choice of test will depend partly on local resources, but both exercise and 4.5% saline have the benefit of exposing the candidate to stimuli that may actually be encountered during scuba diving. Indeed, it is not uncommon for a prospective diver to voluntarily withdraw from dive training after having a significant response to these indirect tests; the implications are all too obvious to them. Another advantage is that treatment with inhaled corticosteroids will reduce bronchial hyper-reactivity to these challenges over several weeks, making them useful indicators of the response to therapy.[114]

It is our practice to strongly suggest that diving is inadvisable for any individual with asthma with positive results of bronchial provocation testing by an indirect method. In these situations, we suggest counseling with regard to the theoretical dangers discussed earlier and the implications of the response to the challenge. We also encourage those who

express great disappointment to seek further treatment advice from a specialist respiratory physician and to consider retesting when better control has been established according to the stepwise approach outlined in Table 5.2. We accept there are data to suggest that some individuals with asthma who would have positive bronchial hyper-reactivity testing results are successfully diving.[115] Nevertheless, we believe there may be a net advantage in identifying and treating such individuals before recommending dive training.

Although a current asthmatic with normal spirometry and a negative bronchial provocation test may be allowed to dive, this does not mean the individual should give no further thought to his or her condition. There are two relevant issues: (1) continuing control and monitoring, and (2) how long to wait after requiring reliever medication. All individuals with active asthma should be strongly encouraged to monitor their peak flow regularly. Opinions differ, but the British Sub-Aqua Club

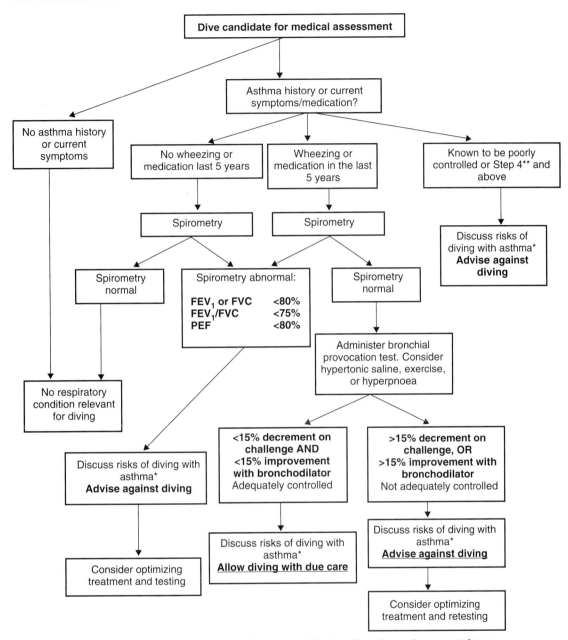

Figure 5.3 A suggested schema for dealing with individuals with asthma who present for an assessment for fitness to dive. *See text for a discussion of appropriate advice. **Step 4 refers to the incremental treatment protocol described in Table 5.3. FEV_1, forced expiratory volume in 1 second; FVC, forced vital capacity; PEF, peak expiratory flow.

guidelines suggest peak expiratory flow estimation twice daily during diving periods and recommend no diving if the peak expiratory flow rate is more than 10% less than their best value.[116] Opinions also differ on how long an individual with asthma should refrain from diving after an episode of wheezing. Glanvill and colleagues[106] examined the reported ac-

tivity of 100 divers with asthma and suggest the current British Sub-Aqua Club guideline of 48 hours appears to be sufficiently restrictive. Finally, we strongly advise divers specifically against taking a reliever medication and diving immediately, but also counsel them not to take this as a recommendation to proceed with a dive when actively wheezing!

Table 5.3   Summary of Available Indirect Methods of Bronchial Provocation Testing

PROVOCATION TEST	BRIEF DESCRIPTION
Hypertonic saline (4.5%)	Candidate inspires a wet aerosol of 4.5% saline for a stepwise increasing time with measurement at each step.
Exercise	Run outside to 80% of predicted maximum for no more than 10 minutes. Perform spirometry 5 minutes after completion of exercise.
Dry air hyperpnea	Hyperpnea of dry air containing 5% CO_2 at room temperature for 6 minutes at a ventilation equivalent to 30 times baseline FEV_1.
Mannitol	Uses a dry mannitol powder aerosol to present an osmotic challenge similar to hypertonic saline.

Readers should perform such tests only after appropriate training and accreditation.
   FEV_1, forced expiratory volume in 1 second.

Chronic Airways Limitation

The term *chronic airways limitation* encompasses emphysema and chronic obstructive airways disease. Few individuals with significant chronic airways limitation present for entry-level diving medical examinations because of limitations in exercise tolerance. In some asymptomatic candidates, chronic airways limitation will be indicated by abnormal spirometry. Such candidates should be advised that they are unlikely to cope with the physical demands of diving, and that diving is likely to involve an unacceptable risk for PBT. There is never likely to be reliable evidence that definitively validates these concerns, but theoretical considerations suggest they are appropriate.

Bullous Disease, Spontaneous Pneumothorax, and Other Problems

Any condition in which bullous disease or subpleural "blebs" are known to be present is considered a contraindication to diving (Table 5.4). If these air-filled spaces do not readily communicate with the airway, there is a risk for PBT and CAGE through shearing forces within the lung, or between the lung and chest wall, particularly during ascent. This risk is largely theoretical, and for obvious reasons, it is unlikely that relevant data will be forthcoming.

Spontaneous pneumothorax is generally regarded as an absolute contraindication to diving. Surgical pleurodesis is commonly undertaken after a second event to prevent further recurrence and has been used to reduce the risks for dysbaric injury in aircrew.[117] However, no good evidence has been reported that this procedure will be protective in diving where the volume changes are potentially much greater and where PBT may be complicated by CAGE. Although the lung may be less likely to collapse, the pleurodesis does not remove the blebs that predispose to PBT. Diving is considered contraindicated after spontaneous pneumothorax, even when a pleurodesis has been performed.

Previous penetrating chest injuries, traumatic pneumothorax, interstitial lung disease, necrotizing pneumonias, and chest surgery where the pleura is entered (and especially where the lung is operated on) are also considered to be conditions where diving is not recommended. In theory, any scar within the lungs may create adjacent areas of nonhomogeneous compliance, promote gas trapping, and predispose the candidate to PBT. Little clinical evidence exists to confirm this view, however, and an honest risk assessment should acknowledge both the theoretical risks and the lack of confirmatory clinical evidence. When asked to advise an experienced diver who has suffered a traumatic or surgical pneumothorax, one approach is to discuss all risks described earlier and then perform a high-resolution CT of the lung to exclude any gross scarring. In assisting the diver to come to a risk versus benefit decision about diving, it has been our practice to suggest that a normal high-resolution CT is compatible with a lower risk for PBT and CAGE; however, this is an entirely theoretical assessment.

Table 5.4   Some Respiratory Conditions Associated with Air Trapping and/or Shearing Forces on Distention

CONDITIONS ASSOCIATED WITH BULLAE, BLEBS, OR DIFFERENTIAL LUNG COMPLIANCE	COMMENTS
Spontaneous pneumothorax	Associated with apical blebs; likely to recur, particularly within 2 years, even without barometric stress
Penetrating chest injury with lung injury or traumatic pneumothorax	Scars in the lung tissue may predispose to pulmonary barotrauma from shearing forces
Chest surgery including any operation where the visceral pleura is breached	Scars in the lung tissue may predispose to pulmonary barotrauma from shearing forces
Interstitial lung diseases, e.g., sarcoid, cystic fibrosis	May be associated with air trapping and significant exercise limitation
Connective tissue disorders, e.g., Marfan's disease, Ehlers–Danlos syndrome	May be associated with apical blebs or variable alveolar compliance
Infections, e.g., tuberculosis	May result in scarring and differential compliance and exercise limitation

Candidates with any of these conditions are generally counseled against diving.

Bleomycin

Bleomycin is an antineoplastic antibiotic that exerts cytotoxic effects by producing free oxygen radicals and inhibiting angiogenesis.[118] The most dramatic adverse effect of this drug is the induction of pneumonitis in about 20% of patients in whom the early mortality rate may be as high as 25%.[119] In vivo studies of concurrent oxygen and bleomycin administration support the concern that use of supplemental oxygen is a potent risk factor for the development of this complication.[120] There is a widespread perception that supplemental oxygen can provoke pulmonary fibrosis many years after bleomycin exposure, but this has not been supported by clinical human data.[121,122] Although the connection between high inspired oxygen pressure and bleomycin-related lung damage is poorly established, it is prudent to clearly advise prospective divers of this potentially fatal complication and to discuss diving with their oncologist.

Diabetes

Diabetes that requires medication has been (and still widely is) considered a contraindication to diving because of the potential for hypoglycemic events, the frequency of co-morbidity such as ischemic heart disease, and the potential for complications of diabetes to be mistaken for DCS.[123-127] Since the late 1990s, however, there has been a gradual softening of attitudes toward diving by individuals with diabetes. Several studies have demonstrated the feasibility of safe blood glucose management by individuals with diabetes who dive,[124,127] and it has become clear that individuals with diabetes are participating in recreational diving regardless of whether the diving medical organizations endorse this.[128] Moreover, notwithstanding the potential for bias in the relevant surveys, they appear to be diving with an incidence of problems similar to that recorded among populations of nondiabetic divers.[128,129]

In 2005, a consensus workshop of experts debated recreational diving by individuals with diabetes and promulgated guidelines for selection and surveillance of divers with diabetes, the scope of diving considered appropriate, and management of blood glucose on the day of diving.[130] The guidelines for selection and surveillance are prefaced by a reminder that the candidate must be suitable for diving in all respects other than suffering diabetes, and recommend an eight-step procedure for evaluation and annual surveillance. Although a detailed discussion of these guidelines is beyond the scope of this chapter, the general aim is to ensure that the prospective diver with diabetes is familiar enough with the disease to understand the relation between various stressors and hypoglycemic reactions, that the likelihood of experiencing development of a hypoglycemic reaction is acceptably low, and that there are no complications of diabetes (e.g., coronary artery disease) that might be incompatible with diving. Any hyperbaric physician who may become involved in the evaluation of diving candidates with diabetes is strongly recommended to purchase the recently published guidelines.[130]

Ear, Nose, and Throat Problems

Clearance to dive must not be given to a candidate who cannot insufflate the middle ear via the eustachian tubes. The paranasal sinuses must also equalize with ambient pressure during compression via their boney ostia. However, the ability to equalize the sinuses is difficult to assess in the office, and problems with sinuses typically present when a candidate performs his or her first open-water dives. The most common cause of temporary inability to "equalize" the middle ear and sinuses is an upper respiratory tract infection. Persistent problems are best dealt with by referral to an appropriate surgeon.

Potential causes of hearing loss in diving were mentioned briefly earlier. These include noise exposure and disorders such as inner-ear barotrauma and DCS. A conundrum that often arises is how to advise the candidate or diver who exhibits significant preexisting hearing loss. No consensus on a definition for "severe" in this context has been reached. Farmer[131] proposes that any loss greater than 20 dB in the speech frequencies 200 to 2000 Hz or a speech discrimination score less than 90% should result in disqualification. In practice, this recommendation is not always followed among occupational divers because disqualification has such profound implications and noise-induced hearing loss is common. When a new diving candidate exhibits significant preexisting hearing loss, he or she should be counseled

about the potential for further loss associated with diving. In candidates who rely heavily on their hearing professionally, such as pilots or musicians, such counseling should occur even if their hearing is perfect. Established divers who exhibit hearing loss should be counseled about the potential for the problem to progress with further exposure to the diving environment and be given advice about ear protection in noisy environments. Finally, we discourage any candidate who is completely deaf in one ear from diving because the functional consequences of an accident involving their good ear are too serious.

Any history of ear surgery should alert the examiner to the possibility of poor eustachian tube function. Most diving physicians agree that a successful tympanic membrane repair is compatible with diving providing eustachian tube function is intact. A candidate with a persistent tympanic membrane perforation or with tympanostomy tubes should not be cleared to dive because there is a risk for infection or troublesome caloric stimulation when water enters the middle ear. Simple mastoidectomy is compatible with diving provided the eustachian tube functions adequately. A radical mastoidectomy or modified radical mastoidectomy leaves the middle-ear space open to the environment and is thus not compatible with diving. A stapedectomy procedure has long been considered to be a contraindication to diving because of concerns over increased risk for inner-ear barotrauma.[3] Based on a retrospective survey that involved 22 patients who dived after stapedectomy,[132] it was concluded that "stapedectomy does not appear to increase the risk of inner ear barotrauma in scuba divers." In our opinion, this report does not establish the relative risk, and we would still discourage patients who had undergone a stapedectomy from diving. There is little experience to date of diving by patients with cochlear implants. Testing of implant components under hyperbaric conditions to 6 ATA demonstrated no problems,[133] and there is anecdote supportive of their use during actual diving.[134] Medical diseases of the vestibulocochlear apparatus that cause vertigo and ataxia, such as Ménière's disease and viral labyrinthitis, are incompatible with diving. However, candidates who have fully recovered after a single episode of labyrinthitis may dive.

Return to diving after middle-ear barotrauma is contingent on the tympanic membrane being intact, the resolution of otoscopic abnormalities, and demonstration of the ability to insufflate the middle-ear space via the eustachian tube. Return to diving after inner-ear barotrauma is also contingent on a full recovery but remains controversial,[135] mainly because of concerns over persisting predispositions. For example, divers with a degree of eustachian tube dysfunction who are forced to Valsalva vigorously to insufflate the middle-ear space are probably at risk for recurrent inner-ear barotrauma. It would be appropriate to counsel such a diver against further diving unless something could be done to improve his or her eustachian tube function. In contrast, return to diving might be appropriate for a fully recovered diver whose event appeared to be attributable to a problem that could be avoided in the future, such as temporary eustachian tube dysfunction caused by an upper respiratory tract infection. Patients must be counseled about the risks of a repeated event, possibly with a worse outcome, including deafness. Although arbitrary, we usually recommend a period of several months with no diving in those candidates for whom a return appears to be appropriate, and longer periods if surgical repair of a perilymph fistula was undertaken.

Neurologic Problems

Epilepsy is a contraindication to diving because of the disastrous consequences of a seizure underwater. Unfortunately, seizure control in daily life cannot be confidently extrapolated into the underwater environment where unique epileptogenic stimuli are encountered. These views are widely accepted, even among contemporary reviewers who advocate participation by individuals with epilepsy in a wide variety of sports.[136] Provided the diagnosis was certain and not complicated by predictors of subsequent nonfebrile seizures,[137] adult candidates with a history of febrile convulsions in childhood may be cleared to dive. A history of a syncopal event without a clear explanation must be investigated, and provided there is no evidence for epilepsy (including a normal EEG) or another significant risk for diving (such as a cardiac arrhythmia), it would be reasonable to permit diving after a suitable interval of observation.

A related concern is how to approach the patient who has had a severe head injury and now wishes to dive. The standardized incidence ratio (indexed to the rate of new unprovoked seizures in the general population) for posttraumatic seizures in mild, moderate, and severe head injuries is 1.5, 2.9, and 17, respectively.[138] After severe head injury, the standardized incidence ratio was 95, 17, 12, 4 for the time periods less than 1 year, 1 to 4 years, 5 to 9 years, and 10 or more years, respectively, indicating that, although the greatest danger period for development of new seizures is in the first year after injury, the risk remains significantly increased for at least 5 to 10 years. The cumulative probability of a new seizure in the severely injury group was approximately 7% at 1 year, 10% at 5 years, and 13% at 10 years. Based on these data, we would attempt to discourage a patient who had suffered a severe traumatic head injury from any recreational diving, and we would not clear such a candidate for occupational diving. For the patient with mild head injury (no fracture, contusion, or bleed, and loss of consciousness or amnesia for no more than 30 minutes), the standardized incidence ratio for new seizures is 3.1 for the first year and 2.1 for the next 4 years, after which there is no increase in risk for new seizures over that for the general population. We consider the absolute risk implied by these figures to be sufficiently small as to justify only a short delay in return to diving provided the candidate is appropriately counseled about risk. Conservative (or risk-averse) patients may consider a 5-year wait to be justified.

For patients with migraine headache without aura, a decision on clearance to dive should be based on the frequency and severity of events. Migraine with a neurologic "aura" raises concerns because an aura phase of a migraine might be mistaken for DCS and result in inappropriate evacuation and treatment. Moreover, some manifestations would compromise safety if they occurred during a dive. In addition, a clear link has been established between migraine with aura and the presence of a significant right-to-left intracardiac shunt, usually via a PFO.[139] The link between a significant PFO and serious neurologic DCS was discussed earlier. The diving physician must interpret this complex inter-relation of pathologies in formulating an approach to these candidates. Our view is that these issues constitute reason enough to refuse clearance to dive. However, after appropriate counseling, these candidates may be a group in whom prospective screening for a PFO is justified because the benefits of PFO closure might extend beyond facilitation of a diving hobby.[140,141]

Obesity

Obesity, usually defined as a body mass index (BMI) greater than 30, is viewed as disadvantageous in diving because it is a predictor of problems such as hypertension and ischemic heart disease, it potentially reduces physical performance in the water, and it has long been considered a risk factor for DCS.[142] Experimental data from human dives show greater bubble formation after dive in subjects with greater percentages of body fat.[59] In addition, observations dating back to Pol and Wattelle[143] have identified obesity as a risk factor for clinical DCS. Lam and Yau[144] have determined risk factors for DCS among 932 caisson workers using multivariate analysis and found that obesity was an independent risk factor with an odds ratio for DCS of 2.2. Some conflicting data remain in the literature, however. For example, Conkin and colleagues[58] did not find BMI to be predictive of venous bubble formation after hypobaric decompression, and an observational study involving 1742 dive training professionals failed to identify a link between risk for DCS and being "overweight."[63] Although it appears reasonable to conclude that obesity is undesirable in diving, it is not clear where to set a threshold BMI for the

purposes of exclusion,[145] or even if exclusion based simply on BMI is appropriate at all. We favor an approach based on the candidate's ability to satisfy the requirements of the functional analysis for diving proposed earlier in this chapter. If a candidate is sufficiently obese or unfit to be incapable of meeting these requirements, the person probably should not be diving. It would also seem prudent to counsel the overweight diver about his or her theoretically increased risk for DCS and the advisability of diving conservative time–depth–ascent rate profiles.

Pregnancy

Diving is not recommended during pregnancy. In part, this is related to the disadvantageous side effects of pregnancy on the female diver, which include nausea and vomiting, the impairment of exercise tolerance that occurs in late pregnancy, and the associated abdominal distension that complicates equipment configuration.[50] However, the major concerns focus on the risk for harm to the fetus from exposure to high oxygen tensions and from DCS. The Undersea and Hyperbaric Medical Society dedicated a workshop to this issue, and the proceedings summarize the relevant in vivo evidence, which is conflicting.[146] Few human data are available. A survey that compared outcomes for 109 women who dived during pregnancy with those for 69 female divers who refrained showed a greater rate of birth defects in those who dived, but the rate remained within that expected for the general population.[147] Insufficient data are available to define the risk of diving during pregnancy, and a conservative recommendation not to dive is considered an appropriate default position.

Psychiatric Disorders

Patients with major depression, bipolar disorder, or psychoses should not dive for reasons that are largely self-evident. Although there are essentially no data that establish greater risk in these groups, it seems plausible that such patients may be less likely to concentrate and function appropriately and more likely to exhibit erratic unpredictable behavior. Perhaps the most troublesome group of "psychiatric" patients in the modern context are those with "mild" depression or "dysthymic" disorders who are treated with selective serotonin reuptake inhibitors. Concerns over diving while taking selective serotonin reuptake inhibitors relate to the psychiatric disorder being treated and to the potential interaction between the drug and diving. These drugs may cause drowsiness (albeit less than caused by tricyclic antidepressants) and may lower the seizure threshold, especially in overdose.[148] Nevertheless, no reports have been published of apparent problems despite what is almost certainly a large number of divers taking them. We would allow diving by a patient taking an selective serotonin reuptake inhibitor provided that the treated mood disturbance was mild before treatment and has been well controlled by the drug, the drug has been used for at least 1 month without evidence of relevant side effects, and the diver understands and accepts the relevant theoretical risks.

Return to Diving after Illness

In general, return to diving after recovery from illness is contingent on full recovery of a functional capacity compatible with safe diving. A prevalent belief among divers is that injury, surgical scarring, or the presence of metal implants will cause perturbation of local perfusion and a predisposition to DCS. Although this cannot be definitively excluded, there is little support for the concern in the literature. We usually advise that return to diving is appropriate once both the treating clinician and the diver agree that the injury is sufficiently recovered to cope with the usual demands of diving. Any wounds should be completely healed.

After DCS, a return to diving should not be contemplated unless the diver makes a complete recovery.[149] Thus, careful clinical examination is important, and investigations may be necessary. For example, residual abnormalities could be detected by electronystagmography in a significant proportion of patients who claimed to be asymptomatic after vestibular DCS.[135] In addition, return to diving is appropriate only if the initial event did not suggest any preexisting predisposition, as would be implied by a serious neurologic event after a dive well inside the limits prescribed by the dive table or computer used. This would require follow-up by a specialist diving physician and would likely justify a range of investigations including a bubble contrast TEE to check for a PFO that readily shunts from right to left. Where there is a complete recovery and no indication of predisposition, a return to diving is appropriate. It is customary to recommend a period of at least 1 month with no diving after recovery from the initial event, although intervals as short as 24 hours have been endorsed if the symptoms were mild.[149] It is also prudent to counsel the patient that no guarantees can be given that a similar DCS event (or worse) will not occur again. If the patient is risk averse, he or she may choose to give up diving. Experienced diving physicians may also provide advice about diving practices that may reduce the risk for future events.

In AGE suspected to involve PBT, decision making is complicated by the possibility that there may be a preexisting anatomic disorder or that the barotrauma may have caused parenchymal scarring that might become a future predisposition. Investigation of these issues using techniques such as high-resolution CT scanning and the related concerns over sensitivity and specificity have been discussed elsewhere. There is no universally accepted policy on return to diving after AGE involving PBT. Our own approach is to discourage further diving after suspected PBT. However, if there is no objective evidence of preexisting or consequent anatomic abnormality and the diver remains highly motivated after counseling about the theoretical risks, then we will allow diving. Once again, a break of at least 1 month is recommended.

CLEARANCE FOR WORK IN HYPERBARIC CHAMBERS

Work in hyperbaric chambers involves compression and decompression. Not surprisingly, many aspects of diving fitness are relevant to hyperbaric chamber occupants, but adoption of a diving fitness standard is excessive. Hyperbaric chamber attendants are vulnerable to ear barotrauma, sinus barotrauma, and PBT, but risks are lower because the pressure changes are much slower and there is precise control that prevents unexpected rapid pressure changes. Attendants breathe the chamber atmosphere (air), and though they are vulnerable to DCS, there are several mitigating factors in comparison with diving. They perform little physical work, which lessens their inert gas uptake; decompressions are slow and highly controlled; and they can safely breathe 100% oxygen during the latter stages of decompression to hasten inert gas elimination. Nevertheless, hyperbaric chamber decompressions can result in venous bubble formation in attendants,[150] and cases of DCS do occur,[151] albeit most commonly at the mild end of the spectrum of severity.

With regard to heart disease, hyperbaric chamber work is more closely related to the myocardial stress of ward duties than diving, and it follows that expectations of functional capacity are correspondingly less rigorous. If a nurse with a history of ischemic or other heart disease is fit for usual duties on a ward, he or she is likely to be medically suitable for hyperbaric chamber work. We believe the issue of PFO should be approached in the same manner as it is for divers. There is no justification for prospective screening of hyperbaric attendants, but a TEE could be considered after an episode of neurologic, inner-ear, or cutaneous DCS.

With regard to respiratory conditions, less concern exists about reactive airways disease than in diving. It is possible to use a β-agonist inhaler in the chamber, and as already mentioned, PBT is less likely given the slow decompression rates involved. Nevertheless, it would not be appropriate for an individual with asthma to work during periods of active wheezing, and total exclusion would still be warranted for candidates with poorly controlled asthma or those who are prone to severe attacks. Exclusion would also be warranted for candidates with a history of spontaneous pneumothorax, complex disease of the pulmonary parenchyma such as sarcoid, obvious bullous disease of the lungs, or with only one lung.

With regard to neurologic problems, some theoretical concerns about epilepsy in the hyperbaric chamber environment remain. Hyperbaric attendants are required to breathe 100% oxygen during the decompression phase of treatments, and these oxygen breathing periods may be protracted in the recompression of divers with DCS. The attendant's dose of oxygen is minimized to reduce the likelihood of an oxygen toxicity seizure, but any preexisting reduction in the seizure threshold may increase risk. However, no confirmatory data have been reported.

With respect to ear, nose, and throat problems, there is an absolute requirement for an ability to insufflate the middle-ear spaces and sinuses, which is in common with diving. We would also recommend that stapedectomy should exclude a candidate from hyperbaric work as it does in diving. In contrast, a radical mastoidectomy would probably not contraindicate hyperbaric exposure because the subject is not immersed.

REFERENCES

1. Brubakk AO, Neuman TS (eds): Bennett and Elliott's Physiology and Medicine of Diving, 5th ed. London, Saunders Publishers, 2003.
2. Russi EW: Diving and the risk of barotrauma. Thorax 53:S20–S24, 1998.
3. Bove AA: Fitness to dive. In: Brubakk AO, Neuman TS (eds): Bennett and Elliott's Physiology and Medicine of Diving, 5th ed. London, Saunders Publishers, 2003, pp 700–717.
4. Navy Department: US Navy Diving Manual Volume 1 Revision 3: Air Diving. Washington, DC, US Government Printing Office, 1996.
5. Elliott D, Edge C: Restricted diving for the unfit. SPUMS J 31:41–44, 2001.
6. Gorman DF: From police to health advisor: The evolution of modern occupational health surveillance. SPUMS J 33:134–139, 2003.

7. Maron BJ, Mitten MJ, Quandt EK, et al: Competitive athletes with cardiovascular disease—the case of Nicholas Knapp. N Engl J Med 339:1632-1635, 1998.

8. Bennett MH: Designing a recreational diving medical for the 21st century. SPUMS J 34:150-152, 2004.

9. Gorman D: Where is for occupational medicine? Int Med J 34:449-450, 2004.

10. Moller L: Risk perception—the behavioral reaction to health risks. In: Moller L (ed): Environmental Medicine. Stockholm, Karolinska Institute, 2001, pp 386-404.

11. Richardson D: The RSTC medical statement and candidate screening model. SPUMS J 30:210-213, 2000.

12. Glen S, White S, Douglas J: Medical supervision of sport diving in Scotland: Reassessing the need for routine medical examinations. Br J Sports Med 34:375-378, 2000.

13. Glen S: Three year follow up of a self certification system for the assessment of fitness to dive in Scotland. Br J Sports Med 38:754-757, 2004.

14. Maron BJ: Sudden death in young athletes—lessons from the Hank Gathers affair. N Engl J Med 329:55-57, 1993.

15. Edmonds C: The Mickey Mouse Medical. SPUMS J 16:3-4, 1986.

16. Ornhagen H: Heath assessment for recreational diving requires special medical competence. Lakartidningen 101:780-786, 2004.

17. Simpson G, Roomes S: Scuba diving medicine examinations in practice: A postal survey. Med J Aust 171:584-586, 1999.

18. Coren S: The law and the diving professional. Santa Ana, Calif, Professional Association of Diving Instructors, 1985.

19. Lehm J, Bennett MH: Predictors of middle ear barotrauma associated with hyperbaric oxygen therapy. SPUMS J 33:127-133, 2003.

20. Uzun C, Adali MK, Tas A, et al: Use of the nine-step inflation/deflation test as a predictor of middle ear barotraumas in sports scuba divers. Br J Audiol 34:153-163, 2000.

21. Bluestone CD: Assessment of Eustachian tube function. In: Jerger J (ed): Handbook of Clinical Impedance Audiometry. New York, American Electromedics Corporation, 1975, pp 127-148.

22. Sim RJ, Youngs RP: Otolaryngological requirements for recreational self-contained underwater breathing apparatus (SCUBA) diving. J Laryngol Otol 121:306-311, 2007.

23. Shupak A, Sharoni Z, Ostfeld E, et al: Pressure chamber tympanometry in diving candidates. Ann Otol Rhinol Laryngol 100:658-660, 1991.

24. Fitzgerald B: A review of the sharpened Romberg test in diving medicine. SPUMS J 26:142-146, 1996.

25. Lee C-T: Sharpening the sharpened Romberg. SPUMS J 28:125-132, 1998.

26. Molvaer OI, Albrektsen G: Hearing deterioration in professional divers: An epidemiological study. Undersea Biomed Res 17:231-246, 1990.

27. Klingmann C, Knauth M, Reis S, et al: Hearing threshold in sport divers: Is diving really a hazard for inner ear function? Arch Otolaryngol Head Neck Surg 130:221-225, 2004.

28. Taylor DM, Lippmann J, Smith D: The absence of hearing loss in otologically asymptomatic recreational scuba divers. Undersea Hyperb Med 33:135-141, 2006.

29. Benton PJ, Francis TJ, Pethybridge RJ: Spirometric indices and the risk of pulmonary barotrauma in submarine escape training. Undersea Hyperb Med 26:213-217, 1999.

30. Tetzlaff K, Reuter M, Leplow B, et al: Risk factors for pulmonary barotrauma in divers. Chest 112:654-659, 1997.

31. Neuman TS, Clausen JL: Recommend caution in defining risk factors for barotrauma in divers. Chest 114:1791-1792, 1998.

32. Leitch DR, Green RD: Recurrent pulmonary barotraumas. Aviat Space Environ Med 57:1039-1043, 1986.

33. Yildiz S, Ay H, Gunay A, et al: Submarine escape from depths of 30 and 60 feet: 41,183 training ascents without serious injury. Aviat Space Environ Med 75:269-271, 2004.

34. Denison DM: Lung function testing of divers. In: Elliott DH (ed): Medical Assessment of Fitness to Dive. Surrey, UK, Biomedical Seminars, 1995, pp 123-133.

35. Linaweaver PG: Commentary in discussion following presentation by O'Hara. In: Vorosmarti J (ed): Fitness to Dive: Proceedings of the Thirty Fourth Undersea and Hyperbaric Medical Society Workshop. Bethesda, Md, Undersea and Hyperbaric Medical Society, 1987, pp 66-67.

36. Mellem H, Emhjellen S, Horgen O: Pulmonary barotrauma and arterial gas embolism caused by an emphysematous bulla in a SCUBA diver. Aviat Space Environ Med 61:559-562, 1990.

37. Miller IL: Should computed tomography of the chest be recommended in the medical certification of professional divers? Br J Sports Med 38:2-3, 2004.

38. Farmer J: Commentary in discussion following presentation by O'Hara. In: Vorosmarti J (ed): Fitness to Dive: Proceedings of the Thirty Fourth Undersea and Hyperbaric Medical Society Workshop. Bethesda Md, Undersea and Hyperbaric Medical Society, 1987, pp 67.

39. Toklu AS, Kiyan E, Aktas S, et al: Should computed chest tomography be recommended in the certification of professional divers? A report of three cases with pulmonary air cysts. Occup Environ Med 60:606-608, 2003.

40. Acott CJ: Prolonged QT syndrome: A probable cause of a drowning death in a recreational scuba diver. SPUMS J 34:209-213, 2004.

41. Short B: Electrocardiographic abnormalities in young athletes and scuba divers [letter]. SPUMS J 35:109, 2005.

42. Elliott DH: Medical evaluation of working divers. In: Bove AA (ed): Bove and Davis' Diving Medicine, 4th ed. Philadelphia, Saunders Publishers, 2004, p 538.

43. Wilmshurst P: Cardiological investigation and assessment (Discussion following paper). In: Elliott DH (ed): Medical Assessment of Fitness to Dive. Surrey, UK, Biomedical Seminars, 1995, p 91.

44. Risberg J: Haematology. In: Elliott DH (ed): Medical Assessment of Fitness to Dive. Surrey, UK, Biomedical Seminars, 1995, pp 190-192.

45. Discussion following presentation by Risberg. In: Elliott DH (ed): Medical Assessment of Fitness to Dive. Surrey, UK, Biomedical Seminars, 1995, pp 193-196.

46. Medical Research Council—Decompression Sickness Panel: Decompression sickness and aseptic necrosis of

bone. Investigations carried out during and after the construction of the Tyne Road Tunnel (1962-1966). Br J Indust Med 28:1-21, 1971.

47. Elliott DH: Commentary following presentation by McCallum. In: Elliott DH, ed. Medical Assessment of Fitness to Dive. Surrey, UK, Biomedical Seminars, 1995, p 189.

48. Johnson W: Osteonecrosis as it concerns the insurance underwriter. In: Beckman EL, Elliott DH (eds): Dysbarism-Related Osteonecrosis. Proceedings of a Symposium on Dysbaric Osteonecrosis. Washington, DC, National Institute for Occupational Safety and Health, 1972, pp 233-234.

49. Jones JP, Neuman TS: Dysbaric osteonecrosis. In: Brubakk AO, Neuman TS (eds): Bennett and Elliott's Physiology and Medicine of Diving, 5th ed. London, Saunders Publishers, 2003, pp 659-679.

50. Parker JL: The Sports Diving Medical. Melbourne, JL Publications, 2002.

51. Gorman D: Health surveillance in the 21st century. SPUMS J 31:39-41, 2001.

52. Walker R: How old is old enough? SPUMS J 33:78-80, 2003.

53. Tsung JW, Chou KJ, Martinez C, et al: An adolescent scuba diver with 2 episodes of diving-related injuries requiring hyperbaric oxygen recompression therapy: A case report with medical considerations for child and adolescent scuba divers. Pediatr Emerg Care 21:681-686, 2005.

54. Mitchell S: Children in diving: How young is too young? SPUMS J 33:81-83, 2003.

55. Richardson D: Children and diving: The recreational-diving training perspective. SPUMS J 33:83-89, 2003.

56. Vandenhoven G, Collard F, Schamp S: Children and diving: Medical aspects. Eight years sports medical follow-up of the first scuba diving club for children in Belgium. SPUMS J 33:70-73, 2003.

57. Caruso JL, Bove AA, Uguccioni DM, et al: Recreational diving deaths associated with cardiovascular disease: Epidemiology and recommendations for pre-participation screening. Undersea Hyperb Med 28(supp):75-76, 2001.

58. Conkin J, Powell MR, Gernhardt ML: Age affects severity of venous gas emboli on decompression from 14.7 to 4.3 psia. Aviat Space Environ Med 74:1142-1150, 2003.

59. Carturan D, Boussuges A, Vanuxem P, et al: Ascent rate, age, maximal oxygen uptake, adiposity, and circulating venous bubbles after diving. J Appl Physiol 93:1349-1356, 2002.

60. Dunford RG, Vann RD, Gerth WA, et al: The incidence of venous gas emboli in recreational diving. Undersea Hyperb Med 29:247-259, 2002.

61. Sulaiman ZM, Pilmanis AA, O'Connor RB: Relationship between age and susceptibility to altitude decompression sickness. Aviat Space Environ Med 68:695-698, 1997.

62. Bradley ME: Metabolic considerations. In: Vorosmarti J (ed): Fitness to Dive. Proceedings of the Thirty Fourth Undersea and Hyperbaric Medical Society Workshop. Bethesda, Md, Undersea and Hyperbaric Medical Society, 1987, pp 98-104.

63. Hagberg M, Ornhagen H: Incidence and risk factors for symptoms of decompression sickness among

male and female dive masters and instructors—a retrospective cohort study. Undersea Hyperb Med 30:93-102, 2003.

64. DAN—Diver's Alert Network. Report on Decompression Illness, Diving Fatalities and Project Dive Exploration (based on 2002 data). Durham, NC, Diver's Alert Network, 2004, p 87.

65. L'Italien G, Ford I, Norrie J, et al: The cardiovascular event reduction tool (CERT): A simplified cardiac risk prediction model developed from the West of Scotland Coronary Prevention Study (WOSCOPS). Am J Cardiol 85:720-724, 2000.

66. Bove AA: Cardiovascular problems and diving. SPUMS J 26:178-186, 1996.

67. Grindlay J, Mitchell S: Isolated pulmonary oedema associated with scuba diving. Emerg Med 11:272-276, 1999.

68. Cross MR: Cardiovascular problems commonly found in divers. In: Elliott DH (ed): Medical Assessment of Fitness to Dive. Surrey, UK, Biomedical Seminars, 1995, pp 77-83.

69. Broome JR, Dick EJ, Axley MJ, et al: Spinal cord hemorrhage in short latency decompression illness coincides with early recompression. Undersea Hyperb Med 22(supp):35, 1995.

70. Wilmshurst PT, Crowther A, Nuri M, et al: Cold-induced pulmonary oedema in scuba divers and swimmers and subsequent development of hypertension. Lancet i:62-65, 1989.

71. Hagen PT, Scholz DG, Edwards WD: Incidence and size of patent foramen ovale during the first 10 decades of life: An autopsy study of 965 normal hearts. Mayo Clin Proc 59:17-20, 1984.

72. Pinto FJ: When and how to diagnose a patent foramen ovale. Heart 91:438-440, 2005.

73. Cross SJ, Evans SA, Thomson LF, et al: Safety of subaqua diving with a patent foramen ovale. Br Med J 304:481-482, 1992.

74. Butler BD, Hills BA: The lung as a filter for microbubbles. J Appl Physiol 47:537-543, 1979.

75. Moon RE, Camporesi EM, Kisslo JA: Patent foramen ovale and decompression sickness in divers. Lancet i:513-514, 1989.

76. Wilmshurst PT, Byrne JC, Webb-Peploe MM: Relation between interatrial shunts and decompression sickness in divers. Lancet 334:1302-1306, 1989.

77. Germonpre P, Dendale P, Unger P, et al: Patent foramen ovale and decompression sickness in sports divers. J Appl Physiol 84:1622-1626, 1998.

78. Wilmshurst P, Bryson P: Relationship between the clinical features of neurological decompression illness and its causes. Clin Sci 99:65-75, 2000.

79. Wilmshurst PT, Pearson MJ, Walsh KP, et al: Relationship between right to left shunts and cutaneous decompression illness. Clin Sci 100:539-542, 2001.

80. Cantais E, Louge P, Suppini A, et al: Right-to-left shunt and risk of decompression illness with cochleovestibular and cerebral symptoms in divers: Case control study in 101 consecutive dive accidents. Crit Care Med 31:84-88, 2003.

81. Klingmann C, Benton PJ, Ringleb PA, et al: Embolic ear decompression illness: Correlation with a right-to-left shunt. Laryngoscope 113:1356-1361, 2003.

82. Torti SR, Billinger M, Schwerzmann M, et al: Risk of decompression illness among 230 divers in relation to the presence and size of patent foramen ovale. Eur Heart J 25:1014-1020, 2004.

83. Reul J, Weis J, Jung A, et al: Central nervous system lesions and cervical disc herniations in amateur divers. Lancet 345:1403-1405, 1995.

84. Knauth M, Ries S, Pohimann S, et al: Cohort study of multiple brain lesions in sport divers: A role of a patent foramen ovale. BMJ 314:701-705, 1997.

85. Schwerzmann M, Seiler C, Lipp E, et al: Relation between directly detected patient foramen ovale and ischemic brain lesions in sport divers. Ann Intern Med 134:21-24, 2001.

86. Schuchlenz HW, Weihs W, Horner S, et al: The association between the diameter of a patent foramen ovale and the risk of embolic cerebrovascular events. Am J Med 109:456-462, 2000.

87. Ries S, Knauth M, Daffertshofer M, et al: Echocontrast TCD-testing for patent foramen ovale in sports divers: A useful test to estimate the risk of accumulating brain lesions. Neurology 50(suppl 4):A445, 1998.

88. Walsh KP, Wilmshurst PT, Morrison WL: Transcatheter close of patent foramen ovale using the Amplatzer septal occluder to prevent recurrence of neurological decompression illness in divers. Heart 81:257-261, 1999.

89. Moon RE, Bove AA: Transcatheter occlusion of patent foramen ovale: A prevention for decompression illness? Undersea Hyperb Med 31:271-274, 2004.

90. Ladd G, Stepan V, Stevens L: The Abacus Project: Establishing the risk of recreational scuba death and decompression illness. SPUMS J 32:124-128, 2002.

91. Gardner M, Forbes C, Mitchell SJ: One hundred cases of decompression illness treated in New Zealand during 1995. SPUMS J 26:222-226, 1996.

92. Ries S, Knauth M, Kern R, et al: Arterial gas embolism after decompression: Correlation with right-to-left shunting. Neurology 52:401-404, 1999.

93. Bove AA: Risk of decompression sickness with patent foramen ovale. Undersea Hyperb Med 25:175-178, 1998.

94. Daniel WG, Erbel R, Kasper W, et al: Safety of transesophageal echocardiography. A multicenter study of 10,419 examinations. Circulation 83:817-821, 1991.

95. Balestra C, Germonpre P, Marroni A: Intrathoracic pressure changes after Valsalva strain and other maneuvers: Implications for divers with patent foramen ovale. Undersea Hyperb Med 25:171-174, 1998.

96. Berdat PA, Chatterjee T, Pfammatter JP, et al: Surgical management of complications after transcatheter closure of an atrial septal defect or patent foramen ovale. J Thorac Cardiovasc Surg 120:1034-1039, 2000.

97. Van Hoesen K, Neuman T: Asthma and SCUBA diving. Immunol Allergy Clin North Am 16:917-928, 1996.

98. Elliott DH (ed): Are asthmatics fit to dive? Bethesda, Md, Undersea and Hyperbaric Medical Society, 1996.

99. Gorman D, Veale A: SPUMS policy on asthma and fitness for diving, 1996. SPUMS online. Available at: http://www.spums.org.au/spums_policy/spums_policy_on_asthma_and_fitness_for_diving. Accessed December 20, 2007.

100. Bove A, Neuman T, Kelsen S: Observations on asthma in the recreational diving population. Undersea Biomed Res 19(suppl):18, 1992.

101. Farrell PJ, Glanvill P: Diving practices of scuba divers with asthma. BMJ 300:166, 1990.

102. Corson KS, Dovenbarger JA, Moon RE, et al: Risk assessment of asthma for decompression illness. Undersea Biomed Res 18:16-17, 1991.

103. Neuman TS, Bove AA, O'Connor RD, et al: Asthma and diving. Ann Allergy 73:344-350, 1994.

104. Dovenbarger JA: DAN Annual Report on Diving Accidents and Fatalities. Durham, NC, Divers Alert Network, 1996.

105. Koehle M, Lloyd-Smith R, McKenzie D, et al: Asthma and recreational SCUBA diving: A systematic review. Sports Med 33:109-116, 2003.

106. Glanvill P, St Leger Dowse M, Bryson P: A longitudinal cohort study of divers with asthma: Diving habits and asthma health issues. SPUMS J 35:18-22, 2005.

107. Edmonds CJ: Asthma and diving. SPUMS J 21:70-74, 1991.

108. Corson KS, Moon RE, Nealen ML, et al: A survey of diving asthmatics. Undersea Biomed Res 19:18-19, 1992.

109. Miller-Larsson A, Selroos O: Advances in asthma and COPD treatment: Combination therapy with inhaled corticosteroids and long-acting beta 2-agonists. Curr Pharm Des 12:3261-3279, 2006.

110. Global Initiative for Asthma (GINA): Global strategy for asthma management and prevention. Bethesda, Md, National Heart, Lung and Blood Institute (NHLBI), 2006.

111. Bousquet J, Jeffery PK, Busse WW, et al: Asthma. From bronchoconstriction to airways inflammation and remodeling. Am J Respir Crit Care Med 161:1720-1745, 2000.

112. Anderson SD, Wong R, Bennett M, et al: Summary of knowledge and thinking about asthma and diving since 1993. Discussion paper for the Thoracic Society of Australia and New Zealand, November 2004. Diving Hyperb Med 36:12-18, 2006.

113. Zhong NS, Chen RC, Yang MO, et al: Is asymptomatic bronchial hyperresponsiveness an indication of potential asthma? A two-year follow-up of young students with bronchial hyperresponsiveness. Chest 102:1104-1109, 1992.

114. Koskela HO, Hyvarinen L, Brannan JD, et al: Responsiveness to three bronchial provocation tests in patients with asthma. Chest 124:2171-2177, 2003.

115. Anderson SD, Brannan J, Trevillion L, et al: Lung function and bronchial provocation tests for intending divers with a history of asthma. SPUMS J 25:233-248, 1995.

116. British Thoracic Society Fitness to Dive Group: British Thoracic Society guidelines on respiratory aspects of fitness for diving. Thorax 58:3-13, 2003.

117. North JH Jr: Thoracoscopic management of spontaneous pneumothorax allows prompt return to aviation duties. Aviat Space Environ Med 65:1128-1129, 1994.

118. Chow LM, Nathan PC, Hodgson DC, et al: Survival and late effects in children with Hodgkin's lymphoma treated with MOPP/ABV and low-dose, extended-field irradiation. J Clin Oncol 24:5735-5741, 2006.

119. Martin WG, Ristow KM, Habermann TM, et al: Bleomycin pulmonary toxicity has a negative impact on the outcome of patients with Hodgkin's lymphoma. J Clin Oncol 23:7614-7620, 2005.

120. Tryka AF, Skornik WA, Godleski JJ, et al: Potentiation of bleomycin-induced lung injury by exposure to

70% oxygen. Morphologic assessment. Am Rev Respir Dis 126:1074-1079, 1982.

121. Donat SM, Levy DA: Bleomycin associated pulmonary toxicity: Is perioperative oxygen restriction necessary? J Urol 160:1347-1352, 1998.

122. Douglas MJ, Coppin CM: Bleomycin and subsequent anaesthesia: A retrospective study at Vancouver General Hospital. Can Anaesth Soc J 27:449-452, 1980.

123. Taylor L, Mitchell S: Diabetes as a contraindication to diving: Should old dogma give way to new evidence? SPUMS J 31:44-50, 2001.

124. Dear Gde L, Pollock NW, Uguccioni DM, et al: Plasma glucose responses in recreational divers with insulin requiring diabetes. Undersea Hyper Med 31:291-301, 2004.

125. Thomas R, McKenzie B: The Diver's Medical Companion. Sydney, Diving Medical Centre, 1981, p 137.

126. Betts JC: Diabetes and diving. Pressure June: 2-3, 1983.

127. Lerch M, Lutrop C, Thurm U: Diabetes and diving: Can the risk of hypoglycemia be banned? SPUMS J 26:62-66, 1996.

128. Dear Gde L, Dovenbarger JA, Corson KS, et al: Diabetes among recreational divers. Undersea Hyperb Med 21(supp):94, 1994.

129. Edge CJ, St Leger Dowse M, Bryson P: Scuba diving with diabetes mellitus—the UK experience 1991-2001. Undersea Hyperb Med 32:27-38, 2005.

130. Pollock NW, Uguccioni DM, Dear G deL (eds): Diabetes and Recreational Diving: Guidelines for the Future. Proceedings of the Undersea and Hyperbaric Medical Society/Divers Alert Network 2005 Workshop. Durham, NC, Divers Alert Network, 2005, pp 1-4.

131. Farmer JC: ENT considerations: Otolaryngologic standards for diving. In: Vorosmarti J (ed): Fitness to Dive: Proceedings of the Thirty Fourth Workshop of the Undersea and Hyperbaric Medical Society. Bethesda, Md, Undersea and Hyperbaric Medicalz Society, 1987, pp 70-79.

132. House JW, Toh EH, Perez A: Diving after stapedectomy: Clinical experience and recommendations. Otolaryngol Head Neck Surg 125:256-260, 2001.

133. Backous DD, Dunford RG, Segel P, et al: Effects of hyperbaric exposure on the integrity of the internal components of commercially available cochlear implant systems. Otol Neurotol 23:463-467, 2002.

134. Kompis M, Vibert D, Senn P, et al: Scuba diving with cochlear implants. Ann Otol Rhinol Laryngol 112:425-427, 2003.

135. Shupak A, Gil A, Nachum Z, et al: Inner ear decompression sickness and inner ear barotrauma in recreational divers: A long-term follow up. Laryngoscope 113:2141-2147, 2003.

136. Howard GM, Radloff M, Sevier TL: Epilepsy and sports participation. Curr Sports Med Rep 3:15-19, 2004.

137. Berg AT, Testa FM, Levy SR, et al: The epidemiology of epilepsy. Past, present and future. Neurol Clin 14:383-398, 1996.

138. Annegers JF, Hauser WA, Coan SP, et al: A population-based study of seizures after traumatic brain injuries. N Engl J Med 338:20-24, 1998.

139. Wilmshurst P, Nightingale S: Relationship between migraine and cardiac and pulmonary right-to-left shunts. Clin Sci (Lond) 100:215-220, 2001.

140. Giardini A, Donti A, Formigari R, et al: Transcatheter patent foramen ovale closure mitigates aura migraine headaches abolishing spontaneous right-to-left shunting. Am Heart J 151:922.e1-e5, 2006.

141. Evans RW, Wilmshurst P, Nightingale S: Is cardiac evaluation for a possible right-to-left shunt indicated in a scuba diver with migraine with aura? Headache 43:294-295, 2003.

142. Mouret GM: Obesity and diving. Diving Hyperb Med 36:145-147, 2006.

143. Pol B, Wattelle T: Memoire sur les effets de la compression de l'air appliqué au creusements des puits a houille. Ann Hyg Lang Fr Med Twtr I:241-279, 1854.

144. Lam TH, Yau KP: Analysis of some individual risk factors for decompression sickness in Hong Kong. Undersea Biomed Res 16:283-292, 1989.

145. McCallum RI, Petrie A: Optimum weights for commercial divers. Br J Ind Med 41:275-278, 1984.

146. Kent MB (ed): Effects of Diving on Pregnancy. Proceedings of the 19th Workshop of the Undersea and Hyperbaric Medical Society. Bethesda, Md, Undersea and Hyperbaric Medical Society, 1978.

147. Bolton M: Scuba diving and fetal well-being: A survey of 208 women. Undersea Biomed Res 7:183-189, 1980.

148. Cuenca PJ, Holt KR, Hoefle JD: Seizure secondary to citalopram overdose. J Emerg Med 26:177-181, 2004.

149. Francis TJR: Criteria for return after decompression illness. In: Elliott DH (ed): Medical Assessment of Fitness to Dive. Surrey, UK, Biomedical Seminars, 1995, p 262.

150. Risberg J, Englund M, Aanderud L, et al: Venous gas embolism in chamber attendants after hyperbaric exposure. Undersea Hyperb Med 31:417-429, 2004.

151. Sheffield PJ, Pirone CJ: Decompression sickness in inside attendants. In: Workman WT (ed): Hyperbaric Facility Safety: A Practical Guide. Flagstaff, Ariz, Best Publishing, 2003, pp 643-663.

Hyperbaric Oxygen Therapy in Newborn Infants and Pediatric Patients

6

Dan Waisman, MD,
Oskar Baenziger, MD,
and Nachum Gall, MD

Newborn infants and children are treated regularly for acute or chronic conditions in hyperbaric facilities throughout the world. In this chapter, we review the indications for hyperbaric oxygen therapy (HBOT) for which scientific evidence has been established and the indications where empiric treatment is still used. Furthermore, we examine the experience gained by different countries and individual hyperbaric centers as an example of the heterogeneity in the use of HBOT. Most studies were performed with adult patients, and most indications for the treatment of children were not established on the basis of studies with infants and children.

In the last two decades, the list of indications for HBOT has begun to be analyzed in a critical manner, to provide a scientific foundation for the usefulness of HBOT in the short and long terms.

The objectives of this chapter are: (1) to provide neonatal and pediatric medical teams, as well as hyperbaric medical and paramedical teams, with basic knowledge of the indications for HBOT, so that they can refer the pediatric patient for treatment; and (2) to describe the special needs of the neonatal and pediatric patient inside the hyperbaric chamber.

When hyperbaric treatment of newborns, infants, children, or adolescents is indicated, close collaboration between the pediatric and the hyperbaric medical teams is essential, to assure adequate care of these patients with special needs in the hyperbaric chamber.

Numerous reports are available in the pediatric, hyperbaric, and general medical literature on children treated with HBOT. However, few reports provide a broader review of specific approaches to the pediatric patient in the hyperbaric chamber.[1-4]

All branches of pediatric medicine—that is, general pediatrician, pediatric intensive care unit (ICU), neonatal ICU, pediatric surgeon, and orthopedic surgeon—may be involved in cases with one of the conditions that can benefit from HBOT.

In this chapter, we emphasize the importance of consultation and collaboration between the pediatrician and the staff of the hyperbaric chamber. This begins in the emergency department, pediatric ICU, or neonatal ICU, where the pediatrician should be capable of recognizing the conditions that may benefit from hyperbaric oxygenation. It continues during the HBOT sessions, with proper management of pediatric patients, especially the critically ill patients, to meet their particular requirements.

Indications relevant to pediatric patients, based on current clinical practice and reviews, are listed in many publications,[2-5] but the accepted indications for HBOT listed by the

Undersea and Hyperbaric Medical Society (UHMS; http://www.uhms.org/Indications/indications.htm) are all relevant to newborn infants and children as well. It needs to be stated that there are no specific scientific or professional committee recommendations concerning the treatment of the neonatal and pediatric population. An excellent source for the review of published studies that have undergone peer review is the Database of Randomised Controlled Trials in Hyperbaric Medicine (http://www.hboevidence.com). In this chapter, we attempt to summarize the results regarding HBOT current to the publication of this textbook, to define what level of evidence justifies such therapy, and outline the information kindly provided by different hyperbaric facilities and medical centers regarding their experience in the treatment of pediatric cases.

Unfortunately, evidence-based treatment using HBOT in the pediatric patient is not abundant. In most cases, the actual number of patients suffering from some acute life-threatening indications (i.e., massive air embolism or gas gangrene) is small. For that reason, the performance of a randomized controlled study may not be possible for many centers. In such cases, collaboration between centers could be a good alternative. In contrast, with relatively frequent indications as carbon monoxide (CO) intoxication or chronic or subacute conditions, the situation is different and a well-designed clinical trial is achievable. For pediatric patients, an urgent need exists to establish clinical and scientific bases that will allow the rational use and administration of HBOT.

DEVICES USED FOR THE TREATMENT OF THE PEDIATRIC PATIENT

Oxygen Delivery and Mechanical Ventilation for Infants and Children

Administration of oxygen inside the chambers has been and still is performed in many different ways. One of the main concerns while providing oxygen under pressurized atmosphere is the "contamination" of the multiplace chamber with increasing oxygen concentrations and the resulting hazards. Many devices have been adapted to provide treatment to noncooperative infants and children to prevent this contamination.

- **Oxyhood:** This is commonly used for adult patients, as well as children, who are uncooperative or have facial deformities, but its use forces the hyperbaric team to do repeated "washouts" of the chamber to reduce oxygen contamination (Fig. 6.1). The number of washouts can be reduced when using a neck ring device that seals better,

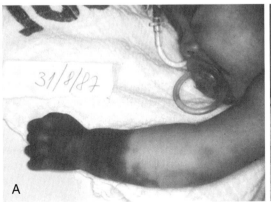 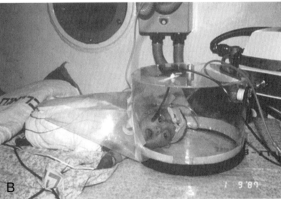

Figure 6.1 *A,* A case of a 6-month-old infant after an iatrogenic intra-arterial fluid infusion. A progressive improvement occurred after twice-daily hyperbaric oxygen treatments and concluded with the amputation of the distal phalanxes. *B,* Treatment was performed using a Perspex-made oxyhood. Frequent air flushes are required to prevent high oxygen concentrations within the chamber using this method. **(See Color Plate 1.)** *(Courtesy Israeli Naval Medical Institute and Dr. Yehuda Melamed.)*

or a device for small infants as designed by Aguiluz and Hill,[6] a mini-oxygen tent.

- **Masks:** The oxygen delivery system is adapted to patient capacity and cooperation. BIBS (Built-in Breathing System) demand masks and free-flow masks are available for nonassisted and cooperative children.
- **Mechanical ventilators:** For the mechanically assisted patient, many types of ventilators are in use in multiplace hyperbaric facilities. In his article, Kot[7] describes in detail the properties required if a ventilator is to be able to provide adequate flow during atmospheric pressure changes in the chamber, and lists the pressure-driven devices used in hyperbaric chambers. Out of his list of 24 types of ventilators that have been tested under hyperbaric conditions, some are capable of providing small volumes to ventilated infants with a weight of less than 5 kg (e.g., Servo 900 C [Siemens-Elema AB, Solna, Sweden], Evita 4 [Dräger Medical AG & Co., Lübeck, Germany]). At the Israel Navy Medical Institute and in the Asaf-Harofeh Medical Center, the Penlon-Oxford pneumatically driven ventilator (Penlon Ltd., Abingdon, Oxfordshire, United Kingdom), which was designed for adults, is in use with an adaptor for pediatric patients. Changes in ventilator settings are performed during HBOT according to volume measurement alterations during pressure changes, oxygen saturation, and blood gas monitoring of the patient. Blood gas monitoring is usually performed in nearby laboratory facilities when the samples are transferred through the chamber's medical air locks.

Airway Management

In any chamber where infants are treated, there must be an appropriate set of equipment for airway management. This includes all sizes of laryngoscope blades, from 0 upward, endotracheal tubes starting from 2.5, and a suction system including a manual device as a backup; appropriate sizes of suction catheters; airways; and, if possible, laryngeal masks. This equipment must be controlled regularly using a checklist procedure.

Monitoring Devices

Multiplace chambers usually can be equipped with all the medical devices required for the treatment of the critically ill patient. Monitoring devices can be inside the chamber if they run on batteries (for fire safety) and have been approved for work under pressure. They can be connected to the patient inside the chamber or, if possible, via specially prepared connections through the chamber wall, to place the monitor outside the chamber. Kot[8] listed numerous devices and equipment manufacturers. These devices include cardiac monitors, invasive and noninvasive blood pressure monitoring, and pulse oximetry, some including transcutaneous Po_2/Pco_2 monitoring and end-tidal CO_2 monitoring. Battery-operated fluid/drug infusion pumps must be available as well.

Drug and Fluid Administration

To provide appropriate care to an infant or child who requires the administration of fluids and drugs (cardiorespiratory or analgesia/anesthesia), an intensivist familiar with the age-specific requirements of the patient must be involved in the treatment. A list of drugs and fluids according to the treatment policies of the supporting neonatal and pediatric ICUs must be prepared in advance to provide real-time practical support to the team inside the chamber. This must be translated into a regular maintenance checklist for drugs and fluids kept inside the multiplace chamber, as well as a table with the dosages and formulation for quick-drip preparation (e.g., dopamine, dobutamine hydrochloride, morphine, midazolam hydrochloride) and preferred fluid management policies.

Thermoregulation

Temperature control inside the chamber must be tight to prevent hypothermia or hyperthermia in the smallest and youngest critically ill patients. Both can be detrimental. Specially designed air-conditioning systems are part of the newer multiplace chambers. Items of clothing that can produce static electricity, as well as any electrical heating devices, are prohibited in the chamber for reasons of fire safety.

Hyperbaric Chambers Used for Newborn Infants and Children

Small monoplace chambers were and are used for the treatment of many conditions in newborns and small infants. In some hyperbaric centers, an adult enters the monoplace chamber together with a ventilated infant to sustain ventilation using a self-inflating ventilation bag (Fig. 6.2). Monoplace chambers such as the type manufactured by Sechrist offer the possibility of mechanical ventilation with the patient inside while the caregivers are outside.

The hyperbaric specialist should consider that the use of monoplace chambers may endanger the patient when the need for airway management is crucial. For a ventilated young patient, caregivers must have the possibility of suctioning the airway when necessary or replacing the endotracheal tube if dislodged (a common scenario in neonatal and pediatric intensive care). A patient who is not ventilated, and is sick, is at risk for development of apnea or aspiration of secretions after vomiting or regurgitation during treatment. When isolated in a chamber, the patients are at extreme risk if these aspects are uncontrolled during treatment, and a sudden decrease in pressure in the chamber for any reason can jeopardize patient health. When treating sick newborn infants and young children, it must be clear that apnea and vomiting are frequent, and precautions must be taken in advance to protect the airway.

In 1966, in a study by Hutchinson and colleagues,[9] published in *The Lancet,* the use of a small hyperbaric chamber for the resuscitation of newborns who failed to breathe effectively 3 minutes after birth was compared with intubation and ventilation with a manual device. The study included 111 newborns in the control group (the intubated

ones) and 107 in the group who received hyperbaric oxygen for 30 minutes at 4 atmospheres absolute (ATA). The study included term and preterm infants, and the reported results showed no significant differences between the groups. Later, on the basis of that article, some authors discussed the effects of transcutaneous oxygenation achieved by HBOT in hypoxic infants. Not surprisingly, in a letter to the editor published in *The Lancet* many years later, Phillip James[10] recalls that the system became known as "the death chamber" in Glasgow, because staff witnessed the demise of several infants locked inside without a clear airway. In his letter, James mentions the need for the provision of artificial ventilation to prevent asphyxia in an infant who fails to breathe.

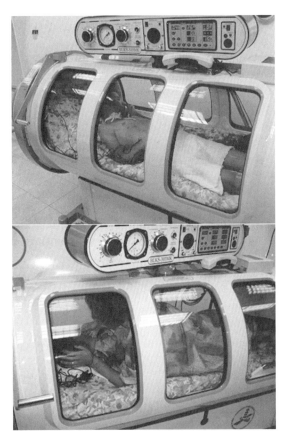

Figure 6.2 Treatment of a tracheostomized spontaneously breathing child with a parent in a monoplace chamber. A tender inside the chamber is necessary during treatment to prevent airway management complications. *(Courtesy Dr. Nachum Gall, Institute of Hyperbaric Medicine and Wound Care Center, Assaf Harofeh Medical Center, Zerifin, Israel.)*

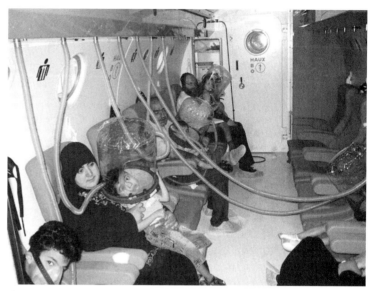

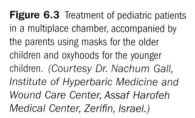

Figure 6.3 Treatment of pediatric patients in a multiplace chamber, accompanied by the parents using masks for the older children and oxyhoods for the younger children. *(Courtesy Dr. Nachum Gall, Institute of Hyperbaric Medicine and Wound Care Center, Assaf Harofeh Medical Center, Zerifin, Israel.)*

Temperature control is possible only in multiplace chambers, where air-conditioning systems are available. When hypothermia or hyperthermia is present, the morbidity and side effects of hyperbaric oxygen treatment for the smaller and younger patients may increase.

Multiplace chambers currently are the ideal way of giving appropriate HBOT to an infant or child. Almost all indications for HBOT in a neonate require airway control and management of the cardiorespiratory status. In older children, great concern no doubt exists about the possible lack of understanding of simple instructions, when alone in a monoplace chamber for an acute indication. In multiplace chambers, neonates and children can be treated for any eventuality and should be accompanied by two caregivers, one of which can be a relative, should the situation require it (Fig. 6.3).

ACCEPTED AND LISTED INDICATIONS FOR HYPERBARIC OXYGEN THERAPY

Indications relevant to pediatric patients, based on current clinical practice, are listed in many publications,[2-5] but the most accepted indications for HBOT are listed by the UHMS, and these are also relevant to newborn infants and children (Table 6.1).

Acute Carbon Monoxide Poisoning

CO is produced by the incomplete combustion of materials that contain carbon. CO poisoning is not uncommon among children and should be considered the possibility of concomitant exposure to cyanide in a CO poisoning.[11-18] The pathophysiology of CO poisoning is discussed in Chapter 15.

Clinical Signs and Symptoms of Acute Carbon Monoxide Intoxication

Clinical signs and symptoms of acute CO intoxication include headache, nausea and vomiting, dyspnea, vision abnormalities, muscular weakness, syncope, convulsions, coma, and death. Children may present with general symptoms such as nausea, vomiting, and diarrhea, and be mistakenly diagnosed as suffering from gastrointestinal disease.[13] Small infants can present with poor feeding, irritability, and vomiting. Many fire victims suffering from smoke inhalation and traumatic injuries may arrive in a coma and need mechanical ventilation. The history of exposure and the measurement of carboxyhemoglobin levels can

Table 6.1 Accepted Indications for Hyperbaric Oxygen Therapy Relevant to Newborn Infants and Children According to the Undersea and Hyperbaric Medical Society/ European Underwater and Baromedical Society

Acute carbon monoxide poisoning
Cyanide poisoning
Arterial (cerebral) gas embolism
Compartment syndrome; acute traumatic peripheral ischemia
Clostridial myonecrosis (gas gangrene) and necrotizing soft-tissue infections
Compromised skin flaps and grafts
Chronic or refractory osteomyelitis
Osteoradionecrosis; radiation-induced soft-tissue injury
Intracranial abscess
Chronic, nonhealing wounds
Decompression sickness
Exceptional blood loss (anemia)

help confirm the diagnosis. When there is unclear symptomatology in an individual patient without a clear history of exposure to a CO source, diagnosis may be difficult, but if the same situation is present in an entire family, diagnosis is much easier.

In a series of 28 pediatric CO exposures, Crocker and Walker[19] found a greater rate of lethargy and syncope at lower carboxyhemoglobin levels than expected, and they suggested that a carboxyhemoglobin level of 15% may be the threshold for neurologic changes in children. This assumption is not fully accepted because a combination of duration of exposure, type of source of CO, and delay between exposure and measurement of the carboxyhemoglobin levels[20] may be confounders.

The concentration of fetal hemoglobin in fetuses, newborns, or older children with hemoglobinopathies may increase susceptibility to CO intoxication because of a higher affinity and longer half-life.

Syndrome of Delayed Neurologic Sequelae

The syndrome of delayed neurologic sequelae (DNS), which can appear from 3 days to 3 weeks after recovery of an acute intoxication, is well known in children.[14,21] It is difficult to determine the incidence of DNS in the pediatric population. Kim and Coe[22] report that the incidence rate of DNS was 10.9% in their series of 107 Korean children with CO poisoning. In their study, DNS was more likely to occur in children presenting with coma than in those not in a coma. Other investigators report much lower incidence rates in children.[23] These variations probably reflect the small numbers of patients studied, the severity of poisoning, age at time of exposure, and baseline intellectual level, as well as the different causes of CO poisoning (e.g., fire victims have concurrent traumatic injuries, such as burns, which may result in hypotension and significant anoxia, and even go through a full resuscitation for cardiorespiratory arrest). This variability probably contributed to Meert and colleagues'[23] conclusions in their retrospective chart review article, in which they state, "Delayed neurologic syndromes are uncommon in children treated with normobaric oxygen"; however, the incidence rate of DNS in their study is 3%, excluding those who died or remained with permanent neurologic sequelae from the beginning. For a further discussion on the indications for treatment and DNS, see Chapter 15.

Treatment of Carbon Monoxide Intoxication in Pregnant Women and Fetal Outcome

Treatment of CO intoxication is indicated in the case of the pregnant patient to prevent neurologic damage to, or death of, both the mother and the fetus. Teratogenesis, neurologic damage, and increased risk for fetal death have been reported as a result of CO intoxication in animal experiments and from clinical data.[24-26] As mentioned earlier, fetal hemoglobin displays much higher affinity for binding CO molecules, thus worsening hypoxia at the cellular level, making the fetus much more susceptible.

Current recommendations are that HBOT should be administered if the mother has neurologic signs, if her carboxyhemoglobin level is greater than 15%, or if there are signs of fetal distress on the monitor.[27,28] The results of animal experiments involving prolonged exposures suggest that there is a possibility of teratogenicity induced by hyperbaric oxygen, but there has been no evidence of this in humans who received HBOT.[29] Concerning teratogenesis, retinopathy of prematurity (ROP), alterations in placental blood flow, and premature closure of the ductus arteriosus, these conditions have not been reported in pregnant women receiving HBOT for CO intoxication.[30] Currently, no clinical evidence exists of adverse effects on the fetus after HBOT in pregnant woman.

Clostridial Myonecrosis (Gas Gangrene) and Necrotizing Soft-Tissue Infections

Gas gangrene is a severe, rapidly progressing infection caused by specific clostridium strains, of which clostridium perfringens is the most common. Their systemic effects are produced by exotoxins, particularly alpha toxin (a lecithinase), which are able to destroy membranes and alter capillary permeability. Gas gangrene is most commonly seen in combat injuries,[31] as a result of soil contamination and entry of foreign bodies.[32] Hypoxic tissues caused by vascular compromise and vast soft-tissue damage provide the anaerobic environment required for the bacteria to proliferate.

A considerable number of cases can be found among the civilian adult and pediatric population, where clostridial myonecrosis may be associated with trauma, surgical procedures, venipunctures, insect bites, diagnostic gynecologic and urologic examinations, parenteral drug abuse, or de novo occurrence in the immunocompromised patient.[33-35]

Atraumatic infection with clostridium septicum has been reported in children suffering from different forms of neutropenia[36-38] (see Chapter 18).

Necrotizing Fasciitis

Necrotizing fasciitis, a rapidly progressive infection of the soft tissues, with typical sparing of the underlying muscle, may be produced by a combination of aerobic and anaerobic flora. Mortality is high, and progression of the disease is usually similar to that of clostridial myonecrosis, although less rapid. This type of infection is more common in immunocompromised adults and patients with diabetes, but it has also been described in neonates in association with omphalitis, necrotizing enterocolitis, varicella, staphylococcal skin infections, and balanitis after circumcision. The use of HBOT has been reported for newborns who experienced development of necrotizing fasciitis of the abdominal wall.[39] However, HBOT for necrotizing fasciitis remains controversial, most reports being retrospective analyses of adult patients.[40,41]

Purpura Fulminans

Purpura fulminans, a life-threatening, mutilating entity, was first described by Hjort.[42] It appears in the form of progressive purpuric lesions of the skin, mainly on the lower limbs, which eventually become necrotic. Purpura fulminans has been described in association with previous infection by varicella or streptococcus; sepsis or septic shock associated with *Escherichia coli, Haemophilus,* or meningococcus; and protein C or protein S deficiency. The development of disseminated intravascular coagulation with small-vessel thrombosis, and endothelial damage with massive capillary leak and bleeding into tissues and skin, may precede the patient's death or lead to peripheral ischemia and limb loss if the patient survives. There have been reports of a mortality rate as high as 90%.[43-47] Treatment of this overwhelming entity consists of the administration of steroids, anticoagulants, protein C concentrate, blood derivates, and antibiotics. Several authors report success in reducing mortality and the level of amputation of the limb by HBOT adjunctive to the intensive care treatment.[48-52] HBOT should be instituted as soon as possible, to reduce the extent of necrosis. The rationale for the use of HBOT is similar to that described for the treatment of acute peripheral ischemia (see Chapter 9) with tissue preservation until the main vascular axis is restored (Fig. 6.4).

Gas Embolism: Cerebral Arterial Gas Embolism

The introduction of air into the arterial system can result in cerebral air embolism, to which we refer because it can lead to severe neurologic damage and death. Signs and symptoms depend on the organ to which blood supply is arrested. Clinical presentation of iatrogenic cerebral arterial gas embolism (CAGE) may include coma, seizures, encephalopathic features, respiratory arrest, and sensory and motor deficits; but in many cases, especially during surgery, it occurs under general anesthesia, thus lacking clinical signs, and can be diagnosed only by the personnel who see the air entering the circulation through the tubing systems (intravenous lines or catheters from cardiac pumps, extracorporeal membrane oxygenator, etc.). These episodes lead to late neurologic sequelae. Sometimes diagnosis is made in a retrospective manner after signs of neurologic deficits after general anesthesia has been stopped.

Most cases of CAGE reported in the literature are iatrogenic, where embolism is the result of an invasive medical procedure or surgery. These include umbilical venous catheterization in newborns, the introduction of central venous lines, neurosurgical procedures, open-heart surgery, and pulmonary barotrauma as a complication of ventilator therapy.[53-55] CAGE may also be seen after diving as a result of pulmonary barotrauma or secondary to acute decompression. Although explosive decompression will probably be a nonexistent event in a pediatric patient, pulmonary barotrauma is potentially possible after the increase in the number of children (8- to 12-year-olds) SCUBA diving in shallow water.

Pulmonary barotrauma is often accompanied by vascular rupture. Air under high pressure can thus enter the systemic arterial vasculature, resulting in CAGE, as well as through the venous side. A large number of venous bubbles are introduced into the systemic circulation, either because of a preexisting right-to-left shunt (such as via a patent foramen ovale) or by overwhelming the pulmonary filtration mechanism.[56-60] This paradoxic arterial embolism in infants, children, or adults with cyanotic heart disease may even occur through peripheral IV lines, by which the air enters the systemic circulation.[61,62] This mechanism

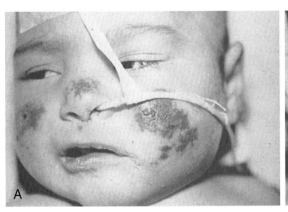
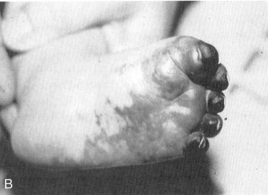

Figure 6.4 *A* and *B,* Progression of necrotic lesions of the face and lower extremities after purpura fulminans that significantly improved after hyperbaric oxygen treatment. **(See Color Plate 2.)** *(Courtesy Israeli Naval Medical Institute and Dr. Yehuda Melamed.)*

makes small infants with cyanotic congenital heart disease particularly susceptible to CAGE. For further discussion of the pathophysiology, diagnosis, and treatment of arterial gas embolism, see Chapter 13.

Unstable infants with congenital cyanotic heart disease are usually cared for in tertiary care centers where HBOT is readily available. If air transportation is necessary, the plane should be pressurized to 1 ATA, or if a helicopter is used, it should fly below 300 m to avoid bubble expansion and clinical deterioration. The hyperbaric physician should be involved in transportation arrangements. The fear of complications related to transportation should not prevent treatment. Permanent neurologic sequelae secondary to arterial gas embolism already exist, whereas transport-related complications are relatively low and are only a potential threat.[63]

Treatment for such complex cases is best performed in multiplace chambers, suitable for treatment with high-pressure capabilities and enough room for a team to provide ongoing intensive care. Monoplace chambers (which have limited pressure capabilities) have been used for arterial gas embolism; but in the case of infants or ventilated patients, its use can jeopardize the patient's safety when close airway supervision is necessary. A study was published confirming that its use in adult patients is safe and successful[64]; however, this approach should be avoided in newborn infants and young children.

Considering that CAGE is a complication that can occur during the treatment of small premature newborns, several aspects regarding their treatment should be taken into account when deciding about the possibility of HBOT: temperature control and active heating in the chamber may be difficult to achieve, ROP is a frequent complication in the very-low-birth-weight premature infant, and the effects of HBOT on the development of this pathology are not fully known. Thus, the initiation of HBOT for a very-low-birth-weight infant with extensive air embolism is still a difficult decision because of the complications and undesirable side effects of the treatment, as well as the possible liability of the teams involved because of the expected complications of severe prematurity, such as ROP and neurologic sequelae.

Refractory Osteomyelitis

Chronic osteomyelitis, which has persisted or recurred after appropriate interventions, or acute osteomyelitis, which fails to respond to intensive medical and surgical treatment within a reasonable period, may benefit from adjunctive HBOT. The therapeutic action of HBOT is associated with the improvement of oxygenation in infected ischemic and hypoxic tissue, thereby enhancing the white blood cell killing index and osteoclast activity, as well as potentiating the antibiotic action of the aminoglycosides. Reviews in the literature report that good results have been achieved with HBOT in the treatment of chronic refractory osteomyelitis in combination with appropriate surgical procedures and antibiotics.[65,66]

In many cases described in the medical literature, chronic protracted osteomyelitis developed in children suffering from debilitating diseases and not after multitrauma or acute hematogenous osteomyelitis. Some cases involved children with familial dysautonomia.[51] Usually, these patients need numerous treatments (up to 100 sessions) with the concomitant antibiotic and surgical care. Treatment needs to be continued until the wound is clean or, in some cases, until the tissue is ready for a skin transplant.

Decompression Sickness

No data in the medical literature concern the susceptibility of children to decompression and bubble formation. Most decompression tables are based on empirical data from animal research or adult divers, but none of the data relates to children. We also know that bubble formation can occur in shallow-water dives, attenuated during exercise. With the increasing accessibility to diving and future developments in aviation and space flight, there is a distinct possibility that pediatricians will be increasingly faced with this kind of problem. A few cases were reported in the literature concerning HBOT for suspected decompression sickness in children after a dive and traveling to higher locations.

Exceptional Blood Loss (Anemia)

Exceptional blood loss, anemia, occurs when sufficient blood is lost to compromise respiratory requirements. The most important consequence of severe anemia is cellular hypoxia as a result of the inadequate delivery of oxygen to tissues. Normally, blood or blood substitutes are infused to correct the deficiency. However, occasionally, a blood transfusion cannot be provided, for example, where there are religious reasons (Jehovah's Witnesses) or in the rare cases where it is difficult to obtain compatible blood for transfusion.

Under these conditions, HBOT is an effective, alternative treatment that can be provided until a more definitive solution is available. The rationale for the use of HBOT is based on the pioneer work of Boerema in the early 1960s. Boerema showed that treatment with HBOT up to 3 ATA sustained life in exsanguinated piglets, the blood was replaced by an acellular saline solution. The amount of oxygen dissolved in the intravascular solution, 6 volume percentage, was enough to sustain life.[67] Other animal studies using HBOT for severe anemia and hemorrhagic shock also showed beneficial results.[68,69]

Most of the clinical reports regarding the use of HBOT in severe anemia deal with Jehovah's Witnesses who seek alternatives to red blood cell transfusion. Hart[70] published several case reports and provided criteria for the selection of patients, as well as indications for HBOT in patients with anemia (systolic pressure lower than 90 mm Hg, alteration of mental status, signs of ischemic bowel, and signs of coronary syndrome). Treatment of severe anemia with HBOT should be performed early to address the accumulating oxygen debt. The use of air brakes is mandatory to prevent oxygen toxicity.[70,71] However, there are no reported cases of hyperbaric treatment in pediatric patients for this indication.

Intracranial Abscess

Brain and intracranial abscesses (epidural and subdural empyemas) in children are a rare but devastating condition. Outcomes have greatly improved with the development of the combination of new antibiotics and guided neurosurgical techniques; actual reported mortality rates of not more than 10%[72,73] have been reported for treatments that combine surgical intervention, correction of the primary source of infection, and long-term use of antibiotics.

The origin of a brain abscess can be hematogenous spread (bacteremia mainly in cyanotic heart disease or an immunocompromised host) or contiguous to a focus of infection (such as sinusitis).[74] The most frequent pathogens isolated from brain abscesses are streptococci, but 25% of the specimens do not grow pathogens.

Treatment including HBOT should be considered when there are multiple abscesses, abscesses in deep inaccessible locations, an immunocompromised host, contraindications for surgery, or when no good clinical response is achieved by initial treatment that included surgery or needle aspiration and wide-spectrum antibiotic treatment.[75]

Kurschel and colleagues[74] report the treatment of five children presenting with brain abscesses, four of them after sinusitis and one in an immunocompromised child with leukemia. All underwent combined and multidisciplinary treatment with favorable outcomes. HBOT was provided in twice-daily sessions at 2.2 ATA in 60-minute sessions. Patients completed a mean of 30 sessions before clinical and radiologic findings resolved. Patients were observed for a mean time of 21 months (range, 7–72 months). No recurrence was observed during that period. The authors concluded that HBOT in children with brain abscesses appears to be safe and effective, even when the abscesses are associated with subdural or epidural empyemas. It provides a helpful adjuvant tool in the usual multimodal treatment of cerebral infections. Multidisciplinary management is recommended to optimize care of these critically ill children.

Radiation and Cancer-Related Complications

The use and effectiveness of hyperbaric oxygen for *radiation-induced bone and soft-tissue complications* has been documented for adult patients.[76-78] Few studies aimed to analyze the results of adjuvant therapy with HBOT for pediatric patients. In a retrospective study, Ashamalla and coworkers[79] describe the outcome of 10 patients who received radiotherapy as children for head, neck, and pelvic cancer, subsequently receiving HBOT for later complications as adults. HBOT was shown to improve outcome when used as a prophylactic measure before maxillofacial or dental procedures that followed radiation therapy, as well as for difficult-to-heal wounds and bone necrosis after radiation therapy for bone and soft-tissue cancer (Ewing sarcoma, rhabdomyosarcoma). Most treatments were successful, and HBOT was shown to be safe, resulting in only a few significant adverse effects.

A trial for the reduction of *bone marrow edema* and *aseptic osteonecrosis* in pediatric patients with acute lymphoblastic leukemia and non–Hodgkin lymphoma was performed.[80] A reduction in pain scores and aseptic osteonecrosis lesions was shown, but no statistical significance was reached in the study.

NONLISTED/NONAPPROVED/ CONTROVERSIAL INDICATIONS FOR HYPERBARIC OXYGEN THERAPY

Hypoxic Ischemic Encephalopathy

The use of HBOT has been suggested as a neuroprotector after acute ischemic injury to the central nervous system, as, for example, after perinatal hypoxic-ischemic encephalopathy. Beneficial effects were shown in an animal model with rat pups subjected to ischemia, where the ischemic event was produced by unilateral carotid artery ligation and inhalation of 8% oxygen mixture.[81]

Empirical clinical experience was gained by many Chinese authors who provided HBOT to asphyxiated newborns within the first hours of the hypoxic-ischemic event. Liu and colleagues[82] evaluated several such publications using a systematic review of the Chinese literature, and their conclusion was that the use of hyperbaric oxygen in term neonates with hypoxic-ischemic encephalopathy reduces mortality and neurologic sequelae. However, most of the studies examined were of low scientific quality compared with western standards, which may introduce an element of bias as to the conclusions.

In an animal model of ischemic-hypoxic encephalopathy, Calvert and coworkers[83] showed that HBOT offered neuroprotection by reducing apoptosis in the injured brain tissue. The studies were performed in rat pups, subjected to unilateral carotid artery ligation followed by 2 hours of hypoxia (breathing 8% oxygen). Apoptotic cell death was examined using the TUNEL (terminal deoxynucleotide transferase-mediated deoxyuridine triphosphate nick-end labeling) staining technique in the tissue of the injured cortex and in the hippocampus tissue. Caspase-3 level (cysteine protease proenzymes subunit) was measured as an example of apoptotic activator. Its expression and activity were found to be increased 18 and 24 hours after the hypoxic-ischemic insult. A single HBOT session (100% oxygen, 3 ATA for 1 hour) was then provided. The results showed a reduction in the enhanced caspase-3 expression and activity, and a reduced number of TUNEL-positive cells were observed in the cortex and hippocampus. These results suggest that the neuroprotective effect of HBOT is at least partially mediated by the reduction in apoptosis. However, the treatment of newborns with oxygen is highly controversial, and there is increasing evidence from experimental work that resuscitation with 100% normobaric oxygen may be associated with an aggravation of cellular injury when compared with resuscitation in air. Some studies showed apparent increased brain injury, demonstrated by the leakage of glycerol in conjunction with a reduced antioxidant capacity in cerebral tissue, in animals resuscitated with 100% oxygen compared with those resuscitated in room air.[84-86]

Hepatic Artery Thrombosis after Liver Transplantation in Children

A case report has been published regarding an infant who underwent an orthotopic liver transplant (OLT) and experienced development of hepatic artery thrombosis.[87] Alteplase (TPA) failed to open the artery, so the child received systemic heparin and HBOT. After six HBOT sessions, the hepatic artery recanalized and the liver function tests returned to normal or near normal. There were no complications to the HBOT, and 1 year after the transplant, the child's liver still functioned normally.

A more extensive study reviewed 375 consecutive pediatric patients who underwent 416 OLTs.[88] Thirty-one patients (7.5%) acquired hepatic artery thrombosis at a mean time of 8.2 days (range, 1–52 days) after OLT. In 17 patients, HBOT was started within 24 hours of hepatic artery thrombosis or immediately after the revascularization attempt and performed twice daily for 90 minutes at 2.4 ATA. Fourteen patients were treated without using HBOT. None of the HBOT-treated patients experienced development of hepatic gangrene. Eight HBOT patients (47%) were bridged to retransplantation at a mean time of 157 days (range, 3–952 days) after initial OLT, and all survived. Mean time to retransplant in the control group was 12.7 days (range, 1–64 days). HBOT was well tolerated without significant complications. Although there was no significant difference in survival or retransplantation rates, HBOT significantly delayed the need for retransplantation.

Cerebral Palsy

Cerebral palsy (CP) is a term that describes a group of motor syndromes resulting from several insults sustained by the brain in early brain development. CP is caused by a broad group of developmental, genetic, metabolic, ischemic, infectious, and other acquired causative factors that produce a common group of neurologic phenotypes. Although it has historically been considered as a static encephalopathy, this term is now inaccurate because of the recognition that the neurologic features of CP often change over time. In addition, although CP is often associated with epilepsy and abnormalities of speech, vision, and intellect, it is the selective vulnerability of the brain's motor system that defines the disorder.[89-91]

CP is a common problem, the worldwide incidence being 2 to 2.5 per 1000 live births. The motor dysfunctions, which are the keystone of this clinical condition, can change with time. The changes are the result of neurologic maturation and are also attributed to continuous physical and behavioral therapy, as well as to corrective surgery.[90-92]

All available treatment, even if it is intensive, has only a moderate effect on the natural course of CP. Therefore, the introduction of HBOT with the theoretical benefit of improving the patient's condition beyond that expected of other treatment was tempting for many hyperbaric centers, as well as for many parents seeking alternative treatment to overcome this irreversible condition. Many severely affected children are already receiving numerous courses of HBOT in various centers worldwide, and even at home with privately purchased small chambers.

What place does HBOT take in the treatment of this condition? Montgomery and coworkers[93] conducted a pilot study using HBOT for infants with CP with encouraging results. The authors report some improvement in gross motor function, fine motor function, spasticity, and parental perception by questionnaire. The information regarding the claimed effects of hyperbaric oxygen and the possible benefit for handicapped children even encouraged a group of parents to establish an association that promotes HBOT for several neurologic conditions.[94]

In 1999, Collet and colleagues[95,96] performed the first multicenter study for CP comparing the use of HBOT with pressurized air. The treated group was given 100% oxygen at 1.75 ATA for 60 minutes, in 20 treatment sessions. The group that received air under pressure (1.3 ATA) received the same number of sessions. By the end of the study, both groups showed improvement in motor and cognitive functions, and the conclusion of the study was that there is no benefit from HBOT in CP. A heated debate between the supporters and the opponents of HBOT then started, as the supporters claimed that exposure to compressed air at 1.3 ATA increases the plasma oxygen tension from 95 to 148 mm Hg. Therefore, the control group underwent a certain degree of hyperoxic treatment, which influenced the results of the study, and for this reason cannot be regarded as a real control group. Currently, there are no conclusive studies that support HBOT for children with CP, and some studies even claim that HBOT may be detrimental for them.[84,97] Some research is ongoing that in due time will contribute to our knowledge on this subject.

When considering HBOT for patients with CP, it is necessary to remember that a significant proportion of the infants and children with this condition have CP related to prematurity or asphyxia. This group of patients is likely to have concomitant hyperactive airways as a result of bronchopulmonary dysplasia and from gastroesophageal reflux. These conditions can increase both the risk for pulmonary barotraumas, because of air trapped during decompression, and the risk for aspiration after vomiting. Fitness to "dive" and a caregiver inside the chamber must be preconditions of HBOT for such complex patients.

Hyperbaric Oxygen Therapy in Autism

Autism is a neurodevelopmental disorder characterized by impairment of social interaction, difficulty with communication, and restrictive and repetitive behaviors.[98] It affects children from all socioeconomic and ethnic backgrounds.[99,100] The cause of the disease is unknown, although a strong genetic component is suspected. Inheritance is complex, with more than one gene being involved.[101] Several risk factors have been shown to be implicated in this disease—maternal obstetric complications,[102] viral infection during pregnancy or in the postnatal period,[103] and immunologic abnormalities[104]—but a specific

causative factor has not been found. MMR vaccine has been thought to be associated with autistic disorders, but this has been disproved.[105]

It has been claimed that patients with autism have anomalies in regional blood flow of parts of the brain. Even in the presence of normal magnetic resonance imaging, a single-photon emission computed tomography scan will show areas of decreased blood flow, most notably in the temporal lobes.[106] This area often correlates with the clinical manifestations of the disease. A relation between decreased intelligence quotient and hypoperfusion of the temporal and frontal lobes has been described in patients with autism.[107] Based on these findings, HBOT has been proposed for the treatment of this spectrum of diseases[108]; in a report on a retrospective analysis of six children with autism who underwent HBOT, improvement in the range of 12% to 22% in some behavioral markers was observed.[108] A description of some anecdotal cases can be found on the Internet, but because no clinical trials are available, recommendations as to the usefulness of this treatment still cannot be made.

SIDE EFFECTS AND COMPLICATIONS REPORTED WITH REGARD TO HYPERBARIC OXYGEN THERAPY IN THE PEDIATRIC PATIENT

The side effects of hyperbaric oxygenation are related to pressure/volume changes and to oxygen toxicity. The most common side effects seen during hyperbaric treatment are those related to the increase of chamber pressure and the resultant volume changes in closed, gas-filled spaces (Boyle's Law). The middle ear, sinuses, and lung are commonly affected by pressure changes. *Middle ear and sinus barotrauma* are the injuries most frequently encountered, especially when congestion is present. They can usually be prevented by coaching the cooperative patient in ways to equilibrate middle-ear pressure and enhance eustachian tube function (swallowing, yawning, chewing, Frenzel or Valsalva maneuvers). Local or systemic decongestants can also be used. When indicated, for example, in the uncooperative young or comatose patient, tympanocentesis needs to be performed before HBOT. In a second report derived from the study on the effect of HBOT on CP patients, Muller-Bolla and coworkers[109] report that middle-ear barotrauma was the most frequent complication in 50% of the children with CP who received HBOT at 1.75 ATA and in 27.8% of the children with CP from the control group who received compressed air at 1.3 ATA. This happened even when children who had a recent episode of acute otitis media were excluded from the study. All children were instructed in the Valsalva technique, and in most cases, an adult was present in the chamber. Ear pain was the second most common side effect of HBOT (3.6% in the HBOT group).

Hypoxemia during the air breathing periods must be tightly controlled and prevented by oxygenation monitoring.[110]

Pulmonary barotrauma during decompression and pulmonary and central nervous system oxygen toxicity are rare, preventable complications during HBOT in the pediatric patient. These entities are discussed in Chapters 13 and 23.

Because of their susceptibility to ROP, preterm infants younger than 35 weeks' postconceptual age should be considered only with caution as candidates for HBOT at present, that is, until more data are available on the effects of HBOT on the developing retina. Funduscopic examination before the final decision before HBOT for a premature infant 32 to 33 weeks gestational age may reveal already developed retinal vessels and, therefore, a low risk for ROP development.

Oxygen has been the most common form of therapy given to newborn infants and children since the 1940s. Despite that, little is still known about how much infants actually need, or how much it is wise to give. A great degree of uncertainty remains in neonatal medicine concerning the use of normobaric oxygen, with a tight balance between oxygen levels and the fluctuation between the development of blindness after ROP with high, or poorly controlled, oxygen saturation level policies, and the increased incidence of CP and greater

mortality in premature low-birth-weight infants following low oxygen saturation policies.[111,112]

There are many animal studies with contradictory results concerning the effects of HBOT on the development of ROP. Torbati and colleagues[113] found that sustained HBOT-induced retinal vasoconstriction in newborn rats, followed by hypoxic-ischemic injury, might result in vascular proliferation, thereby initiating ROP development on return to air. In contrast, in a study performed on rat pups,[114] there were no abnormalities in the structure of the retina and no changes in the protein expression of hypoxia-inducible factor-1α and vascular endothelial growth factor after exposure to hyperoxia for 1 hour at normobaric or hyperbaric pressures; thus, this did not result in the structural changes or abnormal vascularization that is associated with ROP, suggesting that hyperoxia is a safe treatment for hypoxic newborns. However, it is necessary to consider the validity of this model when comparing the retinal development of rat pups with the degree of immaturity of the retina in premature infants.

Hypothermia and Hyperthermia

Thermoregulation and thermoprotection, which are of critical importance for the neonate and the infant, are also difficult to achieve and maintain in the hyperbaric environment. External warming techniques, such as the use of warm blankets or water-filled devices, may be used; heaters are not safe in the chamber.

Transport-Related Complications

In a series of ventilated patients, Keenan and coworkers[63] assessed the rate of complications induced by the management and transport of complex intensive care patients to a hyperbaric chamber for HBOT. They found no significant increase in complications related to this complex procedure.

Nuthall and colleagues[115] report on two patients with CP who experienced complications related to HBOT: one resulting in *aspiration* to the lungs after vomiting in the chamber, and the second with respiratory distress and convulsions caused by a cerebral infarction suspected to be temporally related to HBOT. In both cases, HBOT was related to the pathology in a temporal manner.

PREPARATION OF THE PATIENT BEFORE HYPERBARIC OXYGEN THERAPY

Although many of the complications and problems associated with HBOT are similar for adults and children (see Chapters 22–26), several issues are potentially unique to the pediatric population.

Children as young as 5 years of age can perform a pressure compensation maneuver ("clearing the ears") by closing both nose and mouth and elevating the pressure against a closed glottis. Younger or disoriented children, as well as infants, should undergo myringotomy to prevent middle- and inner-ear barotrauma. Giving an infant a bottle to suck is not a reliable method of equalizing pressure and can delay or jeopardize treatment.

In the majority of children, endotracheal intubation is performed using an uncuffed endotracheal tube. However, if the child is intubated with a low-pressure balloon, the air inside the balloon must be replaced by fluid. The same applies to a urinary bladder catheter.

Sometimes a child is frightened and unwilling to enter the chamber. In such cases, it is advisable to allow a family member to enter the chamber with the patient, after otoscopic examination and a chest radiograph have been performed exactly as for the patient.

Among the other special requirements of the pediatric patient in the hyperbaric chamber is the advance preparation, or adaptation, of medical instruments suited to the patient's age. Suitable oxygen delivery systems must also be made available, such as an oxyhood, or a free-flow or demand mask for the more cooperative child. Mechanical ventilators can be adapted or their settings changed when treating infants, to prevent pulmonary barotrauma.

REPORTS FROM DIFFERENT COUNTRIES ON THE TREATMENT OF THE PEDIATRIC PATIENT

Clinical Experience Reported by Russian Authors

A huge amount of clinical experience in the use of hyperbaric medicine for adults and pediatric patients has been reported by Russian authors. Large hyperbaric facilities have been built at many centers in Russia. Unfortunately, most of this medical experience was reported in a small number of publications, mainly in Russian, and using medical terms and concepts not totally accepted by "Occidental" medicine, or to be more exact, not in accordance with what we today call the more evidence-based medical treatment approach.

Baydin[1] has reported on the experience accumulated at the Russian State Medical University in Moscow with the treatment of 4500 children, including newborns and children up to 15 years of age. The main treatment indications for the use of HBOT related to surgical pathology. He reports that about 5000 HBOT sessions have been conducted in their clinic for this age group. HBOT has been used at their clinics since 1969 using a monoplace chamber under the direction of the Department of Pediatric Surgery and Resuscitation.

The main indications for treatment that Baydin[1] mentions in his review are peritonitis and necrotizing enterocolitis, crush injury and scalping wounds, and after abdominal surgery. HBOT is also mentioned as part of the treatment after resuscitation from cardiac and respiratory arrest.

The outcome for children treated with HBOT for multiple trauma, crush injury, and abdominal surgery was reviewed: 64 children were examined (32 treated with HBOT) after extensive multiple trauma and initial surgical intervention. The group treated with HBOT had faster wound healing, improved general condition, and shorter hospital stays. Extensive studies on wound healing in these patients were performed using the cellular composition of the exudates as markers for improvement. HBOT resulted in a reduction in the number of neutrophils of 19.4% and necrotic cells of 55.2%, as well as an increase in the number of macrophages and fibroblasts, thus shortening the time of wound healing. Baydin reports the treatment of 31 patients after crush injury, but their outcomes are not given in detail. The outcome of a group of 127 children who suffered from purulent peritonitis was compared with 118 control cases. No details of the groups are given, but the outcome is described as favorable for the HBOT group showing 2.8 times fewer postoperative complications, 1.4 times shorter wound healing time, plus shorter times in intensive care and in total hospital stay (1.6 and 1.2 times, respectively).

The same success was reported concerning 28 newborns with postoperative paralytic ileus. Bioelectrical activity of the bowel and functional recovery (general condition, stools) was faster in the treated group than in the control group. The bioelectrical activity of transposed bowel in esophagoplasty for esophageal atresia appeared earlier in the treated group; 75 infants with necrotizing enterocolitis showed earlier improvement in bowel function and 18% lower mortality, with 10 or more sessions depending on the stage of the disease (50% more sessions for stages 2 and 3). In stage 4, with intestinal perforation and peritonitis, HBOT did not show any effect. Because there is no mention of the demographic data of the patients, gestational age, and birth weight, and because necrotizing enterocolitis is more frequent in the range where ROP can occur, these reports raise questions about the possible side effects on the visual outcomes of these infants.

Sixty children who needed surgery for megacolon (there is no mention of the cause) received 8 to 10 sessions of HBOT as preparation for surgery. They did not receive HBOT after surgery. The treated group showed faster resolution of paralytic ileus (80% in the control group vs. 10% in the HBOT group), faster stool passage, fewer days in the ICU, decreased complication rate (5% vs. 35%, respectively),

and no deaths in the HBOT group compared with two deaths in the control group.

As for the use of HBOT during pregnancy and delivery, the authors reviewed a number of indications that are practically nonexistent in occidental medical practice, such as threatened abortion and fetoplacental insufficiency, fetal hypoxia and growth delay in pregnancies of women with heart disease, renal disorders, hypertension, anemia, and fetoplacental insufficiency. These pregnant women received 10 to 12 sessions of HBOT, and favorable outcomes were reported for the pregnancies compared with a control group. Deliveries complicated with toxemia, late gestation, diabetes, or congenital or acquired heart disease were managed inside the hyperbaric chamber, whether by vaginal delivery or by cesarean section, to prevent hypoxia in both the mother and fetus with cardiopulmonary pathology. Almost all of the mentioned cases were presented in medical meetings in the 1980s according to the references in Baydin's chapters,[1] but to the best of our knowledge, none of them was published in indexed medical journals.

It must be noted that no data were given on complications related directly to treatment or to the performance of the procedures inside the chamber (such as the immediate need for advanced procedures for neonatal or maternal resuscitation, infection rates, the need for assistance from more personnel at the scene, etc.). However, a number of the diseases mentioned have a completely different therapeutic approach in the medicine currently practiced in most countries.

Turkey

A total of 47 pediatric patients received HBOT at the Gulhane Military Medical Academy, Haydarpasa Training Hospital, between the years 2002 and 2006. Mean age of the patients was 8.7 ± 5 years (range, 10 months to 17 years). Thirty patients (63%) were treated for acute CO poisoning, whereas the rest of the patients received HBOT for sudden deafness (3 patients, 6%), crush injury (3 patients, 6%), nonhealing wound (2 patients, 4%), hypoxic-ischemic encephalopathy (2 patients, 4%), autism (2 patients, 4%), purpura fulminans (1 patient, 1%), facial nerve paralysis (1 patient, 2%), thermal burn (1 patient, 2%), near drowning (1 patient, 2%), and Perthes disease (1 patient, 2%).[116]

Israel

We reference here reports from two of the four hyperbaric facilities in Israel: Assaf Harofeh Hospital and the Israeli Naval Medical Institute. At Assaf Harofeh Hospital, between the years 1999 and 2005, 65 infants and children were treated with hyperbaric oxygen. A total of 32 (48%) patients were treated for CO intoxication, 7 (11%) for hypoxic brain damage (late treatment), 7 (11%) for CP, 5 (8%) for postirradiation necrosis, 3 (5%) for avascular necrosis, 2 (3%) for nonhealing wound, 2 (3%) for air embolism, 1 (2%) for compartment syndrome, 1 (2%) for brain abscess, 1 (2%) for autism, 1 (2%) for reflex sympathetic dystrophy, 1 (2%) for severe hypotonia (cerebral atrophy), 1 (2%) for acute ischemia (finger), and 1 (2%) for decompression sickness. The median age of this group of patients was 14 years (range, 3–18 years).

At the Israeli Naval Medical Institute, as previously published,[51] by far the most frequent reason for HBOT is related to CO intoxication during wintertime (more than 70% of the pediatric cases treated in this facility). This was followed by crush injury, acute peripheral ischemia, and reimplantation (9% of cases). All the other indications that are listed by the UHMS as accepted indications are mainly sporadic. The median age of the patients is 7.7 years (range, 2 months to 18 years). The policy of treating accepted indications only is still the current practice at this facility.

United States

More than 600 facilities, some hospital based, some military or privately owned, are spread throughout the United States. The practices in the United States are heterogeneous, but official policies are well known and established by regulatory organizations such as the UHMS, which publishes regular reports and position statements (http://www.uhms.org). Even though it is an international association, the statements released by this organization form the bases for many medical institutions and health insurance policies in the United States.

Advertisements in different media by many facilities mainly involved in wound healing treatment also offer treatment for children with CP and recently for those with autism (http://www.geocities.com/aneecp/hbocent.htm).

Canada

Twenty-six hyperbaric facilities are listed for Canada; some of these are public (in hospital, fire service, or naval establishments) and some private. Many of the private centers offer treatment for a wide range of diseases, including CP in children. The private chambers are often not listed at all. In the Vancouver area alone, which has 1,500,000 habitants, there are 6 active hyperbaric chambers. Between 2004 and 2006, 12 patients younger than 16 years received HBOT at the hyperbaric facilities at Vancouver General Hospital: 1 had soft-tissue radionecrosis, 2 had chronic refractory osteomyelitis, and the rest had CO poisoning.[117]

Switzerland, Austria, and Germany

Forty-five hyperbaric facilities are listed in Germany, Austria, and Switzerland; most of these centers offer treatment for the indications listed by the UHMS. There are no reports of HBOT for children apart from the UHMS indications.

SUMMARY

Pediatricians are not always aware of the potential benefit of HBOT in the treatment of the diseases for which it is indicated, whereas the HBOT staff is not always familiar with the specific management requirements of the pediatric patient, especially the critically ill patient. The physician inside the chamber who is caring for a ventilated, critically ill infant or child should have knowledge of this type of treatment, that is, of the required ventilator settings, of intubation or reintubation of the patient, and of medication management. A fundamental need exists for pediatricians and institutions engaged in pediatric health care to be actively involved in the decision-making process regarding HBOT in the pediatric patient. Wise decision making, based on an understanding of the known benefits of this modality, can reduce mortality and the severe sequelae of those diseases for which hyperbaric oxygen is indicated. As in most areas of medicine, we should be able to establish treatments on the basis of clinical and investigational evidence of their effectiveness. This is not always possible, but the tendency to base new modalities, mainly for nonemergency indications, on clinical trials should be encouraged.

REFERENCES

1. Baydin SA: Hyperbaric oxygen therapy in pediatric surgery and hyperbaric oxygenation in obstetrics and neonatology. In: Jain KK (ed): Textbook of Hyperbaric Medicine, 3rd ed. Toronto, Hogrefe & Huber Publishers, 1999, chapters 27 and 31.
2. Thombs PA, Martorano FJ: Hyperbaric medicine in pediatric practice. In: Kindwall EP (ed): Hyperbaric Medicine Practice. Flagstaff, Ariz, Best Publishing Company, 1995, pp 261-275.
3. Santamaria JP, Williams ET III, Desautels DA: Hyperbaric oxygen therapy in pediatrics. Adv Pediatr 42:335-366, 1995.
4. Sukoff MH, Gottlieb SF: Hyperbaric oxygen therapy. In: Nussbaum E (ed): Pediatric Intensive Care, 2nd ed. Mount Kisko, NY, Futura Publishing Company, 1989, pp 483-507.
5. Tibbles PM, Edelsberg JS: Hyperbaric-oxygen therapy. N Engl J Med 334:1642-1648, 1996.
6. Aguiluz L, Hill RK: Alternate method of oxygen delivery for neonatal use. J Hyperb Med 5:259-261, 1990.
7. Kot J: Medical equipment for multiplace hyperbaric chambers. Part II: Ventilators. Eur J Underwater Hyperb Med 7:9-12, 2006.
8. Kot J: Medical equipment for multiplace hyperbaric chambers. Part I: Devices for monitoring and cardiac support. Eur J Underwater Hyperb Med 6:115-120, 2005.
9. Hutchinson JH, Kerr MM, Inall JA, Shanks RA: Controlled trials of hyperbaric oxygen and tracheal intubation in asphyxia neonatorum. Lancet 7444:935-939, 1966.
10. James PB: Hyperbaric oxygen in neonatal care. Lancet 1:764-765, 1988.
11. Zimmerman SS, Truxal B: Carbon monoxide poisoning. Pediatrics 68:215-224, 1981.
12. Gozal D, Ziser A, Shupak A, Melamed Y: Accidental carbon monoxide poisoning. Emphasis on hyperbaric oxygen treatment. Clin Pediatr (Phila) 24:132-135, 1985.
13. Gemelli F, Cattani R: Carbon monoxide poisoning in childhood. Br Med J 291:1197, 1985.
14. Binder JW, Roberts RJ: Carbon monoxide intoxication in children. Clin Toxicol 16:287-295, 1980.
15. Parish RA: Smoke inhalation and carbon monoxide poisoning in children. Pediatr Emerg Care 2:36-39, 1986.
16. Ascone DS, Marcy NE: Non-fire carbon monoxide deaths associated with the use of consumer products: 2002 annual estimates. US Consumer Product Safety Commission (Bethesda, Md). Available at http://www.cpsc.gov/library/data.html. Accessed December 19, 2007.
17. Baud FJ, Barriot P, Toffis V, et al: Elevated blood cyanide concentrations in victims of smoke inhalation. N Engl J Med 325:1761-1766, 1991.
18. Yeoh MJ, Braitberg G: Carbon monoxide and cyanide poisoning in fire related deaths in Victoria, Australia. J Toxicol Clin Toxicol 42:855-863, 2004.
19. Crocker PJ, Walker JS: Pediatric carbon monoxide toxicity. J Emerg Med 3:443-448, 1985.
20. Liebelt EL: Hyperbaric oxygen therapy in childhood carbon monoxide poisoning. Curr Opin Pediatr 11:259-264, 1999.
21. Lacey DJ: Neurologic sequelae of acute carbon monoxide intoxication. Am J Dis Child 135:145-147, 1981.
22. Kim JK, Coe CJ: Clinical study on carbon monoxide intoxication in children. Yonsei Med J 28:266-273, 1987.
23. Meert KL, Heidemann SM, Sarnaik AP: Outcome of children with carbon monoxide poisoning treated with normobaric oxygen. J Trauma 44:149-154, 1998.
24. Ginsberg MD, Myers RE: Fetal brain injury after maternal carbon monoxide intoxication: Clinical and neuropathologic aspects. Neurology 26:15-23, 1976.
25. Muller GL, Graham S: Intrauterine death of the fetus due to accidental carbon monoxide poisoning. N Engl J Med 252:1075-1078, 1955.
26. Koren G, Sharav T, Pastuszak A, et al: A multicenter, prospective study of fetal outcome following accidental carbon monoxide poisoning in pregnancy. Reprod Toxicol 5:397-403, 1991.
27. Ginsberg MD, Myers RE: Fetal brain injury after maternal carbon monoxide intoxication. Clinical and neuropathologic aspects. Neurology 26:15-23, 1976.
28. Van Hoesen KB, Camporesi EM, Moon RE, et al: Should hyperbaric oxygen be used to treat the pregnant patient for acute carbon monoxide poisoning? A case report and literature review. JAMA 261:1039-1043, 1989.
29. Elkharrat D, Raphael JC, Korach JM, et al: Acute carbon monoxide intoxication and hyperbaric oxygen in pregnancy. Intensive Care Med 17:289-292, 1991.
30. Van Hoesen KB, Camporesi EM, Moon RE, et al: Should hyperbaric oxygen be used to treat the pregnant patient for acute carbon monoxide poisoning? A case report and literature review. JAMA 261:1039-1043, 1989.

31. Workman WT, Calcote RD: Hyperbaric oxygen therapy and combat casualty care: A viable potential. Milit Med 154:111-115, 1989.

32. Melamed Y, Bursztein S: Hyperbaric medicine. In: Reis ND, Dolev E (eds): Manual of Disaster Medicine. Civilian and Military. Berlin, Springer-Verlag, 1989, pp 149-160.

33. Kuncir EJ: Necrotizing soft-tissue infections. Emerg Med Clin North Am 21:1075-1087, 2003.

34. Frank G: Musculoskeletal infections in children. Pediatr Clin North Am 52:1083-1106, 2005.

35. Hart GB, Lamb RC, Strauss MB: Gas gangrene: I. A collective review. II. A 15-year experience with hyperbaric oxygen. J Trauma 23:991-1000, 1983.

36. Seidel M, Weiss M, Nicolai T, et al: Gas gangrene and congenital agranulocytosis. Pediatr Infect Dis J 9:437-440, 1990.

37. Bar-Joseph G, Halberthal M, Sweed Y, et al: Clostridium septicum infection in children with cyclic neutropenia. J Pediatr 131:317-319, 1997.

38. Smith-Slates CL, Bourque M, Salazar JC: Clostridium septicum infections in children: A case report and review of the literature. Pediatrics 117:e796-e805, 2006.

39. Sawin RS, Schaller RT, Tapper D, et al: Early recognition of neonatal abdominal wall necrotizing fasciitis. Am J Surg 167:481-484, 1994.

40. Riseman JA, Zamboni WA, Curtis A, et al: Hyperbaric oxygen therapy for necrotizing fasciitis reduces mortality and the need for debridements. Surgery 108:847-850, 1990.

41. Shupak A, Shoshani O, Goldenberg I, et al: Necrotizing fasciitis: An indication for hyperbaric oxygenation therapy? Surgery 118:873-878, 1995.

42. Hjort PF, Rapaport SI, Jorgensen L: Purpura fulminans. Report of a case successfully treated with heparin and hydrocortisone. Review of 50 cases from the literature. Scand J Haematol 1:169-192, 1964.

43. Dudgeon DL, Kellogg DR, Gilchrist GS, Woolley MM: Purpura fulminans. Arch Surg 103:351-358, 1971.

44. Canale ST, Ikard ST: The orthopaedic implications of purpura fulminans. J Bone Joint Surg 66:764-769, 1984.

45. Watson CHC, Ashworth MA: Growth disturbance and meningococcal septicemia. Report of two cases. J Bone Joint Surg 65:1181-1183, 1983.

46. Nogi J: Physeal arrest in purpura fulminans. A report of three cases. J Bone Joint Surg 71:929-931, 1989.

47. Mahasandana C, Suvatte V, Chuansumrit A: Homozygous protein S deficiency in an infant with purpura fulminans. J Pediatr 117:750-753, 1990.

48. Kuzemko JA, Loder RE: Purpura fulminans treated with hyperbaric oxygen. Br Med J 4:157, 1970.

49. Rosenthal E, Benderly A, Monies-Chass I, et al: Hyperbaric oxygenation in peripheral ischaemic lesions in infants. Arch Dis Child 60:372-374, 1985.

50. Dollberg S, Nachum Z, Klar A, et al: Haemophilus influenzae type B purpura fulminans treated with hyperbaric oxygen. J Infect 25:197-200, 1992.

51. Waisman D, Shupak A, Weisz G, Melamed Y: Hyperbaric oxygen therapy in the pediatric patient: The experience of the Israel Naval Medical Institute. Pediatrics 102:E53, 1998.

52. Krzelj V, Petri NM, Mestrovic J, et al: Purpura fulminans successfully treated with hyperbaric oxygen—a report of 2 cases. Pediatr Emerg Care 21:31-34, 2005.

53. Daneman A, Abou-Reslan W, Jarrin J, et al: Sonographic appearance of cerebral vascular air embolism in neonates: Report of two cases. Can Assoc Radiol J 54:114-117, 2003.

54. VanRynen JL, Taha AM, Ehrlich R, Parlette DM: Treatment of cerebral air embolism in the pediatric patient. J Hyperb Med 2:199-204, 1987.

55. Kol S, Ammar R, Weisz G, Melamed Y: Hyperbaric oxygenation for arterial air embolism during cardiopulmonary bypass. Ann Thorac Surg 55:401-403, 1993.

56. Fok TF, Shing MK, So LY, Leung RKW: Vascular air embolism—possible survival. Acta Paediatr Scand 79:856-859, 1990.

57. Stoney WS, Alford WC Jr, Burrus GR, et al: Air embolism and other accidents using pump oxygenators. Ann Thorac Surg 29:336-340, 1980.

58. Marini JJ, Culver BH: Systemic gas embolism complicating mechanical ventilation in the adult respiratory distress syndrome. Ann Intern Med 110:699-703, 1989.

59. Lau KY, Lam PKL: Systemic air embolism: A complication of ventilator therapy in hyaline membrane disease. Clin Radiol 43:16-18, 1991.

60. Banagale RC: Massive intracranial air embolism: A complication of mechanical ventilation. Am J Dis Child 134:799-800, 1980.

61. LeDez KM, Zbitnew G: Hyperbaric treatment of cerebral air embolism in an infant with cyanotic congenital heart disease. Can J Anesth 52:403-408, 2005.

62. Heckmann JG, Lang CJ, Kindler K, et al: Neurologic manifestations of cerebral air embolism as a complication of central venous catheterization. Crit Care Med 28:1621-1625, 2000.

63. Keenan HT, Bratton SL, Norkool DM, et al: Delivery of hyperbaric oxygen therapy to critically ill, mechanically ventilated children. J Crit Care 13:7-12, 1998.

64. Weaver LK: Monoplace hyperbaric chamber use of U.S. Navy Table 6: A 20-year experience. Undersea Hyperb Med 33:85-88, 2006.

65. Kaplan SL: Osteomyelitis in children. Infect Dis Clin North Am 19:787-797, 2005.

66. Mader JT, Adams KR, Wallace WR, Calhoun JH: Hyperbaric oxygen as adjunctive therapy for osteomyelitis. Infect Dis Clin North Am 4:433-440, 1990.

67. Boerema I, Meijne NG, Brummelkamp WH, et al: Life without blood. J Cardiovasc Surg 182:133-146, 1960.

68. Martzella L, Yin A, Darlington D, et al: Hemodynamic responses to hyperbaric oxygen administration in a rat model of hemorrhagic shock. Circ Shock 37:12, 1992.

69. Adir Y, Bitterman N, Katz E, et al: Salutary consequences of oxygen therapy or long-term outcome of hemorrhagic shock in awake, unrestrained rats. Undersea Hyperb Med 22:23-30, 1995.

70. Hart GB: Hyperbaric oxygen and exceptional blood loss anemia. In: Kindwall EP, Whalen HT (eds): Hyperbaric Medicine Practice, 2nd ed. rev. Flagstaff, Ariz, Best Publishing, 2002, pp 744-751.

71. Van Meter KW: A systematic review of the application of hyperbaric oxygen in the treatment of severe

anemia: An evidence-based approach. Undersea Hyperb Med 32:61-83, 2005.

72. Mathisen GE, Johnsos JP: Brain abscess. Clin Infect Dis 25:763-779, 1997.

73. Rosenblum ML, Hoff JT, Norman D, Weinstein PR: Decreased mortality from brain abscesses since advent of computerized tomography. J Neurosurg 49:658-668, 1978.

74. Kurschel S, Mohia A, Weigl V, Eder HG: Hyperbaric oxygen therapy for the treatment of brain abscess in children. Childs Nerv Syst 22:38-42, 2005.

75. Jacoby I: Intracranial abscess. In: Feldmeier JJ (ed): Hyperbaric oxygen 2003. Indications and results. The Hyperbaric Oxygen Therapy Committee report. Kensington, Md, Undersea and Hyperbaric Medical Society, 2003, pp 63-67.

76. Davis JC, Dunn JM, Gates GA, Heimbach RD: Hyperbaric oxygen. A new adjunct in the management of radiation necrosis. Arch Otolaryngol 105:58-61, 1979.

77. David LA, Sandor GK, Evans AW, Brown DH: Hyperbaric oxygen therapy and mandibular osteoradionecrosis: A retrospective study and analysis of treatment outcomes. J Can Dent Assoc 67:384, 2001.

78. Gal TJ, Yueh B, Futran ND: Influence of prior hyperbaric oxygen therapy in complications following microvascular reconstruction for advanced osteoradionecrosis. Arch Otolaryngol Head Neck Surg 129:72-76, 2003.

79. Ashamalla HL, Thom SR, Goldwein JW: Hyperbaric oxygen therapy for the treatment of radiation-induced sequelae in children. The University of Pennsylvania experience. Cancer 77:2407-2412, 1996.

80. Bernbeck B, Christaras A, Krauth K, et al: Bone marrow oedema and aseptic osteonecrosis in children and adolescents with acute lymphoblastic leukaemia or non-Hodgkin-lymphoma treated with hyperbaric-oxygen-therapy (HBO): An approach to cure? BME/AON and hyperbaric oxygen therapy as a treatment modality. Klin Padiatr 216:370-378, 2004.

81. Calvert JW, Yin W, Patel M, et al: Hyperbaric oxygenation prevented brain injury induced by hypoxia-ischemia in a neonatal rat model. Brain Res 951:1-8, 2002.

82. Liu Z, Xiong T, Meads C: Clinical effectiveness of treatment with hyperbaric oxygen for neonatal hypoxic-ischaemic encephalopathy: Systematic review of Chinese literature. BMJ 333:374, 2006.

83. Calvert JW, Zhou C, Nanda A, Zhang JH: Effect of hyperbaric oxygen on apoptosis in neonatal hypoxia-ischemia rat model. J Appl Physiol 95:2072-2080, 2003.

84. Essex C: Hyperbaric oxygen and cerebral palsy: No proven benefit and potentially harmful. Dev Med Child Neurol 45:213-215, 2003.

85. Temesvari P, Karg E, Bodi I: Impaired early neurologic outcome in newborn piglets reoxygenated with 100% oxygen compared with room air after pneumothorax-induced asphyxia. Pediatr Res 49:812-819, 2001.

86. Munkeby BH, Borke WB, Bjornland K, et al: Resuscitation with 100% O2 increases cerebral injury in hypoxemic piglets. Pediatr Res 56:783-790, 2004.

87. Grover I, Conley L, Alzate G, et al: Hyperbaric oxygen therapy for hepatic artery thrombosis following liver transplantation: Current concepts. Pediatr Transplant 10:234-239, 2006.

88. Mazariegos GV, O'Toole K, Mieles LA, et al: Hyperbaric oxygen therapy for hepatic artery thrombosis after liver transplantation in children. Liver Transpl Surg 5:429-436, 1999.

89. Haslam RHA: The nervous system: Cerebral palsy. In: Behrman RE, Kliegman RM, Jenson HB (eds): Nelson Textbook of Pediatrics Online, 17th ed. New York, Elsevier, 2006. Available at http://www.nelsonpediatrics.com.

90. Keogh JM, Badawi N: The origins of cerebral palsy. Curr Opin Neurol 19:129-134, 2006.

91. Mutch L, Alberman E, Hagberg B, et al: Cerebral palsy epidemiology: Where are we now and where are we going? Dev Med Child Neurol 34:547-551, 1992.

92. Lawson RD, Badawi N: Etiology of cerebral palsy. Hand Clin 19:547-556, 2003.

93. Montgomery D, Goldberg J, Amar M, et al: Effects of hyperbaric oxygen therapy on children with spastic diplegic cerebral palsy: A pilot project. Undersea Hyperb Med 26:235-242, 1999.

94. MUMS National Parent-to-Parent Network: Available at www.netnet.net/mums/. Accessed December 19, 2007.

95. Collet JP, Vanasse M, Marois P, et al: Hyperbaric oxygen for children with cerebral palsy: A randomized multi-centre trial. Lancet 357:582-586, 2001.

96. Hardy P, Collet JP, Goldberg J, et al: Neuropsychological effects of hyperbaric oxygen therapy in cerebral palsy. Dev Med Child Neurol 44:436-446, 2002.

97. Rosenbaum P: Controversial treatment of spasticity: Exploring alternative therapies for motor function in children with cerebral palsy. J Child Neurol 18:S89-S94, 2003.

98. Tuchman R: Autism. Neurol Clin 21:915-932, 2003.

99. Rapin I: Autism. N Engl J Med 337:97, 1997.

100. Centers for Disease Control and Prevention: How common is autism spectrum disorder? Available at www.cdc.gov/od/oc/media/pressrel/2007/r070208.htm. February 8, 2007. Accessed December 19, 2007.

101. Risch N, Spiker D, Lotspeich L, et al: A genomic screen of autism: Evidence for a multilocus etiology. Am J Hum Genet 65:493-507, 1999.

102. Glasson EJ, Bower C, Petterson B, et al: Perinatal factors and the development of autism: A population study. Arch Gen Psychiatry 61:618-627, 2004.

103. Wilkerson DS, Volpe AG, Dean RS, Titus JB: Perinatal complications as predictors of infantile autism. Int J Neurosci 112:1085-1098, 2002.

104. Korvatska E, Van de Water J, Anders TF, Gershwin ME: Genetic and immunologic considerations in autism. Neurobiol Dis 9:107-125, 2002.

105. Madsen KM, Hviid A, Vestergaard M, et al: A population-based study of measles, mumps, and rubella vaccination and autism. N Engl J Med 347:1477-1482, 2002.

106. Ohnishi T, Matsuda H, Hashimoto T, et al: Abnormal regional cerebral blood flow in childhood autism. Brain 123:1838-1844, 2000.

107. Hashimoto T, Sasaki M, Fukumizu M, et al: Single-photon emission computed tomography of the brain in autism: Effect of the developmental level. Pediatr Neurol 23:416-420, 2000.

108. Rossignol DA, Rossignol LW: Hyperbaric oxygen therapy may improve symptoms in autistic children. Med Hypotheses 67:216-228, 2006.

109. Muller-Bolla M, Collet JP, Ducruet T, Robinson A: Side effects of hyperbaric oxygen therapy in children with cerebral palsy. Undersea Hyperb Med 33:237-244, 2006.

110. Weaver LK, Churchil SK: Hypoxemia with air breathing periods in U.S. Navy treatment Table 6. Undersea Hyperb Med 33:11-15, 2006.

111. Tin W: Oxygen therapy: 50 years of uncertainty. Pediatrics 110:615-616, 2002.

112. Silverman WA: A cautionary tale about supplemental oxygen: The albatross of neonatal medicine. Pediatrics 113:394-396, 2004.

113. Torbati D, Peyman GA, Wafapoor H, et al: Experimental retinopathy by hyperbaric oxygenation. Undersea Hyperb Med 22:31-39, 1995.

114. Calvert JW, Zhou C, Zhang JH: Transient exposure of rat pups to hyperoxia at normobaric and hyperbaric pressures does not cause retinopathy of prematurity. Exp Neurol 189:150-161, 2004.

115. Nuthall G, Seear M, Lepawsky M, et al: Hyperbaric oxygen therapy for cerebral palsy: Two complications of treatment. Pediatrics 106:e80, 2000.

116. Dr. Senol Yildiz: Department of Underwater and Hyperbaric Medicine, GMMA Haydarpasa Training Hospital, Istanbul, Turkey. Personal communication, September 2006.

117. Dr. David Harrison: VGH Hyperbaric Unit, Vancouver, British Columbia, Canada. Personal communication, September 2006.

Critical Care of Patients Needing Hyperbaric Oxygen Therapy

7

Lindell Weaver, MD

Not all hospital-based hyperbaric medicine departments offer management of critically ill patients. It is imperative that those hyperbaric medicine departments that treat, or offer to treat, critically ill patients have the appropriate equipment, certified personnel, and proximity to important hospital services, so that there is no decrement in the level of care delivered to the critically ill patient. Hyperbaric oxygen therapy (HBOT) is at a disadvantage treating critically ill patients because typical intensive care unit (ICU)–related equipment has not been designed or intended for the care of critically ill patients in the hyperbaric environment.

DEFINITION OF CRITICAL CARE

Critical care may bring up different images. It may include the patient at risk for worsening of his or her condition, with concomitant increase in morbidity and mortality. It may include anyone residing within an ICU. For purposes of this chapter, critical care connotes those patients who are intubated and mechanically ventilated.

DISORDERS TREATED WITH HYPERBARIC OXYGEN THAT MAY OCCUR OR CAUSE CRITICAL ILLNESS

Disorders for which HBOT is indicated[1] that may cause critical illness include severe infections (gas gangrene with myonecrosis and necrotizing fasciitis), acute carbon monoxide poisoning, crush injury, severe decompression sickness, and gas embolism. Hyperbaric oxygen may also be indicated and used in critically ill patients with acute compromised grafts or flaps, osteomyelitis, diabetic lower extremity ulcers, and acute arterial insufficiency. The *Hyperbaric Oxygen Therapy Committee Report* of the Undersea and Hyperbaric Medical Society (www.uhms.org) reviews the indications and rationale for hyperbaric oxygen in several conditions.[1]

Determining whether a critically ill patient needs or will benefit from HBOT must be bal-

anced by the risk of removing and transporting the patient from the well-controlled intensive care environment, as well as the risk of HBOT.[1] Risks to critically ill patients undergoing transport have been well-documented.[2,3] Information exists about methods of reducing intrahospital transport risk.[4] Nevertheless, when the patient is removed from the ICU, unforeseeable risks can ensue. The benefit with HBOT ideally should be apparent from clinical trials and experience.

GAS EXCHANGE AND TREATMENT PROTOCOLS

Various HBOT protocols are used in critically ill patients. The *Hyperbaric Oxygen Therapy Committee Report*[1] provides guidelines about typical treatment pressures and durations. For some disorders, more than one protocol has been described; currently, however, it is unknown whether one is superior to another.

Lung dysfunction, often manifested in critically ill patients, is an important variable that may influence efficacy of treatment. An intubated patient who needs a fractional inspired oxygen concentration (FI_{O_2}) of 0.3 would be expected to have significantly different arterial oxygen tensions at any given dose of hyperbaric oxygen compared with a patient who requires an FI_{O_2} of 0.7.[5] If the patient has a high right-to-left shunt because of profound lung dysfunction or a main-stem intubation, that patient's arterial oxygen tension during hyperbaric oxygen may be far lower than expected.[5,6]

Some centers routinely measure arterial oxygen tensions of intubated patients via indwelling arterial catheters. Continuous monitoring allows careful adjustment of hyperbaric oxygen dose, the amount of positive end-expiratory pressure (PEEP), and the degree of sedation or paralysis. A reasonable goal with modifications is to maintain the arterial oxygen tension during hyperbaric oxygen between 1000 and 1400 torr, a value typically observed when individuals with normal cardiopulmonary function are exposed to HBOT. If the arterial oxygen tension fails to achieve at least 800 torr, it may be prudent to refrain from using HBOT until lung function improves.

The measurement of arterial oxygen tension while patients undergo HBOT can be performed accurately with instrumentation that remains at atmospheric pressure if strict protocols are followed. For example, a validated technique was described using the ABL 330 (Radiometer, Copenhagen, Denmark).[5,7,8] Unfortunately, this instrument is no longer produced, and the manufacturer does not support its maintenance. A newer device, the ABL 525 (Radiometer), did not perform as well as the ABL 330, but for gas tensions less than 1500 torr, it may be adequate for clinical decision making.[9] The new generation ABL 800 may function better, but this has not been validated using hyperbaric tonometry experiments. Clearly, other devices could be investigated and may function adequately, but published validation trials do not currently exist.

TISSUE OXYGEN MEASUREMENTS

In the future, tissue oxygen measurements may be found to be helpful to predict response and outcomes after HBOT. Implantable oxygen sensors exist, but again, clinical trials are lacking.[10]

TRANSCUTANEOUS MEASUREMENTS OF OXYGEN AND CARBON DIOXIDE

Transcutaneous oxygen measurements during HBOT are routine, and Food and Drug Administration–approved devices exist for use in monoplace and multiplace chambers (Tina, Radiometer). The measurement of oxygen tension of patients with ischemic wounds may predict outcome.[11,12] Whether these measurements can be used as surrogates for arterial blood gas measurements has been examined in a small trial of healthy adults. Chest transcutaneous oxygen measurements were found to correlate with arterial oxygen tensions ($R^2 = 0.99$) in 10 healthy subjects. When subjected to HBOT at 1.12 to 3.0 atmospheres absolute (ATA), the transcutaneous oxygen values were less than arterial oxygen tensions by approximately 10%. The transcutaneous carbon dioxide tensions were 2 to 6

torr (0.3–0.8 kPa) greater than the arterial carbon dioxide tensions, but the correlation was moderate ($R^2 = 0.21$).[13]

Chest transcutaneous oxygen and carbon dioxide measurements have been described in 17 critically ill patients undergoing HBOT.[14] Among these patients, 13 were intubated and 8 were receiving continuous infusions of vasoactive drugs to maintain arterial blood pressure and cardiac output. Before HBOT, the patients had a mean arterial oxygen/F_{IO_2} (P/F) ratio of 237 $\pm$ 141, minute ventilation (V_E) of 9.1 $\pm$ 2 L/min, and PEEP of 6.5 $\pm$ 2.4 cm H_2O, and the chest transcutaneous oxygen correlated with arterial oxygen tensions ($R^2 = 0.89$). As with healthy subjects, while undergoing HBOT, these patients demonstrated transcutaneous oxygen values that were less than arterial oxygen tensions by approximately 10%. The transcutaneous carbon dioxide tensions were approximately 10% less than arterial carbon dioxide tensions, although the correlation was moderate ($R^2 = 0.66$).[14] These limited data suggest that, in some critically ill patients, chest transcutaneous oxygen and carbon dioxide measurements may be acceptable for clinical decision making.

HYPOXEMIA AFTER HYPERBARIC OXYGEN THERAPY

Immediately after exposure to hyperbaric oxygen, intubated patients often require a higher F_{IO_2} than before HBOT,[15] hence special attention must be taken to assure that these patients do not become hypoxic. This transient worsening of lung function may be because of atelectasis caused by 100% oxygen (nitrogen washout from the lung) or because of other causative factors of worsening right-to-left shunt fraction. Typically, within a few hours after decompression, lung function returns to prehyperbaric oxygen levels.[5,15]

Hypoxia While Breathing Hyperbaric Air

Some HBOT schedules incorporate intermittent periods of air breathing to reduce the risk for oxygen toxicity.[16,17] Critically ill patients who need supplemental oxygen to maintain adequate arterial oxygen tensions can manifest hypoxemia while breathing hyperbaric air.[18] Monitoring of the patient's arterial oxygen tension is advisable to prevent hypoxemia during hyperbaric air periods. Pulse oximetry measurements would be helpful to monitor for hypoxemia during hyperbaric air breathing, but no devices have received Food and Drug Administration approval for hyperbaric use. Therefore, transcutaneous oxygen monitoring may be useful to monitor for hypoxia during air-breathing periods. Of course, an alternative strategy is to omit air-breathing periods, but this approach must be balanced against the risk for oxygen toxicity.

EQUIPMENT NECESSARY TO TREAT CRITICALLY ILL PATIENTS WITH HYPERBARIC OXYGEN

Hyperbaric medicine departments that treat critically ill patients need similar or identical equipment as is found in an ICU. Ideally, this includes monitors for electrocardiogram, invasive blood pressure, pulse oximetry, and end-tidal carbon dioxide. Although pulse oximetry may not be used inside the chamber, it is important to monitor the arterial oxygen saturation of critically ill patients before and after HBOT. Additional equipment includes defibrillators and crash carts; intubation equipment and a selection of endotracheal tube sizes; tube thoracostomy equipment; suction, central, and arterial catheters; gowns; gloves; and so forth.

MECHANICAL VENTILATORS FOR HYPERBARIC OXYGEN THERAPY OF CRITICALLY ILL PATIENTS

Mechanical ventilation of patients treated with hyperbaric oxygen is hampered because hyperbaric-approved ventilators ex-

hibit marginal performance. For monoplace chamber use, common ventilators include the 500A (Sechrist Industries, Anaheim, Calif) (Fig. 7.1) and the Omni-Vent (Allied Healthcare Products, Inc., St. Louis, Mo; also sold as the MaxO$_2$ and the Magellan) (Fig. 7.2). The 500A performs adequately if the minute ventilation is less than 12 L/min and PEEP values are less than 10 cm H$_2$O.[19] For patients who require higher minute ventilations, the Omni-Vent exhibits better performance.[20] Both ventilators have manual controls for adjusting inspiratory flow, inspiratory time, and expiratory time, but neither has an alarm. Operation of either ventilator with oxygen delivered at a typical hospital headwall pressure (55 pounds per square inch gauge [psig]) severely limits their performance.[19,20] The 500A performance is improved when operated at 80 psig, whereas Omni-Vent performance is improved when operated at 120 psig.[20] Therefore, both venti-

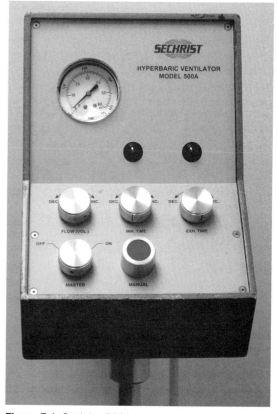

Figure 7.1 Sechrist 500A monoplace hyperbaric ventilator.

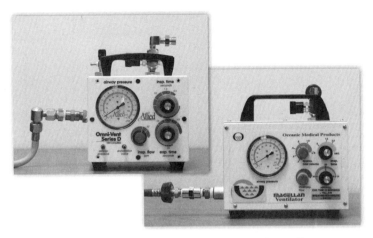

Figure 7.2 Omni-Vent and Magellan hyperbaric ventilators.

lators need a separate high-pressure oxygen source (and air source, if air-breathing periods are provided).

The 500A control module is outside the monoplace chamber, and the patient circuit inside the chamber is connected to a ventilator block (see Fig. 7.1). We do not use the nebulizer and have not encountered inspissated secretions. A peak pressure pop-off valve needs to be adjusted before HBOT. Tidal volumes are measured inside the chamber with a spirometer. Airway pressures are measured inside the chamber on the inspiratory side of the patient airway circuit. Positive expiratory pressure can be applied using continuous positive airway pressure valves (Accu-PEEP; Vital Signs, Totowa, NJ). The ventilator requires one pass-through port. If air-breathing periods are to be provided, special modifications are necessary, as well as two pass-through ports.[21]

The Omni-Vent is located outside the monoplace chamber. High-pressure gas hoses (rated at several hundred psig) are placed between the ventilator inspiratory port and the chamber hatch pass-through (Fig. 7.3). It is important to install a one-way back-check valve in this inspiratory circuit to prevent pulmonary "squeeze" if pressure is lost in this high-pressure hose during the delivery of hyperbaric therapy. As with the 500A, tidal volume is measured with a spirometer, and proximal airway pressures are measured with

a manometer located inside the chamber. The peak pressure "pop-off" is located inside the chamber and adjusted before HBOT. This ventilator requires two pass-through ports, one for the inspiratory circuit and the other for the exhalation valve operation (see Fig. 7.3). Air-breathing periods can be provided by driving the Omni-Vent with air at the appropriate supply pressure.

Disadvantages of the 500A are the limitations with high rates, especially with higher PEEP, and at greater chamber pressures.[19] Disadvantages of the Omni-Vent are sensitive inspiratory time and expiratory time control knobs. A minor turn of either knob may result in a dramatic change in either inspiratory or expiratory time (i.e., tidal volume or respiratory rate, respectively). The Magellan ventilator has been improved in this regard with less sensitive control knobs.

For mechanical ventilation in multiplace chambers, experiences with several ventilators have been reported.[22,23] Devices include the Penlon,[24,25] Monahan 225,[26] Bird,[27] Omni-Vent, a modified Servo 900C, as well as others[28-31] (Folke Lind, MD, PhD, Karolinska Hospital, Stockholm, Sweden, personal communication, February 2006). For ventilators that do not provide tidal volume and respiratory rate information, volume monitors have been modified and attached to the ventilator to monitor minute ventilation of patients

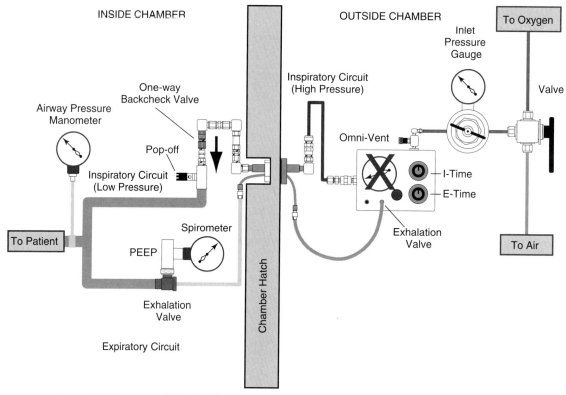

Figure 7.3 Schematic of the Omni-Vent or Magellan with monoplace hyperbaric chambers. PEEP, positive end-expiratory pressure.

treated in multiplace chambers.[32] The Uni-vent, Eagle, Model 754 (Impact Instrumentation, Inc., Caldwell, NJ) passed the U.S. Navy Experimental Diving Unit testing for multiplace chamber operations,[30,31] but it is unknown whether any have been put into use in an HBOT treatment center.

Hypercapnia can occur if there is poor matching of alveolar ventilation to carbon dioxide production. Even with modern-day microprocessor-controlled mechanical ventilators in an ICU setting, hypercapnia canoccur. For patients with acute lung injury or acute respiratory distress syndrome, therapeutic permissive hypercapnia with a low tidal volume strategy reduces mortality.[33] This strategy poses special risks with regard to HBOT, however, because if hypercapnia is maintained or develops during hyperbaric oxygen, the risk for central nervous system oxygen toxicity increases.[34] Many centers customarily sedate intubated patients during HBOT using drugs that are also anticonvulsants (e.g., propofol, lorazepam). When para-

lytic agents are used, it is customary to also provide sedation, but paralysis does raise concern about nonobservable seizure activity.

END-TIDAL CARBON DIOXIDE MONITORING

The end-tidal carbon dioxide levels can be monitored during hyperbaric pressurization in both monoplace[35,36] and multiplace[37,38] chambers. For monoplace chambers, exhaled gas can be passed out through the chamber hatch to the end-tidal carbon dioxide analyzer. Because the patient is compressed and the analyzer is calibrated at atmospheric pressure, the measured end-tidal carbon dioxide values must be "corrected" for interpretation. For example, a patient compressed to 2.0 ATA may have an actual end-tidal carbon dioxide level of 36 torr. Ideally, this value should measure 18 (36/2) with a monitor located at sea-level pressure.[36]

ENDOTRACHEAL TUBES

The endotracheal tube cuff needs to be filled with sterile saline before compression. This is especially true for treating critically ill patients in the monoplace chamber because caregivers do not have access to the endotracheal tube cuff pilot balloon during therapy. The cuff should be filled with saline sufficient to prevent the endotracheal tube from leaking. After hyperbaric oxygen, the patient's oropharynx should be suctioned, and all the saline must be removed and the cuff filled with air, while confirming safe cuff-to-tracheal tube pressures.[39] This is not as critical in a multiplace chamber because air can be added to the cuff as pressurization occurs. If this mode of endotracheal tube care is used, attention must be paid to vent the cuff during decompression.

INTRAVENOUS INFUSION PUMPS

At the time of publication of this textbook, no Food and Drug Administration–approved intravenous (IV) infusion pump for HBOT exists. Monoplace chambers use three IV pumps: IVAC 530, Abbot LifeCare, and Baxter Flo-Guard. (None of these pumps are available from the manufacturers, but may be available from hyperbaric equipment suppliers. See www. uhms.org classifieds for assistance.) The Abbot LifeCare IV pump was approved for monoplace chamber use, but this pump is no longer available. The Baxter Flo-Guard IV pump performs well during monoplace chamber use.[40,41] For the Baxter Flo-Guard pump to infuse fluid against the pressure inside the monoplace chamber, however, the downstream occlusion adjustment plug must be adjusted to activate at 30 to 35 pounds per square inch (psi).[40]

It is important for clinicians guiding IV infusion therapy to patients compressed within monoplace chambers to know that the IV tubing between the IV infusion pump and the chamber hatch is compliant and expands during chamber pressurization. Because of this, a patient will not receive IV drugs at low infusions (≤10 mL/hr) for at least 20 minutes.[40,41] One solution to this problem is withdrawing all of the IV set tubing proximal through the pump so that only a minimal amount of IV set tubing is present between the pump and the chamber door. This IV set tubing can then be connected to hard, pressure, Luer-lock tubing to the IV pass-through (Argon Medical Devices, Inc., Athens, Tex). Alternatively, the low-rate infusion could be piggybacked onto a high-rate infusion.

Several pumps have been used and tested within multiplace chambers.[42-44] One multiplace facility reports adequate performance from the ALARIS Medley IV infusion pump (ALARIS Medical Systems, Inc., San Diego, Calif) (Neil Hampson, MD, personal communication, August 4, 2006). The hyperbaric facility staff should carefully assess any IV infusion pump they contemplate using for performance accuracy, suitability, and safety.[42] Reductions in inotropic support while using syringe pumps to 2.8 ATA have been observed, which could explain hypotension of critically ill patients during compression.[44]

PHYSIOLOGIC MONITORING

Monitoring apparatus and procedures for the monoplace hyperbaric chamber were outlined in Chapter 2. For multiplace chambers, several articles have reviewed physiologic monitoring.[45,46] The monitoring system may be identical to that used elsewhere within the hospital. If different, attention needs to be focused on integrating the monitoring system with the hospital's to streamline transitions to and from the ICU and the hyperbaric chamber. The hospital biomedical department should be involved with establishing connections between the chamber and the monitors located outside the chamber. It is helpful to place a secondary (slave) monitor inside the chamber so that inside attendants can observe physiologic data.

SUCTION

Apparatus and procedures for suctioning in the monoplace hyperbaric chamber were outlined in Chapter 2. Suction can be applied in monoplace and multiplace chambers.[47] Common uses for suction are nasogastric, drains, and vacuum-assisted closure (VAC) devices.[48] VAC devices are commonly used in critically ill patients, such as those with necrotizing fasciitis or open abdomens. Thus providing suction during hyperbaric oxygen is important to prevent loss of the vacuum seal. VAC therapy cleanses and stimulates the wound bed, reduces localized edema, reduces inflammation, reduces pain, and improves local oxygen and nutrient supply to the wound. VAC therapy increases the rate of granulation tissue formation and reduces the number of dressing changes.[49]

TUBE THORACOSTOMIES

Tube thoracostomies, or chest tubes, are placed to evacuate pleural blood, fluid, or air. If the chest tube was placed to evacuate fluid and there was no pneumothorax, the chest tube can drain passively, or it can be attached to suction during HBOT. A one-way Heimlich valve (Bard-Parker Heimich Chest Drain Valve; Becton, Dickinson and Company, Franklin Lakes, NJ) should be placed within the chest tube circuit to prevent a pneumothorax if the evacuation system is inadvertently opened to atmospheric pressure. For patients with drained pneumothoraces, a Heimlich valve must be placed in the pleural drainage circuit, and airway pressures during mechanical ventilation should be minimized. Closed pleural collections systems should be tested before being subjected to hyperbaric pressurization, because some closed drainage collection systems can be damaged and malfunction when subjected to hyperbaric pressure.[50]

PACEMAKERS, INTERNAL CARDIAC DEFIBRILLATORS, AND NERVE AND SPINAL STIMULATORS

Issues that pertain to use of pacemakers, internal cardiac defibrillators (ICDs), and nerve and spinal stimulators in a monoplace chamber are discussed in Chapter 2. For patients with implanted pacemakers, ICDs, or nerve or spinal stimulators, similar concerns apply if treated in either multiplace or monoplace chambers. If a patient has an implanted cardiac pacemaker, the pacemaker manufacturer needs to specify that the device is suitable for hyperbaric compression, and the maximum pressure to which it may be subjected. As discussed in Chapter 2, ICDs may be at risk for ignition if their leads are faulty and the ICD discharges. Until ICD manufacturers indicate their ICDs are safe for use under hyperbaric oxygen conditions, it may be prudent to deactivate the ICD before each HBOT, monitor the patient, and reactivate after HBOT. Personnel and equipment must be available to treat cardiac dysrhythmias during the interval of ICD deactivated. Implanted drug delivery devices and spinal stimulators need to be verified by the manufacturer that they are safe for compression during HBOT. If not, the patient may not be a suitable candidate for HBOT, unless the device can be deactivated.

DEFIBRILLATION AND CARDIOVERSION

Defibrillation and cardioversion can be performed inside the multiplace chamber as long as there is no excess oxygen buildup.[51] For monoplace chamber patients who need defibrillation or cardioversion, these procedures must be done outside the chamber. It is advisable to switch gas supply from oxygen to air while decompressing these patients to hasten dissipation of oxygen from around the hyperbaric chamber door. Patients are cardioverted or defibrillated after opening the chamber hatch and sliding the patient out of the chamber onto the gurney. If switching the chamber gas supply to air is not possible, then 40 seconds or more needs to elapse for oxygen to dissipate before defibrillation.[52] Also, all patient garments must be removed before defibrillation because they, too, will be oxygen enriched and thus increase the risk for fire.

SEDATION

Frequently, critically ill patients are sedated while in the ICU. Thus, these critically ill patients are receiving continuous infusions of narcotics for pain and sedatives for sedation in the ICU as well. Infusions of fentanyl, propofol, and as-needed doses of benzodiazepines will be required during HBOT. Each of these infusions must be on separate pumps and IV sets through the chamber hatch. As mentioned earlier, low-rate infusions require hard, Luer-lock pressure tubing between the IV pump and the chamber hatch to ensure the patient receives these drugs at the desired rates.[40,41]

Before the introduction of propofol, critically ill patients were often paralyzed to facilitate mechanical ventilation inside the monoplace chamber. However, the use of paralytic agents should be avoided whenever possible because of contribution to prolonged neuromuscular weakness.[53,54] However, paralysis may still be necessary (after adequate deep sedation) for patients who have considerable ventilator asynchrony, high risk for self-extubation or harm, or evidence of air trapping, especially if it adversely affects gas exchange.

Restraints

Careful consideration should be given to placement of restraints on sedated, critically ill patients undergoing HBOT. Management decisions are easier in a multiplace chamber because hands-on care is always provided. In the monoplace chamber, it is generally advisable to use restraints because dislodgment of an endotracheal tube, arterial or venous medical lines, or other devices may cause serious harm.

Glucose Control during Hyperbaric Oxygen Therapy

Evidence exists that normalization of blood glucose during critical illness improves outcomes.[55,56] In some patients, discontinuing enteral or parenteral nutrition during hyperbaric oxygen causes tight glucose control to become challenging when nutrition and insulin are reinstituted in the ICU. Therefore, if possible, enteral and parenteral nutrition of critically ill patients during hyperbaric oxygen should be continued. Controlled infusions of insulin to maintain normal glucose values of these patients during HBOT can be used. As stated earlier, low IV infusion rates, such as insulin, require hard, Luer-lock tubing between the IV infusion pump and the chamber hatch,[40,41] or this insulin infusion must be piggybacked into an infusion running at a high rate. Blood can be withdrawn from an arterial catheter or from a central venous catheter to check glucose levels[8] (Fig. 7.4).

Children

Critically ill children can be treated with hyperbaric oxygen in monoplace or multiplace chambers.[57] In one study, hypotension, bronchospasm, hemotympanum, and progressive hypoxemia were noted as complications. However, most complications were deemed manageable by knowledgeable staff.[57] As with adults, critically ill children may require titrated doses of sedation and analgesia during HBOT. Input and, ideally, comanagement by pediatric intensive care are invaluable (see Chapters 2 and 6).

Myringotomies

Differing opinions have been presented regarding whether intubated, sedated patients require prophylactic myringotomies before hyperbaric pressurization.[58-60] It is currently unknown whether prophylactic myringotomies prevent long-term sequelae from inner-ear barotraumas in intubated, sedated patients. A prospective clinical trial is needed to determine whether prophylactic myringotomies of intubated, sedated patients improve ear-related outcomes. If myringotomies are done, thermal[61] or laser[62] myringotomy may be advantageous for middle-ear ventilation, because the placement of tympanostomy tubes in patients treated

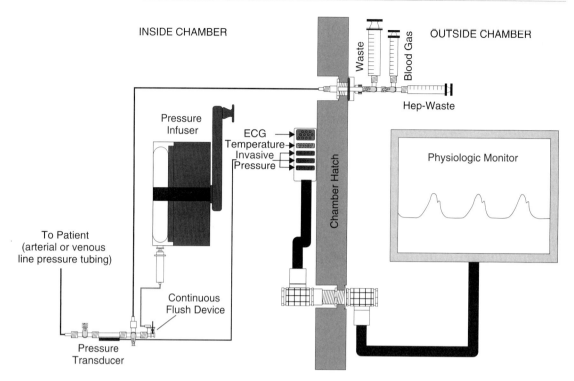

INSIDE CHAMBER   OUTSIDE CHAMBER

Figure 7.4 Setup for withdrawing blood from an arterial catheter and pressure transducer. A four-way stopcock is placed between the pressure transducer and the continuous flush device. The handle of the four-way stopcock is positioned so all ports are open. Hard, pressure, Luer-lock tubing is connected to the stopcock and an intravenous (IV) pass-through, which passes out of the chamber via a hatch pass-through. A stopcock is placed outside the IV pass-through and permits arterial blood to be sampled (Hyperbaric chamber IV extension kit [Part Number: 041600503A], which includes a 3-pound per square inch [psi] check valve, pass-through device, stopcock, and monitoring line; Argon Medical Devices, Inc., Athens, Tex). (For withdrawal of blood from the compressed patient, the 3-psi check valve must be removed.) After sampling, this line should be flushed with sterile saline from outside the chamber. ECG, electrocardiogram.

with hyperbaric oxygen may be excessive.[63] For critically ill patients with brain edema treated with hyperbaric oxygen, prophylactic myringotomies may be important to minimize increases in intracranial pressure during pressurization.[64]

SYSTEMATIC REVIEWS OF CRITICAL CARE AND HYPERBARIC OXYGEN

Information from abstract presentations has reviewed the type of critically ill patients and rates of complications related to hyperbaric oxygen.[65,66] As mentioned earlier, it appears the rate of manageable, hyperbaric-related complications in children may be greater[57] than in the other two studies,[65,66] which include both children and adults.

At Loma Linda, California, from 1981 to 2003, 199 intubated critically ill patients were treated with hyperbaric oxygen in monoplace chambers for necrotizing infections, carbon monoxide poisoning, compromised surgical flaps/grafts, and acute arterial ischemia. No mortality was attributed to this group.[65]

At our own institution from 1986 to 2006, 182 intubated critically ill patients were treated with hyperbaric oxygen in monoplace chambers (representing 1281 hyperbaric oxygen sessions in 61 female and 121 male patients; age, 44 ± 19 [range, 2-83] years).[66] Patients had necrotizing fasciitis, carbon monoxide poisoning, crush injury, gangrene, arterial gas embolism, mucormycosis, arterial insufficiency, failing flaps, osteomyelitis, or radiation necrosis. Myringotomies were done in 66 patients (until 1995), and no myringotomies in 116 since 1995. Of the most recent 108 patients, the Acute Physiology and Chronic Health Evaluation II (APACHE II)[67] score was 17.6 ± 7.5 (range, 6-44). The mean number of separate IV infusions per patient was 3.8 ± 1.8 (range, 1-11). Of 154 patients with outcome data, 27 died from their disease or withdrawal of support. Complications necessitating decompression from the chamber occurred in 35 of 1281 compressions (2.7%). These complications were ventricular tachycardia/fibrillation in 1, hypoxemia with air breathing in 2,[24] arterial line problems in 5, ventilator circuit problems in 8, ventilator malfunctions in 2, seizures in 3, air trapping and hyperinflation with hypotension in 4, inadequate sedation in 5, and arrhythmias in 4 compressions. One additional patient sustained cardiac arrest upon exiting the chamber due to severe hypoxia from acute lung injury from gas embolism.[18]

In an analysis spanning 32 years (10,000 hyperbaric oxygen sessions of patients hospitalized in a critical care unit), reasons for withholding hyperbaric oxygen included hypoxemia requiring an F_{IO_2} greater than 0.50, hypotension requiring vasopressors, hypertension requiring IV vasodilators, hyperthermia, status epilepticus, tension pneumothorax, need for fluidized bed protection, morbid obesity, end-stage malignancy, and concomitant intralipid infusions.[68]

CONCLUSION

Critically ill patients can be treated in both monoplace and multiplace hyperbaric chambers. To deliver safe care to critically ill patients, the chamber environment needs to support critical care, and the staff needs to be trained and experienced in critical care management. Of utmost importance is the consideration of risk versus the benefit of hyperbaric oxygen, and the transport away from the critical care ICU.

ACKNOWLEDGMENTS

I appreciate editorial and schematic and photographic assistance from Kayla Deru, as well as chapter critique by Susan Churchill, NP.

REFERENCES

1. Feldmeier JJ (ed): Hyperbaric oxygen therapy: 2003 committee report. Rev. ed. Kensington, Md, Undersea and Hyperbaric Medical Society, 2003.
2. Waydhas C, Schneck G, Duswald KH: Deterioration of respiratory function after intra-hospital transport of critically ill surgical patients. Intensive Care Med 21:784-789, 1995.
3. Beckmann U, Gillies DM, Berenholtz SM, et al: Incidents relating to the intra-hospital transfer of critically ill patients. An analysis of the reports submitted to the Australian incident monitoring study in intensive care. Intensive Care Med 30:1579-1585, 2004.
4. Shirley PJ, Bion JF: Intra-hospital transport of critically ill patients: Minimising risk. Intensive Care Med 30:1508-1510, 2004.
5. Weaver LK, Howe S: Arterial oxygen tension of patients with abnormal lungs treated with hyperbaric oxygen is greater than predicted. Chest 106:1134-1139, 1994.
6. Weaver LK, Larson-Lohr V: Hypoxemia during hyperbaric oxygen: A case report. Chest 105:1270-1271, 1994.
7. Weaver LK, Howe S, Berlin SL: Normobaric measurement of O_2 tension of blood and saline tonometered under hyperbaric O_2 conditions. J Hyperb Med 5:29-38, 1990.
8. Weaver LK, Howe S: Normobaric measurement of arterial oxygen tension in subjects exposed to hyperbaric oxygen. Chest 102:1175-1181, 1992.
9. Weaver LK, Ershler L, Howe S: Accuracy of the radiometer abl 500 measuring hyperbaric blood gases at atmospheric pressure. Undersea Biomedical Res 19(suppl):105, 1992.
10. Niklas A. Brock D, Schober R, et al: Continuous measurements of cerebral tissue oxygen pressure during hyperbaric oxygenation—HBO effects on brain edema and necrosis after severe brain trauma in rabbits. J Neurol Sci 219:77-82, 2004.
11. Grolman RE, Wilkerson DK, Taylor J, et al: Transcutaneous oxygen measurements predict a beneficial response to hyperbaric oxygen therapy in patients with nonhealing wounds and critical limb ischemia. Am Surg 67:1072-1079, 2001.
12. Fife CE, Buyukcakir C, Otto GH, et al: The predictive value of transcutaneous oxygen tension measurement in diabetic lower extremity ulcers treated with hyperbaric oxygen therapy: A retrospective analysis of 1,144 patients. Wound Repair Regen 10:198-207, 2002.
13. Haberstock D, Weaver LK, Hein S, Howe S: Are transcutaneous oxygen (TCO_2) and carbon dioxide $TCCO_2$) measurements surrogates for arterial oxygen (P_aO_2) and carbon dioxide (P_aCO_2) tensions? Undersea Hyper Med 26(suppl):37, 1999.

14. Weaver LK, Churchill S, Deru K: Transcutaneous oxygen and carbon dioxide tensions compared to arterial oxygen and carbon dioxide tensions in patients. Undersea Hyperb Med 33(5), 2006.

15. Ratzenhofer-Komenda B, Offner A, Quehenberger F, et al: Hemodynamic and oxygenation profiles in the early period after hyperbaric oxygen therapy: An observational study of intensive-care patients. Acta Anaesthesiol Scand 47:554-558, 2003.

16. Clark JM: Extension of oxygen tolerance by interrupted exposure. Undersea Hyperb Med 31:195-198, 2004.

17. Piantadosi CA: A mini-forum on air breaks and O2 toxicity in clinical HBO2 therapy. Undersea Hyperb Med 31:185, 2004.

18. Weaver LK, Churchill S: Hypoxemia with air breathing periods in U.S. NAVY Treatment Table 6. Undersea Hyperb Med 33:11-15, 2006.

19. Weaver LK, Greenway L, Elliott CG: Performance of the Sechrist 500A hyperbaric ventilator in a monoplace hyperbaric chamber. J Hyperb Med 3:215-225, 1988.

20. Churchill S, Weaver LK, Haberstock D: Performance of the Omni-vent mechanical ventilator for use with the monoplace hyperbaric chamber. Undersea Hyperb Med 26(suppl):70-71, 1999.

21. Weaver LK: Air breaks with Sechrist 500A Monoplace Hyperbaric Ventilator. J Hyperb Med 3:179-186, 1988.

22. Gallagher TJ, Smith RA, Bell GC: Evaluation of mechanical ventilators in a hyperbaric environment. Aviat Space Environ Med 49:375-376, 1978.

23. Moon RE, Hart BB: Operational use and patient monitoring in a multiplace hyperbaric chamber. Respir Care Clin N Am 5:21-49, 1999.

24. Saywood AM, Howard R, Goad RF, Scott C: Function of the Oxford Ventilator at high pressure. Anaesthesia 37:740-744, 1982.

25. Lewis RP, Szafranski J, Bradford RH, et al: The use of the Penlon Nuffield 200 in a monoplace hyperbaric oxygen chamber. An evaluation of its use and a clinical report in two patients requiring ventilation for carbon monoxide poisoning. Anaesthesia 46:767-770, 1991.

26. Moon RE, Berguist LV, Conklin B: Monaghan 225 ventilator use under hyperbaric conditions. Chest 89:846-851, 1986.

27. Stahl W, Radermacher P, Calzia E: Functioning of ICU ventilators under hyperbaric conditions—comparison of volume- and pressure-controlled modes. Intensive Care Med 26:442-448, 2000.

28. Risdall JE, Hasan SK: Assessment of the Servo 900C ventilator for use with mixed gas (Heliox) on Royal Navy treatment table 67 [abstract]. Undersea Hyperb Med 31:356-357, 2004.

29. Oberly D, Conley J, Montminy J, Perdrizet G: The use of pressure-control ventilation to mechanically ventilate critically ill adult and pediatric patients [abstract]. Undersea Hyperb Med 32:281, 2005.

30. Stanga DF, Chimiak JM, Beck G: Evaluating the safety, function and use of medical ventilators to provide respiratory support of critically ill patients in the hyperbaric chamber. Undersea Hyperb Med 30:254, 2003.

31. Stanga DF, Beck G, Chimiak JM: Department of Defense, Navy Experimental Diving Unit: Evaluation of respiratory support devices for use in the hyperbaric chamber. Panama City, Fla, Navy Experimental Diving Unit [NEDU] TR 03-18, 2003.

32. Youn BA, Myers RA: Volume monitor for mechanical ventilation in the hyperbaric chamber. Crit Care Med 17:453-454, 1989.

33. The Acute Respiratory Distress Syndrome Network: Ventilation with lower tidal volumes as compared with traditional tidal volumes for acute lung injury and the acute respiratory distress syndrome. N Engl J Med 342:1301-1308, 2000.

34. Clark JM, Thom SR: Oxygen under pressure. In: Bennett PB, Elliott DH (eds): Physiology and Medicine of Diving, 5th ed. London, WB Saunders Company, 2003, pp 358-418.

35. Eskelson MI, Weaver LK, Greenway L: End-tidal CO2 monitoring within the monoplace hyperbaric chamber. Undersea Biomedial Res 16(suppl):18-19, 1989.

36. Haberstock D, Weaver LK, Churchill S: End-tidal CO2 compared to arterial carbon dioxide tension during hyperbaric oxygen therapy [abstract]. Undersea Hyperb Med 32:451-456, 2005.

37. Mummery HJ, Stolp BW, Del Dear G, et al: Effects of age and exercise on physiological dead space during simulated dives at 2.8 ATA. J Appl Physiol 94:507-517, 2003.

38. Arieli R, Daskalovic Y, Eynan M, et al: Use of a mass spectrometer for direct respiratory gas sampling from the hyperbaric chamber. Aviat Space Environ Med 72:799-804, 2001.

39. Galinski M, Treoux V, Garrigue B, et al: Intracuff pressures of endotracheal tubes in the management of airway emergencies: The need for pressure monitoring. Ann Emerg Med 47:545-547, 2006.

40. Ray D, Weaver LK, Churchill S, Haberstock D: Baxter Flo-Gard 6201 Volumetric Infusion Pump for monoplace chamber applications. Undersea Hyperb Med 27:107-111, 2000.

41. Weaver LK, Ray D, Haberstock D: Comparison of three monoplace hyperbaric chamber intravenous infusion pumps. Undersea Hyperb Med 32:451-456, 2005.

42. Lavon H, Shapak A, Tal D, et al: Performance of infusion pumps during hyperbaric conditions. Anesthesiology 96:849-854, 2002.

43. Dohgomori H, Atikawa K, Kubo H: The accuracy and reliability of an infusion pump (STC-3121; Terumo Inst., Japan) during hyperbaric oxygenation. Anaesth Intensive Care 28:68-71, 2000.

44. Story DA, Houston JJ, Millar IL: Performance of the Atom 235 syringe infusion pump under hyperbaric conditions. Anaesth Intensive Care 26:193-195, 1998.

45. Rogatsky GG, Shifren EG, Mayevsky A: Physiologic and biochemical monitoring during hyperbaric oxygenation: A review. Undersea Hyperb Med 26:111-122, 1999.

46. Poulton TJ: Monitoring critically ill patients in the hyperbaric environment. Med Instrum 15:81-84, 1981.

47. Weaver LK: A functional suction apparatus within the monoplace hyperbaric chamber. J Hyperb Med 3:165-171, 1988.

48. Mendez-Eastman S: Use of hyperbaric oxygen and negative pressure therapy in the multidisciplinary care of a patient with nonhealing wounds. J Wound Ostomy Continence Nurs 26:67-76, 1999.

49. Hopf HW, Humphrey LM, Puzziferri N, et al: Adjuncts to preparing wounds for closure: Hyperbaric oxygen, growth factors, skin substitutes, negative pressure wound therapy (vacuum-assisted closure). Foot Ankle Clin 6:661-682, 2001.

50. Walker KJ, Millar IL, Fock A: The performance and safety of a pleural drainage unit under hyperbaric conditions. Anaesth Intensive Care 34:61-67, 2006.

51. Pitkn A: Defibrillation in hyperbaric chambers: A review. J R Nav Med Serv 85:150-157, 1999.

52. Kindwall E: Management of complications in hyperbaric treatment. In: Kindwall EP, Whelan HT (eds): Hyperbaric Medicine Practice, 2nd ed. Flagstaff, Ariz, Best Publishing, 1999, pp 365-375.

53. Burry L, HoSang M, Hynes-Gay P: A review of neuromuscular blockade in the critically ill patient. Dynamics 12:28-33, 2001.

54. Gorson KC: Approach to neuromuscular disorders in the intensive care unit. Neurocrit Care 3:195-212, 2005.

55. Van den Berghe G, Wouters P, Weekers F, et al: Intensive insulin therapy in the critically ill patients. N Engl J Med 345:1359-1367, 2001.

56. Van den Berghe G, Wilmer A, Hermans G, et al: Intensive insulin therapy in the medical ICU. N Engl J Med 354:449-461, 2006.

57. Keenan HT, Bratton SL, Norkool DM, et al: Delivery of hyperbaric oxygen therapy to critically ill, mechanically ventilated children. J Crit Care 13:7-12, 1998.

58. Capes JP, Tomaszewski C: Prophylaxis against middle ear barotrauma in US hyperbaric oxygen therapy centers. Am J Emerg Med 14:645-648, 1996.

59. Churchill S, Weaver LK: Prophylactic myringotomies in intubated patients during hyperbaric oxygen therapy [abstract]. Undersea Hyperb Med 32:240-241, 2005.

60. Presswood G, Zamboni WA, Stephenson LL, Santos PM: Effect of artificial airway on ear complications from hyperbaric oxygen. Laryngoscope 104(11 pt 1):1383-1384, 1994.

61. Potocki SE, Hoffman DS: Thermal myringotomy for eustachian tube dysfunction in hyperbaric oxygen therapy. Otolaryngol Head Neck Surg 121:185-189, 1999.

62. Vrabec JT, Clements KS, Mader JT: Short-term tympanostomy in conjunction with hyperbaric oxygen therapy. Laryngoscope 108(8 pt 1):1124-1128, 1998.

63. Clements KS, Vrabec JT, Mader JT: Complications of tympanostomy tubes inserted for facilitation of hyperbaric oxygen therapy. Arch Otolaryngol Head Neck Surg 124:278-280, 1998.

64. Rockswold GL, Ford SE, Anderson DC, et al: Results of a prospective randomized trial for treatment of severely brain-injured patients with hyperbaric oxygen. J Neurosurg 76:929-934, 1992.

65. Lo T, Sample AS, Christenson D, et al: Mortality associated with hyperbaric oxygen treatment in critically-ill patients [abstract]. Proc Am Thorac Soc 2:A426, 2005.

66. Weaver LK, Churchill S, Deru K: Critical care of patients treated in monoplace hyperbaric chambers, past 20 years. Undersea Hyperb Med 33(5):350-351, 2006.

67. Knaus WA, Draper EA, Wagner DP, Zimmerman JE: APACHE II: A severity of disease classification system. Crit Care Med 13:818-829, 1985.

68. Hart GB, Asciuto TJ, Aksenov IV, et al: Medical contraindications for hyperbaric oxygen treatments in critical care patients. Undersea Hyperb Med 33(5):351-352, 2006.

Physiology ■■■

Pulmonary Gas Exchange, Oxygen Transport, and Tissue Oxygenation

8

Claude A. Piantadosi, MD

The human respiratory system is designed to ensure a supply of molecular oxygen (O_2) sufficient for tissues to meet a wide range of metabolic activities. The system is arranged as a series of compartments linked by the circulation and designed for uninterrupted transfer of O_2 from the inspired gas to cells, where it is consumed principally by mitochondria in the process of cell respiration.[1] Respiration provides most of the energy for cell function through oxidative phosphorylation, which generates adenosine triphosphate (ATP) through stepwise oxidation of glucose and other substrates coupled to the irreversible reduction of O_2 to water.[2]

A large, thin air–liquid interface—imposed between the atmosphere and the blood by

133

the lungs—is composed mainly of the epithelium and capillaries of the alveolar region, which serve as the main site of gas exchange.[3] This pulmonary microcirculation allows for the rapid passage of red blood cells (erythrocytes), which pick up O_2 from the atmosphere and deliver it by the actions of the left heart and arterial circulation to the systemic microcirculation for release and diffusion into tissue. Deoxygenated blood in the venous circulation returns via the right heart and re-enters the lungs, where it releases carbon dioxide (CO_2) captured from cellular metabolism and is replenished with fresh O_2. Thus, the lungs, blood, and circulation comprise an integrated mechanism for continuous delivery of O_2 to the cells for their metabolic activities. A simple in-series compartmental model of the respiratory system illustrating this transport of O_2 and CO_2 to and from the tissue is shown in Figure 8.1.

The function of the erythrocyte as the main carrier of O_2 depends entirely on the hemoglobin (Hb) molecule. Erythrocytes comprise 40% to 45% of the circulating blood volume, and blood Hb concentration is ~14 to 15 grams per deciliter (g/dL).[4] This gives the blood a large O_2 storage capacity, which in combination with the large reserve of the normal heart and circulation for blood flow, is sufficient to deliver enough O_2 to support even heavy exercise.[5] The organization and function of this O_2 transport system is covered in four sections in this chapter beginning with a brief overview of the principles of normal gas exchange and the fundamental capabilities of the respiratory system. These capabilities include significant flexibility in O_2 loading and unloading by red blood cells, the bulk capacity of the O_2 transport system, and the ability to expand the systemic microcirculation. The effects of breathing hyperbaric oxygen (HBO) on this system are then presented, followed by a section on cell metabolism, and, finally, a short synopsis on metabolic CO_2 elimination.

In the presence of lung disease, or with disorders of the heart, circulation, or blood, or in special environments, the O_2 transport

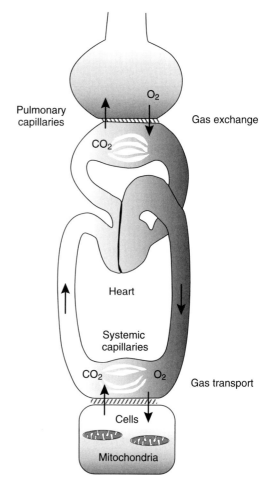

FIGURE 8.1 THE OXYGEN TRANSPORT SYSTEM. Diagram depicts the flow of O_2 from the lungs to the systemic capillaries and the return of CO_2 from cell metabolism to the lungs. The process requires a series of physical links in each direction that includes diffusion → chemical binding → convection → chemical release → diffusion.

system must also adapt to stress to avoid compromise of tissue function from hypoxia and energy failure. Some compromising conditions, whether caused by cardiopulmonary pathology or by an extreme environment, produce critical limitations of O_2 delivery (DO_2) to tissues and therefore interfere with the normal maintenance of cellular energy homeostasis. The nature of such stressors would be fair game for this chapter, but to focus on the physiology, they are discussed only briefly here in the context of the convective O_2 transport system. However, the impact of supplemental O_2 and HBO in particular on physiologic O_2 transport and tissue oxygenation is covered throughout the text for the most relevant clinical conditions and diseases.

PULMONARY VENTILATION AND GAS EXCHANGE

The alveolar region of the human lungs has a surface area of perhaps the size of a tennis court and a thickness of less than 0.5 μm, making it a highly efficient structure for gas exchange.[3] As the lungs are ventilated, inspired gas is conducted through the airways to the airspaces, whereas blood flows through the interfacial pulmonary arteries and alveolar capillaries. To achieve effective alveolar gas exchange in a lung of such geometry and physical dimensions, both processes—ventilation and perfusion—require bulk flow (convection) of gas and liquid, respectively, which is coupled to gas diffusion across the interface.[6]

The composition of alveolar gas is determined by Dalton's Law and the sum of the relevant partial pressures of nitrogen (P_{N_2}), oxygen (P_{O_2}), CO_2 (P_{CO_2}), and water vapor (P_{H_2O}):

$$P_B = P_{N_2} + P_{O_2} + P_{CO_2} + P_{H_2O}$$

where P_B is barometric or atmospheric pressure. Because P_B and P_{N_2} are usually constant, and variations of P_{H_2O} are small, the alveolar gas composition is determined largely by the reciprocal relation between P_{O_2} and P_{CO_2}.[6]

The absolute size of the lungs and the requirement for a large system of conducting airways means that a sizable portion of the total pulmonary ventilation never reaches the alveolar region for gas exchange to occur. For the healthy adult using a tidal breath of 450 mL, about one third of the volume fails to reach the airspaces and is, therefore, unavailable for gas exchange. This 150 mL is the conducting airway volume and is called the *anatomic dead space* ($\dot{V}_D$). The dead space must be subtracted from the total ventilation each minute ($\dot{V}_E$) to compute the alveolar ventilation ($\dot{V}_A$):

$$\dot{V}_A = \dot{V}_E - \dot{V}_D$$

Alveolar ventilation is, therefore, less than total minute ventilation because it mixes with the dead space ventilation. However, all of the CO_2 in the expired gas comes from alveolar ventilation. This means that the volume of CO_2 in the expired gas per minute can be defined by the equation:

$$\dot{V}_{CO_2} = \dot{V}_A \times F_{CO_2}$$

where F_{CO_2} is the fractional CO_2 concentration in the expired gas. Because the P_{CO_2} in the alveolar gas is almost identical to the Pa_{CO_2}, the effective alveolar ventilation is found by

$$\dot{V}_A = \dot{V}_{CO_2}/Pa_{CO_2} \times K$$

where K is a proportionality constant (0.863). This simple equation demonstrates why the Pa_{CO_2} can be used to determine the alveolar ventilation and makes it easy to discern the reciprocal relation between these two parameters—hypoventilation increases the Pa_{CO_2}, whereas hyperventilation decreases it.

It is also important to note that the Pa_{CO_2} depends on the rate of CO_2 production ($\dot{V}_{CO_2}$) and on the dead space volume. The dead space actually has two components: the anatomic component described earlier, and a physiologic component, which is the total volume of lung that does not contribute to CO_2 elimination. The physiologic dead space, usually described by the Bohr equation, is easily derived from the information presented earlier, and in its clinical form is as follows:

$$V_D/V_T = Pa_{CO_2} - P_{E_{CO_2}}/Pa_{CO_2}$$

where V_T is the tidal volume, and $P_{E_{CO_2}}$ is the P_{CO_2} in the expired gas.

Usually, the two components of the dead space, physiologic and anatomic, are roughly equivalent; however, in patients with significant lung disease, the physiologic dead space may be quite a bit larger than the anatomic space because of unequal matching of ventilation and blood flow (perfusion). This unevenness mainly reflects the contributions of lung units with very low blood flow relative to ventilation.

At rest, the alveolar ventilation of the normal human is about 5 L/min, which almost perfectly matches the entire pulmonary blood flow—the cardiac output—of about 5 L/min. Thus, the average or overall ventilation ($\dot{V}_A$) to perfusion ($\dot{Q}$) ratio or $\dot{V}_A/\dot{Q}$ of the human respiratory system is close to 1.0.[5,6] However, the overall $\dot{V}_A/\dot{Q}$ ratio does not account for heterogeneity of ventilation and perfusion, which can be significant. For instance, all lung regions do not receive the same amount of ventilation, and in the upright position, the lower lung zones are better ventilated (and better perfused) than the upper zones, which have greater ventilation than perfusion. The more precisely the lung is able to match ventilation with perfusion, the better will be gas exchange. Indeed, mismatching of ventilation and blood flow is the primary cause of most of the defective gas exchange in patients with lung disease.

Oxygen and CO_2 are exchanged in the terminal respiratory units by simple diffusion across the alveolar-capillary membrane.[1] Gases diffuse from regions of high-to-low partial pressure, and as long as pulmonary ventilation is adequate, O_2 moves from alveolus to capillary blood, and CO_2 from capillary blood to alveolus. The gas exchange in each anatomic unit (local $\dot{V}_A/\dot{Q}$) is averaged to give the overall $\dot{V}_A/\dot{Q}$, and the dispersion of values around the mean determines the heterogeneity of gas exchange. In numeric terms, $\dot{V}_A/\dot{Q}$ regions that have perfusion but no ventilation ($\dot{V}_A/\dot{Q} = 0$) are defined as right-to-left shunts, whereas regions with ventilation but no perfusion ($\dot{V}_A/\dot{Q} = \infty$) are defined as dead space.[6] The magnitude of these extremes and the distribution of high-to-low $\dot{V}_A/\dot{Q}$ ratios determine the values of the Po_2 and Pco_2 in the arterial blood. These principles are illustrated by plotting of the $\dot{V}_A/\dot{Q}$ ratio against actual ventilation or blood flow on a graph (Fig. 8.2).

In general, low $\dot{V}_A/\dot{Q}$ ratios and shunt primarily affect O_2 transfer across the lungs and cause hypoxemia, whereas high $\dot{V}_A/\dot{Q}$ ratios and dead space have more influence on CO_2 elimination and may predispose to hypercapnia. The distribution of $\dot{V}_A/\dot{Q}$ ratios and the effectiveness of gas exchange can be evaluated in several ways, although no method provides an all-inclusive description of pulmonary gas exchange. The simplest approach is to sample arterial blood and alveolar gas and analyze their compositions. Methods that utilize tracer gases and gas exchange models,

such as the multiple inert gas elimination technique, are research tools that are outside the scope of this chapter.[7]

Clinically, the routine assessment of pulmonary gas exchange relies on measurements of the arterial blood gases. The basic information about the adequacy of $\dot{V}_A/\dot{Q}$ matching is provided by arterial Po_2, especially if it is low. And if the inspired O_2 concentration is normal, a low arterial Po_2 indicates the presence of $\dot{V}_A/\dot{Q}$ mismatching or areas of shunt. However, small amounts of shunt and regions of low $\dot{V}_A/\dot{Q}$ may not be reflected in the Po_2. Furthermore, partial pressure of arterial oxygen (Pa_{O_2}) may be low for other reasons, including hypoventilation or low cardiac output. In the clinical setting, the alveolar-to-arterial Po_2 difference (A-aDo_2) must be calculated to properly interpret the arterial blood gases and fully evaluate pulmonary gas exchange.

The A-aDo_2 is more informative than the Pa_{O_2} because it quantitatively accounts for the level of ventilation. The value is calculated from the measurement of Pa_{O_2} and an estimate of the ideal partial pressure of alveolar oxygen (PA_{O_2}) derived from the alveolar gas equation. The alveolar gas equation estimates an ideal PA_{O_2} by simplifying the lungs to a single uniform mathematic compartment as follows:

$$PA_{O_2} = FI_{O_2} (P_B - PH_2O) - PA_{CO_2}$$
$$[FI_{O_2} + 1 - FI_{O_2}/R]$$

where FI_{O_2} is the fractional concentration of inspired oxygen (0.209 in air), P_B is barometric pressure (mm Hg), PH_2O is water vapor pressure at body temperature (47 mm Hg at 37°C), PA_{CO_2} is alveolar Pco_2 (mm Hg), and R the respiratory exchange ratio (0.8 at steady state with a normal diet). To further simplify the calculation, the Pa_{CO_2} can substitute for PA_{CO_2} and the last term reduced to 1/R to give:

$$PA_{O_2} = FI_{O_2} (P_B - PH_2O) - Pa_{CO_2}/R$$

The A-aDo_2 is nonzero, even in the healthy young adults, not because of a diffusion gradient across the pulmonary capillaries, but because small areas of $\dot{V}_A/\dot{Q}$ inequality and minor right-to-left and postpulmonary shunts constitute 2% to 3% of the cardiac output.

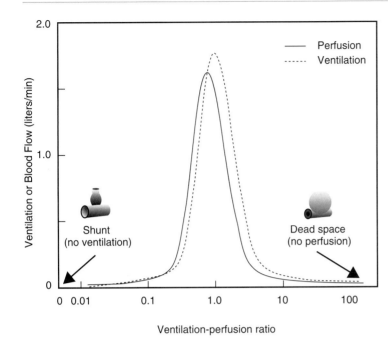

FIGURE 8.2 ALVEOLAR VENTILATION/ PERFUSION ($\dot{V}_A/\dot{Q}$) RATIOS IN THE LUNG. The distribution of $\dot{V}_A/\dot{Q}$ centers around unity for most of the lung's ventilation and blood flow units. *Solid line* represents perfusion; *dotted line* represents ventilation.

Postpulmonary shunts are found normally in the bronchial circulation and the cardiac thebesian veins.[8]

The effect of $\dot{V}_A/\dot{Q}$ mismatching on the A-aD_{O_2} can be shown using a slightly more sophisticated two-compartment lung. If both compartments have identical $\dot{V}_A/\dot{Q}$ ratios (e.g., 0.85), the absence of a diffusion gradient would produce no A-aD_{O_2}. However, if there is a slight $\dot{V}_A/\dot{Q}$ mismatch—assume, for instance, that $\dot{V}_A/\dot{Q}$ is 0.7 in one unit and 1.0 in the other—the overall $\dot{V}_A/\dot{Q}$ will still be 0.85. However, the average $P_{A_{O_2}}$ computed from the one-compartment alveolar gas equation will remain the same. Hence, a small A-aD_{O_2} difference will develop because the unit with a lower $\dot{V}_A/\dot{Q}$ ratio will have less ventilation. The lower ventilation means that the local alveolar and capillary P_{O_2} will also be lower, and that arterial P_{O_2} overall will be reduced slightly. Because the number of low $\dot{V}_A/\dot{Q}$ units tends to increase with age, the A-aD_{O_2} increases with age—in proportion to the decline in P_{O_2}. A normal value for the A-aD_{O_2} is approximately half of the age up to a maximum of 25 to 30 mm Hg.

As inspired P_{O_2} increases, the A-aD_{O_2} also increases because arterial P_{O_2} rises slower than alveolar P_{O_2} because of the impending complete saturation of Hb with O_2 (flattening of the dissociation curve) and elimination of the suppressive effects of $\dot{V}_A/\dot{Q}$ inequality on $P_{a_{O_2}}$. Thereafter, progressive increases in $P_{A_{O_2}}$ with O_2 breathing proportionately increase the A-aD_{O_2}. The effect of O_2 breathing on shunt is nil because, by definition, areas of shunt cannot be ventilated, making it impossible for O_2 to diffuse into the arterial blood. These principles are illustrated in Figure 8.3.

The increase in A-aD_{O_2} with $P_{A_{O_2}}$ makes the value too cumbersome to use clinically unless the patient is breathing room air. However, the A-aD_{O_2} is easily converted to the a/A ratio, which at $P_{a_{O_2}}$ values greater than ~100 mm Hg is constant over a wide range of inspired O_2 concentrations and can be used under hyperbaric conditions. The ratio is taken by dividing the $P_{a_{O_2}}$ into the value of the $P_{A_{O_2}}$ derived from the alveolar gas equation. For instance, at a $P_{a_{O_2}}$ of 90 mm Hg and a $P_{A_{O_2}}$ of 100 mm Hg, the a/A is 0.9 (reference range, 0.8–0.95). During 100% O_2 breathing, $P_{a_{O_2}}$ will increase to close to 600 mm Hg, but the a/A will remain approximately stable. However, the A-aD_{O_2} increases from 10 mm Hg to more than 60 mm Hg!

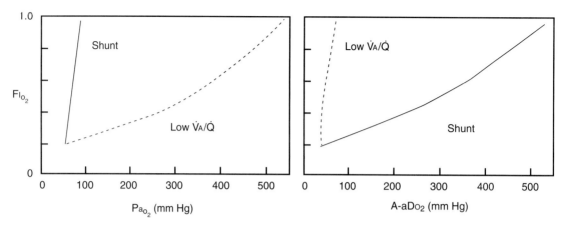

FIGURE 8.3 DIFFERENCES IN RESPONSE TO SUPPLEMENTAL O_2 BREATHING FOR LEFT-TO-RIGHT SHUNT AND ALVEOLAR VENTILATION/PERFUSION ($\dot{V}_A/\dot{Q}$) MISMATCH (low $\dot{V}_A/\dot{Q}$). *Left,* Failure of arterial partial pressure of oxygen (Pa_{O_2}) to increase with increasing fractional concentration of inspired oxygen (FI_{O_2}) in the presence of shunt. *Right,* Greater widening of the alveolar-arterial O_2 difference (A-aD_{O2}) as the FI_{O_2} is increased in the presence of shunt than with low $\dot{V}_A/\dot{Q}$.

The a/A is especially useful for predicting the Pa_{O_2} expected from a change in inspired O_2 concentration in the presence of lung disease. This approach is commonly used in practice to adjust inspired O_2 concentration downward in patients on mechanical ventilation to avoid pulmonary oxygen toxicity. In hyperbaric medicine, the a/A is used to estimate Pa_{O_2} at a specific increased treatment pressure, particularly in patients with significant preexisting lung disease.[9]

The Pa_{O_2} under hyperbaric conditions can be predicted using a room air blood gas and the computed a/A by entering the ratio into the equation:

$$Pa_{O_2} \text{ (predicted)} = FI_{O_2} (760 \times P_{ATA} - P_{H_2O}) - [Pa_{CO_2}/R] \times [a/A_{Air}]$$

where P_{ATA} is the final pressure in atmospheres absolute (ATA). A sample calculation of the predicted Pa_{O_2} under hyperbaric conditions is given below for a patient with a Pa_{O_2} of 70 mm Hg and Pco_2 of 40 mm Hg on room air at sea level who is to receive hyperbaric therapy at 2.5 ATA:

$$Pa_{O_2} \text{ (predicted)} = 1.0 (760 \times 2.5 - 47) - [40/0.8] \times [0.7] = 1262 \text{ mm Hg}$$

The example illustrates that patients with impaired gas exchange at sea level will continue to manifest that impairment under hyperbaric conditions even though the inspired O_2 concentration is increased to high levels. The positive predictive value of a/A_{Air} on Pa_{O_2} has been confirmed in patients in the chamber, and the method is accurate to at least 3 ATA.

OXYGEN TRANSFER FROM ALVEOLAR GAS TO BLOOD

O_2 is transferred from alveolar gas across the pulmonary-capillary membrane into the blood by simple physical diffusion along the concentration gradient between the gas phase and blood plasma and then into the red blood cell where it is bound to Hb. Thus, O_2 transfer represents molecular diffusion across a set of resistances in series, each of which behaves according to Fick's Law of Diffusion.[1] Despite this series of barriers, the overall process occurs rapidly, and for the normal lung under normal conditions, there is no diffusion limitation in pulmonary gas exchange.[6] These principles are illustrated in Figure 8.4.

The diffusion gradient or driving pressure for O_2 across the lungs is determined by the Po_2 difference between mixed venous blood entering the pulmonary capillary and the local PA_{O_2}. At a mixed venous Po_2 of 40 mm Hg and an alveolar Po_2 of 100 mm Hg, this gradient is about 60 mm Hg. Because of the great O_2 capacity of the Hb sink, the Po_2 in the pulmonary capillary blood increases

$$V_{gas} = A/T \times D\ (P_1 - P_2)$$

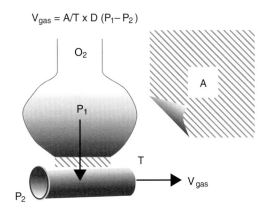

FIGURE 8.4 FICK'S LAW OF DIFFUSION IN THE LUNG. The volume of gas crossing the lung (V_{gas}) is equal to the exchange area (A) divided by the thickness (T) times the diffusion constant (D) times the difference in the gas partial pressure (P), in this case, the P_{O_2}, between the alveolus and the capillary.

quickly and equilibrates with $P_{A_{O_2}}$ over the first one third of the length of the capillary. That is, there is a normal pulmonary capillary reserve of about twofold in residence time that prevents a diffusion limitation. However, disease states that cause pronounced thickening of the alveolar-capillary membrane, such as sarcoidosis, or conditions in which the $P_{A_{O_2}}$ is low and mean capillary transit time is short, such as exercise at high altitude, do produce diffusion impairments (Fig. 8.5).

The structure of the lung is too complex to determine the exact surface area and thickness of the alveolar-capillary barrier for diffusion in vivo; therefore, for clinical purposes, area and thickness are lumped with

an apparent diffusion constant into a single parameter called D_L, or the diffusion capacity of the lung. D_L is usually measured using a tracer gas, such as carbon monoxide (CO), and the D_{LCO} is a standard pulmonary function measurement in modern clinical laboratories.[6] By convention, the D_L is separated into two components on the basis of the work of Roughton and Forster: the in-series resistances of the alveolar-capillary plus erythrocyte membranes ($1/D_M$) and the time required for the chemical reaction and O_2 uptake by Hb ($1/\theta V_c$).[10] In the latter term, θ is the rate constant for the Hb reaction and V_c is the pulmonary capillary Hb volume. The sum of these two components thus represents the overall pulmonary resistance to diffusion or 1 ÷ diffusion capacity:

$$1/D_L = 1/D_M + 1/\theta V_c$$

The Roughton–Forster relation indicates that the membrane and capillary blood volume components of D_L have equal mathematic weights, but V_c turns out to be a more important physiologic factor for O_2 diffusion across the lung (Fig. 8.6). V_c is critical because the amount of Hb in the lung capillaries can vary several fold, for instance, by assuming a supine position or by the dilation and recruitment of capillaries with exercise. These maneuvers substantially increase D_L. Thus, diffusion capacity measurements of the lung are routinely performed upright and at rest, and must be

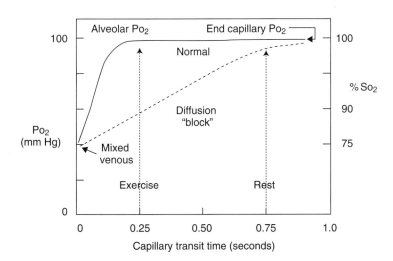

FIGURE 8.5 CAPILLARY TRANSIT TIME AND O_2 SATURATION AT REST AND EXERCISE. Under normal conditions, the erythrocyte transit time through the capillary of about 0.75 second is long enough for hemoglobin to fully equilibrate with partial pressure of alveolar oxygen ($P_{A_{O_2}}$). However, in some pulmonary diseases associated with thickening of the alveolar-capillary membrane, or during exercise at high altitude, a diffusion limitation or "block" can occur.

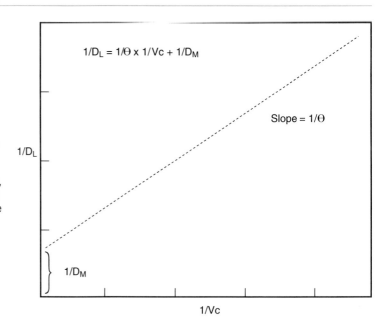

FIGURE 8.6 THE COMPONENTS OF THE DIFFUSION CAPACITY (D_L) OF THE LUNG. To express D_L in a linear form, a double reciprocal is used for the X-Y plot. The capillary hemoglobin concentration is pulmonary capillary hemoglobin volume (V_c), and the rate constant for the O_2-hemoglobin binding reaction is θ. The graph indicates the dependence of D_L on V_c.

corrected for Hb concentration (3.5% per gram of Hb above or below 15 g/dL).

OXYGEN TRANSPORT FROM THE LUNG TO THE SYSTEMIC MICROCIRCULATION

The previous section deals with the diffusive O_2 transfer from the alveoli across the pulmonary microcirculation and into the erythrocyte. This is the first portion of the so-called oxygen cascade by which O_2 moves from the atmosphere to the internal furnace of the cell—the mitochondrion (Fig. 8.7). The physiologic transport of O_2 from pulmonary capillaries to systemic capillaries requires only the physical process of convection.[5] This convective O_2 transport from pulmonary to systemic capillaries is the function of the *distributive circulation*—the heart, aorta, arteries, and arterioles. As in the lung, the main gas exchange region of the systemic circulation resides in the *nutrient* or *microcirculation*, where diffusion again emerges as the physical means of delivering O_2 from capillary to mitochondria.[11]

In the blood, O_2 is transported in bulk by two mechanisms: chemically bound to Hb and dissolved in the blood plasma. The special aspects of dissolved O_2 are covered here in some detail because the principle serves as

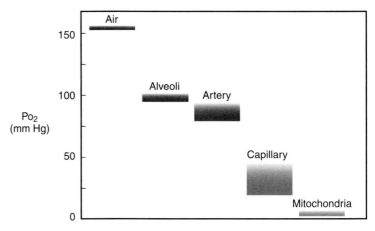

FIGURE 8.7 THE O_2 CASCADE. O_2 is transported down a concentration gradient from the atmosphere to the mitochondrion. The height of the bars indicates the normal partial pressure of oxygen (Po_2) operating range in each compartment. Mitochondrial Po_2 must be less than 1 mm Hg for O_2 to be limiting.

the cornerstone of hyperbaric oxygen therapy (HBOT).[12] However, it is important to remember that the size and high O_2 requirements of even the smallest mammal thwart dissolved O_2 and simple diffusion as reliable means of DO_2 to tissue.[1] Therefore, all mammals and most vertebrates depend on a carrier protein, such as Hb, to supply enough O_2 to the tissues to support aerobic metabolism.

The basal or resting rate of aerobic metabolism in the normal adult—the $\dot{V}O_2$ consumption or $\dot{V}O_2$—is approximately 3 mL O_2 per minute per kilogram body weight. Thus, the average-sized adult man consumes about 250 mL O_2 per minute.[8] Simply put, $\dot{V}O_2$ is the sum of the O_2 utilization of each of the tissues and organs of the whole body. About 90% of this O_2 is used by the terminal mitochondrial electron acceptor, cytochrome c oxidase, which irreversibly reduces it to water.[2] The remaining 10% is consumed by other O_2-requiring enzymes (~8%) and by the incomplete reduction of O_2 to reactive oxygen species (1-2%).

For each 100 mL of molecular O_2 consumed by aerobic metabolism, 70 to 100 mL CO_2 are produced, depending on the type of substrate being oxidized. This means the ratio of CO_2 production to O_2 consumption, called the *respiratory quotient,* varies from 0.7 (protein) to 1.0 (carbohydrate) with an average value of 0.8. It also means that a basal $\dot{V}O_2$ of 250 mL/min will produce 200 mL CO_2.

The time-averaged $\dot{V}O_2$ of the body was used by Fick to perform the first computations of mean cardiac output ($\dot{Q}T$) from the principle of conservation of mass:

$$\dot{Q}T = \dot{V}O_2/[CaO_2 - C\bar{v}O_2]$$

where CaO_2 and $C\bar{v}O_2$ are the arterial and mixed venous O_2 contents, respectively.

The blood O_2 content on each side of the circulation is the sum of the amount of O_2 bound chemically to Hb plus that carried in dissolved form in the plasma. Fick's original equation, however, is now usually written as:

$$\dot{V}O_2 = \dot{Q}T \,[CaO_2 - C\bar{v}O_2]$$

The product of $\dot{Q}T \times CaO_2$ is called the O_2 *delivery* (DO_2), and the quantity $CaO_2 - C\bar{v}O_2$ is the arteriovenous oxygen content difference

($AVDO_2$), which at rest is normally 5 mL/dL or about one fourth of the DO_2.[8] Therefore, the normal O_2 extraction ratio (OER) at rest is about 0.25.

The reference Hb concentration in the blood is ~15 g/dL, and its O_2 carrying capacity is normally ~1.34 mL O_2 per gram.* The amount of O_2 carried by Hb is the product of its concentration [Hb] times the O_2 capacity times the O_2 saturation (SO_2). Therefore, excluding dissolved O_2, fully saturated arterial blood has a CaO_2 about 20.1 mL O_2 per deciliter.

Hb forms a tetramer of two α and two β chains inside the erythrocyte that reversibly and cooperatively binds four O_2 molecules.[4] Cooperative O_2 binding is responsible for the familiar sigmoid shape of the Hb O_2 dissociation curve, which relates O_2 saturation to blood PO_2 (Fig. 8.8). The sigmoid shape of the O_2 dissociation curve facilitates O_2 loading at high PO_2 (flat part of the curve) and O_2 unloading at low PO_2 (steep part of the curve). In addition, the position of the O_2 dissociation curve can be shifted to the left or right with respect to PO_2 by physiologic factors, such as changes in pH, as indicated in Figure 8.8. A shift of the curve to the left increases the O_2 affinity of Hb, for example, with hyperventilation, which increases the rate of O_2 loading in the lungs. A shift of the curve to the right decreases the Hb O_2 affinity, for instance, during metabolic acidosis (Bohr effect), which facilitates O_2 unloading in systemic capillaries. However, the position of the O_2 dissociation curve does not affect the O_2 carrying capacity of Hb. This can be changed only by interfering with the O_2 binding properties of the molecule. The position of the curve determines only the blood O_2 content at a particular PO_2.

The most important influence on the O_2 capacity of the blood is a change in the Hb concentration. Increases in blood Hb concentration lead to polycythemia, which accompanies the response to hypoxemia, whereas decreases in Hb concentration are the hallmark of anemia. Polycythemia and

---

*The value for the O_2 capacity of hemoglobin (Hb) depends on how the measurement is made and varies from 1.34 to 1.39 mL/g. The traditional Huffner constant of 1.34 is used in this chapter.

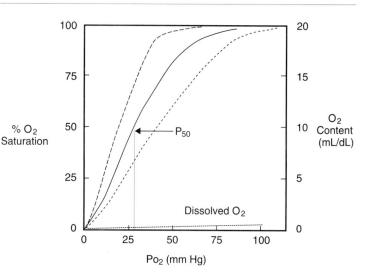

FIGURE 8.8 THE O_2 DISSOCIATION CURVE OF HEMOGLOBIN. The normal curve has a oxygen half-saturation pressure of hemoglobin (P_{50}) of approximately 27 mm Hg (*solid line*). The curve is shifted to the left by alkalosis, hypothermia, carbon monoxide, and low red blood cell (RBC) 2,3-diphosphoglycerate (2,3-DPG). The curve is shifted to the right by acidosis (Bohr effect), fever, and increased RBC 2,3-DPG content.

anemia most often develop slowly and for the purposes of this discussion are considered only at a normal blood volume—under isovolemic conditions. An acute loss of blood (hypovolemia) leads to a decrease in Do_2 from a decline in $\dot{Q}T$, not a decrease in Hb concentration, which remains stable initially and until after compensation by fluid retention or with volume resuscitation.

In general, appropriate polycythemia offsets the decrease in Ca_{O_2} from hypoxemia, which under acute circumstances is compensated for primarily by an increase in cardiac output. Over the long term, polycythemia helps maintain a normal Do_2 by allowing the resting $\dot{Q}T$ to recover toward normal, whereas $\dot{V}o_2$ remains stable. Chronic anemia also increases cardiac output, but Do_2 tends to decline slowly and steadily. Thus, the OER must increase to more than 0.25 to maintain normal $\dot{V}o_2$. In humans, isovolemic anemia to Hb concentrations of about one third of normal (to 5 g/dL) doubles the $\dot{Q}T$ with an increase in OER from 0.25 to about 0.33.[13] The combination of low Ca_{O_2} and high OER means the mixed venous Po_2 decreases to less than 70%.

Interference with the O_2 binding properties of Hb produces anemia-like effects, such as with the formation of *methemoglobin* or *carboxyhemoglobin*. These and other chemical or steric modifications of heme decrease the O_2 capacity of Hb and hence reduce the arterial O_2 content without affecting the circulating Hb concentration. The formation of carboxyhemo-

globin, even though it is reversible, decreases the O_2 capacity of Hb in direct proportion to its concentration because CO avidly binds Hb at more than 200 times the affinity of O_2.

The main function of Hb in O_2 transport can be illustrated by considering the only other mechanism for O_2 carriage in the blood—in dissolved form. The amount of O_2 dissolved in the plasma follows Henry's Law: It is proportional to the O_2 partial pressure in the gas phase and the Bunsen solubility coefficient of plasma. The solubility of O_2 in plasma at body temperature is only 0.0031 mL/mm Hg per 100 mL. Therefore, at sea level and a Pa_{O_2} of 100 mm Hg, the amount of O_2 in plasma is only 0.31 mL/dL.* Because O_2 solubility in plasma is so low, only about 2% of the O_2 in arterial blood is transported as dissolved gas. To meet a basal $\dot{V}o_2$ of 250 mL/min (3 mL/kg/min) solely from dissolved O_2, $\dot{Q}T$ would need to be ~1 L/kg/min, or more than 80 L/min. This is more than double the maximum $\dot{Q}T$ attainable at a normal Hb concentration with exercise at sea level.

Despite the limitations of delivering O_2 in dissolved form, once Hb is saturated, O_2 breathing can only increase blood O_2 content by increasing the amount of O_2 dissolved in plasma. At a Pa_{O_2} of 100 mm Hg or more, the heme O_2 binding sites of Hb are occupied, and the arterial O_2 content, for instance, under

---

*Units of milliliters per deciliter (mL/dL) are sometimes expressed in the clinical literature as volumes percent or vol%.

hyperbaric conditions, increases in direct proportion to Po_2 (Fig. 8.9). For the normal lung, the Po_2 increases by 600 to 700 mm Hg and Ca_{O_2} by about 2 mL/dL for each atmosphere absolute of HBO. Because the body normally extracts about 5 mL/dL O_2 per minute, enough O_2 can be extracted from plasma at 3 ATA to meet metabolic needs. This principle was first demonstrated in 1959 by Boerema, who observed that laboratory animals could survive in the hyperbaric chamber at 3 ATA sans Hb and solely on dissolved O_2 in plasma.[14] These experiments provided the impetus for many of the early studies on clinical HBOT.

Three important principles of tissue oxygenation must be considered before reviewing how O_2 behaves in the microcirculation. The first is that each tissue normally sets its own rate of aerobic metabolism ($\dot{V}o_2$). This fact accounts for the organ-specific range of values in the human body found for blood flow, capillary density, and O_2 extraction. A corollary is that the O_2 supply is normally *not limiting;* in other words, supplemental O_2 administration does not increase the rate of O_2 uptake. Even for maximal exercise, it has been a challenge to show an appreciable benefit of extra O_2 on performance that would demonstrate a critical limitation in the O_2 supply.[15,16]

The second principle is that because the normal arterial O_2 saturation is so high (~98%), an organ can meet an increased oxygen requirement in only two ways—either by increasing Do_2 or by increasing O_2 extraction. The former is usually done by increasing $\dot{Q}T$ (or local blood flow) and the latter by increasing the OER. To achieve maximal rates of O_2 consumption, tissues use both mechanisms.[11] Moreover, the reserves in the system are considerable. For instance, during maximal exercise, $\dot{Q}T$ can increase sixfold and OER threefold.

The third principle is the recognition of a well-defined hierarchy for the distribution of blood flow, which is determined by O_2 availability and metabolic precedence of the various tissues or organs.[5] In general, blood flow through the distributive circulation is regulated by sympathetic constrictor tone and local factors, whereas vessels in the microcirculation are regulated primarily by local metabolic dilators. These regulatory systems are arranged and balanced to match Do_2 optimally with demand (O_2) throughout the body over a range of physiologic conditions.

The relation between Do_2 and $\dot{V}o_2$ previously received a great deal of attention clinically because of evidence that some diseases, such as severe sepsis, may exhibit an abnormal dependence of $\dot{V}o_2$ on Do_2.[17-20] Normally, O_2 is independent of Do_2 until after the blood flow and OER reserves are fully enlisted. For instance, during hemorrhage, $\dot{Q}T$, and hence Do_2, decline progressively, but $\dot{V}o_2$ is preserved until Do_2 is less than ~6 mL/kg (or 400–500 mL/dL). Once this critical threshold is crossed, $\dot{V}o_2$ becomes dependent on Do_2. An optimal $\dot{V}o_2$ can no longer be maintained because neither

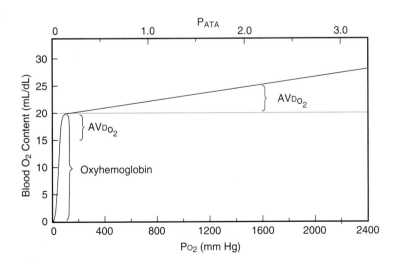

FIGURE 8.9 THE O_2 DISSOCIATION CURVE OF HEMOGLOBIN IN THE HYPERBARIC RANGE. The graph illustrates the effect of dissolved O_2 on the arteriovenous O_2 difference (AVD_{O_2}).

FIGURE 8.10 NORMAL AND
PATHOLOGIC RELATIONSHIPS
BETWEEN OXYGEN DELIVERY (DO_2)
AND CONSUMPTION ($\dot{V}O_2$). Notice that
normally $\dot{V}O_2$ is independent of DO_2 until
low values for O_2 delivery are reached. Under
some pathologic conditions, such as severe
sepsis, the curve can be shifted to the
right and the distinction between the O_2
delivery-independent and -dependent parts
of the curve becomes less distinct.

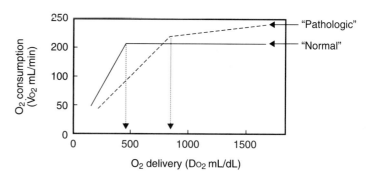

$\dot{Q}_T$ nor OER can be increased further. This principle is illustrated graphically in Figure 8.10.

In diseases that involve severe microcirculatory dysfunction and multiple organ failure, the critical threshold for the dependence of $\dot{V}O_2$ on DO_2 may increase into the reference range of physiologic blood flow regulation and O_2 extraction (see Fig. 8.10). This is called *pathologic O_2 supply dependency* because it deviates from the normal lines of specific OERs. In some cases, $\dot{V}O_2$ supply dependency has turned out to be a mathematic artifact, whereas in others, the observations appear to be correct. The finding implies a widening of the mean intercapillary distance or a compromise in the ability of mitochondria to extract O_2, or both. In any event, attempts to prevent organ failure and improve survival in severe sepsis by intentionally driving up DO_2 with blood transfusions or inotropic agents have been unsuccessful.

SYSTEMIC MICROCIRCULATION AND TISSUE GAS EXCHANGE

The purpose of the systemic microcirculation is to provide a large area for the transfer of nutrients to and removal of waste products from the cells. This function includes, first and foremost, the exchange of O_2 and CO_2. The microcirculation is organized anatomically according to the special characteristics of each tissue or organ, but in general terms, the system is composed of arterioles—vessels of 20 μm or less in internal diameter—as well as the terminal arterioles (metarterioles) and capillaries.[5] Capillary density varies among tissues, but usually, depending on the tissue

type, a cell is no more than 30 to 60 μm away from a capillary.[21] However, capillaries are also rarely perfused continuously; they open and close periodically, for instance, under the control of precapillary sphincters, most notably in relation to local O_2 concentration.[22] Thus, at high rates of O_2 consumption, as PO_2 decreases, the capillaries tend to remain open longer, whereas at low rates of O_2 consumption, the capillaries may be closed much of the time. Moreover, the extraction of O_2 along the length of the capillary means that PO_2 is naturally higher at the arteriolar than at the venule end. It is also observed that the relatively sharp branching angles of different-sized vessels in the microcirculation cause plasma skimming to the smaller vessel. Thus, the microvascular hematocrit routinely declines to less than that in the central vessels by as much as a third.

If one picks a point on a capillary and makes a perpendicular slice through the tissue, as the distance away from the center of the capillary increases, the PO_2 decreases because of O_2 utilization by mitochondria. Plasma O_2 is consumed first, allowing O_2 to diffuse across the erythrocyte membrane, through the plasma layer, through the endothelial cell barrier, and across the cell membrane before it reaches the mitochondria. The main resistance (R) to O_2 diffusion is across the red blood cell membrane and the vascular walls of terminal arterioles and capillaries. Little resistance occurs at the plasma membrane or across mitochondrial membranes. These resistances can be summed and expressed as the reciprocal 1/R, or the conductance (G) of O_2 from capillary to the mitochondrion.[11] The concept is shown in Figure 8.11.

Because of the multiple effects mentioned earlier, the P_{O_2} in tissues is quite variable. Tissue P_{O_2} measurements, for example, using platinum microelectrodes, are also difficult to perform accurately and may be even harder to interpret. Even a single relatively homogeneous tissue shows considerable spatial P_{O_2} heterogeneity, which can be seen by plotting the measurements as a function of their frequency.[23] Thus, a P_{O_2} histogram emerges from which the median and scatter provide an estimate of the O_2 dispersion in the tissue. Sample P_{O_2} histograms of the beating guinea pig heart during air and O_2 breathing are shown in Figure 8.12. The histograms illustrate the effect of O_2 breathing on increasing the median and the dispersion of P_{O_2} in the healthy heart. The pattern is similar among tissues exposed to HBO, although the histograms are shifted even further to the right.

Predictions of tissue P_{O_2} from model calculations are also difficult to interpret and sometimes conflict with experimental measurements. However, since the development of the original cylinder model of Krogh and Erlang for skeletal muscle, models of tissue O_2 distribution have proved instructive for understanding tissue oxygenation.[24] The Krogh–Erlang model makes use of one or more parallel cylinders of highly organized and homogeneous (ideal) tissue, each surrounding a central uniform capillary of known length (L) that can be used to calculate the radius (r) of the P_{O_2} distribution based on diffusion (Fig. 8.13).

The cylinder model is quite simple compared with the morphology of even an elementary capillary network, yet it is highly informative. Most notably, it emphasizes how diffusion limits the movement of O_2 from capillary to tissues, especially at the venous ends of capillaries. In O_2 insufficiency, hypoxia emerges first at the venous end—the so-called lethal corner. Interestingly, living tissues recognize this problem and capillary density tends to be greatest far away from the terminal arterioles.[1] Thus, the microcirculation is not arranged anatomically as parallel cylinders.

The cylinder model does predict correctly the more stringent geometric limits of diffusion at high metabolic rates, as well as the appearance of longer distances for O_2 diffusion when P_{O_2} is high at the capillary entrance (see Fig. 8.13). However, the model overestimates O_2 extraction in the capillary, which can be corrected by building in a precapillary O_2 shunt from arteriole to venule. The presence of a small arteriovenous shunt provides for suitable estimates of venous O_2 saturations in the model, and experimentally, their presence has been seen in a number of living tissues.

As already noted, there are conditions, especially in disease states such as hemorrhage or ischemia, in which O_2 uptake is limited by local D_{O_2} and not by diffusion. Not surprisingly, diffusion models do not fit such perfusion-limited conditions well, even for models that allow different numbers, types, and distributions of capillaries. The variable and intermittent rate of capillary blood flow observed in vivo is also particularly difficult to model, and there are still significant gaps in our understanding of microcirculatory function in disease.

The diffusion models are also informative for understanding the effects of HBOT on living tissue, especially because direct P_{O_2} measurements are technically difficult to make in the chamber, even experimentally. In the 1960s, C. J. Lambertsen measured the arteriovenous O_2

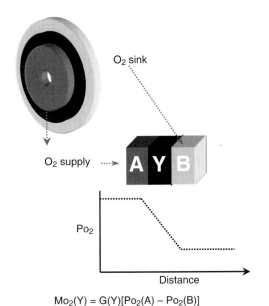

$$M_{O_2}(Y) = G(Y)[P_{O_2}(A) - P_{O_2}(B)]$$

FIGURE 8.11 SLAB DIFFUSION MODEL FOR O_2. M is the mass transport of oxygen across the slab labeled Y; G is the conductance (1/D) of Y where D is the diffusion constant for O_2 (muscle $\sim 1.3 \times 10^{-12}$ mol cm^{-1} min^{-1} mm Hg^{-1}).

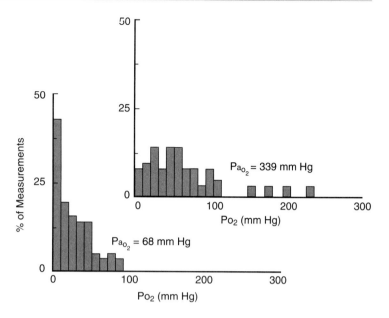

FIGURE 8.12 PARTIAL PRESSURE OF OXYGEN (P_{O_2}) HISTOGRAMS OF THE BEATING GUINEA PIG HEART. *Bottom,* Histogram with the animal breathing room air. *Top,* Histogram with the animal breathing O_2 at sea level. *(Adapted from Schuchardt S: Comparative physiology of the oxygen supply. In: Kessler M, Bruley DF, Clark LC Jr, et al. (eds): Oxygen Supply: Theoretical and Practical Aspects of Oxygen Supply and Microcirculation of Tissue. Baltimore, University Park Press, 1973, pp 223–229, by permission.)*

difference in the cerebral circulation in healthy human subjects and found that even at inspired P_{O_2} of up to 3.5 ATA, jugular venous P_{O_2} rarely exceeded 60 mm Hg (Fig. 8.14).[25] Such profiles indicating high P_{O_2} differences across organ vascular beds are typically caused by the low plasma O_2 solubility and by O_2-induced vasoconstriction. However, the mean capillary P_{O_2} predicted at 3.5 ATA approached 900 mm Hg, an estimate later confirmed experimentally in animals by brain tissue P_{O_2} measurements. Placing these observations into the context of the cylinder model, the fact that HBO arterial-

izes the venous blood means that the radius of diffusion for O_2 into tissue at the venous end of the capillary has been increased to approximately the same level as that of a normal arteriole.[12] This concept is shown in Figure 8.15. Figure 8.15 also demonstrates that the tremendously high values of Pa_{O_2} found under hyperbaric conditions make HBO an exception to the normal rule that partial oxygen pressure in mixed venous blood (Pv_{O_2}) is a good estimate of mean capillary P_{O_2}.[21]

The idea that HBO expands the effective radius of O_2 diffusion in the capillary is useful

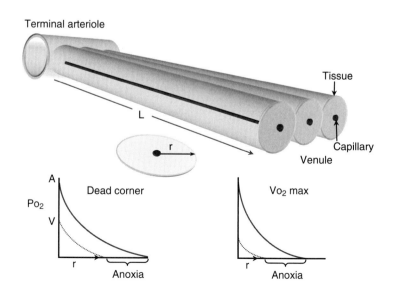

FIGURE 8.13 SCHEMATIC OF THE KROGH CYLINDER MODEL OF TISSUE OXYGENATION. *Left,* Diffusion radii for the arterial and venular ends of the capillary. *Right,* Effect of increased oxygen consumption per minute (Vo_2) on the diffusion radii without an increase in partial pressure of oxygen (P_{O_2}) or blood flow.

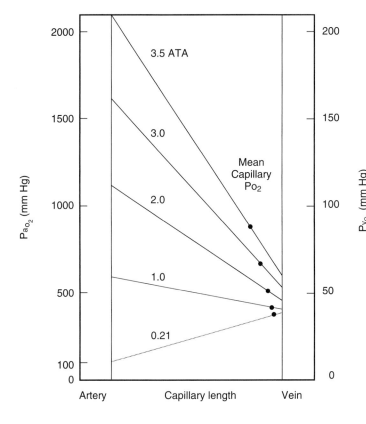

FIGURE 8.14 EFFECT OF O_2 AND HYPERBARIC OXYGEN (HBO) ON ARTERIOVENOUS AND CAPILLARY PARTIAL PRESSURE OF OXYGEN (P_{O_2}) IN THE BRAIN. Note the 10-fold expansion of the scale for the cerebrovenous P_{O_2} values. *Solid circles* indicate the calculated mean capillary P_{O_2}. Pa_{O_2}, partial pressure of arterial oxygen; Pv_{O_2}, partial oxygen pressure in mixed venous blood.

for understanding its therapeutic role in relieving tissue hypoxia when local Do_2 is impaired or when the mean intercapillary distance is increased, for instance, by microcirculatory smooth muscle dysfunction or in the presence of capillary damage or destruction. The latter processes contribute to disordered microcirculatory function in diabetes and in radiated tissues. The concept of an expanded diffusion radius is also useful to help explain the beneficial effect of HBOT in *interstitial edema,* which, in effect, increases the mean intercapillary distance.[26] These principles are illustrated by Figure 8.16.

It should also be remembered that the *maximum* O_2 diffusion distances in tissues are intrinsically short—on the order of a few hundred micrometers—and that the concepts

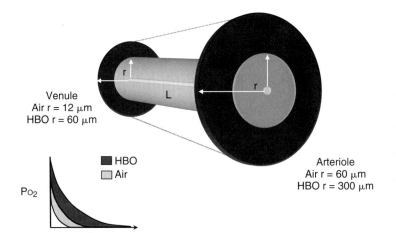

FIGURE 8.15 EFFECTS OF HYPERBARIC OXYGEN (HBO) ON THE CAPILLARY O_2 DIFFUSION RADIUS USING A SIMPLE CYLINDER MODEL. Graph shows partial pressure of oxygen (P_{O_2}) profiles as a function of the initial arteriolar P_{O_2}. r, radius of tissue cylinder before or during HBOT.

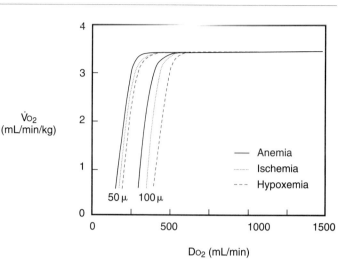

FIGURE 8.16 EFFECT OF INTERCAPILLARY DISTANCE (IC) ON THE CRITICAL O_2 DELIVERY AND CONSUMPTION (D_{O_2}-$\dot{V}_{O_2}$) RELATION. Note that the critical D_{O_2} normally are essentially superimposed for anemia *(solid line)*, ischemia *(dotted line)*, and hypoxemia *(dashed line)* (IC = 50 μ m). The curve, however, may shift to the right, for instance, by doubling IC from the accumulation of the interstitial edema or by failure of capillary recruitment. Whether there is significant separation of the curves under different pathologic conditions remains an open question.

of tissue P_{O_2} discussed earlier do not account for the opposing tendencies by HBOT to suppress $\dot{Q}_T$ and constrict blood vessels. Nevertheless, HBOT clearly improves the oxygenation of both healthy and diseased tissues provided convective D_{O_2} is adequately maintained in the distributive circulation.

Based on the earlier information and before describing organ-specific effects of HBOT, it is helpful to summarize the main physiologic factors that influence P_{O_2} in tissues and their qualitative effects. These factors are listed in Table 8.1. For ease of understanding, Table 8.1 indicates only the independent role of each factor because the effects of combinations are difficult to predict, especially when the combined changes counteract each other. Note, however, that HBOT increases tissue P_{O_2} despite O_2-induced vasoconstriction under most of the listed conditions.

ORGAN-SPECIFIC CIRCULATORY EFFECTS OF HYPERBARIC OXYGEN

The organ-specific circulatory effects of HBO depend on factors related to differences in vascular supply and microcirculatory architecture, such as capillary length and density, as well as the metabolic rate. There are also variable contributions of the autonomic hierarchy of nervous system control over the distributive circulation that protects critical microvascular beds from

hypoxia, for instance, the coronary and cerebral circulations, at the expense of blood flow to the less critical cutaneous and splanchnic beds.[5] Similarly, there are regional differences in the degree of O_2-induced vasoconstriction, although the importance of central autonomic regulatory factors is not as well understood. These differences are summarized in Table 8.2.[27-33]

O_2 induces vasoconstriction most profoundly in the vessels of the brain, retina, and skeletal muscle. The renal vessels also contract in hyperoxia, but hepatic circulatory responses are not robust, presumably because the contribution of blood flow from the low P_{O_2} portal circulation does not allow tissue P_{O_2} to increase under HBOT, as well as in other organs. Skin blood vessels also constrict in HBOT, but cutaneous blood flow responses to HBOT are difficult to quantify precisely because skin blood flow is so sensitive to changes in skin temperature and circulating blood volume. The cardiac responses are discussed later in this chapter. The respiratory muscles actually develop increased blood flow because of accentuated respiratory work from the higher breathing gas density. Nevertheless, as a general rule, O_2 induces smooth muscle contraction in almost all vascular beds, in muscularized vessels of varying diameters and lengths, and on both the arterial and venous sides of the circulation.

The notion that O_2-induced vasoconstriction decreases D_{O_2} and produces hypoxia in some vascular beds is not supported by

Table 8.1 Factors That Influence the Partial Pressure of Oxygen in Tissues

FACTOR	DIRECTION	EFFECT ON TISSUE P_{O_2}	EFFECT OF HBO ON P_{O_2}
Pulmonary shunt	Low*	—	Increase
	High (hypoxemia)	Decrease†	Increase‡
Hematocrit	Increase	Increase§	Increase
	Decrease (anemia)	Decrease	Increase
Position of ODC	Left shift	Decrease‖	Increase
	Right shift (Bohr effect)	Increase	Increase
Metabolic rate	High	Decrease	Increase
	Low	Increase	Increase
Blood flow	High	Increase	Increase
	Low (oligemia or ischemia)	Decrease	No effect or increase
Capillary transit time	Short	Decrease¶	Increase
	Long	Decrease**	No effect or increase
Heterogeneity of perfusion	High	Decrease	Increase
	Low	Increase	Increase
Oxygen shunting	High	Decrease	Small increase
	Low	—	Increase

*Low pulmonary and peripheral shunts for O_2 are normal conditions.
†Hypoxemia from low alveolar ventilation/perfusion ratio ($\dot{V}_A/\dot{Q}$) or hypoventilation will also decrease tissue partial pressure of oxygen (P_{O_2}).
‡Hyperbaric oxygen (HBO) will increase P_{O_2} in the presence of pulmonary shunt through its effects on areas of low $\dot{V}_A/\dot{Q}$, hypoventilation, or normal lung.
§Up to the point where blood viscosity begins to interfere with perfusion; hematocrit > 55%.
‖For normoxia only; in extreme hypoxemia, a left-shifted O_2 dissociation curve (ODC) actually helps O_2 loading in the lungs and may help maintain tissue P_{O_2}.
¶An overly rapid capillary transit time may not allow enough time for O_2 unloading from hemoglobin. This is also the equivalent of peripheral O_2 shunting. A slow transit time is the equivalent of ischemia.
**This is also sometimes called *stagnant hypoxia*.

theory or observation.[34] In fact, there are conditions for which O_2-induced vasoconstriction is desirable, for instance, to reduce edema. This effect may be important in the treatment of brain injuries caused by CO poisoning or arterial gas embolism, decompression sickness involving the spinal cord, and peripherally in the treatment of crush injuries. It has already been noted that the presence of edema increases the mean intercapillary distance and would, therefore, worsen tissue hypoxia in these circumstances.[26]

As mentioned earlier, O_2-induced vasoconstriction is the result of an increase in tissue

Table 8.2 O_2-Induced Vasoconstriction in Different Vascular Beds

TISSUE	RESPONSE	NOTES
Brain	++++	At high partial pressure of oxygen (P_{O_2}), the cerebral circulation "escapes" and blood flow increases before the onset of central nervous system O_2 toxicity
Retina	++++	
Skeletal muscle	++	
Kidneys	++	
Skin	+	Blood flow is more sensitive to temperature and blood volume
Intestines	+	
Liver	−	Contribution from low P_{O_2} in portal venous system likely interferes with O_2-induced vasoconstriction
Heart	++	Blood flow decreases in proportion to decline in cardiac output and myocardial O_2 consumption
Respiratory muscles	Increased blood flow	Higher respiratory work from increased breathing gas density

PO_2, and physiologic events that reduce the tissue PO_2, such as an increase in metabolism, lead to increases in DO_2 through increases in local blood flow, specifically by vasodilation and capillary recruitment. Thus, a worst-case analysis predicts no change in tissue PO_2 during hyperoxic vasoconstriction, even in a hypoxic or ischemic tissue, because of the endogenous dilator mechanisms that oppose the O_2 constrictor effect. Experimentally, this is what is observed; DO_2 is usually increased (or unchanged) by HBOT, and no convincing examples exist for O_2-induced tissue hypoxia.[34] Indeed, O_2-induced vasoconstriction is quite difficult to observe in tissues with compromised microcirculations. Moreover, in the extremities, the extent of the increase in transcutaneous PO_2 during O_2 breathing has been found to be a positive predictor of wound healing.[35]

One possible exception to the principle that HBOT increases tissue PO_2 is the propensity of HBOT to increase cardiac afterload in patients with congestive heart failure. In this condition, HBOT increases the systemic vascular resistance and can place an additional and sometimes dangerous demand on the heart. In a failing heart, such a demand can compromise $\dot{Q}T$ and increase left atrial pressure enough to precipitate pulmonary edema and impair pulmonary gas exchange. Either or both problems can compromise DO_2. In contrast, an ischemic heart may improve its ejection fraction temporarily under hyperbaric oxygenation with an attendant improvement in DO_2. Both salutary and adverse types of cardiac events have been reported clinically.

Indeed, the most prominent physiologic circulatory effect of HBOT appears to be on the heart and manifests as *bradycardia* with a small decrease in $\dot{Q}T$ that is closely proportional to the decline in heart rate.[27,31] The decrease in $\dot{Q}T$ is reflected by appropriate decreases in coronary blood flow and myocardial O_2 uptake. It is unclear whether HBOT has a significant effect on stroke volume. These effects of HBO are also observed during exercise. The mechanism of bradycardia is not fully understood, but direct actions of HBO on the cardiac conduction system and parasympathetic effects of HBO may

both be involved.[36] In any case, hyperbaric bradycardia is a physiologic response and not a harbinger of O_2 toxicity.

It is necessary to emphasize the importance of regional blood flow in setting the tissue PO_2 levels under hyperbaric conditions. Experimentally, the rate of delivery of dissolved O_2 is related linearly to regional blood flow under a range of hyperbaric conditions from at least 2 to 6 ATA (Fig. 8.17). Conversely, preexisting compromise of local blood flow will prevent the appropriate increase in the tissue PO_2 at a particular treatment pressure. In fact, the relief of O_2-induced vasoconstriction using acetylcholine or other vasodilators will substantially increase tissue PO_2 in the healthy brain.[37] Also of particular interest for the brain are observations that at high PO_2, it eventually escapes the effects of O_2-induced vasoconstriction by increasing its nitric oxide ($\cdot NO$) production, which produces the vasodilation that presages the development of central nervous system O_2 toxicity.

The mechanism of O_2-induced vasoconstriction is not yet fully understood. Most investigators agree that O_2 primarily has an indirect instead of a direct action on vascular smooth muscle, and secondary mediators of the constrictor effect have been implicated for a long time.[22,38] A range of candidates have been investigated, but the most impressive effects are those related to the endogenous vasodilator, $\cdot NO$.[39] Although molecular O_2 together with L-arginine is a substrate for the $\cdot NO$ synthases, HBO, at least initially, antagonizes the effects of $\cdot NO$ on vascular tone. This effect is due, in part, to the loss of $\cdot NO$ augmentation of the classical guanylate cyclase mechanism of smooth muscle relaxation.

$\cdot NO$ produced by the endothelium can be scavenged by reacting with locally produced superoxide ($\cdot O_2^-$) to form the peroxynitrite anion ($ONOO^-$).[40] $ONOO^-$ is a weak vasodilator compared with $\cdot NO$, as well as a strong oxidant. At acidic pH, $ONOO^-$ decomposes spontaneously to peroxynitrous acid and a hydroxyl-like species, which react rapidly with biologic macromolecules. The rate of production of vascular extracellular superoxide increases as PO_2 increases, which promotes the paracrine loss of vasorelaxation by

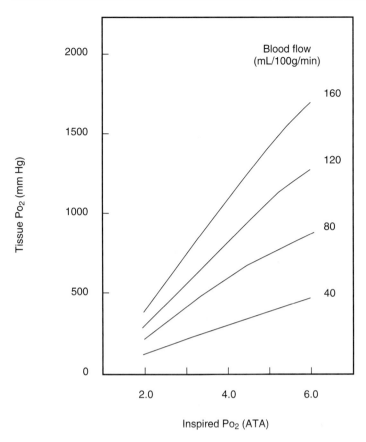

FIGURE 8.17 EFFECT OF CEREBRAL BLOOD FLOW ON BRAIN TISSUE PARTIAL PRESSURE OF OXYGEN (Po₂) UNDER HYPERBARIC CONDITIONS IN THE RAT. *(Data adapted from Demchenko IT, Luchakov YI, Moskvin AN, et al: Cerebral blood flow and brain oxygenation while breathing oxygen under pressure. J Cereb Blood Flow Metab 25:1288–1300, 2005.)*

·NO.[33] Furthermore, it is important to mention that the erythrocyte itself releases vasodilators, including ·NO and ATP. Minute amounts of erythrocyte ·NO are disbursed synchronously with the allosteric release of O_2 from Hb, which serves to relax the smooth muscle and augment local blood flow.[41] This effect is lost under HBOT conditions when Hb allostery is no longer brought into play.[42]

CELLULAR O₂ UTILIZATION

The bulk of the O_2 taken up by the cell is consumed by mitochondria during the process of respiration. Respiration allows cells to consume O_2 to conserve energy in the form of high-energy phosphates from the oxidation of foodstuffs, primarily as ATP.[2] Energy from substrates—carbohydrates, fats, and proteins—is liberated by a sequence of metabolic reactions, which for glucose begins in the cytoplasm with glycolysis. Oxidative metabolism is far more efficient than glycolysis for ATP production, but it depends primarily on the glycolytic end product, pyruvate, which feeds carbon into the citric acid (Krebs) cycle in the mitochondrial matrix. The Krebs cycle generates CO_2 and reduced dinucleotides, nicotinamide adenine dinucleotide (NADH), and flavin adenine dinucleotide ($FADH_2$). These reduced nucleotides are reoxidized by the action of the mitochondrial electron transport (respiratory) chain, and part of the free energy released is conserved by the process of oxidative phosphorylation.

Oxidative phosphorylation couples the transfer of electrons entering the respiratory chain from the Krebs cycle as NADH and $FADH_2$ to ATP synthesis. ATP is the source of energy for almost all of the cell's needs, and its hydrolysis produces primarily adenosine diphosphate and inorganic phosphate, which are then taken up by the mitochondria to regenerate ATP. This process of synthesis, hydrolysis, and resynthesis of ATP is called the *ATP cycle* (Fig. 8.18).

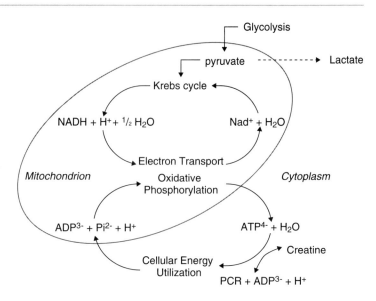

FIGURE 8.18 THE ADENOSINE TRIPHOSPHATE (ATP) CYCLE. The generation of ATP by oxidative phosphorylation in mitochondria is far more efficient than glycolysis; however, the end product of glycolysis, pyruvate, supplies most of the carbon substrate for oxidative phosphorylation. The inability of pyruvate to enter the Krebs cycle, for example, during cellular hypoxia, results in the accumulation of lactate. ADP, adenosine diphosphate; PCR, polymerase chain reaction; Pi, inorganic phosphate.

For the reactions of the ATP cycle to operate, the cell must constantly receive both glucose and O_2. Also, the supply of O_2 for respiration must not be appropriated by other O_2-consuming cellular reactions, including O_2-requiring enzymes and nonspecific biologic oxidations. This is accomplished in design by prioritization of O_2-handling and O_2-consuming reactions, as well as by utilization of the antioxidant defenses. Some antioxidant enzymes, such as the superoxide dismutases, generate hydrogen peroxide (H_2O_2), whereas others, such as catalase and glutathione peroxidase, convert H_2O_2 to water and molecular O_2; thus, a small quantity of O_2 is recovered for use by cell metabolism.[43]

The central strategy of the cell to protect its metabolic O_2 supply is the establishment of an O_2 sink that culminates in the activity of the terminal oxidase of the respiratory chain, cytochrome *c* oxidase, which irreversibly catalyzes the reduction of O_2 to water.[44] The establishment of this sink is illustrated in Figure 8.19, using Hb and myoglobin as O_2 carrier proteins. Although myoglobin participates in cellular O_2 handling, it is not obligatory, even in the working heart, and other O_2 carriers can be found in cells, such as *neuroglobin* and *cytoglobin*. These and perhaps related proteins may be involved in long-sought pathways for facilitated diffusion that preferentially "channel" O_2 to mitochondria.[45,46] In addition, cytochrome *c*

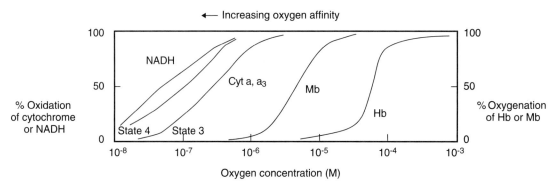

FIGURE 8.19 GENERATION OF A CELLULAR SINK FOR THE UTILIZATION OF MOLECULAR OXYGEN BY MITOCHONDRIA IN TISSUES. Cyt, cytochrome; Hb, hemoglobin; Mb, myoglobin. *(Adapted from Tamura M, Hazuki O, Nioka S, et al: In vivo study of tissue oxygen metabolism using optical and nuclear magnetic resonance spectroscopies. Annu Rev Physiol 51:813–834, 1989, by permission.)*

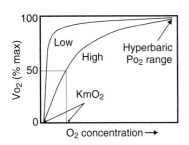

Enzyme	KmO$_2$
Monoamine oxidase	30
Nitric oxide synthase	18
Glucose oxidase	14
Heme oxygenase	10
Xanthine oxidase	10
Tryptophan oxygenase	8
NADPH oxidase	5
Cytochrome c oxidase	0.1

FIGURE 8.20 O$_2$ CONCENTRATION FOR HALF-MAXIMUM ACTIVITY (KmO$_2$) OF CELLULAR ENZYMES (measured in mm Hg). Km is inversely related to O$_2$ affinity (low Km = high affinity). Cytochrome c oxidase has the highest O$_2$ affinity of any enzyme in the body, and O$_2$ is not rate-limiting for cell respiration unless mitochondrial partial pressure of oxygen (Po$_2$) is less than 1 mm Hg. Vo$_2$, oxygen consumption.

oxidase has the highest O$_2$ affinity of any vertebrate enzyme, giving it a privileged place among all of the processes that use O$_2$ in the cell. This principle is illustrated in Figure 8.20.

Molecular O$_2$ is only one of several controls on the rate of respiration of the cell, and as pointed out earlier, it is generally not rate limiting. The single-most important regulatory factor is the adenosine diphosphate concentration, which directly reflects the rate of energy utilization by the cell.[44] Two other important factors are the source of electrons (e.g., NADH) and the availability of inorganic phosphate. All four factors produce the overall rate constant for oxidative metabolism as shown by Figure 8.21. However, notably, the regulation of respiration is not quite so simple because the concentrations of adenosine diphosphate and ATP are themselves regulated parameters.

CARBON DIOXIDE ELIMINATION

The metabolic production of CO$_2$ derives primarily from the reactions of the Krebs cycle in the mitochondria. In the process, the three-carbon pyruvate molecule is broken down into three molecules of CO$_2$ and five molecules of NADH. NADH is reoxidized to NAD$^+$ during the reduction of O$_2$ by the

respiratory chain, and the CO$_2$ is excreted by the cell, carried in the venous blood to the pulmonary capillaries, and eliminated by lung ventilation.[47] CO$_2$ is highly lipid soluble and diffuses rapidly down its concentration gradient from the mitochondria across the cell membrane and into the blood, where it is transported to the lungs. Lung capillary Pco$_2$ is normally greater than P$_{A_{CO_2}}$, and the alveolar ventilation establishes a dynamic equilibrium in which 8% to 10% of the CO$_2$ in the venous blood is removed by its passage through the lungs.[48]

CO$_2$ entering the blood is transported in three ways, as shown in Table 8.3.[6] Most of the CO$_2$ in the blood is present as bicarbonate anion (HCO$_3^-$) formed by the hydration of CO$_2$ by carbonic anhydrase found in high concentrations in the erythrocyte. The enzyme reversibly catalyzes the first of the following two reactions:

$$CO_2 + H_2O \rightarrow H_2CO_2 \rightarrow H^+ + HCO_3^-$$

The catalytic hydration of CO$_2$ occurs rapidly in the erythrocyte during its transit from systemic capillary to the lungs. The reverse reaction, the dehydration of H$_2$CO$_2$ to CO$_2$ + H$_2$O, also catalyzed by carbonic anhydrase, occurs in the erythrocyte during pulmonary CO$_2$ elimination.[47] This process is shown in Figure 8.22.

Overall reaction:

$$\boxed{3ADP + 3P_i + NADH + {}^1/_2O_2} + 4H^+ \rightarrow 3ATP + NAD^+ + 4H_2O$$

Rate control

$$\boxed{[ADP] + [P_i] + [NADH] + [O_2]}$$

Overall rate constant

$$V/V_{max} = 1/k_1/ADP + k_2/P_i + k_3/NADH + k_4/O_2$$

FIGURE 8.21 CONTROL OF CELL RESPIRATION. The overall reaction for oxidative phosphorylation shown in the first reaction is regulated primarily by the concentrations of the four substrates and their respective rate constants.

Table 8.3 Carriage of Carbon Dioxide in Venous Blood

Bicarbonate anion (87%)
Bicarbonate is generated by the reversible hydration of CO_2 catalyzed by the carbonic anhydrase in erythrocytes
Contributes ~58% of the arteriovenous CO_2 difference
Carbamate compounds (8%)
CO_2 reversibly binds nonionized terminal amino groups ($-NH_2$) of blood proteins especially those of hemoglobin, which are not
   ionized at pH 7.40
Contributes ~33% of the arteriovenous CO_2 difference
Dissolved CO_2 (5%)
Blood CO_2 solubility is 0.067 mL/dL/mm Hg at 37°C and follows Henry's Law
Contributes ~9% of the arteriovenous CO_2 difference

The carbon dioxide (CO_2) content of blood is influenced by the hemoglobin concentration and saturation, 2,3-diphosphoglycerate concentration, and pH. Therefore, the estimates of the CO_2 distribution in the blood are approximate. The estimates are for whole blood including the bicarbonate and dissolved CO_2 inside the red blood cells.

CO_2 is also transported in the blood in dissolved form and as carbamate compounds on blood proteins, primarily Hb. The solubility of CO_2 in blood is approximately 20 times greater than the solubility of O_2. This high CO_2 solubility, together with the other two transport mechanisms, gives the CO_2 content curve its exaggerated steepness relative to the oxygen content curve (Fig. 8.23). Although only 5% of the CO_2 in the blood is transported in dissolved form, this component is important in CO_2 exchange because it links the bicarbonate and carbamate pools to each other. Moreover, the high capacity of the blood for CO_2 allows large volumes of CO_2 to be eliminated by the lungs with relatively small changes in P_{CO_2}, thereby minimizing the impact of CO_2 exchange on blood pH.[48]

CO_2 and hydrogen ion (H^+) reversibly bind to uncharged amino groups ($R-NH_2$) in Hb and other proteins. H^+ addition produces ammonium ($R-NH_3^+$), whereas CO_2 binding results in the formation of carbamates ($R-NH\ COO^-$). Carbamates form only on unprotonated NH_2 groups; therefore, the carbamino reaction is pH dependent and increases with alkalosis. Carbamate formation is also influenced by the pK of the NH_2 group and protein α-amino groups that are uncharged at physiologic pH and available to bind CO_2. Nearly all of the blood carbamate formation involves the Hb molecule.[48]

Deoxyhemoglobin compared with oxyhemoglobin contains more unprotonated α-amino groups and binds more CO_2 as carbamate. The difference is called the *oxylabile carbamate* and accounts for the *Haldane effect*, which is defined by the greater CO_2 content at constant P_{CO_2} of deoxygenated than oxygenated blood. When oxyhemoglobin releases O_2 to the tissues, deoxyhemoglobin becomes available to bind CO_2, whereas in the lungs, oxygenation of deoxyhemoglobin facilitates the release of bound CO_2. Hb therefore plays an important

FIGURE 8.22 CARBON DIOXIDE (CO_2) TRANSPORT BY THE ERYTHROCYTE (red blood cell [RBC]). The RBC participates in the carriage of 95% of the metabolic CO_2 to the lungs for excretion. CO_2 is reversibly converted to bicarbonate by RBC carbonic anhydrase or stored as the carbamate on unprotonated amino groups of hemoglobin. As bicarbonate exits the RBC, chloride is exchanged through the Band 3 protein to maintain electroneutrality. The two processes are linked through dissolved CO_2.

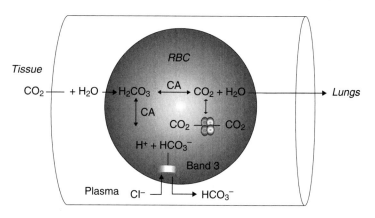

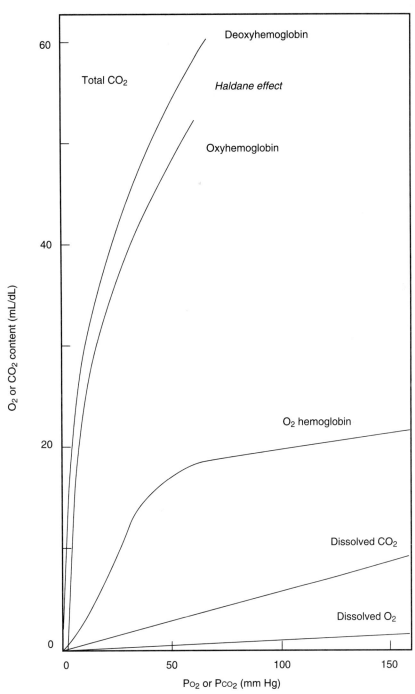

FIGURE 8.23 CARBON DIOXIDE (CO_2) CONTENT CURVES OF BLOOD DRAWN ON THE SAME SCALE AS THE O_2 CONTENT CURVE. The oxylabile carbamate (Haldane effect) is the difference between the two CO_2 content curves. The linear increases in dissolved O_2 and CO_2 as a function of gas partial pressure are also shown for comparison. The difference between the dissolved carbon monoxide (CO) line and the hemoglobin curves is the contribution of the bicarbonate. Po_2, partial pressure of oxygen; Pco_2, partial pressure of carbon dioxide.

role in CO_2 exchange, and the Haldane effect produces about one fourth of the arteriovenous CO_2 content difference.[48]

The influence of O_2 on CO_2 exchange is seen both in carbamate and bicarbonate exchange, and varies as a function of pH, P_{CO_2}, and the concentration of 2,3-diphosphoglycerate, an organic phosphate produced by glycolysis that also increases the oxygen half-saturation pressure of Hb (P_{50}). The maximum pH effect on carbamate formation occurs in the physiologic range, and alkalosis increases the carbamate because of a shortage of protons. The pH sensitivity of CO_2 binding should not be confused with the Bohr effect, which describes the dependence of Hb O_2 affinity on pH.[6] The absence of a Haldane effect would increase both CO_2 tension in tissues and the arteriovenous P_{CO_2} difference; however, CO_2 exchange would still continue.

The implications of the Haldane effect on CO_2 transport during HBOT administration can now be made clear. In the chamber, when venous Hb is nearly saturated with O_2, it does not carry as much CO_2 as carbamate, which causes the Pv_{CO_2} to increase. This effect and the fall in cardiac output during HBOT produce a mild respiratory acidosis. The presence of respiratory acidosis stimulates resting ventilation, and arterial P_{CO_2} tends to remain close to normal. Thus, standard HBOT in the range of 2 to 3 ATA is well tolerated in healthy subjects and by most patients; however, the increased respiratory drive in combination with an increase in breathing gas density in proportion to atmospheric pressure increases the work of breathing. In the presence of obstructive lung disease, or during heavy exercise, this extra respiratory work may not be tolerated and may compromise pulmonary ventilation and CO_2 elimination, leading to a clinically significant respiratory acidosis.

The partial pressures of CO_2 in tissue and blood are also important in HBOT for two other reasons. First, low Pa_{CO_2} tends to constrict systemic blood vessels and may compromise blood flow to sites where it is desirable to augment Do_2. This possibility, however, has not been studied well enough clinically to determine its importance, and it remains conjectural in part because the CO_2 response is not the same in all vascular beds. Second, elevated Pa_{CO_2} increases blood flow in the brain, which will increase central nervous system O_2 toxicity and increase the risk for seizures. Substantial experimental support exists for this possibility in humans.

SUMMARY EFFECTS OF HYPERBARIC OXYGEN ON TISSUE OXYGENATION

The principal effect of HBOT in the therapeutic range is to increase the Po_2 in the tissues by means of dissolved O_2 in blood plasma. In healthy individuals, other effects of HBOT include mild bradycardia, leading to a proportional decline in $\dot{Q}T$ and a small increase in systemic vascular resistance from O_2-induced vasoconstriction. O_2 vasoconstriction increases smooth muscle tone in the medium to small vessels of the arterial and venous circulations, as well as in the microcirculation. This occurs, in part, because O_2 opposes the paracrine effects of the endogenous vasodilator, $\cdot$NO.

An O_2 constrictor response is observed in almost all vascular beds because tissue oxygenation is actively regulated. However, the extent of constriction varies from organ to organ, with the most pronounced effects on the cerebral and coronary circulations, which feed the tissues with the greatest basal aerobic metabolic requirements. The main exception is blood flow to the diaphragm and other respiratory muscles, which must perform greater work because of the increased density of the breathing gas under hyperbaric conditions.

Although HBOT decreases microcirculatory blood flow in healthy tissues, the extra O_2 dissolved in plasma is so great that the tissue Po_2 actually increases. The presence of additional O_2 does not increase $\dot{V}o_2$ unless Do_2 is below the critical threshold for O_2 dependency of aerobic metabolism. In tissues with cellular hypoxia caused by compromised microcirculations, HBOT does not cause significant vasoconstriction, and its administration usually allows temporary restoration of more normal Po_2 values. This response, however, is contingent on the maintenance of adequate convective Do_2 at the arteriolar level.

REFERENCES

1. Weibel ER: The Pathway for Oxygen: Structure and Function in the Mammalian Respiratory System. Cambridge, Mass, Harvard University Press, 1984.

2. Aw TY, Jones DP: Intracellular respiration. In: Crystal RG, West JB, et al. (eds): The Lung: Scientific Foundation, vol 2. New York, Raven Press, 1991, pp 1445-1454.

3. West JB, Wagner PD: Ventilation-perfusion relationships. In: Crystal RG, West JB, et al. (eds): The Lung: Scientific Foundation, vol 2. New York, Raven Press, 1991, pp 1289-1306.

4. Hsia CC: Respiratory function of hemoglobin. N Engl J Med 338:239-247, 1998.

5. Guyton AC, JE Hall: Textbook of Medical Physiology. Unit IV: The Circulation, 10th ed. Philadelphia, WB Saunders, 2000, pp 143-262.

6. West JB: Respiratory Physiology—The Essentials, 7th ed. Philadelphia, Lippincott Wilkins & Wilkins, 2005.

7. Wagner PD, Saltzman HA, West JB: Measurement of continuous distributions of ventilation-perfusion ratios: Theory. J Appl Physiol 36:588-599, 1974.

8. Shapiro BA, Harison RA, Care RD, Templin R: Clinical Applications of Blood Gases, 4th ed. Chicago, Year Book Medical Publishers, 1989.

9. Moon RE, Camporesi EM, Shelton DL: Prediction of arterial PO_2 during hyperbaric treatment. In: Bove AA, Bachrach AJ, Greenbaum LJ (eds): Underwater and Hyperbaric Physiology IX: Proceedings of the Ninth International Symposium on Underwater and Hyperbaric Physiology. Bethesda, Md, Undersea and Hyperbaric Medical Society, 1987, pp 1127-1131.

10. Forster RE: Diffusion of gases across the alveolar membrane. In: Fahri LE, Tenney SM (eds): Handbook of Physiology, The Respiratory System, vol 4. Bethesda, Md, American Physiological Society, 1987, pp 71-88.

11. Popel AS: Theory of oxygen transport to tissue. Crit Rev Biomed Eng 17:257-321, 1989.

12. Saltzman HA: Rational normobaric and hyperbaric oxygen therapy. Ann Intern Med 67:843-852, 1967.

13. Weiskopf RB, Viele MK, Feiner J, et al: Human cardiovascular and metabolic response to acute, severe isovolemic anemia. JAMA 279:217-221, 1998.

14. Boerema I, Meyne NG, Brummelkamp WK, et al: Life without blood. A study of the influence of high atmospheric pressure and hypothermia on dilution of the blood. J Cardiovasc Surg 1:133-146, 1960.

15. Pedersen PK, Kiens B, Saltin B: Hyperoxia does not increase peak muscle oxygen uptake in small muscle group exercise. Acta Physiol Scand 166:309-318, 1999.

16. Webster AL, Syrotuik DG, Bell GJ, et al: Exercise after acute hyperbaric oxygenation: Is there an ergogenic effect? Undersea Hyperb Med 25:153-159, 1998.

17. Cain SM: Oxygen delivery and uptake in dogs during anemic and hypoxic hypoxia. J Appl Physiol 42:228-234, 1977.

18. Morita Y, Chin-Yee I, Yu P, et al: Critical oxygen delivery in conscious septic rats under stagnant or anemic hypoxia. Am J Respir Crit Care Med 167:868-872, 2003.

19. Russell JA, Phang PT: The oxygen delivery-consumption controversy. Am J Respir Crit Care Med 149:433-437, 1994.

20. Schlichtig R: Oxygen delivery and consumption in critical illness. In: Civetta JM, Taylor RW, Kirby RR (eds): Critical Care. Philadelphia, Lippincott-Raven, 1997, pp 337-342.

21. Tenney SM: A theoretical analysis of the relationship between venous blood and mean tissue oxygen pressures. Respir Physiol 20:283-296, 1974.

22. Duling BR: Microvascular responses to alterations in oxygen tension. Circ Res 31:481-489, 1972.

23. Schuchardt S: Comparative physiology of the oxygen supply. In: Kessler M, Bruley DF, Clark LC Jr, et al. (eds): Oxygen Supply: Theoretical and Practical Aspects of Oxygen Supply and Microcirculation of Tissue. Baltimore, Md, University Park Press, 1973, pp 223-229, 1973.

24. Krogh A: The number and distribution of capillaries in muscles with calculations of the oxygen pressure head necessary for supplying the tissue. J Physiol 52:409-415, 1919.

25. Lambertsen CJ: Physiological effects of oxygen inhalation at high partial pressures. Hyperbaric Oxygenation [Publication 1298]. Washington, DC, National Academy of Sciences National Research Council, 1966, pp 13-20.

26. Miller JD, Ledingham IM, Jennett WB: Effects of hyperbaric oxygen on intracranial pressure and cerebral blood flow in experimental cerebral oedema. J Neurol Neurosurg Psychiatry 33:745-755, 1970.

27. Whalen Re, Saltzman HA, Holloway D, et al: Cardiovascular response to hyperbaric oxygenation. Am J Cardiol 15:638-646, 1965.

28. Kioschos JM, Saltzman HA, Thompson HK, et al: The effect of hyperbaric oxygenation upon renal hemodynamics. Am J Med Sci 260:270-278, 1970.

29. Hordnes C, Tyssebotn I: Effect of high ambient pressure and oxygen tension on organ blood flow in conscious trained rats. Undersea Biomed Res 12:115-128, 1985.

30. Bergo GW, Risberg J, Tyssebotn I: Effect of 5 bar oxygen on cardiac output and organ blood flow in conscious rats. Undersea Biomed Res 15:457-470, 1988.

31. Savitt MA, Rankin JS, Elberry JR, et al: Influence of hyperbaric oxygen on left ventricular contractility, total coronary blood flow, and myocardial oxygen consumption in the conscious dog. Undersea Hyper Med 21:169-183, 1994.

32. Abel FL, McNamee JE, Cone DL, et al: Effects of hyperbaric oxygen on ventricular performance, pulmonary blood volume, and systemic and pulmonary vascular resistance. Undersea Hyperb Med 27:67-73, 2000.

33. Demchenko IT, Oury TD, Crapo JD, Piantadosi CA: Regulation of the brain's vascular responses to oxygen. Circ Res 91:1031-1037, 2002.

34. Fortner I, Scafetta N, Piantadosi CA, Moon RE: Hyperoxia-induced tissue hypoxia: A Danger? Anesthesiology 106(5):1051-1055, 2007.

35. Fife CE, Buyukcakir C, Otto GH, et al: The predictive value of transcutaneous oxygen tension measurement in diabetic lower extremity ulcers treated with hyperbaric oxygen therapy: A retrospective analysis of 1144 patients. Wound Repair Regen 10:198-207, 2002.

36 Fagreus L, Linnarsson D: Heart rate in the hyperbaric environment after autonomic blockade. Acta Physiol Scand 9:260-264, 1973.

37. Demchenko IT, Luchakov YI, Moskvin AN, et al: Cerebral blood flow and brain oxygenation while breathing oxygen under pressure. J Cereb Blood Flow Metab 25:1288-1300, 2005.

38. Jackson WF: Arteriolar oxygen reactivity: Where is the sensor? Am J Physiol 253(5 pt 2):H1120-H1126, 1987.

39. Demchenko IT, Boso AE, O'Neill TJ, et al: Nitric oxide and cerebral blood flow responses to hyperbaric oxygen. J Appl Physiol 88:1381-1389, 2000.

40. Rubanyi, GM, Vanhoute PM: Superoxide anions and hyperoxia inactivate endothelium-derived relaxing factor. Am J Physiol 238:H822-H827, 1986.

41. Stamler JS, Jia L, Eu JP, et al: Blood flow regulation by s-nitrosohemoglobin in the physiological oxygen gradient. Science 276:1937-2092, 1997.

42. Allen BW, Piantadosi CA: How do red cells cause hypoxic vasodilation? The SNO-hemoglobin paradigm. Am J Physiol Heart Circ Physiol 291:1507-1512, 2006.

43. Hallwell B, Gutteridge JMC: Oxygen is a toxic gas—an introduction to oxygen toxicity and reactive oxygen species. Free Radicals in Biology and Medicine, 3rd ed. Oxford, UK, Oxford University Press, 1999, pp 1-35.

44. Tamura M, Hazuki O, Nioka S, et al: In vivo study of tissue oxygen metabolism using optical and nuclear magnetic resonance spectroscopies. Annu Rev Physiol 51:813-834, 1989.

45. Longmuir IS: Search for alternative cellular oxygen carriers. In: Jobsis FF (ed): Oxygen and Physiological Function. Dallas, Tex, Professional Information Library, 1977, pp 247-253.

46. Pesce A, Bolognesi M, Bocedi A, et al: Neuroglobin and cytoglobin. Fresh blood for the vertebrate globin family. EMBO Rep 3:1146-1151, 2002.

47. Klocke RA: Carbon dioxide transport. In: Farhi LE, Tenney SM (eds): Handbook of Physiology Gas Exchange. The Respiratory System, vol 4. Bethesda, Md, American Physiological Society, 1987, pp 173-197.

48. Lumb AB: Carbon dioxide. Nunn's Applied Respiratory Physiology, 6th ed. Philadelphia, Elsevier Butterworth Heinemann, 2005, pp 148-165.

Ischemia-Reperfusion Injury and Hyperbaric Oxygen Therapy

9

Basic Mechanisms and Clinical Studies

Jon A. Buras, MD, PhD,
and Lisardo Garcia-Covarrubias, MD

ISCHEMIA-REPERFUSION INJURY: HYPERBARIC OXYGEN AND BASIC STUDIES

Ischemia-Reperfusion Injury and Hyperbaric Oxygen: A Disease of Paradoxes

Ischemia-reperfusion (I/R) injury is defined as an acute interruption in blood flow with subsequent restoration of perfusion creating further tissue damage beyond that observed during the initial ischemic event. This worsening of tissue injury is unexpected, because one would likely predict that reperfusion of ischemic tissue would improve tissue survival rather than create further damage. Oxygen plays a central role in promoting I/R injury through the phenomenon of the "oxygen paradox," as reperfusion of tissue with oxygenated blood greatly enhances subsequent tissue injury as compared with deoxygenated blood (reviewed in Khalil and colleagues,[1] Piper and coworkers,[2] and Hallenbeck and Dutka[3]). This observation is counterintuitive to the logic that ischemic tissue will benefit from restoration of oxygen supplies and oxidative phosphorylation for energy production. Further study suggests that there is a second oxygen paradox, where extreme hyperoxygenation provided by hyperbaric oxygen (HBO) during reperfusion of ischemic tissue prevents subsequent injury (reviewed in Buras[4]). Reactive oxygen species (ROS) appear to represent the central mediator of both oxygen paradoxes, suggesting that there is a dose–response effect attributable to ROS, further solidifying the concept of oxygen as a pharmacologic agent. This chapter discusses the pathophysiology of I/R injury and the role of oxygen in both generating I/R injury and ameliorating it when administered at extreme levels.

Ischemia-Reperfusion Injury: Pathophysiology Overview

The hallmark of I/R injury is extension of damage that occurs after reperfusion of ischemic tissue. I/R injury has been widely observed in experimental animal models and has also been well documented in the human clinical setting of myocardial infarction. During treatment of myocardial infarction, reperfusion by mechanical removal of occlusive coronary artery thrombus allows visible blood flow in large blood vessels. However, flow through the microvasculature remains inadequate, and myocardial function may remain impaired despite successful removal of the initial blockage.[5,6] The continuation of myocardial dysfunction and reperfusion injury has a significant negative effect on clinical outcome with respect to myocardial function and survival.[6,7] The characteristic changes of I/R injury within the microvasculature include arteriolar vasoconstriction, capillary leakage and tissue edema, leukocyte adhesion and extravasation, oxidant production, and reduced energy production (Fig. 9.1).

I/R injury is initiated by an ischemic event, and ischemia, in turn, may be generated by an embolic insult, global hypoperfusion, or isolated compression-crush syndrome. Hypoperfusion of tissue leads to a reduction in the delivery of metabolic substrates, oxygen and glucose, required for adenosine triphosphate (ATP) production. The reduction in ATP ultimately leads to cell death via failure of energy-dependent systems responsible for membrane integrity and maintenance of electrochemical membrane potentials. As energy levels decrease within the cell, cellular processes fail in a somewhat ordered progression dependent on their requirement for ATP. This progression may be reversible to some extent depending on the energy requirement for the cell and tissue in question. The change in oxygen tension

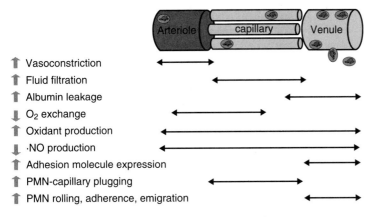

↑ Vasoconstriction
↑ Fluid filtration
↑ Albumin leakage
↓ O₂ exchange
↑ Oxidant production
↓ ·NO production
↑ Adhesion molecule expression
↑ PMN-capillary plugging
↑ PMN rolling, adherence, emigration

Figure 9.1 COMPONENTS OF MICROVASCULAR DYSFUNCTION IN ISCHEMIA-REPERFUSION (I/R) INJURY. Several physiologic parameters within the microvasculature are affected by I/R injury, as shown *(vertical arrows)*. *Horizontal double arrows* demonstrate the primary region affected within the arteriole, capillary, and venule. ·NO, nitric oxide; PMN, polymorphonuclear neutrophil.

in the cell may signal stress responses directly through oxygen-sensing processes.[8,9] Also, the breakdown of ATP to adenosine may play a role in signaling the protective stress response to ischemia.[10] Restoration of energy supplies may prevent complete tissue infarction in the ischemic zone; however, this also creates the environment for reperfusion injury.

Tissue death that occurs by pure ischemia creates a distinct histologic appearance with diffuse pallor noted and preservation of tissue architecture within the ischemic zone on hematoxylin and eosin staining.[11] Reperfusion-mediated tissue death differs histologically, demonstrating disrupted cellular architecture and tissue architecture with notable edema and infiltration of leukocytes, predominantly neutrophils (polymorphonuclear neutrophils [PMNs]). These histologic differences underscore the different mechanisms of tissue injury caused by isolated ischemia as compared with I/R injury.

Reactive Oxygen Species as Initiators and Propagators of Ischemia-Reperfusion Injury

Initiation of I/R injury may be traced to events that occur at the blood-endothelial cell (EC) interface. Central mediators of reperfusion injury are oxygen free radicals or ROS. ROS play a complex role in homeostasis and are normally generated during oxidative phosphorylation in mitochondria. Common ROS formed during metabolism are superoxide

radical and hydrogen peroxide. ROS may be directly toxic to cells through their ability to cause membrane damage via lipid peroxidation and phospholipase activation. ROS may also cause direct DNA and protein damage, further reducing the ability of the cell to generate an appropriate stress response to correct cellular dysfunction. Cells contain a number of antioxidant enzymes that are responsible for decreasing the intracellular ROS concentration. The antioxidant system includes superoxide dismutase, glutathione, several peroxidase enzymes, and catalase.[1] ROS may have a purpose beyond cellular damage, as recent studies have suggested that ROS are involved in a variety of cellular signaling events.[12,13] ROS may function as signaling molecules to activate stress-response pathways.[12] The role of ROS in cellular homeostasis is evolving and extends beyond their original isolated role as mediators of cellular damage. However, it is well established that during reperfusion injury, generation of an excessive amount of ROS is deleterious to tissues, causing loss of membrane integrity, increased levels of apoptosis, and enhanced recruitment of leukocytes to tissues (Fig. 9.2).

During I/R injury, there is a breakdown of the normal housekeeping defenses against ROS (Fig. 9.3). Excess production of ROS may directly damage the enzymes responsible for their clearance, resulting in an overall increase in cellular ROS content. These ROS are then free to react with other molecules such as nitric oxide (·NO) or lipid hydroxyl groups to form more potent or reactive molecules that may be

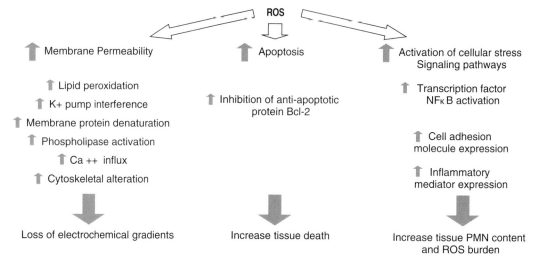

Figure 9.2 ROLE OF REACTIVE OXYGEN SPECIES (ROS) IN ISCHEMIA-REPERFUSION INJURY PATHOPHYSIOLOGY. ROS impact several aspects of cellular physiology enhancing cellular damage and tissue death. NF-κB, nuclear factor κB; PMN, polymorphonuclear neutrophil.

responsible for initiation of chain reaction peroxidation of lipid membranes and denaturation of proteins through nitrosylation (reviewed in Zweier and Talukder[14]) (see Fig. 9.3).

Oxidant damage to the EC enzyme xanthine dehydrogenase, involved in normal purine metabolism, causes conversion to xanthine oxidase that then produces superoxide and hydrogen peroxide during oxidation of the purine metabolite hypoxanthine[14] (Fig. 9.4). The activity of xanthine oxidase further increases the ROS tissue burden, precipitating further tissue damage. The generation of ROS is involved in activating the EC surface to recruit blood

neutrophils (PMNs) to become adherent and ultimately infiltrate through the endothelial barrier into the tissue.

The recruitment of PMNs during reperfusion represents a significant source of ROS because PMNs contain a membrane form of NADPH oxidase that converts NADPH in the presence of molecular oxygen into superoxide radical. Superoxide radicals spontaneously dismutate to form hydrogen peroxide, which combines with halides (such as chloride) via the PMN enzyme myeloperoxidase to form the toxic molecule hypochlorous acid (hypochlorite). The degree of tissue damage

Figure 9.3 ALTERATION OF CELLULAR REACTIVE OXYGEN SPECIES (ROS) GENERATION IN ISCHEMIC-REPERFUSION (I/R) INJURY. During I/R injury, the normal cellular housekeeping systems responsible for removing newly formed ROS are impaired. Resulting superoxide molecules may join with nitric oxide (·NO) to form peroxynitrite (ONOO·), which may further damage cellular structures. PLA$_2$, phospholipase A$_2$; GSSGH, reduced glutathione; SOD, superoxide dismutase.

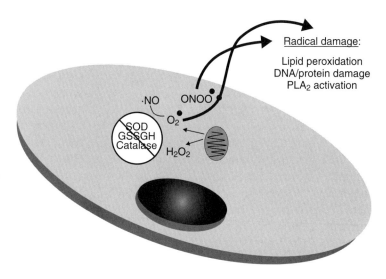

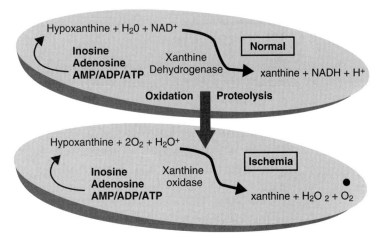

Figure 9.4 ENHANCED REACTIVE OXYGEN SPECIES (ROS) PRODUCTION IN ISCHEMIA-REPERFUSION (I/R) INJURY BY XANTHINE OXIDASE. I/R injury enhances oxidation and proteolysis of xanthine dehydrogenase, causing conversion to xanthine oxidase, further enhancing the ROS-generating capacity of the endothelial cell. ADP, adenosine diphosphate; AMP, adenosine monophosphate; ATP, adenosine triphosphate.

generated by ROS correlates directly with their production. There may be two waves of ROS production during I/R injury, with an early and small increase of ROS generated by the local endothelium, followed by a later, greater, and more sustained production of ROS derived from infiltrating PMNs (Fig. 9.5).

Ischemia-Reperfusion Injury: Effect of Hyperbaric Oxygen on Reactive Oxygen Species Production and Tissue Damage

Reperfusion injury is dependent on the addition of oxygen to previously ischemic tissue. Specifically, exposure to 100% oxygen at 1 atmosphere absolute (ATA) during reperfusion increases ROS-mediated lipid peroxidation and mortality after transient cerebral global ischemia.[15] Based on this observation, it was hypothesized that reperfusion of ischemic tissue with hyperoxygenated blood during hyperbaric oxygen therapy (HBOT) would create a greater amount of tissue damage. Surprisingly, the opposite proved to be true as initial studies of postischemic muscle necrosis demonstrated improved tissue preservation with HBOT.[16,17] Multiple studies specifically evaluating ROS-mediated lipid peroxidation after reperfusion have repeatedly shown a reduction in lipid peroxidation.[18-23] Beneficial outcomes have been documented in these studies despite evidence that HBO may

increase ROS production.[19,24] However, the effect of oxygen-induced ROS is clearly dose dependent, because other studies have demonstrated that exposure to a nonclinical treatment pressure of 4 ATA results in an increase in lipid peroxidation.[25,26]

It is difficult to resolve these conflicting observations; however, in vitro studies using a cell-free system that approximates oxygen tension under relevant hyperbaric conditions suggest that oxygen may actually inhibit lipid peroxidation via the quenching of ROS through oxygen-mediated termination reactions.[27] Another facet of HBO-mediated ROS function suggests that they are required for inhibition of PMN adhesion.[28] In summary, ROS generated by HBOT may have multiple effects on the cellular response to I/R injury, and at the appropriate dose, they are beneficial rather than injurious.

Ischemia-Reperfusion Injury: Hyperbaric Oxygen and Cellular Energetics

I/R injury is considered to disrupt normal cellular metabolism and homeostasis ultimately through interference with energy production. Specifically, ischemia may induce mitochondrial dysfunction such that during reperfusion oxygen no longer serves as a metabolic substrate.[29] The presence of oxygen at the time of reperfusion may then lead to an increase in free radical production.[14,30] Inability to recover

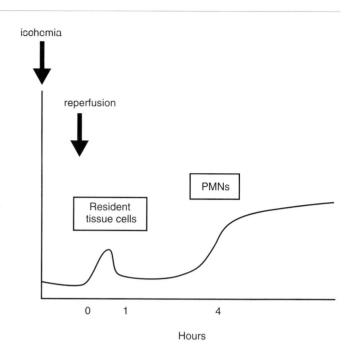

Figure 9.5 HYPOTHETICAL SCHEME FOR REACTIVE OXYGEN SPECIES (ROS) GENERATION AFTER ISCHEMIA-REPERFUSION (I/R) INJURY. During the reperfusion phase of I/R injury, ROS may be generated by resident tissue cells, such as endothelial and supporting parenchymal cells. The total burden of ROS within injured tissue is greatly enhanced and sustained by recruitment of polymorphonuclear neutrophils (PMNs) because of their inherent NADPH oxidase and myeloperoxidase content.

ATP production may ultimately lead to a loss of membrane ionic gradients and cell death.[14,31]

Several studies have shown a beneficial effect of HBOT on preserving cellular homeostasis with respect to ATP levels or energy charge.[20,32,33] In a rat model of hind-limb ischemia for 3 hours immediately followed by HBOT at 2.5 ATA for 45 minutes, the level of ATP present at 5 hours of reperfusion was 50% greater than the I/R group.[32] Lactate production was significantly reduced with HBOT versus ischemic controls, suggesting greater preservation of oxidative phosphorylation apacity.[32] In a model of intestinal I/R utilizing 2 hours of superior mesenteric artery ischemia followed by a 2-hour reperfusion period, ATP and energy charge were assessed.[33] In that study, a single HBOT treatment of 2.0 ATA for 1.5 hours was delivered during the last 1.5 hours of ischemia or immediately on reperfusion. Animals receiving HBOT before reperfusion appeared to gain the greatest benefit as determined by survival at 15 days, although a nonsignificant trend in improved survival was noted in the group receiving HBOT on reperfusion versus I/R controls.[33] The amount of ATP was not significantly different between the HBO-treated and I/R only groups at 30 or 120 minutes of reperfusion, although the HBO-treated groups were not assessed at

similar time points. Energy charge at 30 minutes of reperfusion was significantly greater than I/R-only controls in the group receiving HBOT during the ischemic period.[33] The energy charge in the group receiving HBO during reperfusion did not differ from I/R-only controls; however, this assessment was taken only at 120 minutes of reperfusion, and a comparison among all groups for the 30-minute time point was not performed. In a model of rat hepatic I/R injury, HBO treatment before ischemia was beneficial.[20] In that study, an HBO treatment of 2.5 ATA for 1.5 hours was given before a 1-hour occlusion of the hepatic artery and portal vein followed by 2 hours of reperfusion. ATP levels measured at 2 hours of reperfusion were significantly greater in the HBOT group versus the I/R only controls. Also noted was an inverse correlation between ATP concentration and adherent leukocytes, as well as between ATP concentration and lipid peroxidation.[20]

There may be different explanations for the improvement in cellular energetics in these experiments depending on the timing of HBOT delivery and the specific animal model used. In the intestinal I/R model, venous blood oxygenation was known to be increased and may have functioned to limit ischemia through a type of collateral circulation.[33] Alternatively, in a model without collateral circulation, or when HBOT is applied before injury, the effect may be caused by inhibition of secondary mediators of cell damage such as PMN infiltration or microvascular flow.[20,32,34] It is difficult in vivo to determine mechanistically whether the preservation of cellular energetics by HBOT is due to primary or secondary effects. Further study addressing this specific question is required to clarify the underlying mechanisms.

Neutrophil-Endothelial Cell Adhesion

The adhesion of PMNs to the endothelium is a well-regulated process with respect to both temporal and spatial characteristics (reviewed in Xu and colleagues,[35] Malik and Lo,[36] Aird,[37] Salmi and Jalkanen,[38] and Weber and Koenen[39]). PMNs normally traverse the microvasculature powered by the force of flow. The fixed attachment of PMNs to the endothelium occurs with the reduction of flow inherent in the ischemic event, coupled with interactions between protein receptors and their counterligands that are expressed on the surfaces of both the PMN and the EC. Members of this receptor-ligand class are referred to as cell adhesion molecules (CAMs). Once the PMN has firmly adhered to the endothelium, it traverses the EC barrier into the distal tissue matrix through the process of diapedesis. Diapedesis is dependent both on interaction of CAMs, guiding the PMN to interendothelial gaps, and on chemokines (protein and lipid molecules), forming a chemotactic gradient attracting the PMN to its ultimate distal tissue destination.

The process of PMN trafficking from the microvasculature to distal tissues is often described as a three-step process involving rolling, firm adhesion, and diapedesis (Fig. 9.6).[35] Rolling (so called because of the appearance of the PMN during videomicroscopy) occurs when the PMN makes multiple nonsustained contacts with the endothelium. In this state, the PMN is loosely tethered to the EC surface by forces that transiently overcome the shear force of flow. Enhanced rolling is an early inflammatory event mediated by expression of multiple CAMs including

P-selectin, E-selectin, and intercellular adhesion molecule-1 (ICAM-1) in response to inflammatory mediators and ischemia.[40] P-selectin plays a role in early PMN-EC interaction because it is a premade glycoprotein stored within the Weibel–Palade bodies of ECs and the secretory α-granules of platelets. Cellular activation mobilizes these granules to the membrane surface within 15 minutes of middle cerebral artery (MCA) occlusion, exposing P-selectin to its major ligand, P-selectin glycoprotein ligand-1, present on PMNs.[41-43]

Endothelial activation caused by I/R injury and ROS formation triggers enhanced expression of other CAMs such as E-selectin and ICAM-1 through transcription and translation that is dependent on the activation of the transcription factor nuclear factor-κB.[44] The requirement for new gene expression accounts for the temporal delay in E-selectin and ICAM-1 appearance relative to P-selectin. In a rodent model of MCA occlusion, E-selectin production is noted 2 hours after ischemia and exhibits peak expression at 6 and 12 hours.[42] ICAM-1 expression was increased at 4 hours after MCA I/R injury in the rodent.[45] E-selectin and ICAM-1 bind to their PMN ligands SLe^x/P-selectin glycoprotein ligand-1/CD44 and CD11b/18, respectively, strengthening the bond between the PMN and EC, leading to firm adhesion of the PMN on the EC surface.[46-48] After firm adhesion, the PMN migrates through EC gap junctions via the homotypic interactions among platelet endothelial cell adhesion molecules (PECAMs), present on both the PMN and localized at the EC junctions (reviewed in Cook-Mills and Deem[49]). Platelet endothelial cell adhesion molecule-1–independent diapedesis has been reported; however, this alternative mechanism remains uncharacterized.[50]

The cross talk between PMN and EC during adhesion and transmigration represents a complex process that may be underappreciated. Interaction of the PMN-EC adhesion molecules leads to bidirectional signaling events within each cell type, resulting in cellular activation that further promotes adhesion. Interaction of L- and P-selectin with their respective ligands results in increased avidity

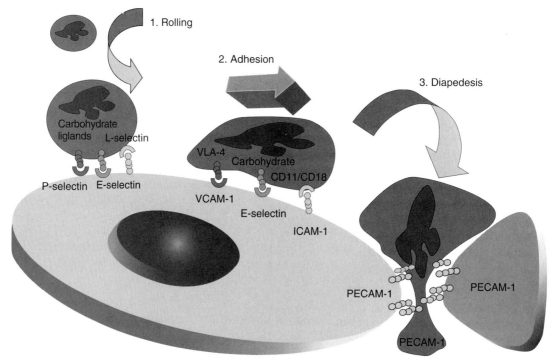

Figure 9.6 PROCESS OF LEUKOCYTE EXTRAVASATION AFTER ISCHEMIA-REPERFUSION (I/R) INJURY. Polymorphonuclear neutrophils (PMNs) enter tissue from postcapillary venules in a stepwise progression regulated by expression of cell adhesion molecules located on both the PMNs and endothelial cell surface. Primary adhesion molecules and their ligands located on endothelial cells and PMNs are shown for each step. ICAM-1, intercellular adhesion molecule-1; PECAM, platelet endothelial cell adhesion molecule; VCAM-1, vascular cell adhesion molecule-1; VLA-4, very-late antigen-4.

of the CD11/18 for ICAM-1.[51-53] Engagement of the E-selectin receptor also leads to phosphorylation of p38 mitogen-activated protein kinase and up-regulation of the CD11/18 complex on the PMN.[54,55]

Using in vivo models of cerebral ischemia, interruption of the PMN-EC interaction has proved beneficial. Interruption of the rolling process by P-selectin blockade by antibody in normal mice or via genetic deficiency in P-selectin knock-out mice results in protection from cerebral infarction.[56] Antibodies that inhibit CD18 have reduced cerebral infarct volumes in baboons.[57] Furthermore, CD18 genetically deficient mice were protected from cerebral ischemia and reperfusion injury, but not permanent ischemia.[58] Similarly, anti–ICAM-1 antibodies have reduced postischemic brain injury in rodents.[59] Mice genetically deficient for ICAM-1 have demonstrated smaller infarct volumes than wild-type mice; however, the number of PMNs recruited to the brain did not differ between

groups.[60,61] These in vivo findings highlight the importance of the PMN-EC interaction in development of cerebral I/R injury and provide one mechanism by which HBOT might be beneficial during acute cerebral I/R injury.

Antiadhesive Mechanisms of Hyperbaric Oxygen in Ischemia-Reperfusion Injury

Early studies that evaluated the protective mechanisms of HBOT during I/R injury were performed by Zamboni and colleagues[34] in a rodent skeletal muscle flap model. In these studies, HBOT was noted to reduce the adhesion of PMNs to injured endothelium by real-time videomicroscopy in vivo. Subsequent studies in a rat model of MCA-mediated I/R injury have shown that HBOT limits cerebral infarct volume and PMN sequestration.[62] Based on these findings, it is possible that HBOT exerts its beneficial effects through interruption of the PMN-EC adhesion mechanism.

Hyperbaric Oxygen and Polymorphonuclear Neutrophil Adhesion

The conclusion that HBOT interferes directly with PMN-endothelium interaction raised the question whether HBOT affected either PMN activation or PMN-specific adhesion molecules. The first PMN-specific adhesion molecule studied was the protein CD11/18. CD11/18 is a heterodimeric protein normally expressed on the PMN surface and is a member of the integrin family of adhesion molecules (reviewed in Xu and colleagues[35]). Three distinct CD11/18 complexes have been described, all containing the same CD18 or b2 integrin subunit, coupled to CD11a, CD11b, or CD11c. The CD11a/18 complex is found on PMNs, monocytes, T cells, and B cells. The CD11b/18 and CD11c/18 complexes are found on both PMN and monocyte cell surfaces. The predominant ligand for CD11a/18 is ICAM-1, located on a variety of cell types including ECs and epithelial cells (reviewed in Xu and colleagues[35] and Kakkar and Lefer[63]). CD11b/18 also binds ICAM-1 but with lower affinity.[64] Both CD11b/18 and CD11c/18 bind to iC3b and fibrinogen. PMN activation increases the avidity of the CD11/18 receptor through phosphorylation events and cytoskeletal alteration.[65]

The first studies evaluating the mechanisms of HBOT and PMN adhesion were conducted using a model of carbon monoxide (CO) poisoning.[18,66] CO poisoning was considered to represent a form of I/R injury as a result of transient cellular ischemia and regional central nervous system hypotension with subsequent reperfusion on CO removal.[66] The transient application of CO in this setting results in several biochemical changes similar to end-artery occlusion I/R injury models including lipid peroxidation, conversion of xanthine dehydrogenase to xanthine oxidase, and intercerebral PMN sequestration.[66] In rats, HBOT was capable of reducing intracerebral PMN accumulation after CO poisoning in a dose-dependent manner with greatest inhibition at 3 ATA.[18] Using an in vitro system of CD18-mediated PMN adherence to nylon columns, HBO was capable of preventing PMN adhesion.[18] This study

was the first to implicate a specific adhesion molecule, CD18, in the antiadhesive mechanism of HBOT. The effect of HBO on adhesion was not irreversible, as demonstrated through restoration of HBO-treated PMN adhesion to nylon after PMN stimulation with phorbol 12-myristate 13-acetate (PMA).[18] Furthermore, in vivo studies demonstrated that HBOT did not prevent CD18-dependent PMN recruitment after glycogen-induced peritonitis.[18]

Subsequent biochemical studies demonstrated that the effect of HBO on CD18 function was mediated by PMN-generated cyclic guanosine monophosphate (cGMP).[28] PMN derived from HBO-treated rats demonstrated reduced adhesion to nylon and was reversible after treatment with PMA, 8-bromo-cGMP (a cGMP analogue), or dithiothreitol.[28] Further experiments using human PMNs demonstrated that HBO inhibits the production of cGMP by the membrane-bound form of guanylate cyclase and does not interfere with the free cytosolic guanylate cyclase.[67] The exact mechanism of how cGMP alters CD11/18 function is unclear; however, it may relate to the subsequent activities of G proteins or cGMP-dependent protein kinase activity, which may regulate interaction of the cytoskeleton and β_2 integrins, as recently suggested.[68,69]

The effect of HBOT on the production of new CD18 molecules has also been studied with less consistent results. The previously described experiments on HBO-only–treated rat and human PMNs found no change in cell surface expression of CD18.[18,67] Similarly, preliminary work has shown that the number of PMN CD18 molecules is not altered by HBOT in a rodent model of skeletal muscle I/R injury.[70] However, other in vivo studies suggest that HBOT decreases new CD18 synthesis on circulating PMN in humans after surgery.[71] Further work is required to determine the effect of HBOT on CD18 expression in the specific setting of I/R injury.

The down-regulation of CD11/18 function represents an attractive hypothesis to explain the beneficial effect of HBOT with respect to the reduction in PMN adhesion. However, limitations exist in accepting this hypothesis as the sole explanation. Although HBOT may be able to decrease CD11/18 function, experiments have shown that this effect may be reversed by activation of PMNs through other pathways.[66,67] It is unknown whether in the setting of I/R injury PMNs may be exposed to other inflammatory mediators, which could then activate CD11/18 through a pathway similar to that activated by PMA, bypassing the HBO protective effect. It is also possible that other CD11/18-independent pathways of cell adhesion are involved in the I/R injury process as suggested by the study described.[18] Finally, most mechanistic HBOT-I/R experimental studies to date have focused on early outcome (Table 9.1); however, the full development of I/R injury extends beyond most of these study periods. For example, in the setting of cerebral I/R injury, the infiltration of leukocytes into injured tissue may occur over a period of 24 to 48 hours.[72] It is unknown whether the HBOT suppression of CD18 function persists throughout the development and maturation of reperfusion injury. Given these caveats, the data thus far strongly suggest that a key mechanism of effect is the HBO-mediated inhibition of CD11/18 function, but further studies in the specific setting of I/R injury are needed to confirm the above findings.

Hyperbaric Oxygen and the Endothelial Cell

Most early work elucidating the antiadhesive mechanisms of HBOT focused on the PMN as described earlier. However, given the importance of the endothelium in mediating PMN adhesion through the tightly regulated expression of CAMs, it seemed likely that HBOT may also influence the EC. Early studies on the oxygen-mediated regulation of EC CAMs focused on ICAM-1.[73] In these studies, prolonged exposure of ECs to oxygen at 1 ATA resulted in enhanced expression of ICAM-1 and PMN adhesion.[73] The first description regarding the effect of HBOT on ICAM-1 expression demonstrated an increase in ICAM-1 within the pulmonary vasculature after exposure at 3 ATA for greater than 4 hours.[74] This information would predict that HBO would enhance PMN ICAM-1–dependent adhesion;

however, this was not the case in the setting of HBO-treated I/R injury.[34] The discrepancy likely relates to the use of toxic oxygen exposures in the former studies,[73,74] rather than the nonoxygen toxic exposures common to clinical and experimental treatment of I/R injury.[34]

In vitro studies specific to EC I/R injury demonstrated that mock ischemia (concurrent hypoxia and hypoglycemia) was capable of inducing expression of ICAM-1 in both bovine and human ECs.[75] In this model system, exposure of I/R-injured ECs to 90 minutes of HBOT at 2.5 ATA reduced expression of ICAM-1 with a concomitant reduction in PMN binding to the EC surface (Figs. 9.7 and 9.8).[75] This finding supports an EC CAM mechanism for HBOT in the setting of I/R injury in vivo. Again, the use of a nonoxygen toxic HBO exposure was required for generating the beneficial suppression of ICAM-1 expression and PMN adhesion.[75] Using the same model system, suppression of I/R-induced ICAM-1 by HBO required ·NO, as the general nitric oxide synthase (NOS) inhibitor L-nitroarginine methyl ester reversed the effects of HBO.[75] In this setting, a single HBO exposure was noted to increase the production of NOS III protein (Fig. 9.9).[75]

Subsequent in vivo I/R experiments in a rodent muscle flap support the in vitro findings on HBO regulation of ICAM-1.[76] HBO administered using a clinically relevant treatment schedule of 2.5 ATA for 90 minutes at the initiation of reperfusion was able to reduce ICAM-1 expression within the flap with an associated reduction in PMN sequestration and improved flap survival.[76] PMN CD18 surface expression was not reduced by HBOT; however, the effect on the avidity of the existing CD11/18 complex was not determined.

Ischemia-Reperfusion Injury: Hyperbaric Oxygen and Nitric Oxide

·NO is a free radical gas (reviewed in Lowenstein and Snyder,[77] Li and colleagues,[78] and Dudzinski and coworkers[79]) that regulates a number of important facets of I/R injury including vascular tone and PMN adhesion

Table 9.1 Selected Hyperbaric Oxygen Use in Ischemia-Reperfusion Injury Model Systems

STUDY	SPECIES	ORGAN	$T_{I/R}$	T_{HBOT}	I_{HBOT}	ATA	OUTCOME MEASURE	EFFECT
Atochin and colleagues[62]	Rat	Brain	2 hr/1.46 hr	45 min	B	2.8	Infarct volume	+
							Neurologic deficit	+
							PMN sequestration	+
Buras and colleagues[75]	Human/bovine	Endothelium	4 hr/20 hr	90 min	A	2.5	ICAM-1 expression	+
							PMN adherence	+
Cabigas and colleagues[118]	Rat	Heart (note I/R done ex vivo)	25 min/180 min	60 min	B	2.0	Infarct size	+
							NOS3 expression	+
							Nitrate production	+
Chen and colleagues[20]	Rat	Liver	1 hr/2 hr	90 min	B	2.5	WBC adherence	+
							Lipid peroxidation	+
							ATP	+
							Blood flow	+
Gurer and colleagues[140]	Rat	Kidney	45 min/24 hr	75 min	B	2.8	GSH levels	NS
							Lipid peroxidation	+
							Histology	+
Hong and colleagues[76]	Rat	Musculocutaneous flap	4 hr/24 hr	90 min	D, A	2.5	Flap survival	+
							CD18 expression	NS
							ICAM-1 expression	+
							PMN sequestration	+
Kihara and colleagues[141]	Rat	Liver	45 min/ 4, 7, 48 hr	1 hr	A	2.5	Survival	+
							Lipid peroxidation	+
							PMN sequestration	+
Mink and Dutka[19]	Rabbit	Brain	10 min/ 75 min	75 min	A	2.8	Lipid peroxidation	+
Nylander and colleagues[32]	Rat	Skeletal muscle	1.5 and 3 hr/5 hr	45 min	A	2.5	ATP	+
							Lactate	+
							Phosphocreatine	+
Sterling and colleagues[142]	Rabbit	Heart	30 min/3 hr	90 min	D, A, DA	2.5	Infarct size	+
Sirsjo and colleagues[103]	Rat	Skeletal muscle	4 hr/1.5 hr and 5 hr	90 min	A	2.5	Blood flow	NS 1 hr, +5 hr
		Skin	4 hr/1.5 hr and 5 hr	90 min	A	2.5	Capillary density	NS 1 hr, +5 hr
Thom[18]	Rat	Brain	2 hr/90 min*	90 min	A	2.5	WBC sequestration	+
							XO production	+
							Lipid peroxidation	+
Yagci and colleagues[143]	Rat	Colon	5-day ischemia	90 min	B, A	2.8	Hydroxyproline	+
							Bursting pressure	+
							Histology	NS
Yamada and colleagues[33]	Rat	Small intestine	2 hr/30 min and 120 min	90 min	D, A	2.0	15-day survival	+D; NS A

Table 9.1 Selected Hyperbaric Oxygen Use in Ischemia-Reperfusion Injury Model Systems—Cont'd

STUDY	SPECIES	ORGAN	$T_{I/R}$	T_{HBOT}	I_{HBOT}	ATA	OUTCOME MEASURE	EFFECT
Yang and colleagues[144]	Rat	Small intestine	60 min/ 30 min	60 min	D	2.8	ATP	NS
							Histology	+D; NS A
							Serum TNF levels	+
Zamboni and colleagues[34]	Rat	Skeletal muscle	4 hr/3 hr	60 min	D, A	2.5	PMN sequestration	+
							WBC adherence	+
							Vasoconstriction	+

*Ischemia induced by carbon monoxide poisoning.
   A, after ischemia; ATA, atmospheres absolute treatment pressure; ATP, adenosine triphosphate; B, before ischemia; D, during ischemia; GSH, glutathione; I_{HBOT}, hyperbaric oxygen treatment relative to ischemia; ICAM-1, intercellular adhesion molecule-1; I/R, ischemia-reperfusion; NOS3, nitric ox ide synthase-3; NS, no significant difference with treatment; PMN, polymorphonuclear neutrophil; t_{HBOT}, duration of hyperbaric oxygen treatment; $t_{I/R}$, ischemia/reperfusion times, respectively; TNF, tumor necrosis factor; WBC, white blood cell; XO, xanthine oxidase; +, beneficial outcome; −, deleterious outcome.

(reviewed in Li and colleagues[78] and Lefer and Lefer[80]). One mechanism of ·NO action is binding to iron in the heme contained within the active site of guanyl cyclase, leading to enzymatic activation and generation of cGMP with subsequent biologic effects. Another mechanism of action is through combination of ·NO with superoxide to form peroxynitrite, which is a one- or two-electron oxidant and nitrating agent (reviewed in Szabo[81] and Donzelli and colleagues[82]). The peroxynitrite-mediated oxidation of biologic molecules is similar to the oxidation mediated by the hydroxy radical; however, the oxidation rate constant for peroxynitrite is 10,000 times slower than the hydroxy radical. Peroxynitrite is toxic to bacteria and eukaryotic cells through its oxidative properties and its ability to nitrate tyrosine residues in cell signaling kinases, transcription factors, and ion channels, which may lead to protein malfunction. However, data suggest that peroxynitrite may also afford a protective effect similar to ·NO during I/R injury at physiologic concentrations.[83,84] It is possible that by combining with superoxide anion ·NO may act as a sink to reduce the contribution of superoxide to further free radical chain reaction propagation.[85] The ultimate effect of ·NO in promoting tissue protection or damage depends on its concentration and the presence of oxidative stress, which may promote peroxynitrite formation.[86]

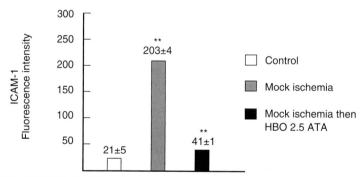

Figure 9.7 HYPERBARIC OXYGEN (HBO) DOWN-REGULATES ENDOTHELIAL EXPRESSION OF INTERCELLULAR ADHESION MOLECULE-1 (ICAM-1). Primary human umbilical vein endothelial cells were exposed to mock ischemia (hypoxia/hypoglycemia) for 4 hours (gray bar), then either normoxia/normoglycemia for 20 hours or 1.5 hours of HBO at 2.5 ATA (black bar), then 18.5 hours of normoxia/normoglycemia. Cells were fixed and immunostained for surface expression of ICAM-1 and analyzed by confocal laser–scanning microscopy. **Significant differences of P, 0.05 by analysis of variance. White bar represents control cells. (Adapted from Buras JA, Stahl GL, Svoboda KK, Reenstra WR: Hyperbaric oxygen downregulates ICAM-1 expression induced by hypoxia and hypoglycemia: The role of NOS. Am J Physiol Cell Physiol 278:C292–C302, 2000, by permission.)

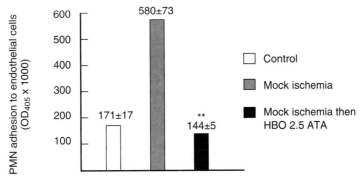

Figure 9.8 HYPERBARIC OXYGEN (HBO) DOWN-REGULATES POLYMORPHONUCLEAR NEUTROPHIL (PMN) ADHESION TO ENDOTHELIAL CELLS AFTER MOCK ISCHEMIA-REPERFUSION INJURY IN VITRO. Primary human umbilical vein endothelial cells (HUVECs) were exposed to mock ischemia (hypoxia/hypoglycemia) for 4 hours *(gray bar)*, then either normoxia/normoglycemia for 20 hours or 1.5 hours of HBO at 2.5 ATA *(black bar)*, then 18.5 hours of normoxia/normoglycemia. Freshly isolated primary PMNs were added to endothelial cell cultures, and adherence was quantified by determining total myeloperoxidase content after washing away nonadherent cells. **Significant differences of $P < 0.05$ by analysis of variance. *White bar* represents control cells. *(Adapted from Buras JA, Stahl GL, Svoboda KK, Reenstra WR: Hyperbaric oxygen downregulates ICAM-1 expression induced by hypoxia and hypoglycemia: The role of NOS. Am J Physiol Cell Physiol 278:C292–C302, 2000, by permission.)*

There are three subtypes of NOS, which are responsible for ·NO production and are designated NOS I, NOS II, and NOS III. NOS isoforms share about 50% amino acid homology, especially at their catalytic sites, and N-terminal variation of the isoforms may be responsible for differential enzyme regulation. All NOS enzymes convert L-arginine to L-hydroxy arginine, and then to L-citrulline with the consumption of NADPH and oxygen and the generation of ·NO. NOS III (also known as endothelial NOS) is predominantly a constitutively produced enzyme found in ECs and fibroblasts. NOS III may also be induced in certain circumstances, for example, by the shear force of flow and hyperoxia.[85,87] The activity of NOS III is mediated through changes in intracellular calcium and calcium-calmodulin.[79] NOS III is responsible for producing the ·NO initially characterized as endothelial-derived relaxing factor and also is responsible for vasodilatation. Studies have shown that inhibition of NOS III promotes the adherence of PMNs to the microvasculature, whereas increased enzyme concentration has an antiadherent effect.[80,88] NOS II (also known as inducible NOS) is an enzyme produced by PMNs, macrophages, and fibroblasts. However, constitutive production of NOS II may also occur. NOS II protein synthesis is induced by lipopolysaccharide, IL-1β, or TNF-α. NOS II activation is not calcium dependent and produces a significantly greater amount of ·NO than does NOS III. Evidence suggests that the ·NO produced by NOS II may reach toxic levels in some cases; as in animal models, selective NOS II inhibition improves outcome and decreases vascular leakage (reviewed in Szabo[81]; also see Laszlo and Whittle,[89] Wei and coworkers,[90] and MacMicking and colleagues[91]). However, the toxicity observed in these models could come through reduction in the concentration of peroxynitrite in favor of superoxide, rather than a directly toxic effect of ·NO.[92] NOS I (also referred to as neuronal NOS) is constitutively expressed and may be induced under certain circumstances. NOS I is found largely within the central nervous system; however, NOS I, as well as a splice variant of NOS I, may also be found in the perivascular environment of larger blood vessels, and its specific contribution to I/R injury is unknown.

Oxygen and HBO are known to affect the production of ·NO, as well as the expression of both NOS III and NOS II. Reports have shown that increases in oxygen tension at 1 ATA lead to an induction of NOS III messenger RNA and protein production.[93,94] Increases in ·NO production were noted by direct measurement in bovine cerebellum after HBO exposure; however, direct analysis of NOS protein levels or

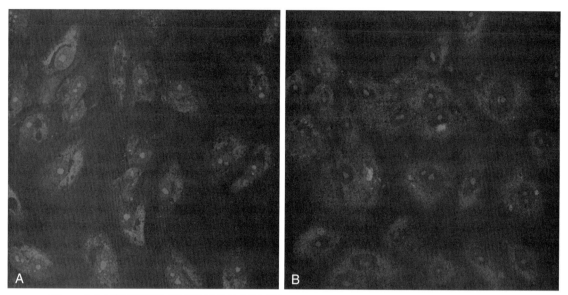

Figure 9.9 HYPERBARIC OXYGEN (HBO) INDUCES NITRIC OXIDE SYNTHASE (NOS) III PRODUCTION AFTER MOCK ISCHEMIA-REPERFUSION INJURY IN VITRO. Primary human umbilical vein endothelial cells (HUVECs) were exposed to mock ischemia (hypoxia/hypoglycemia) for 4 hours, then either normoxia/normoglycemia for 20 hours or 1.5 hours of HBO at 2.5 ATA, then 18.5 hours of normoxia/normoglycemia. Cells were fixed and immunostained for expression of NOS III and analyzed by confocal laser–scanning microscopy (CLSM). Enhanced expression of NOS III after HBO exposure *(B)* can be appreciated relative to control cells *(A)*. **See Color Plate 3** for dual staining image where nucleic acid is stained red with propidium iodide, and NOS III is stained green with a NOS III-specific antibody. *(Adapted from Buras JA, Stahl GL, Svoboda KK, Reenstra WR: Hyperbaric oxygen downregulates ICAM-1 expression induced by hypoxia and hypoglycemia: The role of NOS. Am J Physiol Cell Physiol 278:C292–C302, 2000, by permission.)*

subtype was not performed.[95] HBOT in a zymosan-induced rat shock model significantly reduced serum nitrate/nitrate concentration, reflecting a reduction in the production of ·NO.[96] The source of ·NO was not measured in this study; however, ·NO production in the shock state presumptively originates from inducible NOS.[80] The hypothesis that HBOT may prevent NOS II–specific ·NO production is supported by other in vitro studies showing differential effects of HBOT on the expression of NOS II and NOS III. HBOT has been demonstrated to reduce lipopolysaccharide induction of NOS II transcription in murine macrophages.[97] In a separate study, HBOT was capable of inducing NOS III, but not NOS II, protein production in ECs in an in vitro model of I/R injury (see Fig. 9.9).[75] This same study noted no increase in inducible NOS protein production in a murine macrophage cell line, which is consistent with previous findings.[75] A preliminary in vivo study using a rat model of skeletal muscle I/R detected a trend of in-

creased ·NO production in serum after HBOT; however, this increase was not significant compared with I/R-only control animals.[98]

·NO has been implicated directly in the HBO-mediated suppression of PMN adhesion.[99] In that study, rats were exposed to HBO in the presence or absence of the general NOS inhibitor, L-nitroarginine methyl ester. PMN adhesion to nylon was reduced after HBOT; however, inhibition of ·NO synthesis by L-nitroarginine methyl ester reversed the antiadhesive effect of HBO.[68] It is possible that the ·NO effect mediated by HBO involves the membrane-bound form of guanylate cyclase. Exogenous ·NO is capable of reducing cGMP production from stimulated PMN membrane-bound guanylate cyclase.[99] Furthermore, PMN adhesion may be reduced by ·NO in a dose-dependent manner.[99] These observations suggest that HBOT might alter the adhesive function of PMN CD11/18 by altering ·NO production and resulting in reduced production of cGMP from the membrane-bound form of guanylate cyclase. The source of ·NO responsible for mediating this hypothetical mechanism of HBOT is not currently known. Previous studies have suggested that HBO may increase production of ·NO from NOS I as determined by direct measurements taken adjacent to the abdominal aorta in rats.[100] Measurement of ·NO production in the cerebral cortex during HBO exposure also appears to originate from NOS I, not NOS III, as determined by using NOS knock-out mice.[101] The HBO-induced increase of ·NO production was dependent on the presence of oxidative stress because antioxidants were able to reverse the effect.[100] Also, the effect of HBO was associated with increased influx of intracellular calcium and activity of the heat shock protein Hsp90.[100]

The exact role of HBO regulation of NOS during I/R injury is more difficult to determine. As mentioned earlier, previous in vitro studies have shown that HBO may increase the production of functional NOS III protein.[75] Most recently, preliminary work in a muscle flap I/R injury model has demonstrated an HBO-dependent increase in ·NO from NOS III and an increase in NOS III messenger RNA expression.[102] ·NO clearly plays a significant role in modulating PMN responses to I/R injury, and further work is required to fully understand the mechanisms that regulate ·NO production in this setting.

HBOT improves several markers of microvascular dysfunction after I/R injury (Fig. 9.10). It is possible by extrapolating from existing data to create a unifying hypothesis explaining how the beneficial effect of HBOT in treating I/R injury could be mediated by ·NO (Fig. 9.11). If HBOT is capable of inducing an increase in NOS III protein production in the vascular bed, then it is plausible that in the setting of I/R, calcium influx may increase the amount of NOS III–generated ·NO.[75] Increased ·NO levels may be involved in reducing PMN adhesion through inhibition of CD18 function and down-regulation of endothelial CAM synthesis through suppression of nuclear factor-κB–dependent gene transcription.[75,99] Increased ·NO production in the microvascular bed would also account for the observed vasodilation and preserved capillary flow.[20,34,103] It is intriguing that all of the observed beneficial effects of HBOT may be explained by ·NO bioactivity. Further HBO-I/R studies using ·NO inhibitors in vivo and also specific NOS knock-out mice could confirm the connection between HBO and ·NO production as the primary mechanism responsible for protection in I/R.

Preconditioning

Preconditioning is an interesting phenomenon defined as a pretreatment that renders a tissue resistant to subsequent ischemia. The initial treatment used for preconditioning was actually brief, repeated episodes of ischemia before prolonged I/R, and it has become commonly described as ischemic preconditioning (IP).[104] That study used a canine model with multiple brief periods of myocardial ischemia that limited histologic infarct size after a subsequent sustained ischemic insult. The first human clinical study of IP reported the effects of 2 sequential 90-second coronary occlusions in 19 patients undergoing elective angioplasty of the left anterior descending

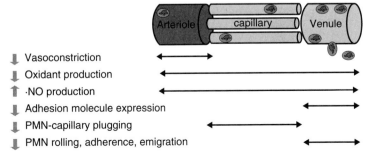

- ⬇ Vasoconstriction
- ⬇ Oxidant production
- ⬆ ·NO production
- ⬇ Adhesion molecule expression
- ⬇ PMN-capillary plugging
- ⬇ PMN rolling, adherence, emigration

Figure 9.10 COMPONENTS OF MICROVASCULAR DYSFUNCTION IN ISCHEMIA-REPERFUSION INJURY IMPROVED BY HYPERBARIC OXYGEN (HBO). Several physiologic parameters within the microvasculature are improved by HBO after I/R injury as listed (*vertical arrows*). *Horizontal double arrows* demonstrate the primary region affected within the arteriole, capillary, and venule.

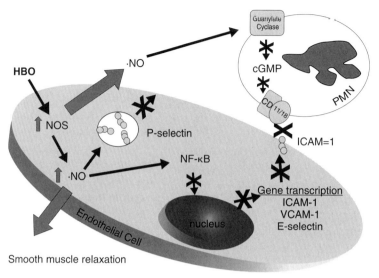

Figure 9.11 UNIFYING MECHANISMS OF HYPERBARIC OXYGEN THERAPY (HBOT) IN ISCHEMIA-REPERFUSION INJURY. HBOT affects both polymorphonuclear neutrophil (PMN) and endothelial cell (EC) components required for rolling and adhesion of PMN to the endothelium. The effects of HBOT may be traced to generation of nitric oxide (·NO) affecting the following processes: (1) cyclic guanosine monophosphate (cGMP) production and CD11/18 function in the PMN; and (2) cell surface expression of P-selectin, local alteration of microvascular blood flow, and cell adhesion molecule expression through potential downregulation of nuclear factor-kB (NF-kB) activation. ICAM-1, intercellular adhesion molecule-1; NOS, nitric oxide synthase; VCAM-1, vascular cell adhesion molecule-1. *(Adapted from Buras J, Reenstra W: Endothelial-neutrophil interactions during ischemia and reperfusion injury: Basic mechanisms of hyperbaric oxygen. Neurol Res 29:127–131, 2007, by permission.)*

coronary artery.[105] The second episode of ischemia caused fewer symptoms and decreased production of myocardial lactate. IP has been described in several tissues such as myocardium, liver, lung, brain, skeletal muscle, kidney, and intestine.[106]

Some of the documented protective effects of IP in the myocardium include preservation of ATP, reduction of lactate accumulation, attenuation of acidosis, decreased generation of ROS, and protection against stunning.[107] In addition to ischemia, preconditioning can be induced pharmacologically.[108] Mechanistically, HBOT may be considered as a potential preconditioning agent because it could induce intracellular oxidant signaling as observed in IP; however, this hypothesis has not yet been proved.

Several protective/adaptive mechanisms to HBOT have been described in the literature. Dennog and colleagues[109] found that a single HBO treatment at 2.5 ATA for 1 hour causes DNA damage in human leukocytes. However, subsequent HBO treatments did not cause further damage, suggesting that the cell increases its antioxidant mechanisms after HBO. The authors also observed that short HBO treatments increased in a stepwise fashion did not cause damage to DNA. In a different study, the same group found rapid repair of HBO-induced DNA damage in blood cells of healthy male volunteers exposed to HBO at 2.5 ATA for 1 hour.[110] Increased production of heme oxygenase-1 has been suggested as an adaptive mechanism to HBO.[111,112] Heme oxygenase-1 appears to be a beneficial host defense mechanism associated with antioxidant properties.[113] Increased production of inducible heat shock protein 70 has been reported after a single treatment of HBO in humans.[114] HBO-induced modulation of other antioxidant mechanisms (catalase and superoxide dismutase) has been described in rat myocardium and skeletal muscle.[115-117] Most recently, HBOT of rats resulted in sustained protection of subsequently isolated hearts subjected to I/R.[118] In that study, NOS III and hsp90 were both increased after HBOT. Furthermore, inhibition of NOS blocked the protective effects of HBOT on infarct size. These experiments were conducted using isolated, perfused hearts during generation of I/R injury. In this setting, the effects of serum components such as complement and clotting factors, circulating leukocytes, and platelets were not assessed. The contribution of these proinflammatory components to I/R in the presence of HBO requires further study. Overall, this study supports the growing hypothesis that ·NO plays a key role in HBOT protection in I/R in both preconditioning and postconditioning situations. The experience with HBOT in clinical preconditioning is limited; however, it has potential to evolve into a useful therapy.

ISCHEMIA-REPERFUSION INJURY: HYPERBARIC OXYGEN AND CLINICAL STUDIES

Numerous basic and animal models have shown beneficial effects of HBO in I/R injury. However, clinical studies remain limited and somewhat controversial. This section reviews the most relevant literature in three specific areas: the brain, the myocardium, and transplantation. The role of HBO in trauma-related I/R injury is discussed in Chapter 20, detailing the role of HBO in crush injury. Relevant studies with the highest level of evidence available in each area are described in Table 9.2.

Brain

Stroke

Interruption of a cerebral artery reduces, but seldom abolishes, the delivery of oxygen to the brain.[119] Histopathologic damage from cerebrovascular occlusion depends on the degree and duration of impaired blood flow or hypoxia.[120] Subsequent to a severe ischemic insult, a central zone exists that necroses and progressively enlarges in a circumferential fashion. A rim of mild to moderately ischemic tissue exists between normally perfused brain and the evolving infarct in which pathophysiologic changes are most dynamic. This rim of

tissue has been called the *ischemic penumbra*, and its viability depends on residual perfusion, presence of collateral vessels, and perfusion pressures.[121] That is, the *ischemic penumbra* represents potentially salvageable tissue. Furlan and colleagues[122] first demonstrated its existence in humans, and they suggest that mapping of its borders might allow for predicting potential for recovery and form a basis to select the most appropriate candidates for therapeutic trials.

It seems logical that HBOT may help to salvage the penumbra in stroke patients and improve the clinical outcome. However, clinical studies have shown mixed results. Despite publication of multiple clinical studies on the use of HBOT in stroke, only three meet the criteria for the highest level of evidence as prospective, randomized, and controlled trials. An extensive review on the literature of HBOT in stroke and traumatic brain injuries demonstrated that a significant number of studies have major methodologic flaws.[123] The three prospective studies are detailed in Table 9.2.

Anderson and investigators[124] reported the first prospective randomized controlled trial in 1991. This investigation included 39 patients with acute ischemic stroke managed in a neurologic intensive care unit and with the contemporary standard of care. Patients were randomized to receive HBOT ($n = 20$) or sham treatments ($n = 19$). The primary outcome measure was a validated graded neurologic examination. A secondary outcome measure was quantification of the volume of infarct measured by head computed tomography. This study was suspended early when an interim analysis showed a trend toward better outcome in the sham group. Of note, the larger infarct volume in the HBOT group begs the question of appropriateness of randomization. One could infer that patients in the HBOT group had a more severe insult. The authors acknowledge frequent deviations from the protocol because of patient instability and other demands of their medical care.

The second study, reported by Nighoghossian,[125] enrolled 34 patients (21 men), between 20 and 75 years old, presenting with a neurologic deficit highly suggestive

Table 9.2 Relevant Clinical Studies on Hyperbaric Oxygen and Ischemia-Reperfusion–Induced Injury

AUTHOR (YEAR)	STUDY DESIGN	PATIENT TRAITS	HBOT PROTOCOL	OUTCOME	BENEFICIAL
STROKE					
Anderson and colleagues (1991)[24]	PRCDB	39 patients (19 HBOT; 20 sham) 20-90 years old with acute ischemic stroke	1 hour at 1.5 ATA every 8 hours. Average time from onset of symptoms until first treatment was 51.8 hours. Average number of treatments per patient was 9.4.	Graded neurologic examination on entry, 5 days, 6 weeks, 4 months, and 1 year after stroke better in sham group. Infarcted area by head CT larger in HBOT group. Study terminated early because of trend favoring sham group.	No
Nighoghossian and colleagues (1995)[125]	PRCDB	34 patients (17 HBOT; 17 sham) 20-75 years old with MCA occlusion and a significant deficit	40 minutes at 1.5 ATA daily. Average time from onset of symptoms until first treatment was 24 hours. Only 13 subjects in the sham group and 14 in the HBOT group completed the 10 planned treatment sessions.	Significant improvement in neurologic exam by graded scales (Orgogozo and Trouillas) in HBOT group. Rankin Scale score did not show any difference.	Yes
Rusyniak (2003)[126]	PRCDB	33 patients (17 HBOT; 16 sham) > 20 years old with ischemic stroke	A single HBO treatment for 1 hour at 2.5 ATA. All HBOT patients completed the protocol.	NIHSS at 24 hours and 90 days. Barthel Index, Rankin Scale score, and Glasgow Scale score at 90 days. No difference between both groups at 24 hours. Sham did better at 90 days.	No
MYOCARDIAL ISCHEMIA					
Thurston and colleagues (1973)[129]	PRC	208 patients (103 HBOT; 105 control) < 70 years old with clinical probability of AMI within 24 hours of admission; patients with more severe conditions were in HBOT group	Continuous cycle of 120 minutes at 2 ATA followed by 60 minutes of normobaric air for 48 hours. Most did not complete planned HBOT protocol.	Death at 3 weeks: HBOT 16.5%; control 22.9% (NS).	Trend favoring HBOT

Study	Type	Patients	HBOT protocol	Results	Significant
Swift and colleagues (1992)[130]	RCB	34 patients (24 HBOT; 10 sham) of average age 58 years with AMI within a week and abnormal wall motion on TEE; 91% were male; 74% received streptokinase	A single treatment at 2 ATA for 30 minutes.	Left ventricular function by TTE and TEE was significantly improved in HBOT group.	Yes
Stavitsky and colleagues (1998)[136]	PRC multicenter	122 patients (59 HBOT; 63 control) of average age 58 years with signs suggestive of AMI admitted within 6 hours of onset of pain; all patients received thrombolytics	Single treatment for 60 minutes at 2 ATA.	Death, serial CPK-MB and ECG, left ventricular ejection fraction (NS). Time to pain relief ($P < 0.001$).	Time to pain relief faster in HBOT group
Sharifi and colleagues (2004)[132]	PRC	61 patients (24 HBOT; 37 control) of average age 64 years with AMI or unstable angina; all patients had to be stable to participate in the study	90 minutes at 2 ATA 1 hour before and immediately after PCI and a second treatment within 18 hours.	Major adverse cardiac events at 8 months significantly less in HBOT group ($P = 0.001$). Restenosis lower in HBOT group ($P < 0.05$) at 8 months.	Yes
Dekleva and colleagues (2004)[133]	PRC	74 patients (37 HBOT; 37 control) of mean age 55 years with first AMI and who had echocardiogram within 24 hours of the onset of pain; all patients received streptokinase	Single treatment within 24 hours of onset of pain at 2 ATA for 60 minutes.	Left ventricular function by serial echocardiograms was significantly improved in HBOT group.	Yes
TRANSPLANTATION					
Mazariegos and colleagues (1999)[139]	Case series with control group	31 pediatric patients (17 HBOT; 14 control) with HAT after liver transplant	90 minutes at 2.4 ATA twice a day started within 24 hours of diagnosis or revascularization attempt for no longer than 2 weeks.	Survival and retransplantation rates similar in both groups. Time to retransplantation longer in HBOT group.	Yes

AMI, acute myocardial ischemia; ATA, atmospheres absolute; CPK-MB, creatine phosphokinase MB; CT, computerized tomography; ECG, electrocardiogram; HBO, hyperbaric oxygen; HBOT, hyperbaric oxygen therapy; MCA, middle cerebral artery; NIHSS, National Institutes of Health Stroke Scale; NS, not significant; PCI, percutaneous coronary intervention; PRC, placebo randomized, controlled trial; PRCDB, placebo randomized, controlled, double-blind trial; RCB, randomized, controlled, blinded trial; TEE, transesophageal echocardiography; TTE, transthoracic echocardiography.

of MCA occlusion. All patients presented within 24 hours of the cerebral event and had a score of less than 80 on the Orgogozo functional scale (0 = completely unresponsive; 100 = no deficit). Once enrolled, all patients received supportive care including low-dose heparin, nursing care, rehabilitation, speech therapy, and occupational therapy. Patients were randomized to HBOT (n = 17) or sham treatments (n = 17). Outcomes included mortality and changes in three healthcare scales (acute assessment scale: Orgogozo [100–0]; Trouillas (0–10); and functional assessment scale: Rankin Scale) that were used to assess neurologic outcome at 6 months and 1 year. A significant difference favoring HBOT was observed at 1 year in the Orgogozo ($P < 0.02$) and Trouillas ($P < 0.03$) scales. No statistical difference was observed in the Rankin Scale.

Rusyniak and colleagues[126] reported a prospective study of the effects of HBOT on acute ischemic stroke in 2003.[126] The study enrolled 33 patients (22 men) presenting to the emergency department within 24 hours of stroke onset, with a deficit on an acute impairment scale—National Institutes of Health Stroke Scale score of less than 23 (30 is maximum disability)—and without evidence of hemorrhage on computed tomography scanning. Those randomized to the HBOT arm received a single session (breathing 100% oxygen for 60 minutes in a monoplace chamber at 2.5 ATA), whereas those in the control arm received a sham treatment (breathing air at 1.14 ATA). Primary outcome measures included the percentage of participants with improvements at 24 hours and 90 days. Secondary measurements included complications of treatment and mortality at 90 days. Outcomes included mortality, adverse effects of treatment, and changes in the National Institutes of Health Stroke Scale at 24 hours and 90 days. Other functional and outcome scales performed in the study were the modified Rankin Scale (90 days) and two outcome scales, the Barthel Index of activities of daily living (90 days) and the Glasgow Outcome Scale (90 days). No statistical difference was found at 24 hours. At 90 days, the sham group did better reaching statistical significance in three of the four scales. It is possible that the poorer outcome in the HBOT group was related to the greater pressure (2.5 ATA) used in the study.

With respect to treatment pressures, Holbach and coworkers[127] determined that HBOT at 1.5 ATA was associated with the most normal respiratory quotient in the brain. That study measured carbohydrate metabolism as an indicator of cerebral well-being in cases of human head trauma and stroke, and found products of anaerobic metabolism at lower and higher pressures.[127] In the clinical arena of cerebral I/R injury, HBOT may exert its impact by mechanisms different than those identified in basic science studies, because greater treatment pressures of 2.0 to 3.0 ATA have been most effective in limiting tissue damage. Another possible explanation is that there are significant differences in tissue responses to HBOT, as well as likely differences between the human and animal species studied. Finally, the timing of HBOT administration during the reperfusion period represents a potentially important factor. Clinical trials cannot match the controlled timing of HBO application in basic science studies after I/R injury. The variation and delay of HBOT in human treatment may alter its effectiveness because the reperfusion window may be narrow. The effectiveness of therapies with respect to the reperfusion window unfortunately is an often overlooked and under-reported phenomenon in I/R injury research and must be considered carefully when interpreting the results of clinical trials.

Myocardium

Cardiac Surgery and Acute Myocardial Infarction

Myocardial reperfusion injury is a phenomenon observed after various procedures such as angioplasty, coronary bypass, and thrombolytic therapy. The clinical application of HBOT in cardiac disease dates back to the 1960s when a personal experience using HBOT in several clinical scenarios including coronary artery occlusion and blue infants with congenital heart disease was presented. In that decade, several clinical publications on HBOT in cardiovascular diseases appeared in highly respected medical journals. Moon and colleagues[128] reported the first human patient treated with HBOT for an acute myocardial infarction (AMI). The patient experienced development of cardiogenic shock refractory to drug therapy that improved significantly when HBOT was given.

Five prospective, randomized, controlled studies published in this area are included in Table 9.2. The first, by Thurston and investigators,[129] recruited 208 patients with a strong clinical probability of AMI. A total of 103 patients received HBOT, and the remaining 105 received standard therapy in a cardiac intensive care unit. The demographics were similar in both groups. However, patients with more severe conditions were allocated to the HBOT group, including seven in cardiogenic shock, all of whom survived. Compliance with the planned HBOT protocol was inconsistent. In addition, 22% of the patients in the HBOT group had limited or no exposure to HBO. Complications from HBOT were infrequent and minor in this study. The authors believed that the trend favoring HBOT justified the routine use of HBOT in myocardial infarction.

The second randomized, controlled trial, by Swift and coworkers,[130] was designed to evaluate the potential for HBOT to improve function in hibernating myocardium (ischemic, viable muscle with the potential to resume contraction if reperfused). The study included 34 subjects within 1 week of AMI. All patients were pressurized at 2 ATA, 10 patients receiving a final gas mixture equivalent to inspired room air at pressure and the remaining 24 receiving 100% oxygen. Each patient underwent transthoracic and transesophageal echocardiography immediately before and after treatments, and a myocardial viability study (thallium scintigraphy) was performed between 3 and 7 days after infarction. Left ventricular function was significantly improved by HBOT compared with the sham group, and there was some overlap with viability as determined by thallium scintigraphy. Interpretation of echocardiography studies was blinded. The authors concluded that HBOT and echocardiography may identify hibernating myocardium and have the potential to predict improvement in left ventricular function with early intervention after infarction.

The Hyperbaric Oxygen Therapy for Myocardial Infarction (HOT MI) study, a multicenter trial that included several hospitals in the United States and Europe, was designed to further assess the benefit of thrombolysis in combination with HBOT in patients with AMI.[131] A single-center pilot study conducted before the multicenter trial showed more rapid resolution of pain and ST-segment changes in patients who received HBOT in addition to thrombolytics.[131] The multicenter trial included 122 patients with AMI admitted within the first 6 hours of onset of pain. Patients were randomized to receive thrombolytics only ($n = 63$) or thrombolytics combined with a single HBO treatment for 120 minutes (2 ATA for 60 minutes plus 30 minutes for compression and 30 minutes for decompression). Outcomes measured included death, serial creatine phosphokinase MB, serial electrocardiograms, time to pain relief, and left ventricular ejection fraction. Only time to pain relief achieved a significant P value (<0.001). Notably, because of the small sample, the study was not conducted in an intention-to-treat basis. The authors recommend a larger sample to attain a sufficient level of statistical evidence.

Sharifi and colleagues[132] reported a study to assess the value of HBOT in inhibiting restenosis after percutaneous coronary intervention in AMI. Based on the invariably disruptive effects of percutaneous coronary intervention in the coronary wall, and the beneficial effects of HBOT in wound healing, the authors hypothesized that adjuvant HBOT would expedite healing of the miniature wounds caused by percutaneous coronary intervention, subsequently decreasing restenosis. This randomized, controlled trial included patients with AMI or unstable angina, 33 patients in the HBOT arm and 36 in the control arm. Eligibility for entering the study included resolution of chest pain and normalization of ST-segment changes. The HBOT group received two treatments. End points were calculated at 8 months and included death, myocardial infarction, coronary artery bypass, revascularization of target lesion, and late angina (after 8 months). Rates of revascularization of target lesion, myocardial infarction, and late angina were statistically lower in the HBOT group. Restenosis was also lower in the HBOT group ($P < 0.05$).

Dekleva and investigators[133] conducted a prospective, randomized trial that examined left ventricular function in patients with AMI treated with streptokinase or streptokinase and HBOT. Patients randomized to the HBOT group received a single treatment within 24 hours of the onset of pain and then serial echocardiograms performed by a blinded interpreter. All patients had similar medical treatment during hospitalization. Patients in the HBOT group had a significant decrease in end-systolic volume index and improved left ventricular ejection fraction. Using the same patient population, the same authors reported no change on left ventricular chamber stiffness in the HBOT arm.

It is somewhat difficult to interpret the results of HBOT effects on clinical studies of myocardial I/R injury because HBOT has been applied during various phases of the reperfusion period. The inconsistency of the timing of applied HBOT makes it impossible to correlate mechanisms and outcomes with the effects observed in basic science studies. This heterogeneity has likely contributed to the conclusion in a review that routine application of HBOT in acute coronary syndrome was not justified.[134] Overall, basic studies suggest that hyperoxia delivered early in the reperfusion phase is beneficial. Recent technology has been developed that is capable of delivering blood, hyperoxygenated to the same degree achieved with HBOT, locally via a catheter-based system.[135] This approach may reduce some of the logistical issues with HBOT after a reperfusion intervention (transfer of patient to the hyperbaric chamber) and still maintain the local beneficial effects of hyperoxia without the systemic effects of oxygen toxicity.[135] Further studies are required to define the mechanistic role of HBOT in myocardial I/R.

Transplantation

HBOT may facilitate organ transplantation through limitation of I/R injury that represents a frequent complication of this procedure. Several positive animal studies on HBOT in transplantation were published in the 1960s. These studies combined hypothermia and HBOT for preservation of solid organs.[136-138] Despite the successful results of these investigations, the use of HBOT in clinical transplantation is limited. A setting that has had some success with adjuvant HBOT is hepatic artery thrombosis in pediatric liver transplant patients. Mazariegos and investigators[139] reported on a series of 31 pediatric patients who experienced development of hepatic artery thrombosis within the first 10 days after a liver transplant. The diagnosis of hepatic artery thrombosis was made by Doppler ultrasound. All patients were treated with intravenous antibiotics and drainage of hepatic abscesses or bile duct strictures and listed for retransplantation. Seventeen patients received adjuvant HBOT started within 24 hours of the diagnosis or immediately after the revascularization attempt. HBOT was given twice a day and continued until resolution of signs of liver ischemia resolved (absence of fever, normalization of liver injury tests, recanalization of hepatic artery collaterals on ultrasound) or for 2 weeks. Fourteen patients constituted a historical control group. Demographics were similar in both groups. Survival and retransplantation rates were similar in both groups. However, HBOT significantly increased the time to retransplantation, and the histopathologic findings of the explanted liver allografts in the HBOT group had less necrosis than the non-HBOT group.

ACKNOWLEDGMENTS

This work was reproduced in part with permission from previous sources including Buras J, Reenstra W: Endothelial-neutrophil interactions during ischemia and reperfusion injury: Basic mechanisms of hyperbaric oxygen. Neurol Res

29:127-131, 2007; and Buras J: Basic mechanisms of hyperbaric oxygen in the treatment of ischemia-reperfusion injury. Int Anesthesiol Clin 38:91-109, 2000.

REFERENCES

1. Khalil AA, Aziz FA, Hall JC: Reperfusion injury. Plast Reconstr Surg 117:1024-1033, 2006.
2. Piper HM, Meuter K, Schafer C: Cellular mechanisms of ischemia-reperfusion injury. Ann Thorac Surg 75:S644-S648, 2003.
3. Hallenbeck JM, Dutka AJ: Background review and current concepts of reperfusion injury. Arch Neurol 47:1245-1254, 1990.
4. Buras J: Basic mechanisms of hyperbaric oxygen in the treatment of ischemia-reperfusion injury. Int Anesthesiol Clin 38:91-109, 2000.
5. Schofer J, Montz R, Mathey DG: Scintigraphic evidence of the "no reflow" phenomenon in human beings after coronary thrombolysis. J Am Coll Cardiol 5:593-598, 1985.
6. Ito H, Maruyama A, Iwakura K, et al: Clinical implications of the 'no reflow' phenomenon. A predictor of complications and left ventricular remodeling in reperfused anterior wall myocardial infarction. Circulation 93:223-228, 1996.
7. Wu KC, Kim RJ, Bluemke DA, et al: Quantification and time course of microvascular obstruction by contrast-enhanced echocardiography and magnetic resonance imaging following acute myocardial infarction and reperfusion. J Am Coll Cardiol 32:1756-1764, 1998.
8. Weir EK, Lopez-Barneo J, Buckler KJ, Archer SL: Acute oxygen-sensing mechanisms. N Engl J Med 353:2042-2055, 2005.
9. Kaelin WG Jr: The von Hippel-Lindau protein, HIF hydroxylation, and oxygen sensing. Biochem Biophys Res Commun 338:627-638, 2005.
10. Sitkovsky MV: Physiological control of immune response and inflammatory tissue damage by hypoxia inducible factors and adenosine A2A receptors. Annu Rev Immunol 22:2101-2126, 2004.
11. Kumar V, Fausto N, Abbas A: Robbins and Cotran Pathologic Basis of Disease, 7 ed. New York, WB Saunders, 2004.
12. Becker LB: New concepts in reactive oxygen species and cardiovascular reperfusion physiology. Cardiovasc Res 61:461-470, 2004.
13. Kevin LG, Novalija E, Stowe DF: Reactive oxygen species as mediators of cardiac injury and protection: The relevance to anesthesia practice. Anesth Analg 101:1275-1287, 2005.
14. Zweier JL, Talukder MA: The role of oxidants and free radicals in reperfusion injury. Cardiovasc Res 70:181-190, 2006.
15. Mickel HS, Vaishnav YN, Kempski O, et al: Breathing 100% oxygen after global brain ischemia in Mongolian Gerbils results in increased lipid peroxidation and increased mortality. Stroke 18:426-430, 1987.
16. Strauss MB, Hargens AR, Gershuni DH, et al: Reduction of skeletal muscle necrosis using intermittent hyperbaric oxygen in a model compartment syndrome. J Bone Joint Surg Am 65:656-662, 1983.
17. Nylander G, Lewis D, Nordstrom H, Larsson J. Reduction of postischemic edema with hyperbaric oxygen. Plast Reconstr Surg 76:596-603, 1985.
18. Thom SR: Functional inhibition of leukocyte B2 integrins by hyperbaric oxygen in carbon monoxide-mediated brain injury in rats. Toxicol Appl Pharmacol 123:248-256, 1993.
19. Mink RB, Dutka AJ: Hyperbaric oxygen after global cerebral ischemia in rabbits reduces brain vascular permeability and blood flow. Stroke 26:2307-2312, 1995.
20. Chen MF, Chen HM, Ueng SW, Shyr MH: Hyperbaric oxygen pretreatment attenuates hepatic reperfusion injury. Liver 18:110-116, 1998.
21. Kawamura S, Yasui N, Shirasawa M, Fukasawa H: Therapeutic effects of hyperbaric oxygenation on acute focal cerebral ischemia in rats. Surg Neurol 34:101-106, 1990.
22. Reitan JA, Kien ND, Thorup S, Corkill G: Hyperbaric oxygen increases survival following carotid ligation in gerbils. Stroke 21:119-123, 1990.
23. Takahashi M, Iwatsuki N, Ono K, et al: Hyperbaric oxygen therapy accelerates neurologic recovery after 15-minute complete global cerebral ischemia in dogs. Crit Care Med 20:1588-1594, 1992.
24. Noda Y, McGeer PL, McGeer EG: Lipid peroxide distribution in brain and the effect of hyperbaric oxygen. J Neurochem 40:1329-1332, 1983.
25. Jerrett SA, Jefferson D, Mengel CE: Seizures, H2O2 formation and lipid peroxides in brain during exposure to oxygen under high pressure. Aerosp Med 44:40-44, 1973.
26. Nishiki K, Jamieson D, Oshino N, Chance B: Oxygen toxicity in the perfused rat liver and lung under hyperbaric conditions. Biochem J 160:343-355, 1976.
27. Doherty P, Pan S, Milloy J, et al: Adenosine deaminase and thymocyte maturation. Scand J Immunol 33:405-410, 1991.
28. Chen Q, Banick PD, Thom SR: Functional inhibition of rat polymorphonuclear leukocyte B2 integrins by hyperbaric oxygen is associated with impaired cGMP synthesis. J Pharmacol Exp Ther 276:929-933, 1996.
29. Hartung KJ, Jung K, Minda R, Kunz W: Mitochondrial respiratory function as indicator of the ischemic injury of the rat kidney. Biomed Biochim Acta 44:1435-1443, 1985.
30. Kilgore KS, Lucchesi BR: Reperfusion injury after myocardial infarction: The role of free radicals and the inflammatory response. Clin Biochem 26:359-370, 1993.
31. Haljamae H, Hagber H, Jennische E: Cellular effects of complete tourniquet ischemia. In: Lewis DH (ed): Induced Skeletal Muscle Ischemia in Man. Basel, Skarger, 1982.
32. Nylander G, Nordstrom H, Lewis D, Larsson J: Metabolic effects of hyperbaric oxygen in postischemic muscle. Plast Reconstr Surg 79:91-97, 1987.
33. Yamada T, Taguchi T, Hirata Y, et al: The protective effect of hyperbaric oxygenation on the small intestine in ischemia-reperfusion injury. J Pediatr Surg 30:786-790, 1995.
34. Zamboni WA, Roth AC, Russell RC, et al: Morphologic analysis of the microcirculation during reperfusion of

ischemic skeletal muscle and the effect of hyperbaric oxygen. Plast Reconstr Surg 91:1110–1123, 1993.

35. Xu H, Gonzalo JA, St Pierre Y, et al: Leukocytosis and resistance to septic shock in intercellular adhesion molecule 1-deficient mice. J Exp Med 180:95–109, 1994.

36. Malik AB, Lo SK: Vascular endothelial adhesion molecules and tissue inflammation. Pharmacol Rev 48:213–229, 1996.

37. Aird WC: Spatial and temporal dynamics of the endothelium. J Thromb Haemost 3:1392–1406, 2005.

38. Salmi M, Jalkanen S: Cell-surface enzymes in control of leukocyte trafficking. Nat Rev Immunol 5:760–771, 2005.

39. Weber C, Koenen RR: Fine-tuning leukocyte responses: Towards a chemokine 'interactome.' Trends Immunol 27:268–273, 2006.

40. Patel KD, Zimmerman GA, Prescott SM, et al: Oxygen radicals induce human endothelial cells to express GMP-140 and bind neutrophils. J Cell Biol 112:749–759, 1991.

41. Moore KL, Varki A, McEver RP: GMP-140 binds to a glycoprotein receptor on human neutrophils: Evidence for a lectin-like interaction. J Cell Biol 112:491–499, 1991.

42. Zhang R, Chopp M, Zhang Z, et al: The expression of P- and E-selectins in three models of middle cerebral artery occlusion. Brain Res 785:207–214, 1998.

43. Vandendries ER, Furie BC, Furie B: Role of P-selectin and PSGL-1 in coagulation and thrombosis. Thromb Haemost 92:459–466, 2004.

44. Kokura S, Yoshida N, Yoshikawa T: Anoxia/reoxygenation-induced leukocyte-endothelial cell interactions. Free Radic Biol Med 33:427–432, 2002.

45. Okada Y, Copeland BR, Mori E, et al: P-selectin and intercellular adhesion molecule-1 expression after focal brain ischemia and reperfusion. Stroke 25:202–211, 1994.

46. Walz G, Aruffo A, Kolanus W, et al: Recognition by ELAM-1 of the sialyl-Lex determinant on myeloid and tumor cells. Science 250:1132–1135, 1990.

47. Zou X, Shinde Patil VR, Dagia NM, et al: PSGL-1 derived from human neutrophils is a high-efficiency ligand for endothelium-expressed E-selectin under flow. Am J Physiol Cell Physiol 289:C415–C424, 2005.

48. Katayama Y, Hidalgo A, Chang J, et al: CD44 is a physiological E-selectin ligand on neutrophils. J Exp Med 201:1183–1189, 2005.

49. Cook-Mills JM, Deem TL: Active participation of endothelial cells in inflammation. J Leukoc Biol 77:487–495, 2005.

50. Schenkel AR, Chew TW, Muller WA: Platelet endothelial cell adhesion molecule deficiency or blockade significantly reduces leukocyte emigration in a majority of mouse strains. J Immunol 173:6403–6408, 2004.

51. Simon SI, Burns AR, Taylor AD, et al: L-selectin (CD62L) cross-linking signals neutrophil adhesive functions via the Mac-1 (CD11b/CD18) beta 2-integrin. J Immunol 155:1502–1514, 1995.

52. Blanks JE, Moll T, Eytner R, Vestweber D: Stimulation of P-selectin glycoprotein ligand-1 on mouse neutrophils activates beta 2-integrin mediated cell attachment to ICAM-1. Eur J Immunol 28:433–443, 1998.

53. Green CE, Pearson DN, Camphausen RT, et al: Shear-dependent capping of L-selectin and P-selectin glycoprotein ligand 1 by E-selectin signals activation

of high-avidity beta2-integrin on neutrophils. J Immunol 172:7780–7790, 2004.

54. Simon SI, Hu Y, Vestweber D, Smith CW: Neutrophil tethering on E-selectin activates beta 2 integrin binding to ICAM-1 through a mitogen-activated protein kinase signal transduction pathway. J Immunol 164:4348–4358, 2000.

55. Hentzen E, McDonough D, McIntire L, et al: Hydrodynamic shear and tethering through E-selectin signals phosphorylation of p38 MAP kinase and adhesion of human neutrophils. Ann Biomed Eng 30:987–1001, 2002.

56. Connolly ES Jr, Winfree CJ, Prestigiacomo CJ, et al: Exacerbation of cerebral injury in mice that express the P-selectin gene: Identification of P-selectin blockade as a new target for the treatment of stroke. Circ Res 81:304–310, 1997.

57. Mori E, del Zoppo GJ, Chambers JD, et al: Inhibition of polymorphonuclear leukocyte adherence suppresses no-reflow after focal cerebral ischemia in baboons. Stroke 23:712–718, 1992.

58. Prestigiacomo CJ, Kim SC, Connolly ES Jr, et al: CD18-mediated neutrophil recruitment contributes to the pathogenesis of reperfused but not nonreperfused stroke. Stroke 30:1110–1117, 1999.

59. Matsuoka A, Shitara T, Okamoto M, Sano H: Transient deafness with iopamidol following angiography. Acta Otolaryngol Suppl 514:78–80, 1994.

60. Soriano SG, Lipton SA, Wang YF, et al: Intercellular adhesion molecule-1-deficient mice are less susceptible to cerebral ischemia-reperfusion injury. Ann Neurol 39:618–624, 1996.

61. Kitagawa K, Matsumoto M, Mabuchi T, et al: Deficiency of intercellular adhesion molecule 1 attenuates microcirculatory disturbance and infarction size in focal cerebral ischemia. J Cereb Blood Flow Metab 18:1336–1345, 1998.

62. Atochin DN, Fisher D, Demchenko IT, et al: Neutrophil sequestration and the effect of hyperbaric oxygen in a rat model of temporary middle cerebral artery occlusion. Undersea Hyperb Med 27:185–190, 2001.

63. Kakkar AK, Lefer DJ: Leukocyte and endothelial adhesion molecule studies in knockout mice. Curr Opin Pharmacol 4:154–158, 2004.

64. Diamond MS, Staunton DE, de Fougerolles AR, et al: ICAM-1 (CD54): A counter-receptor for Mac-1 (CD11b/CD18). J Cell Biol 111:3129–3139, 1990.

65. Valmu L, Fagerholm S, Suila H, Gahmberg CG: The cytoskeletal association of CD11/CD18 leukocyte integrins in phorbol ester-activated cells correlates with CD18 phosphorylation. Eur J Immunol 29:2107–2118, 1999.

66. Thom SR: Leukocytes in carbon monoxide-mediated brain oxidative injury. Toxicol Appl Pharmacol 123:234–247, 1993.

67. Thom SR, Mendiguren I, Hardy K, et al: Inhibition of human neutrophil beta2-integrin-dependent adherence by hyperbaric O2. Am J Physiol 272:C770–C777, 1997.

68. Thom SR: Effects of hyperoxia on neutrophil adhesion. Undersea Hyperb Med 31:123–131, 2004.

69. Wyatt TA, Lincoln TM, Pryzwansky KB: Regulation of human neutrophil degranulation by LY-83583 and L-arginine: Role of cGMP-dependent protein kinase. Am J Physiol 265:C201–C211, 1993.

70. Larson JL, Stephenson LL, Zamboni WA: Effect of hyperbaric oxygen on neutrophil CD18 expression. Plast Reconstr Surg 105:1375-1381, 2000.

71. Ueno S, Tanabe G, Kihara K, et al: Early post-operative hyperbaric oxygen therapy modifies neutrophile activation. Hepatogastroenterology 46:1798-1799, 1999.

72. Akiyama H, Enzan K, Matsumoto J, et al: [Postoperative disturbance of consciousness due to tumor emboli of the orifice of pulmonary artery]. Masui 42:1692-1695, 1993.

73. Bowman CM, Butler EN, Vatter AE, Repine JE: Hyperoxia injuries endothelial cells in culture and causes increased neutrophil adherence. Chest 83:33S-35S, 1983.

74. Shinomiya N, Suzuki S, Hashimoto A, et al: Effect of hyperbaric oxygen on intercellular adhesion molecule-1 (ICAM-1) expression in murine lung. Aviat Space Environ Med 69:1-7, 1998.

75. Buras JA, Stahl GL, Svoboda KK, Reenstra WR: Hyperbaric oxygen downregulates ICAM-1 expression induced by hypoxia and hypoglycemia: The role of NOS. Am J Physiol Cell Physiol 278:C292-C302, 2000.

76. Hong JP, Kwon H, Chung YK, Jung SH: The effect of hyperbaric oxygen on ischemia-reperfusion injury: An experimental study in a rat musculocutaneous flap. Ann Plast Surg 51:478-487, 2003.

77. Lowenstein CJ, Snyder SH: Nitric oxide, a novel biologic messenger. Cell 70:705-707, 1992.

78. Li XA, Everson W, Smart EJ: Nitric oxide, caveolae, and vascular pathology. Cardiovasc Toxicol 6:1-13, 2006.

79. Dudzinski DM, Igarashi J, Greif D, Michel T: The regulation and pharmacology of endothelial nitric oxide synthase. Annu Rev Pharmacol Toxicol 46:235-276, 2006.

80. Lefer AM, Lefer DJ: The role of nitric oxide and cell adhesion molecules on the microcirculation in ischaemia-reperfusion. Cardiovasc Res 32:743-751, 1996.

81. Szabo C: The pathophysiological role of peroxynitrite in shock, inflammation, and ischemia-reperfusion injury. Shock 6:79-88, 1996.

82. Donzelli S, Switzer CH, Thomas DD, et al: The activation of metabolites of nitric oxide synthase by metals is both redox and oxygen dependent: A new feature of nitrogen oxide signaling. Antioxid Redox Signal 8:1363-1371, 2006.

83. Lefer DJ, Scalia R, Campbell B, et al: Peroxynitrite inhibits leukocyte-endothelial cell interactions and protects against ischemia-reperfusion injury in rats. J Clin Invest 99:684-691, 1997.

84. Nossuli TO, Hayward R, Jensen D, et al: Mechanisms of cardioprotection by peroxynitrite in myocardial ischemia and reperfusion injury. Am J Physiol 275:H509-H519, 1998.

85. Nishida K, Harrison DG, Navas JP, et al: Molecular cloning and characterization of the constitutive bovine aortic endothelial cell nitric oxide synthase. J Clin Invest 90:2092-2096, 1992.

86. Walford GA, Moussignac RL, Scribner AW, et al: Hypoxia potentiates nitric oxide-mediated apoptosis in endothelial cells via peroxynitrite-induced activation of mitochondria-dependent and -independent pathways. J Biol Chem 279:4425-4432, 2004.

87. Ahrendt GM, Tantry US, Barbul A: Intra-abdominal sepsis impairs colonic reparative collagen synthesis. Am J Surg 171:102-107, 1996.

88. Kubes P, Suzuki M, Granger DN: Nitric oxide: An endogenous modulator of leukocyte adhesion. Proc Natl Acad Sci USA 88:4651-4655, 1991.

89. Laszlo F, Whittle BJ: Actions of isoform-selective and non-selective nitric oxide synthase inhibitors on endotoxin-induced vascular leakage in rat colon. Eur J Pharmacol 334:99-102, 1997.

90. Wei XQ, Charles IG, Smith A, et al: Altered immune responses in mice lacking inducible nitric oxide synthase. Nature 375:408-411, 1995.

91. MacMicking JD, Nathan C, Hom G, et al: Altered responses to bacterial infection and endotoxic shock in mice lacking inducible nitric oxide synthase. Cell 81:641-650, 1995.

92. Rubanyi GM, Ho EH, Cantor EH, et al: Cytoprotective function of nitric oxide: Inactivation of superoxide radicals produced by human leukocytes. Biochem Biophys Res Commun 181:1392-1397, 1991.

93. Black SM, Johengen MJ, Ma ZD, et al: Ventilation and oxygenation induce endothelial nitric oxide synthase gene expression in the lungs of fetal lambs. J Clin Invest 100:1448-1458, 1997.

94. North AJ, Lau KS, Brannon TS, et al: Oxygen upregulates nitric oxide synthase gene expression in ovine fetal pulmonary artery endothelial cells. Am J Physiol 270:L643-L649, 1996.

95. Rengasamy A, Johns RA: Characterization of endothelium-derived relaxing factor/nitric oxide synthase from bovine cerebellum and mechanism of modulation by high and low oxygen tensions. J Pharmacol Exp Ther 259:310-316, 1991.

96. Luongo C, Imperatore F, Cuzzocrea S, et al: Effects of hyperbaric oxygen exposure on a zymosan-induced shock model. Crit Care Med 26:1972-1976, 1998.

97. Kurata S, Yamashita U, Nakajima H: Hyperbaric oxygenation reduces the cytostatic activity and transcription of nitric oxide synthetase gene of mouse peritoneal macrophages. Biochim Biophys Acta 1263:35-38, 1995.

98. Curry JD, Stephenson L, Zamboni WA: Nitric oxide in skeletal muscle following hyperbaric oxygen therapy in ischemia-reperfusion injury. Undersea Hyperb Med 26:S9, 1999.

99. Banick PD, Chen Q, Xu YA, Thom SR: Nitric oxide inhibits neutrophil beta 2 integrin function by inhibiting membrane-associated cyclic GMP synthesis. J Cell Physiol 172:12-24, 1997.

100. Thom SR, Fisher D, Zhang J, et al: Stimulation of perivascular nitric oxide synthesis by oxygen. Am J Physiol Heart Circ Physiol 284:H1230-H1239, 2003.

101. Thom SR, Buerk DG: Nitric oxide synthesis in brain is stimulated by oxygen. Adv Exp Med Biol 510:133-137, 2003.

102. Baynosa RC, Naig AL, Murphy PS, et al: The effect of hyperbaric oxygen on NOS activity and transcription in ischemia reperfusion injury. Undersea Hyperb Med Supplement, Abstract 89, 2005.

103. Sirsjo A, Lehr HA, Nolte D, et al: Hyperbaric oxygen treatment enhances the recovery of blood flow and

functional capillary density in postischemic striated muscle. Circ Shock 40:9-13, 1993.

104. Murry CE, Jennings RB, Reimer KA: Preconditioning with ischemia: A delay of lethal cell injury in ischemic myocardium. Circulation 74:1124-1136, 1986.

105. Deutsch E, Berger M, Kussmaul WG, et al: Adaptation to ischemia during percutaneous transluminal coronary angioplasty. Clinical, hemodynamic, and metabolic features. Circulation 82:2044-2051, 1990.

106. Pasupathy S, Homer-Vanniasinkam S: Surgical implications of ischemic preconditioning. Arch Surg 140:405-409, 2005.

107. Doents T, Taegtmeyer H: Ischemic preconditioning-from bench to bedside. In: Bayersdorf F (ed): Ischemia-reperfusion injury in cardiac surgery. Georgetown, Tex, Eureka.com/Landes Bioscience, 2001, pp 104-126.

108. Riess ML, Stowe DF, Warltier DC: Cardiac pharmacological preconditioning with volatile anesthetics: From bench to bedside? Am J Physiol Heart Circ Physiol 286:H1603-H1607, 2004.

109. Dennog C, Hartmann A, Frey G, Speit G: Detection of DNA damage after hyperbaric oxygen (HBO) therapy. Mutagenesis 11:605-609, 1996.

110. Speit G, Dennog C, Lampl L: Biological significance of DNA damage induced by hyperbaric oxygen. Mutagenesis 13:85-87, 1998.

111. Rothfuss A, Radermacher P, Speit G: Involvement of heme oxygenase-1 (HO-1) in the adaptive protection of human lymphocytes after hyperbaric oxygen (HBO) treatment. Carcinogenesis 22:1979-1985, 2001.

112. Speit G, Bonzheim I: Genotoxic and protective effects of hyperbaric oxygen in A549 lung cells. Mutagenesis 18:545-548, 2003.

113. Clark JE, Foresti R, Green CJ, Motterlini R: Dynamics of haem oxygenase-1 expression and bilirubin production in cellular protection against oxidative stress. Biochem J 348:615-619, 2000.

114. Dennog C, Radermacher P, Barnett YA, Speit G: Antioxidant status in humans after exposure to hyperbaric oxygen. Mutat Res 428:83-89, 1999.

115. Kim CH, Choi H, Chun YS, et al: Hyperbaric oxygenation pretreatment induces catalase and reduces infarct size in ischemic rat myocardium. Pflugers Arch 442:519-525, 2001.

116. Gregorevic P, Lynch GS, Williams DA: Hyperbaric oxygen modulates antioxidant enzyme activity in rat skeletal muscles. Eur J Appl Physiol 86:24-27, 2001.

117. Nie H, Xiong L, Lao N, et al: Hyperbaric oxygen preconditioning induces tolerance against spinal cord ischemia by upregulation of antioxidant enzymes in rabbits. J Cereb Blood Flow Metab 26:666-674, 2006.

118. Cabigas BP, Su J, Hutchins W, et al: Hyperoxic and hyperbaric-induced cardioprotection: Role of nitric oxide synthase 3. Cardiovasc Res 72:143-151, 2006.

119. Pulsinelli W: Pathophysiology of acute ischaemic stroke. Lancet 339:533-536, 1992.

120. Symon L, Branston NM, Strong AJ, Hope TD: The concepts of thresholds of ischaemia in relation to brain structure and function. J Clin Pathol Suppl 11:149-154, 1977.

121. Astrup J, Siesjo BK, Symon L: Thresholds in cerebral ischemia—the ischemic penumbra. Stroke 12:723-725, 1981.

122. Furlan M, Marchal G, Viader F, et al: Spontaneous neurological recovery after stroke and the fate of the ischemic penumbra. Ann Neurol 40:216-226, 1996.

123. The alternative therapy evaluation committee for the insurance corporation of British Columbia. Brain Injury 17:225-236, 2003.

124. Anderson DC, Bottini AG, Jagiella WM, et al: A pilot study of hyperbaric oxygen in the treatment of human stroke. Stroke 22:1137-1142, 1991.

125. Nighoghossian N, Trouillas P, Adeleine P, Salord F: Hyperbaric oxygen in the treatment of acute ischemic stroke. A double-blind pilot study. Stroke 26:1369-1372, 1995.

126. Rusyniak DE, Kirk MA, May JD, et al: Hyperbaric oxygen therapy in acute ischemic stroke: Results of the Hyperbaric Oxygen in Acute Ischemic Stroke Trial Pilot Study. Stroke 34:571-574, 2003.

127. Holbach KH, Caroli A, Wassmann H: Cerebral energy metabolism in patients with brain lesions of normo- and hyperbaric oxygen pressures. J Neurol 217:17-30, 1977.

128. Moon AJ, Williams KG, Hopkinson WI: A patient with coronary thrombosis treated with hyperbaric oxygen. Lancet 18:18-20, 1964.

129. Thurston JG, Greenwood TW, Bending MR, et al: A controlled investigation into the effects of hyperbaric oxygen on mortality following acute myocardial infarction. Q J Med 42:751-770, 1973.

130. Swift PC, Turner JH, Oxer HF, et al: Myocardial hibernation identified by hyperbaric oxygen treatment and echocardiography in postinfarction patients: Comparison with exercise thallium scintigraphy. Am Heart J 124:1151-1158, 1992.

131. Stavitsky Y, Shandling AH, Ellestad MH, et al: Hyperbaric oxygen and thrombolysis in myocardial infarction: The 'HOT MI' randomized multicenter study. Cardiology 90:131-136, 1998.

132. Sharifi M, Fares W, Abdel-Karim I, et al: Usefulness of hyperbaric oxygen therapy to inhibit restenosis after percutaneous coronary intervention for acute myocardial infarction or unstable angina pectoris. Am J Cardiol 93:1533-1535, 2004.

133. Dekleva M, Neskovic A, Vlahovic A, et al: Adjunctive effect of hyperbaric oxygen treatment after thrombolysis on left ventricular function in patients with acute myocardial infarction. Am Heart J 148:E14, 2004.

134. Bennett M, Jepson N, Lehm J: Hyperbaric oxygen therapy for acute coronary syndrome. Cochrane Database Syst Rev 18:CD004818, 2005.

135. Glazier JJ: Attenuation of reperfusion microvascular ischemia by aqueous oxygen: Experimental and clinical observations. Am Heart J 149:580-584, 2005.

136. Bloch JH, Manax WG, Eyal Z, Lillehei RC: Heart preservation in vitro with hyperbaric oxygenation and hypothermia. J Thorac Cardiovasc Surg 48:969-983, 1964.

137. Blumenstock DA, Lempert N, Morgado F: Preservation of the canine lung in vitro for 24 hours with the use of hypothermia and hyperbaric oxygen. J Thorac Cardiovasc Surg 50:769-774, 1965.

138. Ladaga LG, Nabseth DC, Besznyak I, et al: Preservation of canine kidneys by hypothermia and hyperbaric oxygen: Long-term survival of autografts following 24-hour storage. Ann Surg 163:553-558, 1966.

139. Mazariegos GV, O'Toole K, Mieles LA, et al: Hyperbaric oxygen therapy for hepatic artery thrombosis after liver transplantation in children. Liver Transpl Surg 5:429-436, 1999.

140. Gurer A, Ozdogan M, Gomceli I, et al: Hyperbaric oxygenation attenuates renal ischemia-reperfusion injury in rats. Transplant Proc 38:3337-3340, 2006.

141. Kihara K, Ueno S, Sakoda M, Aikou T: Effects of hyperbaric oxygen exposure on experimental hepatic ischemia. Liver Transpl 11:1574-1580, 2005.

142. Sterling DL, Thornton JF, Swafford A, et al: Hyperbaric oxygen limits infarct size in ischemic rabbit myocardium in vivo. Circulation 88:1931-1936, 1993.

143. Yagci G, Ozturk E, Ozgurtas T, et al: Preoperative and postoperative administration of hyperbaric oxygen improves biochemical and mechanical parameters on ischemic and normal colonic anastomoses. J Invest Surg 19:237-244, 2006.

144. Yang ZJ, Bosco G, Montante A, et al: Hyperbaric O_2 reduces intestinal ischemia-reperfusion-induced TNF-alpha production and lung neutrophil sequestration. Eur J Appl Physiol 85:96-103, 2001.

Pressure Effects on Human Physiology

Jay B. Dean, PhD, and Dominic P. D'Agostino, PhD

OUR PHYSIOLOGIC RANGE OF TOLERABLE PRESSURES

In a general way, the benign or harmful gases (oxygen, carbonic acid, etc.) act on living beings only according to their tension in the surrounding atmosphere, a tension which is measured by multiplying their percentage by the barometric pressure; the increase in one of these factors can be compensated for by the decrease of the other.

—*Paul Bert (1878)*, La Pression Barométrique

English translation by Hitchcock and Hitchcock (1943),[1] *page 1037*

Barometric Pressure

The importance of barometric pressure (P_B) as a physiologic stimulus was first described in 1878 by Paul Bert in his historical tome *Barometric Pressure. Researches in Experimental Physiology.*[1] The fundamental physiologic relation he identified between P_B and the percentage of gas is recounted in the above quotation and can be related to the applications of hyperbaric oxygen therapy (HBOT).[2]

Although the majority of medical problems encountered in hyperbaric medicine and diving medicine are attributed to *increased* gas partial pressures during *descent* (increased P_B; Fig. 10.1) or *decreased* gas partial pressures during *ascent* (decreased P_B), there is always the potential that the change in P_B alone will have an additional effect on the human animal at the level of the organ, tissue, and cell. For example, Boyle's Law predicts that increasing or decreasing the pressure-applied force against the surface of the body will, respectively, decrease or increase the volume of gases contained in our lungs, stomach, and other gas-filled cavities. Changes in P_B will also influence the density of the gases we breathe and, thus, airway resistance during ventilation. At the cellular level, pressurizing the surface of the body will likely produce differential compression of various fine structural, nonfluid components of cells, including the lipid bilayer, cytoskeleton, and membrane-bound proteins, thereby altering various cellular functions.[3,4] In some instances, the physiologic effects of hyperbaric pressure per se are well known, such as in the case of high-pressure nervous syndrome (HPNS), which occurs in deep divers beyond 10 to 15 atmospheres absolute (ATA).[5] In other instances, the physiologic effects of hyperbaric pressure per se are less well known or have yet to be studied and described.[6]

Regarding studies on the effects of hyperbaric pressure per se, there are two general deficiencies that need to be acknowledged and addressed in the field of hyperbaric physiology. First, many investigators do not attempt to run the necessary controls to distinguish between the potential effects of hyperbaric or hydrostatic pressure per se and the narcotic effects of the gas used to pressurize a system.[6] In other words, it is necessary to differentiate the potential effects of hyperbaric N_2 (inert gas narcosis), hyperbaric O_2 (oxidative stress), and CO_2 retention (respiratory acidosis and ultimately neurotoxicity) from the potential effects of hydrostatic or gas compression. Second, the majority of studies that have separated the effects of hyperbaric pressure per se from the narcotic effects of specific gas species,

and their various reaction products (e.g., reactive O_2 and N_2 species, H^+ ions), have used extraordinarily high supraphysiologic levels of pressure in excess of 100 and 200 ATA (many of these studies have been reviewed and are discussed in the literature[4,6-12]). This is especially true of in vitro studies of cellular function at hyperbaric pressure and, in particular, the majority of studies designed to study the cellular and molecular mechanisms underlying HPNS.[7,9-11,13-19] Although such studies are appropriate for understanding the effects of hyperbaric pressure as a thermodynamic intensity parameter,[3,4] it is difficult to extrapolate these data ($>>100$ ATA) to predict the physiologic effects of pressure encountered with HBOT (up to approximately 3 ATA) or in undersea environments (up to approximately 70 ATA)[6,8] (see Fig. 10.1). This is especially true because it appears likely that different signaling mechanisms are involved in expression of cellular barosensitivity depending on the relative range of P_B (small to moderate levels of pressure vs. supraphysiological levels of pressure).[3,4,6] Consequently, the physiologic effects of moderate levels of hyperbaric pressure that are encountered in hyperbaric medicine are only now being elucidated.[20,21]

Because humans live, work, explore, and recreate in a large continuum of P_B-applied forces, which include environments of both gas pressure– and hydrostatic pressure–applied forces, this chapter briefly reviews the range of ambient pressures encompassed by these activities. What then is the range of physiologically tolerable pressures that challenges our human physiology?

Hypobaric Pressure

Much of the world's population lives at or slightly above sea level. Most humans, therefore, are adapted to P_B of approximately 1 ATA or normobaric pressure. Any environment that is defined by P_B significantly less than that at sea level is referred to as a "hypobaric environment." The highest living permanent population of humans recorded live in the Andes Mountains in northern Chile in the

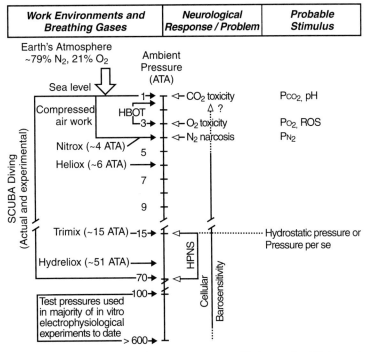

Figure 10.1 Physiologically tolerable hyperbaric pressures encountered by humans breathing air and various hyperbaric gas mixtures *(left)*, the neurologic problems that can result *(middle)*, and the proposed stimulus affecting neuronal function *(right)*. Hyperbaric environments are encountered in hyperbaric oxygen therapy (HBOT), compressed air work (e.g., subterranean tunneling), diving medicine, and disabled submarine accidents. By breathing an assortment of gas mixtures (nitrox, heliox, hydreliox), to avert the narcotic and toxic effects of N_2 and O_2, as well as the direct effects of hydrostatic compression on the central nervous system, humans are able to inhabit hyperbaric environments ranging from more than 1 to approximately 70 atmospheres absolute (ATA) pressure. At extreme hyperbaric pressures (>100 ATA), pressure becomes a tool that can be used to perturb biologic systems (in vitro) by altering protein conformations, membrane fluidity, and configuration of the cytoskeleton. Humans and most mammals, however, have never occupied this extreme range of ambient pressure. The question mark *(?)* emphasizes the point that few studies have examined the effects of moderate levels of hyperbaric pressure per se on cellular barosensitivity, particularly in the range of pressure used during HBOT. HPNS, high-pressure nervous syndrome; Pco_2, partial pressure of CO_2; Pn_2, partial pressure of N_2; Po_2, partial pressure of O_2; ROS, reactive oxygen species; SCUBA, self-contained underwater breathing apparatus. *(Reprinted from Dean JB, Mulkey DK, Garcia III AJ, et al: Neuronal sensitivity to hyperoxia, hypercapnia and inert gases at hyperbaric pressures. J Appl Physiol 95:883–909, 2003, by permission of The American Physiological Society.)*

village of 'Quilcha at 17,500 feet above sea level.[22] Here, P_B has decreased to approximately half of what it is at sea level, or 0.51 ATA. Each day, workers living in 'Quilcha ascend an additional 1500 feet up the mountain to work in the sulfur mines at 19,000 feet (P_B = 0.48 ATA). They do not live at the same altitude as the sulfur mine because it is simply too high to live comfortably on a permanent basis. These high-altitude inhabitants, however, have adapted well to their hypobaric and hypoxic environment at 17,500 feet, as discussed elsewhere.[23-25] This altitude (17,500 feet, P_B 0.51 = ATA), therefore, appears to be the lowest level of P_B-applied force that humans can live at permanently. It is unlikely that the limiting factor that prevents living permanently at higher altitude is hypobaric pressure per se. Rather, it is likely the result of chronic hypoxia and its physiologic consequences for hematocrit, cardiac efficiency, and cardiorespiratory health.[23,25]

For most other people, the only other means of subjecting oneself to even greater hypobaric pressure, for comparatively short periods, is by artificial means using manmade equipment to overcome the oxygen want of high altitude. For example, the summit of

Mount Everest reaches up to an altitude of 29,029 feet where P_B is 0.31 ATA. Although some adventurers and physiologists have reached the summit of Mount Everest without oxygen,[26] most mountaineers who conquer Earth's highest peak require supplemental oxygen to meet the metabolic demands of the climb.[27] Likewise, during World War II, before customary use of pressurized aircraft,[28] aviators ascended to altitudes above 20,000 to 35,000 feet in unprecedented numbers to wage warfare. Without supplemental breathing oxygen, the time for useful consciousness at 26,000 feet was only 4 to 6 minutes; at 30,000 feet, it decreased to only 1 to 2 minutes; and at 38,000 feet, it was a mere 30 seconds or less before the aviator succumbed to hypobaric hypoxia.[29,30] The only way that humans could survive at these altitudes was by breathing pure oxygen with demand oxygen breathing equipment.[29,30] With this method, aviators were exposed to 0.46 ATA at 20,000 feet and 0.24 ATA at 35,000 feet for extended periods, which frequently caused high-altitude decompression sickness.[29,31] To achieve even higher altitudes and survive even lower barometric and oxygen pressures, aviators breathed pure oxygen delivered with positive pressure (+15 to +25 mm Hg) to increase inspired P_{O_2} and maintain consciousness for flight up to 50,000 feet.[32] Today, pressure breathing oxygen masks supply pure oxygen at pressures up to +60 to +70 mm Hg to enable escape from even higher altitudes of 60,000 to 72,000 feet after loss of cabin pressure.[32] In these emergencies, the aviator is equipped with a partial pressure suit to minimize the deleterious effects of low P_B on the body at extreme altitude.[33] Unlike the Chilean residents of 'Quilcha who live permanently at extreme altitude, without benefit of oxygen masks and pressure suits, these adverse hypobaric environments can be penetrated and tolerated for only short periods by pilots wearing survival gear that protect them against the deleterious effects of low pressure–applied forces (decompression sickness), low O_2 content (hypoxia), and extreme cold.

Hyperbaric Pressure

Conversely, hyperbaric pressures in excess of 1 ATA do not occur naturally; that is, humans do not live under hyperbaric conditions. Nonetheless, many medical personnel, military personnel, civilians, and patients routinely encounter hyperbaric conditions in their daily work and recreation practices.[6] For example, today's modern diving gear and breathing gas mixtures enable humans to ascend to great depths, especially when care is taken to avert the physiologic problems of breathing hyperbaric air and oxygen-enriched air, which includes nitrogen narcosis and oxygen toxicity (see Fig. 10.1). As the diver descends beneath sea level, ambient pressure increases to greater than 1 ATA by the weight of the overlying column of water added to that of the Earth's atmosphere. The weight of a column of water at a depth of 33 feet of sea water (fsw; or 10 meters of sea water [msw]) is 1 additional atmosphere. Thus, at 33 fsw, P_B = 2 ATA, which is 1 atmosphere of air pressure plus 1 atmosphere of water pressure. At 66 fsw, P_B = 3 ATA, or 1 atmosphere of air pressure and 2 atmospheres of water pressure; and at 99 fsw, P_B = 4 ATA, or 1 atmosphere of air pressure plus 3 atmospheres of water pressure, and so forth. The effects of true hydrostatic compression of the body can be mimicked in treatment and research hyperbaric chambers by using a gas such as oxygen, air, or helium as the compression medium. In the latter two cases, oxygen is supplied via the breathing gas mixture that is administered to the person/patient in parallel with the gas species or mixture used to compress the chamber.

Using specialized life-support equipment, humans have explored ocean depths as great as 2300 fsw, exposed to a hydrostatic pressure–applied force of approximately 70 ATA.[34] Only a handful of highly trained individuals, however, have encountered such extreme levels of compression. Less severe pressures are the norm for many people who undergo HBOT, which typically reaches a maximum of approximately 3 ATA.[2,35] Dean and colleagues[6] have summarized a variety of normal and catastrophic conditions in which humans encounter moderate levels of hyperbaric pressure that range up to 5 ATA.

To respond to the original question raised earlier—that is, what is the range of physiologically tolerable pressures that challenges our human physiology?—we would have to answer that without benefit of a pressure suit or a pressurized cabin, it ranges from an altitude of approximately 50,000 feet ($P_B = 0.11$ ATA) to a depth of 2300 feet ($P_B = 70$ ATA) beneath the ocean's surface. An approximately 700-fold increase in the P_B-applied force against the body! The caveat is that these extremes in altitude and ocean depth can only be reached and tolerated using specialized oxygen breathing equipment. Obviously, encasing the human body in a pressure suit or pressure cabin, thereby providing further protection against the pressure-applied forces beyond these tolerable extremes, enables humans to exploit even greater altitudes and depths.

Gas Partial Pressures

Although this chapter focuses on the physiologic effects of pressure per se, emphasizing moderate levels of hyperbaric pressure of 5 ATA or less, it is worthwhile to briefly summarize the effects of gas partial pressures on the body. It is only when these additional effects of hyperoxia, narcosis, and respiratory acidosis are controlled for that the effects of hyperbaric pressure alone can be determined in an animal or in vitro biologic system. Because the immediate signs of breathing hyperbaric gases usually manifest as disorders of normal brain function, for example, neurocognition, muscular control, and abnormal cardiorespiratory control, this brief overview focuses on the neurologic effects of hyperbaric gases.

Figure 10.1 shows the broad range of hyperbaric pressure over which the human body can function. It also indicates the type of work environment and threshold barometric or ambient pressures at which particular neurologic problems begin while breathing a specific gas or mixture of gases. The indicated thresholds are approximated from a review of the available literature, and it is important to recognize that interindividual and intraindividual variability exists that depends on other mitigating conditions, such as immersion and CO_2 retention, among other conditions.[6] Figure 10.1 also underscores the fact that both gas partial pressures and hyperbaric pressure per se can affect neurologic function. Presumably, the same can be said for any organ system in the body.

Beginning at sea level ($P_B = 1$ ATA) and descending while breathing air, a person can suffer CO_2 toxicity[36] and N_2 narcosis.[34] Notice that CO_2 toxicity can occur as early as sea level pressure (normobaric pressure) if the fractional concentration of end-tidal CO_2 becomes increased by breathing a gas mixture contaminated with CO_2. Normally, inspired CO_2 has a fractional concentration of essentially zero and an end-tidal CO_2 of approximately 35 to 40 torr. Initially, as inspired CO_2 is increased, cardiorespiratory activity is likewise increased by stimulation of central and peripheral chemoreceptors.[37,38] Continued breathing of up to 10% to 15% CO_2 increases end-tidal CO_2 to 50 to 70 torr, producing confusion, drowsiness, dizziness, irrational behavior, and impaired short-term memory.[36,39] Inspiring 30% CO_2 can produce seizures,[40] and breathing $\geq$70% to 75% CO_2 results in ataxia and anesthesia.[36,41] Extended breathing of more than 70% CO_2 results in death because of narcotic depression of the cardiorespiratory centers.[41,42]

In contrast, nitrogen in air (0.79) is essentially inert, physiologically speaking, until ambient pressure increases to approximately 4 ATA. The relatively higher pressure threshold for N_2 narcosis, as compared with CO_2 toxicity, is thought to be caused by the comparatively lower lipid solubility of N_2 than CO_2 and, thus, lower permeability of the plasma membrane and expansion of the plasma membrane of neurons.[6,43] The effects of hyperbaric N_2 depend on the molecular properties of the gas, whereas the central effects of hyperbaric CO_2 depend on the molecular properties of the gas and its secondary reaction product, H^+ (pH).[6] Obviously, in the case of CO_2, it is difficult to distinguish the effects of pH from those of molecular CO_2 because there is a concomitant parallel change in bicarbonate with protons. Recently, however, Hartzler and colleagues[44] have devised a method for studying the effects of molecular CO_2 on neuronal activity that occurs independently of changes in intracellular pH and bicarbonate concentration, which will help to address this issue.

Figure 10.1 also illustrates that breathing pure oxygen at 3 ATA or less is the standard protocol for HBOT, as discussed elsewhere in this book. What limits the use of hyperbaric oxygen in clinical medicine is the need to avert oxygen toxicity, of which the central nervous system (CNS), pulmonary system, and retina are highly vulnerable.[45] Of these three tissues, CNS oxygen toxicity is the most pressing because it can occur quickly whenever breathing 2 ATA O_2 or more with little to no warning, producing violent seizures.[6,45] Hyperbaric oxygen seizures may be preceded by a series of autonomic, motor, and cardiorespiratory signs, including hyperventilation, dyspnea, bradycardia, and perturbed cardiorespiratory reflexes.[46-48] These signs, however, are not always guaranteed to occur, making it difficult to predict onset of an impending oxygen toxicity event. Although there is likely an effect of molecular oxygen on the physical properties of the plasma membrane of cells, the deleterious effects of protracted hyperbaric oxygen breathing on neurons and their synapses are generally attributed to the formation of various reactive oxygen and nitrogen species and their highly reactive derivatives that can oxidize various proteins and organelles to disrupt normal cellular functions.[6,49]

Finally, Figure 10.1 highlights the effects of hyperbaric pressure per se on the mammalian CNS. Notice that the excitatory effects of hyperbaria on the CNS are manifest after breathing specialty gas mixtures—nitrox, heliox, and hydreliox—to prevent onset of oxygen toxicity, nitrogen narcosis, and HPNS. These gases use various mixtures of nitrogen, helium, and hydrogen for dives made beyond 4 ATA; they are discussed in detail elsewhere.[6,34] Breathing compressed nitrox, heliox, or hydreliox en-

ables a diver to penetrate tremendous depths of up to 70 ATA.[34] What limits diver performance at these depths is the direct effect of hydrostatic compression on the CNS, producing increased neural activity that results in tremors. The constellation of signs that present at P_B greater than 10 to 15 ATA is called HPNS, which has been studied extensively and is reviewed elsewhere.[5,6,34] Figure 10.1 also illustrates that many in vitro studies have focused on ambient pressures in excess of 100 ATA. Comparatively much less work has been done over the range of moderate pressure that humans routinely encounter. The remainder of this chapter addresses the following question: What are the physiologic effects on cells and organ systems of moderate levels of pressure ($\leq$5 ATA), which includes the range of hyperbaric pressure that occurs during HBOT?

COMPRESSION MEDIA

Air and Oxygen: Hyperbaric Oxygen Therapy

Boyle's Law predicts that hyperbaric environments will present many physiologic challenges for gas-filled organs such as the lungs, hollow viscera, and cranial sinuses and cavities, especially when resurfacing from the dive. When exposed to hyperbaric pressure, the soft tissues are believed to behave as a fluid, rapidly transmitting any pressure-applied force against the surface of the body to the various adjoining fluid-filled tissue compartments. This, in turn, is believed to rapidly abolish any hydrostatic pressure gradients across body structures and compartments, but presumably results in hydrostatic compression of the various fluid-filled compartments including the cerebrospinal fluid, vascular system, and extracellular and intracellular fluid compartments in parallel with the exterior of the body.[6] Obviously, under these conditions, it is expected that any effects of hyperbaric pressure per se will be difficult to distinguish from the concomitant increase in alveolar and, thus, tissue Po_2, which, after all, is the rationale for HBOT. The few studies that have been done at pressures associated with HBOT, however, indicate that measurable effects do occur in certain organ systems and cells.

Helium versus Hydrostatic Compression

Immersing the body underwater and breathing with a self-contained breathing apparatus (SCUBA) exposes the body's exterior to true hydrostatic compression. To identify the effects of hyperbaric pressure per se on intact animals (including humans) or, alternatively, reduced tissue and cellular preparations, it is common practice to pressurize the atmosphere surrounding the organism or in vitro tissue preparation with pure helium.[6] In this case, the oxygen required to sustain cellular metabolism and life (normoxia) is supplied in the breathing gas mixture that is delivered in parallel to the organism's lungs. Alternatively, if the study of hyperbaric pressure per se is being done in a reduced tissue/cellular preparation, then oxygen is dissolved in the buffer solution at normobaric pressure and pumped into the hyperbaric chamber and superfused over the submerged tissue/cells maintained in a tissue bath.[6,50] In the latter scenario, on closure of the hyperbaric chamber, all of the air (21% O_2 + 79% N_2) trapped inside the pressure vessel is flushed out and replaced with pure helium (= 0% O_2 and N_2) at normobaric pressure before commencing helium pressurization. Thus, during the ensuing helium compression, no additional oxygen is driven into the superfusate and tissue because the overlying atmosphere inside the chamber is anoxic. All of the oxygen required to sustain the tissue/cells has been dissolved in the superfusate at normobaric pressure before pumping it inside the chamber using a high-pressure liquid chromatography pump. In fact, the anoxic compression medium establishes a diffusion gradient in which oxygen diffuses out the superfusate as it flows over the tissue/cells. This small reduction in O_2 content of the superfusate is offset, however, by the constant delivery of fresh, oxygenated buffer solution to the tissue/cellular preparation.[6,50,51]

How well does helium compression compare with true hydrostatic compression as a method for studying barosensitivity? Helium has the lowest solubility in lipid membranes compared with the other clinically relevant gases (order of increasing lipid solubility: CO_2 >> O_2 > N_2 >>> He).[43] Consequently, it is believed that there are no measurable differences between the two modes of compression over the range of physiologically tolerable pressures.[12,52] Thus, using helium compression under conditions of normoxia is an important experimental protocol for revealing the effects of hyperbaric pressure per se on the body, tissue, and cell, especially in the range of more than 1 to 3 ATA, as used in HBOT.

At much higher levels of hyperbaric pressure, in excess of 100 ATA, helium exerts limited narcotic potency despite its low lipid solubility. Given that this range of pressure exceeds that encountered by humans, it will not be considered further here.[6,8] For a detailed review of helium versus hydrostatic compression as used for basic science research, we refer you to topics in Appendices A through D in Dean and colleagues' article.[6]

PRESSURE-SENSITIVE (BAROSENSITIVE) CELLS

Pressure per se as a Stimulus

Many of the previous studies designed to reveal the cellular and molecular effects of hyperbaric pressure per se have focused on levels of ambient pressure that exceeded the range of physiologically tolerable pressures for humans.[6,8] In these extreme cases, hyperbaric pressure acts as a thermodynamic intensity parameter, which is predicted to affect various thermodynamic reactions, and thus cellular processes.[4,7,9-11] The relations between pressure and both the molar volume change in the free energy reaction and the activation volume for the rate-limiting step of a reaction are reviewed elsewhere.[3,4,6,7] For reactions with small changes in molar volume and activation volume, a large pressure (>100 ATA) will significantly perturb the equilibrium and rate of reaction. At lower levels of pressure, it has been proposed that the thermodynamic and kinetic effects would be too small to cause physiologically relevant changes in the equilibria and rate of reactions.[3,4]

Alternatively, it is hypothesized that a mechanical process that involves localized shear and strain forces between adjoining cellular fine structures will produce differential compression of the nonfluid, fine structural components of cells. For example, the proteins that form the ionic channels and conduct ionic currents and molecules, including water, are affixed and penetrate the lipid bilayers forming the plasma membrane.[53-56] Adjoined to these protein structures is the underlying cytoskeleton.[57] A change in the configuration of one of these fine structures during hydrostatic compression will undoubtedly perturb any adjoining structure to which it is mechanically coupled. In this way, moderate levels of hyperbaric pressure could alter cellular function.[3,4] In this context, it is seems likely that mechanosensitive ion channels are likely candidates for sensing changes in the stress and strain forces exerted between the plasma membrane, ion channels, and cytoskeleton during hydrostatic compression.[58,59] This hypothesis, however, remains to be tested.

Examples of Barosensitive Cells

Physiologic studies of single cells and populations of cells are typically done under in vitro conditions for purposes of physical stability for measurements of cellular function and so the investigator can manipulate the composition of the extracellular fluid that bathes the reduced tissue/cell preparation. One of the reasons that so little information is known about the effects of hyperbaric pressure per se on cellular physiology is that such studies are constrained by the need of a hyperbaric chamber for pressure containment. Thus, the studies become technically challenging because specialized equipment has to be adapted to the pressure vessel. Moreover, the equipment and cellular/tissue preparation must by operated and manipulated by remote control once the chamber is sealed. Similarly, maintaining an anesthetized and instrumented animal inside a sealed pressure vessel is technically feasible but not a simple task.[46,60,61]

Several laboratories have succeeded at adapting cutting-edge cellular research tools to the hyperbaric environment so that new insight is being gained as to the effects of hyperbaric pressure per se on cellular function.[18,19,50,62-67] These same techniques have been used to study CNS oxygen toxicity,[37,51,67-69] nitrogen narcosis,[70,71] and HPNS.[7,16,18,19,72-78] Recalling that many of the early effects of breathing hyperbaric gases present as neurologic dysfunction (see Fig. 10.1), we have focused our own studies of cellular barosensitivity on the electrical signaling of neurons in a rat brain tissue slice preparation.[21] Using this popular in vitro preparation of the CNS, we have found that moderate levels of hyperbaric pressure (helium compression $\leq$ 4 ATA) at constant oxygen, pH, and temperature will stimulate the genesis of action potentials by neurons in the dorsal brainstem (Fig. 10.2A). These changes in action potential generation—the so-called firing rate of the neuron—increase in frequency and correlate with an increase in membrane net conductance; that is, ion channels conducting a net inward depolarizing current are opening and causing increased firing rate.[6,21] Likewise, Figure 10.2B shows a similar response to 20 ATA helium pressure at constant O_2, pH, and temperature. Notice that the greatest change in firing rate occurs early on during the first 1 to 5 ATA of helium compression. The stimulatory effect of hyperbaric pressure is retained during blockade of chemical synaptic transmission (not shown), indicating that barosensitivity is an intrinsic membrane property that is retained in the absence of synaptic input.[21] The significance of barosensitivity in the brainstem remains to be determined, but it may be that these dorsal medullary neurons, which belong to part of the cardioinhibitory center, contribute to the bradycardia caused by pressure per se that has been reported in humans.[20] It is also possible that pressure, like temperature, acts as an environmental stimulus that determines how the organism adapts to changes in its environment.[21,79]

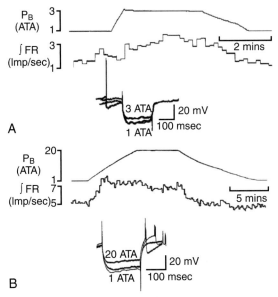

Figure 10.2 Examples of two barosensitive neurons in the solitary complex of the dorsocaudal medulla oblongata (rat brain tissue slice, 300 μm in thickness, 36-37°C) that were stimulated by hyperbaric helium at constant O_2, pH, and temperature, as reported by Mulkey and colleagues.[21] Intracellular recordings from two different neurons showing that 3 (A) and 20 ATA of helium compression (B) decrease input resistance and stimulate neuronal firing rate in a reversible manner. B, The neuron was maximally stimulated during the initial 1 to 5 ATA of helium compression. In these two experiments, input resistance was measured by using brief constant amplitude hyperpolarizing current pulses (superimposed voltage traces in A and B). Based on Ohm's Law (voltage = current × resistance), the change in membrane potential during hyperpolarizing current injection through the microelectrode and across the cell membrane is proportional to the change in input resistance (membrane resistance) and inversely proportional to the membrane conductance. Therefore, the *decrease* in input resistance measured during exposure to hyperbaric pressure per se (using helium) is indicative of an *increase* in net membrane conductance; that is, there is a net opening of membrane channels resulting in depolarization and stimulation of these neurons during helium compression. Action potentials are truncated in membrane potential traces in A and B. *(Reprinted from Dean JB, Mulkey DK, Garcia III AJ, et al: Neuronal sensitivity to hyperoxia, hypercapnia and inert gases at hyperbaric pressures. J Appl Physiol 95:883-909, 2003, by permission of The American Physiological Society.)*

BAROSENSITIVITY OF SYSTEMS PHYSIOLOGY

Although it is clear that many studies have examined the effects of moderate levels of hyperbaric pressure on the body—that is, P_B $\leq$ 5 or 6 ATA—many of these studies did not unequivocally differentiate the physiologic effects of hyperoxia, nitrogen narcosis, or CO_2 retention from those of hyperbaric pressure per se. In addition, many other studies that did focus on the physiologic effects of hyperbaric pressure per se did so using levels of pressure way beyond 5 to 6 ATA. Thus, the following discussion focuses on the most recent work in which the possible physiologic effects of moderate levels of hyperbaria could

be tested. The evidence suggests that hyperbaric pressure of 4 to 6 ATA does have an effect on certain physiologic systems that occurs separately from the effects of gas partial pressure that need to be considered during exposure to pressure and, most importantly, require further study.

Respiration

Hyperbaric environments challenge the respiratory system primarily by increasing the density of inspired and expired gases, and thus causing greater airway resistance. This, in turn, results in an increased work of breathing that decreases work performance during exercise.[80-82] During expiration, increased airway resistance will lead to dynamic compression of airways and larger end-expired lung volume.[82] Under the physical demands of exercise, this often results in dyspnea from respiratory muscle fatigue.[81] In addition, contributing factors such as poor diffusion of gases because of increased gas density causes even greater demands on respiratory muscles. Thus, increased respiratory effort is necessary to sustain ventilation in hyperbaric environments, which causes fatigue of inspiratory muscles and ultimately hypoventilation and CO_2 retention.[82] It is unknown whether respiratory muscles are directly affected by moderate levels of hyperbaric pressure ($\leq$6 ATA) because most muscle studies are done at high levels of hyperbaria (>50 ATA). The limited data suggest that 4 to 6 ATA causes voluntary muscle torque loss and decreased contractile velocity in skeletal muscles.[81] Thus, pressure may attenuate the neural drive for voluntary muscle contraction. No evidence to date, however, demonstrates that hyperbaric pressures at 6 ATA impair myofilament kinetics with tetanic stimulation (i.e., nonvoluntary; 2–40 Hz).[83] In support of this theory is the observation, in isolated in vitro preparations, that pressures as high as 10 MPa (100 ATA) have little effect on muscle structure or function, as measured by Ca^{2+} homeostasis and ionic conductance of sodium and potassium currents. However, supraphysiologic levels of hydrostatic pressure (>20 MPa or >200 ATA) perturb ionic homeostasis and impair muscle contraction.[84]

Cardiovascular System

In humans, an increase in hydrostatic pressure of only 5 ATA causes a significant bradycardia.[20] Mulkey and investigators[21] found that neurons in the dorsal motor nucleus of vagus and nucleus tractus solitarius are stimulated by 4 ATA or less of helium (see Fig. 10.2). Because these neurons are located in part of the cardioinhibitory center in the brainstem, they may underlie the hyperbaric reflex bradycardia that Linnarsson and coworkers[20] reported. Rats, however, exposed to 5 ATA ambient pressure (P_{N_2} = 4.8 ATA; P_{O_2} = 0.2 ATA) demonstrated

an increased myocardial blood flow but no change in unchanged cardiac output, mean arterial pressure, and heart rate.[85] These studies concluded that there was a pressure-dependent increase in myocardial perfusion that occurred independently of gas composition, and that changes were not due to the effect of N_2 or helium. These cardiovascular changes are likely mediated, in part, by a hyperbaric-induced increase in catecholamine secretion.[86,87] In support of this hypothesis is the observation that under hyperbaric conditions the noradrenaline-induced contraction of rat aorta in vitro is greatly enhanced.[88] Furthermore, at lower pressures of sustained hyperbaria (48 hours; 4–11 ATA), nearly all divers experience 24 hours of postdecompression tachycardia (90–108 beats/min), which often persists 24 hours after surfacing.[89] In addition, human studies at relatively high pressures (3.1 MPa, 4.1 MPa) have shown an augmentation of sympathetic nervous system activity, as measured by plasma epinephrine and norepinephrine levels, especially in the early postdive period.[86]

Renal System

Pressure-induced changes in renal physiology are likely to affect cardiovascular function through hemodynamic changes. Hyperbaric diuresis is well documented,[90-93] but few studies have attempted to elucidate the mechanisms for this response. It is well known that atrial natriuretic peptide increases in response to immersion of the body in water[94,95] after activation of atrial stretch from the altered central distribution of intravascular fluid. The pressure-induced hypervolemia from water immersion stimulates atrial natriuretic peptide secretion from the atrial myocytes, which ultimately reduces the water and Na^+ levels so as to decrease (normalize) blood pressure. Diuresis (>500 mL/day) is experienced during "dry" saturation diving (15–50 ATA) and is associated with a decrease in urine osmolality from reduced water reabsorption. This response is characterized by a decrease in antidiuretic hormone, increased aldosterone,[92] and a sharp increase in atrial natriuretic peptide.[90,91,93] The paradoxical increase in aldosterone is triggered from decreased plasma volume that occurs during the initial hyperbaric diuresis. When the pressure-induced decrease in blood pressure is sensed by the stretch receptors located in the atria of the heart, the adrenal gland is stimulated to release aldosterone. Aldosterone normally increases sodium reabsorption from urine, sweat, and the gut, but hyperbaric exposure attenuates this response.[92] Thus, during exposure to hyperbaric pressure, the release of aldosterone fails to adjust osmolarity of the extracellular fluid to normalize blood pressure. These observations suggest that hyperbaric pressure directly affects Na^+ transport in the proximal tubule, but the exact mechanism is unknown. Under normal conditions, aldosterone acts on mineralcorticoid receptors at the distal tubule and increases the permeability of their apical membrane to K^+ and Na^+. Activation of these receptors stimulates basolateral Na^+/K^+ pumps, and the adenosine triphosphate–stimulated phosphorylation of these pumps triggers reabsorption of Na^+ and water into the blood, and secretion K^+ ions into the urine. Thus, hyperbaric pressure could conceivably affect proximal tubular Na^+ transport through a variety of mechanisms, but the mechanism remains largely unknown.

Reproductive System

The effect of hyperbaric pressure on reproductive function is only partially understood, but it is clear that pressure affects male fertility. Moderate levels of hyperbaric pressure (2-5 ATA O_2) have little effect on menstruation,[96] and studies on male rats show little or no effect on testicular function.[97] However, studies in rats exposed to extended levels (24 hours) of 6 ATA have demonstrated significant reductions in blood flow to the testis, epididymis, ventral prostate, and kidneys.[98] In addition, the same study demonstrates that plasma testosterone concentrations were significantly reduced in rats after extended hyperbaric exposure.[98] In humans, exposure to deep saturation dives (>40 ATA) reduces testicular perfusion and overall male reproductive function.[99] Mice exposed to higher pressures (50 ATA) produce sperm with decreased motility and impaired maturation.[100] It is likely that the effect of pressure on male fertility is reversible, and that reduced testicular perfusion is a result of reduced arterial pressure, which is well documented in the literature.[101]

PERSPECTIVE

Our bodies are adapted to live at or near a P_B-applied force of approximately 1 ATA. Humans, however, routinely encounter environments of altered P_B that will affect their physiology by changing the levels of inspired and blood gases, and thus levels of gases dissolved in their tissues and cells. The following question is addressed in this chapter: What additional effects, if any, do changes in P_B have on the body that are related to the effects of pressure alone? Besides affecting the density of gases inspired and the volume of gas in gas-filled organs, are their additional effects of hyperbaric pressure per se on cells and tissues that might need to be considered during the moderate levels of compression that occur during HBOT? Consequently, we have focused our discussion on the effects of moderate levels of hyperbaric pressure per se that humans routinely encounter during HBOT, compressed air work, and routine underwater diving.

Progress toward answering these questions has been slowed in part by study designs that do not unequivocally permit differentiation between the possible effects of hyperbaric pressure per se from the confounding effects of narcosis, oxidative stress, and respiratory acidosis. In other cases, studies that were designed to tease out the physiologic effects of hyperbaric pressure per se have done so using either large levels of hyperbaria that are encountered during mixed-gas technical diving or at even greater levels of hyperbaria that humans do not encounter. Obviously, in the latter case, these studies used various in vitro tissue preparations to study the molecular and cellular effects of hyperbaric pressure per se.

Certainly, future studies should also include the lower, moderate range of pressures because these are what are routinely encountered in hyperbaric medicine.[6]

Accumulating evidence indicates that moderate levels of hyperbaric pressure do indeed affect cellular physiology. The likely mechanisms may involve differential compression of fine structural components of cells such as the plasma membrane, its resident population of proteins that form ion channels and membrane pumps and transporters, and the cytoskeleton that underlies the plasma membrane. The research tools to conduct these studies under hyperbaric conditions have only recently been developed. With technologies such as atomic force microscopy, electrophysiology, and fluorescence microscopy being adapted to hyperbaric chambers, it should be possible to address experimentally these fundamentally important questions about cellular barosensitivity. Accumulating evidence indicates that the effects of moderate levels of hyperbaric pressure can occur centrally, thereby affecting neural control of autonomic regulation at the target organ. In addition, cells at the target organ can be affected. Examples to date indicate that moderate levels of hyperbaric pressure per se affect pulmonary gas diffusion and airway resistance, local tissue blood flow (cardiovascular), neurotransmitter release (cardiovascular), homeostatic mechanisms (renal water resorption), and ionic conductances and electrical signaling (neurons). These findings are encouraging and justify the requirement for additional research on the effects of moderate levels of hyperbaric pressure on the body, tissues, and cells to fully appreciate the physiologic consequences of exposure to pressures used in hyperbaric medicine.

ACKNOWLEDGMENTS

Research from the authors' laboratory leading to many of the ideas summarized here was supported in part by the Office of Naval Research, Undersea Medicine Program.

REFERENCES

1. Bert P: Barometric Pressure. Researches in Experimental Physiology. Columbus, Ohio, FC Long's College Book Company, 1943.
2. Camporesi E: Hyperbaric oxygen therapy: A committee report. Kensington, Md, Undersea and Hyperbaric Medical Society, 1996.
3. Macdonald AG, Fraser PJ: The transduction of very small hydrostatic pressures. Comp Biochem Physiol 122A:13-36, 1999.
4. Macdonald AG: Hydrostatic pressure as an environmental factor in life processes. Comp Biochem Physiol 116A:291-297, 1997.
5. Jain KK: High pressure neurological syndrome (HPNS). Acta Neurol Scand 90:45-50, 1994.
6. Dean JB, Mulkey DK, Garcia III AJ, et al: Neuronal sensitivity to hyperoxia, hypercapnia and inert gases at hyperbaric pressures. J Appl Physiol 95:883-909, 2003.
7. Conti F, Heinemann SH, Stuhmer W: Activation and reaction volumes of ion channels in excitable membranes. In: Jannasch HW, Marquis RE, Zimmerman AM (eds): Current Perspectives in High Pressure Biology. London, Academic Press, 1987, pp 171-179.
8. Halsey MJ: Effects of high pressure on the central nervous system. Physiol Rev 62:1341-1377, 1982.
9. MacDonald AG: The effects of pressure on the molecular structure and physiological functions of cell membranes. Philos Trans R Soc Lond B Biol Sci 304:47-68, 1984.
10. MacDonald AG: The role of membrane fluidity in complex processes under high pressure. In: Jannasch HW, Marquis RE, Zimmerman AM (eds): Current Perspectives in High Pressure Biology. Orlando, Fla, Academic Press, 1987, pp 207-223.
11. Macdonald AG: Ion channels under high pressure. Comp Biochem Physiol 131A:587-593, 2002.
12. Brauer RW, Hogan PM, Hugon M, et al: Patterns of interaction of effects of light metabolically inert gases with those of hydrostatic pressure as such-a review. Undersea Biomed Res 9:353-396, 1982.
13. Wann KT, Macdonald AG: The effects of pressure on excitable cells. Comp Biochem Physiol 66A: 1-12, 1980.
14. Wann KT, Southan AP: The action of anaesthetics and high pressure on neuronal discharge patterns. Gen Pharm 23:993-1004, 1992.
15. Southan AP, Wann KT: Effects of high helium pressure on intracellular and field potential responses in the CA1 region of the in vitro rat hippocampus. Eur J Neurosci 8:2571-2581, 1996.
16. Henderson JV, Gilbert DL: Slowing of ionic currents in the voltage-clamped squid axon by helium pressure. Nature 258:351-352, 1975.
17. Heinemann SH, Conti F, Stuhmer W, et al: Effects of hydrostatic pressure on membrane processes: Sodium channels, calcium channels, and exocytosis. J Gen Physiol 90:765-778, 1987.
18. Tarasiuk A, Grossman Y: High pressure reduces pH sensitivity of respiratory center in isolated rat brainstem. Respir Physiol 86:369-379, 1991.

19. Tarasiuk A, Grossman Y: High pressure modifies respiratory activity in isolated rat brain stem-spinal cord. J Appl Physiol 71:537-545, 1991.

20. Linnarsson D, Ostlund A, Lind F, et al: Hyperbaric bradycardia and hypoventilation in exercising men: Effects of ambient pressure and breathing gas. J Appl Physiol 87:1428-1432, 1999.

21. Mulkey DK, Henderson III RA, Putnam RW, et al: Pressure (<4 ATA) increases membrane conductance and firing rate in the rat solitary complex. J Appl Physiol 95:922-930, 2003.

22. West JB: Highest inhabitants of the world. Nature (Lond) 324:517, 1986.

23. Keys A: The physiology of life at high altitude: The International High Altitude Expedition to Chile 1935. Scientific Monthly 43:289-312, 1936.

24. Keys A, Matthews BHC, Forbes WH, et al: Individual variations in ability to acclimatize to high altitude. Proc R Soc Lond B Biol Sci 126:1-24, 1938.

25. West JB: Permanent residents of high altitude. High Life. A History of High Altitude Physiology and Medicine. New York, Oxford University Press, 1998, pp 194-227.

26. West JB: Climbing Mt. Everest without oxygen: An analysis of maximal exercise during extreme hypoxia. Respir Physiol 52:265-279, 1983.

27. West JB: First ascents of Mt. Everest. High Life. A History of High Altitude Physiology and Medicine. New York, Oxford University Press, 1998, pp 254-290.

28. Lovelace II WR, Gagge AP: Aero medical aspects of cabin pressurization for military and commercial aircraft. J Aeronaut Sci 13:143-150, 1946.

29. Prepared by the Wright Field Aero Medical Laboratory, Engineering Division. Your Body in Flight (T.O. No. 30-105-1). Dayton, Ohio Maintenance Data Section, Maintenance Division, Air Technical Service Command, Wright Field, 1944, pp 1-74.

30. Air Forces Manual No. 34: Notes on the use of oxygen equipment for fighter pilots and P.R.U. (with special reference to the P-38, P-47 and P-51). Washington, DC, Headquarters, US Army Air Forces, 1944, pp 1-60.

31. Fryer DI: Subatmospheric decompression sickness in man (AGARDograph no. 125). Slough: Technivision Services, The Advisory Group for Aerospace Research and Development (AGARD), NATO, 1969, 1-343.

32. Lauritzsen MD, Pfitzner J: Pressure breathing in fighter aircraft for G accelerations and loss of cabin pressurization at altitude—a brief review. Can J Anesth 50:415-419, 2003.

33. Kozloski LD: U.S. Space Gear. Outfitting the Astronaut. Washington, DC, Smithsonian Institution Press, 1994, pp 1-238.

34. Bennett PB: Inert gas narcosis and high pressure nervous syndrome. In: Bove AA (ed): Bove and Davis' Diving Medicine. Philadelphia, WB Saunders Company, 1997, pp 117-130.

35. Tibbles PM, Edelsberg JS: Hyperbaric-oxygen therapy. N Engl J Med 334:1642-1648, 1996.

36. Warkander DE, Norfleet WT, Nagasawa GK, et al: CO_2 retention with minimal symptoms but severe dysfunction during wet simulated dives to 6.8 atm abs. Undersea Biomed Res 17:515-523, 1990.

37. Dean JB, Mulkey DK, Henderson III RA, et al: Hyperoxia, reactive O_2 species, and hyperventilation: O_2-sensitivity of brain stem neurons. J Appl Physiol 96:784-791, 2004.

38. Prabhakar NR: Oxygen sensing by the carotid body chemoreceptors. J Appl Physiol 88:2287-2295, 2000.

39. Morrison JB, Florio JT, Butt WS: Observations after loss of consciousness under water. Undersea Biomed Res 5:179-187, 1978.

40. Woodbury DM, Karler R: The role of carbon dioxide in the nervous system. Anesthesiology 21:686-703, 1960.

41. Coenen AML, Drinkenburg WHIM, Hoenderken R, et al: Carbon dioxide euthanasia in rats: Oxygen supplementation minimizes signs of agitation and asphyxia. Lab Anim 29:262-268, 1995.

42. Danneman PJ, Stein S, Walshaw SO: Humane and practical implications of using carbon dioxide mixed with oxygen for anesthesia or euthanasia of rats. Lab Anim Sci 47:376-385, 1997.

43. Bennett PB, Papahadjopoulos D, Bangham AD: The effect of raised pressure of inert gases on phospholipid membranes. Life Sci 6:2527-2533, 1967.

44. Hartzler LK, Dean JB, Putnam RW: The chemosensitive response of neurons from the locus coeruleus (LC) to hypercapnic acidosis with clamped intracellular pH. Adv Exp Med Biol 605:333-337, 2008.

45. Clark JM, Thom SR: Toxicity of oxygen, carbon dioxide, and carbon monoxide. In: Bove AA (ed): Bove and Davis' Diving Medicine. Philadelphia, Saunders, 1997, pp 131-145.

46. Cragg PA, Drysdale DB, Hamilton JH: Ventilation in intact and glossopharyngeal nerve sectioned anaesthetized rats exposed to oxygen at high pressure. J Physiol (Lond) 370:489-499, 1986.

47. Simon AJ, Torbati D: Effects of hyperbaric oxygen on heart, brain and lung functions in rat. Undersea Biomed Res 9:263-275, 1982.

48. Torbati D, Mokashi A, Lahiri S: Effects of acute hyperbaric oxygenation on respiratory control in cats. J Appl Physiol 67:2351-2356, 1989.

49. D'Agostino, DP, Putnam RW, Dean JB: Superoxide (O_2^-) production in CA1 neurons of rat hippocampal slices exposed to graded levels of oxygen. J Neurophysiol 98:1030-1041, 2007.

50. Dean JB, Mulkey DK: Continuous intracellular recording from mammalian neurons exposed to hyperbaric helium, oxygen, or air. J Appl Physiol 89:807-822, 2000.

51. Mulkey DK, Henderson III RA, Olson JE, et al: Oxygen measurement in brainstem slices exposed to normobaric hyperoxia and hyperbaric oxygen. J Appl Physiol 90:1887-1899, 2001.

52. Wann KT, MacDonald AG, Harper AA, et al: Electrophysiological measurements at high hydrostatic pressure: Methods for intracellular recording from isolated ganglia and for extracellular recording in vivo. Comp Biochem Physiol 64A:141-147, 1979.

53. Lee AG: How lipids affect the activities of integral membrane proteins. Biochim Biophys Acta 1666:62-87, 2004.

54. Cascio M: Connexins and their environment: Effects of lipids composition on ion channels. Biochim Biophys Acta 1711:142-153, 2005.

55. Sperotto MM, May S, Baumgaertner A: Modelling of proteins in membranes. Chem Phys Lipids 141:2-29, 2006.

56. Lindblom G, Grobner G: NMR of lipid membranes and their proteins. Curr Opin Colloid Interf Sci 11:24-29, 2006.

57. Sheetz MP, Sable JE, Dobereiner HG: Continuous membrane-cytoskeleton adhesion requires continuous accommodation to lipid and cytoskeleton dynamics. Annu Rev Biophys Biomol Struct 35:417-434, 2006.

58. Sukharev S, Anishkin A: Mechanosensitive channels: What can we learn from 'simple' model systems? Trends Neurosci 27:345-351, 2004.

59. Martinac B, Kloda A: Evolutionary origins of mechanosensitive ion channels. Prog Biophys Mol Biol 82:11-24, 2003.

60. Demchenko IT, Boso A, Bennett PB, et al: Hyperbaric oxygen reduces cerebral blood flow by inactivating nitric oxide. Nitric Oxide Biol Chem 4:597-608, 2000.

61. Litt L, Xu Y, Cohen Y, et al: Nonmagnetic hyperbaric chamber for in-vivo NMR spectroscopy studies of small animals. Magn Reson Med 29:812-816, 1993.

62. Dean JB, Mulkey DK, Arehart JT: Details on building a hyperbaric chamber for intracellular recording in brain tissue slices. J Appl Physiol 89:807-822, 2000.

63. Fagni L, Hugon M, Folco A, et al: A versatile chamber for microphysiologic studies with gas mixtures under high pressure. Undersea Biomed Res 14:161-168, 1987.

64. Southan AP, Wann KT: Methods for intracellular recording from hippocampal brain slices under high helium pressure. J Appl Physiol 71:365-371, 1991.

65. Henderson JV, Morin RA, Lanphier EH: Apparatus for intracellular electrophysiological measurements at 200 ATA. J Appl Physiol 38:353-355, 1975.

66. Colton JS, Freeman AR: Intracellular measurements in a closed hyperbaric chamber. J Appl Physiol 35:578-580, 1973.

67. King GL, Parmemtier JL: Oxygen toxicity of hippocampal tissue in vitro. Brain Res 260:139-142, 1983.

68. Mulkey DK, Henderson III RA, Putnam RW, et al: Hyperbaric oxygen and chemical oxidants stimulate CO_2/H^+-sensitive neurons in rat brain stem slices. J Appl Physiol 95:910-921, 2003.

69. Colton JS, Colton CA: Effect of oxygen at high pressure on spontaneous transmitter release. Am J Physiol 238:C233-C237, 1978.

70. Bryant HJ, Blankenship JE: Action potentials in single axons: Effects of hyperbaric air and hydrostatic pressure. J Appl Physiol 47:561-567, 1979.

71. Bryant HJ, Blankenship JE: Modification of synaptic facilitation and bursting patterns in Aplysia californica by hyperbaric air. J Appl Physiol 47:568-576, 1979.

72. Fagni L, Soumireu-Mourat B, Carlier E, et al: A study of spontaneous and evoked activity in the rat hippocampus under helium-oxygen high pressure. Electroenceph Clin Neurophysiol 60:267-275, 1985.

73. Fagni L, Zinebi F, Hugon M: Evoked potential changes in rat hippocampal slices under helium pressure. Exp Brain Res 65:513-519, 1987.

74. Fagni L, Zinebi F, Hugon M: Helium pressure potentiates the N-methyl-D-aspartate- and D,L-homocysteate-induced decreases of field potentials in the rat hippocampal slice preparation. Neurosci Lett 81:285-290, 1987.

75. Henderson JV, Lowenhaupt MT, Gilbert DL: Helium pressure alteration of function in squid giant synapse. Undersea Biomed Res 4:19-26, 1977.

76. Conti F, Fioravanti R, Segal JR, et al: Pressure dependence of the potassium currents of squid giant axon. J Membr Biol 69:35-40, 1982.

77. Conti F, Fioravanti R, Segal JR, et al: Pressure dependence of the sodium currents of squid giant axon. J Membr Biol 69:23-34, 1982.

78. Tarasiuk A, Grossman Y, Kendig JJ: Barbiturate alteration of respiratory rhythm and drive in isolated brainstem-spinal cord of newborn rat: Studies at normal and hyperbaric pressure. Br J Anaesth 66:88-96, 1991.

79. Kendig JJ, Grossman Y, Heinemann SH: Ion channels and nerve cell function. In: Macdonald AG (ed): Advances in Comparative and Environmental Physiology, Effect of High Pressure on Biological Systems, vol 17. Berlin, Springer-Verlag, 1993, pp 87-124.

80. Calvet JH, Louis B, Giry P, et al: Effect of gas density variations on respiratory input impedance in humans. Respir Physiol 104:241-250, 1996.

81. Duranti R, Bonetti L, Vivoli P, et al: Dyspnea during exercise in hyperbaric conditions. Med Sci Sports Exerc 38:1932-1938, 2006.

82. Van Liew HD: Mechanical and physical factors in lung function during work in dense environments. Undersea Biomed Res 10:255-264, 1983.

83. Behm D, Power K, White M, et al: Effects of hyperbaric (6 ATA) pressure on voluntary and evoked skeletal muscle contractile properties. Undersea Hyperb Med 30:103-115, 2003.

84. Friedrich O, Kress KR, Ludwig H, et al: Membrane ion conductances of mammalian skeletal muscle in the post-decompression state after high-pressure treatment. J Membr Biol 188:11-22, 2002.

85. Risberg J, Tyssebotn I: Hyperbaric exposure to a 5 ATA $He-N_2-O_2$ atmosphere affects the cardiac function and organ blood flow distribution in awake trained rats. Undersea Biomed Res 13:77-90, 1986.

86. Hirayanagi K, Nakabayashi K, Okonogi K, et al: Autonomic nervous activity and stress hormones induced by hyperbaric saturation diving. Undersea Hyperb Med 30:47-55, 2003.

87. Paul ML, Philp RB: Hyperbaric He but not N_2 augments Ca_2^+-dependent dopamine release from rat striatum. Undersea Biomed Res 16:293-304, 1989.

88. Guerrero F, Lucciano M, Joanny P, et al: Hyperbaric-induced enhancement of noradrenaline-evoked contraction in rat thoracic aorta. Exp Physiol 82:687-695, 1997.

89. Mateev G, Djarova T, Ilkov A, et al: Hormonal and cardiorespiratory changes following simulated saturation dives to 4 and 11 ATA. Undersea Biomed Res 17:1-11, 1990.

90. Goldinger JM, Hong SK, Claybaugh JR, et al: Renal responses during a dry saturation dive to 450 msw. Undersea Biomed Res 19:287-293, 1992.

91. Miyamoto N, Matsui N, Inoue I, et al: Hyperbaric diuresis is associated with decreased antidiuretic hormone and increased atrial natriuretic polypeptide in humans. Jpn J Physiol 41:85-99, 1991.

92. Park YS, Claybaugh JR, Shiraki K, et al: Renal function in hyperbaric environment. Appl Human Sci 17:1-8, 1998.

93. Tao HY, Chen HJ, Zhang H, et al: Urinary ANP, ADH, and electrolyte excretion during saturation-excursion diving to pressures equivalent to 250 and 300 m. Undersea Biomed Res 19:159-169, 1992.

94. Johnston CI, Hodsman PG, Kohzuki M, et al: Interaction between atrial natriuretic peptide and the renin angiotensin aldosterone system. Endogenous antagonists. Am J Med 87:24S-28S, 1989.

95. Weidmann P, Saxenhofer H, Shaw SG, et al: Atrial natriuretic peptide in man. J Steroid Biochem 32:229-241, 1989.

96. Willson JR, Blessed WB, Blackburn PJ: Effect of repeated hyperbaric exposures on the menstrual cycle: Preliminary study. Undersea Biomed Res 11:91-97, 1984.

97. Nakada T, Saito H, Ota K, et al: Serum testosterone, testicular connective tissue protein and testicular histology in rats treated with hyperbaric oxygen. Int Urol Nephrol 18:439-447, 1986.

98. Rockert HO, Damber JE, Janson PO: Testicular blood flow and plasma testosterone concentrations in anesthetized rats previously exposed to air at 6 ATA. Undersea Biomed Res 5:355-361, 1978.

99. Aitken RJ, Buckingham D, Richardson D, et al: Impact of a deep saturation dive on semen quality. Int J Androl 23:116-120, 2000.

100. Fryer P, Gross J, Halsey MJ, et al: Sperm maturation associated with subfertility following hyperbaric exposure of mice. Undersea Biomed Res 13:413-423, 1986.

101. Rogatsky GG, Shifrin EG, and Mayevsky A: Physiologic and biochemical monitoring during hyperbaric oxygenation: A review. Undersea Hyperb Med 26:111-122, 1999.

Oxygen and the Basic Mechanisms of Wound Healing

11

Harriet W. Hopf, MD,
Matthew Kelly, MD,
and Dag Shapshak, MD

Wound healing is a complex process that requires coordinated repair responses including inflammation, matrix production, angiogenesis, epithelization, and remodeling (Fig. 11.1). Many factors may impair wound healing. Systemic factors such as medical comorbidities, nutrition,[1,2] sympathetic nervous system activation,[3] and age[4-6] have a substantial effect on the repair process. Local environmental factors in and around the wound including bacterial load,[7] degree of inflammation, moisture content,[8] oxygen tension,[9] and vascular perfusion[10] also have a profound effect on healing.

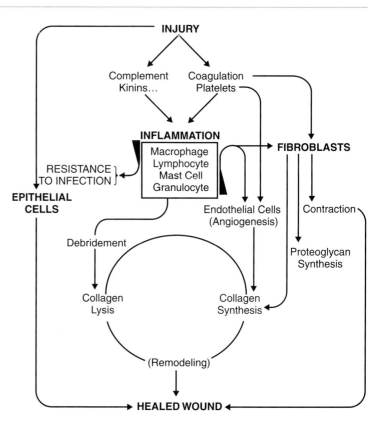

Figure 11.1 Schematic of the processes of wound healing. *(From Zabel DD, Hunt TK: Skin, peritoneum and colonic healing processes. Perspect Colon Rectal Surg 6:191, 1993, by permission.)*

Although all of these factors are important, one of the most critical elements is oxygen supply to the wound. Wound hypoxia impairs essentially all the components of healing.[11]

Although the role of oxygen is usually thought of in terms of aerobic respiration and energy production via oxidative phosphorylation, in wound healing, oxygen is required as a cofactor for enzymatic processes and also is required for signaling mechanisms. Oxygen is a rate-limiting component in leukocyte-mediated bacterial killing and collagen formation because specific enzymes require oxygen at a high partial pressure (at least 40 mm Hg).[12,13] The mechanisms by which the other processes are oxygen dependent are less clear, but these processes also require oxygen at a concentration much greater than that required for cellular respiration (though not necessarily a high volume).[14-17]

Wound hypoxia is a common cause of impaired healing, particularly in lower extremity ulcers. Hyperbaric oxygen therapy (HBOT) is a means of correcting wound hypoxia.[18] In fact, HBOT usually increases wound oxygen well above the physiologic range (>200 mm Hg).[19-21] At these levels, oxygen likely acts as a drug.[22]

This chapter reviews the basic mechanisms of wound healing, with particular emphasis on those for which oxygen is a rate-limiting substrate or are otherwise oxygen dependent. The mechanisms by which hyperbaric oxygen may enhance wound healing, particularly in hypoxic wounds, then are discussed. Evidence related to clinical efficacy and patient selection also are reviewed.

MECHANISMS OF WOUND REPAIR

Initial Response to Injury

A wound is created by disruption of the skin barrier. The injury may be anything that disrupts the local tissue environment, including, for example, thermal, mechanical, antigen, or inflammatory mechanisms, which all act by damaging the microcirculation and causing cell injury. This initiates a complex cascade of cellular and chemical interactions and signaling that ultimately leads to tissue repair.

Wound healing has traditionally been divided into four phases: hemostasis, inflammation, proliferation, and remodeling.[23] Considerable overlap exists between these phases, and the lines separating them are often difficult to distinguish. Each phase is a complex interaction among host cells, contaminants, cytokines, and other chemical mediators that, when functioning properly, lead to repair of injury. These processes are highly conserved across species,[24] indicating the critical importance of the inflammatory response that directs the process of cellular/tissue repair. When any component of healing is impeded, interrupting the orderly progression of repair, a chronic, non-healing wound may result.[25]

Injury damages the local circulation and causes platelets to aggregate and release a variety of substances, including chemoattractants and growth factors.[23] The initial result is coagulation, which prevents exsanguination but also widens the area that is no longer perfused. Platelet degranulation releases platelet-derived growth factor (PDGF), transforming growth factor-β (TGF-β), epidermal growth factor, and insulin-like growth factor-1, which initiate the inflammatory process.[23] Bradykinin, complement, and histamine released by mast cells also perturb the microcirculation. Inflammatory cells (polymorphonuclear leukocytes immediately and macrophages by 24–48 hours) migrate to the wound and are activated in response to endothelial integrins, selectins, cell adhesion molecules, cadherins, fibrin, lactate, hypoxia, foreign bodies, infectious agents, and growth factors.[23] In turn, macrophages and lymphocytes produce more lactate[26] and growth factors (Table 11.1), including insulin-like growth factor-1, leukocyte growth factor, interleukin-1 (IL-1), IL-2, TGF-β, and vascular endothelial growth factor (VEGF).[27] This inflammatory phase is characterized by erythema and edema of the wound edges.

Activated neutrophils and macrophages also release proteases, including neutrophil elastase, neutrophil collagenase, matrix metalloproteinase, and macrophage metalloelastase.[23] These proteases degrade damaged extracellular matrix components to allow their replacement. Proteases also degrade the basement membrane of capillaries to enable inflammatory cells to migrate into the wound.

In wounds, local blood supply is compromised at the same time that metabolic demand is increased. As a result, the wound environment becomes hypoxic and acidotic with high lactate levels.[28,29] This represents the sum of three effects: decreased oxygen supply because of vascular damage and coagulation, increased metabolic demand because of the heightened cellular response (anaerobic glycolysis), and aerobic glycolysis by inflammatory cells.[30,31] Leukocytes contain few mitochondria and develop energy from glucose mainly by production of lactate, even in the presence of adequate oxygen supply.[31] In activated neutrophils, the respiratory burst, in which oxygen and glucose are converted to superoxide, hydrogen ion, and lactate, accounts for up to 98% of oxygen consumption, which increases by up to 50-fold over baseline.[32,33]

Local hypoxia is a normal and inevitable result of tissue injury.[34,35] Hypoxia acts as a stimulus to repair[36] but also leads to poor healing[9] and increased susceptibility to infection.[37,38] Numerous experimental models[38-41] and human clinical experience[42-44] have led to the conclusion that wound healing is delayed in hypoxic wounds. The partial pressure of oxygen in dermal wounds is heterogeneous, ranging from 0 to 10 mm Hg in the central ("dead space") portion of the wound to near arterial adjacent to perfused arterioles and capillaries[34] (Fig. 11.2). The partial pressure of oxygen (Po_2) of a given area depends on diffusion of oxygen from perfused capillaries; thus, wound Po_2 depends on capillary density, arterial partial pressure of oxygen (Pao_2), and the metabolic activity of the cells, with some contribution from shifts in the oxyhemoglobin dissociation curve (e.g., the low wound pH shifts the curve to the right and increases oxygen delivery, whereas decreased wound temperature shifts the curve to the left and decreases oxygen delivery).

Table 11.1 Growth Factors Involved in Wound Healing

GROWTH FACTOR FAMILY	CELL SOURCE	ACTIONS
Transforming growth factor-β (TGF-β): TGF-β1, TGF-β2	Platelets Fibroblasts Macrophages	Fibroblast chemotaxis and activation ECM deposition 　Collagen synthesis 　TIMP synthesis 　MMP synthesis
TGF-β3		Reduces scarring 　Collagen 　Fibronectin
Platelet-derived growth factor (PDGF): PDGF-AA, PDGF-BB, VEGF	Platelets Macrophages Keratinocytes Fibroblasts	Activation of immune cells and fibroblasts ECM deposition 　Collagen synthesis 　TIMP synthesis 　MMP synthesis Neovascularization
Fibroblast growth factor (FGF): acidic FGF, basic FGF, KGF	Macrophages Endothelial cells Fibroblasts	Neovascularization Endothelial cell activation Keratinocyte proliferation and migration ECM deposition
Insulin-like growth factor (IGF): IGF-1, IGF-2, insulin	Liver Skeletal muscle Fibroblasts Macrophages Neutrophils	Keratinocyte proliferation Fibroblast proliferation Endothelial cell activation Neovascularization 　Collagen synthesis ECM deposition Cell metabolism
Epidermal growth factor (EGF): EGF, heparin binding EGF, TGF-α, amphiregulin, beta-cellulin	Keratinocytes Macrophages	Keratinocyte proliferation and migration ECM deposition
Connective tissue growth factor	Fibroblasts Endothelial cells Epithelial cells	Mediates action of TGF-β on collagen synthesis

ECM, extracellular matrix; KGF, keratinocyte growth factor; MMP, matrix metalloproteinase; TIMP, tissue inhibitor of metalloproteinases; VEGF, vascular endothelial growth factor.

From Schulz G: Molecular Regulation of Wound Healing. In: Bryant R, Nix D (eds): Acute and Chronic Wounds: Current Management Concepts, 3rd ed. St. Louis, Mosby Elsevier, 2006, pp 82–99, by permission.

Resistance to Infection

After a disruption of the normal skin barrier, successful wound healing requires the ability to clear foreign material and resist infection. Neutrophils provide nonspecific immunity and prevent infection. Leukocytes migrate in tissue toward the site of injury via chemotaxis, defined as locomotion oriented along a chemical gradient.[23] Chemical gradients can be produced both exogenously and endogenously. Exogenous gradients result from bacterial products present in contaminated tissues. Endogenous mediators include components of the complement system (C5a), products of lipoxygenase pathway (leukotriene B_4), and cytokines

(IL-1, IL-8), together with lactate.[45] Together, these chemical mediators help to organize and control leukocyte invasion, bacterial killing, necrotic tissue removal, and the initiation of angiogenesis and matrix production. In the absence of infection, neutrophils disappear by about 48 hours. Nonspecific phagocytosis and intracellular killing are the major immune pathways activated in wounds.[46]

Neutrophils are the primary cells responsible for nonspecific immunity, and their function depends on a high partial pressure of oxygen.[12,47] This is because reactive oxygen species (ROS) are the major component of the bactericidal defense against wound pathogens.[46] Phagocytosis of the pathogen activates

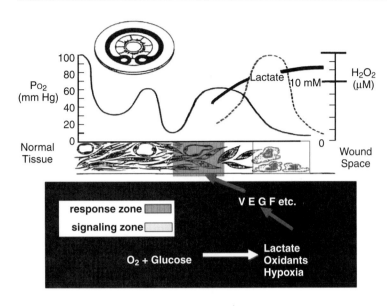

Figure 11.2 The wound module. Cross section of the wound module in a rabbit ear chamber (diagram of chamber is in top left corner). Note that partial pressure of oxygen (Po_2), depicted graphically above the cross section, is highest next to the vessels, with a gradient down to zero at the wound edge. Note also the lactate gradient, high in the dead space and lower (but still above plasma) toward the vasculature. Hydrogen peroxide is present at fairly high concentrations and is also a major stimulus to wound repair.[52] VEGF, vascular endothelial growth factor. *(Modified from Silver IA: The physiology of wound healing. In: Hunt TK, Dunphy JE (eds): Fundamentals of Wound Management. New York, Appleton-Century-Crofts, 1980, p 30, by permission.)*

the phagosomal oxidase (also known as the primary oxidase or nicotinamide-adenosine-dinucleotide phosphate [NADPH]–linked oxygenase), present in the phagocytic membrane, which uses oxygen as the substrate to catalyze the formation of superoxide. Superoxide is bactericidal, but more importantly, it initiates a series of cascades that produce other oxidants within the phagosome that increase bacterial killing capacity (Fig. 11.3). For example, in the presence of superoxide dismutase, superoxide is reduced to hydrogen peroxide (H_2O_2). H_2O_2 combines with chloride and in the presence of myeloperoxidase forms the bactericidal hypochlorous acid (the active ingredient in bleach).[47,48] Because intraphagosomal oxidant production depends on conversion of oxygen to superoxide, the process is exquisitely sensitive to the partial pressure (not content or saturation) of oxygen in the tissue. The Km (the concentration at which half-maximal velocity of the reaction occurs) for the phagosomal oxidase using oxygen as a substrate is 40 to 80 mm Hg.[12] This means that resistance to infection is critically impaired by wound hypoxia and becomes more efficient as Po_2 increases even to high levels (500–1000 mm Hg).[12] Such levels do not occur naturally in tissue but can be achieved by the administration of hyperbaric oxygen.[19-21,49] This is a mechanism for

the benefit of HBOT as an adjunctive treatment for necrotizing infections and chronic refractory osteomyelitis.[50,51]

Oxidants produced by inflammatory cells have a dual role in wound repair. Not only are they central to resistance to infection, but they also play a major role in initiating and directing the healing process. Oxidants, particularly hydrogen peroxide produced via the respiratory burst, increase neovascularization and collagen deposition in vitro and in vivo.[52]

Activated inflammatory cells consume oxygen at a high rate and, coupled with the impaired microcirculation, this results in hypoxia. This is especially true at the center of the wound, where the largest concentration of inflammatory cells is found.[34] Lactate is produced both anaerobically and aerobically, and this results in concentrations of 5 to 10 mm even in well-oxygenated wounds.[53] Lactate is a strong stimulus for collagen secretion and neovascularization.[54,55] Anti-inflammatory steroids impair healing by suppressing inflammation at this step.[56]

Proliferation

The proliferative phase normally begins approximately 4 days after injury, concurrent with a waning of the inflammatory phase. It consists of granulation tissue formation and

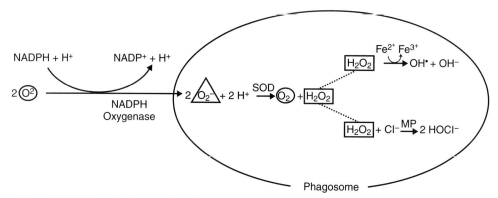

Figure 11.3 Schematic of superoxide and other oxidant production within the phagosome. SOD, superoxide dismutase. *(From Hunt TK, Hopf HW: Wound healing and wound infection. What surgeons and anesthesiologists can do. Surg Clin North Am 77:587–606, 1997, by permission.)*

epithelization. Granulation involves neovascularization and synthesis of collagen and connective tissue proteins.

Neovascularization

New blood vessels must replace the injured microcirculation. Neovascularization proceeds by both angiogenesis and vasculogenesis. Angiogenesis is the phenomenon of new vessel growth via budding from existing vessels. In the setting of wounds, new vessels grow from mature vessels, usually intact, postcapillary venules in the undamaged tissue immediately adjacent to the site of injury. Normally, the oxygen tension in adjacent tissue is sufficient to support this process. The new vessel growth extends and enters into the damaged areas that are typically high in lactate and have a low Po_2. Mature extracellular matrix is required for ingrowth of mature vessels.[57]

In vasculogenesis, bone marrow–derived endothelial precursor cells (EPCs) populate the tissue and differentiate and grow into new vessel tubules. In wounds, these tubules appear in the damaged area before any direct anastomosis with preexisting vessels is made. These tubules must connect with existing vasculature to establish an intact blood supply in the wound. Angiogenesis has long been held to be the primary mechanism for new blood vessel growth in granulation tissue. Recent research, however, has demonstrated that as many as 15% to 20% of new blood vessels are derived from hematopoietic stem cells.[57-59]

Angiogenesis and vasculogenesis both occur in response to similar stimuli, which is some combination of redox stress, hypoxia, and lactate concentration. The specific mechanisms by which they proceed appear to differ somewhat. Angiogenesis involves the movement of endothelial cells in response to three waves of growth factors. The first wave of growth factors comes with the release by platelets of PDGF, TGF-β, insulin-like growth factor-1, and others during the inflammatory phase. The second wave comes from fibroblast growth factor released from normal binding sites on connective tissue molecules. The third and dominant wave comes from VEGF, delivered largely by macrophages stimulated by fibrinopeptides, hypoxia, and the presence of lactate.[60] Although it is usually present, hypoxia is not required for granulation because of constitutive (aerobic) lactate production by inflammatory cells and fibroblasts. In fact, HBOT increases angiogenesis in a mouse model,[17] an effect mediated, at least in part, by stimulation of VEGF production by hyperbaric oxygen.[61] Too little lactate leads to inadequate granulation, whereas levels in excess of about 15 mM (usually associated with excess inflammation or infection) delay granulation.[62] The capillary endothelial response to angiogenic agents (i.e., migration into the wound, tubule formation, and connecting to sources of blood flow) requires oxygen, so that angiogenesis progresses proportional to blood perfusion and Pao_2.[63]

Vasculogenesis occurs in response to similar stressors as angiogenesis. EPCs are mobilized from the bone marrow into the circulation via a nitric oxide (·NO)–mediated mechanism. Tissue hypoxia induces release of VEGF-A, which activates bone marrow stromal nitric oxide synthase (NOS). Increased bone marrow ·NO leads to release of EPCs into the circulation. These circulating EPCs are attracted to the wound via tissue hypoxia-induced upregulation of stromal cell–derived factor-1α. Within the wound, EPCs undergo differentiation and participate in the formation of new blood vessels.

Collagen and Extracellular Matrix Deposition

New blood vessels grow into the matrix that is produced by fibroblasts. Although fibroblasts replicate and migrate mainly in response to growth factors and chemoattractants, production of mature collagen requires oxygen.[13,64,65] Lactate, hypoxia, and some growth factors induce collagen messenger RNA synthesis and procollagen production. Post-translational modification by prolyl and lysyl hydroxylases is required to allow collagen peptides to aggregate into triple helices. Collagen can be exported from the cell only when it is in this triple-helical structure. The helical configuration is also primarily responsible for tissue strength. The activity of the hydroxylases is critically dependent on vitamin C and tissue oxygen tension, with a Km for oxygen of about 25 mm Hg.[13,64-66] Wound strength, which results from collagen deposition, is, therefore, highly vulnerable to wound hypoxia.[9]

Neovascularization and extracellular matrix (primarily collagen) production are closely linked. Fibroblasts cannot produce mature collagen in the absence of mature blood vessels that deliver oxygen to the site. New blood vessels cannot mature without a strong collagen matrix. Mice kept in a hypoxic environment (13% inspired oxygen) develop some new blood vessels in a test wound (with VEGF or lactate added), but these vessels are immature,

with little surrounding matrix, and demonstrate frequent areas of hemorrhage.[17]

Role of Lactate

Although hypoxia has traditionally been viewed as the main stimulus for neovascularization, it is clearly not the sole agent.[67,68] Neovascularization occurs in many circumstances in which energy depletion, or reduced redox potential, is more prominent than hypoxia. Adenosine diphosphoribose ribosylation (ADPR-ribosylation) is a mechanism whereby low redox potential can be sensed and converted into biologic actions including collagen formation, angiogenesis, and induction of cytosolic and nuclear proteins. ADPR mechanisms constitute a link between the metabolic state and gene regulation.[31,57,69,70] When intracellular lactate is at baseline, the NAD^+/NADH ratio favors NAD^+. This works to maintain ADPR in a ribosylated state, thus suppressing collagen gene transcription and inhibiting post-transcriptional collagen hydroxylation, as well as production and post-translational modification of VEGF. When lactate levels increase, the ratio favors NADH, and the inhibition by ribosylated ADPR is interrupted, thus increasing mature collagen production and VEGF activity[71] (Fig. 11.4).

Lactate also mediates neovascularization via hypoxia-inducible factor-1α (HIF-1α). HIF-1α is a helix-loop-helix transcription factor that is composed of a constitutively expressed β subunit and a hypoxia-induced α subunit.[72] HIF-1α was originally identified in a model of hypoxia,[73] but recent research suggests it responds more broadly to redox stress.[57,74] HIF-1α function is regulated by a prolyl hydroxylase. Normally, the enzyme hydroxylates HIF-1α, which leads to its destruction and, therefore, prevents neovascularization. Hypoxia reduces the rate of hydroxylation, thus leading to increased HIF-1α activity and activation of neovascularization pathways.[75]

Hypoxia is not required for HIF-1 α regulation. Lactate stabilizes HIF-1α, even in the presence of oxygen, because lactate and pyruvate bind to and inhibit the HIF prolyl

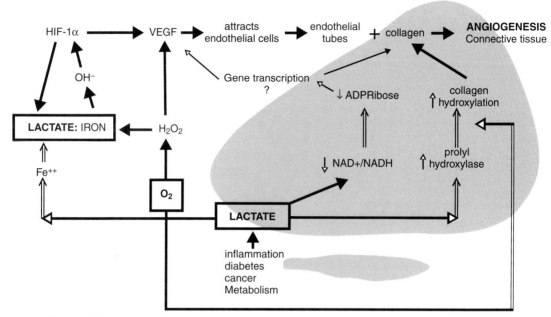

Figure 11.4 Schematic of the mechanisms by which lactate regulates collagen and vascular endothelial growth factor (VEGF) production via control of ribosylation of adenosine diphosphoribose (ADP). HIF-1α, hypoxia-inducible factor-1α. *(Modified from Hunt TK, Aslam RS, Beckert S, et al: Aerobically derived lactate stimulates revascularization and tissue repair via redox mechanisms. Antioxid Redox Signal 9:1115–1124, 2007, by permission.)*

hydroxylases.[76,77] As discussed previously, neutrophils and macrophages in the wound produce lactate aerobically, so that accumulation is not dependent on hypoxia. Regardless of the source, increasing lactate levels from 5 to 15 mmol promotes neovascularization and matrix deposition. This is additive with oxygen[31] (Fig. 11.5). Thus, small increases in lactate level during the acute inflammatory phase may induce blood vessel growth before the development of prolonged hypoxia. In fact, lactate in the presence of oxygen may be an even greater stimulus for neovascularization than hypoxia.[31]

Interestingly, HIF and other growth factors also play important roles in pathologic angiogenesis. Von Hippel–Lindau disease is a hereditary cancer syndrome predisposing carriers to the development of a range of highly vascularized tumors. Von Hippel–Lindau disorder is precipitated by a gene mutation leading to dysfunctional HIF prolyl hydroxylase that results in a decrease in the degradation of HIF. This causes a pathologic accumulation of HIF-1α resulting in increased VEGF

levels and subsequent tumor angiogenesis.[78] Other pathologic processes can produce inappropriate angiogenesis through the same lactate/HIF pathway. For example, diabetic retinopathy is characterized by hypoxic tissues generating lactate and HIF.[79] Increased levels of lactate and HIF lead to increased VEGF levels and subsequent pathologic vessel production in the affected retina. Despite the presence of lactate, as in wounds, hypoxia blocks the essential step of collagen deposition, and these vessels are leaky and poorly functional.

In summary, accumulated lactate, even in the presence of normal or supraphysiologic tissue oxygen concentration, is able to initiate neovascularization and connective tissue synthesis, provided that oxygen is present. This process involves the stabilization of HIF-1α and inactivation of ADPR, which cause an increase in active VEGF and collagen production. However, although lactate is central to normal oxygen homeostasis of tissue, it can also instigate pathologic consequences.

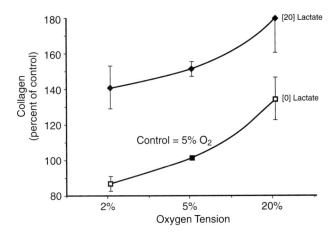

Figure 11.5 Effect of oxygen tension and lactate concentration on collagen synthesis by fibroblasts in vitro. Fibroblasts incubated in 2% (wound hypoxia), 5% (wound normoxia), or 20% (wound hyperoxia) oxygen and 0 or 20 mM lactate were pulsed with tritiated proline. Secretion of hydroxylated collagen into the cell-conditioned medium was then measured. Greater levels of lactate and oxygen increase mature collagen production, with the greatest amount resulting from the combination of high lactate and hyperoxia. *(From Skover GR: Cellular and biochemical dynamics of wound repair: Wound environment in collagen regeneration. Clin Podiatr Med Surg 8:723–756, 1991, by permission.)*

Role of Reactive Oxygen Species/Hydrogen Peroxide

ROS are produced in the wound via the respiratory burst[46] by both phagocytic and nonphagocytic cells. The phagocytic production of ROS and other oxidants via the NADPH-link (phagosomal) oxidase was discussed previously. H_2O_2, produced by dismutation of superoxide, serves as a diffusible signaling messenger and induces neovascularization via increased VEGF expression at levels found in wounds.[80,81] NADPH oxidases are also present in nonphagocytic cells, including fibroblasts, keratinocytes, and endothelial cells.[82] Nonphagocytic cells thus represent a sustained source of low-level H_2O_2 in uninfected wounds. Micromolar levels of H_2O_2 are detectable in both the inflammatory and proliferative phases of wound healing.[74]

An essential subunit of the phagosomal oxidase is p47[phox]. Defects in p47[phox] compromise respiratory burst–dependent oxidant production. Mutations in p47[phox] in humans have been identified as a cause of chronic granulomatous disease, in which an impaired oxidative burst leads to recurrent infections.[83] p47[phox]-deficient mice have impaired healing of excisional wounds.[74] Treatment of the wounds with low-concentration (0.15%) H_2O_2 reverses this defect. Of note, 3% H_2O_2, the commercially available concentration, despite its bactericidal activity, delayed healing in these mice, as it does in human wounds.[84]

Role of Nitric Oxide

·NO is a soluble oxygen radical with a half-life of a few seconds that appears to play a major role in wound repair. ·NO is synthesized from the amino acid L-arginine, molecular oxygen, and NADPH in a reaction catalyzed by the enzyme NOS. The NOSs exist in three isoforms: two constitutive (endothelial and neuronal) isoforms and one inducible. The expression, transcription, and function of the inducible isoform (iNOS) are induced by a variety of cytokines, growth factors, and inflammatory stimuli. Upregulation of iNOS leads to release of high levels of ·NO. Because of the short half-life of ·NO in vivo, ·NO has only a local effect.[85]

iNOS can be expressed in virtually all tissues under the appropriate conditions. The enzyme is synthesized in the early phases of wound healing in response to cytokines, bacteria, bacterial products, and hypoxia. TGF-β and IL-4 increase arginase and inhibit iNOS activity, whereas γ-interferon, IL-1, and lipopolysaccharide increase iNOS.[86] Once formed, iNOS is maintained in an active state by calmodulin bound to the enzyme, allowing it to operate independent of calcium concentrations. This leads to a much larger release of ·NO, limited by substrate and cofactor availability and enzyme concentration.

Expression of iNOS is induced by injury, particularly by platelet degranulation. It peaks by about 48 hours after injury. NOSs require NADPH, oxygen, tetrahydrobiopterin, flavine mononucleotide, and flavine adenosine dinucleotide as cofactors for full activity.[85] Many of the primary effects of ·NO are obvious in the inflammatory phase of wound healing: vasodilation, antimicrobial activity, antiplatelet aggregation activity, and increased vascular permeability.

·NO acts via multiple mechanisms.[87] It reacts with oxygen to form reactive nitrogen-based species.[88] It binds to heme- or metal-containing enzymes such as the heme iron in guanylate cyclase. At the molecular level, ·NO has been shown to act as a signaling molecule that operates via guanylate cyclase to synthesize cyclic guanosine monophosphate. In addition, ·NO acts as a cytostatic/cytotoxic molecule inhibiting cytochromes and aconitase, as well as ribonucleotide reductase. ·NO also regulates gene expression by reacting with the thiol binding site of the transcription factor nuclear factor-κB. By nitrosylating nuclear factor-κB, ·NO prevents binding to the iNOS promoter, suggesting a feedback inhibition mechanism.

Treatment with ·NO donors or dietary arginine or inducing iNOS overexpression increases the collagen content of experimental wounds.[89] Inhibition of iNOS by competitive inhibitors decreases collagen deposition and breaking strength in incisional wounds and impairs healing in other wound models.[90-92] NOS blockade prevents VEGF production, VEGF-induced endothelial cell proliferation, and VEGF-mediated activation of mitogen-activating protein kinase.[93-96]

Induction of ·NO appears to be one mechanism by which HBOT exerts its effects in wounds.[97-99] Gallagher and coworkers[100] demonstrate a defect in the number and function of bone marrow–derived EPCs in streptozotocin-induced diabetic mice. The degree of the defect in EPCs predicts the degree of impairment of wound healing,[100] as well as the development of long-term cardiovascular complications.[97-99] Thom and colleagues[101] demonstrate that HBOT mobilized bone marrow–derived EPCs in human subjects with diabetes. In a murine model, this appears to be mediated via increased ·NO levels within the femoral bone marrow.[102] There appears to be a subpopulation of bone marrow–derived EPCs within the bone marrow available for rapid release to the

circulation in response to ·NO. In a murine model of ischemic wounds, this release of bone marrow–derived EPCs into the circulation increases neovascularization and wound healing in excisional wounds.[100,102] HBOT does not, however, correct the deficit in homing of EPCs to the wound related to decreased stromal cell–derived factor-1α in diabetes.[103]

Epithelization

Epithelization is characterized by replication and migration of epithelial cells across the skin edges in response to growth factors. Cell migration may begin from any site that contains living keratinocytes, including remnants of hair follicles, sebaceous glands, islands of living epidermis, or the normal wound edge. In acute wounds that are primarily closed, epithelization is normally completed in 1 to 3 days. In open wounds, including chronic wounds, healing by secondary intention cannot progress until the wound bed is fully granulated. Like immunity and granulation, epithelization depends on growth factors and oxygen. Silver[104] and Medawar[16] demonstrated in vivo that the rate of epithelization depends on local oxygen. Topical oxygen (applied so that it does not dry out epithelial cells) has been advocated as a method to increase the rate of epithelization.[105] Ngo and investigators[106] demonstrate oxygen-dependent differentiation (21% > 5% > 2%) and cell growth (21% and 5% > 2%) in human keratinocytes in culture. In contrast, O'Toole and coauthors[107] demonstrate that hypoxia increases epithelial migration in vitro. This may be explained, at least in part, by the dependence of epithelization on the presence of a bed of healthy granulation tissue, which is known to be oxygen dependent.

Maturation and Remodeling

The final phase of wound repair is maturation, which involves ongoing remodeling of the granulation tissue and increasing wound tensile strength. As the matrix becomes denser with thicker, stronger collagen fibrils, it becomes stiffer and less compliant. Fibroblasts are capable of adapting to changing mechanical stress and loading. Fibroblasts migrate throughout the matrix to help mold the wound to new stresses. Matrix metalloproteinases and other proteases help with fibroblast migration and continued matrix remodeling in response to mechanical stress. Some fibroblasts differentiate into myofibroblasts under the influence of TGF-β. These cells are contractile. As the myofibroblasts contract, the collagenous matrix crosslinks in the shortened position. This helps to strengthen the matrix and minimize scar size. Contraction is inhibited by the use of high doses of corticosteroids.[108] Even steroids given several days after injury have this effect. In some wounds, where contraction is detrimental, this effect can be beneficial.

Net collagen synthesis continues for at least 6 weeks and up to 6 months after wounding. Over time, the initial collagen threads are reabsorbed and deposited along stress lines, conferring greater tensile strength. Collagen found in granulation tissue is biochemically different from collagen of uninjured skin, and a scar never achieves the tensile strength of uninjured skin. Hydroxylation and glycosylation of lysine residues in granulation tissue collagen leads to thinner collagen fibers. Wound strength also never returns to baseline. At 1 week, a wound closed by primary intention has reached only 3% of the tensile strength of normal skin. By 3 weeks, it is at 30%, and it reaches 80% only after 3 to 6 months.

Some wounds heal to excess. Hypertrophic scar and keloid are common forms of abnormal scarring due to abnormal responses to healing. The distinction between them may be difficult. Hypertrophic scars are common after burns and correlate with the length of time required to close the wound. Rapid healing is less likely to result in excessive scarring. This is one of the strong arguments for early closure and the use of skin substitutes. Early HBOT might also have beneficial effects in burn wounds by accelerating closure. Hypertrophic scars also tend to occur in wounds that cross lines of force in the skin. Hypertrophic scars occur within months or even right after the injury, do not grow beyond the wound edges, and often flatten spontaneously after 1 to 2 years. Hypertrophic scars that do not resolve spontaneously or interfere with function are often best treated surgically with revisions designed to relieve tension. They may also respond to pressure garments, repeated injections of steroids, or to prolonged dressing with thick silicone sheets.

Keloids occur within 1 year after injury and are more common in those of African, Hispanic, or Asian descent, with an incidence rate of 4.5% to 16%. Keloids usually are more painful than hypertrophic scars, pruritic, and grow beyond the edges of the wound without regression. They often occur on the shoulder, upper arm, anterior chest (particularly the presternal area), and upper back, but generally not on hands or below the groin. Recurrence of keloids after excision is common, occurring about 50% to 80% of the time.[109]

Contractures occur when shrinking scars constrict mobility. All scars shrink unless the force of contraction is balanced by stretching forces. In general, prophylactic efforts, braces, physical therapy, stretching, and pressure dressings are the most effective prevention and therapy. Special compression garments can be made. Established contractures that persist or recur are often best treated surgically by flaps, or so-called Z or Y plasties, which relax contractures and interpose normal tissues along the line of contracture.

Nutrition

Skin is the largest and most readily examined organ in the body. It is therefore not surprising that many nutritional deficiencies present with alterations in the skin or in healing. This led to the recognition of the importance of nutrition in wound healing.[2] Nutritional requirements change during the healing process. The initial response to injury is catabolic energy production. This must convert to an anabolic response with protein synthesis for healing to occur. In general, specific nutritional requirements are not well delineated. Recent intake is most important.[110,111]

Proteins are essential for the anabolic phase and are degraded in catabolic states such as sepsis, burns, and major orthopedic injury (e.g., femur fracture). Thus, calculation of the nitrogen balance gives an idea of the amount of protein lost and the required level for replacement. Wound exudates contain large amounts of protein; thus, patients with exudative wounds have increased protein requirements. The major protein of the skin is collagen. Use of specific amino acids has no clear benefit. Arginine, a precursor of proline, and glutamine, a precursor of nucleotide synthesis, both accelerate wound repair when given in doses of 15 to 30 g/day. This appears to be more a pharmacologic than nutritional effect.[89,112]

Scurvy, the nutritional defect induced by vitamin C deficiency, has been recognized since the 15th century, when Portuguese explorer Vasco da Gama described poor healing and hematoma formation in sailors. The British Naval physician James Lind performed the first known randomized, controlled trial in 1747 and demonstrated the efficacy of citrus fruits in preventing scurvy (the cause remained unknown until the description of vitamin C in the 20th century). Vitamin C levels decrease rapidly in patients with major trauma or injury (e.g., long bone fracture), infection, or sepsis; thus, supplemental vitamin C (500 mg twice daily) should be given to patients with extensive wounds or traumatic injuries.[113,114] Vitamin C is a cofactor for prolyl hydroxylase, the same reaction for which oxygen is a rate-limiting substrate.[65] Wound hypoxia thus, to a degree, mimics scurvy.

Vitamin A[115] is a proinflammatory vitamin that is associated with differentiation and growth of the epidermis. Deficiency, although uncommon, is associated with impaired healing. Vitamin A (25,000 IU daily) has been demonstrated to reverse the impaired healing associated with steroid use,[116] diabetes,[117] and radiation.[118] Because it is a fat-soluble vitamin and excess intake is associated with adverse effects, it should be given for only 10 days. Topical vitamin A (available over the counter), applied daily directly to the open wound, is a useful alternative.[119-121]

Vitamin E, a membrane stabilizing, anti-inflammatory vitamin has been shown to *impair* healing in a rat model.[122] Thus, it can be argued that supplemental doses (beyond that found in a standard multivitamin) should be avoided in patients with wounds.

Among trace elements, zinc is the oldest known medicinal treatment and was described by the ancient Egyptians for skin wounds.[112] Zinc is involved in DNA and RNA synthesis. Zinc deficiency impairs healing. There is no evidence, however, that zinc supplementation accelerates healing in patients without a deficiency. However, a short course (220 mg orally daily for 10 days) is reasonable in wound patients to address any unrecognized deficiencies.

Carbohydrates are also necessary for collagen synthesis. It is estimated that a wound 3 cm^2 in surface area and 1 mm in depth requires 10 mg collagen for granulation, which requires 9 Kcal energy to produce (900 cal/1 g collagen).[2,112] Omega-3 fatty acids may modulate the arachidonic acid pathway (inflammatory pathway) and thereby influence wound maturation.[112]

WOUND PERFUSION AND OXYGENATION

Complications of wounds, regardless of the injury that produces them, include failure to heal, infection, and excessive scarring or contracture. Rapid repair has the least potential for infection and excess scarring. The goals for rapid healing, therefore, are to avoid contamination, ensure rapid tissue synthesis, and optimize the immune response. All injuries lead to some degree of contamination that must be controlled by local host defenses. The initial hours after contamination represent a decisive period during which inadequate local defenses may allow an infection to become established.[123] Chronic wounds remain susceptible to infection while they remain open.

Normally, wounds on the extremities and trunk heal more slowly than those on the face. The major difference in these wounds is the degree of tissue perfusion, and thus the wound tissue oxygen tension. As a rule, repair proceeds most rapidly and immunity is strongest when wound oxygen levels are high, and this is achieved only by maintaining perfusion of injured tissue.[124] Ischemic or hypoxic tissue, in contrast, is easily infected and heals poorly, if at all. Wound tissue oxygenation is complex and depends on the interaction of blood perfusion, arterial oxygen tension, hemoglobin dissociation conditions, carrying capacity, mass transfer resistances, and local oxygen consumption. Wound oxygen delivery depends on vascular anatomy, the degree of vasoconstriction, and PaO_2 (see Fig. 11.2).

The standard teaching that oxygen delivery depends more on hemoglobin-bound oxygen (oxygen content) than on PaO_2 may be true of working muscle, but it is not true of wound healing. In muscle, intercapillary distances are small and oxygen consumption is high. Conversely, in subcutaneous tissue, intercapillary distances are large and oxygen consumption is relatively low.[14] In wounds, where the microvasculature is damaged, diffusion distance markedly increases. Peripheral vasoconstriction further increases diffusion distance.[34] The driving force of diffusion is the oxygen concentration, that is, its partial pressure. A high PO_2 is needed to force oxygen into injured and healing tissues, particularly in subcutaneous tissue, fascia, tendon, and bone, the tissues most at risk for poor healing. HBOT increases the diffusion distance of oxygen into the tissue from about 64 mcm (PaO_2 100 mm Hg) to about 247 mcm (PaO_2 2000 mm Hg)[125] by increasing the amount of dissolved oxygen in the plasma.

Although oxygen consumption is relatively low in wounds, it is consumed by processes that require oxygen at a high concentration. As discussed earlier, inflammatory cells use little oxygen for respiration, producing energy largely via the hexose-monophosphate shunt.[12] Most of the oxygen consumed in wounds is used for oxidant production (bacterial killing), with a significant contribution as well for collagen synthesis, angiogenesis, and epithelization. The rate constants (Km) for oxygen for these components of repair all fall within the physiologic range of 25 to 100 mm Hg.[12,13,16,47,64,126]

Because of the high rate constants for oxygen substrate for the components of repair, the rate at which repair proceeds varies according to tissue PO_2 from zero to at least 250 mm Hg.

In vitro fibroblast replication is optimal at a PO_2 of about 40 to 60 mm Hg. Neutrophils lose their ability to kill bacteria in vitro below a PO_2 of about 40 mm Hg.[127,128] These in vitro observations are clinically relevant. "Normal" subcutaneous PO_2, measured in test wounds in uninjured, euthermic, euvolemic volunteers breathing room air, is 65 ± 7 mm Hg.[129] Thus, any reduction in wound PO_2 may impair immunity and repair. In surgical patients, the rate of wound infections is inversely proportional,[37] whereas collagen deposition is directly proportional,[9] to postoperative subcutaneous wound tissue oxygen tension.

High oxygen tensions (>100 mm Hg) can be reached in wounds but only if perfusion is rapid and PaO_2 is high.[124,130] This is true for two reasons. First, subcutaneous tissue serves a reservoir function, so there is normally flow in excess of nutritional needs. Second, wound cells consume relatively little oxygen, about 0.7 mL/100 mL blood flow at a normal perfusion rate.[14,15] At high levels of PaO_2, this small volume can be carried by plasma alone. Contrary to popular belief, therefore, oxygen-carrying capacity, that is, hemoglobin concentration, is not particularly important to wound healing, provided that perfusion is normal.[131] Wound PO_2 and collagen synthesis remain normal in individuals who have hematocrit levels as low as 15% to 18% provided they can appropriately increase cardiac output and vasoconstriction is prevented.[130,133] HBOT can increase wound oxygen tension well above the physiologic range (800–1200 mm Hg), as long as there is some arterial inflow.[19,21,49]

In patients with adequate large-vessel inflow, peripheral vasoconstriction, which results from central sympathetic control of subcutaneous vascular tone, is probably the most frequent and clinically the most important impediment to wound oxygenation. Subcutaneous tissue is both a reservoir to maintain central volume and a major site of thermoregulation. There is little local regulation of blood flow, except by local heating.[134,135] Therefore, subcutaneous tissue is particularly vulnerable to vasoconstriction. Sympathetically induced peripheral vasoconstriction is stimulated by cold; pain; fear; and blood volume deficit;[136,137]

and various medications including smoking (nicotine),[129] β-adrenergic antagonists, and α_1 agonists. In patients undergoing surgery, perioperative hypothermia is common and results from anesthetic drugs, exposure to cold, and redistribution of body heat. Blood loss and increases in insensible losses (third spacing) increase fluid requirements in the perioperative period, thereby leaving the patient vulnerable to inadequate fluid replacement. Thus, vasomotor tone is, to a large degree, under the control of the health-care provider.[136,137]

Prevention or correction of hypothermia[138] and blood volume deficits[139] has been shown to decrease wound infections and increase collagen deposition in patients undergoing major abdominal surgery. Preoperative systemic (forced air warmer) or local (warming bandage) warming have also been shown to decrease wound infections, even in clean, low-risk surgeries such as breast surgery and inguinal hernia repair.[140] Subcutaneous tissue oxygen tension is significantly greater in patients with good pain control than those with poor pain control after arthroscopic knee surgery.[141] Stress also causes wound hypoxia and significantly impairs wound healing and resistance to infection.[142,143] The adverse effects of sympathetic nervous system activation are clearly mediated, in large part, by reducing the partial pressure of oxygen in the injured tissue. Prevention of sympathetic nervous system activation is effective at improving wound healing and resistance to infection largely because it increases wound oxygen tension.

Greif and colleagues[144] demonstrated in a randomized, controlled, double-blind trial that, in warm, well-hydrated patients with good pain control, that is, in well-perfused patients ($n = 500$) undergoing major colon surgery, administration of 80% versus 30% oxygen intraoperatively and for the first 2 postoperative hours significantly reduced the wound infection rate by 50%. Belda and coauthors[145] have replicated these results (significant 40% reduction in surgical site infection) in a randomized, controlled, double-blind trial in 300 colon surgery patients randomized to 80% versus 30% oxygen intraoperatively and

during the first 6 postoperative hours. Surgical and anesthetic management were standardized and intended to support optimal perfusion. Myles and coworkers[146] demonstrated a significant reduction in major postoperative complications, specifically wound infections in 2050 major surgery patients randomized to 80% oxygen versus 30% oxygen in 70% nitrous oxide intraoperatively. A smaller ($n = 165$) randomized, controlled study by Pryor and investigators[147] demonstrated a doubling of surgical site infection in patients randomized to 80% versus 35% oxygen intraoperatively. There were a number of methodological flaws in the study, but more importantly, the two groups of patients were not equivalent, which likely explained the increase in infections seen in the 80% oxygen group. Thus, substantial evidence exists that use of high inspired oxygen intraoperatively and providing supplemental oxygen after surgery in *well-perfused* patients undergoing major abdominal surgery will reduce the risk for wound infection.

Although most data on the value of increasing wound oxygen levels have been obtained in surgical patients and acute wounds, there is growing evidence for the benefit of increased wound perfusion, and thereby oxygenation in chronic wounds as well, even in patients in whom arterial inflow is not compromised. Stotts and Hopf[148] demonstrated that nursing home residents frequently have reduced subcutaneous oxygen levels (<45 mm Hg) and that administration of additional fluid (750 mL extra per day for 3 days) significantly increased wound oxygen. Hopf and colleagues[149,150] demonstrate that reduction of sympathetic outflow with clonidine (a centrally acting α_2 agonist)[149] or percutaneous lumbar sympathetic block[150] increases wound oxygen levels in patients with hypoxic (but not ischemic) lower extremity ulcers. Thus, it appears that reduction of sympathetic outflow by treatment of pain, maintenance of a warm environment for the wound, reduction of stress, and provision of appropriate fluid intake may improve healing in even chronic ulcers.

ROLE OF HYPERBARIC OXYGEN THERAPY IN WOUND HEALING

HBOT was first investigated for use in wound healing because it was thought it would work by increasing oxygen in hypoxic wounds. Indeed, research has shown that it does just that. However, the mechanisms by which HBOT improves healing in hypoxic wounds is far more complicated.

Mechanisms by Which Hyperbaric Oxygen Therapy Improves Wound Healing

HBOT clearly increases wound oxygen concentration, even in ischemic wounds, as long as there is some arterial inflow.[19,21] Although correction of hypoxia is one mechanism by which HBOT improves wound healing, a growing body of research makes it clear that, at the supraphysiologic tissue levels attained under hyperbaric conditions, hyperbaric oxygen acts like a drug, with multiple effects that continue after the treatment ends. Wound oxygen tension decreases rapidly at the end of a treatment, although levels may not completely return to baseline for several hours.[21,49] The brief period of wound hyperoxia does initiate a cascade of events, however, that continue between treatments. For example, recent studies in a murine model and in cultured cells demonstrate the existence of a feed-forward mechanism for HIF-1α activation. Chronic intermittent hypoxia–induced ROS activates HIF-1α, which then promotes persistent oxidative stress, which may further amplify HIF-1 activation and result in an increase in gene expression.[151] As discussed earlier, this increase in HIF leads to an increase in VEGF and promotes neovascularization. It is possible that the cycling of hypoxia and hyperoxia actually contributes to the acceleration of healing seen with HBOT. That question, however, currently cannot be answered because no safe way is available to provide continuous wound hyperoxia at the levels achieved with HBOT.

Wound hyperoxia and specifically HBOT have been shown to increase resistance to infection,[39,50] fibroblast replication and collagen deposition,[152] neovascariztion,[17] and epithelization,[16,153] particularly in hypoxic wounds. There is likely to be a direct effect related to increased availability of oxygen in the wound for these processes. However, it appears likely that the pharmacologic effects of hyperoxia predominate, and that increased neovascularization and hence decreased wound hypoxia between treatments is the major determinant of efficacy.

Resistance to infection appears to relate more directly to the increase in oxygen in the wound during the treatment period. Increased oxygen clearly increases bacterial killing capacity of neutrophils.[12] HBOT also directly potentiates antibiotics, particularly aminoglycosides,[154-156] and suppresses toxin synthesis.[157]

"Pharmacologic" effects of HBOT include:

- Induction of growth factors and growth factor receptors: HBOT increases active VEGF production by macrophages in culture,[158] in wound fluid in a rat model,[61] and in human volunteers. It also up-regulates PDGF receptors.[159] The mechanisms may relate to ·NO, as discussed earlier. HBOT recently has been shown to upregulate basic fibroblast growth factor and hepatocyte growth factor in acutely ischemic hind limbs in a murine model[160]
- Inhibition of neutrophil adhesion: Interaction of neutrophil surface β integrins with intercellular adhesion molecules on the endothelial surface causes neutrophil adhesion. This may be beneficial in allowing neutrophil migration to the wound but may also cause pathological endothelial dysfunction, as in ischemia-reperfusion injury. HBOT inhibits neutrophil β2 integrin function by a localized effect on membrane guanylate cyclase, an effect that appears to be mediated by ·NO[161,162]
- Mobilization of endothelial stem cells from the bone marrow[100]
- Induction of ·NO[162]

The combination of the direct effects of correction of wound hypoxia and the pharmacologic effects of hyperoxia lead to a number of clinically observed benefits:

- More rapid and effective control of infection[163]
- Reduction of ischemia-reperfusion injury[164-166]
- Reduction of pathologic inflammation[161]
- Reduction of edema[167,168]: This effect has widely been attributed to hyperoxia-induced vasoconstriction.[22] However, it seems more likely to result from a reduction in inflammation. Edema is generally caused by "leaky" vessels and venous hypertension, rather than excess arterial flow. Vasoconstriction would reduce arterial inflow. A reduction in inflammation would likely restore integrity to the vessels and thereby reduce edema
- Increased neovascularization and collagen deposition, which together result in increased granulation tissue[17,152,169]
- Increased epithelization[16]
- Increased osteogenesis[170,171]

Clinical Efficacy of Hyperbaric Oxygen Therapy in Wound Healing

Mechanistically, HBOT seems most likely to be of benefit in hypoxic wounds. In fact, Smith and colleagues[20] demonstrate that wounds without significant hypoxia were unlikely to improve during HBOT. The most likely explanation for this is that hypoxia was not the impediment to healing in these patients, and HBOT did not correct the actual impediment. It is possible that hyperoxia could accelerate healing in a normoxic wound, but only in the absence of other impediments to healing. HBOT is an adjuvant treatment. It cannot replace appropriate care, including such therapy as moist wound care, off-loading, debridement, compression, and restoration of arterial inflow. In the absence of proper care, HBOT is unlikely to provide benefit.

The Undersea and Hyperbaric Medical Society recognizes nine indications for HBOT related to wound healing in some capacity (see Table 11.2 for these indications and the likely mechanisms underlying the therapeutic benefit of HBOT). Most of these indications are covered in detail in other chapters of this textbook.

Although it appears reasonable that HBOT should improve healing in patients with hypoxic wounds, almost all of the studies of efficacy of HBOT in chronic wounds to date have evaluated efficacy in healing of ischemic lower extremity ulcers in patients with diabetes (Table 11.3). It is possible that HBOT is specifically useful in diabetic ulcers because of defects unique to those ulcers. For example, diabetic ulcers have been shown to have decreased PDGF and PDGF receptors,[159] and circulating EPCs are known to be reduced in subjects with diabetes.[103] In contrast, Bauer and colleagues[41] demonstrate a similar defect in a murine ischemic ulcer model. Nonetheless, currently, the clinical data support only the use of HBOT to treat ischemic ulcers in patients with diabetes.

Faglia and coworkers[172] performed the largest ($n = 70$) randomized, controlled trial of the efficacy of adjunctive HBOT in reducing major amputation in patients with severe, infected, ischemic diabetic foot ulcers. All patients underwent a standardized evaluation, including angiography if the ankle–brachial index was less than 0.9 or transcutaneous oxygen (see later) was less than 50 mm Hg, initial aggressive surgical debridement, standardized wound care, and optimized medical care. Restoration of arterial inflow by angioplasty or bypass surgery was performed if indicated and possible. Subjects in the treatment arm received HBOT at 2.4 ATA for 90 minutes daily. The decision to perform amputation was made by a consultant surgeon unaware of the study assignment. The treatment group underwent fewer major amputations (treatment group: 3/35 including 2 below-knee amputations and 1 above-knee amputation; control group: 11/33 including 7 below-knee amputations and 4 above-knee amputations; $P = 0.016$). Roeckl-Wiedmann and investigators[173] calculated a number needed to treat value (for the three studies that included major amputation as an outcome: Faglia and coworkers,[172] Abidia and coauthors,[174] and Doctor and colleagues[175]) of four patients to prevent one major amputation.

Table 11.2 Wound Healing–Related Indications for Hyperbaric Oxygen Therapy Recognized by the Undersea and Hyperbaric Medical Society

INDICATION	MECHANISMS FOR EFFICACY
Acute thermal burns	Reduced edema Infection control Increased epithelization and graft take
Clostridial myositis and myonecrosis	Suppression of toxin production Enhanced neutrophil function Antibiotic potentiation
Other necrotizing soft-tissue infections	Enhanced neutrophil function Antibiotic potentiation
Compromised skin grafts*	Increased neovascularization Reduced edema
Compromised flaps*	Amelioration of ischemia-reperfusion injury Reduced edema
Crush injury, compartment syndrome, and other acute ischemias	Amelioration of ischemia-reperfusion injury Reduced edema
Osteoradionecrosis	Increased neovascularization
Soft-tissue radionecrosis	Increased neovascularization
Refractory osteomyelitis	Enhanced neutrophil function Antibiotic potentiation Increased osteogenesis
Problem wounds†	Increased neovascularization Increased collagen deposition Increased epithelization Reduced edema Reduced inflammation Enhanced neutrophil function
Diabetic foot ulcers (Wagner grade 3+)†	Increased granulation Enhanced neutrophil function Reduced edema

*Compromised skin grafts and flaps are treated as a single indication by the Undersea and Hyperbaric Medical Society (UHMS) and Centers for Medicare and Medicaid Services (CMS). They are separated here because the mechanisms underlying the benefit for each differ somewhat.
†The UHMS Hyperbaric Oxygen Therapy Committee Report retained the classification of "Problem Wound" in 2003, although this is likely to evolve toward an indication specifically for hypoxic wounds. CMS reviewed this issue and published a coverage memorandum in 2002 providing coverage for Wagner grade 3 or higher diabetic lower extremity wounds that have not responded to a course of standard therapy.

Although hypoxic wounds may occur in patients without significant peripheral arterial occlusive disease, ischemic wounds are most likely to benefit from HBOT. One randomized, controlled trial[176] demonstrates a more rapid decrease in size in venous leg ulcers (without a significant arterial component) treated with HBOT. Standard therapy of venous leg ulcers includes moist wound care and compression, and these are successful in most patients.[177] HBOT cannot replace compression therapy. It may be useful in selected patients to treat compromised skin grafts, particularly in patients with mixed venous-arterial ulcers, or in patients with uncorrected wound hypoxia despite appropriate compression and edema control.

Standard therapy of pressure ulcers includes pressure relief, debridement, nutritional support, achievement of bacterial balance, and moist wound care.[178] HBOT may be useful in selected patients with compromised skin grafts or flaps, when the ulcer develops at the site of previous radiation or when there is underlying refractory osteomyelitis.

Standard therapy of arterial insufficiency ulcers includes restoration of arterial inflow, followed by debridement and moist wound care.[10] HBOT may benefit patients in whom revascularization is unsuccessful, or is successful but fails to correct wound hypoxia, although this has not been demonstrated, except in such patients who also have diabetes. HBOT may be useful in selected patients with compromised

Table 11.3 Trials of Hyperbaric Oxygen Therapy in Diabetic Foot Ulcers

FIRST AUTHOR, YEAR (COUNTRY)	STUDY DESIGN	N	CONDITION	RESULTS
Doctor,[175] 1992 (India)	RCT	30 (15 HBO, 15 control)	Hospitalized DFU	Above-ankle amputations— HBO: 2/15; control: 7/15; $P < 0.05$ Minor amputations: NS Number of positive cultures decreased in HBO group; $P < 0.05$
Faglia,[172] 1996 (Italy)	RCT	70 (35 HBO, 33 control, 2 lost to follow-up)	Severe, infected, ischemic DFU	Major amputations—HBO 3/35 (8.6%); control: 11/33 (33.3%); $P = 0.016$
Abidia,[174] 2003 (UK)	RCT, double-blind, sham	18 (8 HBO, 8 control; 2 lost to follow-up)	Ischemic DFU, 1–10 mm in diameter	Healing at 12-week follow-up point—HBO: 5/8; control: 1/8
Kalani,[181] 2002 (Sweden)	RCT + CT	38 (17 HBO, 21 control)	DFU	Healing at 3-year follow-up point—HBO: 13/17 (76%); control 10/21 (48%) Amputations—HBO: 2/17 (12%); control: 7/21 (33%)
Kessler,[182] 2003 (France)	RCT	28	Wagner grades 1–3 DFU	HBO: wounds smaller at 2 and 4 weeks, more healed at 2 weeks
Zamboni,[183] 1997 (USA)	CT	10 (5 HBO, 5 control)	DFU	HBO with standard wound care reduced wound size compared with standard wound care alone; $P < 0.05$ At 4–6 months, HBO group had higher rate of complete healing (4/5 vs. 1/5 in control group)
Baroni,[184] 1987 (Italy)	CT	28 (18 HBO, 10 control)	DFU	Healing—HBO: 16/18 (89%); control: 1/10 (10%); $P = 0.001$ Amputations—HBO: 2/18; control: 4/10
Davis,[185] 1987 (USA)	Retrospective review	168 HBO	DFU	118/168 (70%) patients healed at a level providing for bipedal ambulation, 50/168 (30%) required a BKA or AKA, failures in patients with nonbypassable arterial disease at or above ankle
Oriani,[186] 1990 (Italy)	Retrospective comparison	80 (62 HBO, 18 control)	DFU	"Recovery"—HBO: 59/62 (96%); control: 12/18 (67%) Amputation—HBO: 3/62 (5%); control: 6/18 (33%); $P < 0.001$
Wattel,[187] 1991 (France)	Retrospective consecutive review	59 HBO	DFU	52/59 (88%) healed without major amputation, 7/59 (12%) required major amputation, significantly greater $tcPo_2$ values achieved during HBO (786 ± 258 mm Hg vs. 323 ± 214) in success compared with failures
Oriani,[188] 1992 (Italy)	Retrospective consecutive review uncontrolled	151 HBO (may include patients from 1990 series)	DFU	130/151, 86% healed with HBO; 21/115, 14% did not respond to HBO

Table 11.3 Trials of Hyperbaric Oxygen Therapy in Diabetic Foot Ulcers—Cont'd

FIRST AUTHOR, YEAR (COUNTRY)	STUDY DESIGN	N	CONDITION	RESULTS
Stone,[189] 1995 (USA)	Retrospective review Abstract	469 (87 HBO, 382 control)	DFU	Limb salvage—HBO: 72%; control: 53%; $P < 0.002$
Faglia,[190] 1998 (Italy)	Compare	115 (51 HBO, 64 control)	DFU	Major amputations—HBO: 7/51; control: 20/64; $P = 0.012$
Fife,[19] 2002 (USA)	Retrospective review	1144 HBO	DFU	Overall 75% of patients improved with HBO, mean 34 treatments. By Wagner score—I: 100% ($n = 3$); II: 83.1% ($n = 130$); III: 77.2% ($n = 465$); IV: 64.5% ($n = 64.5$%); V: 29.7% ($n = 37$)

AKA, above-knee amputation; BKA, below-knee amputation; DFU, diabetic foot ulcer; HBO, hyperbaric oxygen; NS, not significant; RCT, randomized, controlled trial; tcPo₂, transcutaneous oximetry.

From Warriner RA, Hopf HW: Enhancement of Healing in Selected Problem Wounds, Hyperbaric Oxygen 2003: Indications and Results. In: Feldmeier JJ (ed): The Hyperbaric Oxygen Therapy Committee Report. Kensington, MD, Undersea and Hyperbaric Medical Society, 2003, pp 45-47, by permission.

skin grafts. After revascularization, many patients develop reperfusion injury that delays healing. Mechanistically, this is likely to be ameliorated by HBOT, but clinical trials are required to evaluate efficacy.

Selection of Patients for Hyperbaric Oxygen Therapy for Adjunctive Therapy of Nonhealing Wounds: Transcutaneous Oximetry

Identifying wounds most likely to benefit is paramount for cost-effective application of HBOT. Patients with wounds that fall within a category defined as potentially appropriate for adjunctive HBOT (see Table 11.2) should be evaluated for likelihood of benefit. Hypoxia (i.e., wound $P_{O_2} < 40$ mm Hg) generally best defines wounds appropriate for HBOT—or rather, lack of hypoxia (i.e., wound $P_{O_2} > 40$ to 50 mm Hg) defines wounds not appropriate for HBOT.[19,20,179] Although several tests intended to identify significant wound hypoxia and/or ischemia have been used, including ankle–brachial index, skin perfusion pressure, and laser–Doppler flow, transcutaneous oximetry (tcPo₂) is generally accepted as most valuable in the following ways:

- Predicting failure to heal a wound without intervention
- Predicting failure to heal a planned amputation
- Predicting failure to respond to HBOT
- Predicting and evaluating success of revascularization

Notably, tcPo₂ is a better predictor of failure than success. This underlines the central role of oxygen in wound healing. That is, there is a level of oxygen below which a wound does not have the capacity to heal. Wounds with a P_{O_2} greater than that level, however, are not guaranteed to heal because there is a variety of nonoxygen-related impediments to healing that may prevent the normal progression of repair in the presence of adequate tissue oxygen.

tcPo₂ measurements provide a direct, quantitative assessment of oxygen availability to the periwound skin and an indirect measurement of periwound microcirculatory blood flow. tcPo₂ is a noninvasive measurement in which a small, heated polarographic oxygen electrode is applied to the skin. Normally, little oxygen diffuses through the skin. Heating the probe to 42°C to 45°C increases skin oxygen permeability and enables the measurement. The heated area appears to be small enough that, although blood vessels under the probe become dilated, the stimulus is not sufficient to increase overall blood flow to the limb or skin perfusion outside the probe area.

Wütschert and Bounameaux[42] performed a meta-analysis to determine the ability of tcPo$_2$ measured at sea level with patients breathing room air to predict amputation level, using studies published from 1985 through 1996. There were a total of 615 lower limb amputations (51% in patients with diabetes), and the reamputation rate was 16.4%. Failure was defined as more proximal amputation or extensive (operative) debridement of the stump. They found that 20 mm Hg was the most useful cutoff for failure to heal, with a sensitivity of 82% and specificity of 64%. The positive predictive value (failed to heal) of the 20-mm Hg cutoff was 92%, and the negative predictive value 42%. The accuracy rate was 79%.

tcPo$_2$ is a more effective marker of inadequate wound oxygenation than laser–Doppler assessment or the ankle–brachial index. Thirty-eight studies since 1982 suggest that hypoxia (i.e., inability to heal) should be defined as sea-level room air tcPo$_2$ less than 10 to 40 mm Hg.[10] In general, tcPo$_2$ less than 20 mm Hg is associated with failure to heal, whereas tcPo$_2$ of 20 to 40 mm Hg is associated with delayed healing and greater susceptibility to infection[179] (which may be catastrophic in a hypoxic wound).

Although sea-level room air tcPo$_2$ reliably predicts a failure to heal, it does so only in the context that no intervention (revascularization,

HBOT) is undertaken to correct wound hypoxia. A few studies have suggested that breathing increased inspired oxygen at sea level[179] (usually 10-15 liters per minute via nonrebreather mask or hyperbaric oxygen hood) predicts the likelihood of a response to HBOT, but the most predictive measure appears to be tcPo$_2$ measured at pressure (2-2.4 ATA) in a hyperbaric oxygen chamber breathing 100% oxygen.[19,20,179,180] Although greater elevation of tcPo$_2$ is associated with a greater likelihood of positive outcome, there does not appear to be a therapeutic benefit of 2.4 versus 2.0 ATA.[19] Lack of an increase in tcPo$_2$ to more than 100 mm Hg appears to be an appropriate cutoff for predicting failure to heal, at least in ischemic diabetic foot ulcers (Fig. 11.6). This requirement for achieving supraphysiologic wound oxygen concentration lends support to the argument that restoration of wound normoxia is not the primary mechanism of action of HBOT in healing hypoxic wounds. The failure rate for less than 100 mm Hg is not 100%, however, so it is not unreasonable to give a trial of HBOT (10-15 treatments) to such patients for whom the alternative is amputation.

SUMMARY

Wound repair is a complex process that requires an intact hemostatic and inflammatory response, appropriate matrix formation (largely

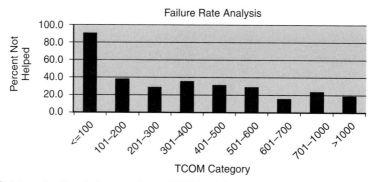

Figure 11.6 Failure rate of hyperbaric oxygen therapy (HBOT) in relation to transcutaneous oximetry (TCOM, or tcPo$_2$) in the chamber at pressure. Failure rate increases as in-chamber tcPo$_2$ decreases. When in-chamber tcPo$_2$ is less than 100 mm Hg, the failure rate is 90%. However, as in-chamber tcPo$_2$ increases to greater than 400 mm Hg, there is little incremental improvement in healing likelihood. *(From Fife CE, Buyukcakir C, Otto GH, et al: The predictive value of transcutaneous oxygen tension measurement in diabetic lower extremity ulcers treated with hyperbaric oxygen therapy: A retrospective analysis of 1,144 patients. Wound Repair Regen 10:198-207, 2002, by permission.)*

collagen) and neovascularization of the injured area, restoration of an intact skin barrier via epithelization, and remodeling to create the strongest possible scar. Although numerous factors, both local and systemic, may impede the progression of an injury through a timely and orderly repair process, inadequate oxygen supply universally prevents or delays healing and puts the patient at high risk for development of an infection. Although arterial occlusive disease is a common cause of impaired wound oxygenation, and thereby impaired wound healing, wounds may become hypoxic despite adequate arterial inflow because of vasoconstriction of vessels feeding the wound or failure of neovascularization within the wound. Common causes of vasoconstriction include cold exposure, inadequate fluid intake, inadequate pain control, and stress, which act via sympathetic nervous system activation. These are all amenable to simple and inexpensive interventions, and correction improves healing. Common causes of impaired neovascularization include soft-tissue radiation injury, diabetes, and wound hypoxia, all of which may be correctable by HBOT. HBOT works by increasing oxygen diffusion into the wound, thereby restoring wound normoxia, and by the pharmacologic action of hyperoxia, which induces stem cell mobilization, up-regulates growth factors and growth factor receptors, and inhibits neutrophil adhesion, among other effects. HBOT should be considered in the management of hypoxic wounds. Currently, clinical trials provide the most support for use in bone and soft-tissue radiation injury, compromised skin grafts and flaps, and ischemic diabetic foot ulcers.

REFERENCES

1. Arnold M, Barbul A: Nutrition and wound healing. Plast Reconstr Surg 117:42S-58S, 2006.
2. Hunt T, Hopf H: Nutrition in Wound Healing. In: Fischer J (ed): Nutrition and Metabolism in the Surgical Patient, 2nd ed. Boston, Little, Brown and Company, 1996, pp 423-441.
3. Jensen JA, Jonsson K, Goodson WH, et al: Epinephrine lowers subcutaneous wound oxygen tension. Curr Surg 42:472-474, 1985.
4. Mogford JE, Sisco M, Bonomo SR, et al: Impact of aging on gene expression in a rat model of ischemic cutaneous wound healing. J Surg Res 118: 190-196, 2004.
5. Mogford JE, Tawil N, Chen A, et al: Effect of age and hypoxia on TGFbeta1 receptor expression and signal transduction in human dermal fibroblasts: Impact on cell migration. J Cell Physiol 190:259-265, 2002.
6. Lenhardt R, Hopf HW, Marker E, et al: Perioperative collagen deposition in elderly and young men and women. Arch Surg 135:71-74, 2000.
7. Robson MC, Mannari RJ, Smith PD, Payne WG: Maintenance of wound bacterial balance. Am J Surg 178:399-402, 1999.
8. Winter GD: Formation of the scab and the rate of epithelisation of superficial wounds in the skin of the young domestic pig. 1962. J Wound Care 4: 366-371, 1995.
9. Jonsson K, Jensen J, Goodson W, et al: Tissue oxygenation, anemia, and perfusion in relation to wound healing in surgical patients. Ann Surg 214:605-613, 1991.
10. Hopf HW, Ueno C, Aslam R, et al: Guidelines for the treatment of arterial insufficiency ulcers. Wound Repair Regen 14:693-710, 2006.
11. Ueno C, Hunt TK, Hopf HW: Using physiology to improve surgical wound outcomes. Plast Reconstr Surg 117:59S-71S, 2006.
12. Allen DB, Maguire JJ, Mahdavian M, et al: Wound hypoxia and acidosis limit neutrophil bacterial killing mechanisms. Arch Surg 132:991-996, 1997.
13. DeJong L, Kemp A: Stoicheiometry and kinetics of the prolyl 4-hydroxylase partial reaction. Biochim Biophys Acta 787:105-111, 1984.
14. Evans NTS, Naylor PFD: Steady states of oxygen tension in human dermis. Respir Physiol 2:46-60, 1966.
15. Hopf H, Hunt T, Jensen J: Calculation of subcutaneous tissue blood flow. Surg Forum 39:33-36, 1988.
16. Medawar PS: The behavior of mammalian skin epithelium under strictly anaerobic conditions. Q J Microsc Sci 88:27, 1947.
17. Hopf HW, Gibson JJ, Angeles AP, et al: Hyperoxia and angiogenesis. Wound Repair Regen 13:558-564, 2005.
18. Sheffield PJ: Tissue Oxygen Measurements. In: Davis JC, Hunt TK (eds): Problem Wounds: The Role of Oxygen. New York, Elsevier, 1988, pp 17-51.
19. Fife CE, Buyukcakir C, Otto GH, et al: The predictive value of transcutaneous oxygen tension measurement in diabetic lower extremity ulcers treated with hyperbaric oxygen therapy: A retrospective analysis of 1,144 patients. Wound Repair Regen 10:198-207, 2002.
20. Smith B, Desvigne L, Slade J, et al: Transcutaneous oxygen measurements predict healing of leg wounds with hyperbaric therapy. Wound Repair Regen 4:224-229, 1996.
21. Rollins MD, Gibson JJ, Hunt TK, Hopf HW: Wound oxygen levels during hyperbaric oxygen treatment in healing wounds. Undersea Hyperb Med 33:17-25, 2006.
22. Fife C: Hyperbaric Oxygen Therapy Applications in Wound Care. In: Sheffield P, Smith A, Fife C (eds): Wound Care Practice. Flagstaff, Ariz, Best Publishing Company, 2004, pp 661-684.
23. Schulz G: Molecular Regulation of Wound Healing. In: Bryant R, Nix D (eds): Acute and Chronic Wounds: Current Management Concepts, 3rd ed. St. Louis, Mosby Elsevier, 2006, pp 82-99.
24. Adams JC: Functions of the conserved thrombospondin carboxy-terminal cassette in cell-extracellular matrix

interactions and signaling. Int J Biochem Cell Biol 36:1102-1114, 2004.

25. Mast B, Schultz G: Interactions of cytokines, growth factors, and proteases in acute and chronic wounds. Wound Repair Regen 4:411-420, 1996.

26. Constant J, Suh D, Hussain M, Hunt T: Wound healing angiogenesis: The metabolic basis of repair. In: Maragoudakis ME (ed): Molecular, Cellular, and Clinical Aspects of Angiogenesis. New York, Plenum Press, 1996, pp 151-159.

27. Dvonch VM, Murphey RJ, Matsuoka J, Grotendorst GR: Changes in growth factor levels in human wound fluid. Surgery 112:18-23, 1992.

28. Heppenstall RB, Littooy FN, Fuchs R, et al: Gas tensions in healing tissues of traumatized patients. Surgery 75:874-880, 1974.

29. Zabel DD, Feng JJ, Scheuenstuhl H, et al: Lactate stimulation of macrophage-derived angiogenic activity is associated with inhibition of poly(ADP-ribos) synthesis. Lab Invest 74:644-649, 1996.

30. Caldwell MD, Shearer J, Morris A, et al: Evidence for aerobic glycolysis in lambda-carrageenan-wounded skeletal muscle. J Surg Res 37:63-68, 1984.

31. Trabold O, Wagner S, Wicke C, et al: Lactate and oxygen constitute a fundamental regulatory mechanism in wound healing. Wound Repair Regen 11:504-509, 2003.

32. Remensnyder JP, Majno G: Oxygen gradients in healing wounds. Am J Pathol 52:301-323, 1968.

33. Klebanoff S: Oxygen metabolism and the toxic properties of phagocytes. Ann Intern Med 93:480-489, 1980.

34. Silver IA: Cellular microenvironment in healing and non-healing wounds. Hunt TK, Heppenstall RB, Pines E, (eds): Soft and Hard Tissue Repair. New York, Praeger, 1984, pp 50-66.

35. Niinikoski J, Hunt TK, Dunphy JE: Oxygen supply in healing tissue. Am J Surg 123:247-252, 1972.

36. Falcone PA, Caldwell MD: Wound metabolism. Clin Plast Surg 17:443-456, 1990.

37. Hopf HW, Hunt TK, West JM, et al: Wound tissue oxygen tension predicts the risk of wound infection in surgical patients. Arch Surg 132:997-1005, 1997.

38. Chang N, Mathes SJ: Comparison of the effect of bacterial inoculation in musculocutaneous and random-pattern flaps. Plast Reconstr Surg 95:527-536, 1982.

39. Knighton DR, Halliday B, Hunt TK: Oxygen as an antibiotic: The effect of inspired oxygen on infection. Arch Surg 119:199-204, 1984.

40. Schwentker A, Evans SM, Partington M, et al: A model of wound healing in chronically radiation-damaged rat skin. Cancer Lett 128:71-78, 1998.

41. Bauer SM, Goldstein LJ, Bauer RJ, et al: The bone marrow-derived endothelial progenitor cell response is impaired in delayed wound healing from ischemia. J Vasc Surg 43:134-141, 2006.

42. Wütschert R, Bounameaux H: Determination of amputation level in ischemic limbs. Reappraisal of the measurement of TcPo2. Diabetes Care 20:1315-1318, 1997.

43. Dowd GS: Predicting stump healing following amputation for peripheral vascular disease using the transcutaneous oxygen monitor. Ann R Coll Surg Engl 69:31-35, 1987.

44. Ito K, Ohgi S, Mori T, et al: Determination of amputation level in ischemic legs by means of transcutaneous

oxygen pressure measurement. Int Surg 69: 59-61, 1984.

45. Beckert S, Farrahi F, Aslam RS, et al: Lactate stimulates endothelial cell migration. Wound Repair Regen 14:321-324, 2006.

46. Babior BM: Oxygen-dependent microbial killing by phagocytes. N Engl J Med 198:659-668, 1978.

47. Edwards S, Hallett M, Campbell A: Oxygen-radical production during inflammation may be limited by oxygen concentration. Biochem J 217:851-854, 1984.

48. Gabig TG, Bearman SI, Babior BM: Effects of oxygen tension and pH on the respiratory burst of human neutrophils. Blood 53:1133-1139, 1979.

49. Sheffield PJ: Measuring tissue oxygen tension: A review. Undersea Hyperb Med 25:179-188, 1998.

50. Mader JT: Phagocytic killing and hyperbaric oxygen: Antibacterial mechanisms. HBO Rev 2:37-49, 1981.

51. Mader JT, Brown GL, Guckian JC, et al: A mechanism for the amelioration by hyperbaric oxygen of experimental staphylococcal osteomyelitis in rabbits. J Infect Dis 142:915-922, 1980.

52. Sen CK, Khanna S, Babior BM, et al: Oxidant-induced vascular endothelial growth factor expression in human keratinocytes and cutaneous wound healing. J Biol Chem 277:33284-33290, 2002.

53. Niinikoski J, Jussila P, Vihersaari T: Radical mastectomy wound as a model for studies of human wound metabolism. Am J Surg 126:53-58, 1973.

54. Hunt TK, Knighton DR, Thakral KK, et al: Studies on inflammation and wound healing: Angiogenesis and collagen synthesis stimulated in vivo by resident and activated wound macrophages. Surgery 96:48-54, 1984.

55. Jensen JA, Hunt TK, Scheuenstuhl H, et al: Effect of lactate, pyruvate and pH on secretion of angiogenesis and mitogenesis factors by macrophages. Lab Invest 54:574-578, 1986.

56. Ehrlich H, Hunt T: Effects of cortisone and vitamin A on wound healing. Ann Surg 167:324-328, 1968.

57. Hunt TK, Aslam RS, Beckert S, et al: Aerobically derived lactate stimulates revascularization and tissue repair via redox mechanisms. Antioxid Redox Signal 9:1115-1124, 2007.

58. Velazquez OC: Angiogenesis and vasculogenesis: Inducing the growth of new blood vessels and wound healing by stimulation of bone marrow-derived progenitor cell mobilization and homing. J Vasc Surg 45(suppl A):A39-A47, 2007.

59. Capla JM, Ceradini DJ, Tepper OM, et al: Skin graft vascularization involves precisely regulated regression and replacement of endothelial cells through both angiogenesis and vasculogenesis. Plast Reconstr Surg 117:836-844, 2006.

60. Schultz G, Grant M: Neovascular growth factors. Eye 5:170-180, 1991.

61. Sheikh AY, Gibson JJ, Rollins MD, et al: Effect of hyperoxia on vascular endothelial growth factor levels in a wound model. Arch Surg 135:1293-1297, 2000.

62. Beckert S, Hierlemann H, Muschenborn N, et al: Experimental ischemic wounds: Correlation of cell proliferation and insulin-like growth factor I expression and its modification by different local IGF-I release systems. Wound Repair Regen 13:278-283, 2005.

63. Knighton DR, Silver IA, Hunt TK: Regulation of wound-healing angiogenesis—effect of oxygen gradients and inspired oxygen concentration. Surgery 90:262-270, 1981.

64. Myllyla R, Tuderman L, Kivirikko KI: Mechanism of the prolyl hydroxylase reaction. 2. Kinetic analysis of the reaction sequence. Eur J Biochem 80:349-357, 1977.

65. Prockop DJ, Kivirikko KI, Tuderman L, Guzman NA: The biosynthesis of collagen and its disorders (first of two parts). N Engl J Med 301:13-23, 1979.

66. Uitto J, Prockop DJ: Synthesis and secretion of under-hydroxylated procollagen at various temperatures by cells subject to temporary anoxia. Biochem Biophys Res Commun 60:414, 1974.

67. Knighton DR, Hunt TK, Scheuenstuhl H, et al: Oxygen tension regulates the expression of angiogenesis factor by macrophages. Science 221:1283-1285, 1983.

68. Constant JS, Feng JJ, Zabel DD, et al: Lactate elicits vascular endothelial growth factor from macrophages: A possible alternative to hypoxia. Wound Repair Regen 8:353-360, 2000.

69. Laato M, Heino J, Gerdin B, et al: Interferon-gamma-induced inhibition of wound healing in vivo and in vitro. Ann Chir Gynaecol 90:19-23, 2001.

70. Wagner S, Hussain MZ, Beckert S, et al: Lactate down-regulates cellular poly(ADP-ribose) formation in cultured human skin fibroblasts. Eur J Clin Invest 37:134-139, 2007.

71. Ghani QP, Wagner S, Hussain MZ: Role of ADP-ribosylation in wound repair. The contributions of Thomas K. Hunt, MD. Wound Repair Regen 11:439-444, 2003.

72. Semenza GL: Regulation of tissue perfusion by hypoxia-inducible factor 1. Exp Physiol 92:988-991, 2007.

73. Wang GL, Jiang BH, Rue EA, Semenza GL: Hypoxia-inducible factor 1 is a basic-helix-loop-helix-PAS heterodimer regulated by cellular O2 tension. Proc Natl Acad Sci U S A 92:5510-5514, 1995.

74. Roy S, Khanna S, Nallu K, et al: Dermal wound healing is subject to redox control. Mol Ther 13:211-220, 2006.

75. Hirota K, Semenza GL: Regulation of hypoxia-inducible factor 1 by prolyl and asparaginyl hydroxylases. Biochem Biophys Res Commun 338:610-616, 2005.

76. Lu H, Dalgard CL, Mohyeldin A, et al: Reversible inactivation of HIF-1 prolyl hydroxylases allows cell metabolism to control basal HIF-1. J Biol Chem 280:41928-41939, 2005.

77. Lu H, Forbes RA, Verma A: Hypoxia-inducible factor 1 activation by aerobic glycolysis implicates the Warburg effect in carcinogenesis. J Biol Chem 277: 23111-23115, 2002.

78. Maxwell PH, Wiesener MS, Chang GW, et al: The tumour suppressor protein VHL targets hypoxia-inducible factors for oxygen-dependent proteolysis. Nature 399:271-275, 1999.

79. Abu El-Asrar AM, Missotten L, Geboes K: Expression of hypoxia-inducible factor-1alpha and the protein products of its target genes in diabetic fibrovascular epiretinal membranes. Br J Ophthalmol 91: 822-826, 2007.

80. Sen CK: The general case for redox control of wound repair. Wound Repair Regen 11:431-438, 2003.

81. Rhee SG: Redox signaling: hydrogen peroxide as intracellular messenger. Exp Mol Med 31:53-59, 1999.

82. Suh YA, Arnold RS, Lassegue B, et al: Cell transformation by the superoxide-generating oxidase Mox1. Nature 401:79-82, 1999.

83. Babior B, Woodman R: Chronic granulomatous disease. Semin Hematol 27:247-259, 1990.

84. Lineaweaver W, Howard R, Soucy D, et al: Topical antimicrobial toxicity. Arch Surg 120:267-270, 1985.

85. Knowles RG, Moncada S: Nitric oxide synthases in mammals. Biochem J 298(pt 2):249-258, 1994.

86. Shearer JD, Richards JR, Mills CD, Caldwell MD: Differential regulation of macrophage arginine metabolism: A proposed role in wound healing. Am J Physiol 272: E181-E190, 1997.

87. Rizk M, Witte MB, Barbul A: Nitric oxide and wound healing. World J Surg 28:301-306, 2004.

88. Stamler JS, Jaraki O, Osborne J, et al: Nitric oxide circulates in mammalian plasma primarily as an S-nitroso adduct of serum albumin. Proc Natl Acad Sci U S A 89:7674-7677, 1992.

89. Barbul A, Lazarou S, Efron D, et al: Arginine enhances wound healing and lymphocyte immune response in humans. Surgery 108:331-337, 1990.

90. Murrell GA, Szabo C, Hannafin JA, et al: Modulation of tendon healing by nitric oxide. Inflamm Res 46:19-27, 1997.

91. Schaffer MR, Tantry U, Gross SS, et al: Nitric oxide regulates wound healing. J Surg Res 63:237-240, 1996.

92. Schaffer MR, Tantry U, Thornton FJ, Barbul A: Inhibition of nitric oxide synthesis in wounds: Pharmacology and effect on accumulation of collagen in wounds in mice. Eur J Surg 165:262-267, 1999.

93. Modolell M, Eichmann K, Soler G: Oxidation of N(G)-hydroxyl-L-arginine to nitric oxide mediated by respiratory burst: An alternative pathway to NO synthesis. FEBS Lett 401:123-126, 1997.

94. Shizukuda Y, Tang S, Yokota R, Ware JA: Vascular endothelial growth factor-induced endothelial cell migration and proliferation depend on a nitric oxide-mediated decrease in protein kinase Cdelta activity. Circ Res 85:247-256, 1999.

95. Noiri E, Hu Y, Bahou WF, et al: Permissive role of nitric oxide in endothelin-induced migration of endothelial cells. J Biol Chem 272:1747-1752, 1997.

96. Noiri E, Lee E, Testa J, et al: Podokinesis in endothelial cell migration: Role of nitric oxide. Am J Physiol 274: C236-C244, 1998.

97. Fadini GP, Miorin M, Facco M, et al: Circulating endothelial progenitor cells are reduced in peripheral vascular complications of type 2 diabetes mellitus. J Am Coll Cardiol 45:1449-1457, 2005.

98. Tepper OM, Galiano RD, Capla JM, et al: Human endothelial progenitor cells from type II diabetics exhibit impaired proliferation, adhesion, and incorporation into vascular structures. Circulation 106:2781-2786, 2002.

99. Loomans CJ, de Koning EJ, Staal FJ, et al: Endothelial progenitor cell dysfunction: A novel concept in the pathogenesis of vascular complications of type 1 diabetes. Diabetes 53:195-199, 2004.

100. Gallagher KA, Goldstein LJ, Thom SR, Velazquez OC: Hyperbaric oxygen and bone marrow-derived endothelial

progenitor cells in diabetic wound healing. Vascular 14:328-337, 2006.

101. Thom SR, Bhopale VM, Velazquez OC, et al: Stem cell mobilization by hyperbaric oxygen. Am J Physiol Heart Circ Physiol 290:H1378-H1386, 2006.

102. Goldstein IJ, Gallagher KA, Bauer SM, et al: Endothelial progenitor cell release into circulation is triggered by hyperoxia-induced increases in bone marrow nitric oxide. Stem Cells 24:2309-2318, 2006.

103. Gallagher KA, Liu ZJ, Xiao M, et al: Diabetic impairments in NO-mediated endothelial progenitor cell mobilization and homing are reversed by hyperoxia and SDF-1 alpha. J Clin Invest 117:1249-1259, 2007.

104. Silver IA: Oxygen tension and epithelialization. Maibach HI, Rovee DT (ed): Epidermal Wound Healing. Chicago, Year Book Medical Publishers, 1972, pp 291.

105. Feldmeier JJ, Hopf HW, Warriner RA 3rd, et al: UHMS position statement: Topical oxygen for chronic wounds. Undersea Hyperb Med 32:157-168, 2005.

106. Ngo MA, Sinitsyna NN, Qin Q, Rice RH: Oxygen-dependent differentiation of human keratinocytes. J Invest Dermatol 127:354-361, 2007.

107. O'Toole EA, Marinkovich MP, Peavey CL, et al: Hypoxia increases human keratinocyte motility on connective tissue. J Clin Invest 100:2881-2891, 1997.

108. Doughty DB: Preventing and managing surgical wound dehiscence. Adv Skin Wound Care 18:319-322, 2005.

109. Fuchs U, Zittermann A, Stuettgen B, et al: Clinical outcome of patients with deep sternal wound infection managed by vacuum-assisted closure compared to conventional therapy with open packing: A retrospective analysis. Ann Thorac Surg 79:526-531, 2005.

110. Haydock D, Hill G: Improved wound healing response in surgical patients receiving intravenous nutrition. Br J Surg 74:320-323, 1987.

111. Goodson WD, Lopez SA, Jensen JA, et al: The influence of a brief preoperative illness on postoperative healing. Ann Surg 205:250-255, 1987.

112. Patel GK: The role of nutrition in the management of lower extremity wounds. Int J Low Extrem Wounds 4:12-22, 2005.

113. Lund C, Levenson SM, Green R, et al: Ascorbic acid, thiamine, riboflavin and nicotinic acid in relation to acute burns in man. Arch Surg 55:557-583, 1947.

114. Levenson SM, Upjohn HL, Preston JA, Steer A: Effect of thermal burns on wound healing. Ann Surg 146:357-368, 1957.

115. Hunt T, Ehrlich H, Garcia J, Dunphy J: Effect of vitamin A on reversing the inhibitor effect of cortisone on healing of open wounds in animals and man. Ann Surg 170:633-641, 1969.

116. Wicke C, Halliday B, Allen D, et al: Effects of steroids and retinoids on wound healing. Arch Surg 135:1265-1270, 2000.

117. Seifter E, Rettura G, Padawer J, et al: Impaired wound healing in streptozotocin diabetes: Prevention by supplemental vitamin A. Ann Surg 194:42, 1981.

118. Winsey K, Simon RJ, Levenson SM, et al: Effect of supplemental vitamin A on colon anastomotic healing in rats given preoperative irradiation. Am J Surg 153:153-156, 1987.

119. Toyama T, Ohura N, Kurita M, et al: Effectiveness of short-contact topical tretinoin in promoting wound healing in db/db mice. Scand J Plast Reconstr Surg Hand Surg 40:329-334, 2006.

120. Paquette D, Badiavas E, Falanga V: Short-contact topical tretinoin therapy to stimulate granulation tissue in chronic wounds. J Am Acad Dermatol 45:382-386, 2001.

121. Haws M, Brown RE, Suchy H, Roth A: Vitamin A-soaked gelfoam sponges and wound healing in steroid-treated animals. Ann Plast Surg 32:418-422, 1994.

122. Ehrlich HP, Tarver H, Hunt TK. Inhibitory effects of vitamin E on collagen synthesis and wound repair. Ann Surg 175:235-240, 1972.

123. Miles A, Miles E, Burke J: The value and duration of defence reactions of the skin to the primary lodgment of bacteria. Br J Exp Pathol 38:79-96, 1957.

124. Gottrup F, Firmin R, Rabkin J, et al: Directly measured tissue oxygen tension and arterial oxygen tension assess tissue perfusion. Crit Care Med 15:1030-1036, 1987.

125. Sheffield P, Smith A: Physiological and Pharmacological Basis of Hyperbaric Oxygen Therapy. In Bakker D, Cramer F (eds): Hyperbaric Surgery: Perioperative Care. Flagstaff, Ariz, Best Publishing, 2002, pp 63-77.

126. Hutton JJ, Tappel AL, Udenfriend S: Cofactor and substrate requirements of collagen proline hydroxylase. Arch Biochem Biophys 118:231-240, 1967.

127. Hohn DC, MacKay RD, Halliday B, Hunt TK: Effect of O2 tension on microbicidal function of leukocytes in wounds and in vitro. Surg Forum 27:18-20, 1976.

128. Jonsson K, Hunt TK, Mathes SJ: Oxygen as an isolated variable influences resistance to infection. Ann Surg 208:783-787, 1988.

129. Jensen JA, Goodson WH, Hopf HW, Hunt TK: Cigarette smoking decreases tissue oxygen. Arch Surg 126:1131-1134, 1991.

130. Hopf HW, Viele M, Watson JJ, et al: Subcutaneous perfusion and oxygen during acute severe isovolemic hemodilution in healthy volunteers. Arch Surg 135:1443-1449, 2000.

131. Hopf H, Hunt T: Does—and if so, to what extent—normovolemic dilutional anemia influence postoperative wound healing? Chirugische Gastroenterologie 8:148-150, 1992.

132. Reference deleted in proofs.

133. Jensen JA, Goodson WH, Vasconez LO, Hunt TK: Wound healing in anemia. West J Med 144:465-467, 1986.

134. Sheffield C, Sessler D, Hopf H, et al: Centrally and locally mediated thermoregulatory responses alter subcutaneous oxygen tension. Wound Repair Regen 4:339-345, 1996.

135. Rabkin JM, Hunt TK: Local heat increases blood flow and oxygen tension in wounds. Arch Surg 122:221-225, 1987.

136. Derbyshire D, Smith G: Sympathoadrenal responses to anaesthesia and surgery. Br J Anaesth 56:725-739, 1984.

137. Halter J, Pflug A, Porte D: Mechanism of plasma catecholamine increases during surgical stress in man. J Clin Endocrin Metab 45:936-944, 1977.

138. Kurz A, Sessler D, Lenhardt R, et al: Perioperative normothermia to reduce the incidence of surgical-wound

infection and shorten hospitalization. N Engl J Med 334:1209-1215, 1996.

139. Hartmann M, Jonsson K, Zederfeldt B: Effect of tissue perfusion and oxygenation on accumulation of collagen in healing wounds. Randomized study in patients after major abdominal operations. Eur J Surg 158:521-526, 1992.

140. Melling AC, Ali B, Scott EM, Leaper DJ: Effects of preoperative warming on the incidence of wound infection after clean surgery: A randomised controlled trial. Lancet 358:876-880, 2001.

141. Akça O, Melischek M, Scheck T, et al: Postoperative pain and subcutaneous oxygen tension [letter]. Lancet 354:41-42, 1999.

142. Rojas IG, Padgett DA, Sheridan JF, Marucha PT: Stress-induced susceptibility to bacterial infection during cutaneous wound healing. Brain Behav Immun 16:74-84, 2002.

143. Horan MP, Quan N, Subramanian SV, et al: Impaired wound contraction and delayed myofibroblast differentiation in restraint-stressed mice. Brain Behav Immun 19:207-216, 2005.

144. Greif R, Akça O, Horn EP, et al: Supplemental perioperative oxygen to reduce the incidence of surgical-wound infection. Outcomes Research Group. N Engl J Med 342:161-167, 2000.

145. Belda FJ, Aguilera L, Garcia de la Asuncion J, et al: Supplemental perioperative oxygen and the risk of surgical wound infection: A randomized controlled trial. Jama 294:2035-2042, 2005.

146. Myles PS, Leslie K, Chan MT, et al: Avoidance of nitrous oxide for patients undergoing major surgery: A randomized controlled trial. Anesthesiology 107:221-231, 2007.

147. Pryor KO, Fahey TJ 3rd, Lien CA, Goldstein PA: Surgical site infection and the routine use of perioperative hyperoxia in a general surgical population: A randomized controlled trial. Jama 291:79-87, 2004.

148. Stotts NA, Hopf HW: The link between tissue oxygen and hydration in nursing home residents with pressure ulcers: Preliminary data. J Wound Ostomy Continence Nurs 30:184-190, 2003.

149. Hopf H, West J, Hunt T: Clonidine increases tissue oxygen in patients with local tissue hypoxia in non-healing wounds. Wound Repair Regen 4:A129, 1996.

150. Hopf H, McKay W, West J, Hunt T: Percutaneous lumbar sympathetic block increases tissue oxygen in patients with local tissue hypoxia in non-healing wounds. Anesth Analg 84:S305, 1997.

151. Semenza GL, Prabhakar NR: HIF-1-dependent respiratory, cardiovascular, and redox responses to chronic intermittent hypoxia. Antioxid Redox Signal 9:1391-1396, 2007.

152. Hunt TK, Pai MP: The effect of varying ambient oxygen tensions on wound metabolism and collagen synthesis. Surg Gynecol Obstet 135:561-567, 1972.

153. Zhao LL, Davidson JD, Wee SC, et al: Effect of hyperbaric oxygen and growth factors on rabbit ear ischemic ulcers. Arch Surg 129:1043-1049, 1994.

154. Adams K, Mader J: Aminoglycoside potentiation with adjunctive hyperbaric oxygen therapy in experimental *Pseudomonas aeruginosa* osteomyelitis. Undersea

and Hyperbaric Medical Society Annual Scientific Meeting, Baltimore, 1987, Abstract 69.

155. Mader JT, Shirtliff ME, Bergquist SC, Calhoun J: Antimicrobial treatment of chronic osteomyelitis. Clin Orthop Relat Res 47-65, 1999.

156. Verklin RM Jr, Mandell GL: Alteration of effectiveness of antibiotics by anaerobiosis. J Lab Clin Med 89:65-71, 1977.

157. Korhonen K, Klossner J, Hirn M, Niinikoski J: Management of clostridial gas gangrene and the role of hyperbaric oxygen. Ann Chir Gynaecol 88:139-142, 1999.

158. Feng J, Gibson J, Constant J, et al: Hyperoxia stimulates macrophage vascular endothelial growth factor (VEGF) production. Wound Repair Regen 6:A252, 1998.

159. Bonomo SR, Davidson JD, Yu Y, et al: Hyperbaric oxygen as a signal transducer: Upregulation of platelet derived growth factor-beta receptor in the presence of HBO2 and PDGF. Undersea Hyperb Med 25:211-216, 1998.

160. Asano T, Kaneko E, Shinozaki S, et al: Hyperbaric oxygen induces basic fibroblast growth factor and hepatocyte growth factor expression, and enhances blood perfusion and muscle regeneration in mouse ischemic hind limbs. Circ J 71:405-411, 2007.

161. Thom SR: Effects of hyperoxia on neutrophil adhesion. Undersea Hyperb Med 31:123-131, 2004.

162. Boykin JV Jr, Baylis C: Hyperbaric oxygen therapy mediates increased nitric oxide production associated with wound healing: A preliminary study. Adv Skin Wound Care 20:382-388, 2007.

163. Bakker D: Pure and mixed aerobic and anaerobic soft tissue infections. HBO Rev 6:65-96, 1985.

164. Zamboni WA, Roth AC, Russell RC, et al: The effect of acute hyperbaric oxygen therapy on axial pattern skin flap survival when administered during and after total ischemia. J Reconstr Microsurg 5:343-350, 1989.

165. Zamboni WA, Roth AC, Russell RC, Smoot EC: The effect of hyperbaric oxygen on reperfusion of ischemic axial skin flaps: A laser Doppler analysis. Ann Plast Surg 28:339-341, 1992.

166. Zamboni WA, Roth AC, Russell RC, et al: Morphologic analysis of the microcirculation during reperfusion of ischemic skeletal muscle and the effect of hyperbaric oxygen. Plast Reconstr Surg 91:1110-1123, 1993.

167. Nylander G, Lewis D, Nordstrom H, Larsson J: Reduction of postischemic edema with hyperbaric oxygen. Plast Reconstr Surg 76:596-603, 1985.

168. Nylander G, Nordstrom H, Eriksson E: Effects of hyperbaric oxygen on oedema formation after a scald burn. Burns Incl Therm Inj 10:193-196, 1984.

169. Marx RE, Ehler WJ, Tayapongsak P, Pierce LW: Relationship of oxygen delivery to angiogenesis in irradiated tissue. Am J Surg 160:519-524, 1990.

170. Niinikoski J, Penttinen R, Kulonen E: Effect of hyperbaric oxygenation on fracture healing in the rat: A biochemical study. Calcif Tissue Res (suppl):115-116, 1970.

171. Penttinen R, Niinikoski J, Kulonen E: Hyperbaric oxygenation and fracture healing. A biochemical study with rats. Acta Chir Scand 138:39-44, 1972.

172. Faglia E, Favales F, Aldeghi A, et al: Adjunctive systemic hyperbaric oxygen therapy in treatment of severe prevalently ischemic diabetic foot ulcer. A randomized study. Diabetes Care 19:1338-1343, 1996.

173. Roeckl-Wiedmann I, Bennett M, Kranke P: Systematic review of hyperbaric oxygen in the management of chronic wounds. Br J Surg 92:24-32, 2005.

174. Abidia A, Laden G, Kuhan G, et al: The role of hyperbaric oxygen therapy in ischaemic diabetic lower extremity ulcers: A double-blind randomised-controlled trial. Eur J Vasc Endovasc Surg 25:513-518, 2003.

175. Doctor N, Pandya S, Supe A: Hyperbaric oxygen therapy in diabetic foot. J Postgrad Med 38:112-114, 111, 1992.

176. Hammarlund C, Sundberg T: Hyperbaric oxygen reduced size of chronic leg ulcers: A randomized double-blind study. Plast Reconstr Surg 93:829-833, 1994.

177. Robson MC, Cooper DM, Aslam R, et al: Guidelines for the treatment of venous ulcers. Wound Repair Regen 14:649-662, 2006.

178. Whitney J, Phillips L, Aslam R, et al: Guidelines for the treatment of pressure ulcers. Wound Repair Regen 14:663-679, 2006.

179. Smart D, Bennett M, Mitchell S: Transcutaneous oximetry, problem wounds and hyperbaric oxygen therapy. Diving Hyperb Med 36:72-86, 2006.

180. Wattel F, Mathieu D, Coget JM, Billard V: Hyperbaric oxygen therapy in chronic vascular wound management. Angiology 41:59-65, 1990.

181. Kalani M, Jorneskog G, Naderi N, et al: Hyperbaric oxygen (HBO) therapy in treatment of diabetic foot ulcers. Long-term follow-up. J Diabet Complicat 16:153-158, 2002.

182. Kessler L, Bilbault P, Ortega F, et al: Hyperbaric oxygenation accelerates the healing rate of nonischemic chronic diabetic foot ulcers: A prospective randomized study. Diabetes Care 26:2378-2382, 2003.

183. Zamboni W: Evaluation of hyperbaric oxygen for diabetic wounds: A prospective study. Undersea Hyperb Med 24:175-179, 1997.

184. Baroni G, Porro T, Faglia E, et al: Hyperbaric oxygen in diabetic gangrene treatment. Diabetes Care 10:81-86, 1987.

185. Davis J: The use of adjuvant hyperbaric oxygen in treatment of the diabetic foot. Clin Podiatr Med Surg 4:429-437, 1987.

186. Oriani G: Hyperbaric oxygen therapy in diabetic gangrene. J Hyperb Med 5:171-175, 1990.

187. Wattel F, Mathieu M, Fossati P, et al: Hyperbaric oxygen in the treatment of diabetic foot lesions: Search for healing predictive factors. J Hyperb Med 6:263-268, 1991.

188. Oriani G, Michael M, Meazza D: Diabetic foot and hyperbaric oxygen therapy: A ten-year experience. J Hyperb Med 7:213-221, 1992.

189. Stone J, Scott R, Brill L, Levine B: The role of hyperbaric oxygen therapy in the treatment of the diabetic foot. Diabetes 44S:71A, 1995.

190. Faglia E, Favales F, Aldeghi A, et al: Change in major amputation rate in a center dedicated to diabetic foot care during the 1980s: Prognostic determinants for major amputation. J Diabet Complicat 12:96-102, 1998.

Indications IV

Hyperbaric Oxygen Therapy for Delayed Radiation Injuries

John J. Feldmeier, DO, FACRO

MAGNITUDE AND NATURE OF THE PROBLEM

It is estimated that currently more than 10 million cancer survivors are alive in the United States.[1] In the United States, more than 1.4 million people are diagnosed annually with invasive, nonbasal, nonsquamous skin cancers.[2] With increasing frequency, patients with cancer receive multimodality therapy to include surgery, radiation, and/or chemotherapy. Approximately 60% of all cancer patients undergo radiation as a component of their treatment at some time during the course of their disease.[3] Ionizing therapeutic radiation is a potent physical entity with dramatic effects in both malignant and surrounding normal tissues.

Untoward reactions to radiation therapy in normal tissues are most frequently classified as either acute reactions or delayed reactions. Acute reactions are pronounced in those normal tissues, such as oral, pharyngeal, gastric, enteric, and colorectal mucosa, which have a high rate of cellular loss and mitosis. In this regard, these tissues mimic malignant tumors that characteristically demonstrate rapid growth with frequent cellular mitoses.

Acute complications occur during or just after the completion of radiation. Acute radiation complications such as acute dermatitis and mucositis (stomatitis, pharyngitis, esophagitis, gastritis, enteritis, and proctitis) can be troublesome. Generally, their severity is related to the total radiation dose and the total time of treatment. They are enhanced in their severity by concurrent chemotherapy. For the most part, they are not dose-limiting within the limits of a typical course of radiation. They are generally self-limited, and when afflicted by such complications, patients are treated symptomatically with special attention to hydration and nutritional support. On rare occasions, acute reactions may be so severe that they evolve into delayed or chronic radiation complications. These complications are termed *consequential effects* of radiation.[4]

A few organ systems such as the lung and the central nervous system may also exhibit subacute reactions (radiation pneumonitis or temporary demyelination leading to Lhermitte syndrome or the somnolence syndrome). These subacute reactions typically occur one to a few months after treatment.

Similarly, for the relatively rarely identified subacute radiation reaction, most resolve with time. Generally, they are treated symptomatically and may require treatment for a longer period than acute reactions. The so-called Lhermitte sign is an indication of a subacute radiation reaction in the spinal cord. It manifests itself by what patients describe as electric-like shocks down the back and into the legs. These symptoms can be induced by flexing the neck anteriorly to stretch the spinal cord. This condition is caused by temporary demyelination of the spinal cord white matter. This condition is usually self-limited, though some believe that it may occur more frequently in those who eventually acquire radiation-induced transverse myelitis. Subacute radiation pneumonitis can also be troublesome. It is more frequently seen when larger volumes of lung are treated with higher doses of radiation. It usually manifests itself in a fashion similar to bronchitis with initially a dry, chronic cough. Some patients with radiation-induced pneumonitis require prolonged courses of corticosteroids and can suffer from profound dyspnea.

This chapter focuses on the use (or prophylactic use) of hyperbaric oxygen therapy (HBOT) for delayed or late radiation injuries. It is these injuries that effectively limit the clinical dose of radiation. They do not resolve over time. They are often progressive and serious and sometimes even lethal. They may occur in patients who have experienced only average or minor acute side effects during and just after their course of radiation. These delayed reactions characteristically occur after a latent period of 6 months or more, and the patient continues to be at risk for such complications for the remainder of their lives. Even years later, delayed radiation complications may develop spontaneously or as the result of surgical wounding, trauma, or a dental extraction within a previously irradiated field. The radiation oncology community is aware of the potential developments of such complications. Tolerance doses have been studied and published with the intent of minimizing the incidence of late complications in critical organs.[5] However, these published tolerance doses may be lower than the dose needed to control the tumor that involves or lies in close proximity to a critical structure. In this case, the tumor is not controlled if the dose is modified downward to prevent complications. The result is an unattractive but unavoidable choice of underdosing the cancer versus a high risk for complications. In addition, some patients exhibit lower tolerance to the effects of radiation therapy and may sustain serious complications even when standard guidelines for radiation dose are followed meticulously. Currently, no reliable biochemical or functional tests exist that can be applied to identify those at unusually significant risk for serious radiation complications at doses generally well tolerated in most patients with cancer.

Radiation oncology patients exhibit a wide range of tolerance to treatment. Although we have identified a few hereditary syndromes that are known to put patients at increased risk for radiation damage, including ataxia-telangiectasia, ataxia-telangiectasia–like disorder, Nijmegen breakage syndrome, and Fanconi's anemia, there are at present no reliable biochemical or functional tests that accurately predict which patients will suffer serious radiation complications at doses well tolerated in the majority of radiation patients. For additional information about those genetic syndromes that place patients at enhanced risks for complications, please consult texts of radiation biology such as Hall and Giaccia's textbook.[6] Additional risk factors for complications include patients who are retreated, those with collagen vascular disorders, and those receiving a higher than standard dose either intentionally or as the result of a treatment dosage error.

Radiation biology and pathology are complex topics. The total dose, dose per treatment, total time of treatment, volume of the tissue irradiated, and the patient's own idiosyncratic, genetically controlled response determine the likelihood and severity for delayed complications. The most recent advances in the technology of radiation therapy include increasingly precise targeting of the tumor in order to avoid normal tissues. The development of these treatment options has required advances in imaging technology, high-powered computers, sophisticated computer algorithms, and treatment machines that can adjust the shape and size of the radiation field continuously as it rotates around the patient. These techniques include three-dimensional conformal radiation therapy, intensity modulated radiation therapy, and stereotactic radiosurgery. At least in part, these targeted therapies are used to reduce the likelihood of radiation-induced injuries. They have also allowed for dose escalation with the intent of improving local tumor control and at the same time avoiding an escalation of radiation-induced complications.[7]

Another strategy that has been widely adopted in radiation oncology clinics across the United States is the use of amifostine as a radioprotector. Amifostine or WR2721 is a drug originally developed to protect U.S. troops from the toxicity of radiation exposure from fallout subsequent to a nuclear bomb. Clinically, it has been applied most frequently in the treatment of head and neck cancer to prevent xerostomia. It has also been applied with success to the prevention of radiation pneumonitis and proctitis. In the latest edition of the textbook *Principles and Practice of Radiation Oncology*,[8] a total of four randomized, controlled trials and nine nonrandomized trials are cited as supporting its application as a prophylaxis for radiation injury. The concern that amifostine might protect the tumor, as well as the intended normal tissues, has not been demonstrated by the accumulated published clinical experience. Amifostine protects against radiation damage by acting as a free radical scavenger. Cellular radiation damage is mediated through free radicals as highly reactive chemical species that cause breaks in the chemical bonds of DNA strands.[9]

THE NATURE OF DELAYED RADIATION INJURY

The pathophysiology of delayed radiation injuries is complex and only incompletely understood. In virtually all tissues that demonstrate deleterious late effects of radiation histologically, we can observe vascular damage characterized by endarteritis. Until quite recently, it was believed that the dominant mechanism for delayed radiation injury in many organ systems was the result of damage to nutrient and oxygen-transporting vasculature.[10] Tissue fibrosis was recognized as an important component of delayed radiation injury but not dominant. It was postulated that when this hypoxia reached a critical level to support cellular metabolism, the damage would result in inadequate or even absent organ function with resultant symptoms.

It had always been a dictum of the radiation oncology community that there was a disconnect and profound difference between acute and delayed radiation reactions. The latest models of delayed radiation injury emphasize the continuity of biochemical effects which begin at the initiation of radiation. Vascular changes are felt to be secondary to the depletion of stem cells and the fibrosis that is induced in radiated tissues. Acute reactions were cellular and related to direct DNA damage. They were mostly epithelial and mucosal. Delayed reactions were vascular and mostly stromal. It is certainly true that some patients experience significant acute radiation reactions without corresponding delayed reactions, and some have serious delayed reactions without ever experiencing notable acute reactions. However, we now appreciate that the spectrum of radiation complications begins at the time of radiation exposure. A new understanding of the nature of delayed radiation injury has recently been postulated and termed the *fibroatrophic effect*. This model is supported by the cellular depletion and exuberant fibrosis that can easily be appreciated with light microscopy of tissue samples taken from patients or experimental animals. In this model, vascular stenosis continues to be a consistent factor in delayed radiation damage. Although there are distinctions and identifiable differences in the nature and site of injury, we have come to appreciate that late radiation damage is initiated with the first treatment. An increase in various biochemical substances including fibrogenetic cytokines is identifiable from the onset of treatment.[11] These have been associated with late radiation damage, and their serial assays and therapeutic suppression may allow for prophylactic interventions. The early demonstration of an increase of those cytokines, which lead to damage or, conversely, a depression of protective cytokines, may identify a group of patients at high risk for late radiation damage. This identification of those at risk before manifestations of frank radiation damage may permit adjustment in the radiation dose and dose frequency or prophylactic pharmacologic intervention. A potential area for future research will include the application of prophylactic interventions to include HBOT during this latent period after radiation but before expressed damage. If a group of reliable predictive assays can be developed and a group at increased risk identified, other therapeutic strategies to prevent radiation damage will also be studied.

A review of the current state of the art in understanding of those biological markers that have been identified and are associated with radiation injury has been published by Fleckenstein and colleagues.[12] These authors report that the most frequently studied cytokine in this regard is transforming growth factor-β. Other cytokines that have been identified as likely to correlate with radiation injury are interleukin (IL)-1, IL-2, IL-4, IL-5, IL-6, IL-7, IL-8, IL-10, IL-12, IL-13, IL-17, tumor necrosis factor-α, granulocyte macrophage colony-stimulating factor, matrix metalloproteinase-3, matrix metalloproteinase-9, and tissue inhibitor of metalloproteinase-1. Most of these correlations have been made in animal models of radiation-induced pneumonitis. For their current utility in managing or preventing radiation injury, the authors state, "[A]t the present time, no reliable and validated predictive assay exists that could definitively be relied on for treatment decision."[12] The authors go on to state their belief that no one single marker for radiation tissue damage is likely to be identified. Figure 12.1 presents a simplified schema for the mechanisms of radiation injury. In spite of the identification of certain promising biochemical markers as discussed earlier, we cannot at this time

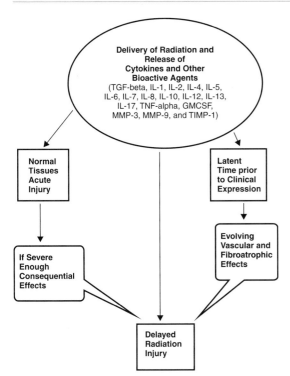

Figure 12.1 Biochemical events resulting in both acute and delayed normal tissue injuries begin at the time of radiation delivery. A latent period exists after radiation before expression of the delayed injuries. During this time, cytokines affect the vascular, fibrotic, and cellular atrophy, leading to manifest injury. If severe enough, acute injury evolves into delayed injury without a distinct latent period that appears injury free. GMCSF, granulocyte macrophage colony-stimulating factor; IL, interleukin; MMP, matrix metalloproteinase; TGF, transforming growth factor; TIMP, tissue inhibitor of metalloproteinase; TNF, tumor necrosis factor.

reliably identify patients who are at high risk for complications.

Current Controversies on Therapy for Radiation Injury

There is no consensus in the radiation oncology community as to an optimal strategy in dealing with serious delayed radiation injuries. Surgical resection and closure with flaps with their blood supply originating outside the radiation field are commonly employed for serious injuries. When surgery is used, serious complications are common and even sometimes lethal. In patients who have already faced cancer therapy including combinations of surgery, chemotherapy, and radiation ther-

apy, this option is unattractive. HBOT has been employed for delayed radiation injury since the 1970s. Its application is not universally accepted by the medical community. Its utilization has usually been predicated on its success in stimulating angiogenesis in hypovascular tissues after radiation. Other pharmacologic interventions are even less well established than HBOT.

Dr. Helen Stone and her colleagues[13] convened a workshop at the National Cancer Institute in September 2000 to explore and discuss options for modifying delayed radiation injuries. A number of experts met to share experiences in applying therapeutic endeavors for various treatment and prophylactic strategies.

A frequent criticism leveled against the evidence supporting HBOT in its role of treatment or prophylaxis against radiation injury is the absence of randomized, controlled clinical trials. Dr. Stone in her previously cited report of the conference conducted by the National Cancer Institute in 2000 mentions several theoretical promising approaches to the treatment and prevention of delayed radiation injuries. None of these had been subjected to phase 3 trials. In a Cochrane review of all nonsurgical interventions for delayed radiation proctitis, Denton and associates[14] could find only six randomized, controlled trials of adequate scientific design to merit inclusion in their analysis. In a review article published in 2007, Delanian and Lefaix[15] discuss current therapies for what they term *radiation-induced fibrosis (RIF) and necrosis*. In this article, the authors briefly discuss their understanding of the pathophysiology of delayed radiation injury, which they subdivide into radiation-induced fibrosis and radiation-induced necrosis. They discuss the application of pentoxifylline, vitamin E, superoxide dismutase, and HBOT alone or in various combinations. For their assessment of the efficacy of HBOT and in light of the recent negative studies by Pritchard and colleagues[16] and Annane and coworkers,[17] they state, "[B]ased on these data, HBOT does not seem to be an effective treatment for RIF." In a discussion of strategies to address delayed radiation injury, these authors present several case series but only two randomized, controlled trials. In the first randomized trial cited, Ferreira and investigators[18] report success in having patients rinse their oral cavities with an oil solution containing vitamin E, resulting in a reduction in mucositis as compared with the placebo group. In another randomized, controlled trial, Gothard and colleagues[19] report no advantage for pentoxifylline and vitamin E in combination as treatment for upper extremity radiation-induced lymphedema. Delanian and Lefaix[15] express their preference for a multidrug regimen in the treatment of delayed radiation injuries that includes pentoxifylline, vitamin E, and clodronate. Their total experience with this combination includes 40 patients with osteoradionecrosis (ORN) and 18 with plexitis who have responded positively with this regimen.

This experience is contrasted with the HBOT experience published by Feldmeier and Hampson[20] in 2002. A total of 74 publications were reviewed, with 67 of them demonstrating successful treatment with HBOT. More than 1000 patient treatment courses were accomplished with HBOT in this review. Despite this large amount of accumulated clinical evidence, no broad support exists in the radiation oncology community for the use of HBOT in the treatment of delayed radiation injury. Delanian and Lefaix[15] made the following statement on the basis of the recent negative trials by Pritchard and colleagues[16] and Annane and coworkers[17]: "HBO today does not seem to be an effective treatment for RIF (radiation-induced fibrosis)."

Early Interactions of Radiation Therapy and Hyperbaric Oxygen: The Era of Radiosensitization

Molecular oxygen available in adequate levels simultaneously at the time of treatment is the most potent and least toxic radiation sensitizer known. The initial clinical application of HBOT to radiation therapy patients was its use as a radiosensitizer. During the 1960s and early 1970s, HBOT was studied as

a radiosensitizer for external beam radiation. Numerous clinical trials (mostly randomized and controlled) were conducted whereby patients undergoing radiation therapy for their malignancies were irradiated through the acrylic hull of monoplace HBOT chambers while at pressure breathing 100% oxygen. A comprehensive review of the experience employing HBOT radiosensitization has recently been published by Bennett and colleagues as part of the Cochrane Collaboration.[21]

Several of these studies demonstrated improvements in local control but not survival, and the practice of HBOT radiosensitization simultaneously with external beam irradiation had been largely abandoned.[22] Since the mid-1990s, several Japanese groups have begun investigating radiation just after HBOT for high-grade brain tumors,[23-26] and the possible effect of HBOT just before irradiation in head and neck cancers as a sensitizer is also the subject of a trial initiated by the Baromedical Research Foundation.[27]

Rationale for Hyperbaric Oxygen as a Treatment for or Prophylaxis against Radiation Injury

Since the 1970s, HBOT has been applied as a therapeutic modality for delayed radiation injury, with its application increasing to the point that about 50% of all patients treated in U.S. hyperbaric centers are treated for radiation injury. HBOT has also been demonstrated to reduce the likelihood of radiation injury when applied as a prophylactic intervention under certain conditions.

Figure 12.1 illustrates a simplified schema whereby radiation at its initiation sets off a complex combination of biochemical events which ultimately can result in significant tissue damage. The three components of damage include the effects of fibrosis, stem cell depletion, and vascular obliteration and narrowing. These, of course, are not independent effects, but instead they combine in a complex fashion to result in delayed radiation toxicity. Figure 12.2 summarizes the known and putative effects of HBOT. A number of researchers have shown HBOT's effect in enhancing vascular density and resultant enhancement of tissue oxygenation within the irradiated tissues. Following is further discussion on the impact of HBOT on fibrosis. Finally, recent evidence suggests that HBOT increases the release and mobilization of stem cells.

The application of HBOT has been most extensively reported in the treatment and prevention of mandibular ORN. HBOT is an effective treatment modality for radiation necrosis because, at least in part, the pathophysiology of this process is vascular and stromal secondary to obliterative endarteritis. HBOT has been shown to induce neovascularization in this hypoxic milieu and to reduce fibrosis in irradiated tissues. Marx[28] has compared the cellularity and vascularity in histologic specimens taken from the same patient before and after HBOT. These demonstrate an increase in vascular density and cellularity after completion of 30 HBOT treatments. Marx[28] has also shown an increase in serial transcutaneous oxygen measurements taken while breathing surface-level air in patients undergoing HBOT for mandibular necrosis.

The importance of the fibroatrophic effect on the incidence and severity of radiation injury has been introduced earlier. Feldmeier and colleagues[29,30] in an animal model of radiation small-bowel injury have shown that HBOT delivered before the manifestation of injury increased the compliance of the small bowel to stretch and reduced the fibrosis of the small bowel as evidenced by a quantitative assessment of collagen content in the tunica media of the bowel wall. The group from the University of Pennsylvania in two publications have demonstrated that HBOT is effective in inducing and mobilizing stem cells by increasing nitric oxide.[31,32] Though not yet proved to be a major effect in radiation injury, a putative impact on stem cell increase within the irradiated field would provide yet another mechanism for a positive therapeutic effect by HBOT in radiation-damaged tissues. Figure 12.2 presents a schematic summarizing the effects of HBOT on radiation injury.

The systematic review by Feldmeier and Hampson[20] (see earlier) analyzes 74 publications

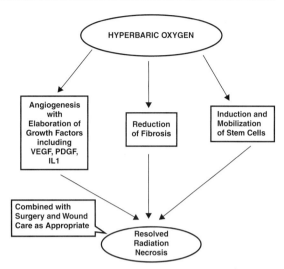

Figure 12.2 Hyperbaric oxygen has been shown to enhance angiogenesis, decrease fibrosis, and mobilize stem cells. All of these effects can counteract the fibroatrophic, avascular, and acellular mechanisms of delayed radiation injury. Especially when bone is involved, appropriate surgical debridement/resection is necessary to resolve injury. IL-1, interleukin-1; PDGF, platelet-derived growth factor; VEGF, vascular endothelial growth factor.

that report the results of HBOT for a wide range of soft tissue and bony necrosis. This review was conducted in an evidence-based fashion. Sixty-seven of these 74 articles reported a positive therapeutic effect. The negative reports were almost all in neurologic injury where, especially in the central nervous system, radiation injuries once fixed are refractory to all interventions. Since this review additional publications have been reported that detail the effects of HBOT on radiation injury. Not all have been positive, and one study, the trial by Annane and coworkers[17] (see earlier discussion and also the detailed discussion later in this chapter), has created considerable controversy in the hyperbaric community because of the authors' and third-party carriers' interpretation of the results. As we show in this chapter, there are several problems with the study design that negate its implications in regard to HBOT for mandibular ORN.

In the following sections, we discuss the application of HBOT to radiation injury on an anatomic or organ system basis. Another logical approach would be to consider soft-tissue radiation injury broadly and, separately, bwony radiation injury. Because of the special nature of neurologic injuries, especially central nervous system injuries, in any scheme, these should be considered separately. In addition, we present some future potential applications of HBOT to the prevention and treatment of radiation injury.

HBOT also has an increasing role when surgery is planned within the irradiated fields. An increasing body of literature exists applying HBOT in a predental and postdental dental implant procedure to enhance the bony integration of the dental implant when placed in irradiated bone.

Site-Specific Applications of Hyperbaric Oxygen to Delayed Radiation Injuries

Mandibular Necrosis

In the 1960s and early 1970s, several reports of partial success in applying HBOT to the treatment for mandibular ORN were published. Success was based on symptom relief, which was in this early experience for the most part partial and often temporary. While stationed at Wilford Hall United States Air Force (USAF) Medical Center, Dr. Robert Marx and his colleagues in collaboration with Davis and his coworkers at the USAF Hyperbaric Medicine Center across town at Brooks Air Force Base developed a staging system and treatment protocol that formally integrated HBOT into the *multidisciplinary* management of mandibular ORN.[28]

The specific recommendations for therapy followed quite logically from the assignment of a patient to a particular stage based on the severity of the patient's mandibular damage. Two key elements are prominent in the Marx[28] protocol for mandibular ORN:

1. An emphasis on presurgical (debridement or resection) HBOT consisting of 30 treatments with an additional 10 treatments after surgery
2. An absolute requirement that necrotic bone be surgically extirpated even if a bony discontinuity and need for reconstruction results

In Marx's[28] protocol, HBOT was administered in a multiplace chamber daily at a pressure of 2.4 atmospheres absolute (ATA) for a total of 90 minutes of 100% oxygen at pressure.

Figure 12.3 displays a schematic depiction of Marx's staging system and the treatments that are direct outgrowth of the stage assignment. The following list represents the staging system that Marx[28] developed to facilitate treatment decisions in the management of mandibular ORN:

a. *Stage I:* These patients have a relatively minor extent of their mandibular necrosis and are believed to require minor debridement to eradicate all necrotic bone. Patients receive 30 HBOT treatments at 2.4 ATA for 90 minutes. If response is good and exposed bone is covering, the patient undergoes 10 more treatments after debridement.

b. *Stage II:* These patients are believed to require more formal surgical debridement but less than a discontinuity procedure. Stage I patients are also advanced to stage II if they are found to require more extensive surgical intervention after the initial 30 HBOT treatments. Debridement is accomplished after 30 HBOT treatments are completed. When formal debridement is adequate to eliminate all necrotic bone, an additional 10 treatments are given after surgery. If patients are found to require resection to ensure removal of all necrotic bone, they are advanced to stage III.

c. *Stage III:* These are patients who have orocutaneous fistula(e), pathologic fracture, or necrosis extending into the inferior cortical border of the mandible at presentation. Stage I and II patients who do not have resolution when treated according to these earlier stages are also advanced to stage III. Thirty HBOT treatments are given followed by resection with 10 postoperative HBOT sessions. After resection, patients are maintained in external fixation to

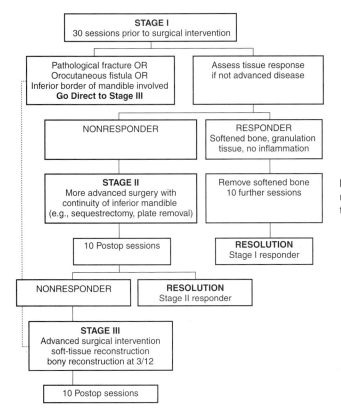

Figure 12.3 The Marx staging and treatment protocol in schematic fashion. See the text for a more complete explanation.

maintain the relation of the temporomandibular joint. About 10 weeks after resection reconstruction was accomplished followed by 10 postreconstructive HBOT sessions. Reconstruction in Marx's series uses freeze-dried cadaver bone obtained from a bone bank and shaped into a carrier tray for the patient's own corticocancellous bone harvested from the iliac crest. External jaw fixation was maintained for 8 weeks after the reconstruction to allow for successful osteogenesis.

Figure 12.4 shows an example of a stage III mandibular ORN. The necrotic process involves the mandible diffusely with extension to the inferior margin of the mandible. The considerable forces placed on the mandible by the muscles of mastication puts such patients at risk for pathologic fracture.

Utilizing the developed protocol discussed earlier, Marx[28] has reported 100% success in the treatment of mandibular ORN. Ultimately, nearly three fourths of his patients require

advancement to treatment in stage III, with resection and reconstruction necessary for resolution. The reconstruction techniques Marx has reported may be considered simplistic compared with more modern surgically complex procedures such as free flap transfers with microvascular anastomoses; however, no reason has been found not to combine the use of free flaps or rotational myocutaneous flaps or any other surgical advances in reconstruction technology with HBOT. For best results as always in combined modality therapies, the best surgical technique for that patient should be combined with the best adjunctive treatment, in this case, HBOT. Reconstruction without HBOT has been reported where the most modern surgical techniques are employed. Several have reported impressive success, but none have been subjected to randomized trials, and reoperation has been required in many cases to achieve success.

Figure 12.5 demonstrates the surgical technique utilized by Marx[28] and reported most frequently in his published series of mandibular resection and reconstruction in the treatment of ORN.

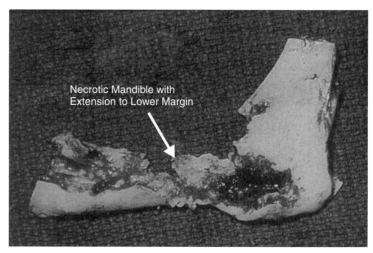

Necrotic Mandible with
Extension to Lower Margin

Figure 12.4 A resected mandible with obvious stage III characteristics. The necrosis extends to the inferior table of the bone. In this case, hyperbaric oxygen must be combined with resection to resolve the process.

A total of 14 publications, including those of Marx,[28] were included in Feldmeier and Hampson's review[20] detailing the experience of applying HBOT to mandibular necrosis. Tobey and Kelly's report[33] was a positive randomized, controlled trial, though numbers were small and details in the report are incomplete. Only 12 patients were enrolled in this study. These patients were treated at 100% oxygen at either 1.2 or 2.0 ATA. The authors state that those patients treated at 2.0 ATA "experienced significant improvement" compared with the control group that received oxygen at 1.2 ATA. No details are given regarding how randomization or outcome determination was made. Indeed, we cannot determine how many patients were assigned to either group. The study was randomized and double blinded in that neither the patient nor the clinician assessing the patient knew to which arm the patient was assigned.

Other than Tobey and Kelly's randomized study,[33] the rest of the publications included in Feldmeier and Hampson's systematic review[20] are case series. Of the 14 publications, only Maier and coauthors' report[34] fails to show a positive impact of HBOT in the treatment of mandibular ORN. In this article, no HBOT is given before surgery. HBOT was added to management of ORN only after an attempt had already been made at surgical correction. Marx[28] had previously established

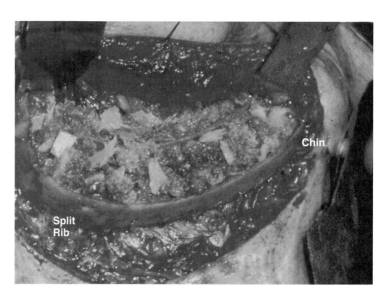

Chin
Split
Rib

Figure 12.5 The Marx technique of reconstruction. After hyperbaric oxygen and resection, the patient is reconstructed with cadaveric bone (in this case, a split rib) serving as the carrier tray for the patient's own corticocancellous bone harvested and placed into the carrier. The patient is kept in external fixation until the graft has ossified. Surgery is done extraorally to prevent infection by introduction of oral flora.
(See Color Plate 4.)

the necessity of preoperative HBOT before any surgical wounding of irradiated tissues.

Since the publication of Feldmeier and Hampson's review[20] there have been additional reports of HBOT in the treatment of mandibular ORN. The negative randomized trial by Annane and coworkers[17] has been the source of controversy in the hyperbaric and head and neck cancer communities. The Annane trial randomized a total of 68 patients with early stage mandibular ORN to either 100% oxygen at 2.4 ATA or mix of oxygen and nitrogen at this pressure, which provided the same partial pressure of O_2 as that breathing air at ground level. Patients received 20 to 30 treatments with only minor curettage planned as surgical intervention. At one-year follow-up, resolution of symptoms was seen in 19% (31) of the HBOT arm and 12% (32) in the control arm. Resolution was defined as absence of pain, coverage of exposed bone, and stabilization of radiographic findings consistent with ORN. Treatment failure was demonstrated by any one of the following: pathologic fracture, bone resorption to the inferior table, cutaneous fistula, or the need for surgical intervention.

It has unfortunately been referenced by many including third-party carriers in excluding HBOT from the management of mandibular ORN. The study design has been the subject of criticism from several circles. The most serious failing of the study was its exclusion of surgery from the management of mandibular ORN. The intent of the study was to determine whether HBOT could be employed as a *solo modality* in the treatment of ORN. Marx[28] had demonstrated two decades earlier that surgical extirpation of necrotic bone to the point of mandibular resection in nearly three fourths of patients was an absolute requirement for the consistently successful treatment of ORN. The need for surgical resection of necrotic bone originally demonstrated by Marx was also confirmed by Feldmeier and coauthors[35] in their review of HBOT in the treatment of radiation-induced necrosis of the chest wall that involved bone.

Several authors[36-38] have responded to the results and conclusions of Annane and coworkers' article.[17] These criticisms include

the failure of the investigators to integrate surgical debridement or resection as needed into the management of mandibular ORN. Moon and colleagues[38] point out that it is possible to deduce that nearly two thirds of the HBOT group of patients received fewer than 22 HBOT treatments. Laden[37] in his response to the Annane article also points out that the control group of patients was at risk for the development of decompression sickness because of the treatment pressure and mix of breathing gases consisting of 9% oxygen and 91% nitrogen.

An editorial by Mendenhall[39] (University of Florida) accompanied the Annane and coworkers' article[17] in the same issue of *Journal of Clinical Oncology.* Dr. Mendenhall, a radiation oncologist, points out that Annane and coworker's study was underpowered, but he still suggests his belief that HBOT is not effective for mandibular ORN.

Additional publications have questioned the efficacy of or at least the need for HBOT in the treatment of mandibular ORN. Gal and his associates[40] have reported a series of 30 patients treated with microvascular reconstruction for stage III ORN. Twenty-one of these patients had had preoperative HBOT and continued to demonstrate persistent disease despite this treatment. At least some had had debridement before referral for definitive management of their radiation injury. Once in the authors' hands, they had the appropriate debridement and reconstruction with free flap reconstruction of their mandibular defect. In the group that had already received HBOT, surgical complications occurred in 52%, whereas in the nonhyperbaric group, similar complications were seen in only 22%. The authors suggest themselves that the HBOT group may have represented a more recalcitrant form of ORN because they were already failures to prior treatment. They also point out that those patients in Marx stage III ORN represent a heterogeneous group with a wide range of injury and outcome.

In a review article by Teng and Futran,[41] the authors suggest that HBOT has no role in the management of either early or advanced ORN. This article is a review and does not present any new clinical experience.

If all of the cases reported in the review by Feldmeier and Hampson[20] are combined (excluding those that Tobey and Kelly[33] reported and noting that Marx's[28] second report includes the 58 patients reported earlier), we find a total of 371 cases of mandibular ORN reported. A beneficial effect is reported in 310 cases, or 83.6%. A better end point for all reports of ORN would be resolution. In the earlier reports, HBOT was not combined with aggressive resection of necrotic bone or with surgical reconstruction of bony discontinuity. Marx reports 100% success, but this successful treatment requires mandibulectomy and reconstruction in the majority of his patients. Dr. Marx has set high standards for what he considers successful results in those patients treated for mandibular ORN. Marx reports success not only with the re-establishment of bony continuity but also requires functional success in that these patients must be able to

wear a denture for both mastication and cosmesis. Figure 12.6 demonstrates the impact that such a reconstruction supported by HBOT can have on patient appearance and quality of life. Nutrition is also a major concern in head and neck patients, who characteristically suffer from nutritional deficiencies. Rehabilitation with dentures is important. The additional negative studies include 22 patients in Gal and associates'[40] article and 31 randomized to HBOT in Annane and coworkers' article.[17]

Hyperbaric Oxygen for Prophylaxis of Osteoradionecrosis

Marx and associates[28] accomplished a randomized, controlled trial that compared penicillin with HBOT before dental extractions as prophylactic strategies to prevent mandibular radiation necrosis in heavily irradiated mandibles.

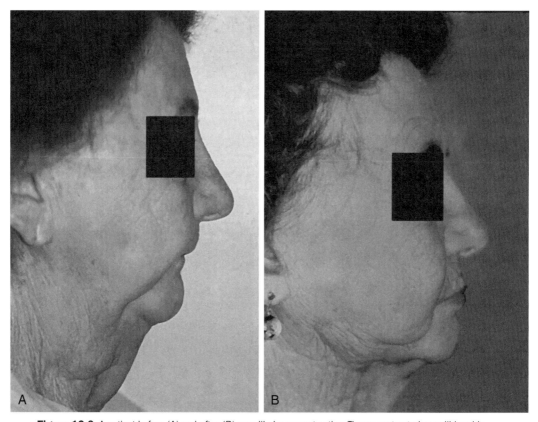

Figure 12.6 A patient before *(A)* and after *(B)* mandibular reconstruction. The reconstructed mandible adds immeasurably to the patient's quality of life and permits denture support, which improves the patient's nutritional status. **(See Color Plate 5.)**

Thirty-seven patients were treated in each group. Mandibular ORN occurred in only 2 of 37 patients (5.4%) in the HBOT group. In the penicillin group, 11 of 37 patients (29.9%) experienced mandibular necrosis.

Besides the Marx[28] controlled trial, two other case series have been published wherein prophylactic HBOT was applied to 53 additional patients before extractions or other surgical procedures in heavily irradiated mandibles and surrounding soft tissues. These two studies have been discussed previously in Feldmeier and Hampson's review.[20] When we combine all the patients from these three reports, we find an incidence of ORN in 4.5% (4/90) of the HBOT prophylaxis group (2/37 from Marx[28]; 1/29 from Vudiniabola[42]; and 1/24 from David[43]). In Marx's control group, the incidence of ORN was 29.9% (11/37).

Recent additional publications not included in the previous review are available. In a prospective but not controlled trial, Chavez and Adkinson[44] present 40 patients treated with HBOT to include 20 pre-extraction and 10 postextraction sessions. In this study at 1 year after extractions, 98.5% of tooth sockets were healed.

Sulaiman and associates[45] from Sloan-Kettering have reported a series of 187 patients who required extractions after radiation therapy. Most of these patients (180) did not receive HBOT prophylaxis, and only 4 of the 180 (2.2%) experienced development of ORN. Most of these patients had received doses of radiation between 6000 and 7000 cGy. The authors attribute this low incidence to their atraumatic surgical technique. They question the need for HBOT in the prophylaxis of ORN for patients who require dental extractions after radiation therapy.

In 2006, Michael Wahl,[46] a dentist in private practice, published a review article in the premier radiation oncology journal *International Journal of Radiation Oncology, Biology and Physics.* The author states, "There is insufficient evidence to support the use of prophylactic HBO treatments ... before extractions or other oral surgical procedures in radiation patients."[46] It is fair to say that recent sentiment as expressed in the above publications and at least in some circles has turned against the need for HBOT for dental extractions in previously irradiated patients. It is also worth noting that the recent negative reports represent a lower level of evidence than the randomized controlled trial accomplished by Marx[28] establishing the role for HBOT in preventing ORN following dental extractions.

Laryngeal Necrosis

Cartilaginous necrosis of the larynx is an uncommon complication of therapeutic radiation. In a well-planned and well-executed course of radiation wherein the larynx is included in the radiation portals, it should occur no more than 1% of the time that the larynx is included in the radiation field. Radiation necrosis of the larynx is more likely to occur when radiation fields are large and when dose per treatment and total dose are large. Neutron radiation is also associated with a greater incidence of laryngeal necrosis.

Four case series and a new case report have been published reporting the impact of HBOT as a treatment for radiation necrosis of the larynx.[47-51] In these five reports, most patients were treated for severe laryngeal necrosis (Chandler grade 3 or 4). Most experts recommend laryngectomy for patients with laryngeal necrosis in Chandler grades 3 or 4. Recurrent or persistent tumor must be ruled out. In some series, when laryngectomy has been done, a majority of patients have been found to have an occult persistence or recurrence of their cancer. Both tumor and chondroradiation necrosis can present with airway compromise, edema, fetid breath, and production of necrotic debris. Biopsy to eliminate the presence of cancer may be necessary. Biopsies, however, must be done with caution and are subject to sampling error. Extensive surgical wounding of already injured tissues may further exacerbate tissue damage.

In the four reports cited, a total of 42 patients were treated. Three in the series by Narzony and investigators[50] had partial laryngectomies. All but six in the combined groups avoided total laryngectomy, and most had good or excellent voice quality with complete resolution of their laryngeal necrosis.

Figure 12.7 presents a photographic series of a patient demonstrating cartilaginous necrosis of the supraglottic larynx. Treatment with predebridement HBOT followed by reconstruction with flap and graft supported by postsurgical HBOT led to resolution of the necrotizing process and preservation of the larynx.

Other Soft-Tissue Necrosis Injuries of the Head and Neck

In the latest version of *Hyperbaric Medicine Practice*,[28] Marx reports his experience in a prospective, controlled trial applying HBOT to support the viability of soft-tissue flaps designed to correct radiation and surgically induced defects in the head and neck in patients who had received at least a 6000-cGy radiation dose. Two groups each were prospectively followed. Eighty patients were studied in each group. The HBOT group received 20 preoperative and 10 postoperative HBOT treatments. Patients were treated at 2.4 ATA for 90 minutes of 100% oxygen. The other group received otherwise identical treatment with surgery by the same surgeon but without any adjunctive HBOT. The groups were compared in regard to wound dehiscence, wound infection, and delayed healing. Marx reported the incidence of these outcome measures in the HBOT group versus the control group in the following fashion: (1) wound infection: 6% versus 24%; (2) wound dehiscence: 11% versus 48%; and (3) delayed wound healing: 11% versus 55%. When we apply the χ^2 test to these results, we obtain highly significant statistical results with *P* values of 0.004, less than 0.0001, and less than 0.0001, respectively, for each of these outcome measures.

Besides the Marx trial, there are four additional published case series reporting HBOT of soft-tissue radiation injuries of the head and neck (excluding the larynx, which has been discussed earlier as a special circumstance). Davis and colleagues[52] report success in 15 of 16 patients treated for soft-tissue radionecrosis of the head and neck. Many of these patients had large, chronic soft-tissue wounds as

a result of their radiation injury. Neovius and colleagues[53] in 1997 reported a series of 15 patients treated with HBOT for wound complications of irradiated tissues. This series was compared with a matched historical control group treated at the same institution without HBOT. In the HBOT group, 12 of the 15 patients healed completely. Among the remaining patients, there was improvement in two and no benefit in the final patient. Only 7 of 15 patients healed in the historical control group. In this group, two patients experienced life-threatening hemorrhage, and 1 of these patients did bleed to death.

Figure 12.8 shows a pictorial series of a patient who had treatment for mandibular necrosis successfully 4 years previously. He continued to smoke, and two additional cancers developed; he was salvaged by surgical resection twice. Surgery was done through the field of radiation with resultant soft-tissue necrosis. Ultimately, he required total laryngectomy and a pectoralis rotational flap to close the resultant soft-tissue defect. In this series of HBOT treatments, he completed 43 treatments in the chamber. His skin graft was lost, but ultimately an excellent granulation base supported epithelial coverage.

Feldmeier and colleagues[54] have reported the successful prophylactic treatment of patients undergoing radical surgical resection for salvage of head and neck cancers after not responding to primary cancer treatment including full-course irradiation. A high incidence of serious surgical complications, including occasional fatalities, has been reported to occur in up to 60% of such previously irradiated patients who underwent surgery without the benefit of HBOT. In this series, with a short course of HBOT (median number of treatments = 12) initiated immediately after surgery, 87.5% of patients had prompt healing without significant complications and with no deaths in the immediate postoperative period.

Narzony and investigators[50] have reported their experience in treating delayed radiation injuries in head and neck cancer. This report includes six patients previously discussed in a review of treatment for laryngeal necrosis. Eight patients in total are reported in this case

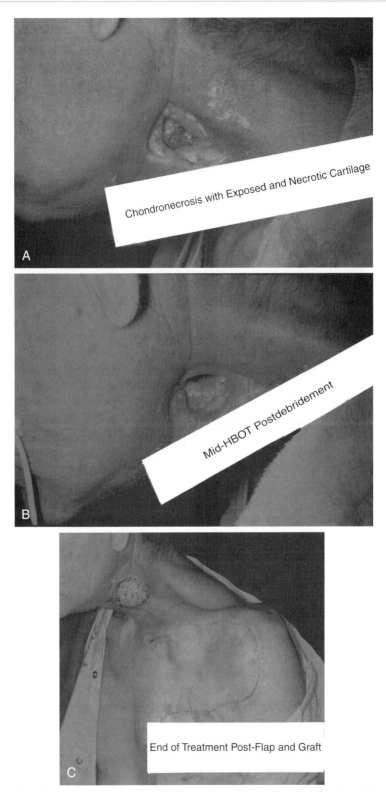

Figure 12.7 *A*, A patient with soft-tissue necrosis including necrosis of the thyroid cartilage. *B*, He received predebridement hyperbaric oxygen therapy (HBOT) followed by closure of the defect with a flap and skin graft. *C*, Additional HBOT was delivered after surgery to enhance graft and flap survival. This type of wound is especially difficult to treat because it is constantly bathed in digestive salivary enzymes. The proximity of the carotid artery also puts the patient at risk for a fatal bleed unless the process is arrested. **(See Color Plate 6.)**

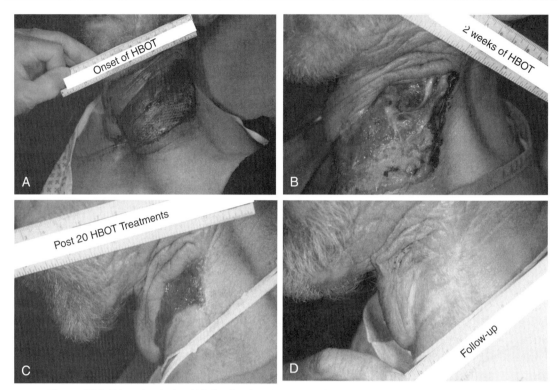

Figure 12.8 This patient had multiple head and neck cancers and required surgical salvage twice after full-course radiation. *A,* Necrosis of skin graft placed after rotational flap. *B,* Wound after about 20 treatments and debridement of graft. *C,* Excellent granulation base and epithelial advancement. *D,* Follow-up about 3 months after completion of treatment. The wound closed without any additional surgery. **(See Color Plate 7.)**

series. The other two include a patient treated for ORN of the temporal bone and a patient treated for soft-tissue necrosis with an esophageal fistula. All patients had resolution of their radiation injury with treatment including surgery in five of the eight to achieve resolution.

Chest Wall Necrosis

Radiation therapy is often applied to malignancies of the thoracic region including lung, breast, certain lymphomas, and esophagus. Because modern radiation has skin-sparing properties, the chest wall is not often treated to full dose during such radiation treatments. In breast cancer, however, the skin and the subcutaneous tissues including ribs usually receive the full or nearly the full prescribed radiation dose. Chest wall injuries due to radiation most often occur as the result of breast cancer. HBOT in this setting has not been extensively reported.

In 1976, Hart and Mainous[74] reported their experience in applying HBOT as an adjunct to skin grafting in six patients with radiation necrosis of the chest wall. All of these patients experienced successful graft take. Feldmeier and his colleagues[33] have reviewed their case series of 23 cases of radiation necrosis of the chest wall. Eight had only soft-tissue necrosis, whereas 15 had a combination of bone and soft-tissue necrosis. Resolution in those with only soft-tissue involvement was 75%. Those with a component of bone necrosis had resolution in only 53%. All of those patients with an element of bone necrosis required resection of the necrotic bone to achieve resolution. When bone is involved, aggressive debridement to include resection of all nonviable bone is required for good results in injuries of the chest wall in the same fashion as demonstrated by Marx[28] many years previously in the treatment of mandibular ORN.

In 1998, Carl and Hartmann[55] published a case study reporting the treatment of a single patient who had experienced long-standing symptomatic breast edema after conservative surgery and postoperative radiation. The patient completed 15 HBOT treatments at 2.4 ATA for 90 minutes of 100% oxygen. The patient experienced complete resolution of pain and edema with the hyperbaric intervention.

In 2001, Carl and colleagues[56] published their experiences in treating 44 patients after lumpectomy with HBOT for complications of radiation including breast pain, edema, fibrosis/fat necrosis, and telangiectasias/erythema. Patients were assessed a numeric score based on a modified Late Effect of Normal Tissue-Subjective Objective Management Analytic (LENT-SOMA) scoring system. Each patient was given a score from 1 to 4 for each of the four categories. Only patients with at least a sum of 8 or at least a pain score of 3 (persistent and intense) pain were included in the analysis. Forty-four women were offered HBOT. Thirty-two accepted treatment, and the other 12 refused treatment and constituted a nonrandomized control group. The authors reported a statistically significant reduction in the post-treatment LENT-SOMA scores in the HBOT group compared with those who did not receive HBOT. Scores for fibrosis and telangiectasia were not decreased. Seven of the 32 women who received HBOT had complete resolution of radiation-induced symptoms.

Radiation Cystitis

Radiation is a frequent treatment for pelvic malignancies including rectal, prostate, and gynecologic malignancies. Fortunately, serious delayed radiation cystitis is not a common complication of pelvic radiation, but it can be a difficult therapeutic challenge. Hemorrhagic cystitis secondary to radiation may require cystectomy if it does not respond to nonsurgical measures such as instillation of formalin or alum. In the previously cited review by Feldmeier and Hampson,[20] 17 articles that discuss the results in applying HBOT to the treatment of radiation cystitis were discussed. Bevers and colleagues' report[57] was

the largest series at that time. It was a prospective but nonrandomized trial. The remainder of the reports are case series. As discussed in the review of Feldmeier and Hampson,[20] Weiss and others have in addition to their original report, an updated report from 1998, included those patients from their original publication. The second article by Lee and coauthors[58] detailing results in 25 patients includes the 20 patients previously reported by the same authors.

Several additional publications addressing this issue have been published since the review by Feldmeier and Hampson[20] cited earlier. Neheman and associates[59] from Israel have reported a series of seven patients treated for hemorrhagic cystitis. All 7 patients received a course of HBOT consisting of a mean number of 30 treatments. Each treatment consisted of 90 minutes of 100% oxygen at 2.0 ATA. All seven patients resolved initially with resolution of their hematuria. Two recurred and were retreated with success after an additional 30 to 37 treatments. One patient with a primitive neuroectodermal tumor died from her malignancy but had had resolution of her hematuria after 20 treatments.

In the largest series to date, Corman and colleagues[60] from Virginia Mason have reported a series of 57 patients in 2003 with an update in 2005 authored by Chong and coworkers[61] that included 3 additional patients. In this series, patients received an average of 33 treatments at 2.36 ATA for 90 minutes of 100% oxygen. Overall, the results were as follows: 18 had complete resolution, 26 had partial resolution, 8 had no change, and 2 had worsening conditions. Eighty percent of those treated had either a total or partial resolution of hematuria. Of the 25 patients who also had clot retention, 6 had complete resolution, 12 had partial resolution, 4 had no change, and 2 had worsening conditions. In the update by Chong and colleagues[61] in 2005, the authors demonstrate the importance of early intervention with HBOT. When treatment was begun within 6 months of onset of hematuria, rates of improvement increased from 80% to 96% and improvement in clot retention improved from 72% to 100%. In this study, outcomes were assessed at least 12 months after completion of HBOT so that a true durable outcome was assessed, avoiding an overestimate of response predicated on early response rates without a determination of longevity of response.

Severe hemorrhagic radiation cystitis can be a life-threatening and quality-of-life limiting disorder. Cheng and Foo[62] have reported their experiences in managing nine refractory cases of hemorrhagic radiation cystitis. Treatment in this series did not include HBOT. Six patients required bilateral percutaneous nephrostomies. Three patients underwent ileal loop diversions of their urinary stream. Four of nine (44%) patients died despite these aggressive surgical interventions. In addition, Li and colleagues[63] have reported a mortality rate of 3.7% due to radiation-induced bladder injury in their retrospective review of 378 patients treated for cervical cancer.

Notably, many of the patients reported in the hyperbaric experience had already not responded to conservative management including continuous irrigation and the instillation of alum or formalin. If we combine the patients reported previously in the publications reviewed by Feldmeier and Hampson[20] to the additional patients reported in these 2 new case reports, we find that of 257 patients treated with HBOT, 196 or 76.3% have had either complete or partial response. A success rate of 76.3% with HBOT is all the more impressive when compared with the reported results with other more aggressive interventions. It is also noteworthy that 18 of 19 publications are positive reports. Only the study by Del Pizzo and coworkers[64] fails to demonstrate a benefit for HBOT. The positive results for HBOT in the treatment of radiation-induced cystitis have been reported by clinicians from several different countries and three different continents.

Radiation Enteritis/Proctitis

Feldmeier and Hampson[20] reviewed 14 publications reporting the published experience in providing HBOT as a component of the management of delayed radiation-induced injuries of the small and large bowel. Nine of these publications were either case reports or case series.

Since the publication of Feldmeier and Hampson's review,[20] several additional clinical reports have been published. Jones and associates[65] from Toronto have reported their experience in treating 10 patients with radiation-induced proctitis. Three of their patients had grade 3 toxicity (bleeding requiring transfusions). The other seven had grade 2 toxicity consisting of rectal pain, diarrhea, or both. Six in this group had rectal bleeding but had not required transfusion. Nine of the 10 patients completed treatment without toxicity. Rectal bleeding resolved in four of nine patients and improved in three other patients; two were nonresponders. Rectal pain completely resolved in three of five patients. Diarrhea resolved completely in one of five patients and improved in three others. Of the 10 patients treated, only 2 did not have detectable improvement with HBOT. Median follow-up was 25 months.

Girnius and coauthors[66] from the University of Cincinnati have published their experiences in the HBOT of nine patients with radiation-induced hemorrhagic proctitis. Three of these patients had had unsuccessful argon plasma coagulation or electrocautery before HBOT. Five had had prior hospitalizations and transfusions. With a median follow-up of 17 months, seven of the nine patients had complete resolution of their symptoms and the other two had a partial response but still had some bleeding.

The largest published experience to date comes from the Virginia Mason group and is documented in two publications.[67,68] Sixty-five patients (37 male and 28 female patients) received HBOT for radiation injury to the gastrointestinal tract. All injuries were documented by endoscopy. Fifty-four of these injuries were to the rectum, whereas 15 patients had injuries to the more proximal alimentary tract (7 small bowel, 6 colon, 6 duodenum, and 4 stomach). The total exceeds 65 because some patients had multiple injuries. Patients received an initial planned course of 30 HBOT treatments at 2.36 ATA for 90 minutes of 100% oxygen. For a subset of patients who demonstrated partial response at 30 treatments, additional treatment varying from 6 to 30 treatments was given. The authors report complete and partial response rates of 43% and 25%, respectively, overall. Results were slightly worse for rectal cancers when analyzed separately with response rates of 65% compared with 73% for the more proximal lesions.

If we combine the studies for the purpose of analysis, the results of HBOT in 197 cases of proctitis, colitis, or enteritis treated with HBOT have been reported. Of these, 80 (41%) have resolved completely and 169 (86%) have had at least a partial response, whereas only 14% have failed to show any response.

The animal studies by Feldmeier and colleagues[29,30] (see earlier discussion of mechanisms by which hyperbaric is effective) demonstrated a decrease in fibrosis in the small bowel of animals subjected to whole abdominal radiation and then treated with prophylactic intent with HBOT. Both histologic and functional assays were accomplished in both study and control animals. The functional assay involved stretching the bowel in a radial fashion to determine compliance. The histologic assay applied a special stain (Mason's trichrome stain) to allow for a quantitative assessment of the amount of fibrosis in the wall of animals that received HBOT compared with animals that did not receive HBOT. In this model, enough time (7 months after radiation) was allowed to pass before the various assays were accomplished to allow for the vascular and fibrotic changes to become established. As discussed earlier, it is characteristic that a latent period of 6 months to several years transpires between the completion of radiation until the appearance of serious delayed radiation damage. The gut, as a hollow tube from mouth to anus, must permit adequate compliance to allow for the passage of food and products of digestion.

Miscellaneous Abdominal and Pelvic Injuries

In an early report of the effects of HBOT on delayed radiation injury, Farmer and colleagues[69] in 1978 included a case report of a single patient with vaginal radiation necrosis. Complete resolution for this injury was accomplished with HBOT. In 1992, Williams and coworkers[70] reported a series of 14 patients treated with HBOT for vaginal necrosis. Thirteen of these patients had complete resolution. One patient required two separate courses of HBOT to

achieve this success. In 1996, Feldmeier and colleagues[71] reported their series of 44 patients treated with HBOT for various radiation-induced injuries of the pelvis and abdomen. Their results in treating enteritis and proctitis have been presented earlier in this chapter. Twenty-six of 31 patients (84%) who were treated with HBOT for delayed radiation injuries of the abdominal wall, groin, perineum, vagina, or pelvic bones and had at least 20 HBOT treatments had complete resolution in this series. Included among these patients were six with vaginal necrosis, and all of these patients experienced complete healing of these lesions.

Fink and colleagues[72] have recently published a series of 14 patients treated with HBOT for a variety of radiation-induced pelvic injuries with HBOT. Six of the 14 had injuries of the vagina or introitus (4 with ulcers, 1 with stenosis, and 1 characterized simply as vaginitis). Many of these patients had injuries to several organ systems simultaneously including proctitis, cystitis, and enteritis. For those treated for vaginal injury either alone or in combination with injury to other organs, the outcome was one resolution, four with greater than 50% improvement, and one patient with less than 50% response. For all patients in this series with a variety of injuries, the authors report a response rate of 71% (at least 50% improvement). Most patients received only 30 HBOT treatments. Only 2 patients in this series received more than 30 treatments at 2.4 ATA. One patient with a necrotic ulcer at the vaginal introitus had complete healing after 40 treatments. The other patient had 37 treatments for radiation proctitis and cystitis with less than 50% response.

When we combine the results of these four series, restricting ourselves to only the vaginal injuries (excluding proctitis and cystitis) reported in Fink and colleagues' article,[72] we find that 45 of 52 (87%) had successful treatment (at least a partial response) with HBOT for injuries of the abdomen and pelvis.

Extremities

Farmer and his colleagues[69] (see earlier) treated a single patient with HBOT for radiation injury of the foot. This patient was not treated successfully.

Feldmeier and colleagues[73] also reported their series of 17 patients treated with HBOT for radiation-induced necrosis of the extremities. Sixteen of these patients had only soft-tissue necrosis, whereas one had elements of ORN and soft-tissue radiation necrosis. In this series, 11 of 13 patients (85%) in whom follow-up was available and who did not have recurrent cancer had complete healing of their necrosis.

Neurologic Radiation Injuries

In their review article, Feldmeier and Hampson[20] present 14 publications wherein HBOT has been applied to radiation-induced neurologic injury. Injuries consisted of necrosis of the brain, transverse myelitis of the spinal cord, optic nerve injury, and brachial plexopathy. Since publication of that review, a few additional studies have been published.

Brain Necrosis

The first reported case of radiation-induced brain necrosis treated with HBOT was published in 1976 by Dr. George Hart,[74] who observed improvement but not resolution. Since the publication of Dr. Hart's report, there have been seven additional publications of HBOT for radiation-induced necrosis of the brain.[75-81] All of these have been case series or case reports. Chuba and coauthors[75] report on 10 children treated for necrosis. All of these children improved initially, whereas five sustained durable improvement. Four patients had died of recurrent tumor by the time of the report. In Leber and colleagues' article,[76] one of two patients had complete resolution of the lesion on magnetic resonance imaging and the other had improvement by magnetic resonance imaging. In the second largest report, by Dear and coworkers,[78] 9 of 20 patients improved with HBOT. Eleven patients had glioblastoma multiforme. In this subgroup, only one patient showed improvement. In part at least, treatment failure in the majority of these 11 patients represents tumor progression in this lethal tumor. Seven of these 11 patients had died before the publication of the report.

Gesell and colleagues[79] have reported 29 patients treated with HBOT for brain necrosis. This is the largest series to date. Neurologic examination improved in 17 (58%) of these patients, and steroid requirements had decreased in 20 patients (69%).

An issue in determining response to HBOT is the significant difficulties in distinguishing radiation necrosis from tumor. Necrosis often causes a mass effect and appears much like a tumor with the anatomic-based imaging modalities of computed tomography and magnetic resonance imaging. Positron emission tomography and magnetic resonance spectroscopy (as metabolically based imaging modalities) are able to make the distinction between tumor and necrosis at least in some cases. Not infrequently, a combination of tumor and necrosis in surrounding normal tissues will be present in a given patient when the patient undergoes craniotomy and resection. A total of 65 patients have been treated in the above listed publications, with improvement reported in 44 patients (68%).

Radiation Myelitis

Transverse radiation myelitis is an exceedingly rare but devastating complication of therapeutic radiation. Initially, symptoms of Brown–Séquard syndrome may be present with loss of motor control on one side and sensation on the contralateral side of the body much like a hemitransection of the spinal cord. Ultimately, the neurologic deficit progresses to become identical to a complete transection of the spinal cord. In addition to the obvious severe impairment of quality of life, transverse myelitis has dire implications for survival with most patients progressing to death within a few months. Fortunately, it is rare. At the University of Florida in the treatment of head and neck cancers, Marcus and Million[82] reviewed their experiences in treating head and neck cancers over 23 years. They report an incidence of myelitis of 2 in 1112 patients, or 0.18%.

The total published clinical experience applying HBOT to radiation myelitis consists of two case series and an additional case report. In 1976, Hart[74] reported a series of five patients, all of whom had improvement in sensory function but no improvement in motor function. Glassburn and Brady[83] in 1977 reported a series of nine patients in whom improvement was seen in six. In 2000, Calabrò and Jinkins[84] reported a single case where the patient experienced progressive improvement after HBOT. Combining all 3 of these publications, of a total of 16 clinical cases reported, 12 patients had some improvement.

In addition to this clinical experience, Feldmeier and colleagues[85] reported an animal study in 1993 where myelitis was delayed in its onset for several weeks in a group of animals that received HBOT 7 weeks after the completion of irradiation. In this study, the conditions of all animals in both the control and the three study groups progressed ultimately to severe myelitis. On review, the dosing scheme was probably so excessive that no durable prevention would be achievable by any means.

In another animal model, Sminia and coauthors[86] investigated whether HBOT given immediately or at intervals of 5, 10, or 15 weeks after an initial fractionated dose of 6500 cGy could prevent the subsequent development of radiation-induced transverse myelitis after an additional single dose of 2000 cGy. In this study, animals were not afforded any radioprotection by the HBOT. The HBOT regimen consisted of 30 daily treatments at 240 kPa (2.4 ATA), each consisting of 90 minutes of 100% oxygen exposure.

Based on this limited clinical and animal experience, it is really impossible to speak with any certainty regarding the effects of HBOT in this disorder. However, because no other therapies have been effective and the consequences are so devastating, the application of HBOT should be considered.

Optic Nerve

Five articles reporting the application of HBOT to the treatment of optic neuritis have been published to date.[87-91] All are either small case series or case reports. Four of the five publications detail positive results for the maintenance or improvement of vision. The three case reports demonstrate strongly positive results with HBOT, whereas the two

small case series give mixed but mostly negative results. In a series of four patients by Guy and Schatz,[87] the two who had prompt treatment (within 72 hours of onset) improved. If treatment was delayed by more than 72 hours, no improvement was detected.

The largest series of 13 patients, by Roden and investigators,[88] showed no improvement in any patient in their series. It should be noted that in this series, no patient initiated treatment sooner than 2 weeks after onset of visual loss, and treatment was initiated as long as 12 weeks after onset of visual loss. Guy and Schatz[87] had shown that HBOT was unlikely to be effective if started more than 72 hours after onset of visual loss. Eleven of 23 patients in this case series were also treated with steroids with doses as high as 1000 mg methylprednisolone daily, which was also ineffective. In a total of 20 patients reported in the above publications who have received HBOT for radiation-induced optic neuritis, improvement has been reported in 7 (35%).

These results taken on the whole are certainly mixed, and a definitive case for HBOT cannot be made in the treatment of radiation-induced optic neuritis. However, because its application in these circumstances can be predicated based on the same mechanistic principles as in brain necrosis and radiation-induced myelitis, and again because there are no other useful strategies and because the implications of progressive optic neuropathy are so dire, treatment based on humanistic considerations should be offered. Treatment must be initiated promptly to be effective.

Brachial Plexus and Sacral Plexus

A single case report by Videtic and Venkatesan,[92] published in 1999, reports a positive outcome in a patient receiving HBOT for a radiation-induced sacral plexopathy.

Pritchard and colleagues[93] have reported the results of a randomized, controlled trial applying HBOT to the treatment of brachial plexopathy. The authors report that the trial did not demonstrate an advantage for the HBOT group compared with a control group based on their primary study end point, warm sensory threshold measurement. However, a careful reading of the Results section of the article reveals that the patients in the study group experienced a decreased rate of deterioration in physical function compared with the control group, and this difference was still statistically significant 12 months after completion of the study. Lymphedema in 6 of 17 HBOT patients improved unexpectedly with no such improvement in the control group.

The observation that lymphedema may be treated effectively by HBOT led to two studies, one by the British group conducting the brachial plexus study and one by the University of South Carolina group.[94,95] The British group enrolled 21 patients in a single arm trial where patients were exposed to 30 treatments of HBOT at 2.4 ATA for 100 minutes. Three of 19 patients had reduction in their arm volume by more than 20%. Six of 13 patients had improved lymphatic drainage as measured by a radioactive isotope clearance study. Eight of 15 patients had at least moderate lessening of induration in the breast, mammary fold or supraclavicular fossa. The mean reduction in arm volume was 7.51% at 12 months. These results were statistically significant.

In the study by Teas and investigators[94] from South Carolina, 10 women who had been irradiated and sustained upper extremity lymphedema received 20 HBOT treatments in a monoplace chamber at 2.0 ATA. Hand lymphedema was reduced an average of 38%, but total lymphedema volume was not reduced. In the eight women who experienced benefit, the improvement was persistent to an average 14.2 months of follow-up. The authors also assayed VEGF-C (the lymphatic vessel growth factor). It increased with HBOT, and these results were statistically significant.

Precautions: Does Hyperbaric Oxygen Enhance Cancer Growth or Recurrence?

Frequently, patients and health-care professionals alike will express a reluctance to consider HBOT as a treatment for radiation injury because of fears that exposure to high-pressure oxygen will increase the likelihood of recurrence or enhance growth in an occult cancer. From a commonsense mechanistic perspective, these concerns would seem reasonable at first glance. After all, HBOT is typically used to stimulate angiogenesis and cellular proliferation in chronic wounds. Feldmeier and associates[96] reviewed this issue initially in 1994 and updated this review in 2003.[97] These review articles considered the published experience in animal models and in clinical experience. Most of the clinical experience was obtained from the era of controlled trials conducted in the 1960s and 1970s wherein HBOT was investigated as a radiation sensitizer. Most of these studies showed no enhancement of cancer recurrence or growth. A few trials reported in this review actually suggest a possible retardation of malignant growth with exposure to HBOT. In the latter of these two reviews, the authors discuss the important differences in control and initiation of angiogenesis in tumors versus healing wounds and postulate that these important differences explain why cancer growth enhancement is not enhanced, whereas wound healing enhancement is seen after hyperbaric oxygen exposure.

Since publication of the Feldmeier reviews, several other authors have reported on this issue. In 2004, Chong and associates[98] reported that in an animal model of transplanted human prostate cancer cells, there was no increase in tumor vessel density, proliferative index, differentiation, or apoptosis markers in animals exposed to HBOT compared with control animals. Six additional investigations have been published including studies of cell cultures, chemically induced murine mammary tumors, xenografts of human head and neck cancers transplanted into experimental animals, and murine colorectal cancer cells transplanted to cause liver metastases.[99-104] None of these publications showed enhanced growth of the cancers being studied. In fact, Granowitz and colleagues' article[102] showed inhibited growth of a human mammary transplanted tumor after exposure to hyperbaric oxygen.

Promising Areas for Additional Research

The prophylaxis of radiation injury with early HBOT is certainly preferable to its treatment after it has become fully developed. The nature of delayed radiation injury with the characteristic latent period between treatment and full expression of the injury provides an opportunity to intervene before its clinical manifestation. It is, however, not practical to treat all 700,000 or so patients who receive therapeutic radiation annually in the United States with prophylactic HBOT. Most patients will not require any therapeutic intervention because they will not demonstrate a degree of radiation injury that is life threatening or quality of life reducing. The development and validation of predictive assays that would reliably identify those at high risk for injury will permit prophylactic intervention. Currently, it is reasonable to consider prophylactic delivery of HBOT to those who have received exceptionally high doses of irradiation either accidentally or intentionally when reirradiation is planned in the setting of salvage therapy where few, if any, other options may be available.

The identification of useful predictive assays for delayed radiation injury will most likely involve the refinement of our understanding of the currently identified fibrogenetic cytokines and the recognition of additional cytokines or other as yet unidentified bioactive reactive chemicals that are generated in response to radiation. Other assays could include functional or metabolic measurements such as transcutaneous oxygen or soft-tissue tonometry or compliance testing.[105]

There has been a renewed interest in revisiting HBOT for its radiation-sensitizing properties. This application is based on sound radiation biology principles. Innovative methods to administer radiation during or just after a session of HBOT have been discussed by several investigators. At the University of Amsterdam at the Children's Cancer Center, researchers have pioneered a technique whereby children with advanced neuroblastoma are infused with a radioactive isotope (MIBG) and then treated with HBOT.[106] The addition of hyperbaric oxygen sensitization has led to much improved response rates. We discussed earlier the interest by several Japanese groups in irradiating high-grade brain tumor patients immediately after HBOT. The Baromedical Research Institute has initiated a protocol for treating head and neck cancer patients with radiation immediately after HBOT.

SUMMARY

HBOT has shown consistent benefit in treating patients with delayed radiation injury when it is applied as a portion of the multidisciplinary management of delayed radiation injury. When it is applied to ORN, management must include surgical extirpation of necrotic bone. We must remember the hard-learned lessons of Marx and others. When surgery is required, the bulk of planned HBOT should come before this surgical intervention. Fruitful areas for future HBOT for the radiation patient should include early prophylactic intervention for those recognized to be at high risk. Additional future applications for HBOT as a radiosensitizer also give great promise. Randomized protocols should establish the efficacy and optimal protocols to be used when using HBOT as a radiation sensitizer. The medical community, especially our youngest colleagues in the 21st century, demands evidence-based guidance when selecting therapeutic endeavors. Currently, the Baromedical Research Institute has taken the lead in providing randomized, controlled studies to establish the role of HBOT for these indications. Ultimately and ideally, reasonably large randomized and multi-institutional trials will support and define the optimal application of HBOT to the treatment and prophylaxis of radiation injury and its use as a radiosensitizer.

REFERENCES

1. Deimling GT, Kahan B, Bowman KF, et al: Cancer survivorship and psychological distress in later life. Psychooncology 11:479, 2002.
2. Jemal A, Thomas A, Siegel R, et al: Cancer statistics, 2007. CA Cancer J Clin 57:43-66, 2007.

3. Perez CA, Brady LW, Halperin EC, Schmidt-Ullrich RK: Preface. In: Perez CA, Brady LW, Halperin EC, Schmidt-Ullrich RK (eds): Principles and Practice of Radiation Oncology, 4 ed. Philadelphia, Lippincott Williams & Wilkins, 2004, pp xix-xx.

4. Dorr W, Hendry H: Consequential late effects in normal tissues. Radiother Oncol 61:223-231, 2001.

5. Emami B, Lyman J, Brown A, et al: Tolerance of normal tissue to therapeutic irradiation. Int J Radiat Oncol Biol Phys 21:109-122, 1991.

6. Hall EJ, Giaccia AJ (eds): Radiobiology for the Radiologist, 6 ed. Philadelphia, Lippincott Williams & Wilkins, 2006, pp 64-65.

7. Mohan R, Low D, Chao KSC, Dong L: Intensity-modulated radiation treatment planning, quality assurance, delivery and clinical application. In: Perez CA, Brady LW, Halperin EC, Schmidt-Ullrich RK (eds): Principles and Practice of Radiation Oncology, 4 ed. Philadelphia, Lippincott Williams & Wilkins, 2004, pp 314-334.

8. Wasserman TH, Chapman JD: Radiation response modulation. In: Perez CA, Brady LW, Halperin EC, Schmidt-Ullrich RK (eds): Principles and Practice of Radiation Oncology, 4 ed. Philadelphia, Lippincott Williams & Wilkins, 2004, pp 663-694.

9. Nias AHW: Reparable damage. An Introduction to Radiobiology, Chirchester, England, John Wiley & Sons, 1990, pp 93-109.

10. Rubin P: Late effects of chemotherapy and radiation therapy: A new hypothesis. Int J Radiat Oncol Biol Phys 10:5-34, 1984.

11. Rubin P, Finkelstein J, Shapiro D: Molecular biology mechanisms in the radiation induction of pulmonary injury syndromes. Int J Radiat Oncol Biol Phys 24:93-101, 1992.

12. Fleckenstein K, Gauter-Fleckenstein B, Jackson IL, et al: Using biological markers to predict risk of radiation injury. Semin Radiat Oncol 17:89-98, 2007.

13. Stone HB, McBride WH, Coleman CN: Meeting report: Modifying normal tissue damage post-irradiation: Report of a workshop by the radiation research program, National Cancer Institute, Bethesda, Maryland, September 6-8, 2000. Radiat Res 157:204-223, 2002.

14. Denton A, Forbes A, Andreyev J, Maher EJ: Non-surgical interventions for late radiation proctitis in patients who have received radical radiotherapy to the pelvis (Cochrane Review). Cochrane Database Syst Rev (1):CD003455, 2002.

15. Delanian S, Lefaix J: Current management for late normal tissue injury: Radiation-induced fibrosis and necrosis. Semin Radiat Oncol 17:99-107, 2007.

16. Pritchard J, Anand P, Broome J, et al: Double-blind randomized phase II study of hyperbaric oxygen in patients with radiation-induced brachial plexopathy. Radiother Oncol 58:279-286, 2001.

17. Annane D, Depondt J, Aubert P, et al: Hyperbaric oxygen therapy for radionecrosis of the jaw: A randomized controlled, double-blind trial from ORN96 Study Group. J Clin Oncol 22:4893-4900, 2004.

18. Ferreira P, Fleck J, Diehl A, et al: Protective effect of alpha-tocopherolin head and neck cancer radiation-induced mucositis: A double blind randomized trial. Head Neck 26:313-321, 2004.

19. Gothard L, Cornes P, Earl J, et al: Double blind placebo-controlled randomized trial of vitamin E and pentoxyfylline in patients with chronic arm lymph-edema and fibrosis after surgery and radiotherapy for breast cancer. Radiother Oncol 73:133-139, 2004.

20. Feldmeier JJ, Hampson NB: A systematic review of the literature reporting the application of hyperbaric oxygen prevention and treatment of delayed radiation injuries: An evidence based approach. Undersea Hyperb Med 29:4-30, 2002.

21. Bennett M, Feldmeier J, Smee R, et al: Hyperbaric oxygenation for tumour sensitisation to radiotherapy. Cochrane Database Syst Rev (4):CD005007, 2005.

22. Kaanders JH: Clinical studies of hypoxia modification in radiotherapy. Semin Radiat Oncol 14:233-240, 2004.

23. Kohshi K, Kinoshita Y, Terrashima H, et al: Radiotherapy after hyperbaric oxygenation for malignant gliomas: A pilot study. Cancer Res Clin Oncol 122:676-678, 1996.

24. Kohishi K, Kinoshita Y, Imada H, et al: Effects of radiotherapy after hyperbaric oxygenation on malignant gliomas. Br J Cancer 80:236-241, 1999.

25. Beppu T, Kamada K, Nakamura R, et al: A phase II study of radiotherapy after hyperbaric oxygenation combined with interferon-beta and nimustine hydrochloride to treat surpratentorial malignant gliomas. J Neurooncol 61:161-170, 2003.

26. Ogawa K, Yoshii Y, Inoue O, et al: Prospective trial of radiotherapy after hyperbaric oxygenation with chemotherapy for high-grade gliomas. Radiother Oncol 67:63-67, 2003.

27. Dick Clarke: Personal communication, January 2006.

28. Marx RE: Radiation injury to tissue. In: Kindwall EP (ed): Hyperbaric Medicine Practice, 2nd ed. Flagstaff, Ariz, Best Publishing, 1999, pp 665-723.

29. Feldmeier JJ, Jelen I, Davolt DA, et al: Hyperbaric oxygen as a prophylaxis for radiation induced delayed enteropathy. Radiother Oncol 35:138-144, 1995.

30. Feldmeier JJ, Davolt DA, Court WS, et al: Histologic morphometry confirms a prophylactic effect for hyperbaric oxygen in the prevention of delayed radiation enteropathy. Undersea Hyper Med 25:93-97, 1998.

31. Goldstein LJ, Gallagher KA, Bauer SM, et al: Endothelial progenitor cell release into circulation is triggered by hyperoxia-induced increases in bone marrow nitric oxide. Stem Cells 24:2309-2318, 2006.

32. Gallagher KA, Liu Z, Xiao M, et al: Diabetic impairments in NO-mediated endothelial progenitor mobilization and homing are reversed by hyperoxia and SDF-1 alpha. J Clin Invest 117:1249-1259, 2007.

33. Tobey RE, Kelly JF: Osteoradionecrosis of the jaws. Otolaryngol Clin North Am 12:183-186, 1979.

34. Maier A, Gaggl A, Klemen H, et al: Review of severe osteoradionecrosis treated by surgery alone or surgery with postoperative hyperbaric oxygenation. Br J Oral Maxillofac Surg 38:173-176, 2000.

35. Feldmeier JJ, Heimbach RD, Davolt DA, et al: Hyperbaric oxygen as an adjunctive treatment for delayed radiation injury of the chest wall: A retrospective review of 23 cases. Undersea Hyperb Med 22:383-393, 1995.

36. Feldmeier JJ, Hampson NB, Bennett M: In response to the negative randomized controlled trial by Annane et al in the treatment of mandibular ORN. Undersea Hyperb Med 32:141-143, 2005.

37. Laden G: Hyperbaric oxygen therapy for radionecrosis: Clear evidence from confusing data [letter]. J Clin Oncol 23:4465, 2005.

38. Moon RE, McGraw TA, Blakey G: Hyperbaric oxygen therapy for radiation necrosis of the jaw: Comments on a randomized study. Undersea Hyperb Med 32:145-146, 2005.

39. Mendenhall WM: Mandibular osteoradionecrosis [editorial]. J Clin Oncol 22:4867-4868, 2004.

40. Gal TJ, Yueh B, Futran ND: Influence of prior hyperbaric oxygen therapy in complications following microvascular reconstruction for advanced osteoradionecrosis. Arch Otolaryngol Head Neck Surg 129:72-76, 2003.

41. Teng MS, Futran ND: Osteoradionecrosis of the mandible. Curr Opin Otolaryngol Head Neck Surg 13:217-221, 2005.

42. Vudiniabola S, Pirone C, Williamson J, Goss ANN: Hyperbaric oxygen in the prevention of osteoradionecrosis of the jaws. Aust Dent J 44:243-247, 1999.

43. David LA, Sandor GK, Evans AW, Brown DH: Hyperbaric oxygen therapy and mandibular osteoradionecrosis: A retrospective study and analysis of treatment outcomes. J Can Dent Assoc 67:384, 2001.

44. Chavez JA, Adkinson CD: Adjunctive hyperbaric oxygen in irradiated patients requiring dental extractions: Outcomes and complications. J Oral Maxillofac Surg 59:518-522, 2001.

45. Sulaiman F, Huryn JM, Ziotolow IM: Dental extractions in the irradiated head and neck patient: A retrospective analysis of Memorial Sloan-Kettering Cancer Center protocols, criteria, and end results. J Oral Maxillofac Surg 61:1123-1131, 2003.

46. Wahl MJ: Osteoradionecrosis prevention myths. Int J Radiation Oncology Biol Phys 64:661-669, 2006.

47. Ferguson BJ, Hudson WR, Farmer JC: Hyperbaric oxygen for laryngeal radionecrosis. Ann Otol Laryngol 96:1-6, 1987.

48. Feldmeier JJ, Heimbach RD, Davolt DA, Brakora MJ: Hyperbaric oxygen as an adjunctive treatment for severe laryngeal necrosis: A report of nine consecutive cases. Undersea Hyperb Med 20:329-335, 1993.

49. Filintisis GA, Moon RE, Kraft KL, et al: Laryngeal radionecrosis and hyperbaric oxygen therapy: Report of 18 cases and review of the literature. Ann Otol Rhinol Laryngol 109:554-562, 2000.

50. Narzony W, Sicko Z, Kot J, et al: Hyperbaric oxygen therapy in the treatment of complications of irradiation in the head and neck area. Undersea Hyperb Med 32:103-110, 2005.

51. Hsu YC, Lee KW, Tsai KB, et al: Treatment of laryngeal necrosis with hyperbaric oxygen therapy: A case report. Kaohsing Med 21:88-92, 2005.

52. Davis JC, Dunn JM, Gates GA, Heimbach RD: Hyperbaric oxygen: A new adjunct in the management of radiation necrosis. Arch Otolaryngol 105:58-61, 1979.

53. Neovius EB, Lind MG, Lind FG: Hyperbaric oxygen for wound complications after surgery in the irradiated head and neck: A review of the literature and a report of 15 consecutive cases. Head Neck 19:315-322, 1997.

54. Feldmeier JJ, Newman R, Davolt DA, et al: Prophylactic hyperbaric oxygen for patients undergoing salvage for recurrent head and neck cancers following full course irradiation [abstract]. Undersea Hyperb Med 25[suppl]:10, 1998.

55. Carl UM, Hartmann KA: Hyperbaric oxygen treatment for symptomatic breast edema after radiation therapy. Undersea Hyperb Med 25:233-234, 1998.

56. Carl UM, Feldmeier JJ, Schmitt G, Hartmann KA: Hyperbaric oxygen therapy for late sequelae in women receiving radiation after breast conserving surgery. Int J Radiat Oncol Biol Phys 49:1029-1031, 2001.

57. Bevers RF, Bakker DJ, Kurth KH: Hyperbaric oxygen treatment for haemorrhagic radiation cystitis. Lancet 346:803-805, 1995.

58. Lee HC, Liu CC, Lin SN: Hyperbaric oxygen therapy in radiation-induced hemorrhagic cystitis—a report of 25 cases. Jpn J Hyperbar Med 29:23, 1994.

59. Neheman A, Nativ O, Moskovitz B, et al: Hyperbaric oxygen therapy for radiation-induced haemorrhagic cystitis. BJU Int 96:107-109, 2005.

60. Corman JM, McClure D, Pritchett R, et al: Treatment of radiation induced hemorrhagic cystitis with hyperbaric oxygen. J Urol 160:2200-2202, 2003.

61. Chong KT, Hampson NB, Corman JM: Early hyperbaric oxygen improves outcome for radiation-induced hemorrhagic cystitis. Urology 65:649-653, 2005.

62. Cheng C, Foo KT: Management of severe chronic radiation cystitis. Ann Acad Med Singapore 21:368-371, 1992.

63. Li A, Sun J, Chao H: Late bladder complications following radiotherapy of carcinoma of the uterine cervix. Zhonghua Fu Chan Ke Za Zhi 30:741-743, 1995.

64. Del Pizzo JJ, Chew BH, Jacobs SC, Sklar GN: Treatment of radiation induced hemorrhagic cystitis with hyperbaric oxygen: Long term follow-up. J Urol 160:731-733, 1998.

65. Jones K, Evans AW, Bristow RG, et al: Treatment of radiation proctitis with hyperbaric oxygen. Radiother Oncol 78:91-94, 2006.

66. Girnius S, Cersonsky N, Gesell L, et al: Treatment of refractory radiation-induced hemorrhagic proctitis with hyperbaric oxygen therapy. Am J Clin Oncol 29:588-592, 2006.

67. Dall'Era MA, Hampson NB, His RA, et al: Hyperbaric oxygen therapy for radiation induced proctopathy in men treated for prostate cancer. J Urol 176:87-90, 2006.

68. Marshall GT, Thirlby RC, Bredfeldt JE, Hampson NB: Treatment of gastrointestinal radiation injury with hyperbaric oxygen. Undersea Hyperb Med 34:35-42, 2007.

69. Farmer JC, Shelton DL, Bennett PD, et al: Treatment of radiation-induced injury by hyperbaric oxygen. Ann Otol 87:707-715, 1978.

70. Williams JAA, Clarke D, Dennis WAA, et al: Treatment of pelvic soft tissue radiation necrosis with hyperbaric oxygen. Am J Obstet Gynecol 167:415-416, 1992.

71. Feldmeier JJ, Heimbach RD, Davolt DA, et al: Hyperbaric oxygen as an adjunctive treatment for delayed radiation injuries of the abdomen and pelvis. Undersea Hyperb Med 23:205-213, 1997.

72. Fink D, Chetty N, Lehm JP, et al: Hyperbaric oxygen therapy for delayed radiation injuries in gynecological cancers. Int J Gynecol Cancer 16:638-642, 2006.

73. Feldmeier JJ, Heimbach RD, Davolt DA, et al: Hyperbaric oxygen in the treatment of delayed radiation injuries of the extremities. Undersea Hyperb Med 27:15-19, 2000.

74. Hart GB, Mainous EG: The treatment of radiation necrosis with hyperbaric oxygen (OHP). Cancer 37:2580-2585, 1976.

75. Chuba PJ, Aronin P, Bhambhani K, et al: Hyperbaric oxygen therapy for radiation-induced brain injury in children. Cancer 80:2005-2012, 1997.

76. Leber KA, Eder HG, Kovac H, et al: Treatment of cerebral radionecrosis by hyperbaric oxygen therapy. Stereotact Funct Neurosurg 70(suppl 1):229-236, 1998.

77. Cirafisi C, Verderame F: Radiation-induced rhombo-encephalopathy. Ital J Neurol Sci 20:55-58, 1999.

78. Dear Gde L, Rose RE, Dunn R, et al: Treatment of neurological symptoms of radionecrosis of the brain with hyperbaric oxygen: A case series. Paper presented at the 35th Annual Undersea and Hyperbaric Medical Society Scientific Meeting. June 28-30, 2002, San Diego, California.

79. Gesell LB, Warnick R, Breneman J, et al: Effectiveness of hyperbaric oxygen for the treatment of soft tissue radionecrosis of the brain. Paper presented at the 35th Annual Undersea and Hyperbaric Medical Society Scientific Meeting. June 28-30, 2002, San Diego, California.

80. Kohshi K, Imada H, Nomoto S, et al: Successful treatment of radiation-induced brain necrosis by hyperbaric oxygen therapy. J Neurol Sci 209(1-2):115-117, 2003.

81. Takenaka N, Imanishi T, Sasaki H, et al: Delayed radiation necrosis with extensive brain edema after gamma knife radiosurgery for multiple cerebral cavernous malformations—case report. Neurol Med Chir (Tokyo) 43:391-395, 2003.

82. Marcus RB Jr, Million RR: The incidence of transverse myelitis after radiation of the cervical spinal cord. Int J Radiat Oncol Biol Phys 19:3-8, 1990.

83. Glassburn JR, Brady LW. Treatment with hyperbaric oxygen for radiation myelitis. In: Smith G (ed): Proceedings of the Sixth International Congress on Hyperbaric Medicine, Aberdeen, Scotland, Aberdeen University Press, 1977, pp 266-277.

84. Calabrò F, Jinkins JR: MRI of radiation myelitis: A report of a case treated with hyperbaric oxygen. Eur Radiol 10:1079-1084, 2000.

85. Feldmeier JJ, Lange JD, Cox SD, et al: Hyperbaric oxygen as a prophylaxis or treatment for radiation myelitis. Undersea Hyperb Med 20:249-255, 1993.

86. Sminia P, Van der Kleij AJ, Carl UM, et al: Prophylactic hyperbaric oxygen treatment and rat spinal cord re-irradiation. Cancer Lett 191:59-65, 2003.

87. Guy J, Schatz NJ: Hyperbaric oxygen in the treatment of radiation-induced optic neuropathy. Ophthalmology 93:1083-1088, 1986.

88. Roden D, Bosley TM, Fowble B, et al: Delayed radiation injury to the retrobulbar optic nerves and chiasm. Clinical syndrome and treatment with hyperbaric oxygen and corticosteroids. Ophthalmology 97:346-351, 1990.

89. Fontanesi J, Golden EB, Cianci PC, Heideman RL: Treatment of radiation-induced optic neuropathy in the pediatric population. J Hyperb Med 6:245-248, 1991.

90. Borruat FXX, Schatz NJJ, Blaser JSS, et al: Visual recovery from radiation-induced optic neuropathy. The role of hyperbaric oxygen therapy. J Clin Neuroophthalmol 13:98-101, 1993.

91. Boschetti M, De Lucchi M, Giusti M, et al: Partial visual recovery from radiation-induced optic neuropathy after hyperbaric oxygen therapy in a patient with Cushing disease. Eur J Endocrinol 154:813-818, 2006.

92. Videtic GM, Venkatesan VM: Hyperbaric oxygen corrects sacral plexopathy due to osteoradionecrosis appearing 15 years after pelvic irradiation. Clin Oncol (R Coll Radiol) 11:198-199, 1999.

93. Pritchard J, Anand P, Broome J, et al: Double-blind randomized phase II study of hyperbaric oxygen in patients with radiation-induced brachial plexopathy. Radiother Oncol 58:279-286, 2001.

94. Teas J, Cunningham JE, Cone L, et al: Can hyperbaric oxygen reduce breast cancer treatment-related lymphedema? A pilot study. J Women's Health 9:1008-1018, 2004.

95. Gothard L, Stanton A, MacLaren J, et al: Non-randomized phase II trial of hyperbaric oxygen therapy in patients with chronic lymphedema and tissue fibrosis after radiotherapy for early breast cancer. Radiother Oncol 70:217-224, 2004.

96. Feldmeier JJ, Heimbach RD, Davolt DA, et al: Does hyperbaric oxygen have a cancer causing or promoting effect? A review of the pertinent literature. Undersea Hyperb Med 21:467-475, 1994.

97. Feldmeier JJ, Carl U, Hartmann K, Sminia P: Hyperbaric oxygen: Does it promote growth or recurrence of malignancy? Undersea Hyperb Med 30:1-18, 2003.

98. Chong KT, Hampson NB, Bostwick DG, et al: Hyperbaric oxygen does not accelerate latent in vivo prostate cancer: implications for the treatment of radiation-induced haemorrhagic cystitis. BJU Int 94:1275-1278, 2004.

99. Stuhr LE, Iverson VV, Straume O, et al: Hyperbaric oxygen alone or combined with 5-FU attenuates growth of DMBA induced rat mammary tumors. Cancer Lett 210:35-40, 2004.

100. Sun TB, Chen RL, Hsu YH: The effect of hyperbaric oxygen on human oral cancer cells. Undersea Hyperb Med 31:251-260, 2004.

101. Shi Y, Lee CS, Wu J, et al: Effects of hyperbaric oxygen exposure on experimental head and neck tumor growth, oxygenation, and vasculature. Head Neck 27:362-369, 2005.

102. Granowitz EV, Tonomura N, Benson RM, et al: Hyperbaric oxygen inhibits benign and malignant human mammary epithelial cell proliferation. Anticancer Res 25:3833-3842, 2005.

103. Daruwalla J, Christophi C: The effect of hyperbaric oxygen therapy on tumour growth in a mouse model of colorectal cancer liver metastases. Eur J Cancer 42:3304-3311, 2006.

104. Haroon AT, Patel M, Al-Mehdi AB: Lung metastatic load limitation with hyperbaric oxygen. Undersea Hyperb Med 34:83-90, 2007.

105. Davis AM, Dische S, Gerber L, et al: Measuring post-irradiation subcutaneous fibrosis: State-of-the-art and future directions. Semin Radiat Oncol 13: 203-213, 2003.

106. Voute PA, van der Kliej AJ, De Kraker J, et al: Clinical experience with radiation enhancement by hyperbaric oxygen in children with recurrent neuroblastoma stage IV. Eur J Cancer 4:596-600, 1995.

Gas Embolism 13
Venous and Arterial Gas Embolism

Karen Van Hoesen, MD, and
Tom S. Neuman, MD, FACP, FACPM

Gas embolism, which is the entry of gas into the vascular system from veins, arteries, or both, is a potentially life-threatening event and can result in serious morbidity and mortality. Venous gas embolism (VGE) occurs when gas enters the venous circulation, usually from iatrogenic causes in the operating room or other invasive medical procedures. VGE may lead to cardiovascular collapse or to paradoxical arterial gas embolism (AGE). AGE is the entry of gas into the pulmonary veins or arterial circulation and most commonly results

257

from pulmonary barotrauma (PBT) while scuba diving. However, gas can be injected directly into the arterial circulation during radiologic procedures and cardiac bypass surgery or transgress through the pulmonary circulation, a patent foramen ovale, or any right-to-left shunt, leading to AGE.

Entry of gas into venous or arterial vessels requires a source of gas (usually the atmosphere or insufflation during arthroscopy or laparoscopy), a breach in the vascular wall, and a pressure gradient that favors entry of gas into the vessel. Although the clinical consequences of VGE and AGE are different, therapeutic interventions may be similar.

VENOUS GAS EMBOLISM

Epidemiology

VGE occurs when air enters the systemic venous system. Because of the increased invasiveness of modern diagnostic and therapeutic technologies, a striking increase in VGE has been reported in the literature. Improvements in end-tidal carbon dioxide and Doppler monitoring confirm that VGE is a common event during surgical procedure.[1] The exact incidence of VGE is unknown because many cases of VGE are subclinical and are unreported. All of the procedures that can lead to VGE have in common an incised vascular bed and a hydrostatic pressure gradient favoring the entry of gas into the vasculature.

Table 13.1 summarizes the surgical and invasive procedures that have been associated with VGE. Neurosurgical procedures have the greatest risk for VGE because of the upright position of the patient during surgery, the position of the brain relative to the heart, and numerous noncompressed venous channels potentially exposed to air.[2] VGE is also common during central venous catheterization and catheter removal.[3-5] Intravascular gas may be introduced during cardiovascular surgery including cardiopulmonary bypass grafting and angioplasty.[6-8] During laparoscopic surgery, air is delivered by positive pressure within the abdominal cavity, increasing the risk for

Table 13.1 Surgical or Invasive Procedures Associated with Gas Embolism

NEUROSURGICAL

Sitting position craniotomies
Posterior fossa procedures
Spinal fusion
Cervical laminectomy

CARDIAC

Cardiovascular surgery
Cardiopulmonary bypass grafting
Angioplasty

PULMONARY

Lung biopsy
Thoracentesis

ORTHOPEDIC

Total hip arthroplasty
Arthroscopy

GASTROINTESTINAL

Laparoscopy
Laparoscopic cholecystectomy
Retrograde cholangiopancreatography
Orthotopic liver transplantation
Percutaneous hepatic puncture

GYNECOLOGIC

Therapeutic abortion
Hysteroscopy
Cesarean delivery

UROLOGY

Transurethral prostatectomy

VGE, which has been reported during laparoscopy[9] and laparoscopic cholecystectomy.[10] Data suggest that VGE is not simply a complication of insufflation, but that surgical manipulation leading to inadvertent open vascular channels causes VGE.[11]

VGE and subsequent AGE have been reported during other surgical procedures including transurethral prostatectomy[12] and lung biopsy.[13-15] Fatal AGE has been associated with endoscopic retrograde cholangiopancreatography.[16] VGE is well described during orthotopic liver transplantation[17,18] and percutaneous hepatic puncture.[19] In addition, VGE is reported as a complication of arthroplasty and arthroscopy.[20-23] VGE can result from obstetric and gynecologic sources including oral sex during pregnancy,[24] therapeutic abortion,[25] hysteroscopy,[26] and cesarean delivery.[27,28] Death from AGE associated with sexual intercourse after vaginal delivery has been reported.[29]

Table 13.2 lists the nonsurgical causes of gas embolism. VGE and AGE can result from nonsurgical procedures including pulmonary overexpansion during mechanical ventilation[30] and during hemodialysis.[31,32] VGE caused by a computed tomography (CT) injector has been reported, but in the majority of cases the air does not arterialize.[33,34] Penetrating chest injuries can allow air to enter the circulation leading to VGE and AGE.[35,36] Massive cerebral air embolism may occur after entrance of air into the circulatory system via ruptured pulmonary vessels during cardiopulmonary resuscitation.[37] Cerebral and coronary gas embolism have occurred from inhalation of pressurized helium[38,39] and ingestion of hydrogen peroxide.[40]

Pathophysiology

The pathophysiology of VGE is related to the volume of gas that enters the vasculature and the rate of accumulation of gas. Rapid entry of gas or large volumes of gas cause increased right pulmonary artery pressures with resultant right ventricular strain.

Pulmonary

The pulmonary circulation and alveolar interface allow for dissipation of intravascular gas. The pulmonary arterioles and capillaries usually act as an effective filter against gas bubbles reaching the systemic circulation. However, the ability of the lung to filter air may be exceeded by rapid introduction of large quantities of air during invasive procedures. In a dog model, Butler and Hills[41] demonstrated that when infused slowly, air bubbles of greater than 22 μm in diameter are filtered by the lungs. However, 30 mL of air injected into a central vein exceeded the filtering capacity of the lung and produced embolization through the left heart and into the arterial circulation.[42,43] Gas bubbles in the pulmonary circulation increase microvascular permeability[44] and can lead to endothelin 1 release from the pulmonary vasculature, causing pulmonary hypertension.[45] Changes in the resistance of the pulmonary vessels lead to ventilation/perfusion mismatch and abnormal gas exchange.[46]

Cardiac

A large volume of gas can strain right ventricular outflow because of migration of the emboli to the pulmonary circulation, increasing pulmonary artery pressure and decreasing pulmonary venous return. Because of diminished pulmonary venous return, there is decreased left ventricular preload, which can lead to compromised cardiac output causing arrhythmias and systemic cardiovascular collapse.[47] Animal experiments estimate the lethal volume of gas as an acute bolus is 0.55 mL/kg in rabbits[48] and 7.5 mL/kg in dogs.[49] From case reports of accidental injections of intravascular air, Toung and colleagues[50] estimate that the lethal volume of gas in an adult human is 200 to 300 mL, or 3 to 5 mg/kg. Such large amounts of gas can cause a gas "air lock" in the right ventricle with complete outflow obstruction, leading to immediate cardiovascular collapse.[47]

Table 13.2 Nonsurgical Causes of Gas Embolism

DIRECT VASCULAR ACCESS

Central venous catheterization and catheter removal
Hemodialysis
CT injector

CHEST TRAUMA

Penetrating chest injuries
Cardiopulmonary resuscitation
Blast injuries

OTHER

Mechanical ventilation
Inhalation of pressurized helium
Ingestion of hydrogen peroxide
Oral sex during pregnancy
Sexual intercourse after vaginal delivery

Paradoxical Embolism

Paradoxical embolization occurs when gas that has entered the venous circulation migrates to the systemic arterial circulation, leading to signs and symptoms of an AGE. The two mechanisms by which this can occur are migration of gas through a right-to-left shunt (i.e., a patent foramen ovale) and overwhelming the pulmonary capillary filtration system.

A patent foramen ovale is found in 27.3% of the general population and 34% of people younger than 30 years at the time of autopsy.[51] When the pressure in the right atrium exceeds the pressure in the left atrium, a hemodynamically important right-to-left shunt occurs and blood flows through the foramen ovale. VGE may cause increased pulmonary artery pressures, as mentioned earlier, leading to elevated right heart pressures, causing gas to pass through a patent foramen ovale and into the systemic circulation.[52-54] In addition, the use of mechanical ventilation and positive end-expiratory pressure may also increase right heart pressures, allowing gas to pass across a patent foramen ovale.

Venous air may also transverse the pulmonary vasculature to enter the arterial circulation. Animal studies demonstrate the presence of intra-arterial bubbles after a large bolus of gas or a small, continuous injection of gas into the venous system.[41,55,56] Butler and Hills[42] have demonstrated arterial embolization of gas after a 30-mL bolus injection of air into a central vein in a dog model. They determined that the physiologic filter of the lung becomes overwhelmed above $0.4 \text{ mL} \cdot \text{kg}^{-1} \cdot \text{min}^{-1}$. Spencer[55] studied a slow venous injection (0.15 mL/kg/min) of gas into the jugular vein of sheep and detected arterial embolization by Doppler in the majority of sheep, none of which had any evidence of cardiac shunts at postmortem examination. Fatal cerebral gas embolisms from large venous gas emboli have been reported in humans without evidence of an intracardiac septal defect.[57,58]

Clinical Manifestations

The clinical manifestations of VGE are dependent on the volume of gas that enters the vasculature and the rate of entrainment of gas. VGE produces cardiovascular, pulmonary, and neurologic sequelae. Symptoms of right heart strain may develop, and tachyarrhythmias and hypotension may occur as cardiac output declines. Awake patients may complain of acute dyspnea, coughing, and chest pain. Pulmonary signs may include rales and wheezing. If the patient is being monitored, such as during anesthesia, decrease in end-tidal carbon dioxide and hypercapnia can be detected.[1] Invasive monitoring may show increased pulmonary airway pressure and central venous pressure. Reduced cardiac output from outflow obstruction, right ventricular failure, or myocardial ischemia can lead to cardiovascular collapse, resulting in cerebral hypoperfusion and altered mental status. The neurologic presentation of venous gas emboli that pass into the arterial circulation and cause cerebral AGE are discussed in the following section.

Diagnosis

The diagnosis of VGE and possible resulting AGE is a clinical diagnosis and requires a high index of suspicion. A sudden loss of consciousness or hemodynamic collapse during or immediately after any invasive procedure that has a risk for gas embolism may indicate a gas embolism. The temporal relation between the injection of air and the sudden development of symptoms must lead the clinician to a presumptive diagnosis of possible gas embolism.

Numerous real-time monitors can be used for the detection of VGE, and many of these are now standard during surgical procedures. Transesophageal echocardiography can visualize intravenous and intracardiac bubbles directly and is the most sensitive monitoring device for VGE.[59] However, its use is limited by the fact that it is invasive and requires expertise and constant monitoring. Precordial

Doppler is the most sensitive of the noninvasive monitors and has been used with success in detecting VGE.[60] Transcranial Doppler ultrasound is highly sensitive for detection of gas that has passed through a right-to-left shunt or a direct AGE and is often used during procedures with a high risk for gas embolism, such as neurosurgical procedures or cardiac surgery.[61,62] A decrease in end-tidal carbon dioxide levels may indicate a change between ventilation and perfusion and may be indicative of a VGE in the pulmonary circulation.[63]

Treatment of Venous Gas Embolism

The treatment for VGE is primarily supportive. Further entry of gas must be prevented. The patient should be placed on 100% oxygen to treat hypoxia and hypoxemia. Supplemental oxygen also reduces the size of the gas embolus by establishing a diffusion gradient to increase the egress of gas from the bubble.[64] Aggressive cardiopulmonary resuscitation may be indicated and has been shown to be effective for massive VGE that results in cardiac arrest.[65] Cardiac massage may force air out of the pulmonary outflow tract into smaller pulmonary vessels and improve blood flow. Both dog models and clinical human evidence have demonstrated the efficacy of cardiac massage.[66] In the case of VGE via a subclavian vein catheter, Coppa and colleagues[67] have recommended advancing the catheter into the heart to withdraw air from the right ventricle. Although some authors have suggested aspiration of air from the right heart percutaneously,[68-70] no data support emergent catheter insertion for aspiration of gas from acute VGE.

Because VGE increases right ventricular afterload resulting in right ventricular failure and a decrease in left ventricular output, inotropic support of the right ventricle may be indicated. Dobutamine and ephedrine have been successfully used in patients with VGE-induced hemodynamic dysfunction.[71,72]

The use of hyperbaric oxygen therapy (HBOT) for the treatment of AGE that results from paradoxical embolism from VGE or gas injected directly into the arterial circulation is discussed in detail in the following section. However, it remains questionable whether HBOT should be used routinely for iatrogenic VGE. Clearly, as mentioned earlier, AGE as a result of VGE should be treated with HBOT, and there are reports suggesting improved outcome.[73-75] As most patients with small VGE (i.e., those of no or minimal hemodynamic consequences) do well with supportive care, HBOT is probably not indicated in those cases. In patients with severe cardiovascular instability, the risks versus benefits of transport to a hyperbaric chamber must be considered, especially because there are no clear data indicating an improved outcome in such patients treated with HBOT.

ARTERIAL GAS EMBOLISM AND PULMONARY BAROTRAUMA

Epidemiology

AGE secondary to PBT ranks second only to drowning as a cause of death in scuba divers.[76,77] In addition, AGE can lead to unconsciousness in the water with subsequent drowning and may be misclassified as a drowning death by pathologists. Any condition that leads to unconsciousness in the water, such as an AGE, an arrhythmia, or hypoglycemia, can result in aspiration of water and subsequent pathologic changes associated with drowning, hence leading to an incorrect diagnosis. AGE may actually be the leading cause of death in scuba divers.[78,79]

PBT caused by overinflation was first reported in cases where bellows were used to provide artificial ventilation around the time of the Civil War,[80] whereas AGE was first described by Polack and Adams in 1932.[81] Currently, the exact incidence of PBT in divers is unknown because cases may be asymptomatic and therefore go undiagnosed. In a group of submarine-escape trainees, 2 of 170 had asymptomatic evidence of extra-alveolar air on chest radiographs after submarine-escape training.[82] In a series of divers with AGE,

Harker and coworkers[83] reported radiographic evidence of PBT in 42%. The incidence of AGE in divers is not known because it may be misdiagnosed. Based on data collected by the Divers Alert Network, approximately 100 cases of AGE occur annually in the United States, Caribbean, and Canada combined.[77]

PBT and secondary AGE occur more frequently in novice or inexperienced divers and are usually associated with panicking in the event of an out-of-air situation or a rapid, uncontrolled ascent.[84] Other specific activities that especially carry a risk for PBT and AGE include submarine-escape training, out-of-air emergency ascent training, and buddy-breathing ascent training.[85,86]

Pulmonary Barotrauma

PBT from diving results from expansion of gas trapped in the lungs during ascent. If a diver does not allow the expanding gas to escape, a pressure differential develops between the intrapulmonary air space and the ambient pressure. The combination of overdistension of the alveoli and overpressurization causes the alveoli to rupture, producing a spectrum of injuries collectively referred to as PBT. Under experimental conditions in fresh chilled human cadavers, a transpulmonic pressure (the difference between the intratracheal and the intrapleural pressures) of 95 to 110 cm H_2O is sufficient to disrupt the pulmonary parenchyma leading to extra-alveolar gas.[87,88]

Breath-holding is the most common cause of PBT and AGE in sport divers. In submarine-escape trainees, breath-holding did not appear to be a major factor, leading to the conclusion that, in the majority of these patients, some intrinsic abnormality of the lungs was the cause of the injury. Review of pulmonary function tests in submarine-escape trainees found that a small forced vital capacity (but still within the reference range) was the only factor that correlated with a risk for PBT.[89] Localized overinflation of the lung from focally increased elastic recoil may occur in divers who ascend at a proper rate.[90,91] Theoretically, if there are focal areas of decreased

compliance in the lungs, the adjacent areas of normal compliance would be subjected to greater forces leading to barotrauma.[92] With immersion in diving, central pooling of blood causes an increase in intrapulmonary blood volume and the lungs become stiffer (less compliant); this decreased compliance of the lung may increase the risk for PBT. This may explain the almost complete absence of case reports of AGE associated with hyperbaric chamber operations.

The exact mechanism of PBT is unclear. There are reports of divers with AGE with no history of breath-holding ascent.[84] Scuba divers with asthma do not appear to have a greater risk for idiopathic AGE than nonasthmatic divers.[93] Tetzlaff and colleagues[94] suggest that, theoretically, divers with preexisting small lung cysts on chest CT scan may be at increased risk for PBT. Currently, in the absence of breath-holding, there does not seem to be a reliable or valid method to accurately predict who is or is not at risk for PBT and subsequent AGE.

Significant change in barometric pressure occurs in shallow water. Boyle's Law dictates greater volume changes for a given change in depth near the surface than at greater depths. Thus, shallow depths are the most dangerous for breath-holding ascents. A pressure differential of only 80 mm Hg (alveolar air) above ambient water pressure on the chest wall, or about 3 to 4 feet of depth under water, is adequate to force air bubbles across the alveolar-capillary membrane. PBT has occurred from breath-holding during ascent from a depth as shallow as 4 feet of water.[95]

The diagnosis of PBT is based on the development of characteristic symptoms after diving. The actual clinical manifestations may take several forms, depending on the course that the extra-alveolar air travels. Once the alveoli rupture, air can remain in the interstitium, causing localized pulmonary injury and alveolar hemorrhage. Air can travel along the perivascular sheaths and dissect into the mediastinum. This air can track superiorly to the neck, resulting in subcutaneous emphysema, and can dissect inferiorly and posteriorly, causing pneumoperitoneum. The air may dissect to the visceral pleura, causing a pneumothorax. If air enters the pulmonary vasculature, it can travel to the heart and embolize systemically, causing AGE. If the volume of air is sufficient, it can completely block the central vascular bed.[96]

Clinical Manifestations of Pulmonary Barotrauma

The clinical manifestations of PBT depend on the location and amount of air that escapes into an extra-alveolar location.

Local Pulmonary Injury

Expanding air can rupture the alveoli, causing localized pulmonary injury and capillary bleeding without other signs of PBT such as pneumomediastinum or AGE. Diffuse alveolar hemorrhage has been described as a rare manifestation of PBT.[97] Symptoms of local pulmonary injury include chest pain, cough, and hemoptysis. A chest radiograph may show evidence of intraparenchymal lung injury and bleeding. Figure 13.1 shows a radiograph of an inexperienced diver who panicked at 60 feet sea water (18 meters sea water) and rapidly ascended to the surface. He never aspirated sea water and had significant hemoptysis on the boat and at a local clinic. His chest radiograph shows diffuse intraparenchymal lung injury and bleeding.

A diver with local pulmonary injury without any evidence of AGE does not require recompression and should be treated with supportive care; however, great care must be taken to assure that the patient did not have a transient episode of neurologic dysfunction immediately after the event because one of the natural histories of AGE is of spontaneous improvement. The neurologic examination that is performed must be so complete as to safely rule out subtler forms of brain injury that might be the consequence of a less obvious AGE. Subtle parietal lobe dysfunction may be the only abnormality detectable on physical examination by the time the patient reaches the hyperbaric chamber.[98] Complaints of hemisensory loss or an episode of transient loss of consciousness should be considered an AGE until proved otherwise.

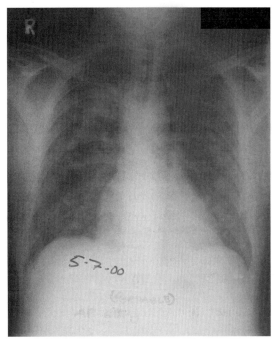

Figure 13.1 Radiograph of diffuse alveolar hemorrhages and intraparenchymal lung injury associated with pulmonary barotrauma.

Pneumomediastinum

Pneumomediastinum or mediastinal emphysema is the most common form of PBT, resulting from pulmonary interstitial air dissecting through the perivascular sheaths of the pulmonary vasculature along bronchi to the mediastinum. The diver may be asymptomatic or complain of substernal chest pain; however, respiratory distress is typically not present. The air can dissect from the mediastinum up to the neck, causing subcutaneous emphysema, and the diver may experience hoarseness and neck fullness. Subcutaneous emphysema may be present and palpated as crepitance under the skin of the neck and anterior chest. In severe cases, the diver may report marked chest pain, dyspnea, and dysphagia.

On physical examination, a crunching sound synchronous with cardiac action may rarely be auscultated (Hamman's sign), and a chest radiograph confirms the diagnosis. Radiographs may show extra-alveolar air in the neck, mediastinum, or both, although with the above findings, radiographs are not necessary to make the diagnosis. Figure 13.2 is a radiograph of a diver who surfaced rapidly and demonstrates

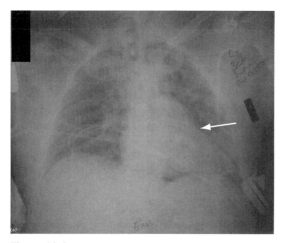

Figure 13.2 Radiograph of air along the left heart showing a reflection of the pleural away from the left border of the heart (see *arrow*). This should not be confused with pneumocardium, which can be seen in fatal cases of arterial gas embolism.

air along the left heart, causing a reflection of the pleural away from the left border of the heart. Subcutaneous air is also seen in the neck. In distinction to clinically obvious PBT, the presence of air on a radiograph may be subtle and should be looked for along the pulmonary artery and aorta, and along the edge of the heart. Figure 13.3 reveals subtle, small air lucency along the left mediastinum on posteroanterior view and posterior to the heart on the lateral view. When doubt exists, computerized tomography is more sensitive than a plain radiograph.

Treatment of pneumomediastinum is conservative, consisting of rest, avoidance of further pressure exposure (including flying in commercial aircraft), and observation. Although there is no standard recommendation

regarding safety of air travel after documented PBT, no data support long periods of refraining from air travel and 1 week is most likely adequate. Supplemental oxygen administration may be useful in severe cases. As mentioned earlier, any transient neurologic symptoms in the presence of pneumomediastinum suggest an AGE and a detailed neurologic examination is indicated. Recompression is indicated only in cases associated with either confirmed or suspected AGE.

Pneumothorax

Pneumothorax is an infrequent manifestation of PBT[83] because it requires that air be vented through the visceral pleura, a path presumably having greater resistance than air tracking through the interstitium. Pneumothorax has been reported to occur in 5% to 10% of cases of AGE.[99] Despite being infrequent, pneumothorax must be considered and excluded whenever PBT or AGE is suspected because recompression can theoretically turn a simple pneumothorax into a tension pneumothorax during ascent in the chamber. Although an untreated pneumothorax is almost universally considered an absolute contraindication to hyperbaric treatment, if a practitioner is so equipped, a tension pneumothorax can be treated by simple venting within a multiplace chamber.

In cases of diving-related pneumothorax, the diver usually describes pleuritic chest pain, breathlessness, and dyspnea, just as in cases of pneumothorax from any other cause. Occasionally, a pneumothorax can be complicated

Figure 13.3 Radiograph of subtle pneumomediastinum of air along the left mediastinum on posteroanterior view *(A)* and posterior to the heart on the lateral view *(B)*.

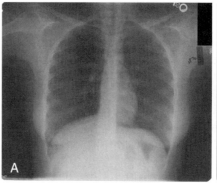
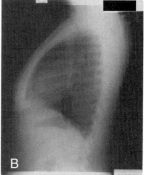

by a large hemothorax. Figure 13.4*A* presents a radiograph of a diver who ran out of air and made a panic ascent; Figure 13.4*B* shows a CT scan of the same diver demonstrating a massive pneumohemothorax.[79] Plain radiographs may confirm the diagnosis; however, as with mediastinal emphysema, a CT scan is more sensitive. Because the majority of diving-related pneumothoraces are small, treatment may consist simply of supplemental oxygen and observation, and repeating the chest radiograph as needed to ensure resolution. Tube thoracostomy is usually reserved for larger pneumothoraces or if the diver is to undergo recompression treatment.

Arterial Gas Embolism

AGE results from air bubbles entering the pulmonary venous circulation from ruptured alveoli. When air is introduced into the pulmonary capillaries, gas bubbles are showered into the left atrium, to the left ventricle, and subsequently into the aorta, where they are distributed throughout the vasculature. In addition, air introduced into the pulmonary vasculature appears to be capable of raising right side pressures so it distributes into the entire central vascular bed (i.e., pulmonary artery, the right ventricle, the superior and inferior vena cavae, and even the subclavian veins). Figure 13.5 shows air in both subclavian vessels from a diver who died of an AGE. The exact mechanism by which gas enters the pulmonary vasculature remains unknown.

Pathophysiology of Arterial Gas Embolism

Much of our understanding of the pathophysiology of AGE is based on experimental models in animals, clinical studies of thromboembolic stroke in humans, and limited clinical series of human AGE victims. There are, however, major differences between the observations made in these animal models and the clinical experience in human victims. Because most of the animal experiments of AGE use a model that injects gas directly into the cerebral vascula-

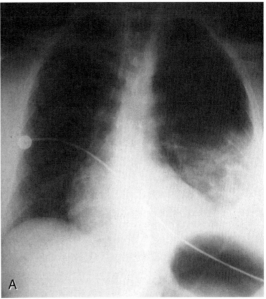

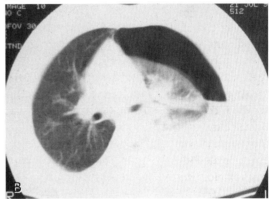

Figure 13.4 *A,* Radiograph of a diver who ran out of air and made a panic ascent. *B,* A computed tomography scan of the same diver demonstrating a massive pneumohemothorax.

ture, caution must be taken in extrapolating these experimental data with the injury produced by PBT-induced AGE in humans.

Animal experiments demonstrate that overdistension of the lung coupled with overpressurization allows gas to enter the circulation,[81] and in a dog model, lung rupture occurs when lung volume approaches three times functional residual capacity.[100] The bubbles entering the aorta pass into the systemic circulation, lodging in small- and medium-sized arteries and occluding the more distal circulation, and the distribution of these bubbles appears to be related to blood flow rather than gravity.[101] Although bubbles can cause

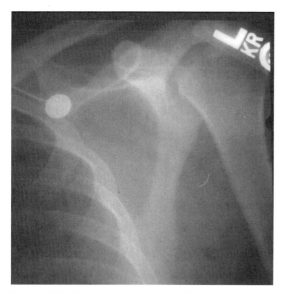

Figure 13.5 Radiograph of a diver who died of an arterial gas embolism showing air in the subclavian artery and vein.

sustained occlusion of the cerebral vasculature, if the gas volume is not sufficient to interfere with the circulation,[102] most bubbles will pass through the cerebral vasculature after varying amounts of delay.[103,104] Occlusive bubbles lodge most frequently in small arterioles with a diameter of 30 to 60 μm, which are found at the junction between the white and the gray matter[105]; thus, this area may be particularly prone to injury from AGE.[106]

A variety of changes is seen in the cerebral and systemic circulation after embolization. Cerebrospinal fluid pressure increases secondary to a reactive hyperemia with a resultant increase in cerebral blood volume.[107-109] Systemic hypertension occurs either by an increase in circulating catecholamines and release of vasopressin[110] or by a brainstem reflex. Vasodilatation occurs and autoregulation of cerebral perfusion is lost, resulting in blood flow that reflects the changes in systemic blood flow and systemic blood pressure. The end result is a further increase in cerebral blood volume. Within 30 to 60 minutes after the injection of air, cerebrospinal fluid pressure decreases[109] and areas of hyperemia develop adjacent to areas of hypoperfusion.[111]

Bubble damage to the vascular endothelium causes the release of vasoactive substances both in the brain and the lung.[112-114]

This combined with platelet and leukocyte aggregation around bubbles[115,116] helps to explain the delayed effects of air embolization on circulatory dynamics,[117] and blood flow can progressively decrease to a level below which neuronal function is compromised or even neuronal death occurs[118,119] despite the return of cerebral circulation after the passage of gas bubbles.

Decompression adversely affects nitric oxide (·NO)–mediated endothelial cell function.[120] Bubbles are known to incite endothelial cell shear stress because of the "negative wake" created as they pass through the circulation and "microstreaming" when a bubble is in close proximity to the endothelial lining.[121,122] Shear stress is a potent activation stimulus for nitric oxide synthase and NADPH oxidase, especially when flow is pulsatile.[123,124]

Experiments with cerebral air embolism demonstrate an immediate opening of the blood–brain barrier after embolization.[125] This increased permeability is short lived and tends to return to normal after several hours.[126] The permeability to large molecules peaks within 60 minutes after embolism, but then falls off rapidly. Permeability to smaller molecules may remain increased for up to 24 hours. Edema appears to be vasogenic rather than cytotoxic in origin, which is usually associated with cerebral ischemia. Neuronal adenosine triphosphate decreases and lactic acid production increases, which may further increase cellular damage.[127,128] The electroencephalogram and evoked potentials become abnormal immediately after embolization.[109]

Air injected directly into the cerebral circulation in animal models results in initial hypertension, ventricular arrhythmias, then hypotension and eventually death.[107] Premature ventricular contractions and runs of ventricular tachycardia occur, but sudden cardiac arrest does not occur. Cardiac arrest develops late only after spontaneous ventilation ceases or circulatory collapse occurs. When air is injected into the left ventricle and coronary arteries, death occurs only after the animals experience development of hypotension and depressed left ventricular function. Again, sudden cardiac arrest does not occur in these animal models[129] in distinction to the clinical course seen in some human victims.

Clinical Manifestations of Arterial Gas Embolism

Clinical manifestations of cerebral air embolism are sudden and occur within minutes of ascent. Approximately 4% of victims of AGE will suffer immediate cardiac respiratory arrest and die. Another 5% will die in the hospital because of consequences of the AGE or severe near-drowning that can accompany AGE. More than half of the remaining victims of AGE will have a complete functional recovery.

Sudden Death Caused by Arterial Gas Embolism

Approximately 4% of divers who suffer an AGE will die immediately, presenting with sudden loss of consciousness, pulselessness, and apnea. These victims are generally not responsive to immediate cardiopulmonary resuscitation or recompression. Previously, the cause of sudden death from AGE was thought to be caused by either reflex arrhythmias from brainstem embolization or myocardial ischemia secondary to coronary artery embolization and occlusion.[107,130] These hypotheses were advanced because earlier experiments, in a dog model, were unable to cause cardiac arrest by injecting air into the left ventricle.[131]

Unfortunately, these proposed mechanisms do not explain what is seen in more recent animal models or clinically in humans. In animal models of AGE, death caused by embolization of the cerebral vasculature occurs only after prolonged periods of embolization and after ventilation is suppressed by the central nervous system dysfunction because of embolization. Similarly, accidental injection of air into the coronary arteries of humans (in catheterization mishaps) does not result in sudden death but rather chest pain, transient hypotension, and ischemic electrocardiographic changes. Furthermore, there is only one case report of a myocardial infarction associated with an AGE,[132] and this

would be expected more frequently if death were due to occlusion of coronary arteries from air. Biochemical evidence for myocardial ischemia in cases of AGE has also not been found.[133]

In human victims who die suddenly of AGE, they die most frequently immediately on surfacing. Autopsies typically reveal large amounts of air in the central vascular bed, particularly in the pulmonary arteries and right ventricle.[134] When one examines radiographs of human victims of AGE who die suddenly, there is complete filling of the central vascular bed with air, including the left ventricle, aorta, carotid arteries, and subclavian vessels.[79,96,134,135] Figure 13.6 is a fatal case of PBT and AGE showing large amounts of air in the central vasculature, filling the cardiac chambers, aorta, carotid arteries, and subclavian vessel. Figure 13.7 is a radiograph of another fatal case of AGE revealing air in the aorta. Thus, it appears that the primary mechanism of cardiac arrest in most cases of AGE is vascular obstruction caused by air leading to pulseless electrical activity.[79,96]

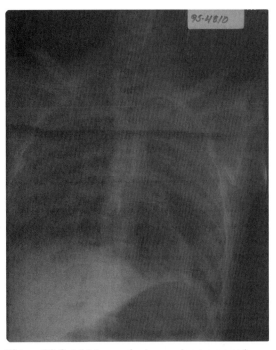

Figure 13.6 A fatal case of pulmonary barotrauma and arterial gas embolism demonstrating air filling the central vasculature including air in the heart, aorta, carotid arteries, and subclavian vessel.

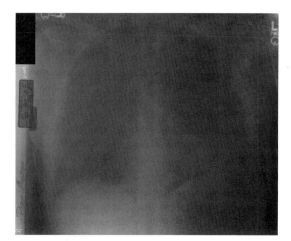

Figure 13.7 Radiograph of a fatal case of arterial gas embolism showing air in the aorta.

Signs and Symptoms of Arterial Gas Embolism

Victims of AGE present with varied neurologic and systemic signs and symptoms depending on the amount and distribution of air. The most common initial neurologic manifestations of AGE include loss of consciousness, stupor, or confusion. Headache, cortical blindness, monoplegia or asymmetric multiplegia, focal paralysis, paresthesias or other sensory disturbances, convulsions, aphasia, visual field defects, and vertigo or dizziness are also frequent findings (Table 13.3). Hemiplegia and other purely unilateral brain syndromes are somewhat less frequent. Paraparesis or paraplegia is extremely unusual and in one large study was reported not to occur.[136] This is not unexpected because paraplegia would require either absolutely bilateral symmetric cortical emboli or isolated emboli to spinal arteries.

As noted previously, many patients improve dramatically between the time they surface and the time they are actually examined at a medical facility. Therefore, the history of the events surrounding the incident should ideally be carefully explored with any individuals who were at the site of the accident. Even though spontaneous improvement is common, some victims of AGE deteriorate secondarily during hyperbaric treatment[137] presumably because of worsening cerebral edema, increased intracranial pressure, and the effect of

Table 13.3 Signs and Symptoms of Patients Presenting with Arterial Gas Embolism

NEUROLOGIC

Loss of consciousness
Stupor and confusion
Unilateral motor and/or sensory changes
Bilateral motor and/or sensory changes
Monoplegia
Asymmetric multiplegia
Focal paralysis
Convulsions
Asphasia
Vertigo
Ataxia
Dizziness
Headache
Dysmetria
Decreased coordination (rapid alternating movements)
Calculation errors
Construction difficulty

VISUAL CHANGES

Cortical blindness
Gaze preference
Homonymous hemianopsia
Nystagmus

PULMONARY

Chest pain
Shortness of breath
Hemoptysis
Crepitus

OTHER

Cardiac arrest
Nausea
Vomiting

vasoactive substances released from the lungs from the initial PBT.[138]

Although the physical findings of AGE are extremely variable, the signs or symptoms should be referable to occlusion of portions of the vasculature of the central nervous system. All patients with suspected AGE should be carefully examined for neurologic deficits because findings can be subtle and require detailed examinations, including testing of cognitive function.[98] Such testing is rarely possible at the dive site, so divers who have a history suggestive of AGE (most commonly a transient loss of consciousness, an episode of blindness, or a period of disorientation after ascending from a dive) but do not manifest any gross symptoms or signs of neurologic injury in the field should be considered to possibly have had an AGE and be referred to a hyperbaric treatment facility.

Because running out of air near the end of a dive is a common cause of AGE in sport scuba divers, there is some degree of gas loading in the tissues; as a result, a combination of AGE and decompression sickness (DCS) can be seen in this setting. The effects of the intravascular gas associated with AGE on diffusion of gas from tissues remains speculative; however, it does appear that AGE can precipitate DCS in divers who are well within the U.S. Navy no-stop limits and who otherwise would not be expected to experience development of DCS.[139,140] Frequently, the DCS occurring in this setting is extremely resistant to the usual forms of therapy. This syndrome has been referred to as Type III DCS[139] or biphasic DCS.[79] The clinical picture of this syndrome is a diver who presents with symptoms of an acute AGE and with treatment improves significantly or recovers completely from the initial presentation. Later, or even during recompression treatment, signs and symptoms of spinal cord DCS develop. Despite further HBOT, recovery can be minimal.

Hematologic and Biochemical Abnormalities

In addition to the effects on the cerebral circulation, AGE produces systemic hematologic and biochemical abnormalities. Gas bubbles are thought to cause direct organ injury, injury to vascular endothelium, or both. Patients with AGE usually present with hemoconcentration, most likely because of third-spacing of fluid due to endothelial injury from intravascular gas damage. The degree of hemoconcentration correlates with the neurologic outcome of the diver.[141] Creatinine kinase (CK) concentration is increased in almost all cases of AGE and also correlates with neurologic outcome of the diver.[133] In this study, all divers who suffered an AGE with peak CK values of less than 1000 units were discharged from the hospital with a completely normal neurologic examina-

tion. The majority of the increased CK concentration is from skeletal muscle (the MM component). CK concentration begins to increase within a few hours after the AGE insult and peaks at approximately 15 hours after the event before declining rapidly over the next 24 to 48 hours. Figure 13.8 demonstrates this temporal relation between AGE and CK. CK-MB level is increased in some cases, and nonspecific electrocardiographic changes can occur[142]; however, true myocardial infarction caused by AGE is extremely rare. Even in cases of AGE with increased CK-MB level, functional studies of the heart show no evidence of wall motion abnormalities after recovery.[133] Increased troponin level has been reported in cases of coronary air embolism not associated with diving.[28,39,143] With the widespread availability to measure troponin, future data will

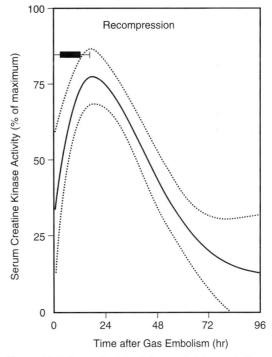

Figure 13.8 Temporal relation between arterial gas embolism and serum creatine kinase activity. The mean serum creatine kinase values in the 12 patients in whom values were determined at least 4 times are expressed as fractions of the peak value and plotted against the time after the occurrence of the arterial gas embolism. The regression line *(solid line)* and 95% confidence intervals *(broken lines)* are shown. *(From Smith RM, Neuman TS: Elevation of serum creatine kinase in divers with arterial gas embolism. N Engl J Med 330:22, 1994, by permission.)*

help to define the importance of these biochemical abnormalities.

Bubbles cause injury to other organs such as
the liver, and increased serum glutamic oxalace-
tic transaminase, serum glutamic pyruvic transaminase, and lactate dehydrogenase levels can
be found in victims of AGE.[144] The increases
in these enzymes correlate with the degree of
increase of CK concentration and reflect the
widespread systemic embolization of gas in
AGE and secondary damage to the endothelium. Despite increases of these enzyme levels,
organ dysfunction usually does not occur.

Radiographic Abnormalities

AGE can lead to loss of consciousness on surfacing, hence there may be evidence of aspiration
on chest radiographs and clinical evidence of
near drowning. Radiographic findings consistent with aspiration can be found in more than
50% of chest radiographs of victims with AGE.
However, radiographic evidence for PBT is seen
in less than half of the victims of AGE.[83] PBT is
most frequently demonstrated as mediastinal
emphysema. Mediastinal gas can be difficult
to detect and, as mentioned earlier, should be
carefully looked for along the borders of the
pulmonary arteries, the aorta (including the
descending aorta), and the heart (see Figs. 13.2
and 13.3). In some cases of pneumomediastinum, the anterior portion of the parietal pleural
displaced off the left heart border has been
reported as pneumopericardium; however,
almost universally, this interpretation is incorrect and the radiologic abnormality is really
pneumomediastinum. Figure 13.9A is a radiograph of pneumomediastinum that was initially
interpreted as pneumopericardium. A CT scan
(see Fig. 13.9B) of the same patient clearly
shows the presence of pneumomediastinum.

Most patients with neurologic injury do
not have clearly defined abnormalities on CT
or a magnetic resonance imaging scan. Rarely,
clear cerebral infarction can be seen on
either CT or magnetic resonance imaging.[145]
Newer magnetic resonance imaging images
and techniques may in the future be shown
to more easily visualize the area of brain
injury in victims of AGE.[146]

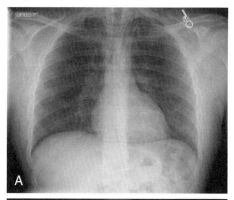

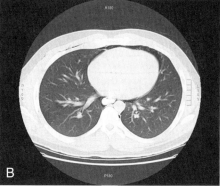

Figure 13.9 *A,* Radiograph of pneumomediastinum that was reported as pneumopericardium. *B,* A computed tomography scan of the same patient clearly demonstrating the presence of pneumomediastinum.

Diagnosis of Arterial Gas Embolism

The diagnosis of AGE is clinical and based on
the diving history, signs, and symptoms. Any
diver who loses consciousness or manifests
symptoms or signs of serious neurologic injury
within minutes of surfacing from a dive must be
considered to have suffered an AGE. Increase of
CK concentration can be helpful in the diagnosis of AGE; however, the initial increase in CK
concentration may not be seen for several
hours after the injury. Hence, if the patient
presents quickly to the hospital or chamber, the
initial CK concentration may be normal. As
mentioned earlier, the presence of mediastinal
air on a chest radiograph in the presence of
neurologic symptoms after a dive is helpful
but occurs in less than 50% of victims with
AGE. Should the CK concentration be normal
12 hours after a neurologic event after surfacing, the hyperbaric medicine practitioner should
consider an alternative diagnosis to AGE.

Treatment of Arterial Gas Embolism

All cases of suspected AGE should be referred for evaluation for possible recompression treatment (HBOT) as rapidly as possible. Early treatment is more likely to be efficacious than delayed treatment,[3,147,148] although there are numerous reports of patients responding to HBOT with delays longer than 6 hours.[149] As noted earlier, the initial manifestations of AGE may spontaneously resolve by the time the victim is examined by medical personnel. Occasionally, a diver has symptoms but no reproducible neurologic deficits on physical examination. Nonetheless, all patients should be referred for hyperbaric consultation and possible hyperbaric treatment if the history is suggestive of AGE because neurologic impairment is difficult to exclude in the acute setting, and waiting to complete definitive diagnostic studies may allow subtle neurologic injuries to become irreversible.[98]

The Divers Alert Network has an on-call diving physician available 24 hours a day, 7 days a week who can assist in triage and arrangement of transport and treatment for all diving injuries. (In the United States, the Divers Alert Network can be contacted at 919-684-8111 or [collect] 919-684-4DAN [4326]. Tell the operator that you have a diving emergency.) The Divers Alert Network's diving medicine consultants provide help with diagnosis and immediate care of the patient, as well as information about the location of the nearest hyperbaric chamber. Before a patient is transferred to the hyperbaric treatment facility, it is appropriate to contact the chamber to determine its availability and the level of staffing.

Prehospital Care

Before recompression, divers with suspected AGE should be given supplemental oxygen at a high flow rate (e.g., 10 L/min) by nonrebreathing face mask to enhance the rate of resolution of inert gas bubbles and treat arterial hypoxemia.[64] Although this makes physiological sense, data to demonstrate that individuals who receive supplemental oxygen compared with individuals who do not have an improved final outcome are lacking.[150] Because victims of AGE may present with hemoconcentration caused by endothelial injury from gas bubbles, it is appropriate to maintain adequate intravascular volume because inert gas cannot be effectively eliminated from tissues or from intravascular bubbles at the arteriolar-capillary level unless adequate capillary perfusion is maintained. In addition, autoregulation of blood flow in the brain is lost after AGE, and cerebral perfusion passively follows systemic blood pressure. Hypotension should be avoided in cases of AGE as in other cases of brain injury. Because AGE can lead to loss of consciousness in the water, the diver may suffer concomitant near drowning and may need airway protection from aspiration of gastric contents secondary to vomiting; however, even severe concomitant near drowning should not be considered a contraindication to HBOT. Furthermore, it should be understood that central nervous system manifestations of AGE can be misinterpreted as being secondary to near drowning. Fortunately, HBOT also provides the near-drowning victim with adequate arterial oxygenation in almost all circumstances.

Historically, much attention was directed toward keeping the patient with AGE in the Trendelenburg position in the field. This was based on anecdotal reports and limited experimental data.[104,151,152] The rationale for keeping the patient with AGE head down was the belief that the weight of the column of blood would force bubbles through the cerebral capillary bed, that the buoyancy of the bubbles would keep them in the aorta or heart, and that the weight of the spinal fluid might compress bubbles in the cord. These benefits were never well demonstrated or experimentally confirmed, and more recent studies showed that the Trendelenburg position did not keep bubbles from being distributed to the systemic circulation and can worsen cerebral edema.[101,153] Patients with AGE should be maintained in a position, both in the field and during transport to an emergency medical treatment facility or recompression chamber, that allows the most access and care of the patient.

If the AGE-stricken diver is first seen at a hospital emergency department or clinic, and if transport to a hyperbaric treatment facility will not be delayed, baseline laboratory, electrocardiographic, and radiographic tests can be obtained before the patient is sent to the chamber. CT or magnetic resonance imaging of the brain should be deferred until after initial hyperbaric treatment unless intracranial hemorrhage or other nondiving injury is suspected. Although delay in hyperbaric treatment theoretically prolongs cerebral ischemia and cellular hypoxia, resulting in significant cerebral edema, data have not demonstrated that a more difficult course of therapy or a worsened outcome ensues. Thus, when there is concern for extra-axial blood or a neurosurgically correctable lesion, the time taken for a simple noncontrast head CT before recompression therapy may be an appropriate clinical decision.

If air medical evacuation is required, the injured diver should ideally be flown in an aircraft pressurized to 1 atmosphere absolute (ATA) during flight. In the case of helicopter evacuation or in the event that an unpressurized aircraft is required, the flight altitude should be maintained as low as possible. All resuscitative measures should be maintained in flight.

Presentation and Management of Arterial Gas Embolism from Nondiving Causes

AGE may occur from paradoxic gas embolism from VGE through a right-to-left shunt, from migration through the pulmonary circulation, or from direct arterial injection of air. The epidemiology and pathophysiology of AGE from nondiving causes is discussed earlier (see Venous Gas Embolism section). The symptoms of AGE in patients undergoing procedures are similar to that in divers and develop suddenly. The clinical presentation is determined by the absolute quantity of gas and the areas of the brain that are affected. Symptoms can range from minor motor weakness and confusion to hemiplegia, convulsion, loss of consciousness, and coma. Abnormal neurologic findings after central venous catheter insertion, manipulation, or removal; surgery; or other invasive procedures should prompt consideration of AGE.

Mental status changes after surgery should raise the suspicion of cerebral ischemia, and AGE should be considered when there is delayed recovery or impaired consciousness after general anesthesia following a surgical procedure that carries a risk for gas embolism. The importance of early HBOT in cases of iatrogenic AGE has been well documented.[73-75]

The diagnosis is based on the temporal relation between the sudden development of neurologic symptoms and the performance of an invasive procedure. Immediate therapeutic measures include the administration of 100% oxygen to reverse cerebral ischemia and to aid in elimination of gas and reduce bubble volume. Cardiopulmonary resuscitation should be performed if necessary, and endotracheal intubation is indicated in somnolent or comatose patients. Patients should be placed in a flat, supine position. Normovolemia should be maintained to optimize the microcirculation. Systemic hypertension after cerebral AGE is common and may promote bubble redistribution; however, prolonged hypertension may lead to increased intracranial pressure and compromise neurologic outcome.

HBOT should be considered in all patients with clinical symptoms of AGE. Numerous case reports demonstrate the potential benefits of HBOT in the presence of iatrogenic AGE.[3,73-75,148,154] Immediate recompression with HBOT has been shown to improve patient outcome[3,148]; however, even delayed treatment (>6 hours) can still have substantial benefits.[149,155] Once cardiac stabilization has been achieved, the patient can be transferred to a hyperbaric chamber. The risks of transportation of an unstable patient to a hyperbaric facility must be considered carefully.

HYERBARIC OXYGEN THERAPY

Mechanisms of Hyperbaric Oxygen Therapy for Arterial Gas Embolism

Although there are no controlled trials of HBOT versus non-HBOT in humans with AGE, the physiologic rationale for its use is overwhelming. A review of a large number of case series of AGE by Dutka[156] clearly demonstrates a worse prognosis without recompression. The rationale for HBOT is both compression of gas bubbles to mechanically clear the cerebral circulation and restore blood flow and hyperoxygenation of ischemic tissues with large volumes of oxygen dissolved in plasma.

HBOT reduces the volume of gas bubbles by increasing ambient pressure.[155] Bubble volume will change in inverse proportion to the ambient pressure. However, the reduction in the various bubble dimensions will depend on the shape of the bubble. A spherical bubble compressed to 6.0 ATA will reduce to 17% of its original volume but only 43% of its original diameter. Cylindrical bubbles will decrease mainly in bubble length.

As partial pressure of oxygen increases in inspired air, the amount of oxygen in solution in plasma increases linearly. For every atmosphere of pressure increase, 1.8 mL/dL oxygen is dissolved in plasma. At 3 atmospheres absolute, approximately 6.8 mL/dL oxygen can be held in solution in plasma. Because normal oxygen extraction at the tissue level is 5 mL/dL (at normal cardiac output), plasma alone can carry enough oxygen to meet the metabolic needs of the tissues. In addition, this increase in oxygen-carrying capacity dramatically increases the driving force for oxygen diffusion. This improvement in oxygen-carrying capacity of plasma and in the delivery of oxygen to tissues offsets the embolic insult to the microvasculature.

Hyperoxia produces a significant diffusion gradient for oxygen into the bubble and for nitrogen out of the bubble. The rate of resolution of a bubble is dependent on the diffusion of nitrogen from a bubble into adjacent tissue or blood and the rate of transport of dissolved gas to the lung. Oxygen is metabolized by the tissues and does not accumulate in tissues as inert gas does. Hence, there is a reduction of the total gas pressure in the tissues surrounding the bubble that enhances the rate of diffusion of inert gas from the bubble into the surrounding tissue (Fig. 13.10). This is referred to as the "oxygen window."[64]

Experimental evidence suggests that HBOT decreases cerebral edema by vasoconstriction.[157,158] HBOT can help prevent cerebral edema by reducing the permeability of blood vessels while supporting the integrity of the blood–brain barrier.[159] Furthermore, HBOT plays a role in protecting tissues from reperfusion injury (see Chapter 9). HBOT antagonizes the β_2-integrin system, which initiates the adherence of neutrophils to postcapillary venule endothelium.[160,161] Reperfusion injury may be inhibited by HBOT via a decrease in leukocyte venular endothelial adherence, release of toxic oxygen species, and arteriolar vasoconstriction; hence, progressive arteriolar vasoconstriction is inhibited.[162] HBOT inhibits intracellular adhesion molecule-1 expression, which plays a role in neutrophil adhesion and ischemia-reperfusion injury.[163] These mechanisms of hyperbaric oxygen are important because neutrophil activity may be responsible for part of the brain injury that is seen after AGE.[164]

Treatment Table Selection

Treatment for AGE had traditionally been with U.S. Navy Table 6A with an initial excursion to 165 feet (6 ATA) for 30 minutes to enhance bubble compression (Fig. 13.11). However, the clinical data that support the use of compression to 6 ATA for AGE are lacking, and many hyperbaric facilities recommend treating patients with AGE at a maximum of 2.82 ATA with U.S. Navy Table 6 (Fig. 13.12). Waite and colleagues[165] show that bubbles in embolized dogs disappeared from cerebral circulation between 3 and 4 ATA; however, Gorman and coworkers[166] demonstrate that only 50% of embolized rabbits had complete clearance of bubbles from the cerebral circulation after compression to 6 ATA. Animal studies with dogs given an intracarotid injection of air showed no additional benefit from compression to 6 ATA compared with 2.82 ATA.[167]

In a scuba diver who already has incurred a significant gas load of nitrogen, treatment with air at 6 ATA may increase nitrogen gas loading in the tissues and could precipitate DCS even during treatment. Signs and symptoms of spinal cord DCS can appear during recompression therapy for AGE as seen in biphasic DCS

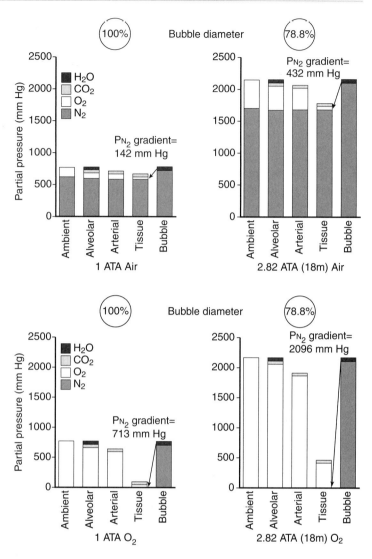

Figure 13.10 Partial pressures of four gases in various locations are shown. Rate of resolution of a bubble will depend on two factors: diffusion of nitrogen from a bubble into adjacent tissue or blood, and the rate of transport of dissolved gas back to the lung (which may be related to tissue phase diffusion, blood flow, and gas solubility). Tissue partial pressures are assumed to be equal to mixed venous values. Partial pressures within the bubble are shown at the time or shortly after bubble formation (before O_2 and CO_2 have diffused into the bubble). The diffusion gradient for nitrogen is greatest while breathing O_2 at 2.82 ATA (atmosphere absolute). This is referred to as the "oxygen window." *(From Moon RE, Gorman DF: Treatment of the decompression disorders. In: Brubakk AO, Neuman TS (eds): Bennett and Elliott's Physiology and Medicine of Diving, 5th ed. London: Saunders, 2003, p 617, by permission.)*

described earlier. If a treatment regimen of 6 ATA is chosen, it is probably wise to select a 50/50 or 60/40 N_2/O_2, or even a helium-oxygen mixture, as the breathing medium to enhance bubble clearance and to minimize further nitrogen gas loading at depth.

Growing evidence exists that recompression to 2.8 ATA on 100% oxygen may be a more effective treatment than initial pressurization to 6 ATA for sports divers because of the typical several-hour delay in getting to a chamber, and thus less need for the higher pressure to compress bubbles and a greater immediate need for tissue oxygenation.[77,167,168]

Patients with AGE can be treated in multiplace or monoplace facilities; the advantage of a multiplace facility is the ability to be pressurized to 6 ATA. Both air and oxygen can be administered to the patient, and direct access to the patient is available. However, patients with AGE have successfully been treated in a monoplace hyperbaric chamber.[169] Current recommendations include initial recompression to 2.82 ATA breathing 100% oxygen. If there is no improvement or clinical deterioration, deeper recompression to 6 ATA can be instituted. If the AGE is iatrogenic or occurs early in the dive such that there is minimal gas loading of the tissue with nitrogen, and the patient is brought to the hyperbaric facility immediately after the injury, then there may be

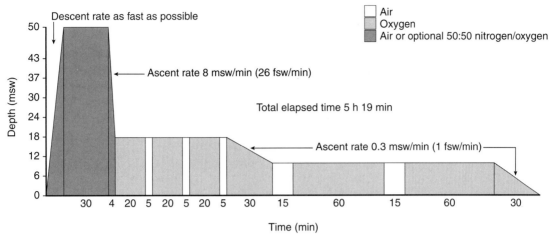

Figure 13.11 U.S. Navy Treatment Table 6A consists of an initial excursion to 6 atmospheres absolute (ATA) or 165 feet sea water (fsw) while the patient breathes either air or a nitrogen/oxygen mixture (60/40 or 50/50). After 30 minutes, the patient is brought to 2.82 ATA (60 fsw) for oxygen breathing identical to U.S. Navy Treatment Table 6. msw, meters sea water. *(From Moon RE, Gorman DF: Treatment of the decompression disorders. In: Brubakk AO, Neuman TS (eds): Bennett and Elliott's Physiology and Medicine of Diving, 5th ed. London, Saunders, 2003, p 624, by permission.)*

benefit to treating the patient at 6 ATA initially with a helium oxygen mixture or a 50/50 or 60/40 N₂/O₂ mixture below 60 feet.

Follow-up Treatments

If the patient has persistent neurologic symptoms after the initial treatment, repetitive hyperbaric treatments daily or twice daily have been performed at a number of facilities. Repeat treatments can be given until the patient has complete relief of symptoms or until there is no further clinical improvement after two consecutive treatments.[170] Once again, the data to demonstrate that patients who receive repetitive treatments compared with those who receive only one have a better long-term outcome are lacking. At most facilities, the majority of patients with AGE rarely are given more than a few treatments. There is no consensus for which treatment table to use for repetitive treatments. U.S. Navy Treatment Tables 5, 6, and 9 have all been recommended for follow-up treatments.

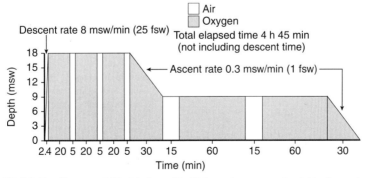

Figure 13.12 U.S. Navy Treatment Table 6 is the most widely used recompression table. Oxygen is administered at 2.82 ATA (60 feet sea water [fsw]) with intermittent air breaks followed by further oxygen breathing at 30 fsw. *(From Moon RE, Gorman DF: Treatment of the decompression disorders. In: Brubakk AO, Neuman TS (eds): Bennett and Elliott's Physiology and Medicine of Diving, 5th ed. London, Saunders, 2003, p 603, by permission.)*

Adjunctive Treatment

Numerous medications have been proposed as adjuncts to recompression and hyperbaric oxygen for the treatment of AGE (e.g., heparin, low-molecular-weight dextran, aspirin, corticosteroids) to prevent the secondary pathophysiologic mechanisms of injury; however, experimental and clinical data do not support the use of any of these for AGE except for lidocaine.

Lidocaine is a Class 1b antiarrhythmic agent and a local anesthetic that appears to have cerebroprotective effects. In animal models of AGE and brain ischemia, lidocaine acts to reduce intracranial pressure and brain edema, preserve neuroelectrical function and brain blood flow, and reduce infarct size.[171,172] Lidocaine given prophylactically reduces brain dysfunction after AGE in cats[173] and improves recovery of brain function in cats and dogs with AGE when given therapeutically.[153,174] Human data are less impressive, because many of the case studies contain patients with both AGE and DCS and there are often delays to treatment.[175,176] Lidocaine has been used in conjunction with hyperbaric oxygen in a case of pure cerebral AGE not related to diving with good results.[38] When lidocaine is used prophylactically during left heart valve surgery, patients had fewer deficits in psychometric test performance after surgery compared with a control group and greater recovery of brain function after surgery.[172] Further human data of lidocaine given as an adjunct to hyperbaric oxygen for the treatment of AGE are needed. Meanwhile, current evidence supports the use of lidocaine as an adjunct to recompression for the treatment of AGE.

Experimental Therapies

New therapies to treat gas embolism are focusing on the interaction between bubble interface and vascular endothelium. Currently, no approved therapeutic drugs directly treat or prevent gas embolism. Surfactants have been proposed to prevent or reduce gas bubble adhesion to the endothelium.[177,178] In in vitro studies, surfactants reduced bubble adhesion force and preserved basic endothelial structure and vasodilatory function by protecting the endothelium from mechanically induced injury. Further research may lead to the potential development of clinical pharmacologic therapy that might preserve or restore blood flow through bubble-embolized vessels to regions of brain or other tissue affected by lodged bubbles.

The use of fluorocarbon derivatives has been suggested for the management of gas embolism. Fluorocarbon emulsions are thought to enhance the reabsorption of bubbles by increasing the solubility of gases in blood. Studies using fluorocarbon FP-43 demonstrate its utility in absorbing air from the circulation.[179] FP-43 reduced the complications of coronary air embolization in dogs.[180] The addition of perfluorocarbon emulsion to the cardiopulmonary bypass prime reduced the incidence and severity of neurologic injury after the formation of massive air embolism during bypass in a swine model.[181] Eckmann and colleagues[182] demonstrate in an in vivo rat model that when a perfluorocarbon emulsion, perftoran, was given in advance of gas embolization, bubbles moved farther into the periphery and cleared from the circulation faster, leading to a 36% reduction in blood flow obstruction. Perftoran given after embolization had no effect, presumably because it could not get past the site of blood flow obstruction.

REFERENCES

1. Mirski MA, Lele AV, Fitzsimmons L, et al: Diagnosis and treatment of vascular air embolism. Anesthesiology 106:164-177, 2007.
2. Porter JM, Pidgeon C, Cunningham AJ: The sitting position in neurosurgery: A critical appraisal. Br J Anaesth 82:117-128, 1999.
3. Murphy BP, Harford FJ, Cramer FS: Cerebral air embolism resulting from invasive medical procedures: Treatment with hyperbaric oxygen. Ann Surg 201:242-245, 1985.
4. Vesely TM: Air embolism during insertion of central venous catheters. J Vasc Interv Radiol 12:1291-1295, 2001.
5. Vignaux O, Borrego P, Macron L, et al: Cardiac gas embolism after central venous catheter removal. Undersea Hyperb Med 32:325-326, 2005.
6. Dib J, Boyle AJ, Chan M, et al: Coronary air embolism: A case report and review of the literature. Catheter Cardiovasc Interv 68:897-900, 2006.

7. Kypson AP, Greenville NC: Sudden cardiac arrest after coronary artery bypass grafting as a result of massive carbon dioxide embolism. J Thorac Cardiovasc Surg 130:936-937, 2005.

8. Sahu MK, Ingole PR, Bisoi AK, et al: Successful management of a case of massive air embolism from cardiopulmonary bypass with retrograde cerebral perfusion in a child. J Cardiothorac Vasc Anesth 20:80-81, 2006.

9. Cottin V, Delafosse B, Viale JP: Gas embolism during laparoscopy: A report of seven cases in patients with previous abdominal surgical history. Surg Endosc 10:166-169, 1996.

10. Khan AU, Pandya K, Clifton MA, et al: Near fatal gas embolism during laparoscopic cholecystectomy. Ann R Coll Surg Engl 77:67-68, 1995.

11. Scoletta P, Morsiani E, Ferrocci G, et al: Carbon dioxide embolization: Is it a complication of laparoscopic cholecystectomy? [Italian] Minerva Chir 58:313-320, 2003.

12. Vacanti CA, Lodhia KL: Fatal massive air embolism during transurethral reception of the prostate. Anesthesiology 74:186-187, 1991.

13. Lattin G Jr, O'Brian W Sr, McCrary B, et al: Massive systemic air embolism treated with hyperbaric oxygen therapy following CT-guided transthoracic needle biopsy of a pulmonary nodule. J Vasc Interv Radiol 17:1355-1358, 2006.

14. Ohashi S, Endoh H, Honda T, et al: Cerebral air embolism complicating percutaneous thin-needle biopsy of the lung: Complete neurological recovery after hyperbaric oxygen therapy. J Anesth 15:233-236, 2001.

15. Tolly TL, Feldmeier JE, Czarnecki D: Air embolism complicating percutaneous lung biopsy. Am J Radiol 150:555-556, 1998.

16. Nayagam J, Ho KM, Liang J: Fatal systemic air embolism during endoscopic retrograde cholangio-pancreatography. Anaesth Intensive Care 32:260-264, 2004.

17. Mazzoni G, Koep L, Starzl T: Air embolism in liver transplantation. Transplant Proc 11:267-268, 1979.

18. Olmedilla L, Garutti I, Perez-Pena J, et al: Fatal paradoxical air embolism during liver transplantation. Br J Anaesth 84:112-114, 2000.

19. Helmberger TK, Roth U, Empen K: Massive air embolism during interventional laser therapy for the liver: Successful resuscitation without chest compression. Cardiovasc Interv Radiol 25:335-336, 2002.

20. Dalsgaard J, Sand NP, Felsby S, et al: R-wave changes in fatal air embolism during bone cementation. Scand Cardiovasc J 35:61-64, 2001.

21. Evans RD, Palazzo MG, Ackers JW: Air embolism during total hip replacement: Comparison of two surgical techniques. Br J Anaesth 62:243-247, 1989.

22. Gruenwald JM: Fatal air embolism during arthroscopy. J Bone Joint Surg B 72:929, 1990.

23. Hedge RT, Avatgere RN: Air embolism during anaesthesia for shoulder arthroscopy. Br J Anaesth 85:926-927, 2000.

24. Bernhardt TL, Goldmann RW, Thombs PA, et al: Hyperbaric oxygen treatment of cerebral air embolism from orogenital sex during pregnancy. Crit Care Med 16:729-730, 1998.

25. Munsick RA: Air embolism and maternal death from therapeutic abortion. Obstet Gynecol 39:688-690, 1972.

26. Tur-Kaspa I: Hyperbaric oxygen therapy for air embolism complicating operative hysteroscopy. Am J Obstet Gynecol 163:680-681, 1990.

27. Davis FM, Glover PW, Maycock E: Hyperbaric oxygen for cerebral arterial air embolism occurring during cesarean section. Anaesth Intensive Care 18:403-405, 1990.

28. Nims M, Hallonquist H, Camann W: Coronary arterial air embolus occurring during cesarean delivery. Int J Obstet Anesth 15:166-169, 2006.

29. Batman PA, Thomlinson J, Moore VC, et al: Death due to air embolism during sexual intercourse in the puerperium. Postgrad Med J 74:612-613, 1998.

30. Avanzas P, Garcia-Fernandez MA, Quiles J: Echocardiographic detection of systemic air embolism during positive pressure ventilation. Heart 89:1321, 2003.

31. Baskin SE, Wozniak RF: Hyperbaric oxygenation in the treatment of hemodialysis-associated air embolism. N Engl J Med 293:184-185, 1975.

32. Yu AS, Levy E: Paradoxical cerebral air embolism from a hemodialysis catheter. Am J Kidney Dis 29:453-455, 1997.

33. Imai S, Tamada T, Gyoten M, et al: Iatrogenic venous air embolism caused by CT injector—from a risk management point of view. Radiat Med 22:269-271, 2004.

34. Price DB, Nard P: Iatrogenic venous air embolism during contrast enhanced computed tomography: A report of two cases. Emerg Radiol 10:147-151, 2003.

35. Smith JM, Richardson JD, Grover FL, et al: Fatal air embolism following gunshot wound of the lung. J Thorac Cardiovasc Surg 72:296-298, 1976.

36. Halpern P, Greenstein A, Melamed Y, et al: Arterial air embolism after penetrating lung injury. Crit Care Med 11:392-393, 1983.

37. Hwang S, Lieu AS, Lin CL, et al: Massive cerebral air embolism after cardiopulmonary resuscitation. J Clin Neurosci 12:468-469, 2005.

38. Mitchell SJ, Benson M, Vadlamudi L, et al: Cerebral arterial gas embolism by helium: An unusual case successfully treated with hyperbaric oxygen and lidocaine. Ann Emerg Med 35:300-303, 2000.

39. Tretjak M, Gorjup V, Mozina H, et al: Cerebral and coronary gas embolism from the inhalation of pressurized helium. Crit Care Med 30:1156-1157, 2002.

40. Ijichi T, Itoh T, Sakai R et al: Multiple brain gas embolism after ingestion of concentrated hydrogen peroxide. Neurology 48:277-279, 1997.

41. Butler BD, Hills BA: The lung as a filter for microbubbles. J Appl Physiol 47:537-543, 1979.

42. Butler BD, Hills BA: Transpulmonary passage of venous air emboli. J Appl Physiol 59:543-547, 1985.

43. Butler BD, Robinson R, Sutton T, et al: Cardiovascular pressures with venous gas embolism and decompression. Aviat Space Environ Med 66:408-414, 1995.

44. Takeoka M, Sakai A, Ueda G, et al: Influence of hypoxia and pulmonary air embolism on lung injury in perfused rat lungs. Respiration 63:346-351, 1996.

45. Tanus-Santos JE, Gordo WM, Udelsmann A, et al: Nonselective endothelin-receptor antagonism attenuates hemodynamic changes after massive pulmonary air embolism in dogs. Chest 118:175-179, 2000.

46. Bove AA, Hallenbeck JM, Elliott DH: Circulatory responses to venous air embolism and decompression

sickness in dogs. Undersea Biomed Res 1:207–220, 1974.

47. Durant TM, Long J, Oppenheimer MJ: Pulmonary (venous) air embolism. Am Heart J 33:269–281, 1947.

48. Munson ES, Merrick HC: Effect of nitrous oxide on venous air embolism. Anesthesiology 27:783–787, 1966.

49. Oppenheimer MJ, Durant TM, Lynch P: Body position related to venous air embolism and associated cardiovascular-respiratory changes. Am J Med Sci 225:362–373, 1953.

50. Toung TJ, Rossberg MI, Hutchins GM: Volume of air in a lethal venous air embolism. Anesthesiology 94:360–361, 2001.

51. Hagen PT, Scholz DG, Edwards WD: Incidence and size of patent foramen ovale during the first 10 decades of life: An autopsy study of 965 normal hearts. Mayo Clin Proc 59:17–20, 1984.

52. Gronert GA, Messick JM, Cucchiara RF, et al: Paradoxical air embolism from a patent foramen ovale. Anesthesiology 50:548–549, 1979.

53. Kubo S, Nakata H: Air embolism due to a patent foramen ovale visualized by harmonic contrast echocardiography. J Neurol Neurosurg Psychiatr 71:555, 2001.

54. Pham Dang C, Pereon Y, Champin P, et al: Paradoxical air embolism from patent foramen ovale in scoliosis surgery. Spine 27:E291–E295, 2002.

55. Spencer MP, Oyama Y: Pulmonary capacity for dissipation of venous gas emboli. Aerosp Med 42:822–827, 1971.

56. Vik A, Brubakk AO, Hennessy TR, et al: Venous air embolism in swine: Transport of gas bubbles through the pulmonary circulation. J Appl Physiol 69:237–244, 1990.

57. Marquez J, Sladen A, Gendell H, et al: Paradoxical cerebral air embolism without an intracardiac septal defect. Case report. J Neurosurg 55:997–1000, 1981.

58. Tommasino C, Rizzardi R, Beretta L, et al: Cerebral ischemia after venous air embolism in the absence of intracardiac defects. J Neurosurg Anesthesiol 8:30–34, 1996.

59. Mammoto T, Hayashi Y, Ohnishi Y, et al: Incidence of venous and paradoxical air embolism in neurosurgical patients in the sitting position: Detection by transesophageal echocardiography. Acta Anaesthesiol Scand 42:643–647, 1998.

60. Boussuges A, Molenat F, Carturan D, et al: Venous gas embolism: Detection with pulsed Doppler guided by two-dimensional echocardiography. Acta Anaesthesiol Scand 43:328–332, 1999.

61. Klotzsch C, Janssen G, Berlit P: Transesophageal echocardiography and contrast-TCD in the detection of a patent foramen ovale: Experiences with 111 patients. Neurology 44:1603–1606, 1994.

62. Stendel R, Gramm HJ, Schroder K, et al: Transcranial Doppler ultrasonography as a screening technique for detection of a patent foramen ovale before surgery in the sitting position. Anesthesiology 93:971–975, 2000.

63. Brechner TM, Brechner VL: An audible alarm for monitoring air embolism during neurosurgery. J Neurosurg 47:201–204, 1977.

64. Van Liew HD, Conkin J, Burkard ME: The oxygen window and decompression bubbles: Estimates and significance. Aviat Space Environ Med 64:859–865, 1993.

65. Ericsson JA, Gottlieb JD, Sweet RB: Closed-chest cardiac massage in the treatment of venous air embolism. N Engl J Med 270:1353–1354, 1964.

66. Yeh PA, Chen HP, Tsai YC, et al: Successful management of air embolism-induced ventricular fibrillation in orthotopic liver transplantation. Acta Anaesthesiol Taiwan 43:243–246, 2005.

67. Coppa GF, Couge TH, Hofstetter SR: Air embolism: A lethal but preventable complication of subclavian vein catheterization. JPEN J Parenter Enteral Nutr 5:166–168, 1981.

68. Artru AA: Venous air embolism in prone dogs positioned with the abdomen hanging freely: Percentage of gas retrieved and success rate of resuscitation. Anesth Analg 75:715–719, 1992.

69. De Angelis J: A simple and rapid method for evacuation of embolized air. Anesthesiology 43:110–111, 1975.

70. Stallworth JM, Martin JB, Postlethwait RW: Aspiration of the heart in air embolism. J Am Med Assoc 143:1250–1251, 1950.

71. Archer DP, Pash MP, MacRae ME: Successful management of venous air embolism with inotropic support. Neuroanesth Intensive Care 48:204–208, 2001.

72. Jardin F, Genevray B, Brun-Ney D, et al: Dobutamine: A hemodynamic evaluation in pulmonary embolism shock. Crit Care Med 13:1009–1012, 1985.

73. Benson J, Adkinson C, Collier R: Hyperbaric oxygen therapy of iatrogenic cerebral arterial gas embolism. Undersea Hyperb Med 30:117–126, 2003.

74. Blanc P, Boussuges A, Henriette K, et al: Iatrogenic cerebral air embolism: Importance of an early hyperbaric oxygenation. Intensive Care Med 28:559–563, 2002.

75. Moon RE, de Lisle Dear G, Stolp BW: Treatment of decompression illness and iatrogenic gas embolism. Respir Care Clin N Am 5:93–135, 1999.

76. McAniff JJ: United States underwater fatality statistics, 1970–82, including a preliminary assessment of 1983 fatalities [Report No. URI-SSR-84-17]. National Underwater Accident Data Center, University of Rhode Island, 1983.

77. Divers Alert Network (DAN): Report on decompression illness and diving fatalities. Durham, NC, DAN, 2005.

78. Powers AT, Bass B, Stewart J, et al: A six-year review of scuba diving fatalities in San Diego County. Undersea Biomed Res 19(suppl):20, 1992.

79. Neuman T: Arterial gas embolism and pulmonary barotrauma. In: Brubakk AO, Neuman TS (eds): Bennett and Elliott's Physiology and Medicine of Diving, 5th ed. London, Saunders, 2003, pp 557–577.

80. Safar P: History of cardiopulmonary-cerebral resuscitation. In: Bircher AW (ed): Cardiopulmonary Resuscitation. New York, Churchill Livingstone, 1989, pp 1–53.

81. Polack B, Adams H: Traumatic air embolism in submarine escape training. US Navy Med Bull 30:165–177, 1932.

82. James RE: Extra-alveolar air resulting from submarine escape training: A post-training roentgenographic survey of 170 submariners [Report No. 550]. Groton, CT, United States Naval Submarine Medical Center, 1968.

83. Harker CP, Neuman TS, Olson LK, et al: The roentgenographic findings associated with air embolism in sport scuba divers. J Emerg Med 11:443–449, 1993.

84. Dick AP, Massey EW: Neurologic presentation of decompression sickness and air embolism in sport divers. Neurology 35:667-671, 1985.

85. Denny MK, Read RC: Scuba-diving deaths in Michigan. JAMA 192:220-222, 1965.

86. Lansche JM: Deaths during ski and scuba diving in California during 1970. Calif Med 116:18-22, 1972.

87. Malhotra MS, Wright HC: The effects of a raised intra-pulmonary pressure on the lungs of fresh unchilled cadavers. J Pathol Bacteriol 82:198-202, 1961.

88. Schaeffer KE, Nulty WP, Carey C, et al: Mechanisms in development of interstitial emphysema and air embolism on decompression from depth. J Appl Physiol 13:15-29, 1958.

89. Benton PJ, Francis TJ, Pethybridge RJ: Spirometric indices and the risk of pulmonary barotrauma in submarine escape training. Undersea Hyperb Med 26:213-217, 1999.

90. Colebatch HJ, Ng CK: Decreased pulmonary disten-sibility and pulmonary barotrauma in divers. Respir Physiol 86:293-303, 1991.

91. Colebatch HJ, Smith MM, Ng CK: Increased elastic recoil as a determinant of pulmonary barotrauma in divers. Respir Physiol 26:55-64, 1976.

92. Francis TJR, Denison DM: Pulmonary barotrauma. In: Lundgren CE, Miller JN (eds): The Lung at Depth. New York, Marcel Dekker, 1999, pp 295-374.

93. Van Hoesen KB, Neuman TS: Asthma and scuba diving. Immunol Allergy Clin North Am 16:917-928, 1996.

94. Tetzlaff K, Reuter M, Leplow B, et al: Risk factors for pulmonary barotrauma in divers. Chest 112:654-659, 1997.

95. Benton PJ, Woodfine JD, Westwood PR: Arterial gas embolism following a 1-meter ascent during helicop-ter escape training: A case report. Aviat Space Environ Med 67:63-64, 1996.

96. Neuman TS, Jacoby I, Bove AA: Fatal pulmonary baro-trauma due to obstruction of the central circulation with air. J Emerg Med 16:413-417, 1998.

97. Balk M, Goldman JM: Alveolar hemorrhage as a mani-festation of pulmonary barotrauma after scuba diving. Ann Emerg Med 19:930-934, 1990.

98. Neuman TS, Hallenbeck JM: Barotraumatic cerebral air embolism and the mental status examination: A report of four cases. Ann Emerg Med 16:220-223, 1987.

99. Pearson RR: Diagnosis and treatment of gas embolism. In: Shilling CW, Carlston CB, Mathias RA (eds): The Physician's Guide to Diving Medicine. New York, Plenum Press, 1984, pp 333-367.

100. Harvey RB, Schilling JA: Relationship between lung pressures and volumes and traumatic air embolism. Fed Proc 13:68, 1954.

101. Butler BD, Laine GA, Leiman BC, et al: Effect of the Trendelenburg position on the distribution of arterial air emboli in dogs. Ann Thorac Surg 45:198-202, 1988.

102. Gorman DF: The redistribution of cerebral arterial gas embolism [PhD thesis]. Sydney, Australia, University of Sydney, 1987.

103. Gorman DF, Browning DM: Cerebral vasoreactivity and arterial gas embolism. Undersea Biomed Res 13:317-335, 1986.

104. Gorman DF, Browning DM, Parsons DW, et al: Distribu-tion of arterial gas emboli in the pial circulation. SPUMS J 17:101-115, 1987.

105. DeReuck J: The corticoangioarchitecture of the human brain. Acta Neurol Belg 72:323-329, 1972.

106. Dutka AJ, Kochanek P, Hallenbeck JM, et al: Air embolism may cause unrecognized ischemia of the gray-white junction. Undersea Biomed Res 15:99-106, 1988.

107. Evans DE, Kobrine AI, Weathersby PK, et al: Cardiovascular effects of cerebral air embolism. Stroke 12:338-344, 1981.

108. De La Torre R, Meredith J, Netsky MG: Cerebral air embolization in the dog. Arch Neurol 6:307-316, 1962.

109. Fritz H, Hossmann KA: Arterial air embolism in the cat brain. Stroke 10:581-589, 1979.

110. Evans DE, Weihl AC, David TD, et al: Effects of cerebral air embolism on circulating catecholamines and angio-tensin. Undersea Biomed Res 6(suppl):30, 1979.

111. Hallenbeck JM, Leitch DR, Dutka AJ, et al: The amount of circumscribed brain edema and the degree of post-ischemic neuronal recovery do not correlate well. Stroke 13:797-804, 1982.

112. Hills BA, James PB: Microbubble damage to the blood-brain barrier: Relevance to decompression sickness. Undersea Biomed Res 18:111-116, 1991.

113. Huang KL, Lin YC: Pharmacologic modulation of pulmonary vascular permeability during air embolism. Undersea Hyperb Med 24:315-321, 1997.

114. Ogston D, Bennett B: Surface-mediated reactions in the formation of thrombin, plasmin and kallikrein. Br Med Bull 34:107-112, 1978.

115. Hallenbeck JM, Leitch DR, Dutka AJ, et al: Prostoglandin I2, indomethacin and heparin promote post-ischemic neuronal recovery in dogs. Ann Neurol 12:797-809, 1982.

116. Neuman TS, Spragg RG, Wohl H: Platelet aggregates following decompression. Undersea Biomed Res 8(suppl):42, 1981.

117. Nossum V, Koteng S, Brubakk AO: Endothelial damage by bubbles in the pulmonary artery of the pig. Under-sea Hyperb Med 26:1-8, 1999.

118. Dutka AJ, Hallenbeck JM, Kochanek P: A brief episode of severe arterial hypertension induces delayed dete-rioration of brain function and worsens blood flow after transient multifocal cerebral ischemia. Stroke 18:386-395, 1987.

119. Helps SC, Parsons DW, Teilly PL, et al: The effect of gas emboli on rabbit cerebral blood flow. Stroke 21:94-99, 1990.

120. Brubakk AO, Duplancic D, Valic Z et al: A single air dive reduces arterial endothelial function in man. J Physiol 566(pt 3):901-906, 2005.

121. Frank X, Li HZ: Negative wake behind a sphere rising in viscoelastic fluids: A lattice Boltzmann investiga-tion. Phys Rev E Stat Nonlin Soft Matter Phys 74 (5 pt 2):056307, 2006.

122. Wu J: Theoretical study on shear stress generated by microstreaming surrounding contrast agents attached to living cells. Ultrasound Med Biol 28:125-129, 2002.

123. Sorop O, Spaan JA, Sweeney TE, et al: Effect of steady versus oscillating flow on porcine coronary arterioles:

Involvement of NO and superoxide anion. Circ Res 92:1344-1351, 2003.

124. Qiu W, Kass DA, Hu O, et al: Determinants of shear stress-stimulated endothelial nitric oxide production assessed in real-time by 4,5-diaminofluorescein fluorescence. Biochem Biophys Res Commun 286:328-335, 2001.

125. Lee JC, Olszewski J: Effect of air embolism on permeability of cerebral blood vessels. Neurology 9:619-625, 1959.

126. Nishimoto K, Wolman M, Spatz M, et al: Pathophysiologic correlations in the blood-brain barrier damage due to air embolism. Adv Neurol 20:237-244, 1978.

127. Levy D, Duffy T: Cerebral energy metabolism during transient ischemia and recovery in the gerbil. J Neurochem 28:63-70, 1976.

128. Scheinberg P, Myer J, Reivich M, et al: Cerebral circulation and mechanism in stroke. Stroke 7:213-233, 1976.

129. Evans DE, Hardenburgh E, Hallenbeck JM: Cardiovascular effects of arterial air embolism. Presented at Workshop on Arterial Air Embolism and Acute Stroke, Toronto, May 13, 1977. Bethesda, MD, Undersea Medical Society, 1977.

130. Cales RH, Humphreys N, Pilmanis AA, et al: Cardiac arrest from gas embolism in scuba diving. Ann Emerg Med 10:589-592, 1981.

131. Geoghegan T, Lam CR: The mechanism of death from intracardiac air and its reversibility. Ann Surg 138:351-359, 1953.

132. Cooperman EM, Hogg J, Thurlbeck WM: Mechanism of death in shallow-water Scuba diving. Can Med Assoc J 99:1128-1131, 1968.

133. Smith RM, Neuman TS: Elevation of serum creatine kinase in divers with arterial gas embolism. N Engl J Med 330:19-24, 1994.

134. Neuman TS, Jacoby I, Olson L: Fatal diving-related arterial gas embolism associated with complete filling of the central vascular bed. Undersea Hyperb Med 21(suppl):95-96, 1994.

135. Williamson JA, King GK, Callanan VI, et al: Fatal arterial gas embolism: Detection by chest radiography and imaging before autopsy. Med J Aust 153:97-100, 1990.

136. Elliott DH, Harrison JAB, Barnard EEP: Clinical and radiological features of eighty-eight cases of decompression barotrauma. In: Schilling CW, Beckett MW (eds): Proceedings of the Vth Symposium on Underwater Physiology. Bethesda, MD, Federation of American Societies for Experimental Biology, 1978, pp 527-536.

137. Pearson RR, Goad RF: Delayed cerebral edema complicating cerebral air embolism: Case histories. Undersea Biomed Res 9:283-296, 1982.

138. Hallenbeck JM: Prevention of postischemic impairment of microvascular perfusion. Neurology 27:3-10, 1977.

139. Neuman TS, Bove AA: Severe refractory decompression sickness resulting from combined no-decompression dives and pulmonary barotrauma: Type III decompression sickness. Underwater and Hyperbaric Physiology IX. Proceedings of the Ninth International Symposium on Underwater and Hyperbaric Physiology, Kobe, Japan, September 1986. Bethesda, MD, Undersea and Hyperbaric Medical Society, 1987, pp 985-991.

140. Neuman TS, Bove AA: Combined arterial gas embolism and decompression sickness following no-stop dives. Undersea Biomed Res 17:429-436, 1990.

141. Smith RM, Van Hoesen KB, Neuman TS: Arterial gas embolism and hemoconcentration. J Emerg Med 12:147-153, 1994.

142. Bove AA, Neuman TS, Smith RM: ECG changes associated with pulmonary barotrauma. Undersea Hyperb Med 22(suppl):55, 1995.

143. Loke GP, Story DA, Liskaser F, et al: Pulmonary arteriovenous malformation causing massive haemoptysis and complicated by coronary air embolism. Anaesth Intensive Care 34:75-78, 2006.

144. Smith RM, Neuman TS: Abnormal serum biochemistries in association with arterial gas embolism. J Emerg Med 15:285-289, 1997.

145. Warren LP, Djang WT, Moon RE, et al: Neuroimaging of scuba diving injuries to the CNS. Am J Roentgenol 151:1003-1008, 1988.

146. Sipinen SA, Ahovuo J, Halonen JP: Electroencephalography and magnetic resonance imaging after diving and decompression incidents: A controlled study. Undersea Hyperb Med 26:61-65, 1999.

147. Moon RE, Gorman DF: Treatment of the decompression disorders. In: Brubakk AO, Neuman TS (eds): Bennett and Elliott's Physiology and Medicine of Diving, 5th ed. London, Saunders, 2003, pp 600-650.

148. Ziser A, Adir Y, Lavon H, Shupak A: Hyperbaric oxygen therapy for massive arterial air embolism during cardiac operations. J Thorac Cardiovasc Surg 117:818-821, 1999.

149. Mader JT, Hulet WH: Delayed hyperbaric treatment of cerebral air embolism. Arch Neurol 36:504-505, 1979.

150. Longphre JM, Denoble PJ, Moon RE, et al: First aid normobaric oxygen for the treatment of recreational diving injuries. Undersea Hyperb Med 43:43-49, 2007.

151. Atkinson JR: Experimental air embolism. Northwest Med 62:699-703, 1963.

152. Van Allen CM, Hrdina LA, Clark J: Air embolism from the pulmonary vein—a clinical and experimental study. Arch Surg 19:567-599, 1929.

153. Dutka AJ: Therapy for dysbaric central nervous system ischemia: Adjuncts to recompression. In: Bennett PB, Moon RE (eds): Diving Accident Management. Bethesda, MD, Undersea and Hyperbaric Medical Society, 1990, pp 222-234.

154. Wherrett CG, Mehran RJ, Beaulieu MA: Cerebral arterial gas embolism following diagnostic bronchoscopy: Delayed treatment with hyperbaric oxygen. Can J Anaesth 49:96-99, 2002.

155. Dexter F, Hindman BJ: Recommendations for hyperbaric oxygen therapy of cerebral air embolism based on a mathematical model of bubble absorption. Anesth Analg 84:1203-1207, 1997.

156. Dutka AJ: Air or gas embolism. In: Camporesi EM, Barker AC (eds): Hyperbaric Oxygen Therapy: A Critical Review. Bethesda, MD, Undersea and Hyperbaric Medical Society, 1991, pp 1-10.

157. Miller JD, Ledingham IM: Reduction of increased intracranial pressure. Comparison between hyperbaric oxygen and hyperventilation. Arch Neurol 24:210-216, 1971.

158. Sukoff MH, Hollin SA, Espinosa OE: The protective effect of hyperbaric oxygenation in experimental cerebral edema. J Neurosurg 29:236-241, 1968.

159. Mink RB, Dutka AJ: Hyperbaric oxygen after global cerebral ischemia in rabbits reduces brain vascular

permeability and blood flow. Stroke 26:2307-2312, 1995.

160. Thom SR: Functional inhibition of leukocyte beta2 interferons by hyperbaric oxygen in carbon monoxide-mediated brain injury in rats. Toxicol Appl Pharmacol 123:248-256, 1993.

161. Thom SR, Mendiguren I, Hardy K, et al: Inhibition of human neutrophil B2-integrin-dependent adherence by hyperbaric oxygen. Am J Physiol 272:C770-C777, 1997.

162. Thom SR: Effects of hyperoxia on neutrophil adhesion. Undersea Hyperb Med 31:123-131, 2004.

163. Buras JA, Stahl GL, Svoboda KK, et al: Hyperbaric oxygen downregulates ICAM-1 expression induced by hypoxia and hypoglycemia: The role of NOS. Am J Physiol Cell Physiol 278:C292-C302, 2000.

164. Helps SC, Gorman DF: Air embolism of the brain in rabbits pretreated with mechlorethamine. Stroke 22:351-354, 1991.

165. Waite CL, Mazzone WF, Greenwood ME, et al: Cerebral Air Embolism. I. Basic Studies. US Naval Submarine Medical Center Report No. 493. Panama City, Fla, US Navy submarine Research Laboratory, 1967.

166. Gorman DF, Browning DM, Parsons DW: Redistribution of cerebral arterial gas emboli: A comparison of treatment regimens. In: Bove AA, Bachrach AJ, Greenbaum LJ Jr (eds): Underwater and Hyperbaric Physiology. IX. Proceedings of the Ninth International Symposium on Underwater and Hyperbaric Physiology. Bethesda, MD, Undersea and Hyperbaric Medical Society, 1987, pp 1031-1054.

167. Leitch DR, Greenbaum LJ Jr, Hallenbeck JM: Cerebral arterial air embolism: I. Is there benefit in beginning HBO treatment at 6 bar? Undersea Biomed Res 11:221-235, 1984.

168. Leitch DR, Green RD: Additional pressurization for treating nonresponding cases of serious air decompression sickness. Aviat Space Environ Med 56:1139-1143, 1985.

169. Weaver LK: Monoplace hyperbaric chamber use of U.S. Navy Table 6: A 20-year experience. Undersea Hyperb Med 33:85-88, 2006.

170. Bennett PB, Moon RE (eds): Diving Accident Management. Bethesda, MD, Undersea and Hyperbaric Medical Society, 1990.

171. Mitchell SJ: Lidocaine in the treatment of decompression illness: A review of the literature. Undersea Hyperb Med 28(3):165-174, 2001.

172. Mitchell SJ, Pellett O, Gorman DF: Cerebral protection by lidocaine during cardiac operations. Ann Thorac Surg 67:1117-1124, 1999.

173. Evans DE, Kobrine AI, LeGrys DC, et al: Protective effect of lidocaine in acute cerebral ischemia induced by air embolism. J Neurosurg 60:257-263, 1984.

174. Evans DC, Catron PW, McDermott JJ, et al: Therapeutic effect of lidocaine after experimental cerebral ischemia induced by air embolism. J Neurosurg 70:97-102, 1989.

175. Drewry A, Gorman DF: Lidocaine as an adjunct to hyperbaric therapy in decompression illness: A case report. Undersea Biomed Res 19:187-190, 1992.

176. Cogar WB: Intravenous lidocaine as adjunctive therapy in the treatment of decompression illness. Ann Emerg Med 29:284-286, 1997.

177. Suzuki A, Eckmann DM: Embolism bubble adhesion force in excised perfused microvessels. Anesthesiology 99:400-408, 2003.

178. Suzuki A, Armstead SC, Eckmann DM: Surfactant reduction in embolism bubble adhesion and endothelial damage. Anesthesiology 101:97-103, 2004.

179. Spiess BD, McCarthy R, Piotrowski D, et al: Protection from venous air embolism with fluorocarbon emulsion FC-43. J Surg Res 41:439-444, 1986.

180. Spiess BD, McCarthy RJ, Tuman KJ, et al: Protection from coronary air embolism by a perfluorocarbon emulsion (FC-43). J Cardiothorac Anesth 1:210-215, 1987.

181. Cochran RP, Kunzelman KS, Vocelka CR, et al: Perfluorocarbon emulsion in the cardiopulmonary bypass prime reduces neurologic injury. Ann Thorac Surg 63:1326-1332, 1997.

182. Eckmann DM, Lomivorotov VN: Microvascular gas embolization clearance following perfluorocarbon administration. J Appl Physiol 94:860-868, 2003.

Decompression 14
Sickness

Richard E. Moon, MD, FACP, FCCP, FRCPC, and Des F. Gorman, MBChB, MD, PhD

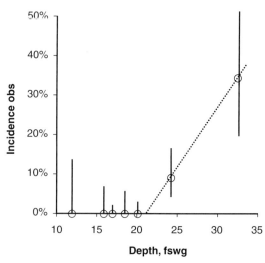

Figure 14.1 DECOMPRESSION SICKNESS (DCS) AFTER DIRECT ASCENT TO THE SURFACE FROM SATURATION. The threshold for DCS is 20 to 25 feet sea water gauge (fswg). obs, observations. *(From Van Liew HD, Flynn ET: Direct ascent from air and N_2-O_2 saturation dives in humans: DCS risk and evidence of a threshold. Undersea Hyperb Med 32:409–419, 2005, by permission.)*

WHAT IS DECOMPRESSION SICKNESS?

Decompression sickness (DCS) is an acute condition that occurs during or shortly after an acute reduction in ambient pressure caused by bubbles. It can be caused by an acute decompression from ground level to altitude or, more commonly, by decompression from a dive or hyperbaric chamber exposure back to ambient pressure. The minimum altitude exposure necessary for DCS is close to 21,200 feet. The minimum depth necessary to produce DCS is estimated from observations of direct decompression to 1 atmosphere absolute (ATA) after a prolonged period at increased pressure (*saturation* exposure). Bubble formation has been observed after a decompression from only 1.35 ATA (11 feet of sea water [fsw]).[1] The minimum pressure change for DCS while breathing air or nitrogen/oxygen mixtures appears to be between 1.6 and 1.76 ATA (20–25 fsw)[2] (Fig. 14.1).

DCS was first observed in the 19th century in compressed air (caisson) workers, hence its original name *caisson disease.* It was also named

the bends, allegedly because some of its original sufferers walked or shuffled in a characteristic forward hunched posture.[3] DCS was later described in divers,[4-6] high-altitude pilots,[7] and astronauts.[8] DCS is a subset of bubble-related diseases, the other being *arterial gas embolism* (AGE). The two conditions are collectively known as *decompression illness.*

PATHOGENESIS

Bubbles

Bubbles in the bloodstream were first reported in 1878 by Bert[9] in experimental animals after decompression from increased ambient pressure. Indirect support for bubbles as the cause of DCS was provided by the observation that the manifestations could be relieved by recompression.[9,10] Bubbles have been observed in autopsied cases of fatal DCS[11] and in the bloodstream of divers after decompression using ultrasound.[12]

Bubbles form within tissues in which the inert gas partial pressure exceeds the pressure within tissue (*autochthonous* bubbles). Bubble formation is believed to be initiated at sites of stable gas micronuclei.[13,14] Such micronuclei could be stabilized against the forces of surface tension by a coating of surfactant.[15] Alternatively, if the gas micronucleus exists in the crevice of a hydrophobic molecule, surface tension would intrinsically tend to stabilize the bubble.

Bubbles can form in the absence of a decrease in ambient pressure when local tissue supersaturation occurs because of a change in breathing gas. This was originally described in a series of divers in a heliox-filled hyperbaric chamber at 7 ATA at Duke University when the breathing gas was switched from heliox to nitrox[16] (see Skin Bends section later in this chapter and also Fig. 14.10). This observation was subsequently observed at the University of Pennsylvania,[17] after which a series of studies led to its understanding. When the ingress into a tissue of a new gas exceeds the egress of a resident gas, the sum of partial pressures can exceed ambient pressure. Isobaric bubble formation has been demonstrated at 1 ATA in experimental animals surrounded by helium while breathing nitrous oxide/oxygen.[18,19]

The presence of bubbles in tissues per se does not imply DCS. Tissue bubbles have been observed radiographically in the absence of symptoms, but only during altitude exposure.[20,21] Bubbles in absence of symptoms in the veins or right heart (venous gas emboli [VGEs]) can be observed commonly using ultrasound after dives.[22,23] The bloodstream is relatively resistant to de novo bubble formation.[24] VGEs are believed to originate in extravascular tissue, possibly muscle, and migrate into the bloodstream where, in the presence of a high inert gas partial pressure, they can enlarge. VGEs are mostly trapped by the pulmonary capillaries, where the gas diffuses into alveoli.

In the presence of a right-to-left shunt, VGEs can enter the left heart, thus becoming AGEs, which are more likely to produce symptoms.[25] Indeed, cross-sectional studies have shown a relation between early onset and neurologic DCS and the presence of a patent foramen ovale (PFO),[26-35] suggesting that arterialized VGE may play a pathophysiologic role

in certain types of DCS, particularly those forms that involve the skin, inner ear, and central nervous system.

Under certain circumstances, VGEs can traverse the pulmonary circulation. Arteriovenous shunt vessels have been demonstrated in normal human lungs,[36] through which 25- and 50-μm diameter microspheres can pass. High exercise cardiac output and pulmonary artery pressure, such as during exercise, may facilitate right-to-left shunting through the lung.[37,38] High bubble rates can also facilitate right-to-left shunting through the lung (Fig. 14.2).

Direct Bubble Effects

Bubbles may cause tissue damage because of direct mechanical effects. Bubble-induced distraction of connective tissue is believed to be the cause of DCS-related pain. Bubbles within and proximal to spinal cord neurons have been described as a possible cause of neuronal dysfunction[39] (Fig. 14.3). Increased intraosseous pressure within the marrow cavity of long bones has been hypothesized as the cause of the pain of limb bends and osteonecrosis that can occur.[40] Increased

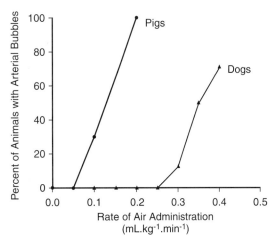

Figure 14.2 ARTERIALIZATION OF VENOUS BUBBLES. The infusion rate at which venous bubbles spill into the arterial circulation is species specific. *(Data for dogs from Butler BD, Hills BA: Transpulmonary passage of venous air emboli. J Appl Physiol 59:543–547, 1985; and data for pigs from Vik A, Brubakk AO, Hennessy TR, et al: Venous air embolism in swine: Transport of gas bubbles through the pulmonary circulation. J Appl Physiol 69:237–244, 1990, by permission.)*

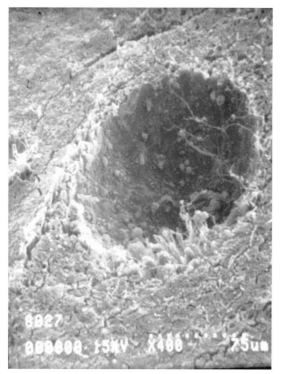

Figure 14.3 SCANNING ELECTRON MICROGRAPH OF AN AUTOCHTHONOUS BUBBLE IN THE SPINAL CORD OF A DOG. *(Courtesy Drs. T. J. Francis and G. H. Pezeshkpour.)*

intramedullary pressure caused by bubble expansion within the spinal cord has been hypothesized as a cause of reduced blood flow.[41] Because the petrous temporal bone surrounding the cochlear-vestibular apparatus is so hard, its fracture by bubbles expanding within lacunae adjacent to the semicircular canals has been hypothesized as the cause of inner ear DCS.[42]

Cellular and Tissue Effects

Endothelial Disruption

Secondary effects of bubbles include endothelial disruption. Bubble–blood vessel interaction strips the endothelial cells from the basement membrane (Fig. 14.4). This then causes loss of endothelial function, including plasma leakage into the interstitium. Indirect evidence for this was observed by Dr. Alphonse Jaminet during construction of the St. Louis bridge (now the Eads Bridge) across the Mississippi River. He observed that caisson workers with DCS had a greater urine specific gravity than asymptom-

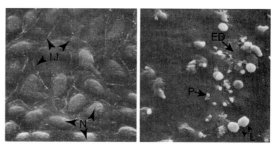

Figure 14.4 ENDOTHELIAL EFFECTS OF BUBBLES. *Left,* Scanning electron microscopy (EM) of luminal surface of jugular vein from control dog. Individual endothelial cells can be seen, outlined by intercellular junctions *(IJ)* and their nuclei *(N)*. There are no adhering blood cells. *Right,* Scanning EM of an area of jugular vein in an animal with severe decompression sickness. There are numerous adhering leukocytes *(L)* and platelets *(P)*. ED, endothelial damage. *(From Levin LL, Stewart GJ, Lynch PR, et al: Blood and blood vessel wall changes induced by decompression sickness in dogs. J Appl Physiol 50:944–949, 1981, by permission.)*

atic men.[43] Cockett and colleagues[44] observed that dogs subjected to severe decompression stress experienced a decrease in plasma volume of up to 35%. In human DCS, damaged endothelium causes a decrease in plasma volume because of extravasation into the interstitium (Fig. 14.5).[45,46] Increased hematocrit level as a measure of plasma volume reduction correlates with the severity of DCS.[47]

Levin's[69] observations were confirmed more recently together with the observation that endothelial relaxation function has been observed in response to substance P[48,49] and acetylcholine.[49]

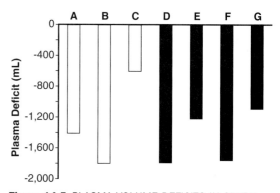

Figure 14.5 PLASMA VOLUME DEFICITS IN SEVEN CASES OF SEVERE ALTITUDE DECOMPRESSION SICKNESS IN HUMANS. *White bars* represent patients who survived; *black bars* represent those who died. *(From Malette WG, Fitzgerald JB, Cockett AT: Dysbarism. A review of thirty-five cases with suggestion for therapy. Aerospace Med 33:1132–1139, 1962, by permission.)*

Heat Shock Protein Expression

DCS in experimental animals induces heat shock protein expression, which appears to provide a degree of prophylaxis against DCS after subsequent pressure exposures.[50]

Complement Activation

Complement activation by bubbles has been observed both in vitro[51,52] and in vivo in experimental animals,[53] and has been proposed as a mechanism in the evolution of DCS. Decomplemented rabbits appear to be resistant to DCS.[53] In humans, erythrocyte-bound C3d increases after repetitive dives, although there does not appear to be a correlation between complement activation and ultrasound bubble score.[54] Some studies have demonstrated a relation between complement activation and susceptibility to DCS in humans[55,56]; however, others have failed to confirm it.[57,58] Complement does not appear to be necessary for bubble-induced endothelial damage.[59] It is possible that the different strength of evidence for a role of complement in rabbit versus human DCS reflects species specificity.

Platelet Activation

Platelets are activated during decompression[60] and are deposited on the surface of intravascular bubbles.[61,62] Platelet numbers are slightly reduced after asymptomatic dives.[63,64] However, the role of the platelet in DCS has been questioned by studies in which platelet inhibition does not appear to be effective in facilitating recovery in animal models of AGE unless combined with full therapeutic anticoagulation with heparin.[65]

Nitric Oxide Production

Recent data implicate nitric oxide as a mediator of bubble formation. Nitric oxide synthase inhibition can increase bubble formation in rats,[66] whereas administration of nitric oxide donors or appropriately timed exercise (a nitric oxide synthase upregulator) before a dive can reduce bubble formation.[67,68] Given the importance of nitric oxide in tissue blood flow regulation, it is likely that these effects are mediated by inert gas washout.

Leukocyte Activation

Considerable evidence implicates the leukocyte in DCS pathophysiology. Leukocytes adhere to both denuded endothelium[69] and bubbles.[70] Leukocytes accumulate in brain areas made ischemic using air emboli,[71] and depletion of neutrophils before air embolism ameliorates the neurologic injury.[72,73]

Organ Effects

Joints and Long Bones

The cause of joint pain due to DCS is unknown. It has been variously speculated that the site of the pain is in ligaments, tendons, the joint space, the marrow, and referred pain from the spinal cord or sensory root. Support for bubbles in the marrow or intramedullary arterioles as a cause is the development of bony infarction in the long bones of some compressed air workers and divers.[74,75]

Spinal Cord

The spinal cord is frequently a target organ in DCS. Proposed mechanisms of bubble formation in the spinal cord include arterial embolization, blood flow reduction due to occlusion by bubbles of the epidural venous plexus (Fig. 14.6) and in situ (autochthonous bubbles;

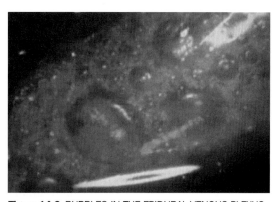

Figure 14.6 BUBBLES IN THE EPIDURAL VENOUS PLEXUS. **(See Color Plate 8.)** *(From Hallenbeck JM: Cinephotomicrography of dog spinal vessels during cord-damaging decompression sickness. Neurology 26:190–199, 1976, by permission.)*

Figure 14.7 SPINAL CORD DECOMPRESSION SICKNESS 1 WEEK AFTER DEVELOPMENT OF QUADRIPARESIS IN A 42-YEAR-OLD MAN WHO MADE A 70 FEET SEA WATER DIVE. *A,* Demyelination can be seen in the long tracts. *B,* Higher magnification view shows hemorrhage in the gray matter. **(See Color Plate 9.)** *(Courtesy Department of Pathology, Duke University Medical Center, Durham, NC.)*

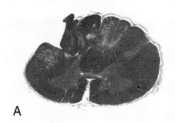
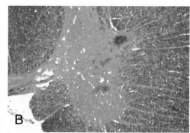

A   B

see Fig. 14.3). Also observed are intramedullary hemorrhage[6,76,77] and demyelination involving the long tracts[78,79] (Fig. 14.7).

Brain

In situ gas bubble formation is believed to be unlikely because of high tissue blood flow and rapid inert gas washout. Hydrogen washout has been measured in the cerebral cortex and has a half-time on the order of 45 seconds.[80] The half-time even in white matter would be only approximately 3 minutes. In addition, cerebral manifestations are usually focal. Therefore, most cerebral manifestations are believed to be caused by bubble emboli, either from pulmonary barotrauma (PBT) or arterialization of VGEs (see later).

Peripheral Nerve

Isolated peripheral nerve manifestations in DCS have rarely been described. This is usually in locations where increased pressure and entrapment could occur,[81,82] although one case report exists of a mononeuropathy involving the medial branch of the deep peroneal nerve.[83]

Lung

High levels of VGEs after decompression cause "chokes," which is associated with radiographic pulmonary edema (Fig. 14.8).[84] Intravenous (IV) bubble infusion also causes pulmonary edema (Fig. 14.9). The mechanism appears to involve leukocytes, which adhere to bubbles[70] (see Fig. 14.9) and accumulate in the lung after VGE.[49]

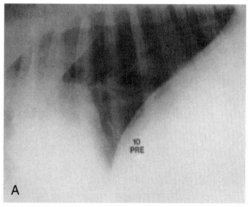

A

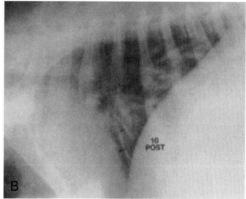

B

Figure 14.8 PULMONARY EDEMA IN A SHEEP WITH "CHOKES" AFTER A 42 FEET SEA WATER (FSW) DIVE FOR 22 HOURS, FOLLOWED BY A SIMULATED ALTITUDE EXPOSURE TO 8000 FEET (0.75 ATMOSPHERE ABSOLUTE [ATA]). *A,* Before dive. *B,* After dive and altitude exposure. Patchy pulmonary infiltrates are consistent with pulmonary edema. *(From Atkins CE, Lehner CE, Beck KA, et al: Experimental respiratory decompression sickness in sheep. J Appl Physiol 65:1163–1171, 1988, by permission.)*

Inner Ear

Inner ear DCS can involve the vestibular apparatus, the cochlea, or both. It was initially believed to occur only in heliox divers, and usually after a gas switch during decompression. However, it does occur in air divers, typically

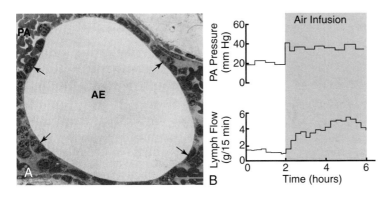

Figure 14.9 *A,* Leukocyte rosette around air bubble in a small pulmonary artery. *B,* Intravenous bubble infusion, causing pulmonary hypertension and increased lymph flow due to pulmonary edema. AE, air embolism; PA, pulmonary artery. *(From Albertine KH, Wiener-Kronish JP, Koike K, et al: Quantification of damage by air emboli to lung microvessels in anesthetized sheep. J Appl Physiol 57:1360–1368, 1984, by permission.)*

after a dive to greater than 60 fsw. The pathophysiology has been ascribed to hemorrhage within the vestibular apparatus caused by vascular occlusion by bubbles,[85] fractures of the bone surrounding the semicircular canals,[42] and gas within the fluids.

Skin and Soft Tissue

Several forms of DCS that involve the skin can occur (see later).

CLINICAL MANIFESTATIONS

DCS is a constellation of symptoms and signs that occurs after a reduction in ambient pressure. Initial symptoms are most commonly paresthesias and joint pain (Fig. 14.10). Mild symptoms may remain stable or progress to more severe manifestations. Serious neurologic symptoms and signs usually occur within 1 hour and can include motor weakness,

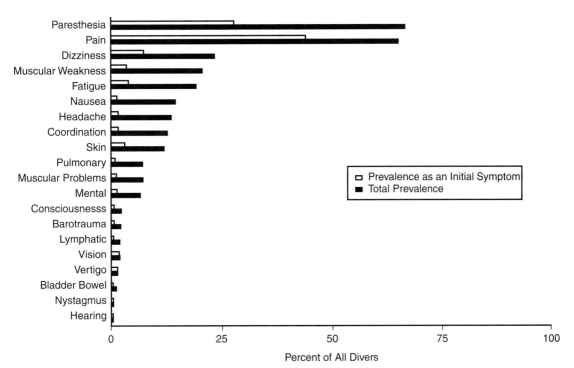

Figure 14.10 SYMPTOMS OF DECOMPRESSION SICKNESS IN RECREATIONAL DIVERS. *White bars represent prevalence as an initial symptom; black bars represent total prevalence. (From the Divers Alert Network Report on Decompression Illness, Diving Fatalities and Project Dive Exploration. Durham, NC, Divers Alert Network, 2005.)*

urinary retention, ataxia, and impaired consciousness. Dyspnea and cough are characteristic of high levels of VGEs, referred to as cardiorespiratory DCS ("chokes").

EVALUATION OF THE PATIENT

DCS is a clinical diagnosis based on history and physical examination.

History

The patient evaluation should include the following information:

- Time of onset and progression of symptoms
- Index of gas burden (e.g., depth–time exposure).
- Evidence of barotrauma, such as rapid or panic ascent, breath-holding during ascent, chest pain, or dyspnea

Severe cases tend to present early after surfacing, whereas minor symptoms can occur after delay. In a published series of 1070 cases of central nervous system (CNS) DCS, symptoms occurred within 10 minutes of surfacing in half of cases and within 3 hours in 90% of cases.[86] Unless there has been an altitude exposure, almost all symptoms occur within 24 hours of surfacing. Pain-only bends tend to have a longer latency; however, around 90% of cases become symptomatic within 6 hours or more of surfacing.[11,87-89] Causes for a diver's symptoms other than DCS should be entertained if the latency between dive and onset of symptoms is prolonged beyond 24 hours. If there has been intervening altitude exposure, onset can be longer, especially after saturation dives.[90,91] Symptoms that occur during compression or at maximum depth cannot be due to DCS. In such cases, one should consider sinus or otic barotrauma, gas narcosis, poisoning from gas contamination (e.g., carbon monoxide), immersion pulmonary edema, or causes unrelated to diving.

An estimate of inert gas uptake can be obtained from the profiles of recent dives, particularly the one immediately before symptom onset. One way to do this is to compare the diver's depth–time profile with a standard decompression table, such as the U.S. Navy Air Decompression Table (from the U.S. Navy Diving Manual,[92] available via the Internet at: http://www.supsalv.org). However, adherence to a standard decompression procedure (table or computer) does not exclude either DCS or AGE. Breath-holding during ascent or a rapid ascent can suggest PBT and intravascular gas, which can occur from depths as shallow as 1 m (3 feet).[93]

Muscle strains and bruises can be mistaken for DCS. Conditions other than DCS that can mimic the disease after a dive include myocardial infarction, subarachnoid hemorrhage, acute disc herniation, complicated migraine, transverse myelitis, vasculitis,[94] multiple sclerosis, carotid dissection,[95] maple syrup urine disease,[96] or neurologic symptoms from fish toxin.[97] Psychiatric disease such as somatoform disorders, factitious disorders, and malingering have been mistaken for DCS.[98-101]

Physical Examination

Pain-Only Bend

Physical examination is usually negative in true pain-only DCS. Signs of joint inflammation are absent, and joint movement rarely alters the pain. Sometimes increasing the local tissue pressure in the affected area may diminish the pain, for example, by having the patient stand up (as in the case of involvement of the legs or hips) or by inflation of a blood pressure cuff placed around the affected area[102]; however, absence of a change in pain does not exclude the diagnosis.

Skin Bends

There are several types of skin bends. The most common type is a nonspecific, erythematous macular eruption, often on the trunk (Fig. 14.11*A*). A rash that is almost specific for DCS is reticulated and known as *cutis marmorata,* or more correctly, *livedo reticularis* (see Fig. 14.11*B*). This rash is sometimes

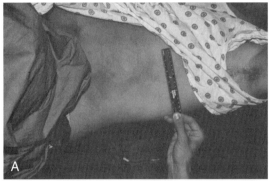

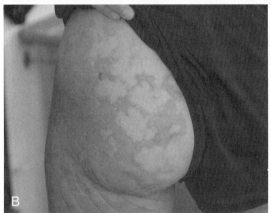

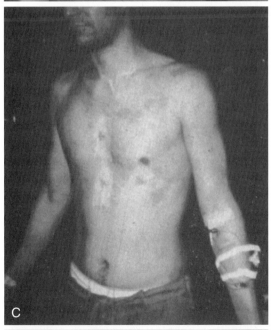

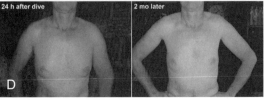

24 h after dive   2 mo later

Figure 14.11 SKIN BENDS. *A,* Nonspecific skin bends in a recreational diver. *B, Cutis marmorata (livedo reticularis)* in a recreational diver. *C,* Urticaria precipitated by breathing 3% oxygen, balance nitrogen at 200 feet sea water in a helium/oxygen environment. *D,* Lymphatic bends 24 hours after onset and 2 months later. **(See Color Plate 10.)** *(C: From Blenkarn GD, Aquadro C, Hills BA, et al: Urticaria following the sequential breathing of various inert gases at a constant ambient pressure of 7 ATA: A possible manifestation of gas-induced osmosis. Aerosp Med 42:141-146, 1971, by permission.)*

associated with neurologic DCS and a PFO.[32] Other types of skin bends include urticaria (see Fig. 14.11*C*), usually associated with a gas switch (see Fig. 14.11*C*). Generalized pruritus without visible rash tends to occur in divers wearing dry suits or after dives in a dry chamber. It is believed to be due to supersaturation of inert gas taken up directly through the skin. Lymphatic bends typically occurs in the trunk and consists of painful swelling (see Fig. 14.11*D*).

Neurologic Decompression Illness

Because AGE and neurologic DCS can be difficult to distinguish, and because the treatment is mostly the same, the term *DCI* rather than *DCS* is used in this section and in the treatment section (see page 294).

Standard evaluation of patients with suspected DCI includes a complete neurologic examination. The time required to obtain a complete neurologic assessment is usually worth a small delay in recompression treatment. It provides a baseline with which to assess evolving manifestations and measure the efficacy of treatment. In the event the diver is deteriorating rapidly, the examination can be abbreviated to the minimum necessary to establish a diagnosis. Sensory abnormalities are often patchy and may not follow the cortical distributions usually seen in patients with hemispheric stroke or standard dermatomal distributions seen in patients with other types of spinal cord injury. Findings are often multifocal, with combinations of cortical, brainstem, spinal cord, and peripheral nerve damage. Abnormalities of gait or tandem gait often predominate, out of proportion to the degree of weakness or sensory abnormality. Two tests of balance with the patient standing barefoot on a hard floor are particularly useful. For the sharpened Romberg test, the patient stands with one foot in front of the other, arms crossed across the chest. The score is the number of seconds balance can be maintained (maximum score, 60). A score of 30 has been proposed as the lower limit of normal.[103] Tandem gait requires the patient to walk heel-to-toe without falling. This can be performed in increasing order of difficulty as follows: with eyes open, walking forward then backward; with eyes closed, forward then backward.

Cardiorespiratory Decompression Sickness

Hypotension, tachycardia, dyspnea, and cough are usually due to massive pulmonary AGE (cardiorespiratory DCS, "chokes"), which may present as a worsening shock state.

Radiography

A chest radiograph is not essential, but it can be useful in patients with DCI[104] to demonstrate barotrauma that may not be detectable on physical examination, such as mediastinal emphysema or small amounts of subcutaneous air. The presence of a pneumothorax may require a chest tube, which is essential if treatment is to be administered in a monoplace chamber. Aspiration of vomitus or salt water, or pulmonary overdistension, can cause focal air-space opacities.[105] Severe VGE, which can result in cardiopulmonary DCS ("chokes"), causes increased pulmonary capillary permeability, which can manifest as pulmonary edema.[106]

Radiographs of the skull and sinuses may occasionally reveal fluid in the paranasal sinuses suggestive of sinus barotrauma. Sinus barotrauma of ascent may also produce tissue gas, which has been observed in the subdural space[107] or in the subcutaneous tissue. Head scanning by both computerized tomography and magnetic resonance imaging is generally not useful in making the diagnosis of neurologic DCI because of a high false-negative rate,[108] although it may be useful if the clinical evaluation suggests alternative diagnoses such as cerebral hemorrhage or thromboembolic stroke. Emission tomography (single-photon emission computed tomography and positron emission tomography) is less sensitive than clinical evaluation[109] or shows nonspecific findings.[110] Limb radiographs can occasionally show soft-tissue gas,[20] but this is neither sensitive nor specific for the diagnosis of DCS.

Neuropsychology

Formal neuropsychological testing can be abnormal in DCS[111,112] and may be more sensitive for the detection of cortical DCI than standard neurologic examination.[113] However, a baseline test is rarely available, a wide variation exists in the normal performance range, and test results are strongly influenced by mood, especially if depressed; education level; the language of the test; alcohol and other drug use; head injuries; and practice.[114] Follow-up studies of divers with DCI, which have cited neuropsychometric abnormalities as the basis of recovery, have overestimated morbidity and confused brain injury in many patients with a post-traumatic stress disorder.[113,115,116]

Neurophysiology

Abnormalities in the electroencephalogram can be found in acute DCI,[113] although it is not a practical test in this setting and an abnormal finding is nonspecific and not useful to follow treatment. Because severe spinal cord DCS often involves the posterior columns, somatosensory-evoked potentials may be abnormal. Somatosensory-evoked potentials are a commonly used end point in animal studies of severe spinal cord DCS.[117-127] However, experience in human DCS reveals that it is not sensitive enough to detect mild abnormalities that can be observed clinically.[108,116,128]

In contrast, both audiometry and vestibular testing are useful to investigate patients with inner ear DCI. Clinical testing of hearing during a physical examination is neither sensitive nor quantitative. For patients with vertigo or ataxia, physical examination is usually inadequate to differentiate vestibular from brainstem or cerebellar pathology. In particular, nystagmus caused by vestibular lesions is typically detectable only with the eyes closed. In inner ear DCS, neurophysiologic testing in the form of electronystagmography with caloric stimulation and air/bone audiography is more sensitive and specific than clinical evaluation. Brainstem auditory-evoked responses interrogate the patient's acoustic pathways from the cochlea to the brainstem and may be useful in the assessment of an uncooperative patient. Inner ear DCS is the only form of DCI in which neurophysiologic testing is more sensitive than clinical examination.[129]

Diagnostic Criteria

In the absence of an unequivocal diagnostic test for DCI, empirical clinical criteria have been used. These have typically included for DCS a minimum depth–time exposure, typical clinical manifestations, and a response to recompression treatment (recognizing that incomplete response to treatment may occur with severe cases or long delays). For AGE, criteria have included evidence of rapid ascent or breath-holding during ascent, short onset time (usually minutes), cerebral manifestations, evidence of PBT, and response to recompression. Insight was gained into the diagnostic criteria actually used by asking undersea medicine experts to diagnose a series of false clinical vignettes.[130] Using this scheme, for the diagnosis of DCS, the most important factors in order of importance were: (1) *a neurologic symptom as the primary presenting symptom,* (2) *onset time of symptoms,* (3) *joint pain as a presenting symptom,* (4) *any relief after recompression,* and (5) *the maximum depth of the last dive.* For the diagnosis of AGE, the top five factors were: (1) *onset time of symptoms,* (2) *altered consciousness,* (3) *any neurologic presenting symptom,* (4) *motor weakness,* and (5) *seizure as the primary presenting symptom.*

A point system for the diagnosis of DCS has been proposed, based on specific clinical markers of DCS, time of onset, and depth–time exposure.[131] It has been tested retrospectively against a clinical series and appears to be relatively specific, though not sensitive. Given the utility of point systems in other areas of medicine, a validated diagnostic tool would be welcome in undersea medicine.

Scoring Systems of Severity and Recovery

One of the most commonly used classifications of DCS was published by Golding and colleagues,[132] who proposed two types: *type I,* pain only; and *type II,* patients with symptoms other than pain or with abnormal physical signs. Over the years this classification has been modified in various ways. Instead of classifying the type of DCS, the current U.S. Navy Diving Manual classifies *symptoms.*[92] Type I symptoms include joint pain (musculoskeletal or pain-only symptoms) and symptoms that involve the skin (cutaneous symptoms) or swelling and pain in lymph nodes. Type II symptoms include neurologic, inner ear (staggers), and cardiopulmonary (chokes) symptoms. In this scheme, type I and II symptoms may be present in the same patient.

The term *type III DCS* was introduced to describe patients who suffered AGE after taking up a significant inert gas load during the earlier part of a dive and who experienced manifestations characteristic of both AGE and neurologic DCS.[133] Previously, these classifications were used to decide treatment; however, this is no longer the case.[92]

Although the traditional classification is often adequate for simple descriptive purposes, the term *type II* encompasses a huge range of severity. For epidemiologic research, a classification or scoring scheme with more gradations is required. Several such scoring systems have been published.[131,134-141]

Summary

Before treating a patient with suspected DCI, the only required components are a medical history and physical examination. Ancillary diagnostic tests such as a blood hemoglobin and chest radiograph may be helpful but are not absolutely required. Although further testing may be indicated (e g , vestibular or auditory), it can be postponed until after initial recompression treatment.

TREATMENT

Natural History if Untreated

The natural history of untreated DCS was provided by authors in the 19th and early 20th centuries. A compressed air environment without recompression facilities was used during construction of the Eads Bridge over the Mississippi River in St. Louis from 1867 to 1874. Of about 600 men employed, there were 91 reported cases of bends, of which 30 were classified as serious; 2 were crippled for life; and there were 13 deaths. Some of the severe cases improved spontaneously,[142] including Dr. Alphonse Jaminet, the physician hired to provide medical support for the men. After spending 2¾ hours at a pressure of 45 pounds per square inch gauge (psig; approximately 31 meters sea water [msw]) and decompressing over 3½ minutes, he experienced epigastric pain, leg weakness, and speech difficulty. Twelve hours later, he began moving his legs and recovered completely.[43,142] Even after introduction of therapeutic recompression, many cases of pain-only bends were untreated and resolved spontaneously.[11]

In pearl divers working around Broome, Australia, 60 of 200 divers with DCS experienced rapid death, and 11 died later (8 of septicemia caused by cystitis and decubitus ulcers, and 3 of meningitis). The majority of the remaining divers recovered spontaneously, with only approximately 10% permanently affected by slight paresis, generally of the anterior muscles of the legs.[6] Spontaneous recovery in 8 of 187 cases of serious DCS was reported in a series collected by the Royal Navy between 1965 and 1984.[143]

First-Aid Treatment

Initial treatment of the injured diver should be similar to the treatment of any patient with a major injury. Attention to airway, breathing, and circulation are paramount. Hypoxemia can occur because of aspiration of water or vomitus, pneumothorax, or cardiorespiratory DCS. The use of supplemental oxygen has two benefits: the treatment of arterial hypoxemia and an enhanced rate of resolution of inert gas bubbles. The fact that O_2 administration can reduce bubble load in DCI was first demonstrated by Bert in the 19th century using experimental animals.[9] The mechanism is believed to be a decrease in tissue inert gas partial pressure and, therefore, a higher diffusion gradient for inert gas from bubble to tissue. Supplemental oxygen, therefore, is routinely recommended. As high an inspired concentration of O_2 as is possible should be administered, preferably using a tightly fitting face mask. Other appropriate interventions may include endotracheal intubation and chest tube insertion to treat pneumothorax.

Systemic capillary leak, coronary artery embolism, or peripheral vasodilation caused by spinal cord injury ("spinal shock") may cause hypotension and tissue hypoperfusion. Fluid administration should be routine, except in isolated cerebral AGE occurring after a short time in shallow water (see later). In cases of cardiorespiratory DCS (chokes) occurring in the field, the benefits of aggressive fluid resuscitation should be weighed against a possible risk for worsening pulmonary edema. In an animal model of chokes, diuretics appear to improve short-term outcome.

For DCS or AGE, recommendations have traditionally included placement of the patient in head-down or left lateral decubitus position. The rationale is based on one study in which dogs were more tolerant of intravenously injected bubbles when placed on their left sides,[144] possibly because in that position the right ventricular outflow tract is inferior to the right ventricular cavity, allowing air to migrate superiorly and prevent obstruction to blood flow. Furthermore, left-sided air injection was more likely to cause death when dogs were embolized in the head-up position compared with supine or head-down position.[145] In another study, head-down position reduced the volume of intra-arterial bubbles in the cerebral vessels because of the hydrostatic effect on intravascular pressure.[146] A case report describes unconsciousness and hypotension after injection of air into the aortic root, which resolved within 1 minute after placing the 63-year-old woman in the vertical head-down position.[147] However, increased brain swelling has been observed when the head-down position is used.[146,148] Moreover, buoyancy appears to have little effect on the distribution or hemodynamic consequences of either arterial[149,150] or venous[151,152] air. For mild cases (e.g., pain-only bends), there is no known reason for body position to be important. For severe cases, the patient should be placed in the best position possible for delivery of care and maintenance of blood pressure, usually supine. Lateral decubitus position may be indicated if the patient is unconscious and does not have a protected airway.

Recompression Therapy

Recompression therapy for caisson disease was first proposed in 1854 by Pol and Wattelle in Europe[10] and then by Andrew Smith, the physician for the Brooklyn Bridge construction in the 1870s[3,153]; however, it was not implemented until 1889 during the Hudson River tunnel construction when Ernest Moir effectively used recompression to reduce the caisson disease death rate.[154] Improved outcome with recompression was then reported in 1896 in England during excavation of the Blackwall Tunnel under the Thames River.[155] Statistical evidence for the benefit of recompression was shown in New York City by Keays,[11] who reported a failure rate of 13.7% in caisson workers with pain treated without recompression versus a 0.5% failure rate with recompression treatment.

Initiation of recompression therapy for divers took much longer. It was not until the 1924 edition of the U.S. Navy Diving Manual[156] that air recompression was recommended. In different settings treatment pressure was based either on the depth of the dive (or a fraction or multiple thereof) or on the depth of relief.[157] During construction of the New York-Queens Midtown Tunnel in 1938, the recommended treatment pressure was equal to that to which the worker was originally exposed, although pressures 5, 10, or

15 psi higher were sometimes used.[158] After reaching the pressure of relief, the consensus at the time favored waiting 20 to 30 minutes before starting decompression.

Oxygen administration was not routinely used until much later, although its scientific rationale had been available since the latter part of the 19th century. In the 1870s, in Paris, Paul Bert first noted that when 100% oxygen was administered to animals after decompression, some of the signs would resolve.[9] He observed that oxygen administration caused resolution of intravascular gas, but that recompression (with air) was necessary to resolve bubbles that had migrated into the central nervous system. Zuntz[159] first suggested using both pressure and oxygen, although he did not have the opportunity to administer it. When it was tried, the initial results, in fact, were somewhat disappointing, probably because it was not administered for long enough.[11]

Choice of Pressure

Compression reduces bubble volume by physical means, such that bubble volume reduces in inverse proportion to ambient pressure. Although the volume may be considerably reduced in this manner, the reduction in the various bubble dimensions will depend on the shape. For example, compression of a spherical bubble to 6 ATA (606 kPa) will reduce bubble volume to just under 17% of the original, but will reduce the diameter by only 43%. Cylindrical bubbles, such as might occur inside a blood vessel, will experience a relatively greater reduction in dimensions, but predominantly in bubble length.

Although a reduction in bubble volume will continue to occur as ambient pressure is increased, several factors limit the maximum compression. Bubble size reduction is asymptotic rather than linear. Progressive recompression will also result in a further uptake of inert gas, unless 100% oxygen is breathed. As a result of this inert gas uptake, symptoms may become even more pronounced during the subsequent decompression.[160] In addition, nitrogen narcosis impairs the performance of chamber tenders at pressures greater than 4 to 6 ATA. Therefore, except under unusual circumstances, conventional (air/oxygen-nitrogen) recompression therapy is limited to 6 ATA (606 kPa).

Canine models have been used to investigate different pressures systematically.[161] After AGE, the investigators tested different pressures varying from 2.8 to 10 ATA breathing air and at 2.8 ATA breathing 100% oxygen. No significant differences were observable in the different rates of recovery, and none of the treatments was better than oxygen administration at 2.8 ATA (60 fsw). In a series of experiments in anesthetized dogs with spinal cord DCS, ambient treatment pressures of 3, 5, and 7 (inspired P_{O_2} = 2 ATA) and 2.8 ATA (inspired P_{O_2} = 2.8 ATA) were tested; results showed no measurable advantage of any pressure.[122]

Oxygen

The effect of 100% O_2 breathing to "wash out" inert gas results in an increased partial pressure gradient for inert gas from inside to outside a bubble. This increases the rate of resolution of tissue gas. Use of O_2 also prevents any additional uptake of inert gas during recompression therapy of decompression illness. HBOT currently represents the standard of care for treatment of DCI.

The initial rationale for hyperbaric oxygen provided by Zuntz[159] was accelerated washout of inert gas and bubble resolution. There are probably additional, possibly more important, mechanisms by which hyperbaric oxygen treats DCI. These include increased oxygen delivery and pharmacologic effects of hyperbaric oxygen such as edema resolution and inhibition of β_2-integrin–mediated neutrophil adhesion to injured endothelium.[162]

In 1939, Yarbrough and Behnke[163] reported the superiority of hyperbaric oxygen in treating DCS, but it was not immediately adopted. It became officially available to the U.S. Navy in 1944[157] but was rarely used. In the Navy oxygen table, 100% O_2 was administered at depths of 60 fsw and shallower, but only for a total of 95 minutes, of which only 30 minutes were spent breathing O_2 at 60 fsw (compared with the current standard of ≥60 minutes). In the 20 years after World War II, the failure rate for the tables used (mostly air) was nearly 30%.[164]

A P_{O_2} of 3 ATA is the greatest ambient pressure at which 100% O_2 administration is practical: central nervous system oxygen toxicity is limiting at higher P_{O_2}. A study of the treatment of spinal cord DCS with different P_{O_2} (from 1–3 ATA) at a constant ambient pressure (5 ATA) revealed the optimum inspired P_{O_2} was 2 to 2.5 ATA.[121] In a follow-up study to compare P_{O_2} of 2.0 ATA with 2.8 ATA, no significant difference in outcome was observed.[123]

Inert Gas

During a therapeutic compression, the use of a different inert gas from the one that was breathed during the dive may facilitate bubble resolution. If the properties of the "therapeutic" inert gas are appropriately chosen such that its rate of transport through tissue is lower than the first, then bubble shrinkage will be accelerated. Helium is approximately 40% less soluble than nitrogen in blood and could therefore facilitate bubble resolution in this way. Anecdotal reports have suggested an advantage of heliox treatment of DCI after nitrogen-oxygen (or air) dives.[165] Although some animal studies of cardiopulmonary decompression illness have failed to demonstrate an advantage of heliox,[166,167] compared with air or oxygen breathing, its administration causes more rapid shrinkage of air bubbles in adipose tissue,[168] spinal cord white matter,[169] tendon, muscle, and aqueous humor.[170] After heliox diving, bubbles tend to grow when air is breathed; shrinkage is fastest with 100% oxygen.[171]

In humans, almost all cases of DCI can be treated at 2.8 ATA (60 fsw), where 100% oxygen is both safe and effective. Choice of an inert gas is important only at greater pressures. Experience with the use of deeper tables in which either nitrogen or helium can be used as the inert gas have not consistently demonstrated an advantage of helium.[172]

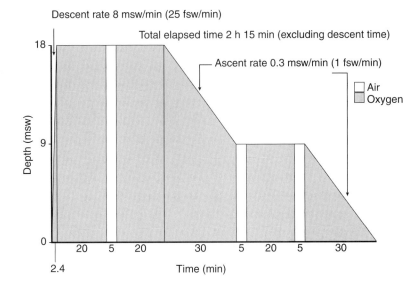

Descent rate 8 msw/min (25 fsw/min)

Total elapsed time 2 h 15 min (excluding descent time)

Ascent rate 0.3 msw/min (1 fsw/min)

☐ Air
☐ Oxygen

Figure 14.12 U.S. NAVY TREAT-MENT TABLE 5. This table is used for pain-only or mild cutaneous symptoms with no neurologic abnormality. If complete relief of symptoms has not occurred within 10 minutes of compressing the patient to 60 feet (18 m), then U.S. Navy guidelines prescribe Table 6. *White areas* denote air; *gray areas* denote oxygen. fsw, feet sea water; msw, meters sea water. *(From Moon RE, Gorman DF: Treatment of the decompression disorders. In: Neuman TS, Brubakk AO (eds): The Physiology and Medicine of Diving. New York, Elsevier Science, 2003, pp 600–650, by permission.)*

Therapeutic Protocols

Recompression schedules for the treatment of DCI consist of a relatively rapid recompression to a specified pressure and then a slow decompression. Oxygen breathing is used as much as possible at ambient pressures of 2.8 ATA (60 fsw) or lower.

Standard U.S. Navy Oxygen Tables

Systematic development and assessment of low pressure ($\leq$60 fsw) oxygen tables was then begun by the U.S. Navy. The initial compression depth was 33 fsw (10 msw) with the diver breathing 100% O_2. If symptoms were relieved within 10 minutes, the chamber was maintained at the same pressure for an additional 30 minutes, then decompressed. Otherwise, the chamber pressure was increased to 60 fsw. A high recurrence rate using the 33 fsw table led to its abandonment and the development of treatment tables requiring an initial recompression to 60 fsw.[164] The new tables were U.S. Navy Tables 5 (Fig. 14.12) and 6 (Fig. 14.13), in which divers were administered 100% O_2 at 60 (18 msw) and 30 fsw (9 msw) continuously, except for short air breaks to reduce O_2 toxicity. Workman's 1968 analysis re-

vealed that these oxygen tables had a high degree of success.[173] Experience since that time has confirmed the initial observations (Table 14.1), and these treatment tables remain the "gold standards" for the treatment of most cases of DCI.[174]

U.S. Navy Table 5 (Royal Navy [RN] Table 61) is used for the treatment of pain-only or skin bends. U.S. Navy Table 6, RN Table 62) is used for the treatment of more severe cases of DCI. Additional periods of O_2 breathing can be added at both 60 (18 m) and 30 feet (9 m). Extensions are prescribed based on the clinical response of the patient as judged by periodic interviews and neurologic examinations during the treatment. The Catalina modification of U.S. Navy Table 6 allows up to eight 20-minute periods of 100% oxygen breathing at 18 msw[175,176] (Fig. 14.14).

Oxygen Tables Designed for Monoplace Use

Monoplace chambers were originally designed without the capability of administering air breaks. Treatments tables within this constraint were developed and tested, and found to be effective for most cases.[177-181]

Kindwall's table for a monoplace chamber without air breaks is as follows[182]:

Pain-only or skin bends:

2.8 ATA (60 feet) for 30 minutes
15-minute decompression to 1.9 ATA (30 feet)
1.9 ATA for 60 minutes
15-minute decompression to 1 ATA

In order to use this schedule, all symptoms must resolve within 10 minutes of reaching 2.8 ATA. If not, the longer table below must be used.

Neurologic DCI, AGE, or pain-only or skin bends that fail to resolve within 10 minutes on the table above:

2.8 ATA (18 m, 60 feet, 26 psig) for 30 minutes
30-minute decompression to 1.9 ATA
1.9 ATA for 60 minutes
30-minute decompression to 1 ATA

If symptoms have not resolved, the table may be repeated after 30 minutes breathing air at 1 ATA.

The monoplace table that Hart[177,178] designed specifies 100% oxygen administration at 3 ATA for 30 minutes followed by 2.5 ATA for 60 minutes.

Short Oxygen Treatment Tables with Excursion to Pressure Greater Than 2.8 Atmospheres Absolute

Different tables were developed in the U.S. Navy for the treatment of AGE, in which it was believed that a higher pressure would be ap-

propriate because of the likelihood of greater gas volume. An experimental study in anesthetized dogs using intracarotid air injection and a skull window technique revealed that all visible bubbles disappeared at a compression depth of 100 fsw,[183] suggesting that this would be an appropriate compression depth for AGE in divers. However, on the basis that fleet diving medical officers would demand a 165 fsw table, U.S. Navy Tables 5A (later abandoned) and 6A (Fig. 14.15), incorporating a 30-minute period of air breathing at 165 fsw (50 msw), were introduced. Many practitioners use 40% to 50%

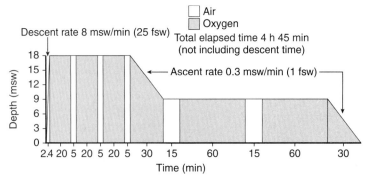

Figure 14.13 U.S. NAVY TREATMENT TABLE 6. Table 6 is used for treatment of neurologic decompression illness and pain-only or mild cutaneous symptoms that are not relieved within 10 minutes of reaching 60 feet (18 m) breathing oxygen. Table 6 can be extended at 60 feet (18 m) and at 30 feet (9 m) if symptoms have not been relieved within the first three oxygen cycles. A modified U.S. Navy Table 6 has been designed at the Catalina Marine Science Center, allowing for up to 5 extensions at 60 fsw (18 msw; see Fig. 14.11). *White areas* denote air; *gray areas* denote oxygen. fsw, feet sea water; msw, meters sea water. *(From Moon RE, Gorman DF: Treatment of the decompression disorders. In: Neuman TS, Brubakk AO (eds): The Physiology and Medicine of Diving. New York, Elsevier Science, 2003, pp 600–650, by permission.)*

Table 14.1 Single Recompression Success Rate of Oxygen Treatment Tables

SOURCE	CASES (N)	TABLE USED	COMPLETE RELIEF (%)	SUBSTANTIAL RELIEF (%)	COMMENTS
Workman[173]	150	USN	85	95.3% after second treatment	
Erde and Edmonds[301]	106	USN	81		
Davis and colleagues[302]	145	USN	98		Altitude DCS
Bayne[303]	50	USN	98		
Pearson and Leitch[304]	28	USN	67	83	
Kizer[305]	157	USN	58	83	Long delays
Yap[306]	58	USN	50	84	Mean delay 48 hours
Gray[307]	812	USN	81	94	
Hart and colleagues[178]	73	Hart Mono-place Table	29 86 (type I) 4 (type II)		Many delayed
Green and colleagues[202]	208	USN	96		All pain only, USN Table 5
Ball[136]	14 11 24	USN	93 (mild cases) 36 (moderate cases) 8 (severe cases)		Many cases with long delays
Smerz and colleagues[185]	89	USN	92		Additional cases treated using deep air tables, similar results
Total	1836		79.2		

DCS, decompression sickness; USN, U.S. Navy.
Adapted from Thalmann ED: Principles of US Navy recompression treatments for decompression sickness. In: Moon RE, Sheffield PJ (eds): Treatment of Decompression Illness. Kensington, MD, Undersea and Hyperbaric Medical Society, 1996, pp 75–95.

oxygen (rather than air, as originally intended) during the 30-minute period at 6 ATA. Comex Table 30 (Fig. 14.16) uses an excursion to 30 m (98 feet), with 50/50 oxygen/helium or oxygen/nitrogen as the breathing gas by mask while the ambient pressure is greater than 2.8 ATA (282 kPa). When this table is used, European practice tends to favor the use of heliox, whereas American experience suggests that nitrogen/oxygen is as efficacious.

Although compression deeper than 2.82 ATA remains in the armamentarium of most navies and offshore commercial diving operators, and many practitioners have observed good clinical results, published evidence for its efficacy is lacking. Animal experiments have thus far failed to find an advantage of Table 6A over Table 6 in models of AGE.[184] In a retrospective review of 14 divers with DCI who had not responded satisfactorily to initial compression to 2.8 ATA (282 kPa) and who were then recompressed to a greater pressure (up to 8.6 ATA, 868 kPa; 76 m, 250 feet), Leitch and Green[160] concluded that additional recompression rarely either altered the clinical course or produced clinically significant improvements. A published series of the routine use of deep initial recompression (up to 8.5 ATA) indicated excellent outcomes but no advantage over standard U.S. Navy Tables.[185] However, anecdotal reports suggest that a small number of divers with DCI who do not respond to treatment at 2.8 ATA (282 kPa) may respond at a higher pressure,[186] particularly if 50/50 or 40/60 oxygen/nitrogen mixtures are used in preference to air at 6 ATA.[187-190]

Deep Tables

Decompression illness during or after short-duration deep dives (usually deeper than 50 m or 165 feet) may benefit from recompression

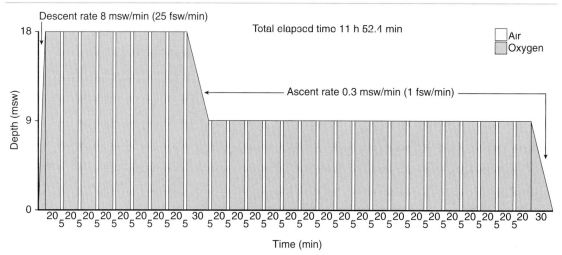

Figure 14.14 CATALINA TREATMENT TABLE. The "Catalina" Table is a modified version of U.S. Navy Treatment Table 6. All oxygen breathing cycles are of 20 minutes in duration followed by 5 minutes breathing air. In its current implementation, shorter versions of this table may be used as follows. After 3 oxygen cycles at 60 feet (18 m), a minimum of 6 cycles are required at 30 feet (9 m; equivalent to U.S. Navy Table 6); after 4 cycles at 60 feet, 9 cycles are required at 30 feet; after 5 to 8 cycles at 60 feet, a minimum of 12 cycles are required at 30 feet. Up to 18 cycles at 30 feet (as shown above) can be used. Tenders must breathe oxygen for 60 minutes at 30 feet and during the decompression to the surface (total, 90 minutes). If there have been fewer than 4 oxygen cycles at 60 feet and fewer than 9 cycles at 30 feet, then only 30 minutes of oxygen breathing is required for the tender at 30 feet in addition to the decompression time (total, 60 minutes), although some practitioners prefer the longer recommendation above. Further treatments can be started only after 12 hours of air breathing at the surface. For further detail on this table, see Pilmanis.[175] *White areas* denote air; *gray areas* denote oxygen. fsw, feet sea water; msw, meters sea water. *(From Moon RE, Gorman DF: Treatment of the decompression disorders. In: Neuman TS, Brubakk AO (eds): The Physiology and Medicine of Diving. New York, Elsevier Science, 2003, pp 600–650, by permission.)*

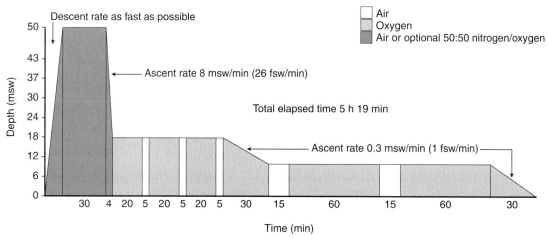

Figure 14.15 U.S. NAVY TABLE 6A. U.S. Navy Table 6A consists of a 30-minute excursion to 6 atmospheres absolute (ATA; 606 kPa; 165 feet, 50 m) while the patient breathes air, followed by an oxygen breathing portion identical to U.S. Navy Table 6. The original rationale of this table was to provide for maximum Boyle's Law compression of gas during the 6 ATA (606 kPa) excursion, followed by bubble resolution augmented by oxygen breathing. It was initially recommended for treatment of arterial gas embolism. Although the U.S. Navy still recommends air as the appropriate breathing gas at 6 ATA, others have used nitrogen-oxygen mixtures (usually 60/40 or 50/50). The advantage of U.S. Navy Table 6A compared with U.S. Navy Table 6 has been called into question by some controlled animal studies in suggesting that compression beyond 2.82 ATA (282 kPa) provides no additional benefit. Nevertheless, clinical experience has suggested that a small percentage of patients may respond to treatment at 6 ATA but fail to do so at 2.8 ATA. The major use of U.S. Navy Table 6A, compared with U.S. Navy Table 6, is likely to be for patients with large volumes of gas treated with short delay. *White areas* denote air; *light gray areas* denote oxygen; *dark gray areas* denote air or optional 50/50 nitrogen/oxygen. fsw, feet sea water; msw, meters sea water. *(From Moon RE, Gorman DF: Treatment of the decompression disorders. In: Neuman TS, Brubakk AO (eds): The Physiology and Medicine of Diving. New York, Elsevier Science, 2003, pp 600–650, by permission.)*

Cx 30₈₆

Cx 30$_{86}$

RECOMPRESS CHAMBER TO 30 METERS ON HELIOX 20/80 or AIR

DEPTH	DURATION	BREATHING MIX		ELAPSED TIME
		PATIENT	ATTENDANT	
30 m	60 min	HELIOX 50/50 60 min ON BIBS	AMBIENT	01h.00
30–24 m	30 min	HELIOX 50/50: 1 BIBS session 25 min ON + 5 min OFF	AMBIENT	01h.30
24 m	30 min	HELIOX 50/50: 1 BIBS session 25 min ON + 5 min OFF	AMBIENT	02h.00
24–18 m	30 min	HELIOX 50/50: 1 BIBS session 25 min ON + 5 min OFF	AMBIENT	02h.30
18 m	60 min	OXYGEN: 2 BIBS sessions 25 min ON + 5 min OFF	AMBIENT	03h.30
18–12 m	30 min	OXYGEN: 1 BIBS session 25 min ON + 5 min OFF	AMBIENT	04h.00
12 m	180 min	OXYGEN: 6 BIBS sessions 25 min ON + 5 min OFF	OXYGEN: 6 BIBS sessions 25 min ON + 5 min OFF	07h.00
12–0 m	30 min	OXYGEN 30 min ON BIBS	OXYGEN 30 min ON BIBS	07h.30

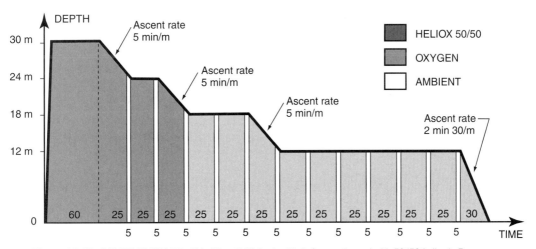

Figure 14.16 COMEX TABLE 30. This 30-m (100-feet) table is frequently used with 50/50 heliox in European diving practice for the initial treatment of decompression illness (Kol S, Adir Y, Gordon CR, et al: Oxy-helium treatment of severe spinal decompression sickness after air diving. Undersea Hyperb Med 20:147–154, 1993). It is also used with 50/50 oxygen/nitrogen. *(From James PB, Imbert J-P, Arnoux G, et al: Comex Medical Book, Revised ed. Marseille, France, Comex SA, 1986.)*

to depths greater than those specified by the standard tables, particularly if there has been significant missed decompression.[191] Examples are the Lambertsen/Solus Ocean Systems Table 7A (Fig. 14.17) and U.S. Navy Treatment Table 8 (Fig. 14.18). Table 8 was designed for treating deep, uncontrolled ascents ("blowups") when more than 60 minutes of decompression has been missed.[192] Another protocol, based on the recommendations of the European Undersea Biomedical Society and the U.K. Association of Diving Contractors, consists of compression to 18 m (60 feet) or depth of relief breathing helium/oxygen. The decompression schedule is shown in Table 14.2. Guidelines for the use of this table are discussed later in the "Closed-Bell and Saturation Diving" section.

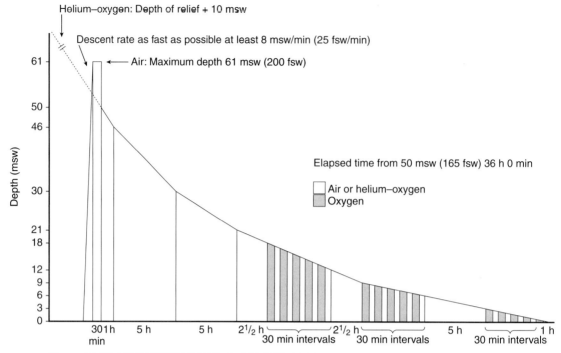

Figure 14.17 LAMBERTSEN/SOLUS OCEAN SYSTEMS TABLE 7A. This table is most commonly used in commercial diving for symptoms that develop at pressure, for recompression deeper than 165 feet (50 m), or when extended decompression is necessary. The patient is held at the treatment depth for 30 minutes. If he or she is breathing air, the depth limit should be 200 feet (61 m). After the 30-minute compression, the patient is decompressed to 165 feet (50 m) in 1 minute, and then the table followed as shown. If the patient is breathing helium/oxygen, he or she should be compressed to depth of relief plus 33 feet (10 m), but not deeper than the bottom depth of the dive. After a 30-minute period at that depth, the chamber should be decompressed to 165 feet at 15 ft/hr (50 m at 4.5 m/hr), and the remainder of the table followed as shown. *White areas* denote air of helium/oxygen; *gray areas* denote oxygen. fsw, feet sea water; msw, meters sea water. *(Reproduced from Moon RE, Gorman DF: Treatment of the decompression disorders. In: Neuman TS, Brubakk AO (eds): The Physiology and Medicine of Diving. New York, Elsevier Science, 2003, pp 600–650, by permission.)*

Saturation Treatment after Shallow Dives

In the event that a patient with significant neurologic symptoms, especially weakness, has incomplete relief of symptoms after a period at 2.8 ATA (282 kPa) during U.S. Navy Table 6, or if there is evidence of deterioration during decompression from that treatment table, then saturation recompression may be an option. This technique consists of maintaining the patient in the hyperbaric chamber at a fixed ambient pressure while administering intermittent enriched O₂ treatment.[188,193] The most straightforward saturation treatment table is U.S. Navy Table 7 because it is designed for a depth (2.8 ATA, 60 fsw) at which air can

be used for the chamber atmosphere without causing pulmonary oxygen toxicity (for details, see U.S. Navy Diving Manual[92]; Fig. 14.19). In this table, the patient is maintained at pressure for a minimum of 12 hours.

Saturation treatments are labor intensive and expensive and require capabilities not available at most chamber facilities, including chamber atmosphere monitoring and maintenance, as well as two inside tenders and two chamber operators constantly on duty. Saturation treatment, therefore, should not be used unless the patient has significant neurologic injury and adequate facilities exist for its implementation. Saturation treatment has not been shown to be more effective than repetitive oxygen tables. Proposed guidelines for saturation treatment

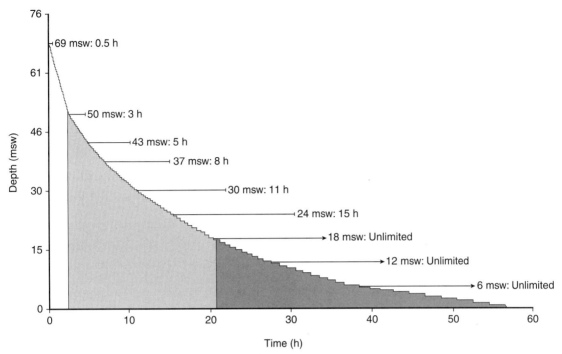

Figure 14.18 U.S. NAVY TREATMENT TABLE 8. Designed for treatment of deep "blowups," in which there has been more than 60 minutes of missed decompression stop time. It can be used in other situations, for example, to compress to a depth greater than 165 feet sea water (fsw; 50 meters sea water [msw]), or to stop decompression between 165 and 60 fsw. Maximum times at each depth are shown; times at 60, 40, and 20 fsw are unlimited; decompression occurs in increments of 2 fsw. When deeper than 165 fsw (50 msw), to reduce narcosis, a 16% to 21% O_2 in helium can be administered. Four treatment cycles, each consisting of 25 minutes of "treatment gas" followed by 5 minutes of chamber air, can be administered deeper than 60 fsw. Treatment gas used deeper than 60 fsw is 40% O_2 in either He or N_2; at 60 fsw (18 msw) or shallower, treatment gas is 100% O_2. For O_2 administration at 60 fsw or shallower, U.S. Navy Treatment Table 7 guidelines are used. Further details can be found in the U.S. Navy Diving Manual.[92] *(From Moon RE, de Lisle Dear G, Stolp BW: Treatment of decompression illness and iatrogenic gas embolism. Respir Care Clin N Am 5:93–135, 1999, by permission.)*

Table 14.2 Therapeutic Table for Use after Helium-Oxygen Bounce Diving

DEPTH	DECOMPRESSION RATE
Deeper than 100 m	1.5 m/hr
100 to 10 m	1.0 m/hr
10 m to surface	0.5 m/hr

From Bennett PB: The Treatment Offshore of Decompression Sickness: European Undersea Biomedical Society workshop. Bethesda, MD, Undersea Medical Society, 1976.

include: (1) major weakness, urethral or anal sphincter dysfunction, cortical symptoms, or altered consciousness; *and* (2) improvement with recompression but incomplete relief at the end of the scheduled period at 2.8 ATA *or* major deterioration in motor strength or

cortical function during decompression from 2.8 ATA while breathing oxygen.

In-Water Recompression

In the absence of a recompression chamber, it may appear logical for the diver with symptoms to recompress himself in the water. Although this may relieve symptoms acutely, it causes further inert gas uptake, which can precipitate more severe decompression illness when the diver eventually surfaces. In-water recompression breathing air has been used successfully.[194-196] Oxygen breathing should be more efficacious, and procedures for in-water recompression while breathing 100% oxygen have been described for use in

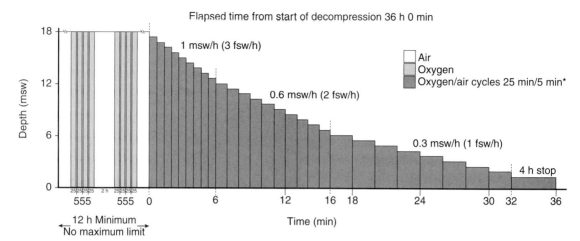

Figure 14.19 U.S. NAVY TREATMENT TABLE 7. This table allows for a prolonged (saturation) stay at 60 feet (18 m). It is used for serious cases of decompression illness that resolve incompletely during one of the standard oxygen tables, or for deterioration during decompression from one of those tables. U.S. Navy guidelines specify that a minimum of 12 hours must be spent at 60 feet, but the maximum duration is not specified. To simplify timekeeping, oxygen breathing periods of 25 minutes are followed by 5 minutes of breathing chamber atmosphere (air). Four oxygen breathing periods are alternated with 2 hours of continuous air breathing; if the patient is conscious, this cycle should be continued until a minimum of eight oxygen breathing periods have been administered. Oxygen breathing periods made before the decision to saturate at 60 feet may be counted. Oxygen breathing periods may be continued to maximize the benefit, but symptoms of pulmonary oxygen toxicity (e.g., pain on inspiration) may require a modification of the above schedule. If the patient is unconscious, oxygen breathing should generally be stopped after a maximum of 24 oxygen breathing periods. *White areas* denote air; *light gray areas* denote oxygen; *dark gray areas* denote oxygen breathing periods of 25 minutes are followed by 5 minutes of breathing chamber atmosphere. *See U.S. Navy Diving Manual[92] for details. *(From Moon RE, Gorman DF: Treatment of the decompression disorders. In: Neuman TS, Brubakk AO (eds): The Physiology and Medicine of Diving. New York, Elsevier Science, 2003, pp 600–650, by permission.)*

locations where chamber recompression is not available.[194,197-200]

Australian guidelines[198,200,201] include the following mandates: (1) oxygen administration (and adequate oxygen supply) via a full face mask, which protects the airway of a semiconscious diver; (2) adequate thermal protection (e.g., wet suit); (3) a rope 10 meters long (a seat or harness may be rigged for support of the diver); (4) an attendant to accompany the diver; and (5) some form of communication among patient, attendant, and surface. Oxygen should be delivered to the diver from a tank on the surface with a nonreturn valve between the supply line and the mask. The initial compression depth is 9 m (30 feet). Time at depth is usually 30 minutes, although this can be extended for 30 or 60 minutes for severe cases. Ascent is at a rate of 12 min/m (4 min/ft). If the symptoms recur, the patient should remain at depth an additional 30 minutes before surfacing. For 12 hours after surfacing the diver should be given 100% oxygen for 1-hour periods, interspersed with similar periods breathing air.

Choice of Treatment Algorithms

Surface-Oriented Diving

Mild Bends or Limb Pain Only

According to U.S. Navy guidelines and common practice, divers with pain-only or skin bends can be treated using U.S. Navy treatment Table 5, provided there are no neurologic abnormalities by history or on examination and if complete relief of symptoms occurs within 10 minutes of compression to 2.8 ATA (282 kPa). Green and colleagues[202] have reviewed a series of cases treated by the U.S. Navy and found that Table 5 is as effective as Table 6 when used according to these guidelines.

Neurologic Decompression Illness

For neurologic DCI, initial compression to 18 msw (60 fsw) while breathing 100% O_2 is recommended.[174] U.S. Navy Table 6 is appropriate treatment for such individuals. Up to two additional periods of O_2 breathing at 60 (18 m; 2.8 ATA, 282 kPa) and 30 feet (9 m; 1.9 ATA, 191 kPa) are allowed according to the U.S. Navy Diving Manual.[92] Further extensions are feasible by using the Catalina Marine Science Center maximum treatment table (see Fig. 14.14).

Some published series suggest that for neurologic DCI, treatment with longer tables (e.g., U.S. Navy Table 6 vs. extended U.S. Navy Table 6) was less efficacious than with shorter tables.[135,143] However, these studies should not be interpreted as indicating that more intensive treatment is less likely to result in a satisfactory result, but rather that divers who do not respond quickly to recompression are more likely to be prescribed an extended treatment.

Clinical experience suggests that AGE will usually respond to U.S. Navy treatment Table 6. Deeper recompressions are recommended only for patients who do not respond at 60 fsw, usually when treatment is initiated quickly after the diver surfaces.

In the event that only a monoplace chamber is available, some hyperbaric physicians have been reluctant to use it for standard recompression table administration because of the difficulty in administrating air breaks. However, tables that Hart and Kindwall have described for monoplace use appear to be effective in most cases.[177-181] Administration of standard U.S. Navy tables in a monoplace chamber requires only a simple modification to install a BIBS (Built-in Breathing System, a mask administration system to allow a chamber occupant to breathe air from a mask).

Closed-Bell and Saturation Diving

The recompression options for those who dive to greater depths than do surface-oriented divers are more complicated. For bends that occur after surfacing, standard oxygen tables are usually effective. Some experts recommend avoiding air recompression, particularly after recently switching from helium/oxygen because, possibly by counterdiffusion, this may lead to a sudden deterioration.[191] However, U.S. Navy practice and commercial diving operations in the Gulf of Mexico include the use of standard therapeutic air/O_2 tables (e.g., U.S. Navy Tables 6, 6A, and 7) for bends that occur after helium/oxygen dives. For symptoms that occur during decompression from a saturation or deep bounce dive, the diver is usually compressed to depth of relief or to the original dive depth. After at least 2 hours at maximum depth, decompression on the schedule in Table 14.2 can be used. Symptoms that occur during decompression from saturation dives are usually minor (generally pain only). Treatment options include combinations of any of the following: (1) administration of O_2-enriched breathing mix (1.5–2.8 ATA), (2) recompression of the chamber, or (3) a temporary halt in the decompression.[203-206] Further details can be found elsewhere.[92,203-209]

Delayed Treatment

The period of delay after which no benefit from hyperbaric treatment can be obtained may be several days long.[210-218] Recompression of a diver is therefore reasonable even up to several days after onset of symptoms. Mild DCS in a remote location, where recompression is not available and immediate evacuation is not feasible, can be managed conservatively. Consensus guidelines for management of such patients are reproduced in Table 14.3.

Timing, Duration of Treatment, and Follow-up Treatment

If complete relief of symptoms is not achieved after a single hyperbaric treatment, repetitive HBOT with daily or twice-daily hyperbaric treatments is recommended until either the patient has experienced complete relief or there is no further incremental improvement as assessed

---

**Table 14.3 Consensus Guidelines for Management of Mild Decompression Sickness
in Remote Locations**

CONSENSUS STATEMENT 1

With respect to decompression illness (DCI), the workshop defines "mild" symptoms and signs as follows:
  - limb pain[1,2]
  - constitutional symptoms
  - some cutaneous sensory changes[3]
  - rash

where these manifestations are static or remitting[4,5] and associated objective neurological dysfunction has been excluded by medical examination.

FOOTNOTES

1. The workshop agrees that severity of pain has little prognostic significance, but acknowledges that severity of pain may influence management decisions independent of the classification of pain as a "mild" symptom.
2. Classical girdle pain syndromes are suggestive of spinal involvement and do not fall under the classification of "limb pain."
3. The intent of "some cutaneous sensory changes" is to embrace subjective cutaneous sensory phenomena such as paresthesiae that are present in patchy or non-dermatomal distributions suggestive of non-spinal, non-specific, and benign processes. Subjective sensory changes in clear dermatomal distributions or in certain characteristic patterns such as in both feet may predict evolution of spinal symptoms and should not be considered "mild."
4. The proclamation of "mild" cannot be made where symptoms are progressive. If the presentation initially qualifies as mild and then begins to progress, it is no longer classified as "mild" (see also Footnote 5).
5. The possibility of delayed progression is recognized, such that the "mild" designation must be repeatedly reviewed over at least the first 24 hours following diving or the most recent decompression, the latter applying if there has been an ascent to altitude. Management plans should include provisions for such progression.

CONSENSUS STATEMENT 2

The workshop accepts that untreated mild symptoms and signs[1] due to DCI are unlikely to progress after 24 hours from the end of diving.[2]

FOOTNOTE

1. Mild symptoms and signs are strictly limited to those defined in Statement 1 and its footnotes.
2. This statement does not hold where there is a further decompression, such as further diving or ascent to altitude, in the presence of mild symptoms.

CONSENSUS STATEMENT 3

Level B epidemiological[1] evidence indicates that a delay prior to recompression for a patient with mild DCI[2] is unlikely to be associated with any worsening of long-term outcome.

FOOTNOTES

1. Levels of evidence in American Family Physician [Internet]. [Leawood(KS)]: American Academy of Family Physicians; c2004 [Cited 2004 Dec 6]. Available at: http://www.aafp.org/x17444.xml
2. "Mild DCI" is limited to those presentations exhibiting only "mild symptoms and signs" strictly as defined in Statement 1 and footnotes.

CONSENSUS STATEMENT 4

The workshop acknowledges that some patients with mild symptoms and signs after diving[1] can be treated adequately without recompression. For those with DCI, recovery may be slower in the absence of recompression.

FOOTNOTE

1. The non-specific reference to "mild symptoms and signs after diving" is intentional. It reflects the fact that the manifestations may or may not be the consequence of DCI. The statement suggests that even if they are the result of DCI, full recovery is anticipated irrespective of the use of recompression, although resolution may take longer. Importantly, "mild symptoms and signs" are strictly limited to those defined in Statement 1 and footnotes. Where symptoms and signs fall outside the spectrum of manifestations herein defined as "mild," standard management and therapy are indicated.

CONSENSUS STATEMENT 5

The workshop acknowledges that some divers with mild symptoms or signs[1] after diving may be evacuated by commercial airliner to obtain treatment after a surface interval of at least 24 hours, and this is unlikely to be associated with worsening of outcome.[2,3,4]

Table 14.3 Consensus Guidelines for Management of Mild Decompression Sickness in Remote Locations—Cont'd

FOOTNOTES

1. "Mild symptoms and signs" are strictly as defined in Statement 1 and footnotes.
2. It should be noted that most favorable experience with commercial airliner evacuations comes from short-haul flights of between 1 and 2 hours duration. There is much less experience with longer flights.
3. It was agreed that provision of oxygen in as high an inspired fraction as possible is optimal practice for such evacuations. In addition, the risk of such evacuation will be reduced by pre-flight oxygen breathing.
4. It was emphasized that contact must be established with a receiving unit at the commercial flight destination before the evacuation is initiated.

From Mitchell SJ, Doolette DJ, Wachholz CJ, et al. (eds): Management of Mild or Marginal Decompression Illness in Remote Locations. Durham, NC, Divers Alert Network, 2005.

by history and physical examination after each subsequent treatment.[174] Most cases reach such an end point after one to two treatments. A small number of patients with severe neurologic DCI do not reach a plateau until 10 to 20 treatments or more have been administered.

Mechanisms for continued improvement with repetitive hyperbaric treatment include persistence of gas bubbles,[219] reduction of edema,[220,221] provision of adequate oxygen delivery to ischemic tissue,[222] and inhibition of neutrophil adhesion to damaged endothelium.[223,224] No general agreement exists on which table to use for such follow-up therapy. A retrospective analysis supported the use of 2.8 versus 2.4 ATA.[225] Other observations have found no advantage.[136]

ADJUNCTIVE MEASURES TO RECOMPRESSION

Although bubble elimination is the primary goal of treatment, there are secondary pathophysiologic mechanisms of injury that may also be amenable to intervention, including capillary leak and endothelial leukocyte accumulation. The role of leukocytes has been demonstrated in brain AGE in dogs and rabbits[73] and DCS in rats.[162,226] It is possible that the mechanism of HBOT may actually be partly due to its effects on these secondary phenomena, such as the accumulation of leukocytes.[223,224,227,228] Guidelines for adjunctive treatments are discussed here and summarized in Table 14.4.

Fluid Administration

The microcirculation is compromised in DCI as a consequence of bubble-induced endothelial damage and consequential plasma extravasation,[44-47,229,230] platelet and leukocyte accumulation, fat embolism, and thrombus formation. Fluid administration is recommended for all cases of DCI. Isotonic IV fluids are preferred because hypotonic fluids can induce cerebral edema. Glucose-containing solutions should be avoided because they may lead to a worsening of neurologic lesions in both brain[231] and spinal cord.[232] Inert gas washout is accelerated by maneuvers that increase central blood volume and cardiac preload, including supine position,[233] head-down tilt,[234] and head-out immersion.[233,234] Aggressive fluid administration may therefore be indicated for DCI, even if there is no significant dehydration.

The efficacy of oral fluids in the treatment of DCI is unknown. However, fluids that contain 60 mM sodium and 80 to 120 mM glucose have been used successfully for rehydration in severe diarrheal illness. Thus, for mild bends, oral fluids may be adequate, or if IV access in the field is not available and the patient is able to tolerate oral intake, oral resuscitation is better than none. However, such rehydration should be avoided in the acute resuscitation of a severely injured diver, particularly if consciousness is impaired.

End points for fluid administration may include standard clinical assessment of intravascular volume, urine output, and blood hemoglobin/hematocrit. Bladder catheterization is recommended for severe cases.

Table 14.4 Undersea and Hyperbaric Medical Society Summary Guidelines for Adjunctive Therapy

	AGE (NO SIG-NIFICANT INERT GAS LOAD)	DCS: PAIN ONLY, MILD	DCS: NEU-ROLOGICAL	DCS: CHOKES	DCS WITH LEG IMMOBILITY (DVT PROPHY-LAXIS)
Aspirin	2B(C)	2B(C)	2B(C)	2B(C)	
NSAIDs	2B(C)	2B(B)	2B(B)	2B(C)	
Surface O$_2$	1(C)	1(C)	1(C)	1(C)	
Anticoagulants, thrombolytics, IIB/IIIA agents	2B(C)	3(C)	2B(C)	2B(C)	1(A)
Corticosteroids	3(C)	3(C)	3(C)	3(C)	
Lidocaine	2A(B)	3(C)	2B(C)	3(C)	
Fluid					
D5W	3(C)	3(C)	3(C)	3(C)	
LR/crystalloid	2B(C)	1(C)	1(C)	2B(C)	
Colloid	2B(C)	1(C)	1(C)	2B(C)	

Class of evidence is shown (level of evidence in parentheses).
The American Heart Association classification is used:
Class 1: Conditions for which there is evidence and/or general agreement that a given procedure or treatment is useful and effective.
Class 2: Conditions for which there is conflicting evidence and/or a divergence of opinion about the usefulness/efficacy of a procedure or treatment.
Class 2A: Weight of evidence/opinion is in favor of usefulness/efficacy.
Class 2B: Usefulness/efficacy is less well established by evidence/opinion.
Class 3: Conditions for which there is evidence and/or general agreement that the procedure/treatment is not useful/effective and in some cases may be harmful.
Level of evidence A: Data derived from multiple randomized, clinical trials.
Level of evidence B: Data derived from a single randomized trial or nonrandomized studies.
Level of evidence C: Consensus opinion of experts.
AGE, arterial gas embolism; DCS, decompression sickness; DVT, deep venous thrombosis; NSAID, nonsteroidal anti-inflammatory drug.
From Moon RE (ed): Adjunctive Therapy for Decompression Illness. Kensington, MD, Undersea and Hyperbaric Medical Society, 2003, by permission.
Additional details are in the full report and are also available via the Internet at: www.uhms.org.

Corticosteroids

Corticosteroids have been used extensively in the treatment of DCI, with some anecdotal support for their use.[235-238] However, analysis of outcome against the single factor of corticosteroid administration has not shown any benefit.[239] Corticosteroids do not improve outcome in animal models of DCI.[125,148,240] High doses that have been tested as a prophylactic regimen in pigs[241] do not protect against severe DCI in this model and are associated with a greater mortality rate. Corticosteroids are therefore not recommended for DCI treatment.

Anticoagulants and Nonsteroidal Anti-inflammatory Drugs

Bubbles can induce platelet accumulation, adherence, and thrombus formation.[242-246] However, as noted earlier, only the triple combination of heparin, indomethacin, and prostaglandin I$_2$ improved somatosensory-evoked potential recovery in a model of AGE.[247] However, improvements were not sustained beyond 4 hours.[248] Furthermore, the combination did not reduce either neutrophil[249] or platelet accumulation in the affected brain.[248]

In patients with leg immobility caused by DCI, thromboembolic disease is a risk. Of 28 consecutive patients with DCI and inability to walk for at least 24 hours because of leg weakness, there was 1 death and 3 cases of life-threatening pulmonary embolism, of which 1 patient died.[250] It is recommended that all DCI patients with major lower limb weakness receive subcutaneous low-molecular-weight heparin. The efficacy of low-molecular-weight heparin has not been demonstrated in this setting. Nevertheless, consensus guidelines include starting enoxaparin 30 mg subcutaneously every 12 hours (or its equivalent) as soon as possible after injury.[251]

Lidocaine

Lidocaine, a local anesthetic and class 1B anti-arrhythmic agent, has several pharmacologic effects in the injured brain, including deceleration of ischemic ion fluxes, reduction of excitotoxic amino acid release and cerebral metabolic rate for oxygen, inhibition of leukocyte adherence and migration, and reduction of intracranial pressure in the injured brain.[252] Lidocaine has been shown to reduce brain dysfunction after air embolism in cats when given prophylactically[253] and to accelerate recovery of brain function in air-embolized cats[254] and dogs[148] when given therapeutically. After AGE in animals, lidocaine has an ameliorative effect in addition to that of hyperbaric oxygen.[148,255] Case reports support the use of lidocaine in human DCS and AGE.[256-259]

No randomized studies of lidocaine have been performed in human DCI. However, in a model of cerebral gas embolism (open-heart surgery), a blinded, randomized study demonstrated that a perioperative lidocaine infusion for 48 hours after anesthesia induction improved neurocognitive outcome at 10 days, 10 weeks, and 6 months after surgery.[260] Improved outcome 9 days after coronary bypass grafting was achieved in another study using a lidocaine infusion limited to the intraoperative period.[261]

If lidocaine is to be used clinically for adjunctive treatment of DCI, an appropriate end point is attainment of a standard therapeutic antiarrhythmic concentration (2-6 mg/L or μg/mL). Therapeutic serum concentrations can typically be attained by an initial IV bolus dose of 1 mg/kg, then subsequent boluses of 0.5 mg/kg every 10 minutes to a total of 3 mg/kg, while infusing continuously at 2 to 4 mg/min. Use of more than 400 mg within the first hour could be associated with major side effects unless the patient is continuously monitored in a medical unit with the appropriate facilities and personnel. In the field, intramuscular administration of 4 to 5 mg/kg will typically produce a therapeutic plasma concentration 15 minutes after dosing, lasting for around 90 minutes. Use of lidocaine infusions commonly produces perioral paresthesias and ataxia. Seizures can also occur. Therefore, prolonged infusion is best performed while the patient is in an intensely monitored environment.

Blood Glucose Control

Injuries to the central nervous system are worsened by hyperglycemia, probably because of increased lactate production and the resulting intracellular acidosis.[262] Evidence in animals[232,263] and humans[264] suggests that the deleterious effect of hyperglycemia is significant above a plasma glucose of about 200 mg/dL (11 mM/L). Administration of even small amounts of IV glucose may worsen neurologic outcome, even in the absence of significant hyperglycemia.[231] Therefore, unless treating hypoglycemia, it is advisable to avoid administering glucose-containing IV solutions. In the presence of CNS injury, whenever possible, plasma glucose should be measured and hyperglycemia treated.[262]

Temperature Control

Mild reductions in body temperature ameliorate CNS injury, and hyperpyrexia worsens it.[265] It is recommended that simple measures be implemented to avoid hyperthermia, by avoiding a hot environment and aggressively treating fever.

Perfluorocarbons

Perfluorocarbon (PFC) emulsions have a high solubility for both oxygen and inert gases, thus increasing oxygen delivery and providing an inert gas sink. Pretreatment of experimental animals with PFCs increases their tolerance to both AGE[266-271] and VGE.[272-274] In a canine preparation, IV PFC administration enhances inert gas washout[275] and improves outcome in DCS.[276-278] After decompression of dogs from air saturation dives, IV PFCs reduce the incidence and severity of DCS.[279,280] If an approved PFC emulsion is released onto the market, it is likely that it will play a role in the treatment of DCI.

Management of Blood Gases

Animal models of AGE have revealed significant increase of ICP and depression of cerebral Po_2.[281] In a pig model, hyperventilation failed to correct these parameters.[282-284] Therefore, in ventilated patients with severe AGE, it is recommended that arterial Pco_2 be maintained within the reference range.

FOLLOW-UP EVALUATION AND RETURN TO DIVING

Even when there are residual symptoms, long-term outcome of DCI is good. In a series of 69 paralyzed divers followed several months after treatment, half were asymptomatic and only one third had manifestations that interfered with activities of daily living.[285] Figure 14.20 shows the outcome over 12 months of 348 recreational divers with DCI.

With regard to returning to diving, most clinicians agree on the following principles[209]:

- Symptoms and signs of DCI should largely have resolved by the completion of treatment.
- At the time of review (at least 4 weeks after the incident for neurological DCS), the diver should have no evidence of neurologic sequelae.
- There should not be any other identifiable risk factors for DCI.

Pulmonary Barotrauma

Before advising a diver that a return to diving after PBT is safe, an explanation should be diligently sought. Many patients do not have an identifiable predisposition,[239,286] although recent data suggest that a high proportion of divers have lung abnormalities detectable by computerized tomography.[287,288] The patient should be questioned about any history of rapid or uncontrolled decompression, breath-holding, recent respiratory tract infection, or other respiratory illness. A chest radiograph

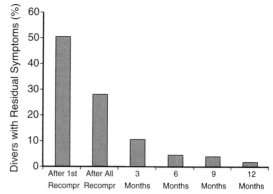

Figure 14.20 TWELVE-MONTH OUTCOME OF 348 CASES OF DECOMPRESSION ILLNESS IN RECREATIONAL DIVERS REPORTED TO THE DIVERS ALERT NETWORK IN 2002. *(Redrawn from Divers Alert Network Report on Decompression Illness, Diving Fatalities and Project Dive Exploration: 2004 Edition. Durham, NC, Divers Alert Network, 2004, p 73, by permission.)*

may show apical bullae or parenchymal scarring,[289] but is usually normal.[104] Computed tomography of the chest is the most sensitive method of excluding bullae.[290] High-resolution computerized tomography chest scans are often abnormal in divers who have normal clinical findings and spirometry.[287-289,291] Low pulmonary compliance and high recoil pressure have been observed in divers with a history of PBT.[292,293] Lower expiratory flow rates at 50% and 25% of vital capacity have been observed in divers after PBT.[294] In both studies, there was considerable overlap between patients and control subjects, and it is quite possible that these findings are the result rather than the cause of the PBT. Spirometry may indicate obstructive disease that could predispose to asthma. If spirometry is normal, repeat testing after exercise with dry gas can reveal airway hyper-responsiveness[295] and can indicate previously undiagnosed asthma, which can predispose to PBT.[296,297]

Decompression Sickness

Fitness to resume diving after DCS is governed by two issues: (1) propensity for recurrence and (2) the effects of cumulative damage caused by a new episode of DCS. Divers may be more likely to suffer recurrences caused by habitual use of provocative depth–time exposures and conditions or by individual physiologic predisposing factors. Speculation also exists that DCS is more likely to occur in tissue damaged by a prior episode, although supporting evidence is anecdotal.

Risk may be reduced if the diver uses more conservative dive profiles (e.g., shorter bottom times, shallower depths, or both).[298] Few identifiable individual predisposing factors have been described. Testing for a PFO is not generally of use unless the following conditions are present: (1) the preceding depth–time profiles are likely to have been associated with VGEs, and (2) the signs and symptoms are severe (i.e., include motor weakness, vertigo, ataxia, or cortical involvement). Any major atrial septal defect is a contraindication to diving.[25] A PFO that requires a Valsalva maneuver to demonstrate it is of uncertain significance. Using occluder devices to close PFOs in divers for the purpose of reducing DCS[299] has not yet been validated.[300]

PBT and AGE can predispose to DCS; thus, an episode of unexpected neurologic DCS should prompt at least a clinical search (by history and physical examination) for causes of PBT. Most physiologic predisposing factors are presumptive and are suggested by several DCS episodes caused by few dives or severity disproportionate to the profile.

Inner ear DCS can become asymptomatic even when there is residual damage. Therefore, during evaluation of divers after inner ear DCS, audiometry and electronystagmography should be performed, even in the absence of residual symptoms.[129]

REFERENCES

1. Eckenhoff RG, Olstad CS, Carrod G: Human dose-response relationship for decompression and endogenous bubble formation. J Appl Physiol 69:914-918, 1990.
2. Van Liew HD, Flynn ET: Direct ascent from air and N_2-O_2 saturation dives in humans: DCS risk and evidence of a threshold. Undersea Hyperb Med 32:409-419, 2005.
3. Phillips JL: The Bends. New Haven, CT, Yale University, 1998.
4. de Méricourt LR: Considérations sur l'hygiène des pecheurs d'éponges. Arch Méd Nav 10:232-234, 1868.
5. Bassett-Smith PW: Diver's paralysis. Lancet 1:309-310, 1892.
6. Blick G: Notes on diver's paralysis. Br Med J 2:1796-1799, 1909.
7. Bendrick GA, Ainscough MJ, Pilmanis AA, et al: Prevalence of decompression sickness among U-2 pilots. Aviat Space Environ Med 67:199-206, 1996.
8. Cowell SA, Stocks JM, Evans DG, et al: The exercise and environmental physiology of extravehicular activity. Aviat Space Environ Med 73:54-67, 2002.
9. Bert P: Barometric Pressure (La Pression Barométrique). Bethesda, MD, Undersea Medical Society, 1978.
10. Pol B, Wattelle TJJ: Mémoire sur les effets de la compression de l'air appliquée au creusement des puits à houille. Ann Hyg Pub Med Leg 2:241-279, 1854.
11. Keays FL: Compressed air illness, with a report of 3,692 cases. Dept Med Publ Cornell Univ Med Coll 2:1-55, 1909.
12. Gillis MF, Karagianes MT, Peterson PO: Detection of gas emboli associated with decompression using the Doppler flowmeter. J Occup Med 11:245-247, 1969.
13. Evans A, Walder DN: Significance of gas micronuclei in the aetiology of decompression sickness. Nature 222:251-252, 1969.
14. Vann RD, Grimstad J, Nielsen CH: Evidence for gas nuclei in decompressed rats. Undersea Biomed Res 7:107-112, 1980.
15. Yount DE: Skins of varying permeability: A stabilization mechanism for gas cavitation nuclei. J Acoust Soc Am 65:1429-1439, 1979.
16. Blenkarn GD, Aquadro C, Hills BA, et al: Urticaria following the sequential breathing of various inert gases at a constant ambient pressure of 7 ATA: A possible manifestation of gas-induced osmosis. Aerosp Med 42:141-146, 1971.
17. Lambertsen CJ, Idicula J: A new gas lesion syndrome in man, induced by "isobaric gas counterdiffusion." J Appl Physiol 39:434-443, 1975.
18. Cowley JR, Allegra C, Lambertsen CJ: Subcutaneous tissue gas space pressure during superficial isobaric counterdiffusion. J Appl Physiol 47:224-227, 1979.
19. Cowley JR, Lambertsen CJ: Isobaric gas counterdiffusion in rabbit eye. J Appl Physiol 47:220-223, 1979.
20. Thomas SF, Williams OL: High-altitude joint pains (bends): Their roentgenographic aspects. Radiology 44:259-261, 1945.
21. Ferris EB, Engel GL, Romano J: The clinical nature of high altitude decompression sickness. In: Fulton JF (ed): Decompression Sickness. Philadelphia, WB Saunders, 1951, pp 4-52.
22. Spencer MP: Decompression limits for compressed air determined by ultrasonically detected bubbles. J Appl Physiol 40:229-235, 1976.
23. Dunford RG, Vann RD, Gerth WA, et al: The incidence of venous gas emboli in recreational diving. Undersea Hyperb Med 29:247-259, 2002.
24. Lee YC, Wu YC, Gerth WA, et al: Absence of intravascular bubble nucleation in dead rats. Undersea Hyperb Med 20:289-296, 1993.
25. Wilmshurst PT, Ellis PT, Jenkins BS: Paradoxical gas embolism in a scuba diver with an atrial septal defect. Br Med J 293:1277, 1986.

26. Moon RE, Camporesi EM, Kisslo JA: Patent foramen ovale and decompression sickness in divers. Lancet 1:513-514, 1989.

27. Wilmshurst PT, Byrne JC, Webb-Peploe MM: Relation between interatrial shunts and decompression sickness in divers. Lancet 2:1302-1306, 1989.

28. Kerut EK, Truax WD, Borreson TE, et al: Detection of right to left shunts in decompression sickness in divers. Am J Cardiol 79:377-378, 1997.

29. Germonpré P, Dendale P, Unger P, et al: Patent foramen ovale and decompression sickness in sports divers. J Appl Physiol 84:1622-1626, 1998.

30. Wilmshurst P, Bryson P: Relationship between the clinical features of neurological decompression illness and its causes. Clin Sci 99:65-75, 2000.

31. Saary MJ, Gray GW: A review of the relationship between patent foramen ovale and type II decompression sickness. Aviat Space Environ Med 72:1113-1120, 2001.

32. Wilmshurst PT, Pearson MJ, Walsh KP, et al: Relationship between right-to-left shunts and cutaneous decompression illness. Clin Sci 100:539-542, 2001.

33. Klingmann C, Knauth M, Ries S, et al: Recurrent inner ear decompression sickness associated with a patent foramen ovale. Arch Otolaryngol Head Neck Surg 128:586-588, 2002.

34. Cantais E, Louge P, Suppini A, et al: Right-to-left shunt and risk of decompression illness with cochleovestibular and cerebral symptoms in divers: Case control study in 101 consecutive dive accidents. Crit Care Med 31:84-88, 2003.

35. Torti SR, Billinger M, Schwerzmann M, et al: Risk of decompression illness among 230 divers in relation to the presence and size of patent foramen ovale. Eur Heart J 25:1014-1020, 2004.

36. Lovering AT, Stickland MK, Kelso AJ, et al: Direct demonstration of 25- and 50-microm arteriovenous pathways in healthy human and baboon lungs. Am J Physiol Heart Circ Physiol 292:H1777-H1781, 2007.

37. Eldridge MW, Dempsey JA, Haverkamp HC, et al: Exercise-induced intrapulmonary arteriovenous shunting in healthy humans. J Appl Physiol 97:797-805, 2004.

38. Stickland MK, Welsh RC, Haykowsky MJ, et al: Intrapulmonary shunt and pulmonary gas exchange during exercise in humans. J Physiol 561:321-329, 2004.

39. Francis TJ, Pezeshkpour GH, Dutka AJ, et al: Is there a role for the autochthonous bubble in the pathogenesis of spinal cord decompression sickness? J Neuropathol Exp Neurol 47:475-487, 1988.

40. Lehner CE, Adams WM, Dubielzig RR, et al: Dysbaric osteonecrosis in divers and caisson workers. An animal model. Clin Orthop 320-332, 1997.

41. Hills BA, James PB: Spinal decompression sickness: Mechanical studies and a model. Undersea Biomed Res 9:185-201, 1982.

42. Fraser WD, Landolt JP, Money KE: Semicircular canal fractures in squirrel monkeys resulting from rapid decompression. Interpretation and significance. Acta Otolaryngol 95:95-100, 1983.

43. Jaminet A: Physical Effects of Compressed Air and of the Causes of Pathological Symptoms Produced on Man by Increased Atmospheric Pressure Employed for the Sinking of Piers in the Construction of the Illinois and St. Louis Bridge. St. Louis, MO, Ennis, 1871.

44. Cockett AT, Nakamura RM, Franks JJ: Delayed shock in experimental dysbarism. Surg Forum 14:7-8, 1963.

45. Malette WG, Fitzgerald JB, Cockett AT: Dysbarism. A review of thirty-five cases with suggestion for therapy. Aerospace Med 33:1132-1139, 1962.

46. Brunner F, Frick P, Bühlmann A: Post-decompression shock due to extravasation of plasma. Lancet 1:1071-1073, 1964.

47. Boussuges A, Blanc P, Molenat F, et al: Haemoconcentration in neurological decompression illness. Int J Sports Med 17:351-355, 1996.

48. Nossum V, Koteng S, Brubakk AO: Endothelial damage by bubbles in the pulmonary artery of the pig. Undersea Hyperb Med 26:1-8, 1999.

49. Nossum V, Hjelde A, Brubakk AO: Small amounts of venous gas embolism cause delayed impairment of endothelial function and increase polymorphonuclear neutrophil infiltration. Eur J Appl Physiol 86:209-214, 2002.

50. Su CL, Wu CP, Chen SY, et al: Acclimatization to neurological decompression sickness in rabbits. Am J Physiol Regul Integr Comp Physiol 287:R1214-R1218, 2004.

51. Ward CA, Koheil A, McCullough D, et al: Activation of complement at plasma-air or serum-air interface of rabbits. J Appl Physiol 60:1651-1658, 1986.

52. Shastri KA, Logue GL, Lundgren CE: In vitro activation of human complement by nitrogen bubbles. Undersea Biomed Res 18:157-165, 1991.

53. Ward CA, McCullough D, Yee D, et al: Complement activation involvement in decompression sickness of rabbits. Undersea Biomed Res 17:51-66, 1990.

54. Zhang J, Fife CE, Currie MS, et al: Venous gas emboli and complement activation after deep repetitive air diving. Undersea Biomed Res 18:293-302, 1991.

55. Ward CA, McCullough D, Fraser WD: Relation between complement activation and susceptibility to decompression sickness. J Appl Physiol 62:1160-1166, 1987.

56. Stevens DM, Gartner SL, Pearson RR, et al: Complement activation during saturation diving. Undersea Hyperb Med 20:279-288, 1993.

57. Hjelde A, Bergh K, Brubakk AO, et al: Complement activation in divers after repeated air/heliox dives and its possible relevance to DCS. J Appl Physiol 78:1140-1144, 1995.

58. Shastri KA, Logue GL, Lundgren CE, et al: Diving decompression fails to activate complement. Undersea Hyperb Med 24:51-57, 1997.

59. Nossum V, Hjelde A, Bergh K, et al: Lack of effect of anti-C5a monoclonal antibody on endothelial injury by gas bubbles in the rabbit after decompression. Undersea Hyperb Med 27:27-35, 2000.

60. Baj Z, Olszanski R, Majewska E, et al: The effect of air and nitrox divings on platelet activation tested by flow cytometry. Aviat Space Environ Med 71:925-928, 2000.

61. Warren BA, Philp RB, Inwood MJ: The ultrastructural morphology of air embolism: Platelet adhesion to the interface and endothelial damage. Br J Exp Pathol 54:163-172, 1973.

62. Lehto VP, Laitinen LA: Scanning and transmission electron microscopy of the blood-bubble interface in

decompressed rats. Aviat Space Environ Med 50:803–807, 1979.

63. Philp RB, Ackles KN, Inwood MJ, et al: Changes in the hemostatic system and in blood and urine chemistry of human subjects following decompression from a hyperbaric environment. Aerosp Med 43:498–505, 1972.

64. Philp RB: A review of blood changes associated with compression-decompression: Relationship to decompression sickness. Undersea Biomed Res 1:117–150, 1974.

65. Hallenbeck JM, Leitch DR, Dutka AJ, et al: Prostaglandin I2, indomethacin and heparin promote postischemic neuronal recovery in dogs. Ann Neurol 12:145–156, 1982.

66. Wisløff U, Richardson RS, Brubakk AO: NOS inhibition increases bubble formation and reduces survival in sedentary but not exercised rats. J Physiol 546:577–582, 2003.

67. Wisløff U, Richardson RS, Brubakk AO: Exercise and nitric oxide prevent bubble formation: A novel approach to the prevention of decompression sickness? J Physiol 555:825–829, 2004.

68. Dujic Z, Duplancic D, Marinovic-Terzic I, et al: Aerobic exercise before diving reduces venous gas bubble formation in humans. J Physiol 555:637–642, 2004.

69. Levin LL, Stewart GJ, Lynch PR, et al: Blood and blood vessel wall changes induced by decompression sickness in dogs. J Appl Physiol 50:944–949, 1981.

70. Albertine KH, Wiener-Kronish JP, Koike K, et al: Quantification of damage by air emboli to lung microvessels in anesthetized sheep. J Appl Physiol 57:1360–1368, 1984.

71. Hallenbeck JM, Dutka AJ, Tanishima T, et al: Polymorphonuclear leukocyte accumulation in brain regions with low blood flow during the early postischemic period. Stroke 17:246–253, 1986.

72. Dutka AJ, Kochanek PM, Hallenbeck JM: Influence of granulocytopenia on canine cerebral ischemia induced by air embolism. Stroke 20:390–395, 1989.

73. Helps SC, Gorman DF: Air embolism of the brain in rabbits pre-treated with mechlorethamine. Stroke 22:351–354, 1991.

74. Jones JP Jr, Neuman TS: Dysbaric osteonecrosis. In: Neuman TS, Brubakk AO (eds): The Physiology and Medicine of Diving. New York, Elsevier Science, 2003, pp 659–679.

75. Walder DN, Elliott DH: Aseptic necrosis of bone. In: Bove AA (ed): Bove and Davis' Diving Medicine. Philadelphia, Saunders, 2004, pp 421–430.

76. Hallenbeck JM: Cinephotomicrography of dog spinal vessels during cord-damaging decompression sickness. Neurology 26:190–199, 1976.

77. Hardman JM: Histology of decompression illness. In: Moon RE, Sheffield PJ (eds): Treatment of Decompression Illness. Kensington, MD, Undersea and Hyperbaric Medical Society, 1996, pp 10–20.

78. Palmer AC, Calder IM, McCallum RI, et al: Spinal cord degeneration in a case of "recovered" spinal decompression sickness. Br Med J (Clin Res Ed) 283:888, 1981.

79. Calder IM, Palmer AC, Hughes JT, et al: Spinal cord degeneration associated with type II decompression sickness: Case report. Paraplegia 27:51–57, 1989.

80. Demchenko IT, Boso AE, Natoli MJ, et al: Measurement of cerebral blood flow in rats and mice by hydrogen clearance during hyperbaric oxygen exposure. Undersea Hyperb Med 25:147–152, 1998.

81. Butler FK Jr, Pinto CV: Progressive ulnar palsy as a late complication of decompression sickness. Ann Emerg Med 15:738–741, 1986.

82. Ball R, Auker CR, Ford GC, et al: Decompression sickness presenting as forearm swelling and peripheral neuropathy: A case report. Aviat Space Environ Med 69:690–692, 1998.

83. Sander HW: Mononeuropathy of the medial branch of the deep peroneal nerve in a scuba diver. J Periph Nerv Syst 4:134–137, 1999.

84. Atkins CE, Lehner CE, Beck KA, et al: Experimental respiratory decompression sickness in sheep. J Appl Physiol 65:1163–1171, 1988.

85. Landolt JP, Money KE, Topliff ED, et al: Pathophysiology of inner ear dysfunction in the squirrel monkey in rapid decompression. J Appl Physiol 49:1070–1082, 1980.

86. Francis TJ, Pearson RR, Robertson AG, et al: Central nervous system decompression sickness: Latency of 1070 human cases. Undersea Biomed Res 15:403–417, 1988.

87. Van Der Aue OE, Duffner GJ, Behnke AR: The treatment of decompression sickness: An analysis of one hundred and thirteen cases. J Ind Hyg Toxicol 29:359–366, 1947.

88. Rivera JC: Decompression sickness among divers: An analysis of 935 cases. Mil Med 129:314–334, 1964.

89. Lam TH, Yau KP: Manifestations and treatment of 793 cases of decompression sickness in a compressed air tunneling project in Hong Kong. Undersea Biomed Res 15:377–388, 1988.

90. Bennett PB, Dovenbarger JA, Bond BG, et al: DAN 1987 diving accident incidence for flying after diving. In: Sheffield PJ (ed): Proceedings of a Workshop on Flying after Diving. Bethesda, MD, Undersea Medical Society, 1989, pp 29–34.

91. Sheffield PJ: Flying after diving guidelines: A review. Aviat Space Environ Med 61:1130–1138, 1990.

92. Navy Department: U.S. Navy Diving Manual. Revision 5. Vol 5. Diving Medicine and Recompression Chamber Operations. NAVSEA 0910-LP-103-8009. Washington, DC, Naval Sea Systems Command, 2005.

93. Benton PJ, Woodfine JD, Westwook PR: Arterial gas embolism following a 1-meter ascent during helicopter escape training: A case report. Aviat Space Environ Med 67:63–64, 1996.

94. Benton PJ, Smith RW: Vasculitis masquerading as neurologic decompression illness. Undersea Hyperb Med 23:189–191, 1996.

95. Nelson EE: Internal carotid artery dissection associated with scuba diving. Ann Emerg Med 25:103–106, 1995.

96. Asola MR: A diver unconscious after gastroenteritis. Lancet 346:1338, 1995.

97. Isbister GK, Kiernan MC: Neurotoxic marine poisoning. Lancet Neurol 4:219–228, 2005.

98. Kemp JH, Munro JG: Munchausen's syndrome simulating caisson disease. Br J Ind Med 26:81–83, 1969.

99. Murphy BP, Davis JC, Henderson DL: Factitious decompression sickness. Aviat Space Environ Med 55:396–397.

100. Massey EW, Moon RE: Pseudo stroke associated with decompression. Undersea Biomed Res 17(suppl):30, 1990.

101. Looi JC, Bennett MH: Munchausen's syndrome presenting as decompression illness. Undersea Hyperb Med 25:235-237, 1998.

102. Rudge FW, Stone JA: The use of the pressure cuff test in the diagnosis of decompression sickness. Aviat Space Environ Med 62:266-267, 1991.

103. Gorman D, Fitzgerald B: An evaluation of the sharpened Romberg's test in diving medicine. Undersea Hyperb Med 21:55, 1996.

104. Harker CP, Neuman TS, Olson LK, et al: The roentgenographic findings associated with air embolism in sport scuba divers. J Emerg Med 11:443-449, 1993.

105. Koch GH, Weisbrod GL, Lepawsky M, et al: Chest radiographs can assist in the diagnosis of pulmonary barotrauma. Undersea Biomed Res 18(suppl):100-101, 1991.

106. Zwirewich CV, Müller NL, Abboud RT, et al: Noncardiogenic pulmonary edema caused by decompression sickness: Rapid resolution following hyperbaric therapy. Radiology 163:81-82, 1987.

107. Goldmann RW: Pneumocephalus as a consequence of barotrauma. JAMA 255:3154-3156, 1986.

108. Moon RE: Diagnostic techniques in diving accidents. In: Bennett PB, Moon RE (eds): Diving Accident Management. Bethesda, MD, Undersea and Hyperbaric Medical Society, 1990, pp 146-154.

109. Lowe VJ, Hoffman JM, Hanson MW, et al: Cerebral imaging of decompression injury patients with ^{18}F-2-fluoro-2-deoxyglucose positron emission tomography. Undersea Hyperb Med 21:103-113, 1994.

110. Staff RT, Gemmell HG, Duff PM, et al: Decompression illness in sports divers detected with technetium-99m-HMPAO SPECT and texture analysis. J Nucl Med 37:1154-1158, 1996.

111. Curley MD, Schwartz HJC, Zwingelberg KM: Neuropsychologic assessment of cerebral decompression sickness and gas embolism. Undersea Biomed Res 15:223-236, 1988.

112. Curley MD, Amerson TL: Use of psychometric testing in decompression illness. In: Moon RE, Sheffield PJ (eds): Treatment of Decompression Illness. Kensington, MD, Undersea and Hyperbaric Medical Society, 1996, pp 152-162.

113. Gorman DF, Edmonds CW, Parsons DW, et al: Neurologic sequelae of decompression sickness: A clinical report. In: Bove AA, Bachrach AJ, Greenbaum LJ Jr (eds): Underwater and Hyperbaric Physiology IX Proceedings of the Ninth International Symposium on Underwater and Hyperbaric Physiology. Bethesda, MD, Undersea and Hyperbaric Medical Society, 1987, pp 993-998.

114. Lezak MD: Neuropsychological Assessment, 3rd ed. New York, Oxford University Press, 1995.

115. Brew SK, Kenny CT, Webb RK, et al: The outcome of 125 divers with dysbaric illness treated by recompression at HMNZS PHILOMEL. SPUMS J 20:226-230, 1990.

116. Murrison AW, Glasspool E, Pethybridge RJ, et al: Neurophysiological assessment of divers with medical histories of neurological decompression illness. J Occup Environ Med 51:730-734, 1994.

117. Leitch DR, Hallenbeck JM: A model of spinal cord dysbarism to study delayed treatment: I. Producing dysbarism. Aviat Space Environ Med 55:584-591, 1984.

118. Leitch DR, Hallenbeck JM: A model of spinal cord dysbarism to study delayed treatment: II. Effects of treatment. Aviat Space Environ Med 55:679-684, 1984.

119. Leitch DR, Hallenbeck JM: Somatosensory evoked potentials and neuraxial blood flow in central nervous system decompression sickness. Brain Res 311:307-315, 1984.

120. Leitch DR, Hallenbeck JM: Remote monitoring of neuraxial function in anesthetized dogs in compression chambers. Electroencephalogr Clin Neurophysiol 57:548-560, 1984.

121. Leitch DR, Hallenbeck JA: Oxygen in the treatment of spinal cord decompression sickness. Undersea Biomed Res 12:269-289, 1985.

122. Leitch DR, Hallenbeck JA: Pressure in the treatment of spinal cord decompression sickness. Undersea Biomed Res 12:291-305, 1985.

123. Sykes JJW, Hallenbeck JM, Leitch DR: Spinal cord decompression sickness: A comparison of recompression therapies in an animal model. Aviat Space Environ Med 57:561-568, 1986.

124. Yiannikas C, Beran R: Somatosensory evoked potentials, electroencephalography and CT scans in the assessment of the neurological sequelae of decompression sickness. Clin Exp Neurol 25:91-96, 1988.

125. Francis TJR, Dutka AJ: Methylprednisolone in the treatment of acute spinal cord decompression sickness. Undersea Biomed Res 16:165-174, 1989.

126. McDermott JJ, Dutka AJ, Koller WA, et al: Effects of an increased PO_2 during recompression therapy for the treatment of experimental cerebral arterial gas embolism. Undersea Biomed Res 19:403-413, 1992.

127. McDermott JJ, Dutka AJ, Koller WA, et al: Comparison of two recompression profiles in treating experimental cerebral air embolism. Undersea Biomed Res 19:171-185, 1992.

128. Murrison A, Glasspool E, Francis J, et al: Somatosensory evoked potentials in acute neurological decompression illness. J Neurol 242:669-676, 1995.

129. Klingmann C, Praetorius M, Baumann I, et al: Barotrauma and decompression illness of the inner ear: 46 cases during treatment and follow-up. Otol Neurotol 28:447-454, 2007.

130. Freiberger JJ, Lyman SJ, Denoble PJ, et al: Consensus factors used by experts in the diagnosis of decompression illness. Aviat Space Environ Med 75:1023-1028, 2004.

131. Grover I, Reed W, Neuman T: The SANDHOG criteria and its validation for the diagnosis of DCS arising from bounce diving. Undersea Hyperb Med 34:199-210, 2007.

132. Golding F, Griffiths P, Hempleman HV, et al: Decompression sickness during construction of the Dartford Tunnel. Br J Ind Med 17:167-180, 1960.

133. Neuman TS, Bove AA: Combined arterial gas embolism and decompression sickness following no-stop dives. Undersea Biomed Res 17:429-436, 1990.

134. Dick AP, Massey EW: Neurologic presentation of decompression sickness and air embolism in sport divers. Neurology 35:667-671, 1985.

135. Bond JG, Moon RE, Morris DL: Initial table treatment of decompression sickness and arterial gas embolism. Aviat Space Environ Med 61:738-743, 1990.

136. Ball R: Effect of severity, time to recompression with oxygen, and retreatment on outcome in forty-nine cases of spinal cord decompression sickness. Undersea Hyperb Med 20:133-145, 1993.

137. Boussuges A, Thirion X, Blanc P, et al: Neurologic decompression illness: A gravity score. Undersea Hyperb Med 23:151-155, 1996.

138. Kelleher PC, Pethybridge RJ, Francis TJ: Outcome of neurological decompression illness: Development of a manifestation-based model [erratum appears in Aviat Space Environ Med 1997 Mar;68(3):246]. Aviat Space Environ Med 67:654-658, 1996.

139. Mitchell SJ, Holley T, Gorman DF: A new system for scoring severity and measuring recovery in decompression illness. SPUMS J 28:89-94, 1998.

140. Pitkin AD, Benton PJ, Broome JR: Outcome after treatment of neurological decompression illness is predicted by a published clinical scoring system. Aviat Space Environ Med 70:517-521, 1999.

141. Holley T: Validation of the RNZN system for scoring severity and measuring recovery in decompression illness. SPUMS J 30:75-80, 2000.

142. Woodward CM: A History of the St Louis Bridge. St Louis, GI Jones, 1881.

143. Green RD, Leitch DR: Twenty years of treating decompression sickness. Aviat Space Environ Med 58:362-366, 1987.

144. Durant TM, Oppenheimer MS, Webster MR, et al: Arterial air embolism. Am Heart J 38:481-500, 1949.

145. Van Allen CM, Hrdina LS, Clark J: Air embolism from the pulmonary vein. Arch Surg 19:567-599, 1929.

146. Atkinson JR: Experimental air embolism. Northwest Med 62:699-703, 1963.

147. Krivonyak GS, Warren SG: Cerebral arterial air embolism treated by a vertical head-down maneuver. Catheter Cardiovasc Interv 49:185-187, 2000.

148. Dutka AJ: Therapy for dysbaric central nervous system ischemia: Adjuncts to recompression. In: Bennett PB, Moon RE (eds): Diving Accident Management. Bethesda, MD, Undersea and Hyperbaric Medical Society, 1990, pp 222-234.

149. Butler BD, Laine GA, Leiman BC, et al: Effects of Trendelenburg position on the distribution of arterial air emboli in dogs. Ann Thorac Surg 45:198-202, 1988.

150. Rodriguez RA, Cornel G, Weerasena NA, et al: Effect of Trendelenburg head position during cardiac deairing on cerebral microemboli in children: A randomized controlled trial [erratum appears in J Thorac Cardiovasc Surg 2001 Mar;121:433]. J Thorac Cardiovasc Surg 121:3-9, 2001.

151. Mehlhorn U, Burke EJ, Butler BD, et al: Body position does not affect the hemodynamic response to venous air embolism in dogs. Anesth Analg 79:734-739, 1994.

152. Geissler HJ, Allen SJ, Mehlhorn U, et al: Effect of body repositioning after venous air embolism. An echocardiographic study. Anesthesiology 86:710-717, 1997.

153. McCullough D: The Great Bridge. New York, Avon Books, 1972.

154. Moir EW: Tunnelling by compressed air. J Soc Arts 44:567-585, 1896.

155. Snell EH: Compressed Air Illness or So-Called Caisson Disease. London, HK Lewis, 1896.

156. Navy Department BoCaR: US Navy Diving Manual. Washington, DC, Government Printing Office, 1924.

157. Acott CA: The development of the minimum pressure oxygen tables. SPUMS J 28:138-143, 1998.

158. Thorne IJ: Caisson disease. JAMA 117:585-588, 1941.

159. Zuntz N: Zur Pathogenese und Therapie der durch rasche Luftdruckänderungen erzeugten Krankheiten. Fortschr Med 15:632-639, 1897.

160. Leitch DR, Green RD: Additional pressurization for treating nonresponding cases of serious air decompression sickness. Aviat Space Environ Med 56:1139-1143, 1985.

161. Leitch DR, Greenbaum LJ Jr, Hallenbeck JM: Cerebral arterial air embolism: II. Effect of pressure and time on cortical evoked potential recovery. Undersea Biomed Res 11:237-248, 1984.

162. Martin JD, Thom SR: Vascular leukocyte sequestration in decompression sickness and prophylactic hyperbaric oxygen therapy in rats. Aviat Space Environ Med 73:565-569, 2002.

163. Yarbrough OD, Behnke AR: The treatment of compressed air illness using oxygen. J Ind Hyg Toxicol 21:213-218, 1939.

164. Goodman MW, Workman RD: Minimal recompression oxygen-breathing approach to treatment of decompression sickness in divers and aviators. Washington, DC, US Navy Experimental Diving Unit Report #5-65, 1965.

165. Douglas JD, Robinson C: Heliox treatment for spinal decompression sickness following air dives. Undersea Biomed Res 15:315-319, 1988.

166. Catron PW, Thomas LB, Flynn ET Jr, et al: Effects of He-O₂ breathing during experimental decompression sickness following air dives. Undersea Biomed Res 14:101-111, 1987.

167. Lillo RS, MacCallum ME, Pitkin RB: Air vs. He-O₂ recompression treatment of decompression sickness in guinea pigs. Undersea Biomed Res 15:283-300, 1988.

168. Hyldegaard O, Madsen J: Influence of heliox, oxygen, and N₂O-O₂ breathing on N₂ bubbles in adipose tissue. Undersea Biomed Res 16:185-193, 1989.

169. Hyldegaard O, Moller M, Madsen J: Effect of He-O₂, O₂, and N₂O-O₂ breathing on injected bubbles in spinal white matter. Undersea Biomed Res 18:361-371, 1991.

170. Hyldegaard O, Madsen J: Effect of air, heliox, and oxygen breathing on air bubbles in aqueous tissues in the rat. Undersea Hyperb Med 21:413-424, 1994.

171. Hyldegaard O, Jensen T: Effect of heliox, oxygen and air breathing on helium bubbles after heliox diving. Undersea Hyperb Med 34:107-122, 2007.

172. Thalmann ED: Principles of US Navy recompression treatments for decompression sickness. In: Moon RE, Sheffield PJ (eds): Treatment of Decompression Illness. Kensington, MD, Undersea and Hyperbaric Medical Society, 1996, pp 75-95.

173. Workman RD: Treatment of bends with oxygen at high pressure. Aerosp Med 39:1076-1083, 1968.

174. Moon RE, Sheffield PJ: Guidelines for treatment of decompression illness. Aviat Space Environ Med 68:234-243, 1997.

175. Pilmanis A: Treatment for air embolism and decompression sickness. SPUMS J 17:27-32, 1987.

176. Moon RE, Dear G de L, Stolp BW: Treatment of decompression illness and iatrogenic gas embolism. Respir Care Clin N Am 5:93-135, 1999.

177. Hart GB: Treatment of decompression illness and air embolism with hyperbaric oxygen. Aerosp Med 45:1190-1193, 1974.

178. Hart GB, Strauss MB, Lennon PA: The treatment of decompression sickness and air embolism in a monoplace chamber. J Hyperb Med 1:1-7, 1986.

179. Kindwall EP, Goldman RW, Thombs PA: Use of the monoplace *versus* multiplace chamber in the treatment of diving diseases. J Hyperb Med 3:5-10, 1988.

180. Kindwall EP: Use of short *versus* long tables in the treatment of decompression sickness and arterial gas embolism. In: Moon RE, Sheffield PJ (eds): Treatment of Decompression Illness. Kensington, MD, Undersea and Hyperbaric Medical Society, 1996, pp 122-126.

181. Cianci P, Slade JB Jr: Delayed treatment of decompression sickness with short, no-air-break tables: Review of 140 cases. Aviat Space Environ Med 77:1003-1008, 2006.

182. Elliott DH, Kindwall EP: Decompression sickness. In: Kindwall EP, Whelan HT (eds): Hyperbaric Medicine Practice. Flagstaff, Ariz, Best Publishing, 1999, pp 433-487.

183. Waite CL, Mazzone WF, Greenwood ME, et al: Cerebral air embolism I. Basic studies. US Naval Submarine Medical Center Report No. 493. Panama City, Fla, US Navy Submarine Research Laboratory, 1967.

184. Leitch DR, Greenbaum LJ Jr, Hallenbeck JM: Cerebral arterial air embolism: I. Is there benefit in beginning HBO treatment at 6 bar? Undersea Biomed Res 11:221-235, 1984.

185. Smerz RW, Overlock RK, Nakayama H: Hawaiian deep treatments: Efficacy and outcomes, 1983-2003. Undersea Hyperb Med 32:363-373, 2005.

186. Thalmann ED: Principles of US Navy recompression treatments for decompression sickness. In: Bennett PB, Moon RE (eds): Diving Accident Management. Bethesda, MD, Undersea and Hyperbaric Medical Society, 1990, pp 194-221.

187. Behnke AR, Shaw LA: The use of oxygen in the treatment of compressed air illness. Navy Med Bull 35:1-12, 1937.

188. Miller JN, Fagraeus L, Bennett PB, et al: Nitrogen-oxygen saturation therapy in serious cases of compressed air decompression sickness. Lancet 2:169-171, 1978.

189. Gorman DF, Browning DM, Parsons DW: Redistribution of cerebral arterial gas emboli: A comparison of treatment regimens. In: Bove AA, Bachrach AJ, Greenbaum LJ Jr (eds): Underwater and Hyperbaric Physiology IX Proceedings of the Ninth International Symposium on Underwater and Hyperbaric Physiology. Bethesda, MD, Undersea and Hyperbaric Medical Society, 1987, pp 1031-1054.

190. Lee HC, Niu KC, Chen SH, et al: Therapeutic effects of different tables on type II decompression sickness. J Hyperb Med 6:11-17, 1991.

191. Barnard EEP, Elliott DH: Decompression sickness: Paradoxical response to recompression therapy. Br Med J 2:809-810, 1966.

192. Navy Department. US Navy Diving Manual. Revision 4. Vol 5. Diving Medicine and Recompression Chamber Operations. NAVSEA 0910-LP-708-8000. Washington, DC, Naval Sea Systems Command, 1999.

193. Silbiger A, Halpern P, Melamed Y, et al: Saturation recompression therapy in a diving accident. Aviat Space Environ Med 54:932-933, 1983.

194. Farm FP Jr, Hayashi EM, Beckman EL: Diving and decompression sickness treatment practices among Hawaii's diving fisherman. Sea Grant Technical Paper UNIHI-SEAGRANT-TP-86-01. Honolulu, HI, University of Hawaii, 1986.

195. Gold D, Geater A, Aiyarak S, et al: The indigenous fisherman divers of Thailand: In-water recompression. Int Marit Health 50:39-48, 1999.

196. Westin AA, Asvall J, Idrovo G, et al: Diving behaviour and decompression sickness among Galapagos underwater harvesters. Undersea Hyperb Med 32:175-184, 2005.

197. Navy Department. US Navy Diving Manual. Revision 3. Vol 1. Air Diving. NAVSEA 0994-LP-001-9110. Flagstaff, Ariz, Best, 1993.

198. Edmonds C: Underwater oxygen treatment of DCS. In: Moon RE, Sheffield PJ (eds): Treatment of Decompression Illness. Kensington, MD, Undersea and Hyperbaric Medical Society, 1996, pp 255-265.

199. Kay E, Spencer M (eds): In-Water Recompression. Kensington, MD, Undersea and Hyperbaric Medical Society, 1999.

200. Edmonds C, Lowry C, Pennefather J, et al: Diving and Subaquatic Medicine. London, Hodder Arnold, 2002.

201. Edmonds C: Australian Underwater Oxygen Treatment of DCS. In: Kay E, Spencer MP (eds): In-Water Recompression Proceedings of the 48th Workshop of the Undersea and Hyperbaric Medical Society. Kensington, MD, Undersea and Hyperbaric Medical Society, 1999, pp 2-15.

202. Green JW, Tichenor J, Curley MD: Treatment of type I decompression sickness using the U.S. Navy treatment algorithm. Undersea Biomed Res 16:465-470, 1989.

203. Barnard EEP: The treatment of decompression sickness developing at extreme pressures. In: Lambertsen CJ (ed): Underwater Physiology Proceedings of the Third Symposium on Underwater Physiology. Baltimore, Williams & Wilkins, 1967, pp 156-164.

204. Hanson RdG, Vorosmarti J Jr, Barnard EEP: Decompression sickness following saturation diving. In: Shilling CW, Beckett MW (eds): Underwater Physiology VI Proceedings of the Sixth Symposium on Underwater Physiology. Bethesda, MD, Federation of American Societies for Experimental Biology, 1978, pp 537-545.

205. Berghage TE: Decompression sickness during saturation dives. Undersea Biomed Res 3:387-398, 1976.

206. Peterson RE: Guidelines for the Gas-Pressure Management of Decompression Sickness and Gas Embolism Occurring during Nitrox and Air Saturation-Excursion Diving [Report No.: National Undersea Research Program Technical Report 89-2]. Rockville, MD, National Oceanic and Atmospheric Administration, 1989.

207. Bennett PB: The Treatment Offshore of Decompression Sickness: European Undersea Biomedical Society Workshop [Report No.: UMS Report 4-9-76]. Bethesda, MD, Undersea Medical Society, 1976.

208. Davis JC, Elliott DH: Treatment of the decompression disorders. In: Bennett PB, Elliott DH (eds): The Physiology and Medicine of Diving, 3rd ed. San Pedro, Calif, Best, 1982, pp 473-487.

209. Moon RE, Gorman DF: Treatment of the decompression disorders. In: Neuman TS, Brubakk AO (eds): The Physiology and Medicine of Diving. New York, Elsevier Science, 2003, pp 600-650.

210. Peirce EC 2d: Specific therapy for arterial air embolism. Ann Thorac Surg 29:300-303, 1980.

211. Greenstein A, Sherman D, Melamed Y: Chokes—favorable response to delayed recompression therapy: A case report. Aviat Space Environ Med 52:558-560, 1981.

212. Kizer KW: Delayed treatment of dysbarism: A retrospective review of 50 cases. JAMA 247:2555-2558, 1982.

213. Myers RAM, Snyder SK, Emhoff TA: Subacute sequelae of carbon monoxide poisoning. Ann Emerg Med 14:1163-1167, 1985.

214. Massey EW, Moon RE, Shelton D, et al: Hyperbaric oxygen therapy of iatrogenic air embolism. J Hyperb Med 5:15-21, 1990.

215. Tolsma KA: Efficacy of delayed treatment of dysbaric disease. Undersea Biomed Res 17(suppl):168, 1990.

216. Dovenbarger JA, Corson K, Moon RE, et al: A review of 33 dive accidents with a delay to treatment of 4 days or greater. Undersea Biomed Res 17(suppl):169, 1990.

217. Rudge FW, Shafer MR: The effect of delay on treatment outcome in altitude-induced decompression sickness. Aviat Space Environ Med 62:687-690, 1991.

218. Ross JAS: Clinical Audit and Outcome Measures in the Treatment of Decompression Illness in Scotland. A report to the National Health Service in Scotland Common Services Agency, National Services Division on the conduct and outcome of treatment for decompression illness in Scotland from 1991-1999. Aberdeen, UK, Department of Environmental and Occupational Medicine, University of Aberdeen Medical School, April 27, 2000.

219. Eckenhoff RG, Osborne SF, Parker JW, et al: Direct ascent from shallow air saturation exposures. Undersea Biomed Res 13:305-316, 1986.

220. Miller JD, Ledingham IM, Jennett WB: Effects of hyperbaric oxygen on intracranial pressure and cerebral blood flow in experimental cerebral oedema. J Neurol Neurosurg Psychiatry 33:745-755, 1970.

221. Sukoff MH, Ragatz RE: Hyperbaric oxygenation for the treatment of acute cerebral edema. Neurosurgery 10:29-38, 1982.

222. Weinstein PR, Anderson GG, Telles DA: Results of hyperbaric oxygen therapy during temporary middle cerebral artery occlusion in unanesthetized cats. Neurosurgery 20:518-524, 1987.

223. Thom SR, Mendiguren I, Hardy K, et al: Inhibition of human neutrophil beta2-integrin-dependent adherence by hyperbaric O_2. Am J Physiol 272:C770-C777, 1997.

224. Thom SR: Effects of hyperoxia on neutrophil adhesion. Undersea Hyperb Med 31:123-131, 2004.

225. Wilson M, Scheinkestel CD, Tuxen DV: Comparison of 14 and 18 meter tables on the resolution of decompression sickness (DCS) in divers. Undersea Biomed Res 16(suppl):87-88, 1989.

226. Martin JD, Beck G, Treat JR, et al: Leukocyte sequestration as a consequence of decompression stress. Undersea Hyperb Med 26(suppl):58, 1999.

227. Zamboni WA, Roth AC, Russell RC, et al: The effect of hyperbaric oxygen on reperfusion of ischemic axial skin flaps: A laser Doppler analysis. Ann Plast Surg 28:339-341, 1992.

228. Zamboni WA, Roth AC, Russell RC, et al: Morphological analysis of the microcirculation during reperfusion of ischemic skeletal muscle and the effect of hyperbaric oxygen. Plast Reconstr Surg 91:1110-1123, 1993.

229. Berry CA, King AH: Severe dysbarism in actual and simulated flight: A follow-up study of five cases. U S Armed Forces Med J 10:1-15, 1959.

230. Smith RM, Van Hoesen KB, Neuman TS: Arterial gas embolism and hemoconcentration. J Emerg Med 12:147-153, 1994.

231. Lanier WL, Stangland KJ, Scheithauer BW, et al: The effects of dextrose infusion and head position on neurologic outcome after complete cerebral ischemia in primates: Examination of a model. Anesthesiology 66:39-48, 1987.

232. Drummond JC, Moore SS: The influence of dextrose administration on neurologic outcome after temporary spinal cord ischemia in the rabbit. Anesthesiology 70:64-70, 1989.

233. Balldin UI, Lundgren CEG, Lundvall J, et al: Changes in the elimination of ^{133}Xe from the anterior tibial muscle in man induced by immersion in water and by shifts in body position. Aerosp Med 42:489-493, 1971.

234. Vann RD, Gerth WA: Physiology of decompression sickness. In: Pilmanis AA (ed): Proceedings of the 1990 Hypobaric Decompression Sickness Workshop. San Antonio, TX, Brooks Air Force Base, Air Force Systems Command AL-SR-1992-0005, 1992, pp 35-51.

235. Fructus X: Treatment of serious decompression sickness. In: Davis JC (ed): Treatment of Serious Decompression Illness and Arterial Gas Embolism: Proceedings of the 20th Undersea Medical Society Workshop. Bethesda, MD, Undersea Medical Society, 1979, pp 37-43.

236. Kizer KW: Corticosteroids in treatment of serious decompression sickness. Ann Emerg Med 10:485-488, 1981.

237. Pearson RR, Goad RF: Delayed cerebral edema complicating cerebral arterial gas embolism: Case histories. Undersea Biomed Res 9:283-296, 1982.

238. Leitch DR, Green RD: Pulmonary barotrauma in divers and the treatment of cerebral arterial gas embolism. Aviat Space Environ Med 57:931-938, 1986.

239. Gorman DF: Arterial gas embolism as a consequence of pulmonary barotrauma. In: Desola J (ed): Diving and Hyperbaric Medicine. Barcelona, Spain, European Undersea Biomedical Society, 1984, pp 348-368.

240. Dutka AJ, Mink RB, Pearson RR, et al: Effects of treatment with dexamethasone on recovery from experimental cerebral arterial gas embolism. Undersea Biomed Res 19:131-141, 1992.

241. Dromsky DM, Weathersby PK, Fahlman A: Prophylactic high dose methylprednisolone fails to treat severe decompression sickness in swine. Aviat Space Environ Med 74:21-28, 2003.

242. Philp RB, Inwood MJ, Warren BA. Interactions between gas bubbles and components of the blood: Implications in decompression sickness. Aerosp Med 43:946-953, 1972.

243. Warren BA, Philp RB, Inwood MJ: The ultrastructural morphology of air embolism: Platelet adhesion to the interface and endothelial damage. Br J Exp Pathol 54:163-172, 1973.

244. Obrenovitch TP, Kumaroo KK, Hallenbeck JM: Autoradiographic detection of ^{111}indium-labelled platelets in brain tissue sections. Stroke 15:1049-1056, 1984.

245. Boussuges A, Succo E, Juhan-Vague I, et al: Plasma D-dimer in decompression illness. In: Marroni A, Oriani G, Wattel F (eds): Proceedings of the XII International Joint Meeting on Hyperbaric and Underwater Medicine. Bologna, Grafica Victoria, 1996, pp 247-250.

246. Boussuges A, Succo E, Juhan-Vague I, et al: Activation of coagulation in decompression illness. Aviat Space Environ Med 69:129-132, 1998.

247. Hallenbeck JM, Leitch DR, Dutka AJ, et al: The amount of circumscribed brain edema and the degree of postischemic neuronal recovery do not correlate well. Stroke 13:797-804, 1982.

248. Kochanek PM, Dutka AJ, Kumaroo KK, et al: Effects of prostacyclin, indomethacin, and heparin on cerebral blood flow and platelet adhesion after multifocal ischemia of canine brain. Stroke 19:693-699, 1988.

249. Kochanek PM, Dutka AJ, Hallenbeck JM: Indomethacin, prostacyclin, and heparin improve postischemic cerebral blood flow without affecting early postischemic granulocyte accumulation. Stroke 18:634-637, 1987.

250. Spadaro MV, Moon RE, Fracica PJ, et al: Life threatening pulmonary thromboembolism in neurological decompression illness. Undersea Biomed Res 19(suppl):41-42, 1992.

251. Undersea & Hyperbaric Medical Society: UHMS Guidelines for Adjunctive Therapy of DCI. In: Moon RE (ed): Adjunctive Therapy for Decompression Illness. Kensington, MD, Undersea & Hyperbaric Medical Society, 2003, pp 184-189.

252. Mitchell SJ: Lidocaine in the treatment of decompression illness: A review of the literature. Undersea Hyperb Med 28:165-174, 2001.

253. Evans DE, Kobrine AI, LeGrys DC, et al: Protective effect of lidocaine in acute cerebral ischemia induced by air embolism. J Neurosurg 60:257-263, 1984.

254. Evans DE, Catron PW, McDermott JJ, et al: Therapeutic effect of lidocaine in experimental cerebral ischemia induced by air embolism. J Neurosurg 70:97-102, 1989.

255. McDermott JJ, Dutka AJ, Evans DE, et al: Treatment of experimental cerebral air embolism with lidocaine and hyperbaric oxygen. Undersea Biomed Res 17:525-534, 1990.

256. Drewry A, Gorman DF: Lidocaine as an adjunct to hyperbaric therapy in decompression illness: A case report. Undersea Biomed Res 19:187-190, 1992.

257. Cogar WB: Intravenous lidocaine as adjunctive therapy in the treatment of decompression illness. Ann Emerg Med 29:284-286, 1997.

258. Mutzbauer TS, Ermisch J, Tetzlaff K, et al: Low dose lidocaine as adjunct for treatment of decompression illness. Undersea Hyperb Med 26(suppl):15, 1999.

259. Mitchell SJ, Benson M, Vadlamudi L, et al: Cerebral arterial gas embolism by helium: An unusual case successfully treated with hyperbaric oxygen and lidocaine. Ann Emerg Med 35:300-303, 2000.

260. Mitchell SJ, Pellett O, Gorman DF: Cerebral protection by lidocaine during cardiac operations. Ann Thorac Surg 67:1117-1124, 1999.

261. Wang D, Wu X, Li J, et al: The effect of lidocaine on early postoperative cognitive dysfunction after coronary artery bypass surgery. Anesth Analg 95:1134-1141, table of contents, 2002.

262. Wass CT, Lanier WL: Glucose modulation of ischemic brain injury: Review and clinical recommendations. Mayo Clin Proc 71:801-812, 1996.

263. Prado R, Ginsberg MD, Dietrich WD, et al: Hyperglycemia increases infarct size in collaterally perfused but not end-arterial vascular territories. J Cereb Blood Flow Metab 8:186-192, 1988.

264. Lam AM, Winn HR, Cullen BF, et al: Hyperglycemia and neurological outcome in patients with head injury. J Neurosurg 75:545-551, 1991.

265. Wass CT, Lanier WL, Hofer RE, et al: Temperature changes of ≥ 1°C alter functional neurological outcome and histopathology in a canine model of complete cerebral ischemia. Anesthesiology 83:325-335, 1995.

266. Menasché P, Pinard E, Desroches AM, et al: Fluorocarbons: A potential treatment of cerebral air embolism in open heart surgery. Ann Thorac Surg 40:494-497, 1985.

267. Spiess BD, Braverman B, Woronowicz AW, et al: Protection from cerebral air emboli with perfluorocarbons in rabbits. Stroke 17:1146-1149, 1986.

268. Spiess BD, McCarthy RJ, Tuman KJ, et al: Protection from coronary air embolism by a perfluorocarbon emulsion (FC-43). J Cardiothorac Anesth 1:210-215, 1987.

269. Menasché P, Fleury JP, Piwnica A: 1985. Fluorocarbons: A potential treatment of cerebral air embolism in open-heart surgery. 1992 update. Ann Thorac Surg 54:392-393, 1992.

270. Cochran RP, Kunzelman KS, Vocelka CR, et al: Perfluorocarbon emulsion in the cardiopulmonary bypass prime reduces neurologic injury. Ann Thorac Surg 63:1326-1332, 1997.

271. Herren JI, Kunzelman KS, Vocelka C, et al: Angiographic and histological evaluation of porcine retinal vascular damage and protection with perfluorocarbons after massive air embolism. Stroke 29:2396-2403, 1998.

272. Tuman KJ, Spiess BD, McCarthy RJ, et al: Cardiorespiratory effects of venous air embolism in dogs receiving a perfluorocarbon emulsion. J Neurosurg 65:238-244, 1986.

273. Spiess BD, McCarthy R, Piotrowski D, et al: Protection from venous air embolism with fluorocarbon emulsion FC-43. J Surg Res 41:439-444, 1986.

274. Zhu J, Hullett JB, Somera L, et al: Intravenous perfluorocarbon emulsion increases nitrogen washout after venous gas emboli in rabbits. Undersea Hyperb Med 34:7-20, 2007.

275. Novotny JA, Bridgewater BJ, Himm JF, et al: Quantifying the effect of intravascular perfluorocarbon on xenon elimination from canine muscle. J Appl Physiol 74:1356-1360, 1993.

276. Lutz J, Herrmann G: Perfluorochemicals as a treatment of decompression sickness in rats. Pflugers Arch 401:174-177, 1984.

277. Spiess BD, McCarthy RJ, Tuman KJ: Treatment of decompression sickness with a perfluorocarbon emulsion (FC-43). Undersea Biomed Res 15:31-37, 1988.

278. Lynch PR, Krasner LJ, Vinciquerra T, et al: Effects of intravenous perfluorocarbon and oxygen breathing on acute decompression sickness in the hamster. Undersea Biomed Res 16:275-281, 1989.

279. Dromsky DM, Spiess BD, Fahlman A: Treatment of decompression sickness in swine with intravenous perfluorocarbon emulsion. Aviat Space Environ Med 75:301-305, 2004.

280. Dainer H, Nelson J, Brass K, et al: Short oxygen pre-breathing and intravenous perfluorocarbon emulsion reduces morbidity and mortality in a swine saturation model of decompression sickness. J Appl Physiol 102:1099-1104, 2007.

281. van Hulst RA, Lameris TW, Hasan D, et al: Effects of cerebral air embolism on brain metabolism in pigs. Acta Neurol Scand 108:118-124, 2003.

282. van Hulst RA, Hasan D, Lachmann B: Intracranial pressure, brain PCO_2, PO_2, and pH during hypo- and hyperventilation at constant mean airway pressure in pigs. Intensive Care Med 28:68-73, 2002.

283. van Hulst RA, Haitsma JJ, Lameris TW, et al: Hyperventilation impairs brain function in acute cerebral air embolism in pigs. Intensive Care Med 30:944-950, 2004.

284. van Hulst RA, Lameris TW, Haitsma JJ, et al: Brain glucose and lactate levels during ventilator-induced hypo- and hypercapnia. Clin Physiol Funct Imaging 24:243-248, 2004.

285. Dovenbarger JA, Uguccioni DM, Sullivan KM, et al: Paralysis in 69 recreational scuba injuries. Undersea Hyperb Med 27(suppl):43, 2000.

286. Elliott DH, Harrison JAB, Barnard EEP: Clinical and radiological features of 88 cases of decompression barotrauma. In: Shilling CW, Beckett MW (eds): Underwater Physiology VI Proceedings of the Sixth Symposium on Underwater Physiology. Bethesda, MD, FASEB, 1978, pp 527-535.

287. Reuter M, Tetzlaff K, Warninghoff V, et al: Computed tomography of the chest in diving-related pulmonary barotrauma. Br J Radiol 70:440-445, 1997.

288. Toklu AS, Kiyan E, Aktas S, et al: Should computed chest tomography be recommended in the medical certification of professional divers? A report of three cases with pulmonary air cysts. Occup Environ Med 60:606-608, 2003.

289. Cable GG, Keeble T, Wilson G: Pulmonary cyst and cerebral arterial gas embolism in a hypobaric chamber: A case report. Aviat Space Environ Med 71:172-176, 2000.

290. Mellem H, Emhjellen S, Horgen O: Pulmonary barotrauma and arterial gas embolism caused by an emphysematous bulla in a SCUBA diver. Aviat Space Environ Med 61:559-562, 1990.

291. Gustafsson E, Svedstrom E, Kiuru A, et al: New classification of divers' lungs with HRCT. Undersea Hyperb Med 26(suppl):41, 1999.

292. Colebatch HJH, Smith MM, Ng CKY: Increased elastic recoil as a determinant of pulmonary barotrauma in divers. Respir Physiol 26:55-64, 1976.

293. Colebatch HJ, Ng CK: Decreased pulmonary distensibility and pulmonary barotrauma in divers. Respir Physiol 86:293-303, 1991.

294. Tetzlaff K, Reuter M, Leplow B, et al: Risk factors for pulmonary barotrauma in divers. Chest 112:654-659, 1997.

295. American Thoracic Society: Guidelines for methacholine and exercise challenge testing-1999: Official statement of the American Thoracic Society. Am J Respir Crit Care Med 161:309-329, 2000.

296. Weiss LD, Van Meter KW: Cerebral air embolism in asthmatic scuba divers in a swimming pool. Chest 107:1653-1654, 1995.

297. Elliott DH (ed): Are Asthmatics Fit to Dive? Kensington, MD, Undersea and Hyperbaric Medical Society, 1996.

298. Vann RD: Mechanisms and risks of decompression. In: Bove AA (ed): Bove and Davis' Diving Medicine, 4 ed. Philadelphia, Saunders, 2004, pp 127-164.

299. Walsh KP, Wilmshurst PT, Morrison WL: Transcatheter closure of patent foramen ovale using the Amplatzer septal occluder to prevent recurrence of neurological decompression illness in divers. Heart 81:257-261, 1999.

300. Moon RE, Bove AA: Transcatheter occlusion of patent foramen ovale: A prevention for decompression illness? Undersea Hyperb Med 31:271-274, 2004.

301. Erde A, Edmonds C: Decompression sickness: A clinical series. J Occup Med 17:324-328, 1975.

302. Davis JC, Sheffield PJ, Schuknecht L, et al: Altitude decompression sickness: Hyperbaric therapy results in 145 cases. Aviat Space Environ Med 48:722-730, 1977.

303. Bayne CG: Acute decompression sickness: 50 cases. JACEP 7:351-354, 1978.

304. Pearson RR, Leitch DR: Treatment of air or oxygen/nitrogen mixture decompression illness in the Royal Navy. J Roy Nav Med Serv 65:53-62, 1979.

305. Kizer KW: Dysbarism in paradise. Hawaii Med J 39:109-116, 1980.

306. Yap CU: Delayed decompression sickness—the Singapore experience. In: Knight J (ed): Proceedings of the Joint SPUMS and the Republic of Singapore Underwater Medicine Conference. SPUMS J 11(suppl):29-31, 1981.

307. Gray CG: A retrospective evaluation of oxygen recompression procedures within the US Navy. In: Bachrach AJ, Matzen MM (eds): Underwater Physiology VIII Proceedings of the Eighth Symposium on Underwater Physiology. Bethesda, MD, Undersea Medical Society, 1984, pp 225-240.

308. Mitchell SJ, Doolette DJ, Wachholz CJ, et al. (eds): Management of Mild or Marginal Decompression Illness in Remote Locations. Durham, NC, Divers Alert Network, 2005.

309. Moon RE (ed): Adjunctive Therapy for Decompression Illness. Kensington, MD, Undersea and Hyperbaric Medical Society, 2003.

310. Butler BD, Hills BA: Transpulmonary passage of venous air emboli. J Appl Physiol 59:543-547, 1985.

311. Vik A, Brubakk AO, Hennessy TR, et al: Venous air embolism in swine: Transport of gas bubbles through the pulmonary circulation. J Appl Physiol 69:237-244, 1990.

312. Divers Alert Network: Report on Decompression Illness, Diving Fatalities and Project Dive Exploration. Durham, NC, Divers Alert Network, 2005.

Carbon Monoxide Pathophysiology and Treatment

15

Stephen R. Thom, MD, PhD

Recent investigations have demonstrated that carbon monoxide (CO) plays a role in normal physiology and has complex effects on metabolism and inflammatory responses. These observations hint at the complexity of pathophysiologic responses from CO exposure. Mechanisms associated with hyperbaric oxygen therapy (HBOT) are similarly complex, and several actions of HBOT have been demonstrated to antagonize or counter adverse effects related to CO poisoning.

Environmental CO contamination from incomplete combustion of carbon-containing substances presents a major public health challenge. Many poisonings could be avoided simply by improved communication of its dangers. This is an international problem, and CO may be responsible for more than half of all fatal poisonings.[1-3] Up-to-date data are difficult to obtain, particularly from developing countries.[4] Continuous surveillance is performed by monitoring all patients hospitalized in some regions[2,5], however, individuals experiencing CO poisoning are often unaware of their exposure because symptoms are nonspecific and mimic those of other illnesses. This contributes to misdiagnosis of a significant number of cases by medical professionals.[6-13] When normalized to regional population densities, fatality rates appear to be approximately 0.5 to 1 per 100,000 people.[2,14-23] The incidence of morbidity from CO is greater than the risk for dying and presents even greater challenges to clinical management.

PATHOPHYSIOLOGY

Synopsis of Pathophysiology

The overview in Figure 15.1 highlights components of CO pathophysiology that are discussed in detail in the following sections. CO enters the body via the lungs, where it interacts with blood elements. In erythrocytes, CO binds to hemoglobin to generate carboxyhemoglobin (COHb). COHb can cause hypoxic stress, and it distributes CO to tissues throughout the body. CO binds to hemoproteins in tissues, the most important of which is cytochrome oxidase. This action can mediate mitochondrial dysfunction with impairments of adenosine triphosphate synthesis and excessive production of reactive O_2 species. Concurrently, platelet-neutrophil aggregation/activation occurs and mediates a separate pathway that leads to tissue damage. Injuries to the heart and brain are a combination of hypoxic/ischemic stress, perivascular damage, and excitotoxicity.

Primary Effects

Hemoglobin Binding

Toxic effects of CO arise after it gains entry to the body via the lungs. Hence, the most important event in CO pathophysiology is hemoglobin binding. Claude Bernard[24] and John Haldane[25] described the hypoxic effects of CO. CO has a high affinity for binding to hemoproteins, and deleterious effects can occur because

of impaired O_2 delivery. The affinity of CO for hemoglobin is more than 200-fold greater than that of O_2, and formation of COHb is well recognized as an effect of CO exposure.[26] Pulmonary CO uptake and the variables that influence the body store of CO and COHb level can be estimated using mathematical models such as the Coburn–Forster–Kane equation (Fig. 15.2).[27] Accurate estimations of CO uptake and distribution require knowledge of 13 parameters (Table 15.1); therefore, clinical utilization of relations such as the Coburn–Forster–Kane equation is fraught with uncertainty.

CO elimination displays an exponential relation.[28-31] Elimination from the body occurs via diffusion across the pulmonary alveolar capillary membrane, and a small amount is directly oxidized to CO_2. The same physiologic variables that influence CO uptake in the body also influence its elimination.

Administration of supplemental O_2 is the cornerstone of treatment for CO poisoning. Oxygen inhalation will hasten dissociation of CO from hemoglobin, as well as provide enhanced tissue oxygenation. Reasonable agreement exists among studies in humans as to the mean COHb half-life ($t_{1/2}$), but the values measured in individuals vary widely.[28-34] This is presumably due to the complex kinetics and differences in variables that influence CO elimination (see Table 15.1). Although not proven, authors have also speculated that the pattern of CO exposure (e.g., whether brief or prolonged, continuous or discontinuous) may contribute to the variability observed in clinical situations.[29,34-36]

The mean COHb $t_{1/2}$ among a group of sedentary human volunteers breathing air was reported to be 320 minutes, but the range was 128 to 409 minutes.[29] In patients breathing 100% high-flow O_2 by mask, Burney and colleagues[32] reported that the mean COHb $t_{1/2}$ was 137 minutes, and Myers and coworkers[34] found the mean COHb $t_{1/2}$ to be 130.5 minutes. Among the 19 individuals studied by Myers' group, the range of COHb $t_{1/2}$ was 27 to 464 minutes (between 21% and 357% of the mean).[34] Weaver and colleagues[31] studied 93 patients treated with 100% O_2 and found a somewhat lower mean COHb $t_{1/2}$ of

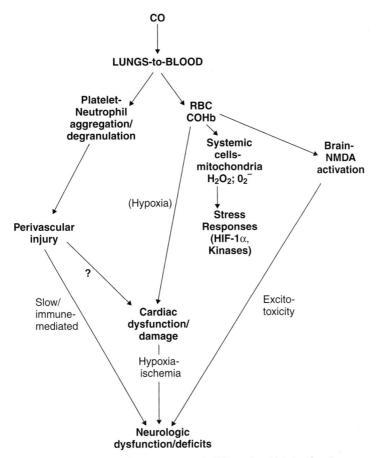

Figure 15.1 Schematic of mechanisms for carbon monoxide (CO)–mediated injuries. Overview on steps that lead to cardiac and brain injuries based on current data. CO causes three concurrent events after its inhalation. It has effects on erythrocyte (red blood cell [RBC]) hemoglobin, circulating platelets, and neutrophils (PMNs). These events mediate cardiac dysfunction and activation of *N*-methyl-ᴅ-aspartate (NMDA) excitatory neurons in the brain. CO rapidly binds to RBC hemoglobin and thus gains entry to the circulation. Hypoxic stress from carboxyhemoglobin (COHb) impairs O_2 delivery, which has an adverse effect on all organs. As brain and heart have the greatest aerobic requirements, they are the first to exhibit dysfunction. Hypoxic stress can cause cardiac injuries and also mediate neuronal loss. Activation of platelets by CO leads to PMN aggregation and degranulation. Myeloperoxidase (MPO) is released to the plasma. Concurrently, activation of NMDA neurons by CO causes neuronal nitric oxide synthase (nNOS) activation, which increases brain nitrite concentration. Endothelium in brain is subjected to oxidative/nitrosative stress by adherent MPO (deposited after PMN degranulation) acting on the increased concentration of nitrite, and this is reflected by nitrotyrosine production. Endothelial cells are activated by MPO-mediated oxidative stress, and they synthesize and express adhesion molecules to which PMN attach. The adherent PMNs release proteases that act on xanthine dehydrogenase. Xanthine oxidase is generated by protease attack on xanthine dehydrogenase, and xanthine oxidase activity generates oxidants that cause brain lipid peroxidation. Adducts form between lipid peroxidation products and myelin basic protein, and render myelin basic protein immunogenic. Lymphocytes are primed because of the altered myelin basic protein and initiate an immunologic response in brain that, in turn, involves activated microglia; learning deficits result from these events. H_2O_2, hydrogen peroxide; HIF-1α, hypoxia inducible factor-1α.

74 minutes, with a range from 26 to 148 minutes.[31] The reduction of COHb $t_{1/2}$ by O_2 has historical importance to the field of hyperbaric medicine because the notion of hastening COHb removal was the initial impetus for considering HBOT in severe poisonings. The mean COHb $t_{1/2}$ decreases to approximately

23 minutes when O_2 is breathed at 3 atmospheres absolute (ATA).[28]

Venous O_2 partial pressure is a useful approximation of mean tissue O_2 tension under normal physiologic conditions.[37] When CO occupies hemoglobin binding sites for O_2, the arterial oxygen content is reduced. CO

$$\exp(-tA/V_bB) = A\,[COHb]_t - B\dot{V}_{co} - PI_{co}/A\,[COHb]_o - B\dot{V}_{co} - PI_{co}$$

$$\text{where:} \quad A = PcO_2/M\,[HbO_2]$$
$$B = 1/DL_{co} + PL/\dot{V}_a$$

Figure 15.2 Coburn-Forster-Kane equation. Units for partial pressures of gases are measured in millimeters of mercury (mm Hg). $[COHb]_0$, carboxyhemoglobin in milliliters of carbon monoxide (CO) per milliliters of blood before exposure; $[COHb]_t$, milliliters of CO per milliliters of blood at time t after exposure; DL_{CO}, diffusing capacity of the lungs for CO in milliliters per minute per millimeter of mercury; $[HbO_2]$, oxyhemoglobin as milliliters of O_2 per milliliters of blood; M, equilibrium constant for reaction of CO with oxyhemoglobin; PcO_2, average partial pressure of O_2 in lung capillaries; PI_{CO}, partial pressure of CO in inhaled air; P_L, barometric pressure minus vapor pressure of water at body temperature; t, exposure duration; $\dot{V}_a$, alveolar ventilation rate per minute; V_b, blood volume in milliliters; $\dot{V}_{CO}$, rate of endogenous CO production.

binding also influences the sigmoidal shape of the oxyhemoglobin dissociation curve, interfering with the release of O_2 to the tissues. The "left" shift of the oxyhemoglobin dissociation curve results in an exaggerated decline in venous O_2 partial pressure.[38] This decreases the amount of O_2 available to tissues so that O_2 tension may be much lower than suggested by the venous O_2 partial pressure during CO poisoning. Partial compensation for the hypoxic stress occurs by increases in microcirculatory blood flow.[39,40]

Decreases in venous O_2 partial pressure have been measured in the brain in response to experimental CO poisoning.[41-44] Similar decreases in venous O_2 tension in animals subjected to CO exposure, hypoxic hypoxia, and anemia have led some investigators to conclude that CO effects are due solely to impairments of O_2 delivery to tissues (e.g., decreases on arterial O_2 content and shift of the oxyhemoglobin dissociation curve).[41-45] This perspective does not take into consideration findings such as modifications in tissue blood flow or the unique effects of CO on intracellular metabolism. When functions other than metabolism are assayed, experimental investigations have noted that pathologic effects cannot be explained by tissue hypoxia from COHb.[46-49] Vasodilation was recently documented in human retinal and choroidal vessels associated with breathing CO sufficient to establish a COHb of approximately 9%.[50]

Table 15.1 Variables Associated with Carbon Monoxide Uptake and Elimination

1. CO concentration in the breathing gas and its relation to partial pressure of oxygen, carbon dioxide, and nitrogen
2. Density of gas mixture breathed
3. Temperature and humidity of the gas breathed
4. Alveolar ventilation
5. Alveolar-pulmonary gradient for CO
6. Cardiac output
7. Pulmonary diffusing capacity for CO
8. Speed of reaction of CO with hemoglobin
9. Quantity and speed of flow of blood in the lung capillaries
10. Hemoglobin and hematocrit values
11. Rate of endogenous CO production
12. Metabolic CO consumption
13. Rate of elimination of CO

CO, carbon monoxide.

Carbon Monoxide–Nitric Oxide–Oxygen Competition

Once CO gains access to body tissues, it can interact with a variety of hemoproteins. Intracellular hemoprotein functions are influenced by the partial pressures of the various ligands: O_2, CO, and the free radical nitric oxide ($\cdot$NO). These gases bind competitively to hemoproteins, thus their effects depend on relative concentrations. This is clinically important because pathophysiologic events can arise because of disturbances in the balance among the ligands, which allows the emergence of alternative reactions. In addition to exogenous sources, CO is also produced in vivo by heme oxygenase enzymes. Production of $\cdot$NO in vivo is mediated by a family of $\cdot$NO synthase

(NOS) isozymes, and ·NO is involved with a wide range of cell-cell communication and metabolic activities.

Experimental evidence has shown that CO will disturb the association between ·NO and hemoproteins. CO increases the steady-state concentration of ·NO in, and around, both platelets and endothelial cells.[51-53] Electron paramagnetic resonance spectroscopy has provided direct evidence that exposure to CO increases the concentration of ·NO in vivo.[54,55] CO does not directly increase activity of NOS enzymes, and CO also does not increase NOS protein concentration in tissues of CO-exposed animals at a time when they exhibit increased ·NO levels.[51-57] In fact, CO partially inhibits NOS activity in animals exposed to 3000 parts per million (ppm; COHb levels of approximately 50%).[51] It appears that CO increases the steady-state level of ·NO because it competes for intracellular sites that normally would bind ·NO.

Whereas CO has weaker affinity for many hemoproteins compared with ·NO or O_2, two chemical parameters are involved with hemoprotein binding: the association and the dissociation rate constants. CO exhibits a relatively slow dissociation constant for many proteins, and this has an important influence on overall kinetics. Moreover, the relative concentrations of the various ligands are often underappreciated. Published values for myoglobin are used in this chapter to illustrate the potential for effects from even a relatively low concentration of environmental CO (Table 15.2).[58]

When the competition between ·NO and CO is considered, the calculated equilibrium constant favors ·NO over CO by a factor of 10^4 when concentrations of CO and ·NO are equal (e.g., ·NO: $1.7 \times 10^7/1.2 \times 10^{-4} = 1.4 \times 10^{11}$;

CO: $0.5 \times 10^6/1.9 \times 10^{-2} = 2.6 \times 10^7$). Under normal physiologic circumstances, it is difficult to predict which ligand may have greater concentration: ·NO because of the activities of the NOS enzymes, or CO because of the activities of heme oxygenase enzymes. Exogenous CO will, however, have a major impact on this balance. Coburn[59] demonstrated that a predictable relation exists between the tissue concentration of CO and blood COHb up to a level of 50%. At a COHb of 7%, the extravascular fluid CO concentration should be approximately 22×10^{-9} M.[59,60] Because CO is freely soluble, a similar concentration is expected to occur inside cells. The rate of ·NO production by endothelial cells (taken as an example because these cells are physically close to delivered CO from the blood) has been estimated to be 1.1×10^{-18} M/cell/min.[61] Therefore, even in a situation where there is a relatively low COHb, the CO concentration may be as much as 10^9 greater than the concentration of ·NO. Therefore, competition is quite feasible.

Perivascular Oxidative Changes

Platelet-neutrophil aggregates and intravascular neutrophil activation occur in association with CO poisoning by an ·NO-dependent mechanism, as illustrated in Figure 15.3.[62] Because CO does not augment NOS activity, these events appear to be a consequence of the competition between CO and ·NO.[51,61] It is well known that ·NO can inhibit platelet-platelet (homotypic) adhesion events, but more complicated interactions occur when considering platelet-neutrophil interactions.[63-65] When activated platelets synthesize ·NO or when platelets are artificially loaded with ·NO-donating compounds, platelet-neutrophil interactions

Table 15.2 Rate Constants for Different Gaseous Ligands with Myoglobin

GAS	ASSOCIATION RATE CONSTANT (M^{-1} SEC^{-1})	DISSOCIATION RATE CONSTANT (SEC^{-1})
·NO	17×10^6	1.2×10^{-4}
CO	0.5×10^6	1.9×10^{-2}
O_2	14×10^6	12

CO, carbon monoxide; ·NO, nitric oxide.

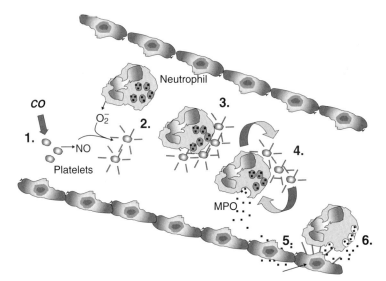

Figure 15.3 Schematic illustrating the carbon monoxide (CO)-mediated intravascular neutrophil activation. *(1)* CO binds to platelet hemoproteins and the resulting competition with intraplatelet nitric oxide (·NO) increases the flux of ·NO that diffuses from platelets. *(2)* Platelet-derived ·NO reacts with neutrophil derived $O_2-\cdot$, creating reactive species that activate platelets. *(3)* The result is formation of platelet-neutrophil aggregates. *(4)* Ongoing interactions between reactive products and adhesion molecules of platelets and neutrophils *(large arrows)* cause firm aggregation and stimulate intravascular neutrophil degranulation and release of myeloperoxidase (MPO) into the bloodstream. *(5)* MPO from neutrophils is deposited along the vascular lining and some is transcytosed to the subendothelial matrix. *(6)* Products from MPO-mediated reactions cause endothelial cell activation that facilitates firm adhesion between neutrophils and the vascular lining, and further neutrophil degranulation. *(Reprinted from Thom SR, Bhopale VM, Han ST, et al: Intravascular neutrophil activation due to carbon monoxide poisoning. Am J Respir Crit Care Med 174:1239–1248, 2006, by permission.)*

are stimulated.[66] This occurs because the liberated ·NO reacts with superoxide anions $(O_2-\cdot)$ generated by nearby neutrophils in the blood to produce the potent oxidizing and nitrating agent peroxynitrite $(ONOO^-)$. $ONOO^-$ will activate platelet adhesion molecules, and this leads to platelet-neutrophil aggregation.[67] This situation is quite close to the effects mediated by CO exposure, because CO increases the ·NO flux from platelets. Platelet-neutrophil aggregates are found in CO-poisoned animals and in patients.[62]

Once a physical linkage between platelets and neutrophils is established, neutrophils exhibit a marked increase in oxidative burst and synthesis of additional reactive ·NO-derived species.[68] For neutrophils to degranulate they must adhere to a surface, typically to platelets or endothelial cells.[69] Primary granules contain elastase, myeloperoxidase (MPO), and lipases. Secondary and tertiary granules contain a number of metalloproteinases, and tertiary granules contain preformed β_2 integrins that facilitate

prolonged adhesion when mobilized to the cell surface. Peroxynitrite can stimulate β_2 integrin expression, but it will not stimulate primary granule release unless neutrophils are adherent to either endothelium or platelets.[68] Once released, MPO can interact with surface β_2 integrins to cause an autoactivation process.[70] Thus, if circulating neutrophils bind with platelets and are activated by substances such as $ONOO^-$, they will degranulate, which may trigger an autoactivation loop.

The interactions between platelets and neutrophils triggered by CO exposure mediate secondary neutrophil activation with intravascular neutrophil degranulation. MPO levels from neutrophil primary granules are significantly increased in plasma of animals and patients with CO poisoning.[62] In animals, the released MPO can be shown to accumulate along the vascular wall.[62] MPO will bind to endothelial cell glycosaminoglycans and can be transcytosed to accumulate in the subendothelial matrix.[71] Once there, MPO catalyzes the reaction between nitrite (the major oxidation product of $\cdot NO$) and H_2O_2 to form nitrogen dioxide ($\cdot NO_2$), which will cause endothelial cell oxidative stress. This is manifested by nitration of protein tyrosine residues and E-selectin expression.[72-76]

Animals exposed to even modest levels of CO ($\sim$50–100 ppm; COHb levels of 4.8–10.6%) exhibit perivascular nitrotyrosine and a capillary leak in aorta, lung, skeletal muscle, and brain.[54-56] CO poisoning also causes oxidation of proteins in mitochondria, plasma, and brain parenchyma.[77-80] $\cdot$NO-mediated oxidative stress is one mechanism for tissue injury by CO, and animal studies point to its crucial role for development of neurologic injuries.[62,80]

Mitochondrial Cytochrome Oxidase Binding

Cytochrome c oxidase (CCO), the terminal enzyme of the mitochondrial electron transport chain, interacts with all three gaseous ligands—O_2, $\cdot$NO, and CO. Reduction of O_2 to water is central to adenosine triphosphate production by mitochondria. Binding of $\cdot$NO to CCO inhibits mitochondrial respiration, and $\cdot$NO has been shown to be a physiologic regulator of cellular O_2 consumption.[81] When cells generate excess amounts of $\cdot$NO (e.g., after inflammatory [type 2] NOS is induced), impairment of mitochondrial function is profound.[82-84] Recently, a similar observation was made pertaining to CO synthesized by intracellular heme oxygenase. CCO binds CO, but much less avidly than $\cdot$NO or O_2. CO can inhibit mitochondrial function, and this becomes particularly notable when cells are subjected to hypoxic conditions. In this setting, endogenously synthesized CO can reduce cellular respiration by as much as 70%.[85]

Exogenous CO can perturb cellular bioenergetics because it inhibits mitochondrial respiration by binding to CCO.[86,87] CO binds only to the reduced form of CCO, and experimental observations with respiring tissues have shown that the CO concentration must be 12- to 20-fold greater than that of O_2 to reduce mitochondrial O_2 uptake by 50%.[88,89] Spectrophotometric evidence of CO binding to CCO in intact animals can be shown when

the circulating COHb level is 50% or more, but it is difficult to detect at lower levels of COHb.[90] Secondary cytochrome changes that occur in response to CO binding by CCO can be shown at much lower CO levels in animals perfused with fluorocarbons rather than blood.[91,92] In contrast with spectrophotometric methods, if free radical production by the mitochondrial electron transport pathway is measured as an index for CO binding to CCO, effects can be seen at quite low environmental CO concentrations ($\sim$50 ppm) even in intact animals.[93]

In brain, CO binding to mitochondrial hemoproteins leads to production of reactive O_2 species in addition to impeding adenosine triphosphate synthesis.[87,90,94,95] Energy production and mitochondrial function are restored after COHb levels decrease, but the transient changes appear to contribute to neuronal necrotic or apoptotic death.[90,96-98] The chronologic aspects of clinical brain injuries are discussed in greater detail later in this chapter.

Exposure to CO can also activate some protein functions. Anti-inflammatory and antiapoptotic effects of CO are well described in the literature, and they appear to be based on activation of several stress-dependent protein kinase pathways.[99-101] Emerging data indicate that cell stress responses are activated via the flux of free radicals generated by CO-mediated mitochondrial disturbances. Reactive species promote activation and stabilization of hypoxia-inducible factor-1α, which regulates genes involved with cell proliferation, differentiation, and survival.[102] In animal models, some of these effects are described as "protective" because they can reduce organ responses to injury. For example, exogenously added CO can reduce experimental ventilator-associated lung injury based on differences in tumor necrosis factor-α elaboration and bronchoalveolar lavage cellularity.[99] In other trials, CO was shown to diminish injuries from shock, postoperative ileus, organ transplantation, and ischemia-reperfusion injuries.[103-110] The levels of CO required to initiate these actions could result in blood COHb levels as high as

20%. Therefore, consideration of iatrogenic CO administration must be tempered against potential organ injuries mediated by alternative mechanisms, as outlined in Figure 15.1.

Alternative Protein Targets for Carbon Monoxide

CO will bind with variable affinity to a variety of heme-containing and also copper-based proteins. A detailed discussion of this topic can be found in Coburn and Forman's review.[89] Some cell proteins, such as cytochrome P450, exhibit such poor CO binding that an interaction is unlikely to have bearing on pathophysiology. Other proteins exhibit moderate binding, but whether inhibition of function has a pathophysiologic effect is unclear. For example, CO binds to myoglobin, a protein involved with O_2 transport within muscle cells. This has been demonstrated in animals exposed to even low CO concentrations, but CO inhibition of myoglobin has not been found to have adverse effects on muscle physiology.[59,111]

Neurotransmission and Excitotoxicity

Neurotransmission

CO has a physiologic role as a neurotransmitter, and whether exogenous CO related to environmental contamination perturbs this function is not clear. Neurotransmission is linked to CO synthesized by the enzyme heme oxygenase-2 (HO-2). Both NOS and HO-2 are found in neural pathways, so there appears to be an overlap. Just as the case for NOS/·NO, no storage organelle for CO exists. HO-2 activated by phosphorylation synthesizes CO and neurotransmission is the result.[112] The protein target for HO-2–generated CO appears to be guanylate cyclase. Neuronal pathways enriched in HO-2 are also enriched in guanylate cyclase, especially olfactory neuronal tissues.[113] HO-2/CO is also involved in regulating stimulated vasopressin secretion from the hypothalamus, it may play a role in long-term potentiation in the hippocampus and supe-

rior cervical ganglion, and peripherally it influences intestinal peristalsis.[114-116]

Excitotoxicity

Increases in excitatory neurotransmitters occur in the brain during CO poisoning.[98,117-119] Whether this response represents a direct effect of CO interacting with neurons or is the result of some other process (e.g., mitochondrial dysfunction/oxidative stress) is unclear. Four types of receptors are activated by excitatory amino acids: N-methyl-D-aspartate (NMDA), metabotropic, D-amino-3-hydroxy-5-methyl-4-isoxazoleproprionic acid, and kainic acid. Glutamate is the major excitatory amino acid in mammalian brains, and NMDA receptor activation, in particular, mediates most excitotoxic neuronal damage.[120] Antagonism of NMDA receptors attenuates CO-mediated neuron degeneration in the hippocampus and reduces the incidence of memory deficiency.[121-124] Toxicity from NMDA activation is closely linked to calcium mobilization, and prophylactic administration of nimodipine, a calcium channel blocker, will inhibit CO-mediated neuronal death, learning impairment, and hippocampal neuropathology.[125] NMDA activation triggers an influx of calcium through both the NMDA channel and neuronal L-type calcium channels, which stimulates neuronal (type I) NOS.[126-128] Production of ·NO in response to excessive NMDA stimulation has been linked to neuronal injury from CO, and it is lower in knockout mice that lack functional genes for neuronal NOS.[124]

Oxidative stress will increase basal (nondepolarized) glutamate release from cortical neurons.[129] Neuron and astrocyte glutamate reuptake transporters are inhibited by reactive oxygen species and peroxynitrite.[130,131] Therefore, oxidative stress as might arise from mitochondrial dysfunction or that triggered via perivascular CO-mediated events may also exacerbate excitotoxicity by diminishing reuptake of glutamate. Arachidonic acid that is released as part of several neuropathological pathways will also inhibit glutamate reuptake, but by a mechanism different from reactive oxygen species, so its effect is additive.[132]

Carbon Monoxide Pathologic Cascade

Animal studies have provided evidence for a progressive pathologic process, or a cascade of events triggered by CO exposure. Figure 15.4 summarizes the steps identified with CO poisoning and shows overlaps among hypoxic/ischemic, excitotoxic, and immune-mediated brain injury.

Intravascular Changes

Events start with CO-mediated alterations in circulating blood elements. Erythrocyte COHb, platelet activation, and platelet-neutrophil interactions are shown within a box to highlight that they occur simultaneously. Processes that lead to neutrophil degranulation were discussed earlier and are shown in Figure 15.3.

Cardiac Dysfunction

The two organs that exhibit the greatest sensitivity to CO are the heart and brain. The common interpretation for their sensitivity is because these organs have the greatest need for oxidative metabolism. Tissues with high rates of O_2 utilization are likely to have steep O_2 gradients in the cells, which would facilitate mitochondrial CO uptake.[133] Once again, however, injuries appear more complex than merely related to hypoxia.[46-49] Animals exposed for 90 minutes to modest CO levels (250 ppm, where the COHb is on the order of 11%) exhibit an increase in coronary perfusion pressure and impaired contractility that lasts for 48 hours.[111] Recent clinical reports have described a high incidence of cardiac injuries in patients with moderate to severe CO poisoning who had normal coronary arteries.[134,135] Impaired respiration caused by CCO binding is a possible mechanism for the cardiac insult from CO, although this should not persist after removal from the CO environment. Oxidative stress resulting from free radical production is yet another possible mechanism, although it has not been demonstrated. Insults mediated by platelet-neutrophil interactions offer an alternative possibility, although this too is not yet proven. Platelet-neutrophil interactions, reduced neutrophil MPO index (MPO/cell), and increased intravascular MPO levels are linked to a heightened risk for acute coronary syndromes.[136-138]

Cardiac dysfunction when COHb levels are severely increased can lead to systemic hypoperfusion that will cause ischemic injuries. Hypoxic and ischemic stresses can also cause neuronal activation.

Neuronal Events

NMDA neurons and neuronal NOS activity are required for development of neurologic sequelae in animal models of CO poisoning.[121,124] The ·NO synthesized in brain in response to CO poisoning leads to greater nitrite levels, and perivascular MPO (the result of the platelet-neutrophil interactions discussed earlier) appears to focus oxidative stress at the vascular lining.[54] This may be the reason the brain is particularly sensitive to CO poisoning. The two processes—perivascular MPO deposition and excitotoxicity—appear to be linked because thrombocytopenic and neutropenic rats exhibit lower NMDA neuronal activation caused by CO poisoning.[124] This suggests that early intravascular events that lead to perivascular deposition of MPO are involved with neuronal activation, and this may create a feedback loop of progressive free radical production.

Changes at the Vascular Wall

Perivascular oxidative stress as was discussed earlier (see Fig. 15.3) leads to inflammation. MPO is deposited along the microvasculature in the brains of animals with CO poisoning and colocalizes with nitrotyrosine.[62] Bands of nitrotyrosine also colocalize with adherent neutrophils, suggesting that oxidative stress from MPO stimulates expression of endothelial adhesion molecules, which

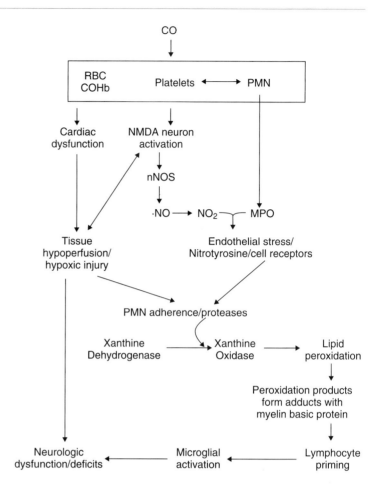

Figure 15.4 Schematic of mechanisms for carbon monoxide (CO)–mediated injuries. Overview on steps that lead to cardiac and brain injuries based on current data. CO causes three concurrent events after its inhalation. It has effects on erythrocyte (red blood cell [RBC]) hemoglobin, circulating platelets, and neutrophils (PMNs). These events mediate cardiac dysfunction and activation of N-methyl-D-aspartate (NMDA) excitatory neurons in the brain. nNOS, neuronal nitric oxide synthase; ·NO, nitric oxide; NO$_2$, nitrite.

interact with neutrophils.[56,61,77] Peroxynitrite has been shown to induce P-selectin expression on endothelial cells and platelets and to stimulate endothelial cells to synthesize E-selectin.[67,139,140] By 45 minutes after experimental CO poisoning, neutrophils adhere firmly to the vasculature via β$_2$ integrins.[51,77,141,142] Concurrent with β$_2$ integrin engagement, neutrophils liberate proteases such as elastase, as well as oxidizing species. In the CO model, neutrophil-derived proteases act on endothelial cell xanthine dehydrogenase (XD) and convert it to xanthine oxidase (XO).[141-143] Several groups have shown that a high local concentration of elastase in the vicinity of adherent neutrophils can convert XD to XO.[144,145] In brain, XD and XO are largely localized to endothelial cells. XO generates reactive species that cause brain lipid peroxidation in response to CO poisoning.[143] The role of XO was shown

because lipid peroxidation does not occur in rats treated with allopurinol or if they are fed a tungsten diet. Although there is no specific XO inhibitor, tungsten feeding inhibits molybdenum-containing enzymes such as XD and XO, and allopurinol inhibits XD and XO (but it can also scavenge reactive nitrogen species). The combination of both manipulations offers the most convincing proof of the role for XO in CO-mediated pathophysiology.

Lipid Peroxidation and Adaptive Immunologic Responses

Aldehydic lipid peroxidation products can react with proteins to render them immunogenic.[146,147] CO poisoning causes adduct formation between myelin basic protein (MBP) and malonylaldehyde, a reactive product of lipid peroxidation. The three-dimensional structure of MBP is modified because of CO poisoning and this triggers an immunologic response.[80] Lymphocytes from CO-poisoned rats (but not control rats) proliferate when exposed to MBP, and activated microglia increase in brains of CO-poisoned rats. Rats made immunologically tolerant to MBP before CO poisoning exhibit acute biochemical changes in MBP because of reactions with lipid peroxidation products, but no proliferative lymphocyte response or brain microglial activation.[80]

The consequences of brain inflammation have been extensively studied in infection processes, but inflammation is also believed to play a role in the pathogenesis of a variety of neurodegenerative disorders.[148-152] Inflammatory cells inflict damage on neighboring cells by releasing a variety of cytotoxic molecules including reactive oxygen and nitrogen species and cytokines. Activated microglia can attack oligodendroglia, and microglial activation has been associated with demyelination processes. In addition, impaired neuronal progenitor cell activity has been found in response to inflammatory insults.[153,154] Activated microglia in hippocampus can inhibit both basal and insult-induced neurogenesis, which impairs learning.[151] The birth of new neurons within the hippocampal region of the brain continues throughout life and correlates closely with learning and memory.[155,156] CO-poisoned rats exhibit a decrement in learning, but this does not occur in immunologically tolerant rats or in rats in which XO was depleted.[80,157] Therefore, acute CO-mediated lipid peroxidation is linked to neuropathology because it precipitates an adaptive immunologic response.

Animal trials may offer insight into some clinical observations related to CO poisoning. Exposure to CO for protracted periods has been suggested to increase risk for suffering neurologic sequelae, although numerous variables may confound the reliability of this association (see Treatment section later in this chapter).[158-160] One experimental model involves exposure to 1000 ppm and then 3000 ppm CO; the sequence of the exposures is important. If reversed, so that animals are first exposed to 3000 ppm CO to cause unconsciousness followed by the 1000 ppm CO "soak," then neutrophil adhe-

sion, XO formation, and brain lipid peroxidation do not occur.[161] Marked oxidative/nitrosative stress occurs during the 3000 ppm CO/loss of consciousness component of the model because of NMDA neuronal activation and ·NO synthesis. It appears that the MPO deposits resulting from neutrophil activation during the CO "soak" act on the nitrite resulting from NMDA activity, and this focuses oxidative stress at the vascular lining. This highlights the multicomponent nature of CO pathophysiology.

CLINICAL PRESENTATION

Signs and Symptoms

Initial symptoms arising because of CO exposure are subtle and nonspecific. With acute exposure to high concentrations, patients may quickly be rendered unconscious. It is more typical, however, for patients to report nonspecific symptoms such as headache, nausea, and dizziness. Clearly, this presentation mimics many ailments, such as a viral syndrome, and may delay diagnosis and identification of a source of environmental CO contamination.[6-13] Although quality and characteristics of headache are variable, it is overwhelmingly the most common manifestation and is reported to occur in 90% of pateints.[32,162]

Numerous investigations have reported subtle alterations of visual and auditory function, alertness, task performance, and learning with exposures to low levels of CO sufficient to cause no more than 5% to 10% COHb.[163-173] These reports have garnered substantial debate because of questions of reproducibility.[174-176] Some more objective observations, such as auditory-evoked potential, suggest that low-level CO can have adverse effects on higher functions. The mechanism(s) behind these effects have not been determined.[177]

Common physical findings include tachycardia and tachypnea; blood pressure changes are variable.[159] Patients with underlying coronary artery disease may suffer reduced exercise tolerance, greater frequencies of premature contractions, and also symptoms of myocardial ischemia even with low COHb levels of 2% to 6%.[46,178-180] Dysrhythmias, cardiomyopathy, myocardial infarctions, and sudden cardiac arrest are reported in victims of severe CO poisoning.[178,181-186] Clinical observations and animal trials suggest that acute mortality from CO poisoning is probably related to cardiac injuries.[178,179,183,184] Some of the cardiac damage arises because of hypoxic stress, particularly in patients with underlying coronary artery disease, but global dysfunction can be seen in those with normal coronary arteries.[134,135] Chronic obstructive pulmonary disease may also decrease exercise tolerance in the face of CO exposure.[187] A rare physical finding is cherry red coloration of the skin. It is much more common to observe superficial blisters in dependent areas when patients have been lying comatose for a period of time.[188,189] This is likely to be a nonspecific finding.

Laboratory Testing

Measurement of COHb by spectrophotometry is the standard method for confirming the diagnosis of CO exposure. Normal levels in nonsmokers are between 0.2% and 0.85% (because of heme oxygenase activity). Smokers often have COHb levels of about 4%, and heavy smokers may have levels of 10%. When evaluating neonates, it is important to know that absorption characteristics of fetal hemoglobin are close to those for COHb and this may cause confusion.[190] For all patients, clinicians should be aware that pulse oximetry is an unreliable method for estimating CO exposure because most instruments cannot discern the difference in spectral characteristics between oxyhemoglobin and COHb.[191]

A correlation exists between development of symptoms such as headache and dizziness and COHb levels on the order of 2% to 10%.[10,11] Unfortunately, no reliable correlation exists for more severe signs and symptoms and COHb level. Absence of objective measures for establishing the severity of CO poisoning remains among the most troublesome aspects of clinical evaluations. Metabolic acidosis, blood lactate, amylase, B-type natriuretic

peptide, and S100 protein from brain have all been examined, but none provides a reliable estimation for severity of poisoning.[192-195] Newer tests such as measurements of plasma MPO and platelet-neutrophil aggregates have not yet been correlated with poisoning severity or prognosis in prospective trials.[62]

Because of the risk for cardiac injuries from CO poisoning, obtaining an electrocardiogram and plasma cardiac markers for injury is prudent. Those who suffer an acute cardiac injury have an increased risk for cardiovascular-related death in the following 10 years.[135] A chest radiograph also should be part of emergency evaluation. This is an obvious point in patients with concurrent smoke inhalation; however, pulmonary vascular congestion and alveolar infiltrates can also occur with isolated exposures to CO because of compromised myocardial function.[185,186]

Neuroimaging

A large number of clinical reports have documented brain computed tomography and magnetic resonance imaging abnormalities after CO poisoning. Lesions have been reported in globus pallidus, putamen, thalamus, caudate, substantia nigra, fornix, hippocampus, corpus callosum, and diffusely throughout the cortex.[196-201] Obviously, neuronal insults mediated by CO are not anatomically discrete. White matter changes can be found in approximately one third of patients with severe poisoning, and lesions in the centrum semiovale are related to worse cognitive outcomes.[202] Imaging studies from several sources suggest that CO neurotoxicity can involve a vascular injury. Vascular abnormalities and atypical coupling between cerebral blood flow and neuronal O_2 demand have been found in CO victims.[203-206] The mechanism(s) for these changes are unknown, but the findings are consistent with animal experimentation showing perivascular CO pathophysiology, as was discussed earlier. Symptomatic recovery from neurologic sequelae may occur in approximately 50% of patients over a span of 2 years, and there are rare reports that evidence of white matter damage may also resolve in these patients.[153,207]

Neurologic Sequelae

Survivors of CO poisoning are faced with potential impairments to cardiac and neurologic function. As discussed earlier, CO poisoning can cause an acute compromise in cardiac function, and survivors exhibit an increased risk for cardiovascular-related death in the following 10 years.[134,135] With regard to neurologic impairments, there is a historical precedence for dividing disorders into "acute/persistent" and "delayed" forms. Some patients exhibit acute abnormalities wherein they have an abnormal level of consciousness and/or focal neurologic findings from the time of initial presentation and never recover. Other patients seem to recover from acute poisoning, but then manifest neurologic or neuropsychiatric abnormalities from 2 days to about 5 weeks after poisoning. Events that occur after a clear or "lucid" interval have been termed "delayed" neurologic sequelae (DNS).

Results from animal studies do not provide a clear distinction between mechanisms responsible for "acute/persistent" and "delayed" sequelae. Several animal studies indicate that "acute/persistent" sequelae arise because of neuronal necrotic or apoptotic death, but this does not necessarily mean that injuries are mediated solely by hypoxia/ischemia versus the events linked to excitotoxicity, perivascular oxidative stress (see Figs. 15.1 and 15.4), or as yet unidentified processes.[61,80,96,97] Moreover, because they occur concurrently, one might expect that pathologic insults for "acute/persistent" and "delayed" sequelae overlap. Thus, there may be more of a continuum of clinical disorders versus distinctly different syndromes. The current practice of dividing neurologic insults based on chronology does not necessarily mean that the underlying mechanisms are different.

Acute/persistent sequelae cover a broad spectrum of abnormalities.[153,207-210] Patients may present in coma, slowly improve their level of consciousness, but never regain their former level of neurologic function. Residual deficits can include dementia, psychosis, chorea, apraxias, amnesia and confabulatory syndromes, cortical blindness, incontinence, or peripheral neuropathies. Some patients will experience development of a Parkinsonian-like syndrome, typically 2 or more weeks after recovering consciousness. Characteristic symptoms of CO-induced Parkinson's disease include bradykinesia, but not a resting tremor.[210]

DNS are characterized clinically by the appearance of neurologic and/or psychiatric symptoms after an asymptomatic time period following the acute stage of CO poisoning. This chronologic pattern of abnormalities can occur after a variety of hypoxic/ischemic injuries such as respiratory arrest, strangling, drug-induced coma, and seizures.[211-213] Whether the same mechanism is responsible for all these injuries is unknown. Documentation of DNS often requires use of neuropsychiatric tests; thus, the apparent incidence depends on methods of detection. Most investigations have found DNS in from 10% to 47% of CO poisoning survivors.[153,214-220] One study reported the incidence as 74%, but testing performed in this trial could not discern performance decrements from depression.[221,222] Because a large proportion of patients had attempted suicide, the conclusions in this study are suspect.

Delayed sequelae often involve neuropsychiatric symptoms such as impaired judgment, poor concentration, disorientation, confusion, coma, depression, cogwheel rigidity, opisthotonic posturing, extremity flaccidity or spasticity, extensor plantar response, and/or a relative indifference to obvious neurologic deficits.[153,208,214-219,223,224] These events can occur despite rapid and appropriate emergency care. Delayed sequelae can also develop in patients who do not suffer from alterations of consciousness during their acute poisoning.[217-219]

TREATMENT

Emergency stabilization of patients should follow standard management practices with provision of a patent airway and support of circulation. Administration of supplemental O_2 is the cornerstone of treatment of CO poisoning. Oxygen inhalation will hasten dissociation of CO from hemoglobin, as well as provide enhanced tissue oxygenation. As discussed earlier, in primary pathology, HBOT causes CO dissociation from hemoglobin to occur at a rate greater than that achievable by breathing pure O_2 at sea-level pressure. In addition, HBOT, but not ambient pressure O_2 treatment, has several actions demonstrated in animal models to be beneficial in ameliorating pathologic events associated with central nervous system injuries. These include an improvement in mitochondrial oxidative processes,[225] inhibition of lipid peroxidation,[226] and impairment of leukocyte adhesion to injured microvasculature.[142] Animals poisoned with CO and treated with HBOT exhibit more rapid improvement in cardiovascular status,[227] lower mortality,[228] and lower incidence of immune-mediated neurologic sequelae.[229] Hypoxic brain injury from CO may be established at time of exposure, and in these situations, HBOT does not appear to alter outcome.[97]

Animal studies have demonstrated several treatments in addition to hyperbaric oxygen (HBO) that may ameliorate CO-mediated injuries. Mortality is reduced by hypothermia treatment.[228] Antagonism of NMDA receptors attenuates CO-mediated neuron degeneration in the hippocampus and reduces delayed memory deficiency.[121,124] Nimodipine, a calcium channel blocker, also inhibits CO-mediated neuronal death, learning impairment, and hippocampal neuropathology.[123] The only treatment option that has been investigated in a controlled manner in clinical trials is HBOT.

Randomized Clinical Trials of Hyperbaric Oxygen Therapy

The clinical efficacy of HBOT for acute CO poisoning has been assessed in five prospective, randomized trials published in peer-reviewed journals.[203,216-218,221] Only one clinical trial satisfies all items deemed to be necessary for the highest quality of randomized, controlled trials.[230] This study, by Weaver and colleagues,[218] reports a randomized, double-blinded, placebo-controlled human clinical trial involving 152 patients. All enrolled patients received treatment with either three sessions of HBOT or normobaric O_2 with sham pressurization to maintain blinding. Critically ill patients were included, with half of enrolled patients having lost consciousness and 8% requiring intubation. The follow-up rate was 95%, with assessments performed by trained examiners and compared with age, sex, and education-controlled norms. The definition of neurologic sequelae, defined a priori, was fulfilled in symptomatic patients by an aggregate performance on six neuropsychological tests that was at least one standard deviation below predicted, or by an aggregate score of two or more standard deviations below expected in asymptomatic individuals. At 6 weeks after poisoning, the cognitive sequelae rate was 25% in patients treated with HBOT compared with 46% of patients treated with normobaric oxygen ($P = 0.007$). When adjusted for cerebellar dysfunction and stratification, the odds ratio was 0.45 ($P = 0.03$; 95% confidence interval, 0.129–0.919).

Chronologically, the next most recent trial, by Scheinkestel and coworkers,[221] reports on 191 patients treated with continuous O_2 by face mask for 3 days after CO poisoning with daily HBOT. Patients with severe poisoning were included, and more than half were comatose. To maintain blinding, patients randomized to the non-HBOT group received "sham" pressure treatments. Additional HBOT (up to six daily sessions total) was performed in patients without neurologic recovery. The primary outcome measure for this trial was testing performed at completion of treatment (3–6 days), not long-term follow-up. This study had a high rate of adverse neurologic outcomes in all patients, regardless of treatment assignment. Neurologic sequelae were reported in 74% of HBOT-treated patients and 68% of control patients. No other clinical trial has approached this degree of neurologic dysfunction. As mentioned earlier, the high incidence is likely to be related to the assessment tool that could not discern true neurologic impairments from poor test-taking related to depression.[222] Suicide attempts with CO represented 69% of cases in this trial. Moreover, 54% of patients were lost to follow-up. Outcomes at 1 month were not reported, but remarks indicated no difference. Multiple statistical comparisons were reported without apparent planning or the requisite statistical correction. Both treatment arms received continuous supplemental mask O_2 for 3 days between their hyperbaric treatments (both true HBOT and "sham"), resulting in greater overall O_2 doses than conventional therapy. Flaws in the design and execution of this study make it impossible to draw meaningful conclusions from the data.

Thom and investigators[217] report a benefit to HBOT in a study of 65 patients with CO poisoning randomized to a single HBO treatment session or mask O_2. This was an unblinded trial, and patients suffered from mild-to-moderate poisoning because those with loss of consciousness were not included. The primary outcome measure was self-reported symptoms of neurologic sequelae combined with deterioration in at least one of six neuropsychological tests occurring during the time when new symptoms occurred. Neuropsychological testing was performed in all patients at 4 weeks after treatment. Sequelae were found in 0% (95% confidence interval, 0–12%) of the patients who received HBOT and 23% (95% confidence interval, 10–42%) of the patients treated with ambient pressure O_2. All patients with reported neurologic sequelae had resolution by 77 days. Limitations in this trial were lack of blinding and selection of a subgroup of patients likely to have suffered less severe poisoning.

A prospective trial by Ducasse and colleagues[203] randomized 26 patients with acute CO poisoning to receive normobaric O_2 (100% oxygen for 6 hours, then 50% oxygen for 6 hours) or HBOT (2 hours at 2.5 ATA, then 4 hours of 100% normobaric O_2, followed by 6 hours of 50% normobaric O_2).[203] Poisoning was accompanied by loss of consciousness in 65% of the patients. Outcome measures included symptoms, electroencephalogram, and cerebral blood flow responses to acetazolamide administration. A significant benefit at 3 weeks was seen in the HBOT group ($P \leq 0.02$). Limitations of this trial included small size, inadequate

allocation concealment, and use of surrogate outcome measures.

Raphael and colleagues[216] studied 343 CO poisoning patients without loss of consciousness who were randomized to one HBOT session or an equivalent duration of mask O_2. This was an unblinded trial and the primary outcome measure was abnormalities noted on a symptom questionnaire, supplemented by physical and neurological examinations in an unspecified number of patients. One month after treatment, 32.2% of patients who received HBOT and 33.8% of control patients reported neurologic symptoms ($P = 0.75$, not significant, χ^2 test), and 97% of patients in each group had resumed their previous occupation. Data from this study were republished with additional subgroup analysis showing no change in outcome.[231] The study has been criticized for using overly broad inclusion criteria, an inadequate regimen for HBOT, long treatment delays, and weak outcome measures.[232,233]

In conclusion, published clinical trials span a broad range in quality. Efficacy of HBOT for acute CO poisoning is well supported in animal trials, and studies provide a mechanistic basis for treatment. In this era of evidence-based medicine, a great deal of emphasis is placed on systematic reviews. Treatment of CO poisoning has undergone a number of these reviews, but the analytic fidelity has been poor. For example, profound flaws in two successive Cochrane Library Reviews have been identified.[234]

Several recent reports have provided additional insight into risks for neurologic sequelae after CO poisoning and the benefit of HBO. Weaver and coworkers[219] reported on a cohort of 238 patients and found that independent risk factors for development of neurologic sequelae include age of 36 years or older, exposure for 24 hours or longer (with or without intermittent exposures), and acute complaints of memory abnormalities. These conclusions were based on univariate analysis, but once subjected to multivariate analysis, only age of 36 years or older and exposure of longer than 24 hours persisted as independent risk factors. The only risk factor where HBOT demonstrated a reduction in incidence of sequelae was for the group aged 36 years or older. The trial was underpowered to reliably assess the benefit of HBOT in those with long-duration CO exposure, but none of five patients exposed for 24 hours or longer manifested neurologic sequelae.[219]

Hopkin and investigators[220] have shown that HBOT is beneficial only in reducing neurologic sequelae among patients who do not possess the apolipoprotein ε4 allele.[220] Because genotype is typically unknown, this report does not provide treatment guidelines, but it will be important for future research. It is well established that the apolipoprotein genotype can have profound effects on risk for a variety of neuropathologic events.[235-238] Whether apolipoprotein ε4 modifies the primary pathophysiologic insults of CO or mechanisms of HBOT is currently unknown.

The preponderance of evidence indicates that HBOT significantly reduces the incidence of neurologic sequelae. Retrospective comparisons indicate that HBOT also diminishes acute mortality.[239] An assessment as to the length of delay from poisoning beyond which there is no chance for benefit from HBOT has not occurred. One trial has remarked that if patients incur a cardiac arrest and are resuscitated, HBOT does not appear to alter the outcome.[240] This finding is consistent with the animal studies where HBOT reduces immune-mediated neurologic injury, but not that mediated by hypoxia.[97,229] In summary, current results support use of HBOT to reduce cognitive sequelae in victims of CO poisoning who have any of the following characteristics: loss of consciousness, exposures for 24 hours or longer, COHb of 25% or greater, and age of 36 years or older.

MATERNAL-FETAL CARBON MONOXIDE POISONING

Maternal CO poisoning is a special clinical situation that is often highly emotionally charged and therefore deserves additional commentary. Maternal symptoms at the time of exposure more closely predict the risk for associated fetal morbidity/mortality than COHb, just as is the case for the general population.[241]

Severe CO poisoning is associated with a maternal mortality rate between 19% and 24%, and a fetal mortality rate between 36% and 67%.[242] When mother and fetus survive, many fetuses subsequently develop somatic and neurologic sequelae, including malformations of limbs, hypotonia and areflexia, persistent seizures, mental and motor disabilities, and microcephaly.[243,244]

Hypoxic stress related to impaired O_2 delivery is an obvious component to fetal distress. Normal fetal arterial partial pressure of O_2 is low, about 20 versus 100 mm Hg for maternal arterial blood. Hence, the fetal O_2 exchange typically occurs near the steep part of the oxyhemoglobin dissociation curve. A small decline in maternal partial pressure of O_2 can cause a precipitous decline in fetal partial pressure of O_2. This physiologic stress occurs more quickly than that associated with CO binding to fetal proteins. Studies with sheep demonstrated that fetal COHb does not reach steady state until approximately 36 to 48 hours, whereas maternal COHb reaches steady state in 7 to 8 hours.[245] The second insult related to fetal COHb is a disturbance in O_2-hemoglobin dissociation curve. Binding by CO causes a left shift of the curve, which increases the hypoxic stress to the fetus. Fetal COHb concentration increases more slowly than does maternal COHb, but once steady state is reached, the fetal level is higher. This is related to the higher affinity fetal hemoglobin has for CO as compared with hemoglobin A. The human fetal-maternal COHb concentration ratio is 1.1 to 1.0[246]; that is, at steady state, the fetal COHb concentration will be 10% to 15% greater than maternal COHb. Although the slow kinetics may be viewed as a protective factor for the fetus, the dynamics work in reverse for CO elimination. The half-life for fetal COHb is nearly twice that for maternal COHb.[245] Therefore, a physiologic basis exists for treating CO poisoning in pregnant women with ambient pressure O_2 for longer than the time it takes to register negligible maternal COHb. Whether complex intravascular processes such as CO-induced platelet-neutrophil aggregation occur in the fetal circulation is unknown.

Anecdotal clinical reports suggest that HBOT may improve fetal outcome.[242,247-252] The only experimental study that addresses the efficacy of HBOT for reducing fetal risk from acute CO poisoning shows a reduction in spontaneous abortion in pregnant rats.[253] No significant extra risks are presented to the fetus or mother due to HBOT when following therapeutic protocols.[254,255] The current recommendations for use of HBOT in pregnant women are the same as those to treat any other patient.

PROLONGED CARBON MONOXIDE EXPOSURE

It is intuitive to suggest that longer durations of CO exposure should increase risk for injury. This association has been supported by some, but not all, clinical studies.[158,159,216-219,220,256]

Epidemiologic investigations suggest that CO pollution is a chronic stressor and correlates with hospital admissions among patients with underlying cardiovascular disease. Unfortunately, these studies are complex, and numerous confounding variables do not allow for an accurate assessment of the incremental effect of CO versus, for example, the effect of small particulates, or NO_2.[257-259]

A separate but related question is whether protracted CO exposure because of indoor pollution poses special risk. A number of publications have addressed the issue of "chronic" CO poisoning. On reviewing this literature, the first notable finding is that there is no accepted definition. In publications dating to the mid-1930s, the effects of prolonged CO exposures have been investigated with the idea that pathophysiologic effects may arise because of repeated or protracted exposure to CO of such low concentration that if there were only a single short-term exposure instance, insignificant or possibly no signs/symptoms may occur.

Animal studies have been performed in rodents, cats, and dogs. Rats and mice exposed to 50 ppm CO for 3 months to 2 years (continuously) showed no change in body weight or hematologic, behavioral, or reproductive characteristics.[260] Rats exposed continuously to

500 ppm CO for 30 or 62 days, achieving COHb 40%, demonstrated no pathologic changes other than cardiac hypertrophy.[261,262] Supfle and investigators[263,264] found that dogs exposed daily to 2000 to 6000 ppm CO for 15 to 20 weeks were more irritable. Dogs exposed to 100 ppm CO for 11 weeks, 5.75 to 7 hours/day, to achieve COHb levels of approximately 20%, exhibited electrocardiographic evidence of cardiac injury and neuropathology at 3 months after exposure.[265] The authors commented that difference between histologic changes in acute and chronic CO appeared to be purely quantitative. Vestibular function studied in cats exposed daily to 40,000 to 60,000 ppm CO for 1 month was found to be unchanged unless blood flow was disturbed by unilateral carotid ligation.[266]

Reports describing human exposures to prolonged or "chronic" CO fall into two general categories: (1) large, carefully documented reports that involve workers exposed to CO daily for years, and (2) case reports or small case series that describe individuals reporting injuries after accidental exposures. An exceptionally detailed study was reported by Lindgren[267] in 1960 that involved 970 Scandinavian workers employed at ironworks, mines, gasworks, or automobile repair shops. Findings among the 970 workers were compared with 432 control subjects who were not employed in areas exposed to contamination by CO. Workers had been employed in "at-risk" sites for up to 4 years. The COHb levels of the workers were as high as 30%, and measured levels of CO in the employment sites ranged from 3.8 to 887 ppm. Subjects were compared with regard to expressed symptoms, neurologic signs, electrocardiogram results, hematologic examination (hemoglobin/hematocrit), and formal psychometric examinations. The author found no higher frequency of abnormalities among the CO-exposed workers than control subjects, except for reversible headaches thought to result from repeated, acute poisonings.

Kruger and coworkers[268] studied a group of 833 ironworks and gasworks employees with COHb values of 0% to more than 10% (>80% of all workers had values of <5%). The authors found an increased incidence of headache but no permanent or function-impairing disorders. No measurements of CO concentrations were taken in the work environments. Komatsu and colleagues[269] studied 153 workers with COHb values between 0% and 30% who had worked in areas where measured CO levels were less than 10 to as high as 1370 ppm. They found greater incidence of reversible headaches and some subjective symptoms but concluded that "workers thought themselves to be healthy without paying attention to their reversible complaints such as headache and forgetfulness."

Ely and coworkers[270] described an incident where a group of workers was exposed to CO from a propane-powered fork-lift truck for 3 months with ambient CO level of ~386 ppm. Acute symptoms such as headache, dizziness, and difficulty with concentration were present in 93% of the 30 cases, and 30% had self-reported residual deficits such as arm/leg numbness 2 years later. A total of 13% reported memory loss at 2 years. Formal neuropsychological evaluations on these cases were not reported.

Beck[271,272] described clinical aspects of "chronic" CO poisoning in several reports. Among those, in a series of 97 patients exposed to CO "repeatedly at sublethal doses...over prolonged periods"(months to 18 years), symptoms were frontal headache, weakness, and "functional nervous and mental symptoms." In an earlier report, he noted some cases suffered headache and polycythemia. He stated that, for most, symptoms resolved in 3 to 4 days, but in some, recovery was longer, and he had one patient for whom symptoms did not reverse in 3 years. Kirkpatrick[273] reported on 26 patients with CO exposures spanning 1 month to 4 years from home furnaces or automobiles. Three patients suffered intervals of unconsciousness, and one patient did not recover fully (residual minor difficulties with balance). In all other patients, symptoms resolved on removal of the CO source.

There are also reports that focused on more unusual ocular or vestibular dysfunction after CO exposures. Whether these are truly manifestations of some low-level protracted exposure is unclear because similar symptoms can arise with more acute poisoning.[274-277] Gilbert and Glasser[278] report, "The prognosis in treated cases of chronic CO poisoning is excellent. In most, symptoms clear in two weeks, and 95% of patients become symptom free within 3 months." Grace and Platt described four cases of repeated CO exposures over days to weeks caused by malfunctioning furnaces. All neurologic signs and symptoms resolved over days after removal from CO (including one patient who lost consciousness).[279] Pavese and colleagues[280] published a clinical report including 8 patients with CO exposures from 12 to 30 days caused by failure of domestic heating systems and COHb levels on admission of 12.5% to 40.8%. One patient presented with mutism, masked face, and cognitive impairment, and these conditions did not improve. No other patients had magnetic resonance imaging abnormalities or neurologic sequelae. Webb and Vaitkevicius[281] described a 73-year-old woman with a 4-month period of confusion and headache caused by a faulty heater. All symptoms resolved over 5 days after the heater was fixed. Foster and coworkers[282] described a 3.5-year-old girl with admissions at 2 and 3 months of age because of respiratory distress, including a period of cyanosis with apnea, associated with up to 4300 ppm CO in a house with a faulty heater. The patient was described as doing well, "thriving," at 6-month follow-up examination. A series of six case reports described symptoms that resolved after removal from environmental CO contamination suspected to have been present for 2 to 20 years.[283]

These reports should not be taken to demonstrate that "chronic" CO exposures pose no risk, but rather that current experience does not support the notion of additive or synergistic injury results from recurrent or protracted exposures. Historical accounts of widespread "chronic" CO exposures during World War II make note that, for most individuals, symptoms resolved with cessation of exposure, but not in all cases.[284] Untoward outcomes are well documented in several reports and case series. Ryan[285] reported a 48-year-old woman exposed to CO at 180 ppm for 3 years who suffered headaches, lethargy, memory problems, and mental confusion. She experienced

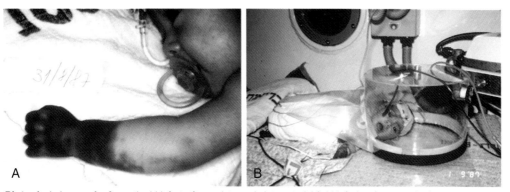

Color Plate 1 *A,* A case of a 6-month-old infant after an iatrogenic intra-arterial fluid infusion. A progressive improvement occurred after twice-daily hyperbaric oxygen treatments and concluded with the amputation of the distal phalanxes. *B,* Treatment was performed using a Perspex-made oxyhood. Frequent air flushes are required to prevent high oxygen concentrations within the chamber using this method. *(Courtesy Israeli Naval Medical Institute and Dr. Yehuda Melamed.)*

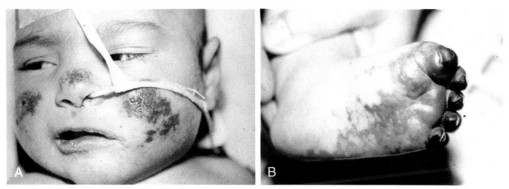

Color Plate 2 *A and B,* Progression of necrotic lesions of the face and lower extremities after purpura fulminans that significantly improved after hyperbaric oxygen treatment. *(Courtesy Israeli Naval Medical Institute and Dr. Yehuda Melamed.)*

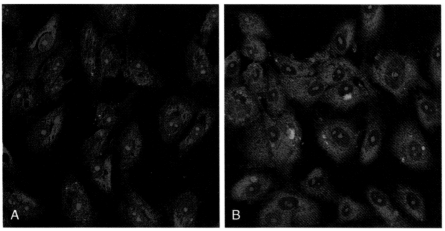

Color Plate 3 HYPERBARIC OXYGEN (HBO) INDUCES NITRIC OXIDE SYNTHASE (NOS) III PRODUCTION AFTER MOCK ISCHEMIA-REPERFUSION INJURY IN VITRO. Primary human umbilical vein endothelial cells (HUVECs) were exposed to mock ischemia (hypoxia/hypoglycemia) for 4 hours, then either normoxia/normoglycemia for 20 hours or 1.5 hours of HBO at 2.5 ATA, then 18.5 hours of normoxia/normoglycemia. Cells were fixed and immunostained for expression of NOS III and analyzed by confocal laser–scanning microscopy (CLSM). Enhanced expression of NOS III after HBO exposure *(B)* can be appreciated relative to control cells *(A).* Nucleic acid is stained red with propidium iodide, and NOS III is stained green with a NOS III–specific antibody. *(Adapted from Buras JA, Stahl GL, Svoboda KK, Reenstra WR: Hyperbaric oxygen downregulates ICAM-1 expression induced by hypoxia and hypoglycemia: The role of NOS. Am J Physiol Cell Physiol 278:C292–C302, 2000, by permission.)*

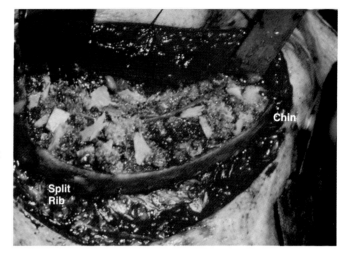

Color Plate 4 The Marx technique of reconstruction. After hyperbaric oxygen and resection, the patient is reconstructed with cadaveric bone (in this case, a split rib) serving as the carrier tray for the patient's own corticocancellous bone harvested and placed into the carrier. The patient is kept in external fixation until the graft has ossified. Surgery is done extraorally to prevent infection by introduction of oral flora.

Color Plate 5 A patient before *(A)* and after *(B)* mandibular reconstruction. The reconstructed mandible adds immeasurably to the patient's quality of life and permits denture support, which improves the patient's nutritional status.

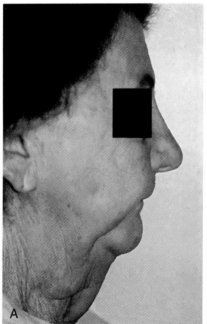

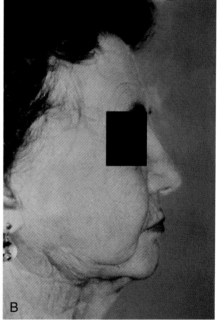

Color Plate 6 Additional HBOT was delivered after surgery to enhance graft and flap survival. This type of wound is especially difficult to treat because it is constantly bathed in digestive salivary enzymes. The proximity of the carotid artery also puts the patient at risk for a fatal bleed unless the process is arrested.

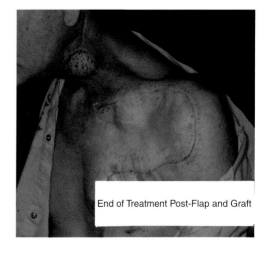

End of Treatment Post-Flap and Graft

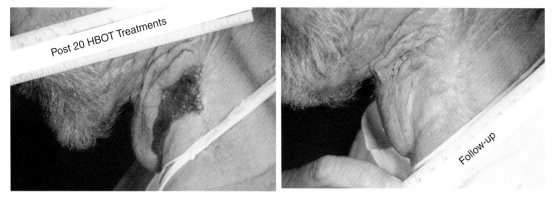

Color Plate 7 *Left,* Excellent granulation base and epithelial advancement. *Right,* Follow-up about 3 months after completion of treatment. The wound closed without any additional surgery.

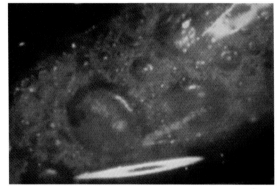

Color Plate 8 BUBBLES IN THE EPIDURAL VENOUS PLEXUS. *(From Hallenbeck JM: Cinephotomicrography of dog spinal vessels during cord-damaging decompression sickness. Neurology 26:190–199, 1976, by permission.)*

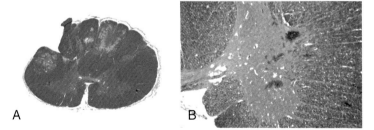

Color Plate 9 SPINAL CORD DECOMPRESSION SICKNESS 1 WEEK AFTER DEVELOPMENT OF QUADRIPARESIS IN A 42-YEAR-OLD MAN WHO MADE A 70 FEET SEA WATER DIVE. *A,* Demyelination can be seen in the long tracts. *B,* Higher magnification view shows hemorrhage in the gray matter. *(Courtesy Department of Pathology, Duke University Medical Center, Durham, NC.)*

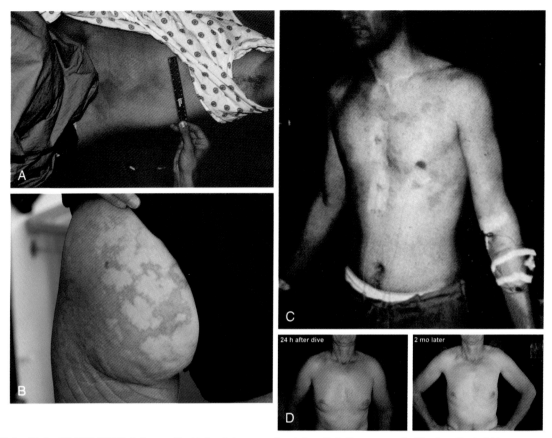

Color Plate 10 SKIN BENDS. *A,* Nonspecific skin bends in a recreational diver. *B, Cutis marmorata (livedo reticularis)* in a recreational diver. *C,* Urticaria precipitated by breathing 3% oxygen, balance nitrogen at 200 feet sea water in a helium/oxygen environment. *D,* Lymphatic bends 24 hours after onset and 2 months later. *(C: From Blenkarn GD, Aquadro C, Hills BA, et al: Urticaria following the sequential breathing of various inert gases at a constant ambient pressure of 7 ATA: A possible manifestation of gas-induced osmosis. Aerosp Med 42:141-146, 1971, by permission.)*

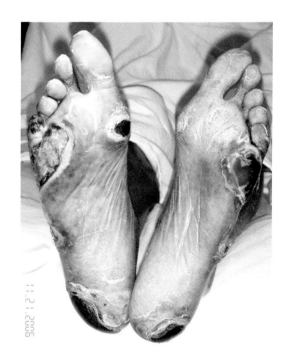

Color Plate 11 An elderly, wheelchair-bound patient whose feet have multiple, bilateral ulcerations due, in part, to unrelieved pressure from inadequate footwear and the wheelchair footrests.

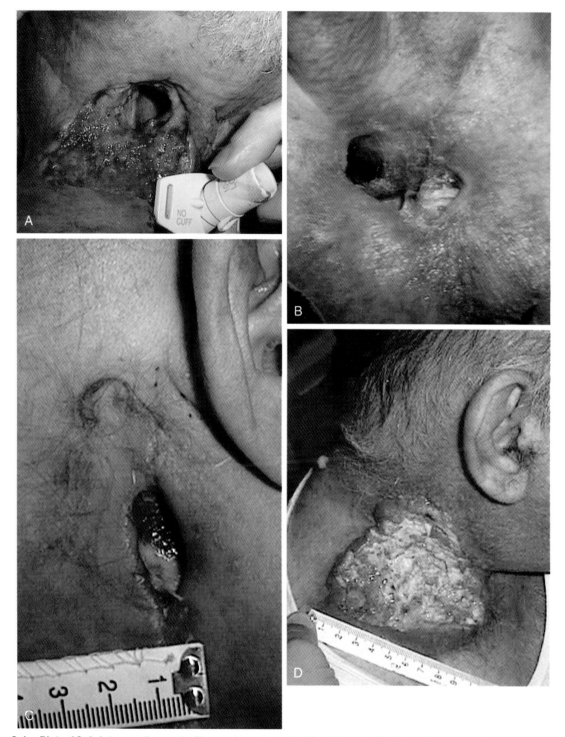

Color Plate 12 Soft-tissue radionecrosis of laryngectomy stomas (A, B) and the neck (C, D) in patients treated for head and neck cancers. The neck sites show ulcerating and fungating presentations.

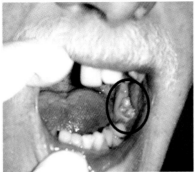
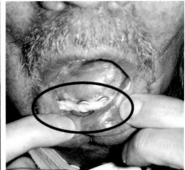
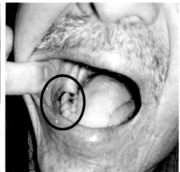

Color Plate 13 Radionecrosis of the mandible presenting with oral lesions corresponding to the necrosis.

Color Plate 14 Serial images of a patient's lateral foot wound as it was reassessed during hyperbaric oxygen therapy. The series shows progressive granulation and contraction of the wound edge.

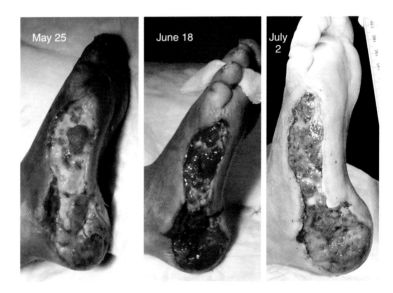

Color Plate 15 A patient's heel wound treated with hyperbaric oxygen therapy shows a robust granulation bed with characteristically smooth, contracting wound edge and the pale, pearly appearance consistent with epithelialization at the edge.

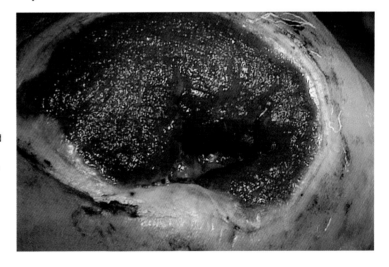

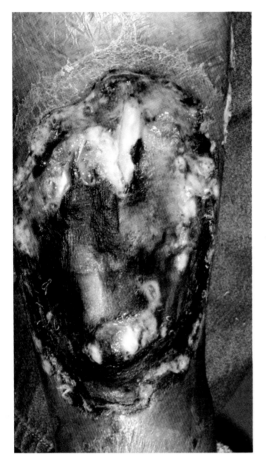

Color Plate 16 A patient's posterior shin arterial ulcer is filled with devitalized tissue and proteinaceous exudates. The exposed tendon at 12 o'clock position suggests osteomyelitis may be present and warrants further clinical evaluation.

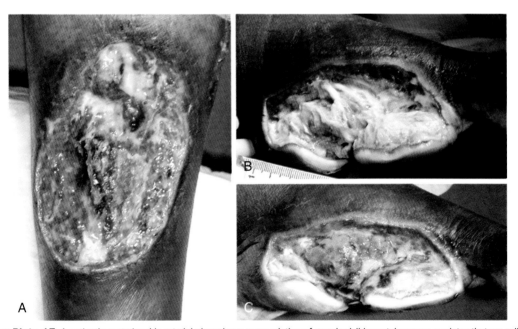

A

B

C

Color Plate 17 A patient's posterior shin arterial ulcer shows accumulation of grossly visible proteinaceous exudates that are yellow *(A)*. Serial images of patient's lateral foot ulcer *(B, C)* show large amounts of pale, devitalized tissue together with some proteinaceous exudates *(B)*, which is reduced with enzymatic debridement *(C)*.

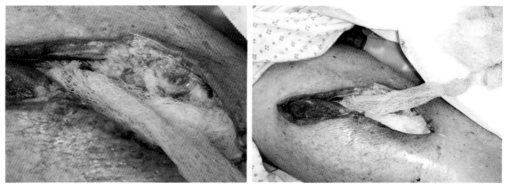

Color Plate 18 A patient's leg wound is packed with roll gauze that has been dampened with normal saline solution. Note that the wound is packed by layering the gauze into the wound, which limits overpacking and allows for atraumatic removal.

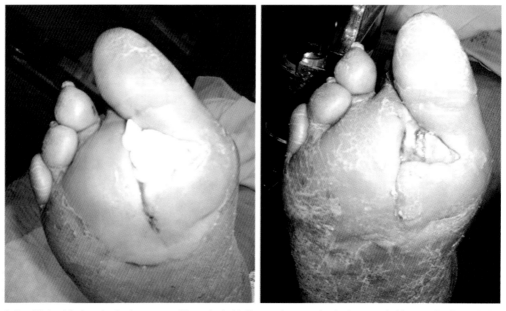

Color Plate 19 A patient's plantar wound is packed with fine mesh gauze that is dampened with normal saline solution.

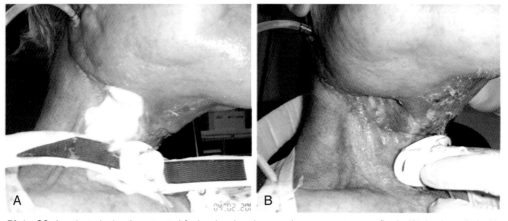

A

B

Color Plate 20 A patient who has been treated for head and neck cancer has an orocutaneous fistula *(A)* that is packed with calcium alginate dressing to manage the fistulous drainage *(B)*.

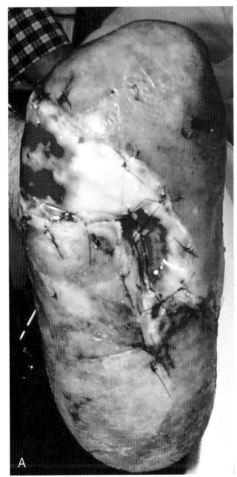

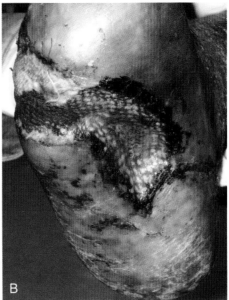

Color Plate 21 A patient with an extensive and complicated plantar foot wound was treated with HBOT. A biomembrane dressing was used to maintain wound moisture, reduce pain, and maintain tissue position *(A)*. The wound healing, by tertiary intent, created a granulated wound bed that was closed using a split thickness skin graft *(B)*.

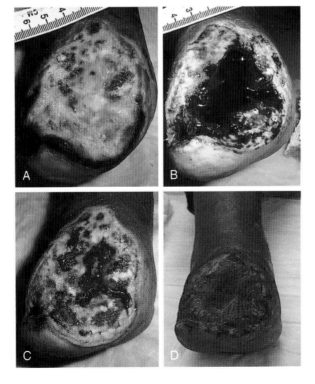

Color Plate 22 Images of an amputation site show devitalized tissue, adherent exudates, and other debris *(A)* that warrant debridement *(B)*. *C,* Some granulation tissue and proteinaceous exudates covering varying portions of the wound bed. *D,* Wound shortly after split-thickness skin graft placement.

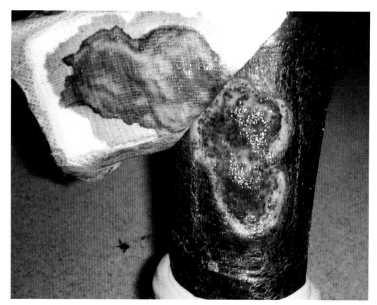

Color Plate 23 A patient with an anterior shin arterial ulcer is being treated with hyperbaric oxygen therapy and use of a papain ointment to debride exudate and support granulation. Note the green color of the ointment visible on the dressing as it is removed and the granulation islands present at the lateral wound borders.

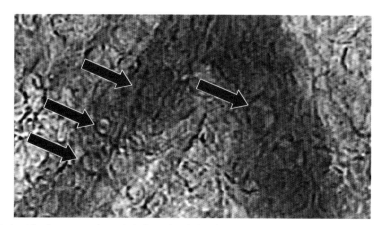

Color Plate 24 Neutrophil adherence to the endothelium of an ischemic postcapillary microvenule at 15 minutes of reperfusion. The leukocytes are marked by arrows and are easily identified by their characteristic size and whitish color.

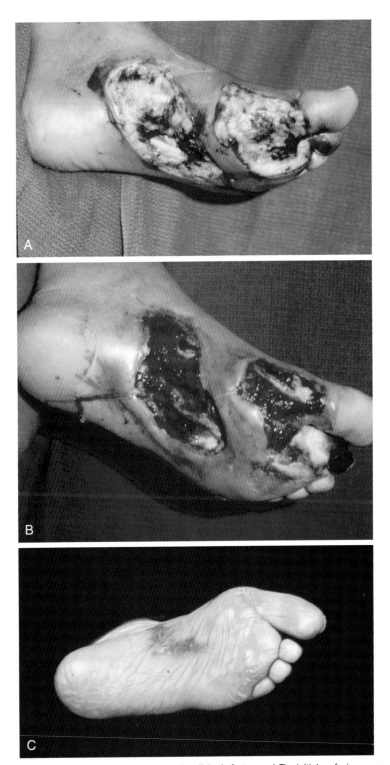

Color Plate 25 *A,* A 78-year-old patient with a limb-threatening diabetic foot wound. The initial perfusion pressure was normal, but transcutaneous partial pressure of oxygen (tcPo$_2$) tension was low. *B,* Wound after initial surgical debridement and after 15 hyperbaric oxygen therapy (HBOT) treatments. *C,* Postoperative follow-up view of wound after 30 HBOT treatments with successful healing. *(Adapted from Zamboni WA: Applications of hyperbaric oxygen therapy in plastic surgery. In: Oriani G, Marroni A, Wattel F (eds): Handbook on Hyperbaric Medicine. New York, Springer, 1995, pp 443–507, by permission.)*

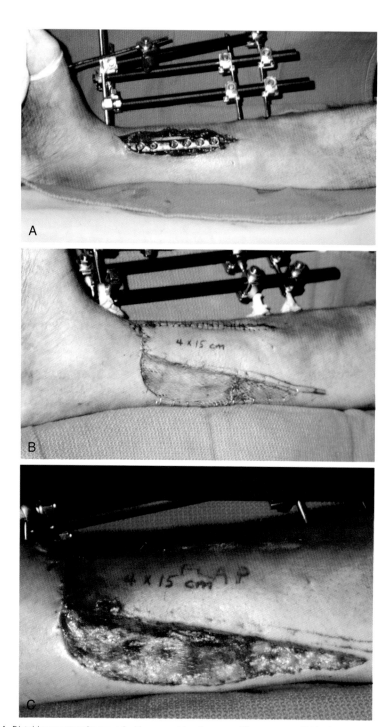

Color Plate 26 *A,* Distal lower extremity wound with exposed hardware requiring coverage. *B,* The hardware has been covered with a local fasciocutaneous flap. *C,* Evidence of compromise and impending necrosis in the distal random portion of the flap. The patient was started on the compromised flap hyperbaric oxygen therapy (HBOT) protocol.

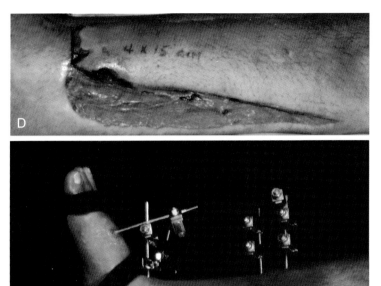

Color Plate 26 *Cont'd D*, Appearance of the flap after 10 treatments with improved appearance of the compromised portion of the flap. *E*, Complete healing was achieved after 20 treatments with salvage of the compromised portion. *(Adapted from Zamboni WA: Applications of hyperbaric oxygen therapy in plastic surgery. In: Oriani G, Marroni A, Wattel F (eds): Handbook on Hyperbaric Medicine. New York, Springer, 1995, pp 443–507, by permission.)*

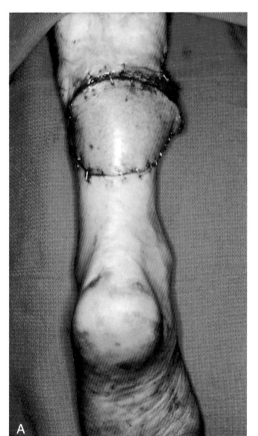

Color Plate 27 *A*, Immediate postoperative view of a free scapular fasciocutaneous flap to cover exposed calcaneal tendon in an unstable burn scar.

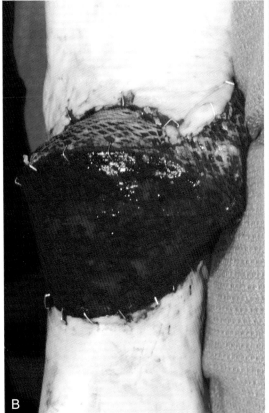

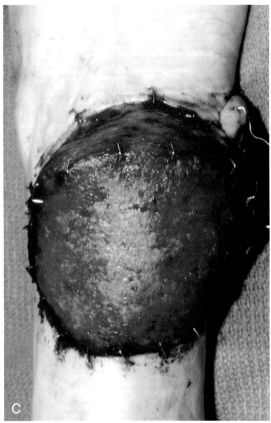

Color Plate 27 *Cont'd B,* Total venous occlusion 12 hours after the free scapular fasciocutaneous flap. Note the dark color of the flap. The patient refused surgery; therefore, immediate leeching and hyperbaric oxygen therapy (HBOT) was initiated. *C,* Flap after 6 days of HBOT with complete survival and establishment of inherent venous drainage. *D,* Six-month follow-up demonstrated stable soft-tissue coverage of the calcaneal tendon. *(Adapted from Zamboni WA: Applications of hyperbaric oxygen therapy in plastic surgery. In: Oriani G, Marroni A, Wattel F (eds): Handbook on Hyperbaric Medicine. New York, Springer, 1995, pp 443–507, by permission.)*

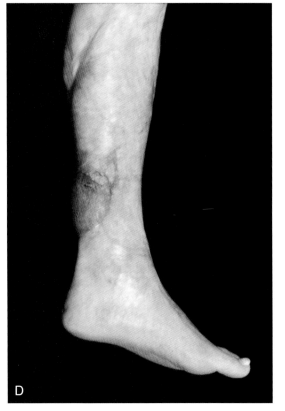

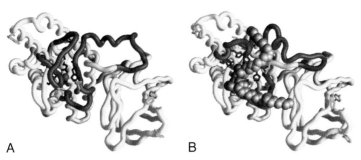

A   B

Color Plate 28 α-Toxin has been crystallized in two distinct conformations. *A* is believed to be catalytically active and so is known as the "open form." The second form, *B,* known as the "closed form," has two loops partially closing the active site and leaving the protein inactive. A short animated loop at the Birkbeck Toxin Structure Group Homepage Web site shows the dynamic opening and closing of the molecule, centered on its binding site. *(From Institute of Structural Molecular Biology, Birkbeck College School of Crystallography, University of London, UK: Available at http://people.cryst.bbk.ac.uk/_bcole04/ambrose.html, by permission. Accessed August 30, 2007.)*

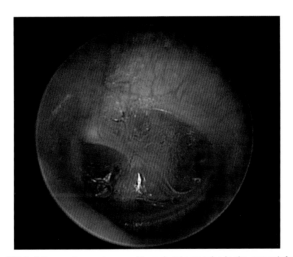

Color Plate 29 Left tympanic membrane with myringotomy tube in the anteroinferior quadrant.

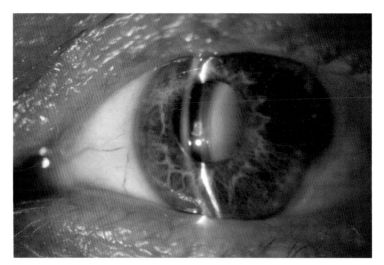

Color Plate 30 Slit-lamp image of a nuclear sclerotic cataract. *(Courtesy Dr. David Harris.)*

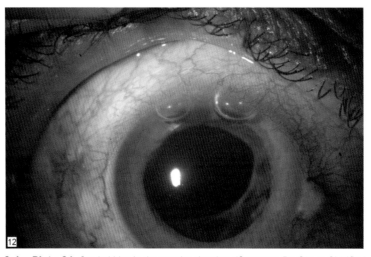

Color Plate 31 Gas bubbles in the anterior chamber. *(Courtesy Dr. Steve Chalfin.)*

one episode of near syncope during this period and had abnormal psychometric test scores when seen 3 months after the faulty furnace was replaced. No further long-term information was reported for this case. Another report involved four individuals with ~3-day exposures to CO, admission COHb levels of 17% to 29%, and no reported loss of consciousness. In studies performed 8 years after the exposure, the individuals were found to have psychiatric, neuropsychological, and IQ deficits thought to be attributable to CO.[286] Another report of seven cases also described long-term, seemingly permanent deficits in patients. This report adds the caveat that evaluations can be particularly challenging because it may be difficult to discern CO-mediated pathology from neuropsychological abnormalities that predated CO poisoning.[287]

In conclusion, despite extensive effort, little evidence has been reported for a syndrome related to "chronic" CO poisoning. Some patients have sustained permanent injuries and manifest persistent deficits. Evidence is lacking, however, to suggest that the injuries were caused by an accumulated "insult" resulting from an extended CO exposure.

REFERENCES

1. National Safety Council: How people died in home accidents, 1981. Accident Facts, 1982 ed. Chicago, National Safety Council, 1982, pp 80-84.
2. Cobb N, Etzel RA: Unintentional carbon monoxide-related deaths in the United States, 1979 through 1988. JAMA 266:659-663, 1991.
3. Mathieu D, Mathieu-Nolf M, Wattel F: Intoxication par le monoxide de carbone: Aspects actuels [Carbon monoxide poisoning: Present aspects]. Bull Acad Natl Med (Paris) 180:965-973, 1996.
4. Chen BH, Hong CJ, Pandey MR, et al: Indoor air pollution in developing countries. World Health Stat Q 43:127-138, 1990.
5. Litovitz TL, Holm KC, Bailey KM, et al: 1991 Annual report of the American Association of Poison Control Centers national data collection system. Am J Emerg Med 10:452-505, 1992.
6. Barret L, Danel V, Faure J: Carbon monoxide poisoning, a diagnosis frequently overlooked. Clin Toxicol 23:309-313, 1985.
7. Dolan MC, Haltom TL, Barrows GH, et al: Carboxyhemoglobin levels in patients with flu-like symptoms. Ann Emerg Med 15:653, 1986.
8. Fisher J, Rubin KP: Occult carbon monoxide poisoning. Arch Intern Med 142:1270-1271, 1982.
9. Grace TW, Platt FW: Subacute carbon monoxide poisoning. JAMA 246:1698-1700, 1981.
10. Heckerling PS, Leikin JB, Maturen A, et al: Predictors of occult carbon monoxide poisoning in patients with headache and dizziness. Ann Intern Med 107:174-176, 1987.
11. Heckerling PS, Leikin JB, Maturen A: Occult carbon monoxide poisoning: Validation of a prediction model. Am J Med 84:251-256, 1988.
12. Heckerling PS, Leikin JB, Terzian CG, et al: Occult carbon monoxide poisoning in patients with neurologic illness. J Toxicol Clin Toxicol 28:29-44, 1990.
13. Kirkpatrick JN: Occult carbon monoxide poisoning. West J Med 146:52-56, 1987.
14. Meredith T, Vale A: Carbon monoxide poisoning. Br Med J 296:77-79, 1988.
15. Gajdos P, Conso M, Korach JM, et al: Incidence and causes of carbon monoxide intoxication: Results of an epidemiological survey in a French department. Arch Environ Health 46:373-376, 1991.
16. Gujer H: Accidental CO poisoning caused by incomplete combustion of liquid gases. Soz Pravantivmed 27:39-42, 1982.
17. Hung D, Deng J, Yang C, et al: The climate and the occurrence of carbon monoxide poisoning in Taiwan. Hum Exp Toxicol 13:493-495, 1994.
18. Kim Y: Seasonal variation in carbon monoxide poisoning in urban Korea. J Epidemiol Comm Health 39:79-81, 1985.
19. Milis L, Lagasse R: Carbon monoxide poisoning in the Brussels metropolitan area. Home survey technics and proposals for action. Arch Belge 47:24-28, 1989.
20. Saunders PJ: Surveillance of non-infectious environmental hazards in the West Midlands. Chemical Incident 1:1, 1996.
21. Taudorf K, Michelsen K: The danger of CO poisoning from gas water heaters. A study of 124 systems and their uses. Ugeskr Laeger 145:3593-3598, 1983.
22. Theilade P: Carbon monoxide poisoning. Five year's experience of a defined population. Am J Forensic Med Pathol 11:219-225, 1990.
23. Thomsen JL, Kardel T: Accidents caused by gas water heaters. Fatalities and a non fatal case. Ugeskr Laeger 145:3598-3600, 1983.
24. Bernard C: An Introduction to the Study of Experimental Medicine [original publication 1865]. New York: HC Greene Dover Publications, 1957.
25. Haldane J: The action of carbonic oxide on man. J Physiol 18:430-462, 1895.
26. Douglas CG, Haldane JS, Haldane JBS: The laws of combination of haemoglobin with carbon monoxide and oxygen. J Physiol (Lond) 44:275-304, 1912.
27. Coburn RF, Forster RE, Kane PB: Considerations of the physiological variables that determine the blood carboxyhemoglobin concentration in man. J Clin Invest 44:1899-1910, 1965.
28. Pace N, Strajman E, Walken EL: Acceleration of carbon monoxide elimination in man by high pressure oxygen. Science 111:652-654, 1950.
29. Peterson JE, Steward RD: Absorption and elimination of carbon monoxide by inactive young men. Arch Environ Health 21:165-171, 1970.

30. Root WS: Carbon monoxide. In: Fenn WD, Rahn H (eds): Handbook of Physiology, vol II, Sect 3. Washington, DC, American Physiological Society, 1965, pp 1087-1098.

31. Weaver LK, Howe S, Hopkins R, et al: Carboxyhemoglobin half-life in carbon monoxide-poisoned patients treated with 100% oxygen at atmospheric pressure. Chest 117:801-808, 2000.

32. Burney RE, Wu S, Meniroff MJ: Mass carbon monoxide poisoning: Clinical effects and results of treatment in 184 victims. Ann Emerg Med 11:394-399, 1982.

33. Jay GD, Tetz DJ, Hartigan CF: Portable hyperbaric oxygen therapy in the emergency department with a modified Gamow bad. Ann Emerg Med 26:707-711, 1995.

34. Myers RAM, Jones DW, Britten JS: Carbon monoxide half-life study. In: Kindwall EP (ed): Proceedings of the Eighth International Congress on Hyperbaric Medicine. Flagstaff, Ariz, Best Publishing, 1987, pp 263-266.

35. Britton JS, Myers RAM: Effects of hyperbaric treatment on carbon monoxide elimination in humans. Undersea Biomed Res 12:431-438, 1985.

36. Wagner JA, Horvath SM, Dahms TE: Carbon monoxide elimination. Respir Physiol 23:41-47, 1975.

37. Forster RE: Carbon monoxide and the partial pressure of oxygen in tissue. Ann NY Acad Sci 174:233, 1970.

38. Tenney SM: A theoretical analysis of the relationships between venous blood and mean tissue oxygen pressure. Respir Physiol 20:283, 1977.

39. Coburn RF: Mechanisms of carbon monoxide toxicity. Prev Med 8:310, 1979.

40. Meilin S, Rogatsky GG, Thom SR, et al: Effects of carbon monoxide on the brain may be mediated by nitric oxide. J Appl Physiol 81:1078-1083, 1996.

41. Doblar DD, Santiago TV, Edelman NJ: Correlation between ventilatory and cerebrovascular responses to inhalation of CO. J Appl Physiol Respir Environ Exercise Physiol 43:455, 1977.

42. Koehler RC, Jones MD, Traystman RJ: Cerebral circulatory response to carbon monoxide and hypoxic hypoxia in the lamb. Am J Physiol 243:H27, 1977.

43. Paulson, OB, Parving HH, Olesen J, et al: Influence of carbon monoxide and of hemodilution on cerebral blood flow and blood gases in man. J Appl Physiol Respir Environ Exercise Physiol 35:111, 1973.

44. Traystman RJ, Fitzgerald RS, Loscutoff SC: Cerebral circulatory responses to arterial hypoxia in normal and chemodenervated dogs. Circ Res 42:649, 1981.

45. Roth RA Jr, Rubin RJ: Comparison of the effect of carbon monoxide and of hypoxic hypoxia. I. In vivo metabolism, distribution and action of hexobarbital. J Pharmacol Exp Ther 199:53, 1976.

46. Arnow WS, Isbell MW: Carbon monoxide effect of exercise-induced angina pectoris. Ann Intern Med 79:392, 1973.

47. Halperin MH, McFarland RA, Niven JI, et al: The time course of the effects of carbon monoxide on visual thresholds. J Physiol 146:583, 1959.

48. Horvath SM, Raven PB, Dahms TE, et al: Maximal aerobic capacity at different levels of carboxyhemoglobin. J Appl Physiol Respir Environ Exercise Physiol 38:300, 1975.

49. Winston JM, Roberts RJ: Influence of carbon monoxide, hypoxic hypoxia or potassium cyanide pretreatment on acute carbon monoxide and hypoxic hypoxia lethality. J Pharm Exp Ther 193:713, 1975.

50. Resch H, Zawinka C, Weigert G, et al: Inhaled carbon monoxide increases retinal and choroidal blood flow in healthy humans. Invest Ophthal Vis Sci 46:4275-4280, 2005.

51. Thom SR, Ohnishi ST, Ischiropoulos H, et al: Nitric oxide released by platelets inhibits neutrophil B_2 integrin function following acute carbon monoxide poisoning. Toxicol Appl Pharmacol 128:105-110, 1994.

52. Thom SR, Ischiropoulos H: Mechanism of oxidative stress from low levels of carbon monoxide, Health Effect Institute Research Report 80. Cambridge, Mass, Health Effects Institute, 1997.

53. Thom SR, Xu YA, Ischiropoulos H: Vascular endothelial cells generate peroxynitrite in response to carbon monoxide exposure. Chem Res Toxicol 10:1023-1031, 1997.

54. Ischiropoulos H, Beers MF, Ohnishi ST, et al: Nitric oxide and perivascular tyrosine nitration following carbon monoxide poisoning in the rat. J Clin Invest 97:2260-2267, 1996.

55. Thom SR, Ohnishi ST, Fisher D, et al: Pulmonary vascular stress from carbon monoxide. Toxicol Appl Pharmacol 154:12-19, 1999.

56. Thom SR, Fisher D, Xu YA, et al: Role of nitric oxide-derived oxidants in vascular injury from carbon monoxide in the rat. Am J Physiol 276(3 pt 2) 45: H984-H992, 1999.

57. Thom SR, Fisher D, Xu YA, et al: Adaptive responses and apoptosis in endothelial cells exposed to carbon monoxide. Proc Natl Acad Sci USA 97:1305-1310, 2000.

58. Gibson QH, Olson JS, McKinnie RE, et al: A kinetic description of ligand binding to sperm whale myoglobin. J Biol Chem 261:10228-10239, 1986.

59. Coburn RF: The carbon monoxide body stores. Ann NY Acad Sci 174:11-22, 1970.

60. Gothert M, Lutz F, Malorny G: Carbon monoxide partial pressure in tissue of different animals. Environ Res 3:303-309, 1970.

61. Schmidt HHHW, Nau H, Wittfoht W, et al: Arginine is a physiological precursor of endothelium-derived nitric oxide. Eur J Pharmacol 154:213-216, 1988.

62. Thom SR, Bhopale VM, Han ST, et al: Intravascular neutrophil activation due to carbon monoxide poisoning. Am J Respir Crit Care Med 174:1239-1248, 2006.

63. Dembinska-Kiec A, Zmuda A, Wenhrynowicz O, et al: P-selectin-mediated adherence of platelets to neutrophils is regulated by prostanoids and nitric oxide. Int J Tissue React 15:55-64, 1993.

64. Hirayama A, Noronha-Dutra AA, Gordge MP, et al: S-nitrosothiols are stored by platelets and released during platelet-neutrophil interactions. Nitric Oxide 3:95-104, 1999.

65. Radomski MW, Palmer RM, Moncada S: Comparative pharmacology of endothelium-derived relaxing factor. Nitric oxide and prostacyclin in platelets. Br J Pharmacol 92:181-187, 1987.

66. Hirayama A, Noronha-Dutra AA, Gordge MP, et al: S-nitrosothiols are stored by platelets and released during platelet-neutrophil interactions. Nitric Oxide 3:95-104, 1999.

67. Brown AS, Moro MA, Masse JM, et al: Nitric oxide-dependent and independent effects on human

platelets treated with peroxynitrite. Cardiovasc Res 40:380–388, 1998.

68. Hirayama A, Noronha-Dutra AA, Gordge MP, et al: S-nitrosothiols are stored by platelets and released during platelet-neutrophil interactions. Nitric Oxide 3:95–104, 1999.

69. Rainger EE, Rowley AF, Nash GB: Adhesion-dependent release of elastase from human neutrophils in a novel, flow-based model: Specificity of different chemotactic agents. Blood 92:4819–4827, 1998.

70. Lau D, Mollnau H, Eiserich JP, et al: Myeloperoxidase mediates neutrophil activation by association with CD11b/CD18 integrins. Proc Natl Acad Sci USA 102:431–436, 2005.

71. Baldus S, Eiserich JP, Mani A, et al: Endothelial transcytosis of myeloperoxidase confers specificity to vascular ECM proteins as targets of tyrosine nitration. J Clin Invest 108:1759–1770, 2001.

72. Brennan ML, Wu W, Fu X, et al: Defining both the role of peroxidases in nitrotyrosine formation in vivo using eosinophil peroxidase and myeloperoxidase-deficient mice, and the nature of peroxidase-generated reactive nitrogen species. J Biol Chem 277:17415–17427, 2002.

73. Baldus S, Eiserich JP, Brennan ML, et al: Spatial mapping of pulmonary and vascular nitrotyrosine reveals the pivotal role of myeloperoxidase as a catalyst for tyrosine nitration in inflammatory diseases. Free Radic Biol Med 33:1010–1019, 2002.

74. Marletta MA, Yoon PS, Iyengar R, et al: Macrophage oxidation of L-arginine to nitrite and nitrate: Nitric oxide is an intermediate. Biochemistry 27:8706–8711, 1988.

75. Sohn HY, Krotz F, Zahler S, et al: Crucial role of local peroxynitrite formation in neutrophil-induced endothelial cell activation. Cardiovasc Res 57:804–815, 2003.

76. Zouki C, Zhang SL, Chan JS, Filep JG: Peroxynitrite induces integrin-dependent adhesion of human neutrophils to endothelial cells via activation of the Raf-1/MEK/Erk pathway. FASEB J 15:25–27, 2001.

77. Thom SR, Fisher D, Manevich Y: Roles for platelet-activating factor and *NO-derived oxidants causing neutrophil adherence after CO poisoning. Am J Physiol Heart Circ Physiol 281:H923–H930, 2001.

78. Thom SR, Kang M, Fisher D, et al: Release of glutathione from erythrocytes and other markers of oxidative stress in carbon monoxide poisoning. J Appl Physiol 82:1424–1432, 1997.

79. Piantadosi CA, Carraway MS, Suliman HB: Carbon monoxide, oxidative stress, and mitochondrial permeability pore transition. Free Radic Biol Med 40:1332–1339, 2006.

80. Thom SR, Bhopale VM, Fisher D, et al: Delayed neuropathology after carbon monoxide poisoning is immune-mediated. Proc Natl Acad Sci USA 101:13660–13665, 2004.

81. Clementi E, Brown GC, Foxwell N, et al: On the mechanism by which vascular endothelial cells regulate their oxygen consumption. Proc Natl Acad Sci USA 96:1559–1562, 1999.

82. Palacios-Callender M, Quintero M, Hollis VS, et al: Endogenous NO regulates superoxide production at low oxygen concentrations by modifying the redox

state of cytochrome c oxidase. Proc Natl Acad Sci USA 101:7630–7635, 2004.

83. Koivisto A, Matthias A, Bronnikov G, et al: Kinetics of the inhibition of mitochondrial respiration by NO. FEBS Lett 417:75–80, 1997.

84. Xu W, Liu L, Charles IG, et al: Nitric oxide induces coupling of mitochondrial signalling with the endoplasmic reticulum stress response. Nat Cell Biol 6:1129–1134, 2004.

85. D'Amico G, Lam F, Hagen T, et al: Inhibition of cellular respiration by endogenously produced carbon monoxide. J Cell Sci 119:2291–2298, 2006.

86. Chance B, Williams GR: The respiratory chain and oxidative phosphorylation. Adv Enzymol 17:65, 1956.

87. Chance B, Erecinska M, Wagner M: Mitochondrial responses to carbon monoxide toxicity. Ann NY Acad Sci 174:193, 1970.

88. Keilin D, Hartree EF: Cytochrome and cytochrome oxidase. Proc R Soc Lond Ser B 27:167, 1939.

89. Coburn RF, Forman HJ: Carbon monoxide toxicity. In: Fishman AP, Farki LE, Geiger SR (eds): Handbook of Physiology. Baltimore, Williams & Wilkins, 1987, pp 439–456.

90. Brown SD, Piantadosi CA: In vivo binding of carbon monoxide to cytochrome c oxidase in rat brain. J Appl Physiol 68:604, 1990.

91. Piantadosi CA, Sylvia AL, Saltzman HA, et al: Carbon monoxide-cytochrome interactions in the brain of the fluorocarbon-perfused rat. J Appl Physiol 58:665, 1985.

92. Piantadosi CA: Spectrophotometry of cytochrome b in rat brain in vivo and in vitro. Am J Physiol 256:C840, 1989.

93. Piantadosi CA, Carraway MS, Suliman HB: Carbon monoxide, oxidative stress, and mitochondrial permeability pore transition. Free Radic Biol Med 40:1332–1339, 2006.

94. Piantadosi CA, Tatro L, Zhang J: Hydroxyl radical production in the brain after CO hypoxia in rats. Free Radic Biol Med 18:603–609, 1995.

95. Zhang J, Su Y, Oury TD, et al: Cerebral amino acid, norepinephrine and nitric oxide metabolism in CNS oxygen toxicity. Brain Res 606:56–62, 1993.

96. Piantadosi CA, Zhang J, Levin ED, et al: Apoptosis and delayed neuronal damage after carbon monoxide poisoning in the rat. Exp Neurol 147:103–114, 1997.

97. Gilmer B, Kilkenny J, Tomaszewski C, et al: Hyperbaric oxygen does not prevent neurologic sequelae after carbon monoxide poisoning. Acad Emerg Med 9:1–8, 2002.

98. Okeda R, Funata N, Song SJ, et al: Comparative study pathogenesis of selective cerebral lesions in carbon monoxide poisoning and nitrogen hypoxia in cats. Acta Neuropathol 56:265–272, 1982.

99. Dolinay T, Szilasi M, Liu M, et al: Inhaled carbon monoxide confers anti-inflammatory effects against ventilator-induced lung injury. Am J Respir Crit Care Med 170:613–120, 2004.

100. Otterbein LE, Bach FH, Alam J, et al: Carbon monoxide has anti-inflammatory effects involving the mitogen-activated protein kinase pathway. Nat Med 6:422–428, 2000.

101. Otterbein LE, Zuckerbraun BS, Haga M, et al: Carbon monoxide suppresses arteriosclerotic lesions associated

with chronic graft rejection and with balloon injury. Nat Med 9:183-190, 2003.

102. Chin BY, Jiang G, Wegiel B, et al: Hypoxia-inducible factor 1α stabilization by carbon monoxide results in cytoprotective preconditioning. Proc Natl Acad Sci USA 104:5109-5114, 2007.

103. Mazzola S, Forni M, Albertini M, et al: Carbon monoxide pretreatment prevents respiratory derangement and ameliorates hyperacute endotoxic shock in pigs. FASEB J 14:2045-2047, 2005.

104. Moore BA, Overhaus M, Whitcomb J, et al: Brief inhalation of low-dose carbon monoxide protects rodents and swine from postoperative ileus. Crit Care Med 6:1317-1326, 2005.

105. Neto JS, Nakao A, Kimizuka K, et al: Protection of transplant-induced renal ischemia-reperfusion injury with carbon monoxide. Am J Physiol 287:F979-F989, 2004.

106. Ameredes BT, Otterbein LE, Kohut LK, et al: Low-dose carbon monoxide reduces airway hyperresponsiveness in mice. Am J Physiol 285:L1270-L1276, 2003.

107. Zuckerbraun BS, Otterbein LE, Boyle P, et al: Carbon monoxide protects against the development of experimental necrotizing enterocolitis. Am J Physiol 289:G607-G613, 2005.

108. Nakao A, Neto JS, Kanno S, et al: Protection against ischemia/reperfusion injury in cardiac and renal transplantation with carbon monoxide, biliverdin and both. Am J Transplant 5:282-291, 2005.

109. Taille C, El-Benna J, Lanone S, et al: Mitochondrial respiratory chain and NAD(P)H oxidase are targets for the antiproliferative effect of carbon monoxide in human airway smooth muscle. J Biol Chem 280:25350-25360, 2005.

110. Emerling BM, Platanias LC, Black E, et al: Mitochondrial reactive oxygen species activation of p38 mitogen-activated protein kinase is required for hypoxia signaling. Mol Cell Biol 25:4853-4862, 2005.

111. Favory R, Lancel S, Tissier S, et al: Myocardial dysfunction and potential cardiac hypoxia in rats induced by carbon monoxide inhalation. Am J Respir Crit Care Med 174:320-325, 2006.

112. Boehning D, Moon C, Sharma S, et al: Carbon monoxide neurotransmission activated by CK2 phosphorylation of heme oxygenase-2. Neuron 40:129-137, 2003.

113. Verma A, Hirsch DJ, Glatt CE, et al: Carbon monoxide: A putative neural messenger. Science 259:381-384, 1993.

114. Alkadhi KA, Al Hijailan RS, Malik K, Hogan YH: Retrograde carbon monoxide is required for induction of long term potentiation in rat superior cervical ganglion. J Neurosci 21:3515-3520, 2001.

115. Zhuo M, Small SA, Kandel ER, Hawkins RD: Nitric oxide and carbon monoxide produce activity-dependent long-term synaptic enhancement in hippocampus. Science 260:1946-1950, 1993.

116. Zakhary R, Poss KD, Jaffrey SR, et al: Targeted gene deletion of hemeoxygenase 2 reveals neural role for carbon monoxide. Proc Natl Acad Sci USA 94:14848-14853, 1997.

117. Hara S, Mukai T, Kurosaki K, et al: Characterization of hydroxyl radical generation in the striatum of free-moving rats due to carbon monoxide poisoning,

as determined by in vivo microdialysis. Brain Res 1016:281-284, 2004.

118. Hiramatsu M, Yokoyama S, Nabeshima T, et al: Changes in concentrations of dopamine, serotonin, and their metabolites induced by carbon monoxide (CO) in the rat striatum as determined by in vivo microdialysis. Pharmacol Biochem Behav 48:9-15, 1994.

119. Newby MB, Roberts RJ, Bhatnagar RK: Carbon monoxide- and hypoxia-induced effects on catecholamines in the mature and developing rat brain. J Pharmacol Exp Ther 206:61-68, 1978.

120. Rothman SM, Olney JW: Excitotoxicity and the NMDA receptor. Trends Neurosci 10:299-302, 1987.

121. Ishimaru HA: Effects of n-methyl-d-aspartate receptor antagonists on carbon monoxide-induced brain damage in mice. J Pharmacol Exp Ther 261:349-352, 1992.

122. Maurice T, Hiramatsu M, Kameyama T, et al: Cholecystokinin-related peptides, after systemic or central administration, prevent carbon monoxide-induced amnesia in mice. J Pharmacol Exp Ther 269:665-673, 1994.

123. Nabeshima T, Katoh A, Ishimaru H, et al: Carbon monoxide-induced delayed amnesia. J Pharmacol Exp Ther 256:378-384, 1991.

124. Thom SR, Fisher D, Zhang J, et al: Neuronal nitric oxide synthase and N-methyl-D-aspartate neurons in experimental carbon monoxide poisoning. Toxicol Appl Pharmacol 194:280-295, 2004.

125. Yang JQ, Qi-Xin Z: Protective effect of nimodipine against cerebral injury induced by subacute carbon monoxide intoxication in mice. Acta Pharmacol Sin 22:423-427, 2001.

126. Bredt DS, Snyder SH: Nitric oxide mediates glutamate-linked enhancement of cGMP levels in the cerebellum. Proc Natl Acad Sci USA 86:9030-9033, 1989.

127. Garthwaite J, Charles SL, Chess-Williams R: Endothelium-derived relaxing factor release on activation of NMDA receptors suggests role as intercellular messenger in the brain. Nature 336:385-388, 1988.

128. Rodriguez-Alvarez J, Lafon-Cazal M, Blanco I, et al: Different routes of Ca^{++} influx in NMDA-mediated generation of nitric oxide and arachidonic acid. Eur J Neurosci 9:867-870, 1997.

129. Gilman SC, Bonner MJ, Pellmar TC: Peroxide effects on [^{3}H]L-glutamate release by synaptosomes isolated from the cerebral cortex. Neurosci Lett 140:157-160, 1992.

130. Trotti D, Rizzini BL, Rossi D, et al: Neuronal and glial glutamate transporters possess an SH-based redox regulatory mechanism. Eur J Neurosci 9:1236-1243, 1997.

131. Trotti D, Rossi D, Gjesdal O, et al: Peroxynitrite inhibits glutamate transporter subtypes. J Biol Chem 271:5976-5979, 1996.

132. Volterra A, Trotti D, Tromba C, et al: Glutamate uptake inhibition by oxygen free radicals in rat cortical astrocytes. J Neurosci 14:2924-2932, 1994.

133. Jones DP, Kennedy FG: Intracellular oxygen supply during hypoxia. Am J Physiol 243:C247, 1982.

134. Satran D, Henry CR, Adkinson C, et al: Cardiovascular manifestations of moderate to severe carbon monoxide poisoning. J Am Coll Cardiol 45:1513-1516, 2005.

135. Henry CR, Satran D, Lindgren B, et al: Myocardial injury and long-term mortality following moderate to

severe carbon monoxide poisoning. JAMA 295:398-402, 2006.

136. Biasucci LM, D'Onofrio G, Liuzzo G, et al: Intracellular neutrophil myeloperoxidase is reduced in unstable angina and acute myocardial infarction, but its reduction is not related to ischemia. J Am Coll Cardiol 27:611-616, 1996.

137. Furman MI, Benoit SE, Barnard MR, et al: Increased platelet reactivity and circulating monocyte-platelet aggregates in patients with stable coronary artery disease. J Am Coll Cardiol 31:352-358, 1998.

138. Ott I, Neumann FJ, Gawaz M, et al: Increased neutrophil-platelet adhesion in patients with unstable angina. Circulation 94:1239-1246, 1996.

139. Zhao S, Zhang Y, Gu Y, et al: Heme oxygenase-1 mediates up-regulation of adhesion molecule expression induced by peroxynitrite in endothelial cells. J Soc Gynecol Investig 11:465-471, 2004.

140. Sohn HY, Krotz F, Zahler S, et al: Crucial role of local peroxynitrite formation in neutrophil-induced endothelial cell activation. Cardiovasc Res 57:804-815, 2003.

141. Thom SR: Leukocytes in carbon monoxide-mediated brain oxidative injury. Toxicol Appl Pharmacol 123:234-247, 1993.

142. Thom SR: Functional inhibition of leukocyte B2 integrins by hyperbaric oxygen in carbon monoxide-mediated brain injury in rats. Toxicol Appl Pharmacol 123:248-256, 1993.

143. Thom SR: Dehydrogenase conversion to oxidase and lipid peroxidation in brain after carbon monoxide poisoning. J Appl Physiol 73:1584-1589, 1992.

144. Phan SH, Gannon DE, Ward PA, et al: Mechanism of neutrophil-induced xanthine dehydrogenase to xanthine oxidase conversion in endothelial cells: Evidence of a role for elastase. Am J Respir Cell Mol Biol 6:270-278, 1992.

145. Wakabayashi Y, Fujita H, Morita I, et al: Conversion of xanthine dehydrogenase to xanthine oxidase in bovine carotid artery endothelial cells induced by activated neutrophils: Involvement of adhesion molecules. Biochim Biophys Acta 1265:103-109, 1995.

146. Steinbrecher UP: Oxidation of human low density lipoprotein results in derivatization of lysine residues of apolipoprotein B by lipid peroxide decomposition products. J Biol Chem 262:3603-3608, 1987.

147. Thiele GM, Tuma DJ, Willis MS, et al: Soluble proteins modified with acetaldehyde and malondialdehyde are immunogenic in the absence of adjuvant. Alcohol Clin Exp Res 22:1731-1739, 1998.

148. Fan LW, Pang Y, Lin PG, et al: Minocycline attenuates lipopolysaccharide-induced white matter injury in the neonatal rat brain. J Neurosci 133:159-168, 2005.

149. McGeer PL, Itagaki S, Boyes BE, et al: Reactive microglia are positive for HLA-DR in the substantia nigra of Parkinson's and Alzheimer's disease brains. Neurology 38:1285-1291, 1988.

150. Montague PR, Gancayco CD, Winn MJ, et al: Role of NO production in NMDA receptor-mediated neurotransmitter release in cerebral cortex. Science 263:973-977, 1994.

151. Ballestas ME, Benveniste EN: Interleukin 1β and tumor necrosis factor α mediated regulation of ICAM-1 gene expression in astrocytes requires protein kinase C. Glia 14:267-278, 1995.

152. Wu DC, Jackson-Lewis V, Vila M, et al: Blockade of microglial activation is neuroprotective in the 1-methyl-4-phenyl-1,2,3,6-tetrahydropyridine mouse model of Parkinson Disease. J Neurosci 22:1763-1771, 2002.

153. Feng R, Rampon C, Tang YP, et al: Deficient neurogenesis in forebrain-specific presenilin-1 knockout mice is associated with reduced clearance of hippocampal memory traces. Neuron 32:911, 2001.

154. Monje ML, Mizumatsu SA, Fike J, et al: Irradiation induces neural precursor-cell dysfunction. Nat Med 8:955-962, 2002.

155. Madsen TM, Kristjansen PEG, Bolwig TG, et al: Arrested neuronal proliferation and impaired hippocampal function following fractionated brain irradiation in the adult rat. Neuroscience 119:635-642, 2003.

156. Shors TJ, Miesegaes G, Beylin A, et al: Neurogenesis in the adult is involved in the formation of trace memories. Nature 410:372-376, 2001.

157. Han S-T, Bhopale VM, Thom SR: Xanthine oxidoreductase and neurological sequelae of carbon monoxide poisoning. Toxicol Lett 170:111-115, 2007.

158. Bogusz M, Cholewa L, Pach J, Mlodkowska KA: Comparison of two types of acute carbon monoxide poisoning. Arch Toxicol 33:141-149, 1975.

159. Choi IS: Delayed neurologic sequelae in carbon monoxide intoxication. Arch Neurol 40:433-435, 1983.

160. Crocker PJ, Walker JS: Pediatric carbon monoxide toxicity. J Emerg Med 3:443-448, 1985.

161. Thom SR: Carbon monoxide-mediated brain lipid peroxidation in the rat. J Appl Physiol 68:997-1003, 1990.

162. Burney RE, Wu S-C, Nemiroff MJ: Mass carbon monoxide poisoning: Clinical effects and results of treatment in 184 victims. Ann Emerg Med 11:394-399, 1982.

163. McFarland RA, Roughton FJW, Halperin MH, Niven JI: The effects of carbon monoxide and altitude on visual thresholds. J Aviat Med 15:381-394, 1944.

164. Halperin MH, McFarland RA, Niven JI, Roughton FJW: The time course of the effects of carbon monoxide on visual thresholds. J Physiol Lond 146:583-593, 1959.

165. McFarland RA: The effects of exposure to small quantities of carbon monoxide on vision. Ann NY Acad Sci 174:301-312, 1970.

166. Abramson E, Heyman T: Dark adaptation and inhalation of carbon monoxide. Acta Physiol Scand 7:303-305, 1944.

167. Luria SM, McKay CL: Effects of low levels of carbon monoxide on visions of smokers and nonsmokers. Arch Environ Health 34:38-44, 1979.

168. Von Restorff W, Hebisch S: Dark adaptation of the eye during carbon monoxide exposure in smokers and nonsmokers. Aviat Space Environ Med 59:928-931, 1988.

169. Hudnell HK, Benignus VA: Carbon monoxide and exposure and visual detection thresholds. Neurotoxicol Teratol 11:363-371, 1989.

170. Beard RR, Wertheim GA: Behavioral impairment associated with small doses of carbon monoxide. Am J Public Health 57:2012-2022, 1967.

171. O'Donnell RD, Chikos P, Theodore J: Effects of carbon monoxide exposure on human sleep and psychomotor performance. J Appl Physiol 31:513-518, 1971.

172. Stewart RD, Newton PE, Hosko MJ, Peterson JE: Effect of carbon monoxide on time perception. Arch Environ Health 27:155-160, 1973.

173. Wright GR, Shephard RJ: Carbon monoxide exposure and auditory duration discrimination. Arch Environ Health 33:226-235, 1978.

174. Otto DA, Benignus VA, Prah JD: Carbon monoxide and human time discrimination: Failure to replicate Beard-Wertheim experiments. Aviat Space Environ Med 50:40-43, 1979.

175. Benignus VA: Importance of experimenter-blind procedure in neurotoxicology. Neurotoxicol Teratol 14:45-49, 1993.

176. Benignus VA: Behavioral effects of carbon monoxide: Meta analyses and extrapolations. J Appl Physiol 76:1310-1316, 1994.

177. Amitai Y, Zlotogorski Z, Golan-Katzav V, et al: Neuropsychological impairment from acute low-level exposure to carbon monoxide. Arch Neurol 55:845-848, 1998.

178. Anderson EW, Andelman RJ, Strauch JM: Effects of low-level carbon monoxide exposure on onset and duration of angina pectoris. Ann Intern Med 79:46-50, 1973.

179. Allred EN, Bleecker ER, Chaitman BR, et al: Short-term effects of carbon monoxide exposure on the exercise performance of subjects with coronary artery disease. N Engl J Med 321:1426-1432, 1989.

180. Sheps DS, Herbst MC, Hinderliter AL, et al: Production of arrhythmias by elevated carboxyhemoglobin in patients with coronary artery disease. Ann Intern Med 113:343-351, 1990.

181. Marek Z, Piejko M: Circulatory failure in acute carbon monoxide poisonings. Forensic Sci 1:419-425, 1972.

182. Hubalewska A, Pach D, Pach J, et al: Clinical status of carbon monoxide poisoned patients and the results of rest 99mTc-MIBI and 99mTc-Amiscan heart scintigraphy performed in the acute phase of intoxication and stress-rest 99mTc-MIBI scintigraphy six months later. Przegl Lek 61:213-216, 2004.

183. Scharf SM, Thames MD, Sargent RK: Transmural myocardial infarction after exposure to carbon monoxide in coronary-artery disease. N Engl J Med 291:85-86, 1974.

184. Cramlet SH, Erickson HH, Gorman HA: Ventricular function following acute carbon monoxide exposure. J Appl Physiol 39:482-486, 1975.

185. Swank G, Jain AC, Morise AP, Schmidt S: Carbon monoxide poisoning: A case report of reversible cardiomyopathy. W V Med J 100:228-231, 2004.

186. Johnson CD: Carbon monoxide toxicity with neurological and cardiac complications. Bol Asoc Med PR 97:315-322, 2005.

187. Kurt TL, Mogielnicki RP, Chandler JE: Association of the frequency of acute cardiorespiratory complaints with ambient levels of carbon monoxide. Chest 74:10-14, 1978.

188. Myers RA, Snyder SK, Emhoff TA: Subacute sequelae of carbon monoxide poisoning. Ann Emerg Med 14:1163-1167, 1985.

189. Torne R, Soyer HP, Leb G, et al: Skin lesions in carbon monoxide intoxication. Dermatologica 183:212-215, 1991.

190. Perrone J, Hoffman RS: Falsely elevated carboxyhemoglobin levels secondary to fetal hemoglobin. Acad Emerg Med 3:287-289, 1996.

191. Hampson NB: Pulse oximetry in severe carbon monoxide poisoning. Chest 114:1036-1041, 1998.

192. Sokal JA, Kralkowska E: The relationship between exposure duration, carboxyhemoglobin, blood glucose, pyruvate and lactate and the severity of intoxication in 39 cases of acute carbon monoxide poisoning in man. Arch Toxicol 57:196-199, 1985.

193. Takahashi M, Maemura K, Swada Y: Hyperamylasemia in acute carbon monoxide poisoning. J Trauma 22:311-314, 1982.

194. Brvar M, Mozina H, Osredkar J, et al: S100B protein in carbon monoxide poisoning: A pilot study. Resuscitation 61:357-360, 2004.

195. Pach D, Gawlikowski T, Targosz D, et al: B-type natriuretic peptide plasma concentration in acutely poisoned patients. Przegl Lek 62:465-467, 2005.

196. Ferrier D, Wallace CJ, Fletcher WA, et al: Magnetic resonance features in carbon monoxide poisoning. Can Assoc Radiol J 45:466-468, 1994.

197. Tuchman RF, Moser FG, Moshe SL: Carbon monoxide poisoning: Bilateral lesions in the thalamus on MR imaging of the brain. Pediatr Radiol 20:478-479, 1990.

198. Kawanami T, Kato T, Kurita K, et al: The pallidoreticular pattern of brain damage on MRI in a patient with carbon monoxide poisoning. J Neurol Neurosurg Psychiatry 64:282, 1998.

199. Porter SS, Hopkins RO, Weaver LK, et al: Corpus callosum atrophy and neuropsychological outcome following carbon monoxide poisoning. Arch Clin Neuropsychol 17:195-204, 2002.

200. Kesler SR, Hopkins RO, Weaver LK, et al: Verbal memory deficits associated with fornix atrophy in carbon monoxide. J Int Neuropsychol Soc 7:640-646, 2001.

201. Gale SD, Hopkins RO, Weaver LK, et al: MRI, quantitative MRI, SPECT and neuropsychological findings following carbon monoxide poisoning. Brain Injury 13:229-243, 1999.

202. Parkinson RB, Hopkins RO, Cleavinger HB, et al: White matter hyperintensities and neuropsychological outcome following carbon monoxide poisoning. Neurology 58:1525-1532, 2002.

203. Ducasse JL, Celsis P, Marc-Vergnes JP: Non-comatose patients with acute carbon monoxide poisoning: Hyperbaric or normobaric oxygenation? Undersea Hyperb Med 22:9-15, 1995.

204. Maeda Y, Kawasaki Y, Jibiki I, et al: Effect of therapy with oxygen under high pressure on regional cerebral blood flow in the interval form of carbon monoxide poisoning: Observation from subtraction of technetium-99m HMPAOSPECT brain imaging. Eur Neurol 31:380-383, 1991.

205. Shimosegawa E, Hatazawa J, Nagata K, et al: Cerebral blood flow and glucose metabolism measurements in a patient surviving one year after carbon monoxide intoxication. J Nucl Med 33:1696-1698, 1992.

206. Silverman CS, Brenner J, Murtagh FR: Hemorrhagic necrosis and vascular injury in carbon monoxide poisoning: MR demonstration. AJNR Am J Neuroradiol 14:168-170, 1993.

207. Sohn YH, Jeong Y, Kim HS, et al: The brain lesion responsible for parkinsonism after carbon monoxide poisoning. Arch Neurol 57:1214-1218, 2000.

208. Ginsberg MD, Myers RE, McDonagh BF: Experimental carbon monoxide encephalopathy in the primate. II. Clinical aspects, neuropathology, and physiologic correlation. Arch Neurol 30:209-216, 1974.

209. Lapresle J, Fardeau M: The central nervous system and carbon monoxide poisoning, II. Anatomical study of brain lesions following intoxication with carbon monoxide. Prog Brain Res 24:31-74, 1967.

210. Choi IS: Parkinsonism after carbon monoxide poisoning. Eur Neurol 48:30-33, 2002.

211. Ginsberg MD: Delayed neurological deterioration following hypoxia. Adv Neurol 26:21-44, 1979.

212. Roychowdhury S, Maljian JA, Galetta SL, et al: Postanoxic encephalopathy: Diffusion MR findings. J Comput Assist Tomogr 22:992-994, 1998.

213. Dooling EC, Richardson P: Delayed encephalopathy after strangling. Arch Neurol 33:196-199, 1976.

214. Gorman DF, Clayton D, Gilligan JE, et al: A longitudinal study of 100 consecutive admissions for carbon monoxide poisoning to the Royal Adelaide Hospital. Anaesth Intensive Care 20:311-316, 1992.

215. Mathieu D, Nolf M, Durocher A, et al: Acute carbon monoxide poisoning risk of late sequelae and treatment by hyperbaric oxygen. Clin Toxicol 23:315-324, 1985.

216. Raphael JC, Elkharrat D, Guincestre MCJ, et al: Trial of normobaric and hyperbaric oxygen for acute carbon monoxide intoxication. Lancet 1:414-419, 1989.

217. Thom SR, Taber RL, Mendiguren II, et al: Delayed neuropsychological sequelae following carbon monoxide poisoning and its prophylaxis by treatment with hyperbaric oxygen. Ann Emerg Med 25:474-480, 1995.

218. Weaver LK, Hopkins RO, Chan KJ, et al: Hyperbaric oxygen for acute carbon monoxide poisoning. N Engl J Med 347:1057-1067, 2002.

219. Weaver LK, Valentine KJ, Hopkins RO: Carbon monoxide poisoning: Risk factors for cognitive sequelae and the role of hyperbaric oxygen. Am J Resp Crit Care Med 2007;176:491-497.

220. Hopkin RO, Weaver LK, Valentine KJ, et al: Apolipoprotein E genotype and outcome with and without hyperbaric oxygen in acute carbon monoxide poisoning. Am J Resp Crit Care Med 176:1001-1006, 2007.

221. Scheinkestel CD, Bailey M, Myles PS, et al: Hyperbaric or normobaric oxygen in acute carbon monoxide poisoning: A randomised controlled clinical trial. Med J Australia 170:203-210, 1999.

222. Schiltz KL: Failure to assess motivation, need to consider psychiatric variables, and absence of comprehensive examination: A skeptical review of neuropsychologic assessment in carbon monoxide research. Undersea Hyperb Med 27:48-50, 2000.

223. Remick RA, Miles JE: Carbon monoxide poisoning: Neurologic and psychiatric sequelae. Can Med Assoc J 117:654-657, 1977.

224. Schulte JH: Effects of mild carbon monoxide intoxication. Arch Environ Health 7:524-530, 1963.

225. Brown SD, Piantadosi CA: Recovery of energy metabolism in rat brain after carbon monoxide hypoxia. J Clin Invest 89:666-672, 1991.

226. Thom SR: Antagonism of carbon monoxide-mediated brain lipid peroxidation by hyperbaric oxygen. Toxicol Appl Pharmacol 105:340-344, 1990.

227. End E, Long CW: Oxygen under pressure in carbon monoxide poisoning. J Ind Hyg Toxicol 24:302-306, 1942.

228. Peirce EC, Zacharias A, Alday JM Jr, et al: Carbon monoxide poisoning: Experimental hypothermic and hyperbaric studies. Surgery 72:229-237, 1972.

229. Thom SR, Bhopale VM, Fisher D: Hyperbaric oxygen reduces delayed immune-mediated neuropathology in experimental carbon monoxide poisoning. Toxicol Appl Pharmacol 213:152-159, 2006.

230. Junker C, Egger M, Schneider M, et al: The CONSORT statement. JAMA 276:1876-1877, 1996.

231. Raphael JC, Chevret S, Driheme A, et al: Managing carbon monoxide poisoning with hyperbaric oxygen [abstract]. J Toxicol Clin Toxicol 42:455-456, 2004.

232 Brown SD, Piantadosi CA: Hyperbaric oxygen for carbon monoxide poisoning [letter]. Lancet 2:1032, 1989.

233. Gorman DF, Gilligan JEF, Clayton DG: Hyperbaric oxygen for carbon monoxide poisoning [letter]. Lancet 2:1032, 1989.

234. Logue C: The Cochrane Library—Feedback. Available at: http://www.cochranefeedback.com/cf/cda/citation. do?id=9569#9569. Accessed November 27, 2006.

235. Aamar S, Saada A, Rotshenker S: Lesion-induced changes in the production of newly synthesized and secreted apo-E and other molecules are independent of the concomitant recruitment of blood-borne macrophages into injured peripheral nerves. J Neurochem 59:1287-1292, 1992.

236. Saunders AM, Strittmatter WJ, Schmechel D: Association of apolipoprotein E allele epsilon 4 with late-onset familial and sporadic Alzheimer's disease. Neurology 43:1467-1472, 1993.

237. Friedman G, Froom P, Sazbon L: Apolipotrotein E-epsilon 4 genotype predicts a poor outcome in survivors of traumatic brain injury. Neurology 52:244-248, 1999.

238. McCarron MO, Muir KW, Nicoll JA: Prospective study of apolipoprotein E genotype and functional outcome following ischemic stroke. Arch Neurol 57:1480-1484, 2000.

239. Goulon MA, Barios M, Rapin M, et al: Intoxication oxy carbonee at anoxie aique par inhalation de gay de charbon et d'hydrocarbures. Ann Med Interne (Paris) 120:335-339, 1969 [English translation: J Hyperbaric Med 1:23-41, 1986].

240. Hampson NB, Zmaeff JL: Outcome of patients experiencing cardiac arrest with carbon monoxide poisoning treated with hyperbaric oxygen. Ann Emerg Med 38:36-41, 2001.

241. Caravati EM, Adams CJ, Joyce SM, et al: Fetal toxicity associated with maternal carbon monoxide poisoning. Ann Emerg Med 17:714-717, 1988.

242. Elkharrat D, Raphael JC, Korach JM, et al: Acute carbon monoxide intoxication and hyperbaric oxygen in pregnancy. Intensive Care Med 17:289-292, 1991.

243. Norman CA, Halton DM: Is carbon monoxide a workplace teratogen? A review and evaluation of the literature. Ann Occup Hyg 34:335-347, 1990.

244. Ginsberg MD, Myers RE: Fetal brain injury after maternal carbon monoxide intoxication. Neurology 26:15-23, 1976.

245. Longo LD, Hill EP: Carbon monoxide uptake and elimination in fetal and maternal sheep. Am J Physiol 232: H324-H330, 1977.

246. Longo LD: The biological effects of carbon monoxide on the pregnant woman, fetus, and newborn infant. Am J Obstet Gynecol 129:69-103, 1977.

247. Brown DB, Mueller GI, Golich FC: Hyperbaric oxygen treatment for carbon monoxide poisoning in pregnancy: A case report. Aviat Space Environ Med 63:1011-1014, 1992.

248. Gabrielli A, Layon AJ: Carbon monoxide intoxication during pregnancy: A case presentation and patho-physiologic discussion, with emphasis on molecular mechanisms. J Clin Anesth 14:876-882, 1995.

249. Hollander DI, Nagey DA, Welch R, et al: Hyperbaric oxygen therapy for the treatment of acute carbon monoxide poisoning in pregnancy. A case report. J Reprod Med 32:615-617, 1987.

250. Koren G, Sharav T, Pastusazk A, et al: A multicenter, prospective study of fetal outcome following accidental carbon monoxide poisoning in pregnancy. Reprod Toxicol 5:397-403, 1991.

251. Ledingham IM, McBride TI, Jennett WB, et al: Fatal brain damage associated with cardiomyopathy of pregnancy with notes on caesarean section in a hyperbaric chamber. Br Med J 4:285-287, 1968.

252. Van Hoesen KB, Camporesi EM, Moon RE, et al: Should hyperbaric oxygen be used to treat the pregnant patient for acute carbon monoxide poisoning? JAMA 261:1039-1043, 1989.

253. Cho SH, Yun DR: The experimental study on the effect of hyperbaric oxygen on the pregnancy wastage of rats with acute carbon monoxide poisoning. Seoul J Med 23:67-75, 1982.

254. Gilman SC, Greene KM, Bradley ME, et al: Fetal development: Effects of simulated diving and hyperbaric oxygen treatment. Undersea Biomed Res 9:297-304, 1982.

255. Jennings RT: Women and the hazardous environment: When the pregnant patient requires hyperbaric oxygen therapy. Aviat Space Environ Med 58:370-374, 1987.

256. Pracyk JB, Stolp BW, Fife CE, et al: Brain computerized tomography after hyperbaric oxygen therapy for carbon monoxide poisoning. Undersea Hyperb Med 22:1-7, 1995.

257. Yang W, Jennison BL, Omaye ST: Cardiovascular disease hospitalization and ambient levels of carbon monoxide. J Toxicol Environ Health A 55:185-196, 1998.

258. Linn WS, Szlachcic Y, Gong H, et al: Air pollution and daily hospital admissions in metropolitan Los Angeles. Environ Health Perspect 108:427-434, 2000.

259. Andersen ZJ, Wahlin P, Raaschou-Nielsen O, et al: Ambient particle source apportionment and daily hospital admissions among children and elderly in Copenhagen. J Expo Sci Environ Epidemiol 17:625-636, 2007.

260. Stupfel M, Bouley G: Physiological and biochemical effects on rats and mice exposed to small concentrations of carbon monoxide for long periods. Ann NY Acad Sci 174:342, 1972.

261. Bambach GA, Penney DG, Negendank WG: In situ assessment of the rat heart during chronic carbon monoxide exposure using nuclear magnetic resonance imaging. J Appl Toxicol 11:43-49, 1991.

262. Penney DG, Giraldo AA, Van Egmond EM: Chronic carbon monoxide exposure in young rats alters coronary vessel growth. J Toxicol Environ Health 39:207-222, 1993.

263. Supfle K, Hofman P, May J: Hygienische studien uber kohlenoxyd. Zeitschr fur Hyg 115:623-633, 1933.

264. Supfle K, Hofman P, May J: Tierexperimentelle untersuchungen uber die chronische wirkung der auspuffgase von kraftfahrzeugen. Arch Hyg 112:84-88, 1934.

265. Lewey FH, Drabkin DL: Experimental chronic carbon monoxide poisoning in dogs. Am J Med Sci 208:502-511, 1944.

266. Floberg LE: Vestibular symptoms in carbon monoxide poisoning after unilateral ligation of the common carotid artery. Acta Otolaryngol Suppl 106:1-55, 1953.

267. Lindgren SA: A study of the effect of protracted occupational exposure to carbon monoxide. Acta Med Scand 167(suppl 356):1-105, 1960.

268. Kruger PD, Zorn O, Portheine F: Probleme akuter und chronischer Kohlenoxyd-Vergiftungen. Arch Gewerbepath 18:1-44, 1960.

269. Komatsu FS, Handa S, Ishii H, et al: The effect of prolonged exposure to carbon monoxide on human health. Med J Shinshu University 3:165-177, 1958.

270. Ely EW, Moorehead B, Haponik EF: Warehouse workers' headache: Emergency evaluation and management of 30 patients with carbon monoxide poisoning. Am J Med 98:145-155, 1995.

271. Beck HG: The clinical manifestations of chronic carbon monoxide poisoning. Ann Clin Med 5:1088-1096, 1926.

272. Beck HG: Slow carbon monoxide asphyxiation. JAMA 107:1025-1029, 1936.

273. Kirkpatrick JN: Occult carbon monoxide poisoning. Western J Med 146:52-56, 1987.

274. Shahbaz HM, Ray J, Wilson F: Carbon monoxide poisoning and sensorineural hearing loss. J Laryngol Otol 117:134-137, 2003.

275. Trese MT, Krohel GB, Hepler RS: Ocular effects of chronic carbon monoxide exposure. Ann Ophthalmol 11:536-538, 1980.

276. Stockard-Sullivan JE, Korsak RA, Webber DS, Edmond J: Mild carbon monoxide exposure and auditory function in the developing rat. J Neurosci Res 74:644-655, 2003.

277. Harbin TJ, Benignus VA, Muller KE, Barton CN: The effects of low-level carbon monoxide exposure upon evoked cortical potentials in young and elderly men. Neurotoxicol Teratol 10:93-100, 1988.

278. Gilbert GJ, Glaser GH: Neurologic manifestations of chronic carbon monoxide poisoning. N Engl J Med 261:1217-1220, 1959.

279. Grace TW, Platt FW: Subacute carbon monoxide poisoning. JAMA 246:1698-1700, 1981.

280. Pavese N, Mapolitano A, DeIaco G, et al: Clinical outcome and magnetic resonance imaging of carbon monoxide intoxication. A long term follow-up study. Ital J Neurol Sci 20:171-178, 1999.

281. Webb C, Vaitkevicius PV: Dementia with a seasonal onset secondary to carbon monoxide poisoning. J Am Geriatr Soc 45:1281-1282, 1997.

282. Foster M, Goodwin SR, Williams C, Loeffler J: Recurrent acute life-threatening events and lactic acidosis caused by chronic carbon monoxide poisoning in an infant. Pediatrics 104:e34-e39, 1999.

283. Knobeloch L, Jackson R: Recognition of chronic carbon monoxide poisoning. Wis Med J 98:26-29, 1999.

284. Tvedt B, Kjuus H: Chronic CO poisoning. Use of generator gas during the Second World War and recent research. Tidsskr Nor laegeforen 117:2454-2457, 1997.

285. Ryan CM: Memory disturbances following chronic, low-level carbon monoxide exposure. Arch Clin Neuropsychol 5:59-67, 1990.

286. Dunham M, Johnstone B: Variability of neuropsychological deficits associated with carbon monoxide poisoning: Four case reports. Brain Injury 13:917-925, 1999.

287. Myers RAM, DeFazio A, Kelly MP: Chronic carbon monoxide exposure: A clinical syndrome detected by neuropsychological tests. J Clin Psychol 54:555-567, 1998.

Management of Chronic Wounds

Sarah H. Kagan, PhD, RN

OVERVIEW

Care of people who have chronic wounds is a complex activity. It requires drawing together detailed considerations of a patient's physio-

logic state with variations in human behavior that demand meticulous assessment; an array of interventions encompassing physiologic to social issues; and performing consistent, repetitive evaluations. Evidence to support the methods of assessment, the types of interventions, and outcome measurement is often scant and requires careful judgment for application. Technologies for local wound care proliferate rapidly and are marketed aggressively, though often without compelling evidence. This profusion of interventions without substantiating evidence and a framework for application of these interventions within a comprehensive plan of care often complicates or diffuses the impact of any single intervention including hyperbaric oxygen therapy (HBOT).

This chapter proposes a best practices approach using available evidence to manage chronic wounds. The goal is to create a comprehensive plan of care and a best practices approach on the basis of careful evaluation. As aspects of wound healing physiology, contributing pathophysiology, and interventional technologies evolve and develop, the opportunities for successful intervention increase. Risks also exist, however, because given the complex nature of chronic wound management, the possibilities of unexpected interactions, adverse events, and contraindications expand. The correct diagnosis, reasonable goals, judicious treatment, and consistent evaluation help to balance these threats and improve prospects of success. Assessment, intervention, and evaluation of chronic wounds are influenced by factors such as systemic disease, localized pathology, malnutrition, the phase of wound healing, and the microenvironment and macroenvironment of the wound. Patients who are engaged in their own care are more likely to participate in and understand the therapeutic plan for their care. Thus, an evaluation should be made regarding a patient's capacity and desire for self-care, the family and community support available, and behavior that may influence nutrition, perfusion, and repeated wounding.

CLINICAL APPROACH

Chronic wound management and local wound care require a clinical approach that integrates detailed knowledge of pathophysiology with a broad understanding of psychologic, behavioral, and social antecedents, as well as the ramifications of chronic wounds. The phrase "wound care" belies the complexity of the problem, and more appropriately should be stated as "care of the person with the chronic wound." Tacit omission of the person from care that is implied by the phrase "wound care," combined with a singular focus on the wound itself, overlooks systemic aspects of the problem. Such thinking also jeopardizes the likelihood of reaching the correct diagnosis, to achieve reasonable goals, to provide judicious treatment, and to produce consistent evaluations. For example, misjudging the capacity of the person to heal a chronic wound despite repetitive injury from a poorly functioning assistive device or uncontrollable pathology generates an unreasonable plan of care that is likely to fail.

Chronic wound management is well framed by placing the person with the chronic wound—the patient—at the center of care. This central position reinforces the patient's rights and responsibilities and optimizes interactions among the patient and the interdisciplinary team members. With the patient and

not the wound centrally placed, comprehensive assessment, intervention, and evaluation strategies emerge. Discrete elements in the plan of care can then be created and linked to one another. Possible interactions among interventions, contraindications, pharmaceuticals, required devices, and settings necessary for the implementation of a care plan may then be more easily identified. Unexpected and relative contraindications occur often during care. Complications that must be considered include the physical visibility of the wound, pain, psychologic discomfort, impact on quality of daily life, and the human and financial resources required for the wound care plan. Finally, with care centered on the patient and not solely on the wound itself, the interdisciplinary team and the contributions of each team member may be delineated and relationships to the patient and other providers specified.

The complex and intricate nature of chronic wound care is best managed by an interdisciplinary team.[1] The nature of the team and its members are varied. Interdisciplinary teams must match the needs of the patient population with the dynamics, culture, work habits, and collaborations of the team members. Considerable interest and literature on composition of comprehensive wound care clinics and marketable interdisciplinary teams exists. This literature lacks overwhelming argument or evidence for a narrowly defined team makeup and spurs ongoing debate. Consequently, the approach proposed here presupposes an interdisciplinary team composed of members who possess the requisite clinical skills to meet the needs of a patient population. Table 16.1 lists potential members of the interdisciplinary wound care team.

Interdisciplinary chronic wound management necessitates integrating evidence, skill, and interaction to create a comprehensive plan for wound healing. A comprehensive plan is easily structured by applying basic principles to reach the correct diagnosis, to achieve reasonable goals, to provide judicious treatment, and to produce consistent evaluations. Diagnosis and goal setting are produced through analysis of available data, and the selection of treatment components, in turn,

Table 16.1 Interdisciplinary Team Members

Hyperbaric Oxygen Therapy Physician
Registered Nurse Specializing in Hyperbaric Oxygen Therapy
Primary Care Provider
· Physician or Nurse Practitioner
Certified Wound Ostomy and Continence Nurse
· Tissue Viability Nurse in the United Kingdom
Registered Dietitian
Nutrition Support Specialist
· Nurse Practitioner or Physician if dietitian does not
  specialize
Speech Language Pathologist
Surgical Subspecialists
· Plastic Surgeon
· Vascular Surgeon
· General Surgeon
Dermatologist
Infectious Disease Specialist
Radiologist
Physiatrist
Geriatrician/Geriatric Advanced Practice Nurse
Physical Therapist
Occupational Therapist
Social Worker
Nursing or Health-Care Assistant
Chaplain or Spiritual Advisor
Mental Health Professional
· Psychiatric Advanced Practice Nurse
· Psychiatrist
· Psychologist

hinge on that analysis. Evaluation procedures rely on an analysis consistent with the scientific evidence and use processes created by interdisciplinary team members.

PATIENT ASSESSMENT

Patient assessment should begin with a full patient interview and physical examination. Addressing systemic concerns before examining the wound reinforces the patient as the focus of care and commonly gleans information important to accurate diagnosis and reasonable goal setting. Interviews with family or other informal caregivers complete the data collection process and further support goals and intervention plans.

Systemic Assessment

Systemic diseases and conditions, as well as global functional impairment, commonly create or contribute to chronic wounds. Consideration of all pathologies, nutritional needs, and functional status may reveal other causative or contributing factors. The treatment of these factors can influence the overall likelihood of healing. As a result, systemic assessment is an important corollary to wound assessment and is necessary to diagnosis and goal setting.

Functional assessment and interaction with the environment is likewise a component of systemic assessment. Questioning the patient about daily activities and observing movement in the clinical setting can gauge mobility. Use of assistive devices should be noted. For example, use of a wheelchair may create physical pressure (e.g., friction with a foot rest adjacent to an arterial ulcer) that contributes to the development of and inability to heal a chronic wound (Fig. 16.1). The evaluation should also include a falls assessment[2]; this history can be used to identify falls prevention and home safety interventions, and further to trigger referral to appropriate specialists as needed. Assessment of mental functional status should complement the appraisal of physical functional status. Recognition of mental status abnormalities should lead to formal assessment if this has not been done previously.

Laboratory studies are essential to complete systemic assessment. Studies should investigate status of primary and comorbid diseases, nutritional status, immunocompetence, and infection if it is suspected on physical examination. Although there is no agreed-on screening battery of laboratory tests, an initial evaluation of a patient with a chronic wound should probably include a complete blood cell count, serum albumin, serum prealbumin, assessment of renal function, and evaluation of glucose tolerance. It is worth remembering that albumin has a long half-life, making it better suited for assessing the patient's long-term nutritional status, whereas prealbumin with its short half-life is more useful to assess response to nutritional

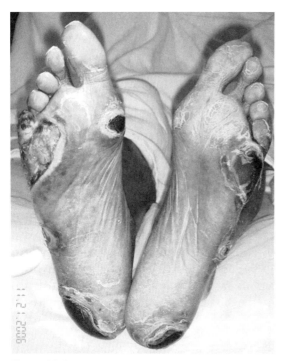

Figure 16.1 An elderly, wheelchair-bound patient whose feet have multiple, bilateral ulcerations due, in part, to unrelieved pressure from inadequate footwear and the wheelchair footrests. **(See Color Plate 11.)**

supplementation over time. Other laboratory studies may also be indicated on the basis of the presence of known or suspected disease.

Analysis of these data offers the opportunity to consider all possible causes and contributors to a given process. These data may also trigger connections to psychosocial concerns. Associated pathology may become more clearly evident on examination of the systemic data in advance of local wound assessment.

Wound Assessment

Detailed description of the extent of tissue involvement together with the dimensions, depth, and anatomy of the destruction are the hallmark of skillful wound assessment. Careful wound assessment may uncover details critical to making the correct diagnosis. As Ayello's[3] aptly titled article "What Does the Wound Say?" reminds us, clinicians must listen carefully to what the wound says. Many authors offer clear, well-developed wound

assessment guidelines and schemas.[4-7] Available schemas include broadly based discussion of assessment features, assessment guides, templates, and mnemonic acronyms. Although such literature may offer appealing advantages in systematizing data collection and ensuring detailed documentation, little comparative evidence exists to suggest that one format is linked to improved outcomes. Rather, systematic collection and attention to core variables including dimensions, anatomy, appearance, exudates, and periwound tissues are the mainstays of wound assessment. Misuse of categoric systems that serve as shorthand to describe wounds is common among those who are inexperienced and should be avoided. For example, it is better to describe the wound appearance and level of tissue involvement versus using a label with staging or other nomenclature (e.g., the National Pressure Ulcer Advisory Panel's description of wound stages is available online at: http://www.npuap.org/documents/NPUAP2007_PU_Def_and_Descriptions.pdf) because clinically relevant details are omitted when reporting stage as a primary description. Fundamentally, assessment must include and record information that describes the wound as completely as possible. Wound assessment also requires prior study and familiarity with features of diseases and conditions that cause wounds of a particular type. In addition, appropriate assessment requires the appreciation of the characteristics typical of common chronic wounds (e.g., pressure ulcers, arterial ulcers, venous stasis dermatitis and ulceration, diabetic neuropathic foot ulcers). Assessment of patients referred for HBOT also necessitates familiarity with characteristics of less common wounds that are more often treated with HBOT (e.g., soft-tissue radiation necrosis, osteoradionecrosis) (Figs. 16.2 and 16.3).

Evidence of wound healing should also be carefully and repetitively assessed including recognition of ongoing healing by secondary intention (Fig. 16.4). Contraction is often indicated by smoothed and rounded wound edges. Granulation tissue is identified by its characteristic red, granular appearance or initial emergence of small areas of granulation,

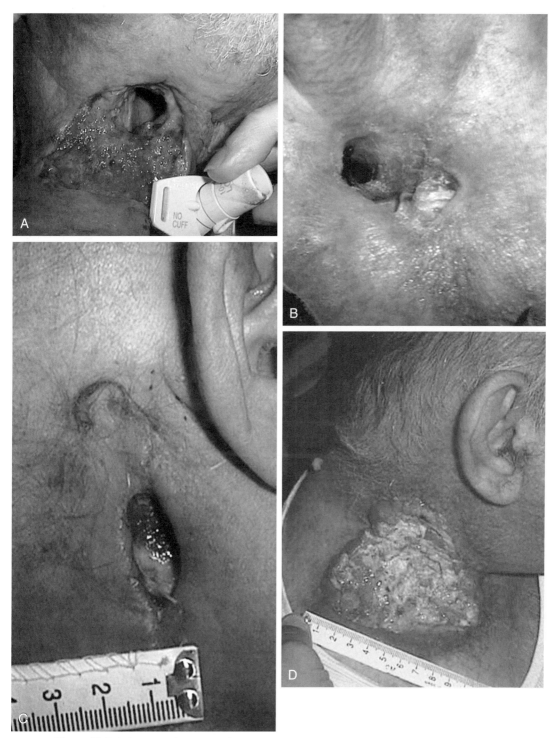

Figure 16.2 Soft-tissue radionecrosis of laryngectomy stomas *(A, B)* and the neck *(C, D)* in patients treated for head and neck cancers. The neck sites show ulcerating and fungating presentations. **(See Color Plate 12.)**

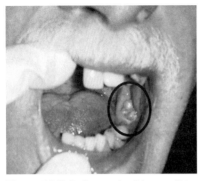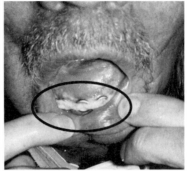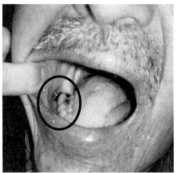

Figure 16.3 Radionecrosis of the mandible presenting with oral lesions corresponding to the necrosis. **(See Color Plate 13.)**

sometimes termed *islands*. Epithelialization requires deliberate further attention to the wound edges; the epithelializing wound edge in healing by secondary intent is classically termed *pearly* with a mounded, pale pink or white, shiny appearance (Fig. 16.5). Absence of these features or presence of devitalized tissue, accumulated exudates, or other debris is indicative of poor healing (see Fig. 16.5). The presence and character of gross debris and exudates are also important details of wound appearance. Color, consistency, texture, and the extent of and adherence to the wound bed are important descriptors. Characteristics of surrounding, or periwound, tissue including color, texture, and integrity are essential to gauging the full extent of the wound and the processes that created it. Assessment must then encompass the visible wound and periwound tissue. Finally, evidence of prior treatment including past surgeries, old scars from healing by secondary intention, and more unusual findings including staining from biomedical or alternative treatment and dressing materials (e.g., zinc oxide residue, silver dressing stains, and marks from coining) offer important information about prior treatment and further the clinician's understanding of the patient's knowledge.

Wound and Periwound Tissue Measurement

Many tools are available to measure chronic wound dimensions.[6,8] Extant tools, intended for research or practice, measure not only wound dimensions but surface area and volume, tissue interface pressures, and wound impact on quality of life.[6,8-13] Other tools record or categorize qualitative wound ap-

Figure 16.4 Serial images of a patient's lateral foot wound as it was reassessed during hyperbaric oxygen therapy. The series shows progressive granulation and contraction of the wound edge. **(See Color Plate 14.)**

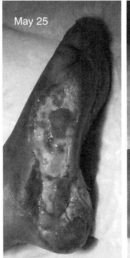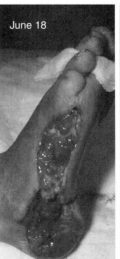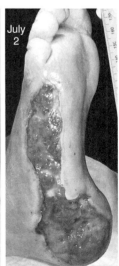

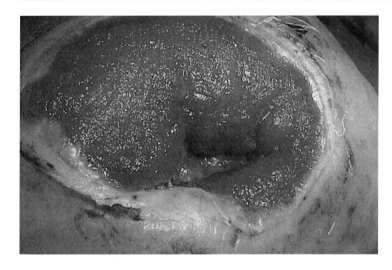

Figure 16.5 A patient's heel wound treated with hyperbaric oxygen therapy shows a robust granulation bed with characteristically smooth, contracting wound edge and the pale, pearly appearance consistent with epithelialization at the edge. **(See Color Plate 15.)**

pearance.[8,14] The relation between the use of such tools and patient outcomes lacks comprehensive and rigorous investigation. Furthermore, the use of these devices may entail significant cost because the use of devices may not be supported by current evidence and limited reimbursement may limit utility. Table 16.2 lists measurement methods and tools, outlining advantages and disadvantages shown in current investigation.

Clinical Studies and Imaging

Studies that clarify local effects of disease such as vascular studies (e.g., pulse volume recordings, interpretation of ankle–brachial indices, and angiograms in arterial disease) or tissue biopsy for diagnosis (e.g., definitive diagnosis of cutaneous, vascular, or rheuma-tological disease) are best undertaken in consultation with specialist team members with appropriate expertise. Studies to assess the local wound environment are generally limited to wound cultures[15-18] and transcutaneous oxygen measurement.[19-23] Issues of technique and utility deserve attention.

Wound cultures for bacteria are performed with tissue obtained from surgical biopsy and topical swabs. Although clinical wisdom has long held that swab cultures will reveal nothing more than normal flora and contaminants together with possible pathogens, recent research supports utility of this practice if performed correctly.[16,17,24] Sibbald and colleagues[25] together with Gardner and coauthors[24] underscore the care with which a swab culture, using the technique that Levine and investigators[18] outlined, must be collected.

Table 16.2 Wound Measurement Methods

TYPE	METHOD	FEATURES
TWO-DIMENSIONAL	Linear measurement	Inexpensive; quantitative only and is least reliable method[11]
	Acetate tracing	Inexpensive; can be reliable but is quantitative only; improved with addition of planimetry[6,8,10,11]
	Full-scale photography or planimetry plus acetate tracings	Requires investment in software and hardware including camera; reliable[8,10,11]
	Full-scale photography with photogrammetry	Requires investment in software and hardware including camera; reliable[8,10,11]
THREE-DIMENSIONAL	Full-scale photography with stereophotogrammetry	Requires investment in software and hardware including camera; reliable[8,10,11,13]
	Digital image analysis software for full-scale photography, including light pattern analysis	Requires investment in software and hardware including camera[8,9]

Levine's technique is semiquantitative, requires collection over one square centimeter of tissue, and differs markedly from other techniques using wound exudates or a simple Z-shaped swab pattern.[24] Gardner and coauthors[24] emphasize the need for further study to ensure comparability with biopsy culture results based on quantitative definitions of infection and threshold titers. The potential value of correctly obtained swab cultures cannot be dismissed as surgical biopsy for culture is invasive and may pose clinically relevant risks for some patients. Evidence of infection from the patient's history and physical and the relative risk of empiric treatment based on interpretation of these data should be weighed when considering the method of culture.

Measurement of the partial pressure of oxygen at the wound may assist with a prediction of the likelihood to achieve healing.[19-21,26-28] The importance of oxygen in wound healing stems from classic work performed by Hunt and others and supports the use of HBOT.[29-33] Variations in local and systemic perfusion, oxygen-carrying capacity, and oxygen consumption (including effects of systemic infection) all influence the wound environment and healing.[19,27,31,34] Most significantly, oxygen tension in the wound itself has profound effects on infection, complications such as dehiscence, and ultimately whether a wound may fail to heal.[19,35,36] Hence, a number of investigators have measured partial pressure of oxygen at the wound bed using noninvasive transcutaneous techniques to explore the associations between these values and outcomes.[20,21,26-28,37] Studies conducted using a set of pathologic models that center on impaired arterial perfusion and common clinical outcomes (i.e., amputation and wound healing) collectively suggest that a transcutaneous partial pressure of oxygen ($tcPo_2$) of around 40 to 50 mm Hg is the point above which healing occurs.[19,20,26,28] The relation between $tcPo_2$ and clinical wound healing in situations other than those with a primary arterial source (e.g., osteoradionecrosis and radiation-induced tissues changes) has not been evaluated. Furthermore, how the oxygen environment of normally healing wounds such as acute surgical wounds differs from that of chronic wounds remains unclear.[27] For example, although examination of acute wounds that heal reveals a relative decline in $tcPo_2$, whether similar changes occur in chronic wounds lacks evidentiary support.[27] Finally, the interplay among dressings and devices used adjunctively to prepare the wound bed during HBOT that may influence alterations in $tcPo_2$ are unexplored. Hence, little guidance exists about how sequential measurements of $tcPo_2$ should be used for assessment and intervention in chronic wound management. Nonetheless, given the evidence that suggests the predictive capacity of $tcPo_2$, the noninvasive nature of the technique, and its reliability, the use of $tcPo_2$ measurement is perhaps worthwhile in creating a comprehensive wound assessment. The availability and cost of the technology balance this decision.

The presence of exposed bone within a wound, the presence of significant periwound tissue changes including bogginess and fluctuance, and the presence of foreign bodies in and adjacent to the wound bed warrant clinical evaluation that includes a variety of imaging techniques.[38,39] Exposed bone or skeletal structures, or other clinical evidence that suggests osteomyelitis (e.g., presence of long-standing gaps in granulation tissue or tracts and sinuses involving the wound bed) mandates comprehensive work-up to exclude this possibility (Fig. 16.6). The availability of positron emission tomography has enhanced the ability to detect osteomyelitis. Termaat and colleagues'[39] recent review and meta-analysis reveals the utility of positron emission tomography and leukocyte scintigraphy over other imaging techniques in diagnosing osteomyelitis. Whether these more advanced technologies will provide important clinical information compared with lower cost imaging techniques may require additional consultation.

Psychosocial Concerns

The experience of having chronic wounds is inherently complex. A patient's behavior and psychosocial status may influence healing through direct or indirect means.[40-42] Smoking

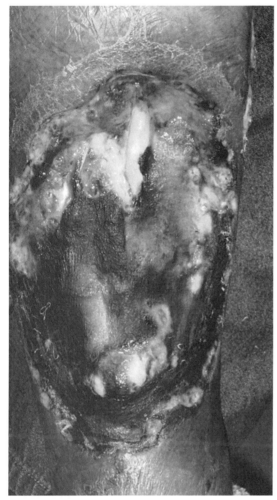

Figure 16.6 A patient's posterior shin arterial ulcer is filled with devitalized tissue and proteinaceous exudates. The exposed tendon at 12 o'clock position suggests osteomyelitis may be present and warrants further clinical evaluation. **(See Color Plate 16.)**

tobacco, for example, appears to influence wound healing.[32,43,44] The patient may experience prototypical unpleasant sensations such as pain or pruritus or may experience development of unexpected hypesthesia or anesthesia.[45] These symptoms can handicap interpersonal and larger social role functions.[41,42] The initial patient assessment should explore behavior, psychosocial concerns, and function, as well as knowledge of the current condition. In addition, behavioral assessment is indicated when self-injury, whether intentional or incidental, may be at hand. The patient's and family's knowledge of the disease process influences all aspects of care from assessment

(e.g., ability to provide accurate history) through goal setting (e.g., capacity to understand clinically realistic goals) to intervention (e.g., self-care ability). Family members who are primary caregivers should be included in initial psychosocial assessment. The basic assessment may be used to trigger referral and follow-up with a mental health professional when evidence of major mental health concerns are present.[46,47]

Only a few instruments emphasize psychosocial impacts of chronic wounds through health-related quality-of-life measurements or more focal investigations such as wound pain.[6,48,49] The MEASURE system[6] notably includes suffering in the wound assessment, but only within a larger set of variables. The Cardiff Wound Impact Schedule[48,49] has been tested in groups of patients with limited types of chronic wounds but is not yet in widespread use.

Wound Environment

There is a growing body of knowledge on the chronic wound environment at microscopic and macroscopic levels, and how this environment influences healing.[25,36,50-56] The well-accepted maxim of keeping a wound *clean, moist, and protected* speaks to the importance of wound environment for promoting healing.[57,58] These principles of *clean, moist, and protected* have been dissected to reveal elements of promotion, benefit, harm, and balance at cellular and molecular levels.[59] Furthermore, the impact of gross debris in the wound bed is increasingly well described[60-62] (Fig. 16.7). Discrete elements in the environment and their impact on it, the physiology of healing, and the pathophysiology of delayed or impaired healing in chronic wounds are now better understood and can be considered in clinical chronic wound management.[25,51,54,55,59-61,63-67]

Chronic wound management relies on estimations of the wound environment. Knowledge of normal wound healing physiology (see Chapter 11) and pathophysiology of chronic wounds provides the groundwork for consideration of the wound environment at both microscopic and macroscopic levels.

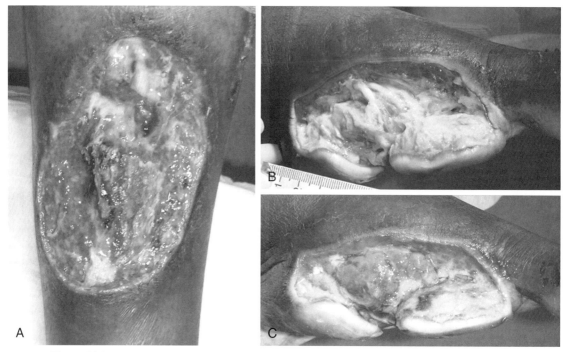

Figure 16.7 A patient's posterior shin arterial ulcer shows accumulation of grossly visible proteinaceous exudates that are yellow *(A)*. Serial images of patient's lateral foot ulcer *(B, C)* show large amounts of pale, devitalized tissue together with some proteinaceous exudates *(B)*, which is reduced with enzymatic debridement *(C)*. **(See Color Plate 17.)**

Interventions are designed on the basis of available evidence, clinical hypotheses in the absence of direct evidence, and clinical judgment grounded in best practices. The phase of wound healing may be assessed by macroscopic features of wound appearance, characteristics (such as color) of the wound bed, and consistency or odor of exudates. Clinical assessment of the microscopic wound environment lacks sensitivity and specificity. Cytokines, proteases, and bacterial load are primary factors in the microscopic wound environment together with the cell groups active in the three phases of wound healing. Other variables in the wound history may also suggest characteristics of the microenvironment. These include the chronologic age of the patient, comorbidities, diet (including protein or protein-calorie malnutrition and specific nutritional deficiencies), injuries, time without clinical evidence of healing, failure to heal, and clinical progression and regression in healing.[50] Inherent threats to wound healing, such as senescence with changes in cellular replication, and elements of the pathophysiol-

ogy and history of the chronic wound, such as high concentrations of matrix metalloproteinases, are now understood to shape the microenvironment of the wound and to create clinically significant alterations in healing.[50,59]

Clinical assessment of the wound environment may trigger additional investigation and generate refined hypotheses. For example, a surgical wound that dehisces after nearly complete re-epithelialization without evidence of infection may suggest malnutrition. Further assessment and investigation to confirm this hypothesis may then disclose possible vitamin A deficiency with links to long-term use of drugs metabolized in the liver and direct nutritional supplementation.[36] Similarly, assessing a foul odor emanating from a chronic wound that is worse when debris accumulates may suggest pathologic bacterial colonization or infection.[25,66] Further assessment and investigation to confirm this hypothesis may reveal poor perfusion to the wound bed and a high likelihood of anaerobic infection. Pursuing this line of thought still further leads to consideration of local and systemic evidence of infection and evaluation of treatment options that acknowledge poor perfusion and implications for systemic drug delivery as well as concerns about antibiotic resistance and nonpharmacologic options such as dressings that contain bactericidal concentrations of silver.[25] Such sequential refinement of hypotheses about the wound environment using clinical data and available evidence directs intervention for management of chronic wounds.

INTERVENTION

Interventions for chronic wound management encompass systemic, local, and psychosocial techniques. Growing interest in paradigms of health beyond allopathic traditional medicine has given rise to testing a variety of techniques less familiar within the classical medical tradition. Psychosocial techniques for supporting the patient and caregiver may augment systemic and local interventions. Among the most important psychosocial interventions is patient and family education. All interventions included in a plan for management should meet several standards. First, interventions should optimize the wound environment, beginning with the maxim of *clean, moist, and protected,* and extending to correction of pathophysiologic characteristics in the wound environment. Second, interventions should match available scientific evidence to objective assessment data. Third, interventions should adhere to current best practices and clinical judgment when scientific evidence is lacking. Finally, interventions should adhere to principles of patient-centered wound management. Table 16.3 outlines these principles and their rationale.

Local interventions begin with the maxim of a *clean, moist, and protected* wound. For example, a wound must be free of debris to match the maxim of clean. Furthermore, the microlevel wound environment requires maintaining microbiologic balance and control of pathogenic overcolonization to meet the needs of the inflammatory wound healing phase.[25,36,59] Wound moisture should be maintained to satisfy requirements of the cells active during the

inflammatory, proliferative, and remodeling phases of wound healing. Similarly, wounds must be protected to maintain cellular activity and avoid destructive physical forces.

The match between *clean, moist, and protected*—noting that these principles generally apply throughout healing in most wounds—and the phases of wound healing offers a clinically useful guide to local care. Product and device choices are often driven by familiarity and comfort, not by analysis of data supporting their use. Products and devices create specific macrolevel and microlevel effects in the wound environment. For example, cotton gauze wet with normal saline solution provides moisture to the wound, although the effect is not constant and is affected by wound moisture (Fig. 16.8). It also abrades the wound and disturbs the microscopic structure such as a biofilm in the bed.[25,59] Easy to use, but lacking technologic sophistication, a normal saline solution on gauze may theoretically be used to clean a chronic wound and maintain moisture if applied with appropriate technique and sufficient frequency (see Fig. 16.8). Thus, although this dressing has potential utility across phases of wound healing and supports the maxim "clean, moist, and protected," it is a relatively difficult and expensive dressing to use to achieve these aims.[68] Principles of patient-centered wound management suggest consideration of other options. Likewise, topical antibiotic agents, such as bacitracin zinc and polymyxin B sulfate ointment with or without neomycin, are commonly applied to maintain a moist wound and to reduce slough or adherent debris in the wound bed. The thought behind their use is to prevent infection, thereby reducing tissue sloughing that is often confused with pus. However, the antibiotics in these agents can produce local sensitivity and overgrowth of organisms such as *Candida albicans.* The petrolatum carrier in these products will prevent infection equally well as the antibiotics themselves, and it creates a barrier under which some autolysis may occur.[69-71] Similarly, devices such as negative-pressure wound therapy have microlevel and macrolevel influence on the wound environment. Negative-pressure wound therapy improves

Table 16.3 Criteria for Selection of Local Wound Care Products

CRITERIA	RATIONALE
Comfortable	Uses techniques and technologies that are well tolerated and adapted to anatomy, function, and personal preference
Commonly available	Provides continuity with home and institutional care
	Access through providers, pharmacies, or medical supply houses without protracted search and excessive cost
Easily used	Enables efficient care by clinicians or family caregivers without difficult work, discomfort, or distress to the patient
	Relies on supportive measures to mitigate workload, discomfort, and distress entailed by necessary interventions
Cost-effective	Prevents an undue financial burden on the patient and family
	Ensures appropriate resource utilization for institutions

local perfusion, manages exudates, and removes bacterial colonies in the exudate to optimize the microscopic environment.[29] The application of this device also balances the general moisture level of the wound and provides physical protection to the wound bed.

Pairing products and devices with the wound environment is complicated by the rapid proliferation of merchandise by the wound care industry. Marketing can sway clinicians, who may be influenced by overly enthusiastic interpretations of available clinical articles or research reports offered by device and product detailers. Often, evidence is inadequate and is outpaced by new and updated versions of products and devices. Successful pairing requires careful examination of products and devices, wound assessment data, and patient characteristics.

Wound Dressings

The treatment of a wound almost always requires application of a physical dressing to manage wound moisture, contain topical agents or otherwise manipulate the microenvironment, and protect the wound and possibly periwound tissue. Dressings for chronic wounds are accomplished using clean technique and a variety of products. Classical products such as cotton gauze and petrolatum gauze are inexpensive and have a number of characteristics such as absorptive capacity, texture, and flexibility that allow them to be used in a variety of ways (Fig. 16.9). More modern products such as composites that absorb proteases or absorptive hydrofiber or calcium alginate dressings, although more

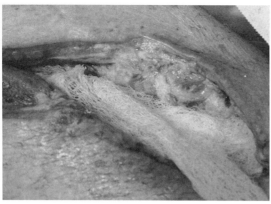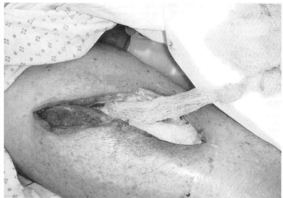

Figure 16.8 A patient's leg wound is packed with roll gauze that has been dampened with normal saline solution. Note that the wound is packed by layering the gauze into the wound, which limits overpacking and allows for atraumatic removal. **(See Color Plate 18.)**

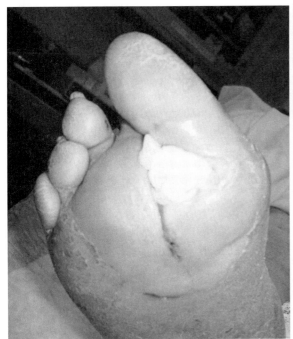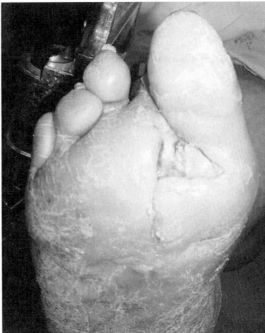

Figure 16.9 A patient's plantar wound is packed with fine mesh gauze that is dampened with normal saline solution. **(See Color Plate 19.)**

expensive, may have specific properties that make them more desirable agents. Consideration of the product composition, its designed and approved use, and the evidence supporting that use should be considered to achieve a match between the characteristics of the wound and the dressing selected.

Managing wound moisture involves assessment of wound exudate and drainage. The characteristics of the exudate and the volume and pattern of drainage are assessed to determine whether the wound lacks moisture or whether the wound bed is overly wet and excessive drainage risks maceration of periwound tissue. Interestingly, wound moisture is measured only at a qualitative level in clinical practice. No evidence points to optimal moisture as measured by any particular method; however, extremes in the range require management.

Products that supplement wound moisture are most often delivered as an irrigant (e.g., normal saline or lactated Ringer's solution) or a gel. Hydrogels use base materials such as glycerin to counteract evaporation. Furthermore, they create consistency that eases application and maintains placement. A gel, for example, stays in a wound more easily and

without a carrier such as gauze than an irrigant, which will dry more rapidly. Hydrophilic and humectant ointments may also be used to enhance moisture in a wound bed by creating a barrier film that prevents evaporation of wound fluid. Among the most common agents in these ointments are glycerin, lanolin, and urea. Their use encompasses the range of treatment from dry desquamation caused by radiation dermatitis to autolytic debridement of an eschar.[72] They are less often used to maintain moisture in clean but dry wounds where hydrogels have come into standard use. Finally, dressings that adhere to the wound and provide a physical barrier that prevents evaporation of wound fluids can also be used to maintain a moistened dry wound bed. These dressings rely on an extended dwell time to prevent significant evaporation, combined with clinically significant amounts of wound fluid exuded over a period of days to create a wet wound environment. Hydrocolloid and transparent film dressings are ubiquitous in most clinical settings and generally familiar to clinicians.

In contrast with wounds with a dry wound bed, wet wounds present the opposite challenge of absorbing and holding excessive drainage so that the wound remains moist but is neither dry nor macerated. To achieve this, an absorptive product must absorb and hold drainage without returning it to the wound bed or periwound skin. Cotton gauze, although able to absorb fluid, lacks capacity to hold it over time. Products such as calcium alginate or hydrofiber dressings absorb and hold moisture over time far better than gauze and benefit from widespread use (Fig. 16.10). Hydrophilic foam dressings are newer additions to the absorptive category. These products are familiar in many settings where people who have chronic wounds are treated.

Mechanical devices can also be helpful in managing exudate and underlying edema. Although the consideration of edema and lymphedema management is beyond the scope of this chapter, the devices used to treat lymphedema and other edema bear mention. Short stretch bandages, other compression dressings such as an Unna's boot, and negative pressure wound therapy may be beneficial in relieving edema and managing exudate over time. Both compression and negative suction may be temporarily difficult for patients to tolerate given the expected increase in exudate and drainage that may initially occur. Patient support and education are even more important if these devices are selected as part of therapy.

Manipulation of the wound microenvironment with dressings offers new, targeted options for local intervention. Use of topical agents such as topical antibiotics has long been part of local wound care, implemented without extensive evidence and relying on practice patterns and empiric understanding of colonizing pathogens.[73] In a critical review, Howell-Jones[73] summarizes the evidence for topical antimicrobial drugs and concludes that sufficient evidence supports the utility of agents such as silver sulfadiazine. These agents are widely available, active against many common pathogens, and inexpensive. Cho[74] warns about possibly delayed healing and addresses it through a preliminary, in vitro intervention model. The advent of dressings that deliver biologically active silver for microbicidal effect have resulted in the proliferation of many products with various forms of silver. Warriner and Burrell[75] and Sibbald and colleagues[25] offer summaries of silver delivery systems in dressings and commercially available products. Considerations including dwell time, cytotoxicity, and ease of use are reviewed by Sibbald and colleagues.[25] Warriner and Burrell's[75] analysis of conflicting literature provides clinical guidance in product selection based on the conclusion that silver concentration appears to be critical to efficacy. Notably, the classic silver preparations, silver sulfadiazine and silver nitrate, together with the nanocrystalline silver preparations (namely, Acticoat products; Smith and Nephew, Largo, Fla) exceed the threshold concentration of 35 mg/L established in their summary.[75] These products

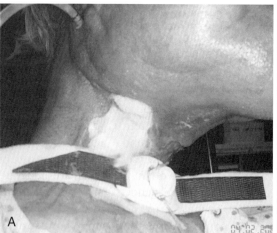 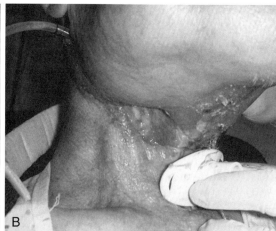

Figure 16.10 A patient who has been treated for head and neck cancer has an orocutaneous fistula *(A)* that is packed with calcium alginate dressing to manage the fistulous drainage *(B)*. **(See Color Plate 20.)**

have the further advantage of being less expensive than many others. Other considerations, such as cost-effectiveness and cytotoxicity, as outlined by Sibbald and colleagues,[25] and concerns about resistance warrant careful attention particularly as use of these dressings become more commonplace.[75,76]

Physical protection of the wound bed is achieved easily with consideration of the mechanical properties of available dressings. Primary and cover dressings that adhere to or are secured to intact periwound tissue provide some cushion against minor trauma including friction and remain in place through the planned dwell time of the dressing (Fig. 16.11). Any number of common and inexpensive, as well as new and often more expensive, products have these characteristics and can be used in wound dressings to protect the wound. In addition, products may have other characteristics that may be useful in achieving the aims of local care. Thus, products such as composite, moisture-proof, layered pads (e.g., known in health-care vernacular as ABD pads) that can be secured with tape can serve as an effective protector, as can soft silicone products (e.g., Mepilex; Mölnlycke, Göteborg, Sweden) that use silicone to be adherent without using an adhesive. ABD pads are relatively nonadherent and comfortable to use but awkward if smaller dressings are required because they fray when cut. However, these pads carry topical agents easily, allowing medications to be spread on the pad and delivered to the wound with a "no-touch" technique that is helpful when patients experience extreme pain on manipulation. Likewise, soft silicone dressings are available in a variety of types that offer wicking to transfer the exudate of wet wounds and occlusive cover dressings that help maintain moisture in a drier wound. Their use can also limit pain in wound care and optimize the wound microenvironment.

Wound Irrigation and Debridement

Irrigation of chronic wounds classically generates substantial clinical controversy. Irrigant cytotoxicity was the vogue topic of the 1980s, and selection of nontoxic agents for irrigation and routine cleansing has become standard in wound care practice.[63,66] Although agents such as dilute povidone-iodine, acetic acid, sodium hypochlorite solution, and hydrogen peroxide undergo further, incidental investigation in wound care research, little compelling evidence exists to argue for their use above normal saline solution or lactated Ringer's solution as standard wound irrigants.[63,77-81] Use of irrigants is further complicated by the delivery and mechanics of irrigation. Tissue trauma with forceful local irrigation is generally not considered helpful in chronic wound management. However, hydrotherapy—as less targeted irrigation with agitation using a container that accommodates the affected anatomy—continues to receive some attention despite lack of any research to support use.[82,83] Although clinical judgment regarding specific application of irrigants for particular patients may vary (e.g., for patients who cannot tolerate any force of stream or who are sensitive to irrigant temperature), available literature offers no more compelling guidance other than routine use of normal saline solution or lactated Ringer's solution. The use of tap water in home care and the use of hydrogen peroxide or soap to "dis-incrust" wound and periwound tissues followed by flooding of a nontoxic irrigant are likely warranted to act as a mild mechanical debriding agent.[63]

Debridement is as controversial a clinical topic as any in chronic wound management (Fig. 16.12). It merges and magnifies issues of clinician training, specialty, skill, and preference. Research addressing the comparative value of sharp mechanical, gross mechanical, enzymatic, osmotic, autolytic, hydrotherapy, and biologic methods is limited in scope and quality.[60-63,84-87] Sharp mechanical debridement is often considered the gold standard against which other methods are judged[60]; however, little evidence supports this standard as a universal rule for management of all chronic wounds. Sharp debridement provides rapid, selective removal of large amounts of nonviable tissue.[63] These attributes make it an

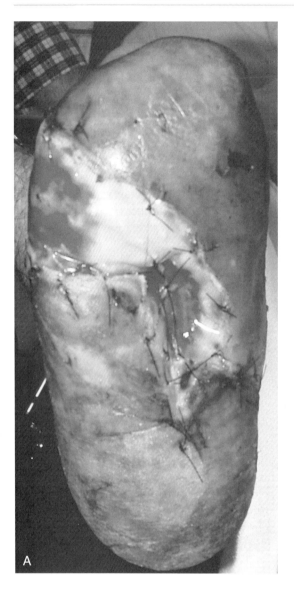

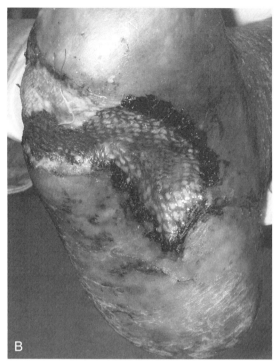

Figure 16.11 A patient with an extensive and complicated plantar foot wound was treated with HBOT. A biomembrane dressing was used to maintain wound moisture, reduce pain, and maintain tissue position (A). The wound healing, by tertiary intent, created a granulated wound bed that was closed using a split thickness skin graft (B). **(See Color Plate 21.)**

advantageous method to use in situations where rapid removal is desired by virtue of physiologic threat or bioburden (namely, infection or abscess), pain associated with infection, or inability to tolerate or withstand a delayed method (e.g., allergy to enzymatic ointments, poor self-care, limited funds for topical agents). Sharp debridement also has the advantage of being easily performed by appropriately trained clinicians. Recently, methods viewed as traditional in some societies and complementary or alternative in Western care have been reviewed and examined.[86,88] Although some of these methods have been easily integrated into traditional care (namely, papain), others including honey, sugar, maggots—often called *biotherapy*—have not gained wide acceptance.[86,88] Evidence supporting these traditional or complementary methods may or may not adhere to a Western clinical research paradigm; however, research is being conducted with greater frequency, compounding the choices and options in debridement. Again, careful examination of effects on the microlevel and macrolevel wound environment and principles of patient-centered care guides selection among a panoply of options. Thus, a patient with continued accumulation of soft slough, no known allergies, well-controlled or minimal wound pain, strong motivation for self-care, and prescription coverage is likely an excellent candidate for debridement using a papain ointment (Fig. 16.13). Conversely, use of maggots, although a physiologically sound choice for debridement, may be personally and socially unacceptable in most Western settings.[86]

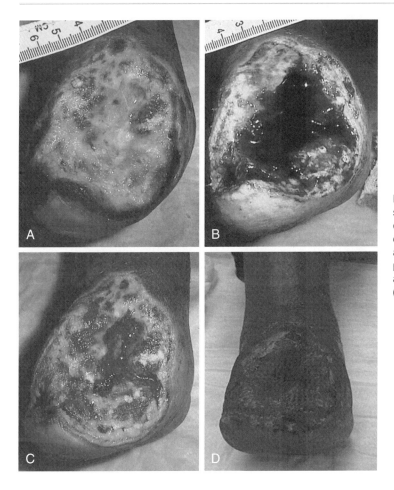

Figure 16.12 Images of an amputation site show devitalized tissue, adherent exudates, and other debris *(A)* that warrant debridement *(B)*. *C,* Some granulation tissue and proteinaceous exudates covering varying portions of the wound bed. *D,* Wound shortly after split-thickness skin graft placement. **(See Color Plate 22.)**

Antibiotic Therapy

Management of infection mandates careful integration of systemic and local data with available options and evaluation of risks to the patient. Options for treatment include sharp debridement, topical antibiotics, dressing preparations that include biologically active silver, and systemic antibiotics. Sharp debridement of devitalized, nonviable tissue and noncellular debris offers rapid reduction of bacterial load.[89] Topical antibiotics available range from common over-the-counter preparations including bacitracin zinc or polymyxin B to prescription drugs such as silver sulfadiazine or mupirocin. Concerns about adverse reactions such as cutaneous sensitivity, microbial resistance, and delayed wound healing with these agents warrant consideration.[74,90] Biologically active silver is a potentially valuable antimicrobial therapy, especially in high-risk patients who may have

difficulty responding to infection and frequently incur chronic wounds. The choice of topical agents may incorrectly receive less attention than systemic therapies. Options are many and should be matched to specific assessment data and weighed against available institutional data on sensitivity, resistance, and epidemiology.[53,66,76,91,92]

Systemic antibiotic therapy requires a clear analysis and well-timed care, particularly in the immunocompromised patient, whether delivered orally or parenterally.[53,66] However, although there are numerous reports of drug trials to support specific antibiotics, the evidence to support drug choice in chronic wound care is sharply limited.[93] Available evidence points to a wide variety of pathogens including commonly suspected *Staphylococcus aureus* and *Pseudomonas aeruginosa,* as well as less common pathogens.[94] Howell-Jones and colleagues[95] report an important

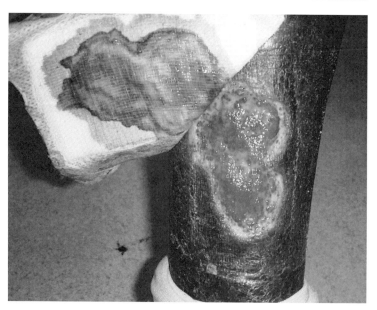

Figure 16.13 A patient with an anterior shin arterial ulcer is being treated with hyperbaric oxygen therapy and use of a papain ointment to debride exudate and support granulation. Note the green color of the ointment visible on the dressing as it is removed and the granulation islands present at the lateral wound borders. **(See Color Plate 23.)**

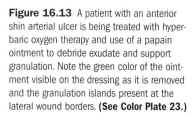

study of prescribing patterns for antibiotic use in chronic wound treatment in a primary care setting. As might be expected, patients with chronic wounds received far more antibiotics than did patients without wounds. However, as Howell-Jones and colleagues[95] point out, the microbiologic rationale for patterns of prescription is not evident, thus suggesting that practice patterns are idiosyncratic and clearly influenced by inadequate evidence. That, combined with ever increasing concerns about resistant organisms (always in the context of differentiating between contamination and frank infection), suggests caution in prescribing for individual patients. It also requires that attention be paid to prescribing patterns and the clinical response of patients in general.[94,96] In addition, wound perfusion may influence drug delivery such that drug concentrations at the wound bed may be inadequate to treat the source of infection. Hernandez[96] summarizes evidence for systemic antibiotic use in chronic wound management. He provides a detailed analysis to guide management. Finally, although there is growing interest and research on complementary therapeutics that fall outside traditional Western care for infection, scant evidence is available in support of such interventions over antibiotic use that is supported by a large body of cumulative data.[88,97-99]

Manipulation of Wound Microenvironment

The ability to manipulate the microscopic wound environment has recently progressed to molecular strategies. Local agents that supply exogenous growth factors (namely, platelet-derived growth factor-bb in a hydrogel carrier—becaplermin [Regranex]; Ortho-McNeil Pharmaceutical, Inc., Raritan, NJ) and absorb excess matrix metalloproteinases (e.g., Promogran; Ethicon, Inc., Somerville, NJ) are now widely available in practice, despite some challenges with cost and coverage. However, these products illustrate the current gap in translational science. Cross and Mustoe[54] emphasize the mismatch between bench science that reveals the role of platelet-derived growth factor in wound healing and the commercially prepared platelet-derived growth factor-bb for use in wound care, the promise of which remains unfulfilled. This may, in part, be because of the challenges of conducting in vivo wound care studies and achieving systematized, standard wound care protocols.[54] The focus on dressings that manage protease concentration is far less than that which platelet-derived growth factor-bb received in the clinical community. Another treatment modality that has been widely adopted without evidence of its efficacy is negative pressure therapy (namely, V.A.C.; KCI, San Antonio, Tex),[100] despite some findings that include a possible increase in bacterial burden.[55] Negative pressure wound therapy was rapidly adopted on the basis of initial hypotheses about mechanism of action, early positive results, and clinically impressive case series, often supported by industry funding.[83,101] The device fast gained popularity in treating a wide variety of wounds deemed slow or difficult to close.[83,102] Although such clinical success is important, many questions about this clinically complex, costly intervention remain unanswered. This underscores the dilemmas inherent to in vivo wound studies eluded to by Cross and Mustoe.[54]

Systemic treatment encompasses a large portion of chronic wound management and includes several components. Issues of disease, nutrition, behavior, and psychosocial disturbances influence wound healing directly or indirectly. Treatment of systemic or local effects of disease to cure or control underlying pathology of the chronic wound is fundamental to successful wound management.[23,103-105] Examples of these interventions and treatments range from diabetic management, incorporating blood glucose control, weight management, and exercise, to peripheral venous disease management, encompassing pharmacotherapy to manage thrombus formation and mechanical control of peripheral edema.[3,23,103-106]

Nutritional Supplementation

Maintenance of macronutrients and micronutrients, correction of protein and calorie malnutrition, and dehydration require careful ongoing clinical evaluation and the use of appropriate laboratory data. This attention is necessary to avoid threats to wound healing and the patient's general health. Correction of protein deficits should take into consideration the relatively inapparent losses in wound exudates and nonviable tissue load. Concomitantly, fluid loss and potential dehydration necessitates a qualitative estimation of fluid loss in dressings and may

also require laboratory assessment of a patient's hydration status. Correction for caloric needs and expenditure, as well as consideration of fat supplementation, together with protein and fluid supplementation, complete the macronutrient profile for nutritional therapies. Use of standard nutritional supplementation equations and support of a registered dietitian familiar with care of patients with chronic wounds enhances precision in macronutrient intervention for chronic wound management.[7,107-112] Micronutrient deficiencies, support, and supplementation remain a focus for research in nutrition and wound healing.[109] Currently available evidence suggests that supplementation with zinc and vitamin C is effective for patients with intact renal function and nutrient deficiencies.[109,113-115] Arginine is receiving fair attention, but evidence to support supplementation in clinical practice remains limited.[108,109,113,116] Vitamin A supplementation may be supported in certain circumstances (namely, deficiency determined by exclusion based on clinical presentation of delayed inflammation or compromised remodeling and chronic use of medications metabolized by the liver).[108] Vitamin E supplementation should be viewed with skepticism given insubstantial evidence and suggestion that large doses may disrupt the inflammatory phase of healing.[108,111] The utility of other micronutrient supplementation, although often regarded with popular acclaim, generally requires substantially more evidence before translation into practice.[109,117]

Medication Interactions and Polypharmacy

Scrutiny of current medications for side effects is necessary because they may alter the wound healing response. This also includes topical or systemic medications used directly in wound management because many patients with chronic wounds are older and at risk for drug–drug interactions and side effects.[30,118] Specific consideration of pain medication must be included in any medication profile for chronic wound management.[40,45,119] Care must be taken to guard against undertreatment of pain, particularly in older adults in whom unrelieved or partially treated pain may have become a way of life. In addition, local pain relief medication and nonpharmacologic interventions should be considered.[45,120]

Psychosocial Intervention

Many elements of chronic wound management have behavioral and psychosocial dimensions that must be treated in tandem with goals for wound care. For example, stoicism about pain and fears of dependency on pain medication are common and may limit successful management if inadequately addressed as problems with treatment adherence and other concerns arise. Thus, these issues require astute assessment and timely intervention. Medications may be used effectively to support psychosocial care and counseling. They are especially useful in controlling addictive behaviors such as smoking or psychological reactions to treatment or to the wound itself. Problems such as claustrophobia, anxiety (which can be caused by HBOT), and depression should similarly be addressed. Tobacco use and cessation, although relatively poorly understood in relation to specific molecular aspects of wound healing, requires a clear plan for cessation. Available evidence and understanding of physiologic effects of smoking in particular compel intervention for cessation to improve wound management.[31,32,43,44] Ongoing wound treatment regimens may interfere with mental health counseling or behavioral therapies that may appear to be too burdensome to an already overwhelmed patient. Psychosocial interventions should be tied directly to ongoing patient assessments and use all available sources for treatment.

EVALUATION

Effective evaluation of chronic wound management requires frequent reassessment. Goals are predicated on systematic appraisal and expectations for progress. Inconsistent wound care that lacks a systematic approach jeopardizes the evaluation process and warrants zealous quality control. Similarly, clinicians should know and acknowledge their own practice patterns to ensure a systematic approach within and across patient cases. Expectations that are unmet with little or no progress toward goals should generate questions. Questions that arise and puzzle clinicians in the care of specific patients suggest re-examination. Researchable questions commonly arise in this process and can trigger quality monitoring, program evaluations, and clinical or basic research depending on the available resources.

REFERENCES

1. Mostow EN: Wound healing: A multidisciplinary approach for dermatologists. Dermatol Clin 21:371-387, 2003.
2. Rubenstein LZ: Falls in older people: Epidemiology, risk factors and strategies for prevention. Age Ageing 35:ii37-ii41, 2006.
3. Ayello EA: What does the wound say? Why determining etiology is essential for appropriate wound care. Adv Skin Wound Care 18:98-111, 2005.
4. Fleck CA: Wound assessment parameters and dressing selection. Adv Skin Wound Care 19:364-370, 2006.
5. Grey JE, Enoch S, Harding KG: Wound assessment. BMJ 332:285-288, 2006.
6. Keast DH, Bowering CK, Evans AW, et al: MEASURE: A proposed assessment framework for developing best practice recommendations for wound assessment. Wound Repair Regen 12:S1-S17, 2004.
7. Kagan SH, Baum ED, Chalian AA: An algorithm for local non-surgical management of complicated wounds in head and neck cancer patients. ORL Head Neck Nurs 23:13-19, 2005.
8. Goldman RJ, Salcido R: More than one way to measure a wound: An overview of tools and techniques. Adv Skin Wound Care 15:236-243, 2002.
9. Krouskop TA, Baker R, Wilson MS: A noncontact wound measurement system. J Rehabil Res Dev 39:337-345, 2002.
10. Gethin G, Cowman S: Wound measurement comparing the use of acetate tracings and Visitrak digital planimetry. J Clin Nurs 15:422-427, 2006.
11. Haghpanah S, Bogie K, Wang X, et al: Reliability of electronic versus manual wound measurement techniques. Arch Phys Med Rehabil 87:1396-1402, 2006.
12. Lucas C, Classen J, Harrison D, De H: Pressure ulcer surface area measurement using instant full-scale photography and transparency tracings. Adv Skin Wound Care 15:17-23, 2002.
13. Langemo DK, Melland H, Olson B, et al: Comparison of 2 wound volume measurement methods. Adv Skin Wound Care 14:190-196, 2001.

14. Localio RA, Margolis DJ, Kagan SH, et al: Use of photographs for the identification of pressure ulcers in elderly hospitalized patients: Validity and reliability. Wound Repair Regen 14:506-513, 2006.

15. Miller PL, Matthey FC: A cost-benefit analysis of initial burn cultures in the management of acute burns. J Burn Care Rehabil 21:300-303, 2000.

16. Slater RA, Lazarovitch T, Boldur I, et al: Swab cultures accurately identify bacterial pathogens in diabetic foot wounds not involving bone. Diabet Med 21:705-709, 2004.

17. Bill TJ, Ratliff CR, Donovan AM, et al: Quantitative swab culture versus tissue biopsy: A comparison in chronic wounds. Ostomy Wound Manage 47:34-37, 2001.

18. Levine NS, Lindberg RB, Mason AD Jr, Pruitt BA Jr: The quantitative swab culture and smear: A quick, simple method for determining the number of viable aerobic bacteria on open wounds. J Trauma 16:89-94, 1976.

19. Niinikoski JHA: Clinical hyperbaric oxygen therapy, wound perfusion, and transcutaneous oximetry. World J Surg 28:307-311, 2004.

20. Niinikoski J: Hyperbaric oxygen therapy of diabetic foot ulcers, transcutaneous oximetry in clinical decision making. Wound Repair Regen 11:458-461, 2003.

21. Grolman RE, Wilkerson DK, Taylor J, et al: Transcutaneous oxygen measurements predict a beneficial response to hyperbaric oxygen therapy in patients with nonhealing wounds and critical limb ischemia. Am Surg 67:1072-1080, 2001.

22. Hopf HW, Hunt TK, West JM, et al: Wound tissue oxygen tension predicts the risk of wound infection in surgical patients. Arch Surg 132:997-1005, 1997.

23. Hopf HW, Ueno C, Aslam R, et al: Guidelines for the treatment of arterial insufficiency ulcers. Wound Repair Regen 14:693-710, 2006.

24. Gardner SE, Frantz RA, Saltzman CL, et al: Diagnostic validity of three swab techniques for identifying chronic wound infection. Wound Repair Regen 14:548-557, 2006.

25. Sibbald RG, Woo K, Ayello EA: Increased bacterial burden and infection: The story of NERDS and STONES. Adv Skin Wound Care 19:447-463, 2006.

26. Smith BM, Desvigne LD, Slade JB, et al: Transcutaneous oxygen measurements predict healing of leg wounds with hyperbaric therapy. Wound Repair Regen 4:224-229, 1996.

27. McPhail IR, Cooper LT, Hodge DO, et al: Transcutaneous partial pressure of oxygen after surgical wounds. Vasc Med 9:125-127, 2004.

28. Ballard JL, Eke CC, Bunt TJ, Killeen JD: A prospective evaluation of transcutaneous oxygen measurements in the management of diabetic foot problems. J Vasc Surg 22:485-492, 1995.

29. Hopf HW, Humphrey LM, Puzziferri N, et al: Adjuncts to preparing wounds for closure: Hyperbaric oxygen, growth factors, skin substitutes, negative pressure wound therapy (vacuum-assisted closure). Foot Ankle Clin 6:661-682, 2001.

30. Wicke C, Halliday B, Allen D, et al: Effects of steroids and retinoids on wound healing. Arch Surg 135:1265-1270, 2000.

31. Jonsson K, Jensen JA, Goodson WH 3rd, et al: Tissue oxygenation, anemia, and perfusion in relation to wound healing in surgical patients. Ann Surg 214:605-613, 1991.

32. Jensen JA, Goodson WH, Hopf HW, Hunt TK: Cigarette smoking decreases tissue oxygen. Arch Surg 126:1131-1134, 1991.

33. Hunt TK, Linsey M, Grislis H, et al: The effect of differing ambient oxygen tensions on wound infection. Ann Surg 181:35-39, 1975.

34. Whitney JD: Supplemental perioperative oxygen and fluids to improve surgical wound outcomes: Translating evidence into practice. Wound Repair Regen 11:462-467, 2003.

35. Tandara AA, Mustoe TA: Oxygen in wound healing—more than a nutrient. World J Surg 28:294-300, 2004.

36. Ueno C, Hunt TK, Hopf HW: Using physiology to improve surgical wound outcomes. Plast Reconstr Surg 117:59S-71S, 2006.

37. Rich K: Transcutaneous oxygen measurements: Implications for nursing. J Vasc Nurs 19:55-61, 2001.

38. Ertugrul MB, Baktiroglu S, Salman S, et al: The diagnosis of osteomyelitis of the foot in diabetes: Microbiological examination vs. magnetic resonance imaging and labelled leucocyte scanning. Diabet Med 23:649-653, 2006.

39. Termaat MF, Raijmakers PGHM, Scholten HJ, et al: The accuracy of diagnostic imaging for the assessment of chronic osteomyelitis: A systematic review and meta-analysis. J Bone Joint Surg Am 87:2464-2471, 2005.

40. Broadbent E, Petrie KJ, Alley PG, Booth RJ: Psychological stress impairs early wound repair following surgery. Psychosom Med 65:865-869, 2003.

41. Rudge T: Skin as cover: The discursive effects of 'covering' metaphors on wound care practices. Nurs Inq 5:228-237, 1998.

42. Rudge T: Situating wound management: Technoscience, dressings and 'other' skins. Nurs Inq 6:167-177, 1999.

43. Kuri M, Nakagawa M, Tanaka H, et al: Determination of the duration of preoperative smoking cessation to improve wound healing after head and neck surgery. Anesthesiology 102:892-896, 2005.

44. Manassa EH, Hertl CH, Olbrisch R-R: Wound healing problems in smokers and nonsmokers after 132 abdominoplasties. Plast Reconstr Surg 111:2082-2089, 2003.

45. Stotts NA, Puntillo K, Bonham Morris A, et al: Wound care pain in hospitalized adult patients. Heart Lung 33:321-332, 2004.

46. Ventura J, Liberman RP, Green MF, et al: Training and quality assurance with the structured clinical interview for DSM-IV (SCID-I/P). Psychiatry Res 79:163-173, 1998.

47. Steiner JL, Tebes JK, Sledge WH, Walker ML: A comparison of the Structured Clinical Interview for DSM-III-R and clinical diagnoses. J Nerv Ment Dis 183:365-369, 1995.

48. Acquadro C, Price P, Wollina U: Linguistic validation of the Cardiff Wound Impact Schedule into French, German and US English. J Wound Care 14:14-17, 2005.

49. Price P, Harding K: Cardiff Wound Impact Schedule: The development of a condition-specific questionnaire to assess health-related quality of life in patients with chronic wounds of the lower limb. Int Wound J 1:10-17, 2004.

50. Medina A, Scott PG, Ghahary A, Tredget EE: Pathophysiology of chronic nonhealing wounds. J Burn Care Rehabil 26:306-319, 2005.

51. Lohmann R, Zemlin C, Motzkau M, et al: Expression of matrix metalloproteinases and growth factors in diabetic foot wounds treated with a protease absorbent dressing. J Diabetes Complicat 20:329-335, 2006.

52. Chandan KS, Khanna S, Gordillo G, et al: Oxygen, oxidants, and antioxidants in wound healing. An emerging paradigm. Ann N Y Acad Sci 957:239-249, 2002.

53. McGuckin M, Goldman R, Bolton L, Salcido R: The clinical relevance of microbiology in acute and chronic wounds. Adv Skin Wound Care 16:12-25, 2003.

54. Cross KJ, Mustoe TA: Growth factors in wound healing. Surg Clin North Am 83:531-545, 2003.

55. Weed T, Ratliff C, Drake DB: Quantifying bacterial bioburden during negative pressure wound therapy: Does the wound VAC enhance bacterial clearance? Ann Plast Surg 52:276-280, 2004.

56. Toy LW: Matrix metalloproteinases: Their function in tissue repair. J Wound Care 14:20-22, 2005.

57. Dyson M, Young S, Pendle CL, et al: Comparison of the effects of moist and dry conditions on dermal repair. J Investig Dermatol 91:434-439, 1988.

58. Chen WYJ, Rogers AA, Lydon MJ: Characterization of biologic properties of wound fluid collected during early stages of wound healing. J Investig Dermatol 99:559-564, 1992.

59. Fleck CA: Differentiating MMPs, biofilm, endotoxins, exotoxins, and cytokines. Adv Skin Wound Care 19:77-81, 2006.

60. Granick M, Boykin J, Gamelli R, et al: Toward a common language: Surgical wound bed preparation and debridement. Wound Repair Regen 14:S1-S10, 2006.

61. Attinger CE, Janis JE, Steinberg J, et al: Clinical approach to wounds: Debridement and wound bed preparation including the use of dressings and wound-healing adjuvants. Plast Reconstr Surg 117:72S-109S, 2006.

62. Williams D, Enoch S, Miller D, et al: Effect of sharp debridement using curette on recalcitrant nonhealing venous leg ulcers: A concurrently controlled, prospective cohort study. Wound Repair Regen 13:131-137, 2005.

63. Ayello EA, Cuddigan JE: Debridement: Controlling the necrotic/cellular burden. Adv Skin Wound Care 17:66-78, 2004.

64. Stotts NA, Hunt TK: Managing bacterial colonization and infection. Clin Geriatr Med 13:565-573, 1997.

65. Mertz PM, Ovington LG: Wound healing microbiology. Dermatol Clin 11:739-747, 1993.

66. Wysocki AB: Evaluating and managing open skin wounds: Colonization versus infection. AACN Clin Issues 13:382-397, 2002.

67. Edwards R, Harding KG: Bacteria and wound healing. Curr Opin Infect Dis 17:91-96, 2004.

68. Armstrong MH, Price P: Wet-to-dry gauze dressings: Fact and fiction. Wounds: A Compendium of Clinical Research and Practice 16:56-62, 2004.

69. Smack DP, Harrington AC, Dunn C, et al: Infection and allergy incidence in ambulatory surgery patients using white petrolatum vs bacitracin ointment. A randomized controlled trial. JAMA 276:972-977, 1996.

70. Campbell RM, Perlis CS, Fisher E, Gloster HM: Gentamicin ointment versus petrolatum for management of auricular wounds. Dermatol Surg 31:664-669, 2005.

71. James WD: Use of antibiotic-containing ointment versus plain petrolatum during and after clean cutaneous surgery. J Am Acad Dermatol 55:915-916, 2006.

72. Pelle MT, Miller OF 3rd: Debridement of necrotic eschar with 40% urea paste speeds healing of residual limbs and avoids further surgery. Arch Dermatol 137:1288-1290, 2001.

73. Howell-Jones RS, Wilson MJ, Hill KE, et al: A review of the microbiology, antibiotic usage and resistance in chronic skin wounds. J Antimicrob Chemother 55:143-149, 2005.

74. Cho Lee A-R, Leem H, Lee J, Chan Park K: Reversal of silver sulfadiazine-impaired wound healing by epidermal growth factor. Biomaterials 26:4670-4676, 2005.

75. Warriner R, Burrell R: Infection and the chronic wound: A focus on silver. Adv Skin Wound Care 18(suppl 1):2-12, 2005.

76. Percival SL, Bowler PG, Russell D: Bacterial resistance to silver in wound care. J Hosp Infect 60:1-7, 2005.

77. Burks RI: Povidone-iodine solution in wound treatment. Phys Ther 78:212-218, 1998.

78. Kozol RA, Gillies C, Elgebaly SA: Effects of sodium hypochlorite (Dakin's solution) on cells of the wound module. Arch Surg 123:420-423, 1988.

79. Lawrence JC: The use of iodine as an antiseptic agent. J Wound Care 7:421-425, 1998.

80. Niedner R: Cytotoxicity and sensitization of povidone-iodine and other frequently used anti-infective agents. Dermatology 195:89-92, 1997.

81. Wilson JR, Mills JG, Prather ID, Dimitrijevich SD: A toxicity index of skin and wound cleansers used on in vitro fibroblasts and keratinocytes. Adv Skin Wound Care 18:373-378, 2005.

82. Burke DT, Ho C, Bchir MB, et al: Effects of hydrotherapy on pressure ulcer healing. Am J Phys Med Rehabil 77:394-398, 1998.

83. Hess CL, Howard MA, Attinger CE: A review of mechanical adjuncts in wound healing: Hydrotherapy, ultrasound, negative pressure therapy, hyperbaric oxygen, and electrostimulation. Ann Plast Surg 51:210-218, 2003.

84. Bale S: A guide to wound debridement. J Wound Care 6:179-182, 1997.

85. Alvarez OM, Fernandez-Obregon A, Rogers RS, et al: Chemical debridement of pressure ulcers: A prospective, randomized, comparative trial of collagenase and papain/urea formulations. Wounds: A Compendium of Clinical Research and Practice 12:15-25, 2000.

86. Mumcuoglu KY: Clinical applications for maggots in wound care. Am J Clin Dermatol 2:219-227, 2001.

87. Steed DL: Debridement. Am J Surg 187:S71-S74, 2004.

88. Pieper B, Caliri MHL: Nontraditional wound care: A review of the evidence for the use of sugar, papaya/papain, and fatty acids. J Wound Ostomy Continence Nurs 30:175-183, 2003.

89. Falabella AF: Debridement and wound bed preparation. Dermatol Ther 19:317-325, 2006.

90. Kresken M, Hafner D, Schmitz F-J, Wichelhaus TA: Prevalence of mupirocin resistance in clinical isolates of Staphylococcus aureus and Staphylococcus epidermidis:

Results of the Antimicrobial Resistance Surveillance Study of the Paul-Ehrlich-Society for Chemotherapy, 2001. Int J Antimicrob Agents 23:577-581, 2004.

91. Kallehave F, Gottrup F: Topical antibiotics used in the treatment of complex wounds. J Wound Care 5:158-160, 1996.

92. Spann CT, Tutrone WD, Weinberg JM, et al: Topical antibacterial agents for wound care: A primer. Dermatol Surg 29:620-626, 2003.

93. Jeffcoate WJ: The evidence base to guide the use of antibiotics in foot ulcers in people with diabetes is thin, but what are we going to do about it? Diabet Med 23:339-340, 2006.

94. Abdulrazak A, Ibrahim Bitar Z, Ayesh Al-Shamali A, Ahmed Mobasher L: Bacteriological study of diabetic foot infections. J Diabet Complicat 19:138-141, 2005.

95. Howell-Jones RS, Price PE, Howard AJ, Thomas DW: Antibiotic prescribing for chronic skin wounds in primary care. Wound Repair Regen 14:387-393, 2006.

96. Hernandez R: The use of systemic antibiotics in the treatment of chronic wounds. Dermatol Ther 19:326-337, 2006.

97. Gregory SR, Piccolo N, Piccolo MT, et al: Comparison of propolis skin cream to silver sulfadiazine: A naturopathic alternative to antibiotics in treatment of minor burns. J Altern Complement Med 8:77-83, 2002.

98. Molan PC: The role of honey in the management of wounds. J Wound Care 8:415-418, 1999.

99. Subrahmanyam M: A prospective randomised clinical and histological study of superficial burn wound healing with honey and silver sulfadiazine. Burns 24:157-161, 1998.

100. Page JC, Newswander B, Schwenke DC, et al: Retrospective analysis of negative pressure wound therapy in open foot wounds with significant soft tissue defects. Adv Skin Wound Care 17:354-364, 2004.

101. Philbeck TE, Whittington KT, Millsap MH, et al: The clinical and cost effectiveness of externally applied negative pressure wound therapy in the treatment of wounds in home healthcare Medicare patients. Ostomy Wound Manage 45:41-50, 1999.

102. Leininger BE, Rasmussen TE, Smith DL, et al: Experience with wound VAC and delayed primary closure of contaminated soft tissue injuries in Iraq. J Trauma 61:1207-1211, 2006.

103. Whitney J, Phillips L, Aslam R, et al: Guidelines for the treatment of pressure ulcers. Wound Repair Regen 14:663-679, 2006.

104. Steed DL, Attinger C, Colaizzi T, et al: Guidelines for the treatment of diabetic ulcers. Wound Repair Regen 14:680-692, 2006.

105. Robson MC, Cooper DM, Aslam R, et al: Guidelines for the treatment of venous ulcers. Wound Repair Regen 14:649-662, 2006.

106. Jeffcoate WJ, Price P, Harding KG, International Working Group on Wound Healing and Treatments for People with Diabetic Foot Ulcers: Wound healing and treatments for people with diabetic foot ulcers. Diabetes Metab Res Rev 20:S78-S89, 2004.

107. Whitney JD, Heitkemper MM: Modifying perfusion, nutrition, and stress to promote wound healing in patients with acute wounds. Heart Lung 28:123-133, 1999.

108. Scholl D, Langkamp-Henken B: Nutrient recommendations for wound healing. J Intraven Nurs 24:124-132, 2001.

109. Arnold M, Barbul A: Nutrition and wound healing. Plast Reconstr Surg 117:42S-58S, 2006.

110. Langemo D, Anderson J, Hanson D, et al: Nutritional considerations in wound care. Adv Skin Wound Care 19:297-298, 2006.

111. Posthauer ME: The role of nutrition in wound care. Adv Skin Wound Care 19:43-54, 2006.

112. Williams JZ, Barbul A: Nutrition and wound healing. Surg Clin North Am 83:571-596, 2003.

113. Desneves KJ, Todorovic BE, Cassar A, Crowe TC: Treatment with supplementary arginine, vitamin C and zinc in patients with pressure ulcers: A randomised controlled trial. Clin Nutr 24:979-987, 2005.

114. Berger MM, Shenkin A: Update on clinical micronutrient supplementation studies in the critically ill. Curr Opin Clin Nutr Metab Care 9:711-716, 2006.

115. Doerr TD, Marks SC, Shamsa FH, et al: Effects of zinc and nutritional status on clinical outcomes in head and neck cancer. Nutrition 14:489-495, 1998.

116. Stechmiller JK, Childress B, Cowan L: Arginine supplementation and wound healing. Nutr Clin Pract 20:52-61, 2005.

117. Alleva R, Nasole E, Di Donato F, et al: alpha-Lipoic acid supplementation inhibits oxidative damage, accelerating chronic wound healing in patients undergoing hyperbaric oxygen therapy. Biochem Biophys Res Commun 333:404-410, 2005.

118. Enoch S, Grey JE, Harding KG: Non-surgical and drug treatments. BMJ 332:900-903, 2006.

119. Jorgensen B, Friis GJ, Gottrup F: Pain and quality of life for patients with venous leg ulcers: Proof of concept of the efficacy of Biatain-Ibu, a new pain reducing wound dressing. Wound Repair Regen 14:233-239, 2006.

120. Blanke W, Hallern BV: Sharp wound debridement in local anaesthesia using EMLA cream: 6 years' experience in 1084 patients. Eur J Emerg Med 10:229-231, 2003.

Compromised Grafts and Flaps

17

William A. Zamboni, MD, FACS, and Richard C. Baynosa, MD

The use of flaps and grafts has become an indispensable tool in the armamentarium of the reconstructive surgeon. Traditionally in the realm of the plastic surgeon, the use of simple grafts and flaps has become prevalent in numerous surgical specialties including general surgery and head and neck surgery. As the surgeon's experience with grafts and flaps increases, the use of hyperbaric oxygen therapy (HBOT) as an adjunct for success will inevitably play a role. Most plastic surgeons will have expertise in the use of grafts and flaps for reconstruction, but few will have knowledge of hyperbaric medicine. In contrast, the hyperbaric medicine physician will be an expert in the indications and uses of hyperbaric therapy but may not be familiar with the definitions, classifications, and principles of using grafts and flaps for reconstruction. The purpose of this chapter is to give an overview of HBOT use in compromised grafts and flaps to allow a multidisciplinary approach to the problem.

HBOT is unnecessary in the support of routine, uncompromised grafts or flaps. However, the appropriate use of HBOT has been shown to be extremely useful in the successful salvage of compromised grafts and flaps.[1-3] The rationale for appropriate HBOT for compromised grafts and flaps should be based on scientific and clinical research whenever possible. This chapter discusses the definition, classification, and diagnosis of compromised grafts and flaps. In addition, the proper indications for the use of HBOT based on available scientific and clinical literature are reviewed. This should assist both the surgeon and the hyperbaric physician in acquiring the necessary background to successfully utilize HBOT for flap or graft salvage using a calculated, multidisciplinary approach.

DEFINITIONS, CLASSIFICATIONS, AND PATHOPHYSIOLOGY

Simple Grafts versus Composite Grafts

A *graft* is a tissue that is completely separated from the donor tissue bed and all vascular connections. By definition, the nonvascularized graft must rely on ingrowth of new blood vessels from the recipient bed for adequate blood supply. Grafts rely on the nutrients and growth factors present in the recipient bed to meet their metabolic requirements for the first few days until angiogenesis occurs. During this initial period, there will be a low oxygen tension within the graft area. It is therefore essential that the graft recipient bed be of optimal condition to allow successful take of the graft.

Grafts may be classified as simple or composite. *Simple grafts* are composed of a single tissue type, whereas composite grafts consist of two or more tissue types. The classic example of the simple graft is the skin graft. Other types of simple tissue grafts include cartilage, bone, and fat. *Composite grafts* are made up of more than one tissue and may contain subcutaneous fat, cartilage, and full-thickness skin. Because composite grafts generally contain multiple tissue types, they have an inherently higher metabolic requirement and, therefore, are more susceptible to ischemic insult than simple grafts.

Flap Classification Based on Blood Supply

A *flap* by definition is a vascularized piece of tissue that remains attached to its donor blood supply or becomes revascularized via microsurgical anastomoses to recipient vessels, as is the case with free tissue transfers. Because flaps are vascularized tissues, they may be classified on the basis of the origin of their blood supply. Flaps classified by blood supply may be random or axial. Because HBOT for compromised flaps involves enhancing oxygenation of troubled circulation, understanding the underlying blood supply for a particular flap is of critical importance.

Random flaps receive their blood supply indirectly from the subdermal vascular plexus and not directly from a specific blood vessel (Fig. 17.1). Classically, random flaps are raised and transferred on the basis of a length-to-width ratio of 2:1.[4] Random flaps are inherently more sensitive to ischemia than axial flaps because of their less robust blood supply. A limitation of the random flap is its restricted arc of rotation where any excessive tension will compromise blood supply to the flap. Compromise and distal necrosis in a random flap are typically the result of an improper flap design.

Axial flaps receive their blood supply on the basis of a named blood vessel. This allows the flap to be designed longer and narrower than a random flap. In addition, because the flap can be isolated on the pedicle artery and vein alone, the flap has a consistent blood supply that will typically have a larger arc of rotation than a random flap. Flaps that are isolated on the supplying artery and vein alone are referred to as *pedicle flaps*. Distal compromise or necrosis in axial flaps usually results from trying to transfer tissue outside of the defined arterial supply of the pedicle or an intrinsic problem with the pedicle such as kinking or external compression.

In addition to local pedicle flaps, distant flaps can be either pedicle based or free. Distant flaps are staged axial flaps that receive their name because the recipient site is at a distant site. These flaps are unique in that they require adequate growth of new blood supply from the recipient site into the distal end of the flap before division of the proximal donor pedicle. The timing of division of the proximal pedicle is crucial because the flap will not survive unless adequate angiogenesis has occurred from the recipient site to provide

RANDOM/RANDOM CUTANEOUS PATTERN SKIN FLAPS

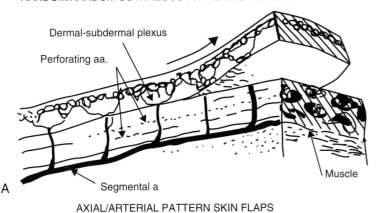

Dermal-subdermal plexus

Perforating aa.

A   Segmental a

AXIAL/ARTERIAL PATTERN SKIN FLAPS

Figure 17.1 Classic classification of skin flaps. *A*, Random pattern flaps. *B*, Axial pattern flaps. a, artery; aa, arteries; v, vein.

Muscle

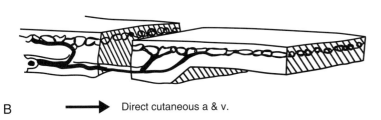

B   Direct cutaneous a & v.

blood circulation to the flap. This will typically take approximately 3 to 4 weeks. The classic example of this flap is the groin flap based on the superficial circumflex iliac vessels. Free flaps are also axial-type flaps, the recipient sites of which are at locations distant to the donor site. In contrast with distant pedicle flaps, however, the donor pedicle vessels are isolated, transected, and then reanastomosed to recipient vessels in proximity to the recipient wound site. Advantages of this technique include a robust blood supply, a single-stage procedure, and the multiple possibilities for donor sites for a given defect. Disadvantages include increased technical difficulty and the potential for complications at the anastomotic sites. Free flaps exposed to prolonged ischemia are also at risk for ischemia-reperfusion (IR) injury (Table 17.1).

Flap Classification Based on Tissue Type

Flaps may also be classified on the basis of their tissue composition. Flaps may be composed of skin, muscle, fascia, or bone. Alternatively, flaps can be designed with a combination of these tissues such as musculocutaneous, fasciocutaneous, or osteofasciocutaneous flaps. Knowledge of the tissues that compose a flap leads to an understanding of the ischemic tolerance of the flap. Skin has an extremely high tolerance for ischemia, whereas muscle is much more susceptible. In addition, skeletal muscle is at risk for IR injury once circulation is restored.

As mentioned earlier, HBOT is unnecessary and is not recommended for the success of normal, well-designed grafts or flaps. Thourani and colleagues[5] demonstrated a greater than 90% success rate for 599 skin grafts in 233 consecutive patients on a variety of suitable graft beds over a 2-year period. Similar results can be expected with well-designed flaps performed by technically capable surgeons. Over a 14-year period using free flaps in 346 patients for reconstruction of head and neck tumor extirpations, Podrecca and investigators[6] demonstrated a 95% success rate in patients with a mean age of 57 years. It is when flaps become compromised that HBOT may be prudently used as a successful adjunct for flap salvage. Recognizing the pathophysiology and clinical manifestations of the compromised graft or flap is therefore of

Table 17.1 Flap Classification Based on Blood Supply

FLAP TYPE	DESCRIPTION
Random	No direct arterial blood supply; blood supply is by the dermal and subdermal plexus
Axial	Blood supply is directly from a specific artery
Local	The employment of adjacent tissue for flap use
Distant	The employment of distant tissue for flap use
Pedicle	Describes a flap raised and based on an intact arterial and venous blood supply
Free	Describes a flap in which the arterial and venous blood supply is divided and reattached to another location by microsurgical anastomosis

the utmost importance for the surgeon and hyperbaric physician to critically evaluate and appropriately prescribe the use of HBOT.

Ischemia, Ischemia-Reperfusion, and the Microcirculation

Ischemia is the usual cause of graft and flap compromise. Ischemia results in an inadequate supply of oxygen to meet the metabolic demands of the graft or flap. Tissue hypoxia results in overall poor wound healing secondary to multiple factors. The neutrophil and macrophage both require oxygen to function during the inflammation phase of wound healing where they play a crucial role in killing microorganisms and preventing infection.[7] In addition, during the repair and remodeling stages of wound healing, oxygen is required by fibroblasts for collagen synthesis and is important ultimately for remodeling and collagen cross-linking.[8] The lack of oxygen in the hypoxic wound, therefore, can lead to problems with chronic infection and delayed wound healing. HBOT is effective in reversing these effects in the proper clinical situations.

Oxygen delivery to tissues is defined by the equation:

$$\text{Oxygen delivery (D}_{O_2}) = CO \times [(1.34 \times \text{Hgb} \times Sa_{O_2}) + (0.003 \times Pa_{O_2})]$$

where CO = cardiac output; Hgb = hemoglobin level; Sa_{O_2} = arterial oxygen saturation; and Pa_{O_2} = partial pressure of oxygen in arterial blood. The term of the equation $1.34 \times Hgb \times Sa_{O_2}$ represents the contribution of hemoglobin to oxygen concentration. In the

second term of the equation, 0.003 represents the solubility of oxygen in plasma at the normal body temperature of $37^\circ C$. Therefore, the term of the equation $0.003 \times Pa_{O_2}$ represents the expected concentration of dissolved oxygen.[9] During normal respiration, the amount of oxygen dissolved in plasma is insignificant. With HBOT, however, oxygen tensions are increased 10 to 13 times above their normal level, and the oxygen-carrying capacity of the blood via plasma is increased by 25%.[10] This increase is inconsequential for normal tissue. However, problem wounds and compromised grafts and flaps often have partially occluded capillaries secondary to microthrombi that restrict the passage of red blood cells.[11] Yet plasma is still able to flow through these capillaries, making the dissolved oxygen in plasma significant. Krogh[12] has shown that in these capillaries that contain only plasma at 2 atmospheres of pressure (ATA), the oxygen concentration on the arterial side is increased fourfold and O_2 concentration on the venous side is increased twofold in comparison with normal inspired air. This effectively allows the plasma to be capable of carrying enough oxygen to meet the needs of the ischemic tissue without hemoglobin-bound oxygen.[13]

IR injury may result from prolonged ischemia time with free flaps or after the restoration of blood flow to the flap after complete arterial occlusion. The mechanism of IR injury revolves around the production of oxygen-derived free radicals.[14,15] These free radicals are extremely toxic to all biologic substances and result in cell death secondary to lipid peroxidation and propagation of more free radicals. Neutrophils are an important source of these

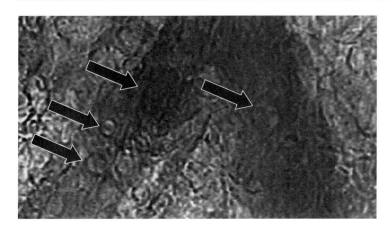

Figure 17.2 Neutrophil adherence to the endothelium of an ischemic postcapillary microvenule at 15 minutes of reperfusion. The leukocytes are marked by *arrows* and are easily identified by their characteristic size and whitish color. **(See Color Plate 24.)**

oxygen free radicals in IR injury. Research on the effects of IR on the microcirculation in skeletal muscle demonstrates significant neutrophil adhesion to postcapillary venules during reperfusion[16-18] (Fig. 17.2). These adherent leukocytes release oxygen free radicals, causing injury to the vascular endothelium, which leads to tissue edema. In addition, severe vasoconstriction of precapillary arterioles occurs, exacerbating the low flow state.[19,20,23] The resultant ischemia coupled with the edema leads to progressive tissue hypoxia, and ultimately to flap necrosis and failure.

HBOT has been shown experimentally to attenuate the effects of IR injury and reduce tissue necrosis in both skin flaps and skeletal muscle.[1,21,22] Using a rat gracilis muscle model, Zamboni and coworkers[23] studied the effect of HBOT on the microcirculatory morphology during IR. This study specifically evaluated leukocyte endothelial adherence and vasoactivity via measurement of precapillary arteriole diameters. Examining the microcirculation of the gracilis muscle in this model, the authors demonstrated a significant reduction of leukocyte adherence to postcapillary venules in tissue treated with HBOT both during and immediately after 4 hours of ischemia. In addition, the progressive arteriolar vasoconstriction was also inhibited by HBOT administered during and up to 1 hour after reperfusion. Subsequent studies have shown that the neutrophil adhesion associated with IR injury is dependent on the β_2 integrin (CD18 chain) on the neutrophil membrane surface.[24,25] More recent work has shown

that the beneficial effects of HBOT on IR injury are mediated by nitric oxide via a nitric oxide synthase pathway, and that vascular endothelial growth factor is an important early initiator of this effect.[26-30] The pathophysiology of ischemia and IR injury is discussed in further detail in Chapter 9.

DIAGNOSIS AND TREATMENT OF THE COMPROMISED GRAFT

Although skin grafts and composite grafts are often classified together with compromised flaps, these two entities are different from a physiologic standpoint. As described earlier, all flaps by definition have an inherent blood supply, whereas skin and composite grafts are avascular tissues that depend on the quality of the recipient bed for revascularization. Therefore, the diagnosis of a compromised graft begins with proper assessment of the recipient wound bed. Indeed, the most effective treatment for the compromised graft is *prevention*. Unlike the treatment for compromised flaps that may be salvaged with HBOT after surgery, the goal for successful grafting is in preparing the hypoxic, compromised recipient bed *before* placement of the graft.

Recognizing the Problem Wound Bed

Appropriate diagnosis of the problem wound requires the physician to determine the cause of nonhealing. Numerous factors can delay wound healing. This section focuses on diagnosing the problem wound recipient bed that will lead to compromised graft take without proper adjunctive treatment.

As mentioned earlier, the ultimate cause of a compromised graft is ischemia. Poor tissue perfusion and oxygenation results in a hypoxic wound bed that will be inadequate for proper graft take. The diagnosis of a hypoxic wound bed begins with a complete history and physical examination. Essential components of the history include duration of the defect, changes in wound size, associated trauma or infections, history of radiation exposure, previous surgeries, current wound care, and any comorbidities such as diabetes, peripheral vascular disease, connective tissue disorders, or use of immunosuppressants and steroids. Physical examination should focus on wound location, size, depth (including types of tissue involved or bone exposure), peripheral pulses, and signs of infection. Quantitative tissue cultures are warranted in wound beds that are suspected of being infected or in chronic wounds that have history of recurrent infections. Wounds with greater than 10^5 colony-forming units per gram of tissue are, by definition, infected and will not allow successful graft take.[31] Determination of ankle–brachial index will give a quick and fairly reliable estimation of lower extremity perfusion. A low ankle–brachial index suggests poor distal extremity blood flow and should be evaluated by a vascular surgeon for a reconstructible lesion. The presence or absence of granulation tissue also provides clues to the adequacy of wound perfusion. A well-oxygenated, healthy wound will have beefy, red granulation tissue present, whereas a hypoxic wound will have pale, friable, or nonexistent granulation.

Lower extremity wounds are widely prevalent and necessitate the evaluation of both tissue perfusion and tissue oxygenation. The assessment of ischemia begins with noninvasive arteriole Doppler studies including an ankle–brachial index. This workup may also include examination of segmental and toe pressures in addition to transcutaneous oximetry. Segmental and toe pressures assess tissue perfusion, whereas transcutaneous oximetry examines tissue oxygenation, and these measures should generally be part of the routine evaluation of any nonhealing wound. Normal wounds require a value of at least 50 mm Hg for toe pressure and transcutaneous partial pressure of oxygen tension ($tcPo_2$) to heal adequately and sustain a graft. Values between 30 and 50 mm Hg are considered marginal, and a $tcPo_2$ or toe pressure less than 30 mm Hg indicates that the wound bed will not likely heal or sustain a graft without adjunctive treatment.[32] The necessity of evaluating both oxygenation and perfusion is illustrated in the ischemic diabetic foot wound. In diabetic lower extremity wounds, it is not unusual to see segmental and toe pressures that are normal or slightly increased while simultaneously exhibiting a low $tcPo_2$. This may be explained physiologically by multiple factors including the noncompressible, calcified vessels and poor microcirculation that characterize patients with diabetes.[2,33] In effect, these values suggest adequate large-vessel perfusion but poor oxygenation of the wound bed possibly secondary to problems with the microcirculation, potentially explaining the difficulties with healing.

Another cause of impaired wound healing that results in a hypoxic wound bed is radiation therapy. Radiation can have both acute and chronic effects on the skin and underlying tissue. Acute effects include erythema, desquamation, and ulceration. Delayed and chronic effects include thickening and fibrosis of the affected tissue, telangiectasias, necrosis, and tumorigenesis. Radiation damage affects the blood vessels of the affected skin, resulting in a hypoxic wound bed. In addition, the oxygen gradient decreases from the wound edge to the center of the radiated wound at such a gradual rate that the typical hypoxic stimulus for angiogenesis is not initiated.[34] Studies of the microvasculature in irradiated tissue demonstrate evidence of endarteritis obliterans on histologic examination.[35,36] All of these factors result in a hypoxic wound bed that characteristically has poor formation of granulation tissue.

Management of the Hypoxic, Compromised Wound Bed

Management of the hypoxic wound bed in preparation for a graft involves control of infection and correction of perfusion and oxygenation deficiencies. Control of infection includes surgical debridement of all necrotic and infected tissue when necessary and the proper use of topical antimicrobial wound dressings. When quantitative wound cultures can reliably demonstrate less than 10^5 colony-forming units of bacteria per gram of tissue, the wound can be safely considered free of infection and suitable for grafting. In the evaluation of tissue perfusion, a vascular surgery consultation, with arteriogram or magnetic resonance angiography as warranted, will help to rule out a vascular lesion that may be treated with bypass or dilation and stenting. If the patient has no reconstructible vascular lesion, an evaluation for the efficacy of HBOT is indicated.

HBOT may be a useful adjunct in preparation of the compromised wound bed for grafting if the oxygen tension within the tissue can be increased to therapeutic levels.[2,32,37,38] To determine whether HBOT will be effective for a compromised wound bed, an oxygen challenge is indicated. Many authors have conducted studies with an oxygen challenge breathing 100% normobaric oxygen. Critical values of tcPo$_2$ used to predict healing range from 50 to 100 mm Hg to an increase of more than 10 mm Hg after inhalation of 100% oxygen.[37,39-42] The wide range of values used with 100% oxygen make this criterion less than optimal. In fact, patients with a minimal 100% O_2 mask response will respond with significant increase in tcPo$_2$ in the hyperbaric chamber. Strauss and investigators[43] have conducted studies examining tcPo$_2$ measurements with HBOT and wound healing and found that an increase in tcPo$_2$ to greater than 200 mm Hg during HBOT at 2.5 ATA resulted in wound healing in more than 80% of problem wounds regardless of room air measurements. Quigley and Faris[44] used tcPo$_2$ measurements to determine the severity and clinical progression of peripheral vascular disease and demonstrated

that values less than 40 mm Hg were associated with poor ulcer healing in patients with diabetes. Therefore, in the absence of a reconstructible vascular lesion, if the wound tcPo$_2$ is less than 40 mm Hg, the wound should be considered hypoxic and treatment with HBOT is recommended.[32] If the tcPo$_2$ increases to greater than 200 mm Hg while undergoing HBOT, the wound bed has an excellent chance of producing enough granulation tissue to support a graft and may potentially go on to complete healing[45] (Fig. 17.3). In these patients, HBOT should be continued, preferably on an outpatient basis, with daily treatments of 100% oxygen at 2.4 ATA for 90 minutes five times per week. Repeat wound tcPo$_2$ measurements should be documented routinely on a weekly basis with the patient breathing room air and at least 12 hours after an HBOT treatment. Once tcPo$_2$ levels are greater than 40 mm Hg, HBOT can be discontinued and routine wound care should be continued until surgery can be scheduled for graft placement.

Rationale for Hyperbaric Oxygen Treatment of the Compromised Graft

The most effective treatment for the compromised graft is prevention with good surgical planning and proper preparation of an adequate wound bed. However, situations may occur where the recipient wound bed ischemia is unrecognized or harvest of a composite graft is larger than what can reasonably be sustained by the recipient bed. Although these situations are not encouraged and can be avoided with good surgical judgment and operative planning, HBOT has been advocated by some as a salvage therapy for the compromised graft.[1-3,37] Some corroborating studies in the literature that involve the use of HBOT in compromised grafts are presented here.

In 1967, Perrins and Cantab[46] conducted the only controlled clinical study specifically evaluating the use of HBOT for success of split-thickness skin graft (STSG) take after surgery. Their study was a prospective, randomized, blinded trial of 48 patients undergoing split-thickness skin graft with 50% of the

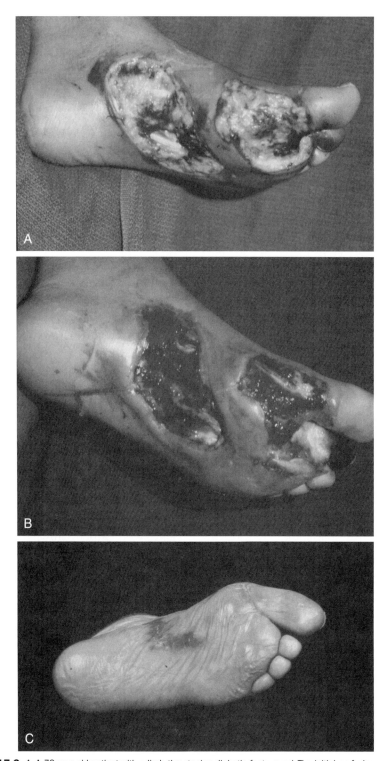

Figure 17.3 *A,* A 78-year-old patient with a limb-threatening diabetic foot wound. The initial perfusion pressure was normal, but transcutaneous partial pressure of oxygen (tcPo$_2$) tension was low. *B,* Wound after initial surgical debridement and after 15 hyperbaric oxygen therapy (HBOT) treatments. *C,* Postoperative follow-up view of wound after 30 HBOT treatments with successful healing. **(See Color Plate 25.)** *(Adapted from Zamboni WA: Applications of hyperbaric oxygen therapy in plastic surgery. In: Oriani G, Marroni A, Wattel F (eds): Handbook on Hyperbaric Medicine. New York, Springer, 1995, pp 443–507, by permission.)*

patients receiving HBOT after surgery and 50% serving as control subjects. HBOT was administered for 2 hours at 2.0 ATA on the evening of the operation and then twice daily for 3 days. Complete graft take was defined as greater than 95% total surface area. A significant 29% improvement in graft survival of the HBOT group occurred in comparison with the control group. The HBOT group had 64% of patients achieving complete take, whereas this was true in only 17% of the control group. Furthermore, 100% of patients in the HBOT group achieved greater than 60% take, whereas only 64% of the control group sustained *at least* 60% take of their split-thickness skin grafts. It is unclear why the overall graft survivals in this study were so low when most plastic surgeons would expect greater than 90% take of a split-thickness skin graft with an adequate recipient bed. Although the cause behind the apparent graft compromise in this study is uncertain, this trial clearly demonstrates a benefit to postoperative HBOT.

In contrast with skin grafts, no prospective, randomized clinical trials have evaluated the efficacy of HBOT for compromised composite grafts. There are, however, multiple case reports and controlled animal experiments that provide information. Three separate case studies with a total of eight patients demonstrated successful take of large composite grafts ranging from 1.7 to 2.2 cm after treatment with HBOT at 2.0 ATA twice a day until complete graft take.[47-49] In a separate series of six patients, Friedman and colleagues[50] performed nasal reconstructions with large composite ear lobule grafts up to 1.5 cm. HBOT was used because the shaping of the composite grafts adversely affected the normal vascular architecture of the graft. All grafts ultimately showed complete take.

Controlled animal studies have had some conflicting results. McFarlane and Wermuth[51] demonstrated that large composite musculocutaneous grafts in rats treated with HBOT for 2 hours/day at 3.0 ATA could be salvaged. Half of the grafts in the experimental group had partial necrosis and half had complete graft survival, whereas all control grafts had complete necrosis. Zhang and coworkers[52] demonstrated a significant 57% increased surface area survival in 1.0 × 0.5 cm composite rat ear grafts treated with HBOT compared with control subjects. Other studies have not been as promising. Both Rubin and investigators[53] and Lim and coauthors[54] examined the benefits of HBOT on large 4-cm × 2-cm skin and cartilage composite grafts in rabbits. Both studies demonstrated a slightly greater percentage of graft survival than control animals, but the results were not significant and the final survival rates would not be clinically meaningful—30.5% for the first trial and 15.4% for the second trial. Mazolewski and colleagues[55] investigated the use of HBOT on rat ear composite graft survival but found no significant effect on grafts larger than 1 cm. It is clear from these conflicting results that further research and clinical trials are warranted to clearly demonstrate the effects of HBOT on composite graft survival.

DIAGNOSIS OF THE COMPROMISED FLAP AND CRITERIA FOR USE OF HYPERBARIC OXYGEN THERAPY

The compromised flap is a specific entity that requires an accurate diagnosis for proper and successful treatment. Unfortunately, an all too common scenario occurs when a truly compromised flap is allowed to progress steadily to signs of necrosis. Usually, it is at this point that the surgeon consults the hyperbaric physician in hopes that HBOT can save the flap. Regrettably, once the flap has demonstrated signs of necrosis, this typically obviates the use of HBOT because it cannot salvage dead tissue. To prevent disappointment and a poor outcome, three major points must be considered in the successful management of the compromised flap. The three keys to successful treatment of the compromised flap are listed in Table 17.2.

It is crucial for the plastic surgeon to immediately recognize the signs of a compromised flap, to correctly assess the cause, and to quickly consult the hyperbaric physician. The hyperbaric physician must be able to accurately diagnose the cause of flap compromise to initiate the proper protocol for successful flap salvage.

Table 17.2 Keys to Successful Management of the Compromised Flap

1. Accurate diagnosis of the specific flap problem
2. Expedient initiation of hyperbaric oxygen therapy
3. Good, open communication between the surgeon and the hyperbaric physician

Clinical Manifestations of the Compromised Flap

The technique of flap monitoring is both an art and a science. As such, there are both clinical and nonclinical modalities available to the physician to diagnose flap compromise. Nonclinical adjuncts to physical examination include monitoring via Doppler probe (internal or external), laser Doppler scanning, transcutaneous oximetry (tcPo$_2$), temperature and pH probes, fluorescein injection and mapping, color duplex imaging, lactic acid monitoring with microdialysis, and photoplethesmography.[56] Many authors have found these monitoring devices useful in the postoperative period and have reported successful salvage of flaps on the basis of abnormal readings, sometimes even before clinical signs were apparent.[57-66] However, although these methods undoubtedly have merit, none is without its own drawbacks, including false-negative and false-positive results. Moreover, no technique has gained universal acceptance. It has been well documented that circulation disturbances, edema within the flap, motion or vibration of the tissue or probe, partial probe detachment, accumulation of clot on the probe, or intrinsic mechanical failure can all cause a false sense of security or unnecessary return to the operating room.[67-70]

In general, clinical evaluation provides the best method for monitoring and diagnosis of the compromised flap.[71] Careful clinical evaluation of all flaps after surgery should include assessment of color, capillary refill, temperature, and bleeding to pinprick. These four parameters can help to diagnose the majority of flap problems and significantly contribute to flap salvage. In a review of 150 consecutive cases out of Memorial Sloan-Kettering Cancer Center, Hidalgo and Jones[72] demonstrated the efficacy of clinical monitoring and the role of aggressive, early surgical re-exploration to increase flap survival from 90% to 98%. A wealth of clinical and experimental studies (see reviews in the following sections) has demonstrated that HBOT is a useful adjunct for salvage of compromised flaps in the proper settings. The recommended clinical criteria for the use of HBOT in flap salvage are presented in Table 17.3.

The cause of flap compromise can be divided into technical and nontechnical factors. Technical problems can be caused by several factors including improper flap design, closure with tension, pedicle or tissue damage, hematoma causing external compression, or prolonged operative ischemia. Nontechnical causes of flap compromise include arterial vasospasm, flap edema, postoperative infection, and patient deterioration. In general, flap compromise can be classified into one of five general categories:

1. Random ischemia
2. Low arterial inflow
3. Total arterial occlusion
4. Partial venous congestion
5. Total venous occlusion

Table 17.3 Criteria for the Appropriate Use of Hyperbaric Oxygen Therapy in Flap Salvage

1. The flap problem must be defined.
2. There must be some documented perfusion of the flap.
3. The treatment should make physiologic sense and be based on the available research and clinical literature.
4. Treatment should be initiated only after appropriate surgical measures of salvage have been considered.
5. The time to initiation of treatment should be minimal.

From Zamboni WA: Applications of hyperbaric oxygen therapy in plastic surgery. In: Oriani G, Marroni A (eds): Handbook on Hyperbaric Medicine. New York, Springer, 1995, pp 443-507.

For each of these categories, the following sections outline the pathophysiology, clinical signs, and treatment, together with the research and clinical experience behind the rationale for using HBOT in the salvage of compromised flaps.

Random Ischemia

Random flaps have an indirect blood supply that makes these flaps the most vulnerable to ischemia. However, with the growing advances in flap design and the continuously developing knowledge of the cutaneous blood supply, including perforating vessels, the choice of flaps for reconstruction has undergone significant evolution. The availability of axial flaps and the ongoing refinements with microsurgery and free tissue transfers allow the reconstruction of almost all defects without reliance on random blood supply.

Nevertheless, situations occur when a designed flap does not go entirely as planned. When an axial flap is inadvertently elevated at a length that exceeds the vascular territory supplied by the artery, this situation effectively creates a random extension of the axial flap. Compromise and necrosis of the random flap will invariably occur at the distal portion of the flap. Another scenario that may be encountered is premature division of a distant pedicle flap. As discussed earlier, a distant flap requires the growth of new blood supply from surrounding tissues into the distal end of the flap before division of the proximal pedicle. When divided prematurely before sufficient vascular ingrowth, this flap essentially behaves as a compromised random flap. Clinically, random ischemia presents within the first 24 hours after surgery[71] with a progressively dusky appearance that ultimately becomes fairly well demarcated and may be associated with epidermolysis (Fig. 17.4).

Many published experimental studies have evaluated the efficacy of HBOT for random flap compromise.[73-91] The majority of these experimental trials have demonstrated a beneficial response with an approximately 15% to 30% improvement in survival with HBOT compared with no treatment. HBOT has also been shown in some experimental models to be synergistic with other adjuncts including pentoxifylline, tocopherol, superoxide dismutase, nicotinamide, and catalase, with improvements in flap survival of 45% to 65% compared with control subjects.[92-94] In addition to the animal studies, some retrospective clinical investigations have shown a benefit to flap salvage with HBOT.[95,96] In these studies, approximately 50% of those treated achieved 100% flap recovery, with many more achieving marked improvements. One such study by Ueda and coauthors[97] demonstrates the benefit of HBOT not only in the distal, compromised portion of axial flaps, but also in ischemic distant flaps such as the forehead flap. The efficacy of HBOT was linked to the timing of the onset of therapy, with those treated early achieving the greatest benefit.

As demonstrated by the available experimental and clinical literature, loss of the compromised portion of a random flap can be minimized with timely HBOT. Although random flap compromise may not be recognized until 24 to 48 hours after surgery, HBOT should be initiated as soon as any visible signs are present. The recommended clinical treatment regimen consists of HBOT for 90 to 120 minutes at 2.0 to 2.5 ATA twice a day for 48 to 72 hours as outlined in the most recent *Hyperbaric Oxygen Therapy Committee Report*.[98] This schedule should be followed with daily treatments until complete healing is achieved. This protocol can often require a total of 20 to 30 treatments to obtain satisfactory flap salvage, and utilization review should be performed after 20 treatments.

Low Arterial Inflow

Low arterial inflow can occur in pedicle and free flaps from a few different causes. This situation may arise if edema in the tissues around the pedicle is partially obstructing inflow. Partial arterial obstruction may also occur secondary to postoperative hematoma around the pedicle. A third cause can be when the pedicle artery is subject to intermittent vasospasms. Accurate diagnosis of low

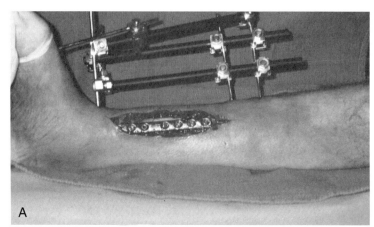

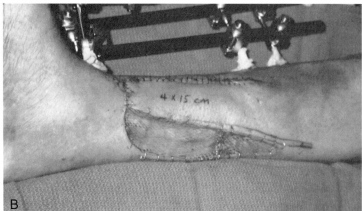

Figure 17.4 *A,* Distal lower extremity wound with exposed hardware requiring coverage. *B,* The hardware has been covered with a local fasciocutaneous flap. *C,* Evidence of compromise and impending necrosis in the distal random portion of the flap. The patient was started on the compromised flap hyperbaric oxygen therapy (HBOT) protocol. *D,* Appearance of the flap after 10 treatments with improved appearance of the compromised portion of the flap.

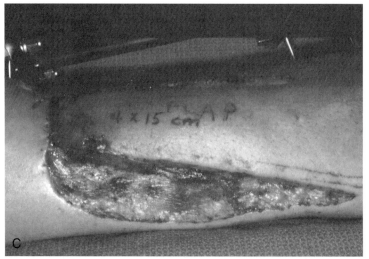

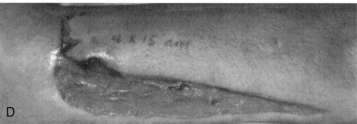

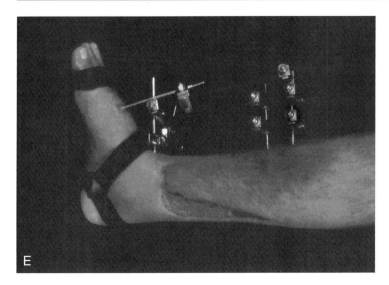

Figure 17.4 *Cont'd E,* Complete healing was achieved after 20 treatments with salvage of the compromised portion. **(See Color Plate 26.)** *(Adapted from Zamboni WA: Applications of hyperbaric oxygen therapy in plastic surgery. In: Oriani G, Marroni A, Wattel F (eds): Handbook on Hyperbaric Medicine. New York, Springer, 1995, pp 443–507, by permission.)*

arterial inflow is predominantly a clinical one. The most notable aspects of physical examination that can help differentiate low arterial inflow from other pedicle-related causes of flap compromise include flap color, temperature, and capillary refill[71,99] (Table 17.4).

The clinical presentation of low arterial inflow in the compromised flap is essentially one of a pale pink flap that demonstrates slow capillary refill. This slow capillary refill may be intermittent if the cause is sporadic vasospasm. The flap will also feel cool to touch secondary to the compromised inflow to the tissue. The primary treatment for low arterial inflow is surgical re-exploration. The goal of operative intervention should be to ensure that a hematoma, anatomic kinking, or twisting of the pedicle is not present. In addition, the presence of edema or excessive tension of wound closure compromising arterial inflow may also be discovered. If no surgically treatable condition is found on exploration and low arterial inflow persists, then HBOT is indicated. The treatment should encompass a multimodality approach when necessary. If arterial vasospasm is suspected, vasodilators should be administered. In addition, dextran and pentoxifylline can be given for rheologic purposes.[71,100-102] The recommended HBOT clinical protocol is similar to random ischemia and involves treatment twice a day for 48 to 72 hours followed by daily treatments until flap compromise is resolved[98] (Table 17.5).

Total Arterial Occlusion

Total arterial occlusion is a postoperative flap complication that is devastating but easily recognizable. On clinical examination, the flap devoid of arterial inflow is pale white with complete absence of capillary refill. This flap will also be cold to touch.

Table 17.4 Clinical Findings in Compromised Flaps

LOW ARTERIAL INFLOW	PARTIAL VENOUS CONGESTION	RANDOM ISCHEMIA
Pale pink	Dusky pink	Progressively dusky
Slow capillary refill	Brisk capillary refill	Epidermolysis
Cool	Cool	
TOTAL ARTERIAL OCCLUSION	**TOTAL VENOUS OCCLUSION**	**ISCHEMIA-REPERFUSION INJURY**
Pale white	Dark blue	Delayed, dark patchy areas
Absent capillary refill	Absent capillary refill	Random distribution
Cold	Cold	

Table 17.5 Recommended Treatment Protocols

CAUSATIVE FACTORS OF COMPROMISE	HYPERBARIC OXYGEN THERAPY PROTOCOL	NECESSARY ADJUNCTS
Random ischemia	2.0–2.5 atmospheres absolute (ATA) for 90–120 minutes twice a day for 48–72 hours, then followed by daily treatments until full healing is achieved*	Consider use of vasodilators, dextran, or pentoxifylline.
Low arterial inflow	2.0–2.5 ATA for 90–120 minutes twice a day for 48–72 hours, followed by daily treatments until full healing is achieved	Primary treatment is surgical re-exploration. If no correctable cause is found, then start HBOT. Consider use of vasodilators, dextran, or pentoxifylline.
Total arterial occlusion	2.0–2.5 ATA for 90–120 minutes every 8 hours for the first 24 hours, followed by treatment every 8–12 hours for the next 48 hours	Surgical re-exploration is mandatory to restore inflow. HBOT should be started only if perfusion is documented.
Partial venous congestion	2.0–2.5 ATA for 90–120 minutes twice a day for 7–10 days until venous outflow is reestablished	Initial treatment is medicinal or chemical leeching. HBOT may be used to help support the flap.
Total venous congestion	2.0–2.5 ATA for 90–120 minutes every 8 hours for the first 24 hours, followed by treatment every 12 hours until venous outflow is reestablished	Primary treatment is surgical re-exploration to resolve venous obstruction. If surgery is not possible, HBOT combined with leeching may allow flap salvage.
Ischemia-reperfusion injury	2.0–2.5 ATA for 90–120 minutes every 8 hours for the first 24 hours, followed by treatment every 8–12 hours for the next 48 hours	Consider use of vasodilators, pentoxifylline, dextran, or aspirin.

*Treatment times and pressures vary depending on type of hyperbaric oxygen therapy (HBOT) facility available and patient status, among other factors.

Furthermore, the flap will not bleed to pinprick. A number of potential causes of inflow obstruction exist. Low arterial inflow can progress to complete obstruction with progressive edema or hematoma compressing the pedicle. There may also be severe anatomic kinking or twisting of the pedicle preventing flow to the flap. Intraoperatively, there may have been intrinsic damage to the arterial pedicle of the flap. If the flap is a free tissue transfer, thrombosis at the arterial anastomotic site can also cause total arterial occlusion. After diagnosis of this cause of flap compromise, the primary treatment goal is immediate surgical re-exploration. Primary therapy with HBOT is not indicated before surgical exploration. In addition, if no flow can be reestablished after surgical intervention, the benefits of the increased partial pressure of oxygen dissolved in plasma cannot access the microcirculation and HBOT will not likely be effective.[2]

However, if the arterial problem is corrected surgically and the flap has sustained a significant period of warm ischemia, then HBOT is indicated after surgery after reestab-lishment of arterial inflow. The initial treatment should be administered soon after surgery if the patient remains stable after surgery under close observation in the recovery room. The clinical rationale behind HBOT for the compromised flap in this situation is to prevent further insult to the flap from subsequent IR injury after reestablishing inflow. The recommended clinical treatment protocol is therefore similar to that used to treat acute traumatic ischemia. HBOT should be initiated at 2.0 to 2.5 ATA for 90 to 120 minutes every 8 hours for the first 24 hours. This should be followed with HBOT every 8 to 12 hours for the next 48 hours.[98] Treatments can be discontinued when clinical signs of complete flap viability are present. Clinical experience suggests that, in most cases, the expected IR injury after reestablishment of inflow to the compromised flap can be reversed by early HBOT. In addition, our experience has shown that it is rarely necessary to administer treatment for more than 72 hours unless flap compromise persists and as long as the initial treatment is initiated within 4 hours after surgery.

Many experimental studies on animals have been conducted to mimic the situation of complete arterial occlusion with subsequent reperfusion. Studies conducted on rat skin and musculocutaneous flaps subjected to total arterial occlusion by clamping of the vascular pedicle and then treated with HBOT demonstrated a significant increase in flap survival compared with control animals.[103-105] Zamboni and coworkers' studies[105] on microcirculation used laser–Doppler flowmetry to demonstrate that treatment with HBOT produced a significant increase in microvascular perfusion of rat skin flaps subjected to 8 hours of ischemia.

Partial Venous Congestion

Partial venous congestion is one of the most common causes of compromise in pedicle axial flaps. As in the previous scenarios, the diagnosis is made by clinical examination. Partial venous congestion presents as a flap that is cool to touch and dusky pink. Contrary to arterial problems, flaps with venous congestion demonstrate brisk capillary refill. The cause for congestion, however, may be a mechanical cause similar to that of arterial compromise including pedicle compression from hematoma or edema, anatomic kinking or twisting of the pedicle vein, or a wound closure with excessive tension resulting in compression. In addition to mechanical causes, there are also other intrinsic causes of venous congestion.

At times in axial flaps, the inherent venous drainage is inadequate due to the choke system between the capillary beds and lack of crossing venous branches.[106-108] The choke system refers to the reduced-caliber ("choke") arteries and arterioles that lead to the capillary beds that are matched on the venous side by avalvular venules that permit bidirectional flow and allow equilibration of flow and pressure to and from the capillaries.[109] Disruption of the venous portion of this system during flap elevation may lead to subsequent congestion secondary to inadequate venous drainage. In addition, the operative planning of the flap may result in the development of reverse venous drainage such as in the reverse radial forearm flap. In these cases, a transient congestion of the flap occurs until the venous outflow can be reestablished through branches and valve blowout of the venae comitantes. These cases typically will resolve without therapeutic intervention. For other causes of venous congestion, initial treatment consists of medicinal or chemical leeching. HBOT can be used as an adjunctive treatment to help support the flap while appropriate venous outflow is being reestablished. This usually occurs within 7 to 10 days. The recommended clinical protocol should be started within 4 hours of recognition of venous congestion and consists of HBOT at 2.0 to 2.5 ATA for 90 to 120 minutes every 12 hours for 7 to 10 days until the signs of venous congestion resolve.[98]

Total Venous Occlusion

Total venous occlusion can occur in pedicle flaps from the same causes as arterial compromise. These include compression from hematoma, twisting, or kinking of the pedicle. In the case of free flaps, thrombosis of the venous anastomosis is more common than arterial thrombosis.[71] Experimental models comparing primary arterial and venous ischemia have suggested that venous ischemia is more deleterious to flap survival.[110-112] The venous occlusion congests the entire microcirculation and ultimately leads to arterial thrombosis followed by complete necrosis of the flap. The flap suffering from total venous occlusion will be dark blue with absent capillary refill. The tissue will be cold to touch because there is no flow within the flap. As with the previous causes of flap compromise, the initial treatment consists of emergent surgical exploration to resolve the cause of thrombosis.

The use of HBOT alone for total venous occlusion is not recommended and has been shown to be ineffective.[113] The use of HBOT in a rat axial skin flap model of total venous occlusion did not improve the 100% necrosis rate of control flaps.[113,114] The results of these experimental studies show that HBOT may play a role, however, in combination with the appropriate adjunctive therapy and in the proper clinical scenario (Fig. 17.5). In the

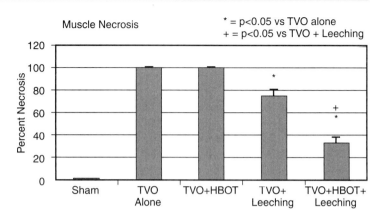

Figure 17.5 Experimental studies examining compromised flaps with total venous occlusion (TVO) demonstrate no change in percentage necrosis with hyperbaric oxygen therapy (HBOT) alone. However, HBOT in combination with leeching demonstrated a significant decrease in percentage necrosis of the flap in comparison with either HBOT or leeching alone. *$P < 0.05$ versus TVO alone; +$P < 0.05$ versus TVO and leeching.

senior author's (W. A. Z.) clinical experience with cases where surgical intervention is not an option secondary to poor patient condition or patient refusal, flap salvage is possible with a regimen consisting of medicinal leeching and HBOT (Fig. 17.6). If flap compromise is diagnosed early enough and arterial inflow remains present, the use of leeches can provide sufficient venous outflow. This combined with the supplemental oxygenation of HBOT has been shown experimentally to have an added positive effect on flap survival.[114] The recommended clinical HBOT protocol consists of treatments at 2.0 to 2.5 ATA for 90 to 120 minutes every 8 hours for 48 hours, followed by treatments every 12 hours for 7 to 10 days until the flap restores its own venous outflow.[98]

Ischemia-Reperfusion Injury

Free flaps represent a unique situation and are extremely susceptible to compromise for the first 24 to 72 hours. Because of the technical demands and precise microsurgery required to perform these reconstructions, the tissue frequently undergoes a period of primary ischemia. If this period is prolonged before revascularization to the recipient vessels, the free tissue transfer is subject to compromise secondary to both the long primary ischemia and subsequent IR injury. This IR injury is typically heterogeneous rather than global and presents clinically with delayed, dark, and patchy areas in a random distribution. As described earlier, IR injury may be reversible in its early stages with prompt HBOT. Using an animal free-flap model, Kaelin

and colleagues[115] demonstrated that the salvage rate in flaps which were made ischemic 18 to 24 hours before revascularization could be increased 40% to 60% with HBOT.

Situations that involve postoperative arteriovenous compromise or occlusion can further

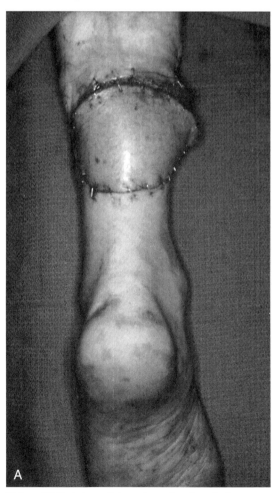

Figure 17.6 *A,* Immediate postoperative view of a free scapular fasciocutaneous flap to cover exposed calcaneal tendon in an unstable burn scar.

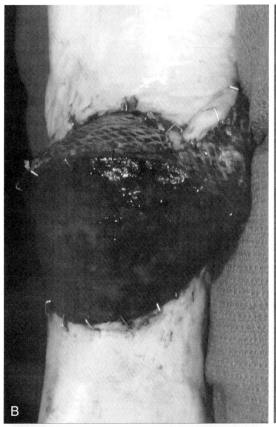

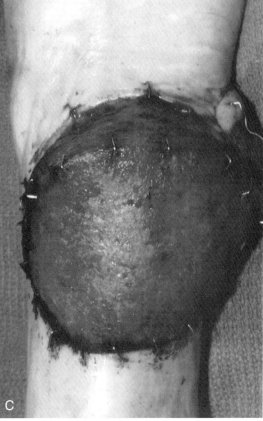

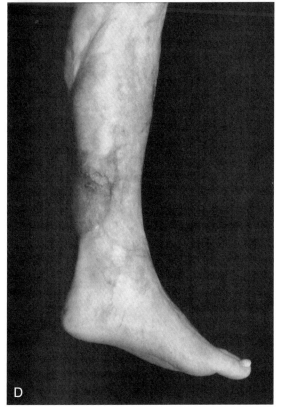

Figure 17.6 *Cont'd B,* Total venous occlusion 12 hours after the free scapular fasciocutaneous flap. Note the dark color of the flap. The patient refused surgery; therefore, immediate leeching and hyperbaric oxygen therapy (HBOT) was initiated. *C,* Flap after 6 days of HBOT with complete survival and establishment of inherent venous drainage. *D,* Six-month follow-up demonstrated stable soft-tissue coverage of the calcaneal tendon. **(See Color Plate 27.)** *(Adapted from Zamboni WA: Applications of hyperbaric oxygen therapy in plastic surgery. In: Oriani G, Marroni A, Wattel F (eds): Handbook on Hyperbaric Medicine. New York, Springer, 1995, pp 443–507, by permission.)*

complicate matters by introducing a period of secondary ischemia to the free tissue transfer. Even if the initial operation was successfully performed without prolonged initial ischemia, any secondary ischemia will have a negative impact on flap survival. It is well established that secondary ischemia contributes to poor outcome and is a significant factor in flap failure.[71] Revascularization of free flaps subjected to secondary ischemia also places the tissue at greater risk for IR injury. In addition, secondary ischemia tends to produce a more severe form of reperfusion injury than primary ischemia.[71,116] Necrosis and failure of a free flap is a significant loss for the microsurgeon and the patient because the initial defect to be reconstructed still exists and is compounded by donor-site morbidity, as well as the underlying psychosocial implications of unsuccessful surgery. Fortunately, HBOT has been shown in multiple experimental and clinical studies to benefit free flap salvage after a secondary ischemic insult. Animal studies have demonstrated the value of HBOT in the successful treatment of flaps subjected to secondary ischemia.[117-119] Waterhouse and investigators' clinical study[120] documents a significant enhancement in the salvage of replants and free flaps with secondary ischemia by HBOT. In this controlled, retrospective review, patients with greater than 6 hours of primary ischemia or any degree of secondary ischemia were examined. The salvage rates of free tissue were increased from 46% in the control patients to 75% in those treated with HBOT. The timing of HBOT in this study was particularly significant with regard to a successful result. Those patients treated within 24 hours of revascularization demonstrated a 100% salvage rate compared with a 0% salvage rate for patients who received HBOT more than 72 hours after reperfusion. These findings correlate with the knowledge that the major effects of IR injury occur within the first 7 hours after reperfusion.[121,122] After this period, it is clear that there is a component of irreversible injury. The timing of HBOT after revascularization after prolonged ischemia and secondary ischemia is critical in the salvage of these flaps and the prevention of IR injury.

Clinical experience has confirmed the results of the experimental and clinical studies. Indeed, in our experience, free flaps compromised by prolonged primary ischemia or secondary ischemia have responded dramatically to HBOT with complete salvage in most cases if the start of treatment is timely. It is therefore critical for timely diagnosis and selection of those patients who will benefit from HBOT. Any patient undergoing a free tissue transfer with a primary ischemia time greater than 4 hours is a candidate for prompt postoperative HBOT. This is especially true of free flaps composed of composite tissues or muscle. In addition, any free flap that must be re-explored secondary to any arteriovenous pedicle com-

promise as described in the previous sections has undergone an associated secondary ischemia and HBOT should be considered after successful revascularization. The recommended protocol consists of HBOT at 2.0 to 2.5 ATA for 90 to 120 minutes every 8 hours for 24 hours, followed by treatments every 8 to 12 hours for the next 48 hours.[98] Continuous clinical re-evaluation must be undertaken to ensure adequate response and to rule out further arteriovenous anastomotic problems. If HBOT is started in an expedient manner, severe IR injury may be avoided and treatment past 72 hours is rarely necessary.

RATIONALE FOR THE USE OF HYPERBARIC OXYGEN THERAPY IN COMPROMISED GRAFTS AND FLAPS

As described in the previous sections, a wealth of literature evaluating the effect of HBOT on the prevention and salvage of compromise grafts and flaps has been published. These studies involve both experimental basic science and clinical trials in a multitude of different situations. Increasingly in recent years, the literature regarding HBOT research has become more scientific and less anecdotal. Generally, the majority of these articles have shown a beneficial response. In addition, the scientific body of evidence allows the development of indications, contraindications, and protocols for the successful use of HBOT.

Yet in the new era of evidence-based medicine, an increasing emphasis is placed on the results of meta-analysis and randomized, double-blind, controlled clinical trials to guide therapeutic decision making. There are prospective, randomized trials regarding the use of HBOT as an adjunct for healing in chronic foot wounds of patients with diabetes and for irradiated tissues. A search of the Cochrane reviews demonstrates positive recommendations on the use of HBOT for foot ulcers of patients with diabetes and for late radiation tissue injury.[38,123] These studies validate the use of HBOT in preparation of problem wound beds for grafting.

However, no controlled, randomized clinical trials for the use of HBOT in compromised grafts and flaps have been reported. Although there are significant amounts of evidence to warrant the institution of these trials, the relative unpredictability and paucity of the clinical situations in which HBOT is warranted would make a meaningful randomized study difficult to conduct in a single institution. The use of HBOT for compromised grafts and flaps may be considered controversial by those intent on basing their treatment recommendations on only interventions backed by randomized, controlled trials. Yet many authors reject this narrow-minded view and insist that the effectiveness of an intervention be judged relative to consequences of nonintervention.[124] Indeed, two separate studies by Concato and colleagues[125] and Benson and Hartz[126] published in the *New England Journal of Medicine* demonstrate that well-designed observational studies do not differ significantly in their treatment recommendations. Until clear-cut clinical data are available, we must base our clinical recommendations on the overwhelmingly supportive randomized, controlled animal experiments and clinical studies while taking into account the risks, benefits, and cost of HBOT. In general, HBOT is a low-risk, well-tolerated therapy in properly screened patients. The contraindications and risks of HBOT are outlined in Chapter 26 and should be reviewed before clinical intervention.

Many benefits of HBOT for prevention and treatment of graft and flap compromise are clear and have been illustrated previously. One advantage to HBOT that has not yet been discussed is its efficacy in comparison with other available methods of treatment for compromised grafts and flaps. Although numerous alternative methods have been attempted to salvage grafts and flaps, few have been routinely successful or applicable in clinical settings. Some animal studies using oxygen free radical scavengers, antioxidants, and thrombolytics alone or in combination with HBOT have had varying success.[127-130] However, these basic science results have not resulted in any clinical acceptance or documented benefits. Therefore, few alternatives for graft and flap salvage are available. Given the infrequent risks, documented benefits, and lack of proven alternatives, it would appear questionable to withhold HBOT for an appropriately selected patient solely on the basis of a lack of prospective, randomized clinical trials.

When examining the relative cost of HBOT versus the cost of graft/flap failure, reoperation, and prolonged hospital stay, not to mention the psychosocial cost of therapeutic failure, the case for HBOT in the salvage of grafts and flaps is further bolstered. In one proposed hypothetical situation in which Nemiroff[131] compared the cost of an unsuccessful flap versus flap salvage, the cost savings of HBOT become clear. For flap failure, the hypothetical cost that Nemiroff[131] described for the year 1999 would be an additional $5,000 to $10,000 in surgical and assistant's fees alone, as well as an additional $10,000 to $20,000 in increased hospitalization and monitoring fees assuming an additional 1 to 2 weeks of hospital care with initial postoperative intensive care unit monitoring. This does not take into account the possibility of a second compromised flap, the additional donor site morbidity, and the psychosocial impact on the patient. Given the increased cost in hospital care and surgical fees combined with inflation, this cost would be significantly greater in current clinical practice. In comparison, the cost of 10 to 20 hyperbaric treatments for flap salvage would be roughly $5,000 to $10,000 given an approximate cost of $500 per HBOT treatment. It is clear from analyzing the risks, benefits, alternatives, and cost that HBOT is a viable and cost-effective adjunct in the salvage of compromised grafts and flaps.

SUMMARY

The information in this chapter should serve as a guide for any hyperbaric physician and plastic surgeon or other subspecialty surgeon who will encounter the compromised graft or flap in practice. As emphasized at the beginning of this chapter, the use of HBOT is not indicated for routine, well-planned grafts or flaps. The clinical benefit of HBOT arises from the treatment of compromised grafts and flaps. It must be emphasized that accurate and prompt diagnosis of the flap or graft problem with early HBOT is the key to a successful outcome and salvage of the compromised graft or flap. The available evidence from experimental animal studies and clinical trials combined with an analysis of the risks, benefits, and cost savings allow the recommendation of HBOT protocols in properly selected patients at risk for compromised grafts or flaps. However, a need still exists for future prospective, randomized clinical trials and systematic reviews to further solidify the therapeutic recommendations of HBOT for the prevention and treatment of compromised grafts and flaps.

REFERENCES

1. Friedman HI, Fitzmaurice M, Lefaivre JF, et al: An evidence-based appraisal of the use of hyperbaric oxygen on flaps and grafts. Plast Reconstr Surg 117(suppl):175S-190S, 2006.
2. Zamboni WA: Applications of hyperbaric oxygen therapy in plastic surgery. In: Oriani G, Marroni A (eds): Handbook on Hyperbaric Medicine. New York, Springer, 1995, pp 443-507.
3. Nemirof PM: HBO in skin grafts and flaps. In: Kindwall EP, Whelan HT (eds): Hyperbaric Medicine Practice, 2nd ed. Flagstaff, Ariz, Best Publishing, 1999, pp 795-811.
4. Mathes SJ, Hansen SL: Flap classification and applications. In: Mathes SJ (ed): Plastic Surgery: General Principles, vol 1, 2nd ed. Philadelphia, Saunders/Elsevier, 2006, pp 365-482.
5. Thourani VH, Ingram WL, Feliciano DV: Factors affecting success of split-thickness skin grafts in the modern burn unit. J Trauma 54:562-568, 2003.
6. Podrecca S, Salvatori P, Squadrelli Saraceno M, et al: Review of 346 patients with free-flap reconstruction following head and neck surgery for neoplasm. J Plast Reconstr Aesthet Surg 59:122-129, 2006.
7. Johsson K, Hunt TK, Mathes SJ: Oxygen as an isolated variable influences resistance to infection. Ann Surg 208:783-787, 1988.
8. Niinikoski J, Hunt TK: Oxygen and healing wounds: Tissue-bone repair enhancement. In: Oriani G, Marroni A (eds): Handbook on Hyperbaric Medicine. New York, Springer, 1995, pp 485-508.
9. Marino PD: Respiratory gas transport. In: Marino PD (ed): The ICU Book. Baltimore, Md, Lippincott Williams & Wilkins, 1998, pp 19-31.
10. Bassett BE, Bennett PB: Introduction to the physical and physiological bases of hyperbaric therapy. In: Hunt TK, Davis JC (eds): Hyperbaric Oxygen Therapy. Durham, NC, Undersea Medical Society, 1977, pp 11-24.
11. Bigelow WG: The microcirculation. Some physiological and philosophical observations concerning the peripheral vascular system. Can J Surg 7:237-250, 1964.
12. Krogh A: The number and distribution of capillaries in muscle with calculations of oxygen pressure head necessary for supplying the tissue. J Physiol 52.409, 1919.
13. Boerema I, Meijne NG, Brummelkamp WK, et al: Life without blood. A study of the influence of high atmospheric pressure and hypothermia on dilution of the blood. J Cardiovasc Surg 1:133-146, 1960.
14. Angel MF, Ramasastry SS, Swartz WM, et al: Free radicals: Basic concepts concerning their chemistry, pathophysiology, and relevance to plastic surgery. Plast Reconstr Surg 79:990-997, 1987.
15. Russel RC, Roth AC, Kucan JO, et al: Reperfusion injury and oxygen free radicals. A review. J Reconstr Microsurg 5:79-84, 1989.
16. Granger DN, Benoit JN, Suzuki M, et al: Leukocyte adherence to venular endothelium during ischemia-reperfusion. Am J Physiol 257:G683-G688, 1989.
17. Goldbeg M, Serafin D, Klitzman B: Quantification of neutrophil adhesion to skeletal muscle venules following ischemia-reperfusion. J Reconstr Microsurg 6:267-270, 1990.
18. Messina LM: In vivo assessment of acute microvascular injury after reperfusion of ischemic tibialis anterior muscle of the hamster. J Surg Res 48:615-621, 1990.
19. Wang WZ, Anderson G, Firrell JC: Arteriole constriction following ischemia in denervated skeletal muscle. J Reconstr Microsurg 11:99-106, 1995.
20. Siemionow M, Wang WZ, Anderson G, et al: Leukocyte-endothelial interaction and capillary perfusion in ischemia/reperfusion of the rat cremaster muscle. Microcirc Endothelium Lymphatics 7:183-197, 1991.
21. Kaelin CM, Im MJ, Myers RA, et al: The effects of hyperbaric oxygen on free flaps in rats. Arch Surg 125:607-609, 1990.
22. Nylander G, Lewis D, Nordstrom H, et al: Reduction of postischemic edema with hyperbaric oxygen. Plast Reconstr Surg 76:596-603, 1990.
23. Zamboni WA, Roth AC, Russell RC, et al: Morphological analysis of the microcirculation during reperfusion of ischemic skeletal muscle and the effect of hyperbaric oxygen. Plast Reconstr Surg 91:1110-1123, 1993.
24. Thom SR: Functional inhibition of leukocyte B² integrins by hyperbaric oxygen in carbon monoxide-mediated brain injury. Toxicol Appl Pharm 123:248-256, 1993.
25. Zamboni WA, Stephenson LL, Roth AC, et al: Ischemia-reperfusion injury in skeletal muscle: CD18-dependent neutrophil-endothelial adhesion and arteriolar vasoconstriction. Plast Reconstr Surg 99:2002-2007, 1997.
26. Jones S, Wang WZ, Nataraj C, et al: HBO inhibits IR-induced neutrophil CD18 polarization by a nitric oxide mechanism. Undersea Hyperb Med 35(suppl):75, 2002.
27. Baynosa RC, Khiabani KT, Stephenson LL, et al: The effect of hyperbaric oxygen on nitric oxide synthase and vascular endothelial growth factor expression in ischemia reperfusion injury. J Am Coll Surg 199(suppl):S65, 2004.
28. Baynosa RC, Naig AL, Murphy PS, et al: The effect of hyperbaric oxygen on NOS activity and transcription in ischemia reperfusion injury. J Am Coll Surg 200(suppl):S57-S58, 2005.

29. Ellis CM, Hansen BK, Baynosa RC, et al: Hyperbaric oxygen decreases neutrophil adherence in ischemia reperfusion by a VEGF-dependent mechanism. J Am Coll Surg 200(suppl):S57, 2005.

30. Zhang Q, Gould L, Chang Q: Mechanism of hyperbaric oxygen on ischemic tissue healing. J Am Coll Surg 200(suppl):S58, 2005.

31. Heggers JP: Defining infection in chronic wounds: Methodology. J Wound Care 7:452-456, 1998.

32. Zamboni WA, Browder LK, Martinez J: Hyperbaric oxygen and wound healing. In: Phillips LG (ed): Clinics in Plastic Surgery—Wound Healing. Philadelphia, Saunders, 2003, pp 67-75.

33. Clark MG, Barrett EJ, Wallis MG, et al: The microvasculature in insulin resistance and type 2 diabetes. Semin Vasc Med 2:21-31, 2002.

34. Burns JL, Mancoll JS, Phillips LG: Impairments to wound healing. Clin Plast Surg 30:47-56, 2003.

35. Reinisch JF, Puckett CL: Management of radiation wounds. Surg Clin North Am 64:795-802, 1984.

36. Rudolph R, Utley J, Woodard N, et al: The ultrastructure of chronic radiation damage in rat skin. Surg Gynecol Obstet 151:171-178, 1981.

37. Niinikoski JH: Clinical hyperbaric oxygen therapy, wound perfusion, and transcutaneous oximetry. World J Surg 28:307-311, 2004.

38. Kranke P, Bennett M, Roeckl-Wiedmann I, et al: Hyperbaric oxygen therapy for chronic wounds. Cochrane Database Syst Rev 1:CD004123, 2004.

39. Sheffield PJ: Tissue oxygen measurements. In: Davis JC, Hunt TK (eds): Problem Wounds: The Role of Oxygen. New York, Elsevier, 1988, pp 17-51.

40. Sheffield PJ: Measuring tissue oxygen tension: A review. Undersea Hyperb Med 25:179-188, 1998.

41. Hayward TR, Volny J, Golbranson F, et al: Oxygen inhalation-induced transcutaneous PO2 changes as a predictor of amputation level. J Vasc Surg 2:220-227, 1985.

42. Matos LA, Nunez AA: Enhancement of healing in selected problem wounds. In: Kindwall EP, Whelan HT (eds): Hyperbaric Medicine Practice, 2nd ed. Flagstaff, Ariz, Best Publishing, 1999, pp 813-849.

43. Strauss MB, Bryant BJ, Hart GB: Transcutaneous oxygen measurements under hyperbaric oxygen conditions as a predictor for healing of problem wounds. Foot Ankle Int 23:933-937, 2002.

44. Quigley FG, Faris IB: Transcutaneous oxygen tension measurements in the assessment of limb ischemia. Clin Physiol 11:315-320, 1991.

45. Niinikoski J: Hyperbaric oxygen therapy of diabetic foot ulcers, transcutaneous oximetry in clinical decision making. Wound Repair Regen 11:458-461, 2003.

46. Perrins DJ, Cantab MB: Influence of hyperbaric oxygen on the survival of split skin grafts. Lancet 1:868-871, 1967.

47. Gonnering RS, Kindwall EP, Goldmann RW: Adjunct hyperbaric oxygen therapy in periorbital reconstruction. Arch Ophthalmol 104:439-443, 1986.

48. Nichter LS, Morwood DT, Williams GS, et al: Expanding the limits of composite grafting: A case report of a successful nose replantation assisted by hyperbaric oxygen therapy. Plast Reconstr Surg 87:337-340, 1991.

49. Rapley JH, Lawrence WT, Witt PD: Composite grafting and hyperbaric oxygen therapy in pediatric nasal tip reconstruction after avulsive dog-bite injury. Ann Plast Surg 46:434-438, 2001.

50. Friedman HI, Stonerock C, Brill A: Composite ear-lobe grafts to reconstruct the lateral nasal ala and sill. Ann Plast Surg 50:275-281, 2003.

51. McFarlane RM, Wermuth RE: The use of hyperbaric oxygen to prevent necrosis in experimental pedicle flaps and composite skin grafts. Plast Reconstr Surg 37:422-430, 1966.

52. Zhang F, Cheng C, Gerlach T, et al: Effect of hyperbaric oxygen on survival of the composite ear graft in rats. Ann Plast Surg 41:530-534, 1998.

53. Rubin JS, Marzella L, Myers RA, et al: Effect of hyperbaric oxygen on the take of composite skin grafts in rabbit ears. J Hyperb Med 3:79, 1988.

54. Lim AA, Wall MP, Greinwald JH: Effects of dimethylthiourea, melatonin, and hyperbaric oxygen therapy on the survival of reimplanted rabbit auricular composite grafts. Otolaryngol Head Neck Surg 121:231-237, 1999.

55. Mazolewski MC, Zamboni WA, Haws MJ, et al: Effect of hyperbaric oxygen on composite graft survival in a rat ear model. Undersea Hyperb Med 22:50, 1995.

56. Furnas H, Rosen JM: Monitoring in microvascular surgery. Ann Plast Surg 26:265-272, 1991.

57. De la Torre J, Hedden W, Grant JH, et al: Retrospective review of the internal Doppler probe for intra- and postoperative microvascular surveillance. J Reconstr Microsurg 19:287-290, 2003.

58. Yuen JC, Feng Z: Monitoring free flaps using the laser Doppler flowmeter: A five-year experience. Plast Reconstr Surg 105:55-61, 2000.

59. Mathieu D, Neviere R, Pellerin P, et al: Pedicle musculocutaneous flap transplantation: Prediction of final outcome by transcutaneous oxygen measurements in hyperbaric oxygen. Plast Reconstr Surg 91:329-334, 1993.

60. Smith AR, Sonneveld GJ, Kort WJ, et al: Clinical applications of transcutaneous oxygen measurements in replantation surgery and free tissue transfer. J Hand Surg 8:139-145, 1983.

61. Khouri RK, Shaw WW: Monitoring of free flaps with surface-temperature recordings: Is it reliable? Plast Reconstr Surg 89:495-499, 1992.

62. Dunn RM, Kaplan IB, Mancoll J, et al: Experimental and clinical use of pH monitoring of free tissue transfers. Ann Plast Surg 31:539-545, 1993.

63. Denneny JC, Weisman RA, Silverman DG: Monitoring free flap perfusion by serial fluorometry. Otolaryngol Head Neck Surg 91:372-376, 1983.

64. Schon R, Schramm A, Gellrich NC, et al: Color duplex sonography for the monitoring of vascularized free bone flaps. Otolaryngol Head Neck Surg 129:71-76, 2003.

65. Udesen A, Lontoft E, Kristensen SR: Monitoring of free flaps with microdialysis. J Reconstr Microsurg 16:101-106, 2000.

66. Futran ND, Stack BC, Hollenbeak C, et al: Green light photoplethysmography monitoring of free flaps. Arch Otolaryngol Head Neck Surg 126:659-662, 2000.

67. Hallock GG: A "true" false-negative misadventure in free flap monitoring using laser Doppler flowmetry. Plast Reconstr Surg 110:1609-1611, 2002.

68. Heller L, Levin LS, Klitzman B: Laser Doppler flowmeter monitoring of free-tissue transfers: Blood flow in normal and complicated cases. Plast Reconstr Surg 107:1739-1745, 2001.

69. Kaufman T, Granick MS, Hurwitz DJ, et al: Is experimental muscle flap temperature a reliable indicator of its viability? Ann Plast Surg 19:34-41, 1987.

70. Raskin DJ, Nathan R, Erk Y, et al: Critical comparison of transcutaneous pO2 and tissue pH as indices of perfusion. Microsurgery 4:29-33, 1983.

71. Vedder NB: Flap physiology. In: Mathes SJ (ed): Plastic Surgery: General Principles, vol 1, 2nd ed. Philadelphia, Saunders/Elsevier, 2006, pp 483-506.

72. Hidalgo DA, Jones CS: The role of emergent exploration in free-tissue transfer: A review of 150 consecutive cases. Plast Reconstr Surg 86:492-498, 1990.

73. Kernahan DA, Zingg W, Kay CW: The effect of hyperbaric oxygen on the survival of experimental skin flaps. Plast Reconstr Surg 36:19-25, 1965.

74. McFarlane RM, Wermuth RE: The use of hyperbaric oxygen to prevent necrosis in experimental pedicle flaps and composite skin grafts. Plast Reconstr Surg 37:422-430, 1966.

75. McFarlane RM, DeYoung G, Henry RA: Prevention of necrosis in experimental pedicle flaps with hyperbaric oxygen. Surg Forum 16:481-482, 1965.

76. Wald HI, Georgiade HG, Angelollo J, et al: Effect of intensive hyperbaric oxygen therapy on the survival of experimental skin flaps in rats. Surg Forum 19:497-499, 1968.

77. Champion WM, McSherry CK, Goulian D: Effect of hyperbaric oxygen on the survival of pedicled skin flaps. J Surg Res 7:583-586, 1967.

78. Niinikoski J: Viability of ischemic skin in hyperbaric oxygen. Acta Chir Scand 136:567-568, 1970.

79. Niinikoski J: Viability of ischemic skin flaps in hyperbaric oxygen. Proceedings of the 5th International Hyperbaric Conference 1:244, 1974.

80. Arturson G, Khanna NN: The effects of hyperbaric oxygen, dimethyl sulfoxide and complamin on the survival of experimental skin flaps. Scand J Plast Reconstr Surg 4:8-10, 1970.

81. Jurell G, Kaijser L: Influence of varying pressure and duration of treatment with hyperbaric oxygen on the survival of skin flaps. Scand J Plast Reconstr Surg 7:25-28, 1973.

82. Manson PN, Im MJ, Myers RA, et al: Improved capillaries by hyperbaric oxygen in skin flaps. Surg Forum 31:564-566, 1980.

83. Tan CM, Im MJ, Myer RA, et al: Effects of hyperbaric oxygen and hyperbaric air on the survival of island skin flaps. Plast Reconstr Surg 73:27-30, 1984.

84. Nemiroff PM, Merwin GE, Brant T: Effects of hyperbaric oxygen and irradiation on experimental skin flaps in rats. Otolaryngol Head Neck Surg 93:485-491, 1985.

85. Caffee HH, Gallagher TJ: Experiments on the effects of hyperbaric oxygen on flap survival in the pig. Plast Reconstr Surg 81:751-754, 1988.

86. Esclamado RM, Larrabee WF, Zel GE: Efficacy of steroids and hyperbaric oxygen on survival of dorsal skin flaps in rats. Otolaryngol Head Neck Surg 102:41-44, 1990.

87. Frigerio D, Lovisetti G, Lovisetti L: Effect of hyperbaric oxygenation on the survival of experimental skin flaps in rats. Proceedings of the 10th International Congress of Hyperbaric Medicine, p. 199, 1990.

88. Zamboni WA, Roth AC, Russell RC, et al: The effect of hyperbaric oxygen therapy on axial pattern skin flap survival when administered during and after total ischemia. J Reconstr Microsurg 5:343-347, 1989.

89. Ramon Y, Abramovich A, Shupak A, et al: Effect of hyperbaric oxygen on a rat transverse rectus abdominis myocutaneous flap model. Plast Reconstr Surg 102:416-422, 1998.

90. Pellitteri PK, Kennedy TL, Youn BA: The influence of invasive hyperbaric oxygen therapy on skin flap survival in a swine model. Arch Otolaryngol Head Neck Surg 118:1050-1054, 1992.

91. Champion WM, McSherry CK, Goulian D: Effect of hyperbaric oxygen on the survival of pedicled skin flaps. J Surg Res 7:583-586, 1967.

92. Nemiroff PM: Synergistic effects of pentoxifylline and hyperbaric oxygen on skin flaps. Arch Otolaryngol Head Neck Surg 114:977-981, 1988.

93. Stewart RJ, Moore T, Bennett B, et al: Effect of free-radical scavengers and hyperbaric oxygen on random-pattern skin flaps. Arch Surg 129:982-987, 1994.

94. Collins TM, Caimi R, Lynch PR, et al: The effects of nicotinamide and hyperbaric oxygen on skin flap survival. Scand J Plast Surg 25:5-7, 1991.

95. Perrins DJD: The effect of hyperbaric oxygen on ischemic skin flaps. In: Grabb WC, Myers MB (eds): Skin Flaps. Boston, Little, Brown, 1975, pp 53-63.

96. Bowersox JC, Strauss MB, Hart GB: Clinical experience with hyperbaric oxygen therapy in the salvage of ischemic skin flaps and grafts. J Hyperb Med 1:141, 1986.

97. Ueda M, Kaneda T, Takahashi H, et al: Hyperbaric oxygen therapy of ischemic skin flaps: Clinical and experimental study. Proceedings of the 9th International Symposium on Underwater Hyperbaric Physiology by the Undersea and Hyperbaric Medical Society, p. 823, 1987.

98. Zamboni WA, Shah HR: Skin grafts and flaps (compromised). In: Feldmeier JJ (ed): Hyperbaric Oxygen 2003. Indications and Results—The Hyperbaric Oxygen Therapy Committee Report. Dunkirk, Md, Undersea and Hyperbaric Medical Society, 2003, pp 101-108.

99. Alizadeh K, Disa JJ: Flap loss, infections, and other complications. In: Greer SE, Benhaim P, Lorenz HP, et al. (eds): Handbook of Plastic Surgery. New York, Marcel Dekker, 2004, pp 15-18.

100. Rothkopf DM, Chu B, Bern S, et al: The effect of dextran on microvascular thrombosis in an experimental rabbit model. Plast Reconstr Surg 92:511-515, 1993.

101. Pomerance J, Truppa K, Bilos ZJ, et al: Replantation and revascularization of the digits in a community microsurgical practice. J Reconstr Microsurg 13:163-170, 1997.

102. Takayanagi S, Ogawa Y: Effects of pentoxifylline on flap survival. Plast Reconstr Surg 65:763-767, 1980.

103. Tomur A, Etlik O, Gundogan NU: Hyperbaric oxygenation and antioxidant combination reduces ischemia-reperfusion injury in a rat epigastric island skin-flap model. J Basic Clin Physiol Pharmacol 16:275-285, 2005.

104. Hong JP, Kwon H, Chung YK, et al: The effect of hyperbaric oxygen on ischemia-reperfusion injury:

An experimental study in a rat musculocutaneous flap. Ann Plast Surg 51:478-487, 2003.

105. Zamboni WA, Roth AC, Russell RC, et al: The effect of hyperbaric oxygen on reperfusion of ischemic axial skin flaps: A laser Doppler analysis. Ann Plast Surg 28:339-341, 1992.

106. Boyd JB, Taylor GI, Corlett R: The vascular territories of the superior epigastric and the deep inferior epigastric systems. Plast Reconstr Surg 73:1-16, 1984.

107. Carramenha E, Costa MA: An anatomic study of the venous drainage of the transverse rectus abdominis myocutaneous flap. Plast Reconstr Surg 79:208-213, 1987.

108. Blondeel PN, Arnstein M, Verstraete K: Venous congestion and blood flow in free transverse rectus abdominis myocutaneous and deep inferior epigastric perforator flaps. Plast Reconstr Surg 106:1295-1299, 2000.

109. Taylor GI, Ives A, Dhar S: Vascular territories. In: Mathes SJ (ed): Plastic Surgery: General Principles, vol 1, 2nd ed. Philadelphia, Saunders/Elsevier, 2006, pp 317-364.

110. Hjortdal VE, Hauge E, Hansen ES: Differential effects of venous stasis and arterial insufficiency on tissue oxygenation in myocutaneous island flaps: An experimental study in pigs. Plast Reconstr Surg 93:375-385, 1992.

111. Hjortdal VE, Sinclair T, Kerrigan CL, et al: Arterial ischemia in skin flaps: Microcirculatory intravascular thrombosis. Plast Reconstr Surg 93:375-385, 1994.

112. Hjortdal VE, Sinclair T, Kerrigan CL, et al: Venous ischemia in skin flaps: Microcirculatory intravascular thrombosis. Plast Reconstr Surg 93:366-374, 1994.

113. Kenneaster DG, Zamboni WA, Stephenson LL: Effect of hyperbaric oxygen on axial skin flaps subjected to total venous occlusion. Undersea Hyperb Med 21(suppl):53, 1994.

114. Lozano DD, Stephenson LL, Zamboni WA: Effect of hyperbaric oxygen and medicinal leeching on survival of axial skin flaps subjected to total venous occlusion. Plast Reconstr Surg 104:1029-1032, 1999.

115. Kaelin CM, Im MJ, Myers RA, et al: The effects of hyperbaric oxygen on free flaps in rats. Arch Surg 125:607-609, 1990.

116. Angel MF, Mellow CG, Knight KR, et al: Secondary ischemia time in rodents: Contrasting complete pedicle interruption with venous obstruction. Plast Reconstr Surg 85:789-793, 1990.

117. Stevens DM, Weiss DD, Koller WA, et al: Survival of normothermic microvascular flaps after prolonged secondary ischemia: Effects of hyperbaric oxygen. Otolaryngol Head Neck Surg 115:360-364, 1996.

118. Gampper TJ, Zhang F, Mofakhami NF, et al: Beneficial effect of hyperbaric oxygen on island flaps subjected to secondary venous ischemia. Microsurgery 22:49-52, 2002.

119. Wong HP, Zamboni WA, Stephenson LL: Effect of hyperbaric oxygen on skeletal muscle necrosis following primary and secondary ischemia in a rat model. Surg Forum 47:705-707, 1996.

120. Waterhouse MA, Brown R, Zamboni WA, et al: The use of HBO in compromised free tissue transfer and replantation: A clinical review. Undersea Hyperb Med 20(suppl):64, 1993.

121. Zamboni WA: The microcirculation and ischemia-reperfusion: Basic mechanisms of hyperbaric oxygen. In: Kindwall EP, Whelan HT (eds): Hyperbaric Medicine Practice, 2nd ed. Flagstaff, Ariz, Best Publishing, 1999, pp 779-794.

122. Olivas TP, Saylor TF, Wong HP, et al: Timing of microcirculatory injury from ischemia reperfusion. Plast Reconstr Surg 107:785-788, 2001.

123. Bennett MH, Feldmeier J, Hampson N, et al: Hyperbaric oxygen therapy for late radiation tissue injury. Cochrane Database Syst Rev 3:CD005005, 2005.

124. Smith GCS, Pell JP: Parachute use to prevent death and major trauma related to gravitational challenge: Systematic review of randomized controlled trials. Br Med J 327:1459-1461, 2003.

125. Concato J, Shah N, Horwitz RI: Randomized, controlled trials, observational studies, and the hierarchy of research designs. N Engl J Med 342:1887-1892, 2000.

126. Benson K, Hartz AJ: A comparison of observational studies and randomized, controlled trials. N Engl J Med 342:1878-1886, 2000.

127. Gurlek A, Celik M, Parlakpinar H, et al: The protective effect of melatonin on ischemia-reperfusion injury in the groin (inferior epigastric) flap model in rats. J Pineal Res 40:312-317, 2006.

128. Hirigoyen MB, Prabhat A, Zhang WX, et al: Thrombolysis at a controlled pressure prolongs the survival of skin flaps treated with superoxide dismutase. J Reconstr Microsurg 12:195-199, 1996.

129. Suzuki S, Yoshioka N, Isshiki N, et al: Involvement of reactive oxygen species in post-ischaemic flap necrosis and its prevention by antioxidants. Br J Plast Surg 44:130-134, 1991.

130. Stewart RJ, Moore T, Bennett B, et al: Effect of free-radical scavengers and hyperbaric oxygen of random pattern skin flaps. Arch Surg 129:982-987, 1994.

131. Nemiroff PM: HBO in skin grafts and flaps. In: Kindwall EP, Whelan HT (eds): Hyperbaric Medicine Practice, 2nd ed. Flagstaff, Ariz, Best Publishing, 1999, pp 795-811.

Clostridial Myositis, Necrotizing Fasciitis, and Zygomycotic Infections

Irving Jacoby, MD, FACP, FACEP, FAAEM

CLOSTRIDIAL MYOSITIS AND MYONECROSIS

Clostridial myositis and associated myonecrosis, commonly known as *gas gangrene,* is a severe, limb- and life-threatening necrotizing infection, characterized by a dramatic, rapidly progressive infection of soft tissues and development of manifestations of toxin-induced cellular injury, systemic toxicity, and rapidly spreading muscle necrosis.[1] It is a classic toxin-induced infectious disease and one of several rapidly progressive necrotizing infections.

Causative Factors

Clostridial myositis infection is caused by an anaerobic, spore-forming, gram-positive rod commonly found in decaying organic material within soil, in the gastrointestinal tract of mammals, and at times in sea sediments. The organism classically identified with myositis and myonecrosis is *Clostridium perfringens.* Historically, it has gone by the names of *Bacillus perfringens* (1898), *Bacterium welchii, Bacterium emphysematosa,* and *Clostridium welchii* (1900). The Clostridia genus contains the spore-forming, gram-positive anaerobic bacteria. There are five groups of *C. perfringens,* designated A through E, based on the pattern of combination of the four major lethal toxins (designated $\alpha, \beta, \epsilon,$ and ι) produced by the organisms.[2] These five biotypes are associated with different diseases of humans and animals. Each of the five biotypes produces α-toxin, with type A producing particularly large amounts. Many of the clinical manifestations are due to the actions of α-toxin, but as many as 12 toxins may be released during infection. Other species of toxin-producing Clostridia that cause gas gangrene are *C. novyi, C. septicum, C. histolyticum, C. fallax, C. sordellii,* and *C. bifermentans.*

Despite being classified as an anaerobe, *C. perfringens* can grow freely in oxygen tensions up to 30 mm Hg, which is an oxygen level that can be found in human tissue, and even in some environments up to 70 mm Hg.

In general, anaerobic organisms do not grow in an oxygen milieu because of low activity levels of enzymes that scavenge and degrade oxygen radicals. These antioxidant enzymes include superoxide dismutases and catalases, which are hydrogen peroxide–degrading enzymes. Hyperbaric oxygen therapy (HBOT) at 2 to 3 atmospheres absolute (ATA), by increasing tissue oxygen tensions to greater than 30 mm Hg, has been demonstrated to stop spore germination and to inhibit bacterial growth in a bacteriostatic fashion. Higher levels of oxygen may be bactericidal, but hyperbaric oxygen alone has no effect on formed α-toxin. α-Toxin is normally cleared by the kidney.

Gas production is thought to be caused by glycolysis by bacteria. Carbon dioxide (CO_2) and water are the natural end products of aerobic metabolism. Theoretically, CO_2 rapidly dissolves in aqueous-based tissue fluid and should rarely accumulate in tissues. Incomplete oxidation by anaerobic and facultative bacteria can produce gases that are not as readily water soluble and can accumulate in tissues. Measurement of the gas within infected muscle tissues from a patient with diabetes with *Clostridium septicum* infection was reported as 5.9% H_2, 3.4% CO_2, 74.5% N_2, and 16.1% O_2.[3] The gas produced within tissues is visible on radiographs and computed tomography (CT) scans in approximately half of reported cases.

Risk Factors

Historically, gas gangrene occurred in war wounds because of the considerable risk factors attendant to contamination of wounds that occur on the battlefield. These include involvement of direct open trauma to muscle and its vascular supply, and to the contamination of such wounds with foreign material. High-velocity bullets and explosive missiles cause "shock-wave" damage surrounding the actual physical pathway taken by the foreign material, increasing the risk for having poorly perfused tissue surrounding the open wound site from penetrating injury, compared with lower-velocity bullets or open wounds from falls and motor vehicle collisions. In combat, infantry soldier wounds are more likely to be contaminated with dirt and pieces of uniform material, and injuries may occur in fields of battle that were contaminated by soil and animal manure. Treatment of the initial wound is said to be the most important factor in the prevention of this complication of war wounds.[4] Extensive review of the occurrence of gas gangrene in the history of America's wars has been well described.[5]

In the civilian population, Clostridial myositis and myonecrosis is more likely to occur in patients after trauma, especially in wounds with poorly perfused muscle. The most frequent kinds of trauma include motor vehicle collisions and farming accidents with open fractures, followed by crush injuries, industrial accidents, and gunshot wounds.[3] It is also seen in patients with diabetes mellitus and vasculopathy, appearing in the presence of chronic, nonhealing wounds, foot ulcers, and sacral decubitus infections. Another major group of patients at risk is the postoperative abdominal surgery patient group with intraabdominal sepsis, because the organisms are normally present in the intestine. The most common surgical procedures it follows are those involving colon resection and biliary tract surgery. In the majority of cases when Clostridia are isolated in the surgical setting, they are likely to be present in mixed cultures, are present as secondary invaders, and may not be producing toxin. Having a gastrointestinal focus of cancer appears to be a risk factor for infection with *C. septicum,* a particularly virulent species. Cases are also reported in patients with burns,[6] and clusters have been reported in intravenous drug users. Gas gangrene of the uterus occurs in the setting of septic abortions[7] but is also reported after delivery[8] or after surgical procedures.[9]

The toxins elaborated by *C. perfringens* are the hallmark of the disease (Table 18.1). The toxins are known to be extracellular enzymes. Of these, the most significant ones are believed to be α-toxin, a Zn^{+2} metalloenzyme, phospholipase C, which splits lecithin and the phosphoglycerides of choline, ethanolamine, and serine present in eukaryotic cell membranes,[10] and θ-toxin, also known as *perfringolysin O,* which

Table 18.1 Main Toxins Elaborated by *Clostridium perfringens* and Their Biologic Effects

α-Toxin: lethal,* lecithinase, necrotizing, hemolytic, cardiotoxic
β-Toxin: lethal,* necrotizing
δ-Toxin: lethal,* hemolysin
ε-Toxin: lethal,* permease
θ-Toxin: lethal,* hemolysin, cytolysin, leukostatic
ι-Toxin: lethal,* necrotizing
κ-Toxin: lethal,* collagenase, gelatinase, necrotizing
λ-Toxin: protease
μ-Toxin: hyaluronidase
ν-Toxin: lethal,* deoxyribonuclease, hemolytic, necrotizing
φ-Toxin: hemolysin, cytolysin

*"Lethal" based on injection into mice.
Modified from Gas gangrene. Available at: http://www.emedicine.com/med/topic843.htm, by permission.

is a hemolysin. Since the 1940s, α-toxin has been suspected to be the major virulence determinant of gas gangrene on the basis of studies with supernatant fluid from cultures of *C. perfringens.* In the mid-1990s, loss of virulence was demonstrated when an allelic-replacement mutant in a virulent strain of *C. perfringens* was constructed, tested in a murine gas gangrene model, and shown to have eliminated virulence.[11] The mutant strain showed loss of virulence, and the foot swelling, blackening, and muscle necrosis normally seen in the control mice were almost completely absent when they were challenged with the α-toxin deficient strain. When the gene was reintroduced into the mutant to re-encode for α-toxin, the virulence properties were restored. The protein has been determined to have two functional domains: (1) the N-terminal domain possessing phospholipase C activity and (2) the C-terminal domain, which binds to eukaryotic cell membranes[12] (Fig. 18.1).

α-Toxin attacks phospholipids in micellar or monodispersed forms. Most phospholipids biologically are present in cell membranes, and cells still undergo lysis when exposed to adequate levels of α-toxin.[13] Additional effects of α-toxin are also evident. Sublytic quantities of α-toxin have been shown to activate the arachidonic acid cascade.[14] This cascade results in production of prostaglandins, thromboxanes,

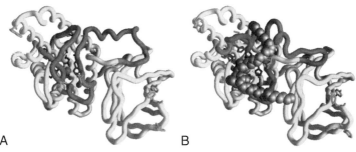

Figure 18.1 α-Toxin has been crystallized in two distinct conformations. *A* is believed to be catalytically active and so is known as the "open form." The second form, *B*, known as the "closed form," has two loops partially closing the active site and leaving the protein inactive. A short animated loop at the Birkbeck Toxin Structure Group Homepage Web site shows the dynamic opening and closing of the molecule, centered on its binding site. **(See Color Plate 28.)** *(From Institute of Structural Molecular Biology, Birkbeck College School of Crystallography, University of London, UK: Available at http://people.cryst.bbk.ac.uk/~bcole04/ambrose.html, by permission. Accessed August 30, 2007.)*

and leukotrienes, which are involved in inflammatory processes. Thromboxanes have been shown to be involved in platelet aggregation in this setting,[15] resulting in decreased blood flow to tissues.[16] Titball theorizes that "it is possible to envisage the situation where α-toxin diffuses away from the initial site of infection into adjacent healthy tissues, and the resultant reduction in blood supply to these tissues then provides the appropriate conditions for the spread of the infection into these tissues."[17]

Another major effect of clinical relevance of α-toxin is the suppression of the cellular inflammatory response by lysis of leukocytes and blockage of the migration of leucocytes into tissue spaces, causing them to accumulate along the walls of blood vessels.[9] The observation of the paucity of white blood cells in areas of infection was first made in 1917 by two military surgeons who had managed battlefield cases of gas gangrene in World War I and who noted that leukocytes are generally conspicuous by their absence in involved muscle tissue.[18] Similar observations have been made repeatedly in clinical reports. Demonstration of the alteration of the traffic of neutrophils to infected tissue because of impaired neutrophil diapedesis caused by large aggregates of adherent platelets induced by phospholipase C was reported by Bryant and colleagues.[19] Furthermore, the stimulated synthesis of platelet-activating factor and prostacyclin, two

vasoactive lipids, was demonstrated in human endothelial cells in response to the presence of α-toxin and subsequent protein kinase C activation. These cultured endothelial cells exhibited enhanced neutrophil adhesion in response to α-toxin, which was mediated through the platelet-activating factor receptor and P-selectin.[20] The effect of hyperbaric oxygen on adhesion molecules P-selectin and β_2 integrin has been demonstrated in scenarios ranging from carbon monoxide poisoning[21] and decompression sickness[22] to reperfusion injury,[23] and thus is an area that should be further studied in the setting of α-toxin–induced leukocyte aggregation to assess additional mechanisms of the positive effect of hyperbaric oxygen. These responses to α-toxin may contribute to localized and systemic manifestations of gas gangrene, including enhanced vascular permeability, localized neutrophil accumulation and clumping, and myocardial dysfunction. In rabbit models, α-toxin induces cardiovascular collapse by direct inhibition of myocardial contractility.[24]

Hemolysis is reported during episodes of Clostridial bacteremia, another effect of phospholipase C. Structural correlates with cytotoxic and hemolytic effects have been reported, and the structure of the toxin has been described by Naylor and colleagues.[25] ε-Toxin is considered responsible for increased vascular permeability and edema.

Clinical Presentation

The incubation period of gas gangrene from time of injury to onset of symptoms is usually 1 to 4 days, although the range can be short as 6 hours and as long as 3 weeks.[26] The first complaint by a patient is usually sudden unrelenting pain at the site of the wound, although some patients report the symptom of heaviness or pressure. These may occur in the absence of any significant clinical findings. Within hours, rapid appearance and progression of tense edema, pallor, and tenderness occur. Typically, tenderness is out of proportion to the physical findings. The skin color progressively changes to a coppery bronze or magenta. Hemorrhagic bullae and subcutaneous emphysema may ensue, although they are not seen in half of the cases. The finding of gas roentgenographically is suggestive, but it is not a requirement for the diagnosis of Clostridial myositis and is not diagnostic because infection with other organisms may also produce gas. Over time, an insipid thin, brownish, greenish, yellow or black exudate may be present, with a "sweetish" or "mousy" odor, not the overwhelming putrid odor of standard anaerobic infections. There is loss of contractility of the affected muscle. Gram stain of the discharge may show the characteristic gram-positive rods (although sometimes the organism may stain poorly and appear gram variable, as mixed gram-positive and gram-negative rods). The hallmark appearance of the Gram stain is described as a paucity of white blood cells, which may either be seen as ghost smudges, after lysis by α- and/or θ- and other toxins, or may not be seen at all because of loss of diapedesis induced by α-toxin. Fluid in bullae from a patient with nontrauma-related *C. septicum* infection was examined by Stevens and colleagues.[27] The typical Gram stain showed many gram-positive rods without leukocytes. Although they found no α- or θ-toxins in the fluid in their assay, they were able to demonstrate adverse effects of the fluid on neutrophil viability, appearance, and function, including decreased chemotaxis and phagocytosis.

The margins of the infection may extend at a rapid rate, and in fulminant cases, can be measured at several inches per hour. Patients appear toxic, with marked tachycardia and the development of hypotension, but they often have intact sensorium until late in the infection. Fever may be low grade or absent. The affected tissue will not bleed easily, if at all, because of ischemia. Extension onto the trunk is a marker for much greater mortality rates, and debridement becomes more complex than if extremity involvement alone is present. Bacteremia may occur in 15% of patients. Later complications include massive hemolysis, hypotension, acute renal failure, and metabolic acidosis. Hemolysis of the entire circulating red cell mass has been reported at least once.[28]

Differential Diagnosis

Other clinical situations that can mimic gas gangrene include other significant necrotizing infections, such as crepitant cellulitis; mixed aerobic/anaerobic necrotizing cellulitis; non-Clostridial myositis and myonecrosis, usually caused by mixed aerobic-anaerobic organisms or group A β-hemolytic streptococci; necrotizing fasciitis; infection secondary to *Vibrio vulnificus,* particularly in patients with underlying liver disease exposed to sea water; and zygomycotic gangrenous cellulitis secondary to fungal organisms of the *Mucorales* and *Entomophthorales* families. In the neonate with omphalitis, it may be difficult to differentiate between Clostridial myositis and necrotizing fasciitis, but even neonates as young as 5 to 7 days should still be considered treatable with HBOT.[29]

Treatment

Standard therapy has historically consisted of antibiotics and surgery. Antibiotic selection is typically directed at the Clostridial organisms responsible for this infection. High-dose intravenous sodium penicillin G has been the standard antibiotic recommended for many years, but data appear to demonstrate that survival may not be improved when penicillin alone is used, and evidence exists that toxin production is not reduced by penicillin. The observation has been made that use of antibiotics that have additional activity that blocks protein synthesis, a step needed to manufacture toxins, would be a physiologic advantage in treating this infection. In Stevens and colleagues' study,[30] inhibition of α-toxin activity was noted by the antibiotics clindamycin, metronidazole, tetracycline, rifampin, and chloramphenicol, but not by penicillin. Doses recommended for sodium penicillin (rather than potassium penicillin, because of the risk for hyperkalemia from breakdown of muscle tissue and subsequent renal insufficiency) are 24 million units per day, divided as 2 million units every 2 hours intravenously or 4 million units every 4 hours intravenously, plus 600 mg clindamycin every 6 hours to 900 mg every 8 hours intravenously. Additional broader-spectrum coverage will likely be required initially to cover other potential organisms such as gram-negative rods. It is reasonable to include clindamycin as part of any regimen used because of its effects on ribosomes to limit or block protein synthesis.

Surgical debridement is an essential part of the management of gas gangrene. Elimination of infected, dead tissues is important as a way to eliminate an infectious source of toxin and to open up the tissues to air. The addition of hyperbaric oxygen is also now recognized as essential in shutting off further α-toxin production and allowing whatever toxin that has already accumulated to be cleared by the body. What remains controversial is the order in which these modalities should be accomplished. There are those who advocate getting the patient to the operating room as soon as possible to perform a wide debridement, whereas others believe that the patient should go the hyperbaric chamber first, either to reduce toxicity, or to assist in defining the edges of viable tissue when the patient does go to the operating room for a more limited debridement, or in the situation when proceeding to the operating room is delayed more than the time needed to complete a hyperbaric treatment. What the literature does support is that clinical responses appear to be improved the earlier that HBOT can be started, in conjunction with initial conservative surgery. Results decline progressively when hyperbaric oxygen treatments are delayed. In the Amsterdam experience of Bakker[31] from 1960 through 1985, of 409 patients with gas gangrene, 361 survived during the active phase of the disease, which is an 11.1% mortality rate (48/409); 325 patients were long-term survivors, with the additional 36 deaths due to causes other than gas gangrene (pulmonary embolism, myocardial infarction, and metastatic colon carcinoma were the leading causes). The group with the greatest mortality (8/28) was already in septic shock when admitted. The group of 257 patients with gas gangrene associated with trauma, mainly of the extremities, had a mortality rate of only 7.0% overall, and if they survived to receive 4 hyperbaric treatments, the mortality rate was only 4.3%. In the group that had proximal extremity or truncal infection contracted after surgery, consisting of 124 patients, the mortality rate was 17.7% from gas gangrene overall, but only 13.7% if they lived to receive 4 hyperbaric treatments. Of the total of 48 deaths, all died within the first 24 hours after the start of hyperbaric therapy, before the fourth session. If patients survived to receive four treatments, given in the first 24 to 28 hours after onset of the first treatment, there were no further deaths. This is in contrast with the historical mortality rate of 50% to 90%.

Rationale for Use of Hyperbaric Oxygen Therapy

HBOT was first conceived by Brummelkamp and colleagues[32] as a treatment modality for anaerobic gas gangrene infections in 1960. In 1964, Van Unnik[33] reported the inhibition of the production of α-toxin by HBOT, in four clinical isolates of *C. perfringens.* Kaye[34] showed a bactericidal effect of oxygen at levels of 1400 mm Hg. Demello and coworkers[35] showed a reduction in the rate of germination of heat-activated spores under hyperbaric oxygen conditions. One of the first animal trials that demonstrated the role of hyperbaric oxygen in an animal model is that of Demello and coworkers,[36] who treated animals injected with a known amount of Clostridial organisms and a traumatized leg. They then treated the animals with antibiotics, surgery, and hyperbaric oxygen, singly, in combinations of two modalities, and with all three modalities. The best results occurred using all three modalities. The triple regimen resulted in 95% salvage of the animals, whereas the next best was only a 70% rate of survival using surgery and antibiotics but without hyperbaric oxygen. Additional animal studies have also shown substantial reduction in morbidity and mortality after Clostridial infection, when used either prophylactically or therapeutically.[37-40]

Clinical studies in humans have demonstrated reductions in human morbidity and mortality around the world. Unsworth and Sharp[41] report on an 11-year experience of 73 patients managed with hyperbaric oxygen in Australia and Papua New Guinea. Seven deaths were attributed to the gas gangrene, for a mortality rate of 9.6%. They concluded that conservative surgery with HBOT preserved as much limb or tissue as possible. Rudge[42] presented a review of 20 clinical studies with a total of more than 1200 patients in whom hyperbaric oxygen was used and reported a cumulative mortality rate of 23%. Desola and coauthors[43] from Barcelona report a series of 85 confirmed cases. Lower limb infection accounted for 71.8% of cases, perineal foci in 8.2%, and abdominal origin in 18.8%. A total of 44.7% of cases were in shock at admission. In only 12.9% of cases was death thought to be directly related to the gas gangrene. Deaths related to the disease occurred within 3 days of presentation. Treatments were at 3 ATA. Korhonen and coworkers[44] report a case series of 53 patients from multiple hospitals in Finland. Treatments were done mostly at 2.5 ATA, with the observation made that hyperbaric oxygen decreased the systemic toxicity and prevented further extension of the infection.

Several details are important to note when comparing human studies. One is to ascertain the treatment tables used. Because the level of the partial pressure of oxygen (Po_2) appears to be important in bacterial killing and shutting off toxin, the higher treatment pressures in the range of 2.8 to 3.0 ATA would be much preferable to the 2.0 or 2.4 ATA sometimes used for more routine wound management protocols. The location of the gas gangrene, whether disease is limited to an extremity, involves the torso, or both, is also extremely important when comparing morbidity and mortality statistics. The much greater mortality of gas gangrene when the torso is involved will skew data when such cases are part of a series and thus should be dissected out when a series combines the cases. A good example of this is the series by Altemeier and Fullen,[45] who reported a 14.7% mortality rate using only antibiotics and "aggressive surgery" and claimed that, because of aggressive surgical technique, including high amputations, this was as good as the death rates reported with HBOT. However, on analysis of the types of cases he reported, one can see that his entire series consisted of cases of traumatic gas gangrene of the extremities, while he compared his results with those that combined extremity and torso involvement. If the results of the cases to which he compared his cases were analyzed by reviewing only those involving extremity involvement, the mortality rate of 7% was half that of Altemeier.[45] The amputation rate is also reduced by half.

Additional mechanisms of action of HBOT that are likely to be beneficial in gas gangrene include hyperoxic vasoconstriction, which would lead to reduction of edema and improved perfusion to swollen ischemic tissue, and hyperoxic protection of areas immediately adjacent to the margins of the infected areas, which would reduce or eliminate the progressive onset of acidosis that would be permissive to conditions conducive to toxin formation. Thus, a ring of bolstered tissue perfusion is created around the area of myositis, tending to limit its extension. Enhancement of phagocytosis has been demonstrated under hyperbaric conditions, which would also tend to augment defenses against *C. perfringens*.

The current use of HBOT consists of 100% oxygen at 3.0 ATA pressure for 90 minutes, with 5-minute air breaks between each

30-minute period of oxygen breathing, per treatment, and delivering 3 treatments within the first 24 hours, followed by twice-daily treatments for the next 2 to 5 days, until the progression of infection appears to have ceased, demarcation of the wounds appears to be proceeding, and the patient shows resolution of clinical toxicity.[46,47] Rationale of the repetitive treatments during the first day or two recognizes that because the first hyperbaric treatments may not be lethal to the organisms, there may be regrowth of the organisms between those initial treatments, with further elaboration of α-toxin and other toxins. Thus, the repetitive treatments are performed to prevent recrudescence of signs and symptoms of the infection before it is well controlled.

Advantages of HBOT include more rapid resolution of the toxic state of the patient; reduction in the mortality rates seen; salvage of major joint levels; and reduction in amputation rates, in extremity involvement. The cost benefit of these advantages far outweighs the cost and effort involved.

Although some authors claim that HBOT remains controversial because of lack of randomized, controlled studies comparing HBOT versus no HBOT, other authors have concluded that the comparison with historic and untreated series of patients would make it unethical to perform a randomized clinical trial on patients, thereby denying a well-substantiated adjunctive treatment for a disease with a high rate of morbidity and mortality to a patient,[48] particularly if it is a readily available modality at a treating institution. In addition, there are, in fact, no randomized, controlled trials of using surgical debridement and antibiotics alone, without HBOT, and thus the argument against using HBOT for that reason cannot be seriously entertained. For those patients diagnosed with Clostridial myositis and myonecrosis at a facility that does not have a chamber, the dilemma of whether to transfer the patient to a facility with a hyperbaric chamber and delay initial surgery or proceed to surgery before transfer, possibly leading to a scenario of having to transfer a decompensated patient, is a real one, and such cases should be dealt with on an individual, case-by-case basis, in consultation with a surgical and hyperbaric team at a referral center, so as to minimize extended transfer times and facilitate time to both hyperbaric treatment and surgical opening of the infected tissue.

NECROTIZING FASCIITIS

Necrotizing fasciitis is an acute, potentially fatal infection of the superficial and deep fascia of the skin and soft tissues, which progresses to ischemic dermal necrosis after involvement of the dermal blood vessels that traverse the fascial layers. The popular media refer to this entity as infection with "flesh-eating bacteria."

Causative Factors

Necrotizing fasciitis was initially described and named "hemolytic streptococcal gangrene" by Meleney[49] in 1924. He described an illness characterized by gangrene of subcutaneous tissues, followed by rapid necrosis of the overlying skin from involvement of the blood vessels supplying the skin, which are found in the affected fascial layers. All his patients grew hemolytic streptococci on cultures, and the patients were all seriously ill. Surgical extirpation appeared to be the therapeutic approach. Reference to this entity as necrotizing fasciitis appears around the time of Wilson's report.[50] The characteristic level of infection is at the deep fascia, and infection with necrosis is noted to spread along fascial planes. Because blood vessels that supply overlying skin travel thru fascia, it is the involvement of these vessels by infection that leads to rapid progression to dermal necrosis. Microbiologically, groups A, C, or G β-hemolytic streptococci can be isolated from tissue specimens in 50% to 90% of case series, with one or two more organisms often also accompanying the streptococci in up to half the cases. The occurrence of *Staphylococcus aureus* plus anaerobic streptococci is also known as Meleney's synergistic gangrene. Necrotizing fasciitis is also reported to be caused by community-acquired strains of methicillin-resistant *S. aureus* alone.[51]

Risk Factors

The most common risk factors associated with necrotizing fasciitis are traumatic breaks in the skin, most commonly lacerations, insect bites, burns, deep abrasions, or after surgery, particularly those involving bowel perforations. Diabetes appears to be a strong risk factor, as are obesity, alcoholism, smoking, and intravenous drug abuse. Reports of necrotizing fasciitis as a result of infection of otherwise typical lesions of chickenpox have been published.[52] An association with the use of nonsteroidal anti-inflammatory agents has also been suggested.[53,54] Nonsteroidal anti-inflammatory drugs are cyclo-oxygenase inhibitors and may have an adverse effect on neutrophil killing and cell-mediated immunity. Nonsteroidal anti-inflammatory drugs are reported to inhibit monocyte superoxide production.[55]

Most common sites of occurrence of necrotizing fasciitis are the lower extremities, whereas an increased incidence in the upper extremities is seen in the parenteral drug abuse population. However, any location of the body can be affected, including the abdominal wall of neonates, in association with omphalitis.[56] Involvement of the scrotum and perineum in the male body is known as Fournier's gangrene, which is essentially necrotizing fasciitis of the superficial perineal fascia, also known as Colles' fascia, which can spread infection to the penis and scrotum via Buck's fascia or Dartos' fascia, or Scarpa's fascia, which connects to, and can spread infection to, the abdominal wall. Perianal or perirectal infection may also spread into these areas, and undrained or inadequately drained perirectal abscesses are often cited as a source of Fournier's gangrene. Perineal necrotizing fasciitis can also occur in the female body. Diabetes mellitus remains a strong risk factor in this particular form of necrotizing fasciitis as well. Fournier's gangrene is more likely to have multiple mixed organisms cultured, par-ticularly Enterobacteriaceae, group D streptococci, and anaerobic organisms such as *Bacteroides fragilis.*

Clinical Presentation

The patient with necrotizing fasciitis will typically present with an acute combination of pain and swelling, which may or may not be accompanied by fever and chills. There may already be a focus of cellulitis apparent, but in some instances early on, there may be few skin changes, putting the physician in the situation of a patient with a painful body part without much else to go on. In some patients, there may be pain out of proportion to the skin findings, which may not be unexpected considering that the initial level of infection is the fascia, not necessarily the skin. In others, manifestations of a large phlegmon may be quite obvious, although at times the area of phlegmon may have been assumed to be cellulitis and not a more serious form of infection. Pain may proceed to numbness, as a result of compression of nerves that also pass through the fascia. With time, however, the infection will rapidly proceed to cause areas of blistering and bullae formation. Hints of darkening of the skin may appear as perfusion decreases, until obvious areas of dermal ischemia appear, making the skin appear dusky, grayish, or frankly black. On exploration of the process, a clinical diagnosis can be confirmed at the time of biopsy or debridement, when the fascia is grossly observed by the surgeon to be necrotic, and will give way easily to a probing finger or surgical clamp, giving the sensation of "thunking" of the skin against the underlying muscle layers, instead of remaining tight and crisply defined. It has been suggested that limbs of patients with necrotizing fasciitis, as opposed to those with cellulitis only, may be observed to have markedly reduced tissue oxygen saturations as measured by near-infrared spectroscopy throughout the involved site, with oxygen saturations in the 52% ± 18% range, compared with control measurements of 86% ± 11% in uninvolved sites.[57]

In the neonate, necrotizing fasciitis of the abdominal wall can be seen as a complication of omphalitis in 10% to 16% of cases[58] and appears to carry more than a 50% mortality rate even when treated with aggressive debridement of involved skin, subcutaneous tissue, and fascia.[59]

A number of diagnostic observations have been made to enable confirmation of the diagnosis of necrotizing fasciitis. Frozen section soft-tissue biopsy early in the evolution of a suspect lesion may provide definitive diagnosis.[60] CT scan findings are also revealing. Asymmetric fascial thickening that was at least twice the contralateral side and associated with fat stranding was seen in 80% of 20 patients with necrotizing fasciitis. Gas tracking along fascial planes was seen in 55% of patients, characteristically did not involve muscle, and was not associated with abscess formation.[61] The authors note that the areas of black, gangrenous skin were far smaller than the widespread infection in the underlying fascial planes. Also of note was that 7 of the 20 patients had associated deep space abscesses that required immediate surgical drainage, which demonstrates the need for CT studies to assess extent of disease, particularly in patients who do not appear to be responding to therapy.

Magnetic resonance imaging also demonstrates the distribution of affected tissue well, is able to differentiate fluid and gas through differential signal intensities, and is useful in differentiating cellulitis from necrotizing fasciitis, after injection of gadolinium contrast. But in a study of 15 patients, magnetic resonance imaging overestimated the extent of deep fascial involvement in one patient who had only cellulitis, after intramuscular injections that showed up on magnetic resonance imaging as thickening of both superficial and deep fascia of the deltoid muscle.[62]

Cultures of deep tissue at the time of debridement are imperative because up to 75% of patients in some series have demonstrated polymicrobial causative agents.

Amputation rates of up to 50% are reported without hyperbaric therapy. Mortality rates in reported series range from 30% to 66% without the use of hyperbaric oxygen, with mortality often associated with delayed diagnosis, underlying immunocompromise, septic shock, and

severe underlying metabolic abnormalities. In a small group of neonatal omphalitis patients with abdominal wall necrotizing fasciitis, 5 of 7 cases died, for a mortality rate of 71%. The two patients who did survive, both of whom were administered HBOT, were noted to have resolved their systemic sepsis more rapidly and had healthier granulation tissue on the perimeter of the debridement. Neither survivor treated with hyperbaric oxygen required any further debridements before their wounds were closed.

Gozal and coworkers[63] treated patients with combined antibiotics, radical surgery, and hyperbaric oxygen, and reduced the historic mortality rate from 38% to 12.5%. Of 29 patients reported retrospectively by Riseman and colleagues,[64] 12 were treated by surgical debridement and antibiotics only, and 17 received HBOT in addition. Both groups had similar parameters of age, race, sex, wound bacteriology, and antimicrobial therapy. Body surface area was also similar. However, perineal involvement (53% vs. 12%) and septic shock (29% vs. 8%) were more common in the hyperbaric group, yet the overall mortality rate was significantly lower at 23% versus 66% in the non-HBOT group. In addition, only 1.2 debridements per patient in the HBOT group were performed versus 3.3 debridements per patient in the surgery plus antibiotics-only group.

Differential Diagnosis

Clearly, a goal when making the diagnosis of necrotizing fasciitis is to make it as early as possible so as to be able to start appropriate treatments and avoid rapid spreading and the onset of sepsis. Time is tissue. The main differential diagnoses include standard cellulitis, which may be a precursor of necrotizing fasciitis in some cases, and erysipelas, with its erythematous, well-delineated border. Additional entities that should be considered include Clostridial myositis and myonecrosis; non-Clostridial myositis and myonecrosis; toxic shock syndrome, which may accompany necrotizing fasciitis; phycomycotic gangrenous cellulitis; mixed aerobic/anaerobic necrotizing cellulitis; toxic epidermal necrolysis, also known as Lyell's disease, usually caused by exposure to particular medications; and Staphylococcal scalded skin syndrome, also known as Ritter's disease, caused by exfoliative toxins produced by Staphylococci, with the latter two entities being most common in neonates and children younger than 5 years. In the neonate with omphalitis, violaceous discoloration of the skin appears to be a strong marker for the emergence of necrotizing fasciitis. Cutaneous anthrax may present with a blackened central area and surrounding edema.

Treatment and Rationale for Use of Hyperbaric Oxygen Therapy

Hypoxia is known to impair phagocytosis by polymorphonuclear leukocytes.[65] After an infective process is initiated, metabolic products of aerobic and anaerobic metabolism tend to reduce the oxidation-reduction potential (E_h), leading to a decline in pH, which creates a milieu for growth of strict and facultative anaerobic organisms. When the blood supply to the skin is affected by involvement within a phlegmon, with edema and necrosis in the deep fascial layers in which they reside, the decreased perfusion pressure and ischemia predispose to progression and advancement of the infectious process within the skin and subcutaneous tissues. Quantities of gas within tissues are frequently seen in both gas gangrene and necrotizing fasciitis.

HBOT can reduce the amount of hypoxic leukocyte dysfunction that occurs within an area of infection and provide oxygenation to otherwise ischemic areas, thus limiting the spread and progression of infection. In cases where the antibiotic being used requires oxygen for transfer across cell walls, HBOT can act to enhance antibiotic penetration into target bacteria. This has been demonstrated for aminoglycosides and Pseudomonas.

Numerous studies have continued to demonstrate the beneficial effect of HBOT in the management of necrotizing fasciitis. Wilkinson and Doolette[66] report a 5-year retrospective

cohort Australian study of 44 patients with necrotizing soft-tissue infection, between 1994 and 1999, analyzing the primary outcome of survival to hospital discharge and secondary outcomes of limb salvage and long-term survival after hospital discharge. Logistic regression analysis determined the strongest association with survival was the intervention of HBOT ($P = 0.02$). HBOT increased survival with an odds ratio of 8.9 (95% confidence interval, 1.3–58.0) and a number needed to treat to benefit of 3. HBOT also reduced the incidence of amputation ($P = 0.05$) and improved long-term outcome ($P = 0.002$). In the series by Escobar and investigators,[67] there were no further amputations beyond those already done before transfer, once HBOT was initiated in their series of 42 patients. The negative study by Brown and coauthors[68] that purports to be a multicenter retrospective review of treatment at 3 facilities over 12 years, of 54 patients, had numerous discrepancies in the demographics of their 2 groups. Half of the HBOT group of 30 patients, all from 1 institution, were noted to have Clostridial infections, whereas the non-HBOT group had only 4 of 24 patients (17%) with Clostridial infection. Six of the 30 patients in the HBOT group are noted to have the diagnosis of Clostridial myositis and myonecrosis, whereas only 1 of the non-HBOT patients were so diagnosed. Hence, this clearly shows the same diseases were not being compared in that study. In addition, as is pointed out in a subsequent letter to the editor,[69] 80% of the patients received 4 or fewer treatments, the remaining 20% received between 5 and 7 treatments, and the timing of these treatments is not specified. If the guideline of treating three times in the first 24 hours were followed, and then twice per day until the patient is stable and shows no relapse of toxicity between treatments, the gas gangrene patients in this study were treated for less than a day and a half, which is a shorter period than most other studies, and the others were treated for about 2 days. In Wilkinson's study,[66] patients received a median of eight treatments, which is more than that received by the patient with the greatest number of treatments in Brown and coauthors' study.[68] The authors state that the mortality difference between the two groups (9/30, or 30% of the HBOT group, vs. 10/24, or 42% in the non-HBOT group) was not statistically significant. Thus, Brown and coauthors' study[68] should not be used as an argument that the use of hyperbaric oxygen for truncal necrotizing fasciitis is "controversial" because these mortality statistics are not comparable, with a different mix of diagnoses in the two, compounded by the fact that the numbers themselves are small. Furthermore, the study does not add to the literature of necrotizing fasciitis involving the limbs and other nontruncal sites.

Fortunately, Fournier's gangrene cases in the literature are usually studied and reported as a distinct group. Hollabaugh and coworkers[70] report a retrospective series of 26 cases from the University of Tennessee's five hospitals. Of the 15 patients with identifiable sources for their infections, 8 had urethral disease or trauma, 5 had colorectal disease, and 2 had penile prostheses. All patients were managed with prompt surgical debridement and broad-spectrum antibiotics. Procedures performed included urinary diversion, fecal diversion, and multiple debridements. Fourteen of the 26 were additionally treated with hyperbaric oxygen. The HBOT group had a mortality rate of 7% versus 42% in the non-HBOT group ($P = 0.04$), with a combined overall mortality rate of 23%. The one patient who died while receiving HBOT had been progressing well without evidence of ongoing infection but suffered an acute myocardial infarction not thought to be related to the underlying disease process. In the non-HBOT group, deaths were usually attributed to ongoing or fulminant sepsis. Relative risk for survival was 11 times greater in the group receiving HBOT. This study did not show a decrease in the number of debridements by HBOT but was confounded because of the larger number of patients who died and thus were not able to get further debridements. Delay to treatment was not a factor in the different groups.

Additional series include that of the group from Genoa, Italy,[71] which treated 11 patients

without any deaths, and all delayed corrective procedures healed without infectious complications. Another 33 patients were reported in a series from Turku, Finland.[72] These patients were treated at 2.5 ATA, in conjunction with antibiotics and surgery. Three patients died, for a mortality rate of 9%. Hyperbaric oxygenation was observed to reduce systemic toxicity, prevent extension of the necrotizing process, and increase demarcation, improving overall outcomes. Two of the three patients who died were moribund on arrival to their facility. Management included diverting colostomies for those patients with a perirectal or perineal source, and orchiectomy, although sometimes reported in all series, is not routinely done because the blood supply to the testes is from the spermatic vessels, which do not perfuse the scrotum and penis. Suprapubic cystostomy was indicated and performed when the source of the infection was genitourinary.

Because of the difficulty in making direct comparisons of clinical series, a Fournier's gangrene severity index score was developed[73] to assess a number of variables rather than the presence of the disease itself. The score uses degrees of deviation from normal of physiologic variables to generate a score that correlates with patient mortality. It is clear that the amount of disease, related by some to body surface area of involvement, may be a significant variable. The Duke University analysis of 50 consecutive patients seen at their institution over a 15-year period had a 20% overall mortality rate.[74] Three statistically significant predictors of outcome were identified when examined using univariate analysis: extent of infection, depth of the necrotizing infection, and treatment with hyperbaric oxygen. However, the same data using multivariate regression analysis identified the extent of the infection as the only statistically significant independent predictor of outcome in the presence of other covariables. Patients with disease involving a body surface area of 3.0% or less all survived. The numbers of patients with disease extent greater than 3%, where hyperbaric oxygen would thus be expected to play a role, became smaller, and with small numbers of patients, the power of the study to demonstrate a significant response was not present. The *P* value for statistical significance for HBOT was 0.06 using multivariate analysis.

With such strong case series evidence of reductions in morbidity and mortality for necrotizing fasciitis and the subset of Fournier's gangrene, it is difficult to envision ever seeing a controlled, double-blinded study of HBOT.

The recommended HBOT protocol for necrotizing fasciitis includes initiating therapy at 2.0 to 2.5 ATA pressure for 90 minutes of oxygen given twice a day for mild-to-moderate cases, until there appears to be no further extension of necrosis in previously debrided areas and infection is "controlled."[75] Some hyperbaric specialists may switch to once-daily treatments once the patients appear stabilized to be sure that the process does not flare up again before stopping treatment completely. HBOT does not substitute for standard wound care, debridement of necrotic tissue, use of antibiotics directed at the expected range of organisms, and goal-directed management of sepsis.

OTHER NECROTIZING BACTERIAL INFECTIONS

Non-Clostridial Myonecrosis

Non-Clostridial myonecrosis is a particularly aggressive soft-tissue infection that clinically acts much like the Clostridial myositis syndrome, with widespread involvement of muscle and fascia. It has also been called "synergistic necrotizing cellulitis."[76] It is differentiated from necrotizing fasciitis by the muscle involvement, although infection from necrotizing fasciitis, if left to progress, will ultimately spread into muscle and may be indistinguishable from non-Clostridial myositis at that point. Organisms described to be involved include the anaerobic *Peptococcus* species, *Peptostreptococcus* species, and *Bacteroides* species, often mixed with aerobic members of the *Enterobacteriaceae*.[77] Clinically, the patient will present with exquisite local tenderness, minimal skin changes, and drainage

of "dishwater" pus from skin surface ulcerations, which become enveloped in blue–gray gangrene. Most patients are quite ill systemically. Half of the patients are bacteremic. Gas can also be seen. This is often described as the entity when Fournier's gangrene extends onto the abdominal wall and pelvis, involving muscle and fascia alike. Treatment remains surgical debridement. Because there is a frequent component of anaerobic organisms in this entity, it would appear reasonable to use the same rationale as for treatment of necrotizing fasciitis and a similar treatment protocol.

Crepitant Anaerobic Cellulitis

The category of crepitant anaerobic cellulitis encompasses both Clostridial and non-Clostridial skin infection. There is abundant tissue gas, but no fascial or muscle involvement. When Clostridial species are present in this situation, the conditions are not conducive to toxin formation and the patient will lack marked systemic toxicity. It is most commonly reported after local trauma to the lower extremities in patients with vascular insufficiency. Organisms reported include *Clostridium* species, *Peptococcus* species, *Peptostreptococcus* species, *Bacteroides* species, and *Enterobacteriaceae*. Gas formation causes the typical "crepitance" palpable within the skin. Antibiotics and surgical therapy in normal hosts is usually adequate therapy. HBOT should be considered in compromised hosts and in those failing to respond. Mortality rate is given at around 10%.

Progressive Bacterial Gangrene

Progressive bacterial gangrene is a subacute process, characterized by slowly progressive dermal ulceration, usually found on the abdominal wall or thorax. It was first described by Cullen[78] in a patient after drainage of an appendiceal abscess. It does not extend to deep fascia. It usually develops at a surgical site, such as a colostomy or ileostomy site. The area around the wound becomes erythematous, swollen, and tender, with progression to induration. A central purple area develops and then proceeds to slough off as the lesion enlarges and develops a granulation area centrally, surrounded by a gangrenous margin. The pathologic lesion is said to be related to progressively expanding infection created by the synergism between aerophilic and anaerobic/microaerophilic bacteria. It is thought to be similar to, or identical to, Meleney's ulcer, which has as its hallmark a progressive, slowly extending rim of necrosis, which may tunnel subcutaneously and spread in an occult fashion. It is also seen after lymph node surgery in the neck, axilla, or groin. HBOT has been shown to lead to improvement when other standard therapies have failed.[79]

ZYGOMYCOTIC GANGRENOUS CELLULITIS

In the immunocompromised population, infection with opportunistic organisms is not an uncommon occurrence. Opportunistic organisms typically do not cause disease in normal host patients, but because of particular deficits in the immune response of various categories, these otherwise unusual organisms become common findings in the abnormal host population. Until now the discussion has centered on bacterial and bacterial toxin–induced diseases, but fungal organisms may also become significant pathogens in that population of patients. A significant virulence factor of these organisms is their characteristic invasion of blood vessels, causing ischemia, hypoxia, and progressive necrosis of tissue, thus creating a niche that would physiologically appear to be amenable to alteration through the use of HBOT.

Causative Factors

Zygomycosis is the name given to the group of fungal infections caused by pathogenic molds belonging to the class Zygomyces, in the phylum Zygomycota. The term *Phycomycosis* has also been used, but it is less commonly used

today. The class Zygomyces is further divided into two orders, *Mucorales* and *Entomophthorales*. The Mucorales usually cause infections that are acute in onset, aggressive, rapidly progressive, and angio-invasive. These infections are commonly called *Mucormycoses.* In the family Mucoraceae within the order Mucorales are organisms of the genera *Absidia, Apophysomyces, Mucor, Rhizomucor,* and *Rhizopus.* Additional, less common families include Cunninghamellaceae with organisms of the single genus *Cunninghamella,* and Saksenaea, with the single genus *Saksenaea,* and others.[80] Organisms in the order *Entomophthorales* are *Conidiobolus coronatus* and *Basidiobolus ranarum.* These produce a group of infections that tend to be more indolent but clearly pathologic and chronically progressive. They typically do not invade blood vessels, although some recent reports suggest that this may occur at times.

Risk Factors

The recognized risk factors for Zygomycoses are numerous. The leading risk factor appears to be diabetes mellitus, particularly in the setting of ketoacidosis or uncontrolled hyperglycemia. It is reported that 70% of cases of rhinocerebral Zygomycosis occur in the setting of ketoacidosis.[81] The acidotic environment is said to be ideal for fungal growth, whereas white blood cell activity is inhibited in the hyperglycemic environment.[82-84] It has been shown that acidosis disrupts the inhibitory activity of sera against fungal growth by interrupting the capacity of transferrin to bind iron, which would normally keep it from being available to the fungal species.[85] Another group of patients at risk are those with iron overload syndromes who are at risk for more significant infections because of the presence of greater levels of iron, a growth factor for most bacteria and fungi capable of synthesizing endogenous metal chelators, or siderophores, or in patients on metal chelators, such as dialysis patients receiving deferoxamine[86,87] for removal of aluminum. Because deferoxamine is normally cleared by the kidney, levels of the drug remain high in the dialysis population, prolonging the time that iron bound to it can be utilized by the fungi. Other susceptible patients are those with underlying malignancies, especially leukemias; patients with neutropenia; solid organ and bone marrow transplant patients; and patients who are actively or passively immunosuppressed. Patients who have been taking broad-spectrum antibiotics may have fungal overgrowth, which is also a risk factor. The organisms are ubiquitous fungi, and they commonly inhabit decaying matter such as common garden soil. Introduction of infection is often related to antecedent trauma.[88] A history of exposure to organisms through farm accidents or trauma in the garden would not be unusual. Gastrointestinal involvement is associated with extreme malnutrition and is also related to oral ingestion of spores of the organisms. About 5% of patients appear to have no risk factors whatsoever.

Clinical Presentations

The most common manifestations of Zygomycosis are sinusitis, rhinocerebral infection, soft-tissue infection, pneumonia, gastrointestinal involvement, and disseminated infection. In the sinusitis and rhinocerebral forms of the infection, initial symptoms would be similar to routine sinusitis, with sinus pain, congestion, and drainage. The infection then accelerates, extending into adjacent structures and tissues, with development of erythema, progressing to violaceous or dusky to frankly black tissue in the nares, turbinates, palate, or orbit. The organisms appear to have a predilection for invasion of arteries, lymphatics, and nerves. Invasion of vascular structures leads to a fibrin reaction and development of a Mucor thrombus within vessels, which leads to infarction. The infarcted tissue becomes acidotic and permissive for even further fungal ingrowth and proliferation. Lack of perfusion prevents antibiotic penetration into affected tissues. Extension into adjacent periorbital and orbital structures is often found even early on. Clinical manifestations can include periorbital edema, tearing, and proptosis, and involvement of the optic nerve will be marked by blurring, followed by loss of vision. Abnormalities of eye movement may occur as markers of cranial nerve involvement. Extension can also move inferiorly into the hard palate via the maxillary sinuses; black, necrotic ulcers may be found on the palate, and the nasal turbinates may appear black and necrotic. Infection may extend into the cranial vault, either via the ethmoid sinus and through the cribriform plate, or through the orbital apex into the area of the cavernous sinus, producing the orbital apex syndrome, consisting of ophthalmoplegia and Vth cranial nerve involvement, progressing to cavernous sinus thrombosis, and thrombosis of the internal carotid artery, resulting in major hemispheric stroke and altered consciousness. Because of the propensity for angio-invasion, fungemia can occur, disseminating the infection systemically. Rhinocerebral mucormycosis has a high mortality rate. Standard treatment consists of the antifungal antibiotic amphotericin B lipid complex or liposomal amphotericin B, in a dose of 5 mg/kg daily and surgical debridement when indicated. Survivors have usually had earlier diagnosis and surgical debridements.

Pulmonary involvement is the second most common type of Zygomycosis overall, seen particularly in patients with leukemia and lymphoma.[89] Isolated solitary nodular lesions, lobar involvement, cavitary lesions, and disseminated lesions have all been reported.[90] Erosion of the fungus into the mediastinal structures, particularly the pulmonary artery, with massive hemoptysis, is a fatal occurrence. Wedged infarctions of the lung may be seen, as a manifestation of thrombosed pulmonary vessels, from angio-invasion.[91]

One of the manifestations of cutaneous infection includes a rapidly progressive, ascending, necrotizing infection consistent with necrotizing fasciitis, which can involve an extremity or the torso. Aerial hyphae can sometimes be grossly visualized in wounds infected with Zygomycosis organisms, as a loose, whitish cottony exudate covering the surface of open wounds. Risk factors for the development of cutaneous and subcutaneous involvement include various types of breakdown of the skin barrier, including puncture wounds, other trauma, and burn wounds. Mortality rates of 30% to 70% are reported in necrotizing fasciitis with these organisms, depending on the underlying condition associated with the infection. Because diabetic ketoacidosis is a treatable condition, reversal of the acidosis affords an opportunity for the host response to reconstitute, and thus may have a decreased mortality compared with patients with nonreversible conditions.

The gastrointestinal syndrome is characterized by abdominal pain and distention, associated with nausea and vomiting. Fever and hematochezia may occur. Stomach, ileum, and colon are most commonly affected. Most such diagnoses are made after death, but, if suspected, may require laparotomy to manage the bowel infarctions that may occur.[92]

Differential Diagnosis

On initial presentation, rhinocerebral mucormycosis may be misidentified as the more common routine bacterial sinusitis because of usual gram-positive or anaerobic organisms, although there should not be any necrotic lesions in those cases. However, once evidence of necrosis is apparent, or in the proper clinical settings, there should be no hesitation in ordering a biopsy, looking for the various fungal forms, which are quite characteristic wide, nonseptate hyphae branching off at right angles; signs of angio-invasive processes also should be sought. Affected tissue usually has neutrophilic infiltrates and inflammatory vasculitis is seen, involving both arteries and veins. Cultures for routine aerobic, anaerobic, and fungal organisms should always be sent. Cavernous sinus thrombosis can occur as an extension of suppurative, usually Staphylococcal, facial cellulitis or abscess, but there would not be the typical lesions in the nose or sinuses. Radiologic studies, such as plain films or CT scans, may show more extensive bone necrosis than was anticipated. Orbital cellulitis and bacterial osteomyelitis of the frontal bone or orbit are other entities that may clinically resemble this form of Zygomycosis.

Lung involvement may be nonspecific and can look like other cases of atelectasis, pneumonia, granulomatous disease, or particularly in patients with cancer, infection caused by *Aspergillus* species. Use of radiologic studies may hasten the diagnosis. In a retrospective analysis of CT findings in 16 cases of pulmonary Zygomycosis versus 29 cases of invasive pulmonary aspergillosis at the University of Texas M.D. Anderson Cancer Center,[93] logistic regression analysis of clinical characteristics demonstrated that concomitant sinusitis and voriconazole prophylaxis were significantly associated with pulmonary Zygomycosis; CT scan findings of multiple ($\geq$10) nodules and pleural effusion were both independent predictors of pulmonary Zygomycosis, suggesting potential clues in differentiating the two types of infections. Pulmonary mucormycosis can also be confused with standard pulmonary embolism. Gastrointestinal disease must be differentiated from other bowel infections, perforation, and Staphylococcal necrotizing enterocolitis, seen in infants.

Rationale for Use of Hyperbaric Oxygen Therapy

From a physiologic viewpoint, mechanistic steps are only now being discovered to explain the virulence and invasiveness of the filamentous fungi in causing disease. Each of these mechanisms, as discovered, would be well worth testing in the presence of hyperbaric oxygen to assess potential roles for HBOT. Filamentous fungi are aerobic; thus, it is not expected that there would be a direct effect on fungi under clinical hyperbaric conditions.

HBOT in the setting of Zygomycosis could be beneficial in a number of ways. The angio-invasive character of these infections creates areas of hypoxia, ischemia, and subsequent necrosis, which will directly affect neutrophilic killing of organisms, as phagocytosis becomes inefficient. Areas of tissue that are ischemic due to partial loss of perfusion can be made normoxic during hyperbaric therapy and can restore immune mechanisms that have become dysfunctional because of hypoxia.

The neutrophil has a significant role in defending against filamentous fungi, despite the larger size of the hyphae. Engulfment by neutrophils and damage to hyphae is correlated with response to infection. Both mononuclear and polymorphonuclear white cells of normal hosts kill *Rhizopus* by generation of oxidative metabolites and cationic peptide defensins.[94-96] Comparison of antifungal function of human polymorphonuclear leukocytes against hyphae of *Rhizopus oryzae* and *Rhizopus microsporus,* the most frequently isolated Zygomycetes, with that of *Absidia corymbifera* has shown that oxidative burst responses by polymorphonuclear neutrophils and polymorphonuclear leukocyte–induced hyphal damage were significantly lower in response to the *Rhizopus* species than to the *Absidia* species, and that hyphal damage increased when polymorphonuclear leukocytes were incubated with interferon-γ and granulocyte-macrophage colony-stimulating factor.[97] Mouse bronchoalveolar macrophages prevent germination of spores in vitro and in vivo in a murine model, and this ability is blocked by corticosteroid therapy. Correction of hypoxia for such critical cells should enhance oxidative killing of fungi. The significant hallmark of Zygomycoses is their ability to invade blood vessels, causing blood vessel inflammation, thrombosis, and tissue necrosis in many different tissues, and subsequent hematogenous dissemination to other organs. Penetration of endothelial cells lining blood vessels must be a key step in the pathophysiology of Zygomycosis. Studies examining these steps are crucial in defining additional steps to treat infection, by blocking fungal dissemination. It has been demonstrated that *Rhizopus oryzae* spores adhere to subendothelial matrix proteins better than hyphae, but spores and hyphae adhere equivalently to human umbilical vein endothelial cells.[98] Phagocytosis of *Rhizopus oryzae* by endothelial cells was also shown to damage the endothelial cells, raising the question of whether such steps could be related to subsequent thromboses. Hyperbaric oxygen research has not begun to delve into these neutrophil and fungal/endothelial interactions, but research is sorely needed.

Much of the surgery required to manage the necrotizing aspects of infection involving sinuses, orbit, and skull is quite deforming, and the addition of hyperbaric oxygen to wound management would facilitate generation of granulation tissue, epithelialization, and bone healing. In addition, there are other nonspecific mechanisms that are still being worked out for several forms of sepsis, which appear to be positively affected by HBOT.[99,100]

Standard therapy involves the use of antifungal antibiotics and definitive debridement of necrotic tissue. Hyperbaric oxygen clinical studies to date have generally been either isolated case reports or retrospective case series and literature reviews. John and colleagues[101] report such a literature review of 28 published cases that had received HBOT. Among the Mucorales isolates, there were 11 cases of *Rhizopus* species, followed by 3 cases of *Apophysomyces* species, and 2 cases each of *Mucor* and *Absidia*. Three isolates from Entomophthoramycoses were *Conidiobolus* species. Risk factors in these patients were a spectrum of the typically seen range, with 17 of 28 (61%) having diabetes, 10 of whom had ketoacidosis; 5 patients (18%) acquired their infections after trauma; 1 patient was taking systemic steroids; 3 (11%) patients had hematologic malignancies or bone marrow transplants; and 3 (11%) patients had no known risk factors for Zygomycosis. Overall survival rate was 86%, which encompassed a 94% survival rate in patients with diabetes but only a 33% survival rate in patients with hematologic malignancies or bone marrow transplants. All patients except for two had also been administered amphotericin B. Despite the range of cases, all groups were small, and there were no control cases with which to compare the case responses.

In a larger series of all cases of Zygomycosis found in the literature since 1885, 929 cases of Zygomycosis were reported and analyzed by Roden and colleagues.[102] Survival rates were reported by type of treatment received. Forty-four patients were identified as having received HBOT; 64% of these patients survived. Other treatments identified and survival rates were as follows: amphotericin B deoxycholate recipients—324 survivors of 532 patients (61%); amphotericin B lipid formulation—80 survivors of 116 patients (69%); itraconazole, ketoconazole, or posaconazole—10 survivors of 15 patients (67%); no antifungal therapy—59 survivors of 333 patients (18%); surgery alone—51 survivors of 90 patients (57%); surgery plus antifungal therapy—328 survivors of 470 patients (70%); granulocyte colony-stimulating factor—15 survivors of 18 patients (83%); granulocyte transfusion—2 survivors of 7 patients (29%); and no therapy—8 survivors of 241 patients (3%). Major difficulties arise with these data, particularly because these studies usually do not differentiate between intent-to-treat studies and salvage therapy when standard treatment appears to be failing, whether the cases related to use of antibiotics, surgery, or HBOT. This is an observed difficulty in interpreting large numbers of individual case reports and series.[103] The case that Bentur and colleagues[104] reported of mucormycosis of the fourth finger of the hand, in a patient with diabetes with ketoacidosis, is such a case, where HBOT is begun only after other modalities, including amphotericin B, amputation of the affected finger, followed by wide debridement of the hand, and fasciotomy of the forearm have been tried and the disease continues to progress. After receiving 29 hyperbaric treatments, the infection appears improved, and the patient went on to heal her wounds. Similarly, the case of an *Entomophthorales* infection in the medial orbit of an 18-month-old is another example of HBOT used as salvage therapy[105] in conjunction with radical surgery, when the organism was found to be resistant to all available antifungal antibiotics. Thus, any future database of cases of Zygomycoses treated with HBOT should document classification of cases by whether hyperbaric oxygen was used as an early adjunct, at the time of initial institution of therapy, or as "rescue" or "salvage" therapy. In addition, hyperbaric oxygen would normally be considered an adjunct to use of antibiotics and indicated surgery, and such subgroup analysis was not done in Roden and colleagues' report.[102] It is unfair to compare

the results if HBOT were started at the time of diagnosis, as opposed to later on, when an initial course of antibiotics and surgical debridement has been determined to have failed, and infection is progressing and considered to be refractory, and then to start HBOT as a salvage step. A strong argument for controlling for such variables in different studies is well advised because when one uses a salvage intervention, such as a new antibiotic, in the way that hyperbaric oxygen is sometimes used, the question of how much of the effect is attributable to the commencement of therapy and how much is attributable to the natural history of partially treated disease can rarely be separated out.[106] In the setting of a rare, relatively unusual infection, it is a given that randomized studies would be unrealistic, and these authors recommend that carefully selected, matched, contemporaneous control subjects are likely to be the most useful alternative. Although these comments were made in reference to use of newer antifungal antibiotics, the same observations would apply to the analysis of HBOT.

Treatment

Antibiotic treatment should be commenced with an amphotericin B preparation. The fungus is relatively refractory to standard medical therapy; thus, maximally tolerated doses of amphotericin B deoxycholate should be used, usually 1.0 to 1.5 mg/kg per day. Lipid complex forms of amphotericin B doses are better tolerated, and doses are higher. The dose of amphotericin B lipid complex (Abelcet) and liposomal amphotericin B (AmBisome) is 5 mg/kg per day. It has been observed that the use of voriconazole as fungal prophylaxis in the hematopoietic stem call transplant population is a risk factor for development of Zygomycosis[107] and should be avoided. Other currently available azoles, such as ketoconazole, itraconazole, fluconazole, or miconazole, are not efficacious either. Posaconazole, a newer extended spectrum oral azole, has demonstrated in vitro and in vivo activity against Zygomycetes and has been used as salvage therapy for 24 patients with Zygomycetes infections who were intolerant of, or whose infections were resistant to, standard antifungal therapy.[108] Surgical debridement should be considered, based on area of involvement, and sequential debridements may be necessary to control spread. Frozen-section guided debridement has been advocated to assure adequate margins.[109] Reconstructive surgery may also be necessary once the infection has been cleared. Intense management of the underlying predisposing cause of infection is also a marker for successful therapy. In patients with diabetes with reversible acidosis, recovery rates are greater than in those patients with underlying malignancy and immunosuppression. Immunosuppressive drugs should be reduced in dosage or discontinued if possible during attempts to control the infection.

HBOT should be considered as adjunctive therapy and does not replace adequate antifungal therapy. There are no clinical data that might suggest a specific treatment pressure to use in the setting of Zygomycosis infection. It would be appropriate to commence HBOT early in the course, rather than as salvage therapy, in the 2.4 to 3.0 ATA range of pressures, twice a day during the acute phase of the illness, to enhance the immune response to the fungal hyphae and protect borderline ischemic areas from progression of ischemia to necrosis. Many of the successful cases have been treated with up to 30 treatments, although there are no controlled studies that would suggest a specific treatment course or pressure. Because of the rarity of the infection, it is unlikely that a prospective, controlled trial could ever be done at a single institution; thus, adequate data would likely require multicenter studies, controlling for intent-to-treat versus salvage therapy timing of hyperbaric therapy, depth and duration of treatments, as well as extent of infection at time of diagnosis, number of debridements necessary, and category of pre-disposing factor, together with other standard parameters.

REFERENCES

1. Bakker DJ: Clostridial myonecrosis. In: Davis JC, Hunt TK (eds): Problem Wounds: The Role of Oxygen. New York, Elsevier Science Publishing, 1988, pp 153-172.
2. Smith LDS, Williams BL: The Pathogenic Anaerobic Bacteria, 3rd ed. Springfield, IL, Charles C. Thomas Publishers, 1984, pp 101-114.
3. Chi CH, Chen KW, Huang JJ, et al: Gas composition in Clostridium septicum gas gangrene. J Formosa Med Assoc 94:757-759, 1995.
4. Brown PW, Kinman PR: Gas gangrene in a metropolitan community. J Bone Joint Surg 56A:1445-1451, 1974.
5. Bellamy RF, Zajtchuk R: The management of ballistic wounds of soft tissue. In: Zajtchuk R, Jenkins DP, Bellamy RF, Quick CM (eds): Textbook of Military Medicine, Part I: Warfare, Weaponry and the Casualty: Conventional Warfare-Ballistic, Blast and Burn Injuries. Washington, DC, Office of the Surgeon General, Department of the Army, United States of America, 1991, pp 163-220.
6. Davies DM: Gas gangrene as a complication of burns. Scand J Plastic Reconstruct Surg 13:73-75, 1979.
7. Decker WH, Hall WH: Treatment of abortions infected with Clostridium welchii. Am J Obstet Gynecol 95:394-399, 1966.
8. Browne JT, Van Derhor AH, McConnell TS, Wiggins JW: Clostridium perfringens myometritis complicating Cesarean section: Report of 2 cases. Obstet Gynecol 28:64-69, 1966.
9. Lorber B: Gas gangrene and other Clostridium-associated diseases. In: Mandell GL, Bennett JE, Dolin R (eds): Mandell, Douglas and Bennett's Principles and Practice of Infectious Diseases, 6th ed. Philadelphia, Elsevier/Churchill Livingston, 2005, pp 2828-2838.
10. Stevens DL, Bryant AE: The role of Clostridial toxins in the pathogenesis of gas gangrene. Clin Infect Dis 35(suppl 1):S93-S100, 2002.
11. Awad MM, Bryant AE, Stevens DL, Rood JI: Virulence studies on chromosomal alpha-toxin and theta-toxin mutants constructed by allelic exchange provide genetic evidence for the essential role of alpha-toxin in Clostridium perfringens-mediated gas-gangrene. Mol Microbiol 15:191-202, 1995.
12. Titball RW, Rubidge T: The role of histidine residues in the alpha toxin of Clostridium perfringens. FEMS Microbiol Lett 56:261-265, 1990.
13. Titball RW: Gas gangrene: An open and shut case. Microbiology 151:2821-2828, 2005.
14. Gustafson C, Tagesson C: Phopholipase-C from Clostridium perfringens stimulates phopholipase-A2-mediated arachidonic acid release in cultured intestinal epithelial cells. Scand J Gastroenterol 25:363-371, 1990.
15. Bryant AE, Chen RY, Nagata Y, et al: Clostridial gas gangrene. II. Phospholipase C-induced activation of platelet gpIIbIIIa mediates vascular occlusion and myonecrosis in Clostridium perfringens gas gangrene. J Infect Dis 182:808-815, 2000.
16. Bryant AE, Chen RY, Nagata Y, et al: Clostridial gas gangrene. I. Cellular and molecular mechanisms of

microvascular dysfunction induced by exotoxins of *Clostridium perfringens.* J Infect Dis 182:799-807, 2000.

17. Titball RW: Gas gangrene: An open and shut case. Microbiology 151:2822, 2005.

18. McNee JW, Dunn JS: The method of spread of gas gangrene into living muscle. Br Med J 1:727-729, 1917.

19. Bryant AE, Bayer CR, Aldape MJ, et al: *Clostridium perfringens* phospholipase C-induced platelet/leukocyte interactions impede neutrophil diapedesis. J Med Microbiol 55:495-504, 2006.

20. Bunting M, Lorant DE, Bryant AE, et al: Alpha toxin from *Clostridium perfringens* induces proinflammatory changes in endothelial cells. J Clin Invest 100:565-574, 1997.

21. Thom SR: Functional inhibition of neutrophil β2 integrins by hyperbaric oxygen in carbon monoxide mediated brain injury. Toxicol Appl Pharmacol 123:248-256, 1993.

22. Martin JD, Thom SR: Vascular leukocyte sequestration in decompression sickness and prophylactic hyperbaric oxygen therapy in rats. Aviat Space Environ Med 73:565-569, 2002.

23. Thom SR, Mendiguren I, Hardy KR, et al: Inhibition of human neutrophil β2 integrin-dependent adherence by hyperbaric oxygen. Am J Physiol 272:C770-C777, 1997.

24. Stevens DL, Troyer BE, Merrick DT, et al: Lethal effects and cardiovascular effects of purified α- and θ-toxins from *Clostridium perfringens.* J Infect Dis 157:272-279, 1988.

25. Naylor CE, Eaton JT, Howells A, et al: Structure of the key toxin in gas gangrene. Nat Struct Biol 5:738-746, 1998.

26. Weinstein L, Barza MA: Gas gangrene. N Engl J Med 289:1129-1131, 1973.

27. Stevens DL, Musher DM, Watson DA, et al: Spontaneous, nontraumatic gangrene due to Clostridium septicum. Rev Infect Dis 12:286-296, 1990.

28. Dean HM, Decker CL, Baker LD: Temporary survival in Clostridial hemolysis with absence of circulating red cells. N Engl J Med 277:700-701, 1967.

29. Powers AT, Jacoby I, Lynch FP, et al: Adjunctive use of HBO for Clostridial myonecrosis in the newborn. Underwater and Hyperbaric Physiology IX: Proceedings of the 9th International Symposium on Underwater and Hyperbaric Physiology. Kobe, Japan September 1986. Bethesda, MD, Undersea and Hyperbaric Medical Society, 1987, pp 1087-1092.

30. Stevens DL, Maier KA, Mitten JE: Effect of antibiotics on toxin production and viability of *Clostridium perfringens.* Antimicrob Agents Chemother 31:213-218, 1987.

31. Bakker DJ: Clostridial myonecrosis. In: Davis JC, Hunt TK (eds): Problem Wounds: The Role of Oxygen. New York: Elsevier Science Publishing, 1988, pp 168-170.

32. Brummelkamp WH, Hogendijk J, Boerema I: Treatment of anaerobic infections (Clostridial myonecrosis) by drenching the tissues with oxygen under high atmospheric pressure. Surgery 49:299-302, 1961.

33. Van Unnik AJM: Inhibition of toxin production in *Clostridium perfringens* in vitro by hyperbaric oxygen. Antonie van Leeuwenhoek 31:181-186, 1965.

34. Kaye D: Effect of hyperbaric oxygen on Clostridia in vitro and in vivo. Proc Soc Exp Biol Med 124:360-366, 1967.

35. Demello FJ, Hashimoto T, Hitchcock CR, Haglin JJ: The effect of hyperbaric oxygen on the germination and toxin production of *Clostridium perfringens* spores. In: Wada J, Iwa JT (eds): Proceedings of the 4th International Congress on Hyperbaric Medicine. Baltimore, Williams & Wilkins, 1970, p 270.

36. Demello FJ, Haglin JJ, Hitchcock CR: Comparative study of experimental *Clostridium perfringens* infection in dogs treated with antibiotics, surgery, and hyperbaric oxygen. Surgery 73:936-941, 1973.

37. Kelley HG, Pace WG: Treatment of anaerobic infections in mice with hyperpressure oxygen. Surg Forum 14:46-47, 1963.

38. Klopper PJ: Hyperbaric oxygen treatment after ligation of the hepatic artery in rabbits. In: Boerema I, Brummelkamp WII, Meijne NG (eds): Clinical Application of Hyperbaric Oxygen. Amsterdam, Elsevier, 1964, pp 31-35.

39. Hill GB, Osterhout S: Experimental effects of hyperbaric oxygen on selected clostridial species I. in vitro and II. In vivo studies in mice. J Infect Dis 125:17-35, 1972.

40. Muhvich KH, Anderson LH, Mehm WJ: Evaluation of antimicrobials combined with hyperbaric oxygen in a mouse model of clostridial myonecrosis. J Trauma 36:7-10, 1994.

41. Unsworth IP, Sharp PA: Gas gangrene: An 11-year review of 73 cases managed with hyperbaric oxygen. Med J Austr 140:256-260, 1984.

42. Rudge FW: The role of hyperbaric oxygenation in the treatment of clostridial myonecrosis. Mil Med 158:80-83, 1993.

43. Desola J, Escolé E, Moreno E, et al: Combined treatment of gaseous gangrene with hyperbaric oxygen therapy, surgery and antibiotics. A national cooperative multicenter study. Med Clin (Barcelona) 94:641-650, 1990.

44. Korhonen K, Klossner J, Hirn M, Niinikowski J: Management of clostridial gas gangrene and the role of hyperbaric oxygen. Ann Chir Gynaecol 88:139-142, 1999.

45. Altemeier WA, Fullen WD: Prevention and treatment of gas gangrene. JAMA 217:806-813, 1971.

46. Heimbach RD, Boerema I, Brummelkamp WH, Wolfe WG: Current therapy of gas gangrene. In: Davis JC, Hunt TK (eds): Hyperbaric Oxygen Therapy. Bethesda, MD, Undersea Medical Society, 1977, pp 153-165.

47. Bakker DJ: Clostridial myonecrosis. In: Feldmeier J (ed): Hyperbaric Oxygen 2003. Indications and Results— The Hyperbaric Oxygen Therapy Committee Report. Kensington, MD, Undersea and Hyperbaric Medical Society, 2003, pp 19-25.

48. Peirce EC: Gas gangrene: Review and update. Surg Rounds 7:17-25, 1984.

49. Meleney FL: Hemolytic streptococcus gangrene. Arch Surg 9:317-364, 1924.

50. Wilson B: Necrotizing fasciitis. Am Surg 18:426-431, 1952.

51. Miller LG, Perdreau-Remington F, Rieg G, et al: Necrotizing fasciitis caused by community-associated methicillin-resistant *Staphylococcus aureus* in Los Angeles. N Engl J Med 352:1445-1453, 2005.

52. Brogan TV, Nizet V, Waldhausen JHT, et al: Group A streptococcal necrotizing fasciitis complicating primary varicella: A series of fourteen patients. Pediatr Infect Dis J 14:588-594, 1995.

53. Rimailho A, Riou B, Richard C, Auzepy P: Fulminant necrotizing fasciitis and nonsteroidal anti-inflammatory drugs. J Infect Dis 155:143-146, 1987.

54. Zerr DM, Alexander ER, Duchin JS, et al: A case-control study of necrotizing fasciitis during primary varicella. Pediatrics 103:783-790, 1999.

55. Bell AL, Adamson H, Kirk F, et al: Diclofenac inhibits monocyte superoxide production ex vivo in rheumatoid arthritis. Rheumatol Int 11:27-30, 1991.

56. Sawin RS, Schaller RT, Tapper D, et al: Early recognition of neonatal abdominal wall necrotizing fasciitis. Am J Surg 167:481-484, 1994.

57. Wang T-L, Hung C-R: Role of tissue oxygen saturation monitoring in diagnosing necrotizing fasciitis of the lower limbs. Ann Emerg Med 44:222-228, 2004.

58. Lally KP, Atkinson JB, Wooley MM, Mahour GH: Necrotizing fasciitis: A serious sequela of omphalitis in the newborn. Ann Surg 199:101-103, 1984.

59. Sawin RS, Schaller RT, Tapper D, et al: Early recognition of neonatal abdominal wall necrotizing fasciitis. Am J Surg 167:481-484, 1994.

60. Stamenkovic I, Lew PD: Early recognition of potentially fatal necrotizing fasciitis: The use of frozen-section biopsy. N Engl J Med 310:1689-1693, 1984.

61. Wysoki MG, Santora TA, Shah RM, Friedman AC: Necrotizing fasciitis: CT characteristics. Radiology 203:859-863, 1997.

62. Schmid MR, Kossman T, Duewell S: Differentiation of necrotizing fasciitis and cellulitis using MR imaging. Am J Roentgenol 170:615-620, 1998.

63. Gozal D, Ziser A, Shupak A, et al: Necrotizing fasciitis. Arch Surg 121:233-235, 1986.

64. Riseman JA, Zamboni WA, Curtis A, et al: Hyperbaric oxygen therapy for necrotizing fasciitis reduces mortality and the need for debridements. Surgery 108:847-850, 1990.

65. Mandell G: Bactericidal activity of aerobic and anaerobic polymorphonuclear neutrophils. Infect Immun 9:337-341, 1974.

66. Wilkinson D, Doolette D: Hyperbaric oxygen treatment and survival from necrotizing soft tissue infection. Arch Surg 139:1339-1345, 2004.

67. Escobar SJ, Slade JB, Hunt TK, Cianci P: Adjuvant hyperbaric oxygen therapy (HBO2) for treatment of necrotizing fasciitis reduces mortality and amputation rate. Undersea Hyperb Med 32:437-443, 2006.

68. Brown DR, Davis NL, Lepawsky M, et al: A multicenter review of the treatment of major truncal necrotizing infections with and without hyperbaric oxygen therapy. Am J Surg 167:485-489, 1994.

69. Monestersky JH, Myers RAM: Hyperbaric oxygen treatment of necrotizing fasciitis [letter]. Am J Surg 169:187-188, 1995.

70. Hollabaugh RS, Dmochowski RR, Hickerson WL: Fournier's gangrene: Therapeutic impact of hyperbaric oxygen. Plast Reconstr Surg 101:94-100, 1998.

71. Pizzorno R, Bonini F, Donelli A, et al: Hyperbaric oxygen therapy in the treatment of Fournier's disease in 11 male patients. J Urol 158:837-840, 1997.

72. Korhonen K, Him M, Niinikoski J: Hyperbaric oxygen in the treatment of Fournier's gangrene. Eur J Surg 164:251-255, 1998.

73. Laor E, Palmer LS, Tolia BM: Outcome prediction in patients with Fournier's gangrene. J Urol 154:89-92, 1995.

74. Dahm P, Roland FH, Vaslef SN, et al: Outcome analysis in patients with primary necrotizing fasciitis of the male genitalia. Urology 56:31-36, 2000.

75. Lepawsky M: Necrotizing soft tissue infections. In: Feldmeier JJ (Chair and Ed.): Hyperbaric Oxygen 2003. Indications and Results—The Hyperbaric Oxygen Therapy Committee Report. Kensington, MD, Undersea and Hyperbaric Medical Society, 2003, pp 69-78.

76. Stone HH, Martin JD: Synergistic necrotizing cellulitis. Ann Surg 175:702-711, 1972.

77. Bessman AN, Wagner W: Nonclostridial gas gangrene. JAMA 233:958, 1975.

78. Cullen TS: A progressively enlarging ulcer of abdominal wall involving the skin and fat, following drainage of an abdominal abscess, apparently of appendiceal origin. Surg Gynecol Obstet 38:579-582, 1924.

79. Ledingham IM, Tehrani MA: Diagnosis, clinical course and treatment of acute dermal gangrene. Br J Surg 62:364-372, 1975.

80. Chayakulkeeree M, Ghannoum MA, Perfect JR: Zygomycosis: The re-emerging fungal infection. Eur J Clin Microbiol Infect Dis 25:215-229, 2006.

81. McNulty JS: Rhinocerebral mucormycosis: Predisposing factors. Laryngoscope 92:1140-1143, 1982.

82. Bagdade JD, Root RK, Bulger RJ: Impaired leukocyte function in patients with poorly controlled diabetes. Diabetes 23:9-15, 1974.

83. Nielson CP, Hindson DA: Inhibition of polymorphonuclear leukocyte respiratory burst by elevated glucose concentration. Diabetes 38:1031-1035, 1989.

84. Alexiewicz JM, Kumar D, Smogorzewski M, et al: Polymorphonuclear leukocytes in non-insulin dependent diabetes mellitus: Abnormalities in metabolism and function. Ann Intern Med 123:919-924, 1995.

85. Artis WM, Fountain JA, Delcher HK, Jones HE: A mechanism of susceptibility to mucormycosis in diabetic ketoacidosis: Transferrin and iron availability. Diabetes 31:1109-1114, 1982.

86. Windus DW, Stokes TJ, Julian BA, Fenves AZ: Fatal Rhizopus infections in hemodialysis patients receiving deferoxamine. Ann Intern Med 107:678-680, 1987.

87. Boelaert JR, Van Roost GF, Vergauwe PL, et al: The role of deferoxamine in dialysis-associated mucormycosis: Report of three cases and review of the literature. Clin Nephrol 29:261-266, 1988.

88. Cocanour CS, Miller-Crouchett P, Reed RL, et al: Mucormycosis in trauma patients. J Trauma 32:12-15, 1992.

89. Tedder MJ, Spratt JA, Anstadt MP, et al: Pulmonary mucormycosis: Results of medical and surgical therapy. Ann Thorac Surg 57:1044-1050, 1994.

90. Ribes JA, Vanover-Sams CL, Baker DJ: Zygomycetes in human disease. Clin Microbiol Revs 13:236-301, 2000.

91. Murray HW: Pulmonary mucormycosis with massive fatal hemoptysis. Chest 68:65-68, 1975.

92. Michalak DM, Cooney DR, Rhodes KH, et al: Gastrointestinal mucormycosis in infants and children: A cause of gangrenous intestinal cellulitis and perforation. J Pediatr Surg 15:320-324, 1980.

93. Chamilos G, Marom EM, Lewis RE, et al: Predictors of pulmonary zygomycosis versus invasive pulmonary aspergillosis in patients with cancer. Clin Infect Dis 41:60–66, 2005

94. Diamond RD, Haudenschild CC, Erickson III NF: Monocyte-mediated damage to Rhizopus oryzae hyphae in vitro. Infect Immun 38:292–297, 1982.

95. Waldorf AR: Pulmonary defense mechanisms against opportunistic fungal pathogens. Immunol Ser 47:243–271, 1989.

96. Waldorf AR, Ruderman N, Diamond RD: Specific susceptibility to mucormycosis in murine diabetes and bronchoalveolar macrophage defense against Rhizopus. J Clin Invest 74:150–160, 1984.

97. Gil-Lamaignere C, Simitsopoulou M, Rollides E, et al: Interferon-γ and granulocyte-macrophage colony-stimulating factor augment the activity of polymorphonuclear leukocytes against medically important zygomycetes. J Infect Dis 191:1180–1187, 2005.

98. Ibrahim AS, Spellberg B, Avanessian V, et al: Rhizopus oryzae adheres to, is phagocytosed by, and damages endothelial cells in vitro. Infect Immun 73:778–783, 2005.

99. Imperatore F, Cuzzocrea S, De Lucia D, et al: Hyperbaric oxygen therapy prevents coagulation disorders in an experimental model of multiple organ failure syndrome. Intensive Care Med 32:1881–1888, 2006.

100. Buras JA, Holt D, Orlow D, et al: Hyperbaric oxygen protects from sepsis mortality via an interleukin-10-dependent mechanism. Crit Care Med 34:2624–2629, 2006.

101. John BV, Camilos G, Kontoyiannis DP: Hyperbaric oxygen as an adjunctive treatment for Zygomycosis. Clin Microbiol Infect 11:515–517, 2005.

102. Roden MM, Zaoutis TE, Buchanan WL, et al: Epidemiology and outcome of Zygomycosis: A review of 929 reported cases. Clin Infect Dis 41:634–653, 2005.

103. Almyroudis NG, Konoyiannis DP, Sepkowitz KA, et al: Issues related to the design and interpretation of clinical trials of salvage therapy for invasive mold infection. Clin Infect Dis 43:1449–1455, 2006.

104. Bentur Y, Shupak A, Ramon Y, et al: Hyperbaric oxygen therapy for cutaneous/soft-tissue Zygomycosis complicating diabetes mellitus. Plast Reconstr Surg 102:822–824, 1998.

105. Temple ME, Brady MT, Koranyi KI, Nahata MC: Periorbital cellulitis secondary to Conidiobolus incongruous. Pharmacotherapy 21:351–354, 2001.

106. Powers JH: Salvage therapy trials in fungal disease: Challenges and opportunities. Clin Infect Dis 43: 1456–1459, 2006.

107. Trifilio SM, Bennett CL, Yarnold PR, et al: Breakthrough Zygomycosis after voriconazole administration among patients with hematologic malignancies who receive hematopoietic stem-cell transplants or intensive chemotherapy. Bone Marrow Transplant 39:425–429, 2007.

108. Greenberg RN, Mullane K, van Burick J-AH, et al: Posaconazole as salvage therapy for Zygomycosis. Antimicrob Agents Chemother 50:126–133, 2006.

109. Langford JD, McCartney DL, Wang RC: Frozen section-guided surgical debridement for management of rhino-orbital mucormycosis. Am J Ophthalmol 124:265–267, 1997.

Hyperbaric Oxygen Therapy in Chronic Osteomyelitis

Juha Niinikoski, MD, PhD

CHAPTER OUTLINE

Hyperbaric oxygen therapy (HBOT) has been used for chronic refractory osteomyelitis as an adjunctive therapy by many groups.[1-9] Treatment for osteomyelitis includes radical surgical debridement, locally applied antibiotic beads, and systemic antibiotic therapy.[2,5,7,8] Bone grafts can be used to fill bone defects after debridement. The term *refractory osteomyelitis* is applied to bone infections that fail to respond despite adequate surgical and antibiotic therapy. Classically, the treatment of chronic refractory osteomyelitis requires an experienced orthopedic surgeon and an infectious diseases specialist. The surgeon debrides the infected area by removing any dead, ischemic, or otherwise devitalized tissues. Quite frequently, a plastic or reconstructive surgeon is needed to cover tissue defects and debrided tissues by means of microvascular soft-tissue flaps. Bacterial cultures of the infected bone should be obtained during the surgical interventions. Culture results help in the selection of the appropriate antibiotic coverage against the pathogenic organisms involved.[10,11]

Adjunctive HBOT can play an integral role in the management of refractory osteomyelitis. The Cierny–Mader classification system (Table 19.1) is currently widely used as a guide to determine candidates for adjunctive HBOT.[5,10,11] In this system, osteomyelitis is classified in four stages: stage 1 (medullary), stage 2 (superficial), stage 3 (localized), and stage 4 (diffuse). The patient's host status is also included in this classification. Patients are classified as follows: normal host (A), compromised host (B), or treatment is worse than the disease (C). Appropriate candidates for HBOT fall in classes 3B and 4B. Patients who benefit

Table 19.1 Cierny–Mader Staging System

ANATOMIC TYPE

Stage 1—Medullary osteomyelitis
Stage 2—Superficial osteomyelitis
Stage 3—Localized osteomyelitis
Stage 4—Diffuse osteomyelitis

Physiologic Class

A Host—Normal host
B Host—Systemic compromise (Bs)
        Local compromise (Bl)
        Systemic and local compromise (Bls)
C Host—Treatment worse than the disease

SYSTEMIC OR LOCAL FACTORS THAT AFFECT IMMUNE SURVEILLANCE, METABOLISM, AND LOCAL VASCULARITY

Systemic (Bs)	Local (Bl)
Diabetes mellitus	Major vessel compromise
Renal, hepatic failure	Small- and medium-vessel disease
Malnutrition	Extensive scarring
Chronic hypoxia	Arteritis
Immunosuppression or immune deficiency	Radiation fibrosis
Malignancy	Chronic lymphedema
Immune disease	Venous stasis
Extremes of age	Neuropathy
	Tobacco abuse (2 packs/day)

From Mader J, Shirtliff M, Calhoun J: The use of hyperbaric oxygen in the treatment of osteomyelitis. In: Kindwall EP, Whelan HT (eds): Hyperbaric Medicine Practice, 2nd ed. rev. Flagstaff, Ariz, Best Publishing Company, 1999, pp 603–616, by permission.

from adjunctive HBOT include those who have preexisting conditions, such as diabetes mellitus, peripheral vascular disease, or extensive soft-tissue scarring that prevents adequate wound coverage. Patients who are immunocompromised or malnourished may also gain benefit from HBOT. Some evidence suggests the outcome of patients with inadequate debridement, poor vascularity, or poor soft-tissue reconstruction may be improved with the use of adjunctive HBOT[10] or in those instances where the patient refuses additional surgery.

EXPERIMENTAL STUDIES

Bone Oxygen Tension

After early clinical studies showed some benefit from HBOT in severe cases of osteomyelitis,[1] several controlled animal studies have confirmed and extended the perceived clinical effect. Niinikoski and Hunt[12] measured bone oxygen tensions in experimental *Staphylococcus aureus* osteomyelitis in rabbits by using implanted Silastic tube tonometers. The oxygen tensions in the medullary canal of the infected tibias were 10 to 20 mm Hg and markedly lower than those in the control tibias (30–45 mm Hg), which suggests that the healing of the osteomyelitic processes was retarded, at least partly, by an extremely unfavorable oxygen environment. The oxygen supply of infected bones could be increased to reference range by systemic hyperoxia during breathing of pure oxygen at 1 atmosphere pressure (ATA). Later studies demonstrated that the decreased oxygen tension typically associated with bone infections could be increased to reference or supranormal levels by using HBOT. Esterhai and colleagues[13] showed that, under atmospheric conditions, the oxygen tension in osteomyelitic tibias reached only 17 mm Hg, whereas in normal bone on the contralateral side, the oxygen tension was 32 mm Hg. During breathing of normobaric oxygen, readings were about 100 mm Hg for normal bone but only 18 mm Hg for infected bone. Using HBOT at 2 ATA pressure, both infected and uninfected bone reached partial pressure of oxygen (Po_2) values of almost 200 mm Hg. In Mader and coworkers' studies,[14,15] a standard rabbit model with diffuse *S. aureus* osteomyelitis of the tibia was used. The animals were treated at 2 ATA oxygen pressure. Oxygen tensions were measured using a mass spectrometer in normal and infected tibias before and during HBOT. Hyperbaric oxygenation increased the oxygen tensions in both the normal and osteomyelitic bone. Under ambient conditions, the oxygen tension in osteomyelitic bone was 23 mm Hg, whereas in normal bone the oxygen tension was 45 mm Hg. HBOT increased the oxygen tension to 104 mm Hg in osteomyelitic bone and to 322 mm Hg in normal bone. The low oxygen tensions in infected bones are probably secondary to hypoperfusion and inflammation. Hypoperfusion is a direct effect of increased intramedullary pressure in the bone. Increased pressure results when pus and other debris fill the Haversian system and medullary canal.[10]

Oxygen and Microbicidal Mechanisms

Oxygen is essential to cellular defense mechanisms in the body because oxygen radicals derived from molecular oxygen are important agents in bacterial killing. Polymorphonuclear leukocytes contain NADP-linked oxygenase that is activated during phagocytosis. This enzyme is the first step in a cycle in which various oxidants are produced from ambient oxygen. After activation, a "respiratory" or "oxidative burst" follows during which molecular oxygen is reduced in large quantities to superoxide radicals. These radicals are then sequestered in the phagosomes, where they and other oxidants derived from them kill

bacteria by oxidizing cell membranes.[16] In polymorphonuclear leukocytes, the phagocytic killing of aerobes is decreased under low oxygen tensions[17] (see Chapter 11). Using an *S. aureus* model, Mader and coworkers[15] showed a proportional relation between the oxygen tensions and the phagocytic killing ability. At the tension found in osteomyelitic bone, 23 mm Hg oxygen, there was a reduced capacity of phagocytes to kill bacteria, as compared with their bactericidal ability at normal bone oxygen tensions of 45 mm Hg. Increasing the oxygen tension to 109 mm Hg, the tension found in osteomyelitic bone under HBOT conditions, further augmented the ability of the phagocytes to kill bacteria. It was also shown that increasing the oxygen tension to 150 and 760 mm Hg generated killing of the greatest number of *S. aureus* bacteria. These findings were confirmed by other studies and extended to bacteria such as *Escherichia coli*, Proteus species, and *Pseudomonas aeruginosa*.[18-20] In summary, HBOT has been shown to be effective as adjunctive therapy in several animal models of chronic osteitis.[14,15,21]

Oxygen and Bone Repair

The discovery that oxygen is an essential nutritional ingredient of healing has stressed the importance of adequate oxygen supply. Fibroblasts cannot synthesize collagen or migrate to the injured area when oxygen tensions are less than 20 mm Hg. Conversely, increasing tissue oxygen tensions to levels greater than 100 mm Hg allows a return to normal function.[16,22] The fibroblasts are then able to produce collagen that forms a protective matrix for tissue repair. After their differentiation from fibroblast-like mesenchymal cells, osteoblasts lay down a layer of immature, coarse fibrillar bone. This immature bone tissue is then replaced by mature lamellar bone that is functionally reconstructed by resorption and deposition by osteoclasts and osteoblasts. Basset and Herrmann[23] showed that variations in the oxygen supply in vitro can alter the type of tissue that differentiates in a culture of multipotent mesenchymal cells. Hyperoxia caused a differentiation to osseous tissue, whereas hypoxia resulted in cartilage formation. Makley and his associates[24] found that fracture healing in air at 0.5 atmosphere of pressure was markedly reduced in unacclimatized animals. Studies by Penttinen and his associates[25] report that acute tissue hypoxia retards the regeneration of bone by reducing both the synthesis of the collagenous matrix and mineralization. HBOT has been found to stimulate the healing of fractures. Coulson and his colleagues[26] observed that fractured femurs of rats treated for 2 hours once daily under 3 ATA oxygen had a greater uptake of radioactive calcium and a higher breaking strength than the control fractures in rats kept at atmospheric pressure. Yablon and Cruess[27] demonstrated by autoradiography with tritiated thymidine that all phases of fracture repair were accelerated under the influence of HBOT. In contrast, when the daily duration of hyperbaric treatment was extended from 4 to 6 hours/day at 2 ATA of oxygen, breaking strength was reduced, as Wray and Rogers[28] described. The influence of intermittent hyperbaric oxygenation on the chemical composition of the callous tissue in the healing fractured tibias of rats was reported by Penttinen and coworkers.[29] Exposure of rats to pure oxygen at 2.5 ATA for 2-hour periods twice daily resulted in increased formation of callous tissue; enhanced accumulation of calcium, magnesium, phosphorus, sodium, potassium, and zinc; and accelerated formation of collagen and other proteins in the fracture calluses as compared with control rats at atmospheric pressure. However, the mechanical strength of healing fractures in the HBOT group showed no difference from the control rats. Barth and colleagues[30] also demonstrated the beneficial effects of HBOT on bone healing by showing that the metaphyseal defects in the cortices of rat femurs were healed by primary ossification when rats were treated with once-daily hyperbaric oxygen treatments for 90 minutes at 2 ATA. This group of rats also appeared to have accelerated bone repair and vessel ingrowth compared with control rats. When the HBOT was given twice daily, the defects healed through enchondral ossification;

the bone repair and vessel ingrowth were retarded, and the osteoclastic activity was upregulated. Thus, it appears that the end result of sustained hyperoxygenation is a development of repair process that is rich in collagen but structurally weak.[10,22] Therefore, based on animal models, maximal bone healing may be achieved when HBOT is provided within the optimal range: once-daily treatments for 90 to 120 minutes at 2 to 3 ATA.[10,11]

Oxygen and Antibiotics

Aminoglycosides have been used in the treatment of gram-negative aerobic infections.[10] This class of antibiotics includes gentamicin, tobramycin, amikacin, and netilmicin. However, like other antibiotics, a therapeutic limitation is their inability to penetrate into necrotic or devitalized tissues, as well as their diminished activity under low oxygen tensions.[31,32] An hypoxic environment also unfavorably affects the activity of other antibiotics such as vancomycin, quinolones, trimethoprim/sulfamethoxazole, and nitrofurantoin.[33] Mader and his coworkers[15,34] have shown that with HBOT the bactericidal activity of the aminoglycosides is enhanced. The bactericidal activity of tobramycin was improved against *Pseudomonas aeruginosa* when oxygen tensions were increased above hypoxic levels. Comparing tobramycin alone, HBOT alone, and the two combined, it was shown that adjunctive HBOT enhanced eradication of the *Pseudomonas aeruginosa* from osteomyelitic bone.[34] Trimethoprim/sulfamethoxazole and nitrofurantoin also show augmented antibacterial activity in elevated oxygen environments.[33] Mendel and coworkers[35] used a standard rat model of *S. aureus*–induced osteomyelitis to compare the effects of HBOT, a local antibiotic carrier (gentamicin-containing collagen sponge), and the combination of HBOT with a local antibiotic carrier. For the induction of osteomyelitis, a defined *S. aureus* suspension was inoculated into the medullary cavity. Arachidonic acid was used as a sclerosing agent. With that procedure an infection rate of more than 95% was attained. Each of the treatment modalities resulted in a significant therapeutic effect with a reduction in organisms of tibial bone. The effect was most marked using a 4-week combination therapy with local application of the gentamicin-containing sponge and additional HBOT. In 9 of 11 animals, bacteria were no longer detectable in the processed bone substance.

CLINICAL STUDIES

Although the physiologic and pathophysiologic basis for the use of HBOT in chronic refractory osteomyelitis is well established, the number of clinical variables involved in this chronic infection makes evidence-based clinical investigations difficult or nearly impossible. Individual variations in the extent and location of the infected bone, the status of the surrounding tissue, the microorganisms involved, antibiotic therapy, the presence of coexisting diseases, the timing and form of surgical intervention, and the unpredictable time course of the disease all render the planning and development of randomized, controlled clinical trials impracticable.[10,11]

As early as 1965, Slack and his associates[1] reported clinical improvement in five patients with chronic osteomyelitis when treated with HBOT at 2 ATA. They found that hyperbaric oxygenation could favorably influence the course of persistent sinus tracts in chronic osteomyelitis and noted most lesions would heal, at least temporarily. It could not be determined whether the beneficial effects were achieved by influencing the oxygen tension of the infected area, inhibiting growth of the organisms, potentiating the action of antibiotics, or an interrelation of these factors.

Morrey and his coworkers[3] also studied a group of patients with chronic refractory osteomyelitis. All patients had a persistent infection of at least 1 month in duration, did not respond favorably to at least one surgical debridement, had received at least 2 weeks of parenteral antibiotics, and had been managed for at least 1 year. The patients were then treated with additional surgery, antibiotics, and HBOT, with a success rate of 85%. The cause of the 15% failure rate was attributed to inadequate surgical management. In other series of patients with refractory osteomyelitis treated with adjunctive HBOT, success rates ranged from 60% to 89%.[4,6,36,37]

Chen and associates[38] investigated the clinical results of HBOT for chronic refractory osteomyelitis of the femur. In this retrospective study, 13 patients with chronic refractory osteomyelitis of the femur were treated with adjunctive HBOT. The most common infecting microorganism was *S. aureus*. All cases were classified as stage 3 or 4 osteomyelitis according to the Cierny–Mader classification. Adequate surgical debridement and parenteral antibiotic treatment were conducted. The number of operations before HBOT was 4.6. HBOT at 2.5 ATA for 120 minutes was administered for 5 days per week in all patients for an average of 50 days. The average number of hyperbaric treatments was 32.2. The average follow-up period was 22 months, ranging from 12 to 42 months. Complete eradication of infection with no recurrence of infection was noted in 12 of the 13 patients. One patient did not respond to the treatment; thus, the success rate of the treatment regimen was 92%. The authors conclude that HBOT is an effective and safe adjunctive therapy for the management of chronic refractory osteomyelitis of the femur provided that patients have received adequate surgical debridement and appropriate antibiotic treatment.

In a study by Kemmer and associates,[11] 54 of 79 patients (68%) with chronic osteomyelitis of the extremities and with a follow-up period of more than 24 months (24–60 months) showed sustained resolution of refractory chronic osteomyelitis. Most of these patients had undergone multiple unsuccessful treatments over more than 3 years (some up to 20 years) in other clinics. The dropout rate in patients with chronic osteomyelitis, because of the patient's refusal to have additional surgery or to continue HBOT beyond about 15 treatments, was about 20%.

Davis[37] demonstrated sustained resolution of chronic refractory osteomyelitis in 89% of 38 patients. Aitasalo and coworkers[39] report a similar success rate with osteomyelitis of the mandible.

Esterhai and coworkers[6] conducted a controlled study on 28 patients in which both groups received adequate debridement surgery and antibiotics, and 1 group received adjunctive HBOT. No differences in the results were found between these groups. However, the effects of adjunctive HBOT could not be evaluated because of the problems with patient compliance with regard to surgical management.

To establish the success rate of combined therapy for tibial osteomyelitis, Maynor and coworkers[40] reviewed all cases of this infection treated with surgery antibiotics and HBOT between 1974 and 1991 at Duke University Medical Center. The median delay from diagnosis of osteomyelitis to initiation of HBOT was 12.5 months. Of 34 patients in whom follow-up data were complete, 27 were male and 7 female with a mean age of 27.9 years. Patients received an average of 8.3 surgical procedures and 35 HBOT sessions. Twenty patients received free vascularized muscle flaps as part of therapy. Of 26 patients with 24 months of follow-up after treatment, 21 remained drainage free. At 60 months and 84 months after treatment, 12 of 15 and 5 of 8 patients, respectively, were drainage free. After more than 84 months, patients who had received muscle flaps were more likely to be drainage free than patients who had received only debridement, and this difference approached statistical significance. An overview of clinical articles focusing on HBOT in chronic refractory osteomyelitis is given in Table 19.2.

COST-EFFECTIVENESS

When compared with high costs of prolonged hospitalization, antimicrobial therapy, and additional surgical procedures, HBOT has demonstrated reasonable cost-effectiveness. In 1987, Strauss[41] reported that in most patients with complicated refractory osteomyelitis, an average of $115,000 (US) was spent on each patient for surgery and hospitalization before any HBOT was administered. Once HBOT was used in conjunction with surgery and antimicrobial therapy, the total cost to treat these patients, who did not respond to their previous care, was reduced to $20,000 per patient. This cost-effectiveness can be achieved only if the hyperbaric specialists, surgeons, and infectious-disease consultants agree on a specified protocol.[10] In Europe, the current average cost of treatment in chronic refractory osteomyelitis is estimated to be about 800,000 euros per patient.[11] Therefore, all treatment options warrant critical consideration to treat and control this form of infection.

CONCLUSION

A certain consensus exists between the major hyperbaric medical societies worldwide regarding the use of adjuvant HBOT in chronic refractory osteomyelitis. Considering the difficulties in performing randomized, controlled clinical studies in this disease, and on the basis

Table 19.2 Clinical Articles on Adjunctive Hyperbaric Oxygen Therapy in Chronic Refractory Osteomyelitis

REFERENCES	YEAR	SUCCESS RATE
Slack and colleagues[1]	1965	5/5
Depenbusch and colleagues[36]	1972	35/50
Davis[37]	1977	63/89
Morrey and colleagues[3]	1979	34/40
Davis and colleagues[4]	1986	34/48
Aitasalo and colleagues[39]	1998	26/33
Maynor and colleagues[40]	1998	21/26
Chen and colleagues[38]	2004	12/13
Kemmer and colleagues[11]	2006	54/79

of the evidence obtained from both experimental studies and clinical experience, HBOT can be recommended as an adjuvant therapy in cases with chronic refractory osteomyelitis, when previous therapy including appropriate antibiotics for 6 weeks and at least one surgical intervention has failed. Treatment protocols based on animal models should use HBOT at 2 to 2.5 ATA with treatment times of 90 to 120 minutes on a once-daily basis.

REFERENCES

1. Slack WK, Thomas DA, Perrins DJD: Hyperbaric oxygenation in chronic osteomyelitis. Lancet 1:1093-1094, 1965.
2. Waldvogel FA, Medoff G, Schwartz MN: Osteomyelitis: A review of clinical features, therapeutic considerations and unusual aspects. N Engl J Med 282:198-206, 1970.
3. Morrey BF, Dunn JM, Heimbach RD, et al: Hyperbaric oxygen and chronic osteomyelitis. Clin Orthop 144:121-127, 1979.
4. Davis JC, Heckman JD, DeLee JC, et al: Chronic nonhaematogenous osteomyelitis treated with adjuvant hyperbaric oxygen. J Bone Joint Surg 68A:1210-1217, 1986.
5. Cierny G, Mader JT: Approach to adult osteomyelitis. Orthop Rev 16:259-270, 1987.
6. Esterhai JL Jr, Pisarello J, Brighton CT, et al: Adjunctive HBOT in the treatment of chronic refractory osteomyelitis. J Trauma 27:763-768, 1987.
7. Mader JT, Hicks SA, Calhoun J: Bacterial osteomyelitis. Adjunctive HBOT. Orthop Rev 18:581-585, 1989.
8. Mader JT, Adams KR, Wallace WR, et al: Hyperbaric oxygen as adjunctive therapy for osteomyelitis. Infect Dis Clin North Am 4:433-440, 1990.
9. Calhoun JH, Cobos JA, Mader JT: Does hyperbaric oxygen have a place in the treatment of osteomyelitis? Orthop Clin North Am 22:467-471, 1991.
10. Mader J, Shirtliff M, Calhoun J: The use of hyperbaric oxygen in the treatment of osteomyelitis. In: Kindwall EP, Whelan HT (eds): Hyperbaric Medicine Practice, 2nd ed. rev. Flagstaff, Ariz, Best Publishing Company, 1999, pp 603-616.
11. Kemmer A, Stein T, Hierholzer C: Persistent osteomyelitis. In: Mathieu D (ed): Handbook on Hyperbaric Medicine. Dordrecht, The Netherlands, Springer, 2006, pp 429-449.
12. Niinikoski J, Hunt TK: Oxygen tensions in healing bone. Surg Gynecol Obstet 134:746-750, 1972.
13. Esterhai JL Jr, Clark J, Morton HE, et al: The effect of hyperbaric oxygen on oxygen tension within the medullary canal in the rabbit tibia osteomyelitis model. J Orthop Res 4:330-336, 1986.
14. Mader JT, Guckian JC, Glass DL, et al: Therapy with hyperbaric oxygen of experimental osteomyelitis due to *Staphylococcus aureus* in rabbits. J Infect Dis 138:312-318, 1978.
15. Mader JT, Brown GL, Guckian JC, et al: A mechanism for the amelioration by hyperbaric oxygen of experimental staphylococcal osteomyelitis in rabbits. J Infect Dis 142:915-922, 1980.
16. Niinikoski J: Physiologic effects of hyperbaric oxygen on wound healing processes. In: Mathieu D (ed): Handbook on Hyperbaric Medicine. Dordrecht, The Netherlands, Springer, 2006, pp 135-145.
17. Hohn DC, MacKay RK, Halliday B, et al: The effect of oxygen tension on the microbicidal function of leukocytes in wounds and in vitro. Surg Forum 27:18-20, 1976.
18. McRipley RJ, Sbarra AJ: Role of phagocyte in host-parasite interactions. J Bacteriol 94:1417-1424, 1967.
19. Mandell G: Bactericidal activity of aerobic and anaerobic polymorphonuclear neutrophils. Infect Immun 9:337-341, 1974.
20. Knighton DR, Halliday B, Hunt TK: Oxygen as an antibiotic. A comparison of inspired oxygen concentration and antibiotic administration on in vivo bacterial clearance. Arch Surg 121:191-195, 1986.
21. Hart GB: Refractory osteomyelitis. In: Feldmeier JJ (ed): The HBOT committee report 2003. Kensington, Md, Undersea and Hyperbaric Medical Society, 2003, pp 79-85.
22. Mainous EG: Osteogenesis enhancement utilizing HBOT. HBO Rev 3:181-185, 1982.
23. Basset CAL, Herrmann I: Influence of oxygen concentration and mechanical factors on differentiation of connective tissues in vitro. Nature 190:460-461, 1961.
24. Makley JT, Heiple KG, Chase SW, et al: The effects of reduced barometric pressure on fracture healing in rats. J Bone Joint Surg 49A:903-914, 1967.
25. Penttinen R, Rantanen J, Kulonen E: Fracture healing at reduced atmospheric pressure. A biochemical study with rats. Acta Chir Scand 138:147-151, 1972.
26. Coulson DB, Ferguson AB Jr, Diehl RC Jr: Effect of hyperbaric oxygen on the healing femur of the rat. Surg Forum 17:449-450, 1966.
27. Yablon IG, Cruess RL: Effect of hyperbaric oxygenation on fracture healing in rats. J Trauma 8:186-202, 1968.
28. Wray JB, Rogers LS: Effect of hyperbaric oxygenation upon fracture healing in the rat. J Surg Res 8:373-378, 1968.
29. Penttinen R, Niinikoski J, Kulonen E: Hyperbaric oxygenation and fracture healing. A biochemical study with rats. Acta Chir Scand 138:39-44, 1972.
30. Barth E, Sullivan T, Berg E: Animal model for evaluating bone repair with and without adjunctive HBOT: Comparing dose schedules. J Invest Surg 3:387-392, 1990.
31. Sheffield PJ: Tissue oxygen measurements with respect to soft-tissue wound healing with normobaric and hyperbaric oxygen. HBO Rev 6:18-46, 1985.
32. Cierny G: Classification and treatment of adult osteomyelitis. In: Evarts CM (ed): Surgery of the Musculoskeletal System. New York, Churchill Livingstone, 1990, pp 4337-4379.
33. Park MK, Myers RAM, Marzella L: Oxygen tensions and infections: Modulation of microbial growth, activity of antibiotics, and immunologic responses. Clin Infect Dis 14:720-740, 1992.
34. Mader JT, Adams KR, Couch LA, et al: Potentiation of tobramycin by hyperbaric oxygen in experimental *Pseudomonas aeruginosa* osteomyelitis. Presented at the 27th Interscience Conference on Antimicrobial Agents and Chemotherapy, 1987, New York.

35. Mendel V, Simanowski HJ, Scholz HC: Synergy of HBO2 and a local antibiotic carrier for experimental osteomyelitis due to *Staphylococcus aureus* in rats. Undersea Hyperb Med 31:407–416, 2004

36. Depenbusch PL, Thompson RE, Hart GB: Use of hyperbaric oxygen in the treatment of refractory osteomyelitis: A preliminary report. J Trauma 12:807–812, 1972.

37. Davis JC: Refractory osteomyelitis of the extremities and axial skeleton. In: Davis JC, Hunt TK (eds): Hyperbaric Oxygen Therapy. Bethesda, Md, Undersea Medical Society, 1977, pp 217–227.

38. Chen CE, Ko JY, Fu TH, Wang CJ: Results of chronic osteomyelitis of the femur treated with hyperbaric oxygen: A preliminary report. Chang Gung Med J 27:91–97, 2004.

39. Aitasalo K, Niinikoski J, Grenman R, et al: A modified protocol for early treatment of osteomyelitis and osteoradionecrosis of the mandible. Head Neck 20:411–417, 1998.

40. Maynor ML, Moon RE, Camporesi EM, et al: Chronic osteomyelitis of the tibia: Treatment with hyperbaric oxygen and autogenous microsurgical muscle transplantation. J South Orthop Assoc 7:43–57, 1998.

41. Strauss MB: Refractory osteomyelitis. J Hyperb Med 2:147, 1987.

Crush Injuries

20

Justification of and Indications for Hyperbaric Oxygen Therapy

Michael B. Strauss, MD,
FACS, AAOS, and
Lisardo Garcia-Covarrubias, MD

BACKGROUND

Spectrum of Crush Injuries

Crush injury is a term used to describe a spectrum of injuries to the body. The injuries may primarily involve soft tissues or bony elements; often it is a combination of the two. What differentiates crush injuries from other types of injuries to the musculoskeletal system is the severity. The severity of injury may range from minor with minimal contusion of soft tissue with or without a related fracture to limb threatening with nonviable soft tissue and associated complex fractures (Table 20.1). As the severity of injury increases, the likelihood of successful outcomes decreases. At a certain point, the tissue damage is so great that successful healing becomes unlikely and limb amputation is necessary. Unfortunately, no universally accepted classification system is available to encompass the spectrum of crush injury. Gustilo and Williams[1] and Johansen and colleagues[2] have generated classifications (see discussion in the next section) that predict outcomes for open fractures and limb survival, respectively, but clinical judgment remains the common final denominator for making decisions about the management of crush injuries.

Challenges of Crush Injuries

Crush injury is a significant challenge to our health-care system, in terms of both management and expenditures. As a cause of trauma-service hospital admissions, crush injury is a diagnosis in about one fifth of the admissions to Level I trauma centers.[3] For complex crush injuries, initial hospitalizations are typically prolonged and rehospitalizations are frequently required to manage the residual complications. The costs and period of convalescence can be a significant challenge to the health-care system and devastating to the patient. The leading causes of crush injury are motor

Table 20.1 Severity of Crush Injuries and Associated Fractures

| TISSUE INVOLVED | MILD | SEVERITY | | |
		MODERATE	SEVERE	LIMB THREATENING*
Skin and subcutaneous tissues	Intact, but contused	Severely contused	Lacerated, questionable viability of margins	Avulsed, nonviable
Muscles	Contused	Severely contused†	Lacerated, torn, questionable viable	Avulsed, nonviable
Neurovascular structures	Intact	Paresthesias, dysesthesias	Injured, but intact or repairable‡	Lacerated and/or avulsed, severe neurologic deficits
Bone	Intact or nondisplaced fracture	Closed, comminuted, minimally displaced fracture	Markedly comminuted and displaced	Severely comminuted and displaced; missing portions

*Appropriate to refer to as a "mangled extremity" (see Johansen and colleagues[2] for further discussion).
  †Presentation for a skeletal-muscle compartment syndrome.
  ‡Prophylactic fasciotomies for postrevascularization swelling of ischemic muscles.

vehicle accidents, gunshot/munition (especially in the combat arena) wounds, and falls.[3] Even with optimal management, outcomes of crush injury are frequently less than desirable with an inverse relationship between good outcomes and the severity of injury. This generates the question whether outcomes even with state-of-the-art surgical and orthopedic interventions can be improved in those patients who have such severe crush injuries that poor outcomes are the expectation.

Hyperbaric Oxygen and Crush Injuries

Hyperbaric oxygen therapy (HBOT) has been used as an adjunct for the management of crush injuries for more than 30 years, but infrequently, inconsistently, and most often not in "mainstream" trauma management. Predominantly in crush injuries, it is used as a "last resort" when complications arise such as a failing flap or uncontrolled infection develop in a crush injury site, and then only if a hyperbaric chamber is in the vicinity. If complications arise, they are attributed to the severity of the injury because the orthopedic and surgical interventions were within the standards of practice. Whereas the indications for surgical and orthopedic interventions are usually clearly defined on the basis of the examination of the patient and imaging studies, the indications for HBOT tend to be subjective and, unfortunately, mostly reactive. That is, HBOT is utilized only after a complication has arisen. Another consideration that often is not appreciated is that the more impaired the host—for example, from increasing age, shock, peripheral artery insufficiency, smoking, among other factors— the more likely complications will arise from injuries of similar severities.[2]

Questions about Using Hyperbaric Oxygen Therapy for Crush Injuries

With this background, two questions arise with respect to using HBOT for the management of crush injuries. First, is there evidence-based information, both basic science and clinical, that justifies the use of HBOT for crush injuries? Sec-

ond, can classification systems, both for injury severity and competency of the host, be used to objectify the indications for using HBOT for crush injuries? This chapter answers both questions; it substantiates the use of and defines the specific indications for HBOT in crush injuries.

CLASSIFICATION SYSTEMS FOR CRUSH INJURIES

Clinical Judgment

Three classification systems provide guidelines for the management of crush injuries. Clinical judgment based on experience is the factor most frequently used by trauma surgeons and orthopedists. The result is a classification of crush injuries along a continuum of word descriptions from mild to moderate to severe to the point of being limb threatening (see Table 20.1). Mild injuries are expected to heal with minimal interventions and the absence of complications. Uniformly good results are anticipated in moderate injuries with appropriate surgical and orthopedic interventions. However, the host status needs to be factored into this group, and if complications arise, they can usually be attributed to an impaired host status. Finally, severe injuries are those where there is a high likelihood that complications will arise. Clinical findings for this group include: (1) loss of soft tissues, (2) marginally viable soft tissues, (3) major arterial injury, (4) missing bone, (5) markedly comminuted and/or displaced fractures, and (6) massive contamination or combinations of these findings. As more and more of these findings accompany the injury, complications such as nonunion, refractory osteomyelitis, loss of function, and limb amputation increase predictably. Primary or delayed amputation is required in the worse-case scenarios. This outcome increases in direct proportion to the degree of host impairment.

Gustilo Grading of Open Fractures

The Gustilo classification[1,4] is widely used by traumatologists. It is based on the amount of soft-tissue injury associated with an open fracture. In grade I fractures, the open wound occurs from inside-to-out and there is minimal associated soft-tissue injury. Gustilo and co-workers[4] subsequently reported that complications are only slightly greater than for similar type closed fractures. Grade II fractures have associated soft-tissue injuries of the laceration, skin avulsion type, and in healthy hosts, healing complications are only slightly greater than in the similar closed fracture.[4] Gustilo Type III open fractures have a crush component. After review of his initial observations, Gustilo found it necessary to subdivide the Type III fractures into A, B, and C groups because each has such different outcomes.[4] In grade III-A open fractures, sufficient soft tissue exists to cover the bone/fracture site after debridement has been completed. In grade III-B open fractures, exposed bone remains after the initial debridement, thereby requiring secondary coverage/closure procedures or allowing the wound to heal by secondary intention. In grade III-C open fractures, there is a concomitant injury to the major blood supplies to the extremity. In the healthy host, complication rates in the 50% range are observed in Gustilo Types III-B and III-C open fracture-crush injury even with optimal standard of practice surgical and orthopedic interventions.[4] Criticisms of the Gustilo classification system include poor interobserver reliability and the observation that serious crush injuries and fractures with or without blood vessel injury can occur in the absence of open wounds, such as is often seen in closed fractures and joint dislocations.

Mangled Extremity Severity Score

Another classification for crush injuries was generated by Johansen and colleagues[2] to provide objective criteria for justifying primary amputation in the mangled extremity. Four assessments—(A) skeletal/soft-tissue injury, (B) limb ischemia, (C) shock, and (D) age—are graded on varying whole-number scales from 0 to 2 (e.g., shock) to 1 to 4 (e.g., skeletal/soft-tissue injury). The higher the number, the more serious the problem is

for each assessment. The authors proposed that a Mangled Extremity Severity Score (MESS) of 7 or greater provided objective criteria for and justified primary limb amputation. Although use of the MESS score appears to be limited to a few academic trauma centers, the score does take into consideration not only the extent of the injury, but also the host status as reflected by shock, perfusion, and patient age. Obviously, MESS scores of 7 or greater are those that correspond to the most serious injury—to the point of being limb threatening for the clinical classification system and the ones described as "severe" Type III-B and/or III-C injuries in the Gustilo classification.

Host Status

The importance of host status as a predictor of outcomes may be as important as the severity of the injury and the quality of care provided. Cierney and coauthors[5] appreciated this when they added a host status subclassification to a standard classification of osteomyelitis. They proposed a three-level host classification: A = normal host; B = compromised host (subclassified as "S" for systemic and "L" for local); and C = inappropriate host for surgical interventions, that is, the infection is so mild or the cure might be worse than the disease. Unfortunately, its narrow scope provides only limited applications to crush injuries. Nonetheless, it did provide somewhat objective criteria for using HBOT for refractory osteomyelitis. For example, if the host was compromised (B host) and a sequestrum was present, they recommended HBOT be used as an adjunct to surgical and antibiotic management. With this precedent, the first author generated a host status score that is simple to use (similar to the five-criteria 0-to-10-point Apgar score used in assessing the vitality of the newborn), objective, and applicable not only to crush injuries, but also to a variety of surgical and orthopedic conditions including refractory osteomyelitis and problem wounds (Table 20.2). Integration of the crush injury classification systems with the host-function

Table 20.2 Host-Function Score (Strauss)

ASSESSMENT	GRADE*		
	2 POINTS	1 POINT	0 POINTS
Age, yr[†]	<40	40-60	>60
Ambulation[‡]	Community	Household	None
Cardiac/renal status (whichever gives the lower score)	Normal is acceptable	Impaired	Decompensated/end stage
Smoking/steroid use (whichever gives the lower score)	None	Past	Current
Neurologic impairment	None	Some	Severe

To determine host-function score, sum the points for each assessment. Score interpretations are as follows: healthy host—8 to 10 points; impaired, but compensated host—4 to 7 points; decompensated host—0 to 3 points.
*Half points may be used between the whole number grade points to indicate the findings are mixed or intermediate between two findings.
[†]Subtract half a point if diabetes or collagen vascular disease coexists.
[‡]Subtract half a point if walking aids are used.

score provides criteria for making decisions regarding whether HBOT is indicated for crush injuries (Fig. 20.1).

PATHOPHYSIOLOGY OF CRUSH INJURIES

Macroscopic Injury to Tissues

Crush injuries have macroscopic, microscopic, and biochemical components. The components are interrelated, and especially for the microscopic and biochemical components, a predictable cascade of events occurs. Two factors, edema and hypoxia, unify the pathophysiology (Fig. 20.2). Macroscopic components of crush injuries include damage to soft tissues, interruption of nerve and blood supplies, and fractures. The clinical examination supplemented with imaging studies is usually sufficient to define

the extent of the macroscopic injury and classify the injury into one of the types described previously (see Fig. 20.1). Each level of tissue provides clues as to the seriousness of the injury (see Table 20.1). For example, from the external appearance of the skin, contusion, ischemia, and avulsion are readily appreciated. Palpation provides information about injury to the deeper soft tissues such as swelling, cavitation, and hematoma formation, as well as the neurovascular status of the extremity distal to the injury. Inspection of alignment, testing for stability, and radiographs demonstrate the location, amount of comminution, and/or the displacement of the fracture. More involved imaging techniques (computerized tomography, magnetic resonance imaging, angiography, magnetic resonance angiography, and/or nuclear medicine scans) may be necessary to supplement the physical examination and plain radiographs when additional information is required.

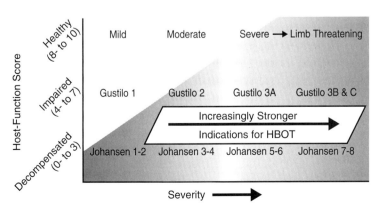

Figure 20.1 Integration of the host-function score and crush injury classifications systems as indications for hyperbaric oxygen therapy (HBOT). The more compromised the host, the greater the indication for using HBOT as an adjunct for the management of crush injuries. The shaded area indicates the authors' recommendations for using HBOT in crush injuries. As the severity of the injury increases (moving to the right side of the figure), the indications become even stronger because predictable complication rates are so high with "standard of practice" surgical and medical interventions alone.

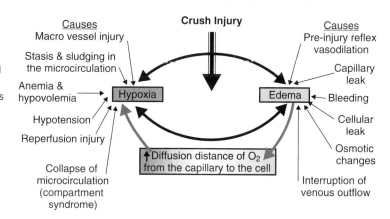

Figure 20.2 The self-perpetuating effect of hypoxia and edema in contributing to the pathophysiology of crush injury. Hypoxia and edema are the common final denominators of crush injury pathophysiology. Many causes contribute to each. Hypoxia is compounded by the limited diffusion distance of O_2 from the capillary to the cell. As the cycle continues, the injury progresses, especially wound hypoxia, which becomes a strong argument for using hyperbaric oxygen therapy.

Kinetic Energy Transfer

Damage from crush injuries occurs because of the transfer of kinetic energy from an object to the tissue. The object may be stationary and the body parts the source of the kinetic energy, such as being hurled from a motorcycle and hitting the ground, or vice versa, such as a bumper injury from a moving motor vehicle striking the leg of a stationary pedestrian. The kinetic energy transfers can be enormous. For comparison purposes, the kinetic energy transfer of stepping off a 1-foot curb and fracturing a hip may be as little as 50 foot pounds. For a pedestrian versus car bumper injury, the kinetic energy transfer to tissues can be 200 times greater, or 10,000 foot pounds. This enormous transfer of energy may immediately destroy the soft tissues that receive the brunt of the energy transfer. Typically, a gradient of injury results from uninjured to nonviable tissue (see Fig. 20.1). The tissues in between may have various degrees of injury. Outcomes largely rest on how these intermediately injured tissues are handled, a target area for HBOT that is discussed in the next section.

Seriousness of Injury

Intact skin in the injury area is not always a sign that the deep tissues are not seriously injured. Some injuries may be deceptive, especially around the knee joint where dislocations, displacement of bony fragments, and/or cavitation can cause much more severe injury than superficial inspection may suggest. These are the types of injuries that are prone to neurovascular damage. Blood vessels and nerves cross joints in protective sheaths or tunnels that allow little displacement yet permit bending through the range of motion of the joint. Generally, the neurovascular injury can be appreciated from the examination, but its precise location must be ascertained with imaging studies such as angiography to determine what vascular interventions are required. The skeletal muscle-compartment syndrome is another condition where the external appearance of the injury site may be deceptive and not reflect the seriousness of the underlying injury. This is especially the situation in closed fractures of the leg and the forearm.

Microcirculation Pathophysiology

Direct Injury

Well-described pathologic events in crush injuries occur at the microcirculation level. The insults can be direct, indirect, or a combination of the two. Direct injury causes physical disruption of the microcirculation caused by the energy exchange from the injury. This causes bleeding and edema into the tissue spaces and renders the tissues supplied by the microcirculation devoid of a blood supply. If the tissues are not immediately destroyed by the energy exchange, they may ultimately succumb to an ischemic death from the lack of blood supply. This is manifested by demarcation between viable and dead tissues that may take several days to several weeks to be fully appreciated. The physical trauma of direct injury can also contribute to the cascade of events that occur at the biochemical level such as alterations in the flux of fluids and electrolytes into and out of the cell.[6]

Indirect Injury

Indirect microscopic events occur in both the microcirculation and the tissues themselves (see Fig. 20.2). In the microcirculation, sludging of cellular elements, as well as platelets and stasis, occurs from physical, sublethal trauma to the vessel walls, slowing of blood flow caused by bleeding and shock, external compression on the vessel walls from swelling, and reperfusion injury.[6,7] External compression of the vessel walls and eventual collapse of the microcirculation defines the pathophysiology of the skeletal muscle-compartment syndrome. Edema accumulates because of physical trauma coupled with the response of tissues to ischemia. The cells comprising the tissues are no longer able to hold their intracellular water, resulting in fluid leakage into the extracellular tissue. Edema is the clinical manifestation of this indirect microcirculation effect.

A physiologic response to ischemia is regional vasodilation in the intact vasculature proximal to the injury. Although, at first consideration, increased blood flow to an ischemic area would seem desirable, with injury to the microcirculation, it can be counterproductive for two reasons. First, if the continuity of the blood vessel is disrupted, bleeding occurs into the tissues. Second, if there is stasis in the microcirculation, the blood within the vessel essentially has no place to go. The consequences are an increased pressure head for transudation and edema formation. Once stasis occurs, a cascade of events results with clotting, Rouleaux formation of red blood cells, and initiation of a variety of biochemical events.[8] In essence, the unifying factor of the microscopic injury is that of a hypoxic insult to tissues. Consequently, supplementation of tissue oxygenation is a desirable intervention and something that HBOT offers.

Biochemical, Cellular, and Molecular Aspects

The pathophysiology of crush injury at these levels includes events caused by direct mechanical stress and events triggered by reperfusion of the tissue. If direct trauma to the muscles is severe enough, rhabdomyolysis occurs.[7] In normal muscle tissue, there is a low concentration of sodium and a high concentration of calcium. Mechanical disruption of the cell (by direct trauma as in a crush injury) opens stretch-activated channels in the muscle cell membrane, resulting in the influx of fluid and electrolytes including sodium and calcium.[6] The cell becomes edematous, and the increased intracellular concentration of calcium activates cytoplasmic proteases that lead to the degradation of fibrillar proteins and decreased adenosine triphosphate production because of inhibition of cellular respiration.[7] With loss of the energy source to drive the sodium pump, the cell will swell until it bursts.[7] This further contributes to the microcirculation pathophysiology described previously.

Ischemia-Reperfusion Injury

Ischemia-reperfusion (IR) injury is a biochemical injury that is mediated by complex mechanisms including a variety of different cells and proinflammatory compounds (Table 20.3). It exerts local and systemic effects that are proportional to the ischemic time and the amount of affected tissue.[8,9] The degree of injury also depends on the specific tissue involved; obviously, some tissues are more tolerant to ischemia than others.[10] For example, after 2 hours of ischemia, skeletal muscle sustains minimal structural damage and completely recovers its metabolic functions once its blood supply is restored; however, after 7 hours of ischemia, severe, irreversible muscle injury is the outcome.[11] IR injury is a predictable response in higher organisms when tissues sustain a transient interruption of blood flow. Although on superficial inspection it appears destructive, the teleologic effect appears to be that of

Table 20.3 Inflammatory Mediators

CELLULAR ELEMENTS	PHYSIOLOGICALLY ACTIVE SUBSTANCES	ENZYME AND HORMONE-LIKE	ELEMENTS AND MOLECULES
Endothelium	Adhesion molecules	Cytokines (proinflammatory)	Calcium
Leukocytes	Complement (alternate pathway)	Leukotrienes	Reactive oxygen species
Macrophages	Prostaglandins	Phospholipases	(superoxides, hydrogen
Platelets		Proteosomes	peroxide, peroxynitrite)
		Thromboxanes	Nitric oxide

isolating irreversibly damaged tissues from the rest of the organism, thereby preserving the organism at the expense of the IR-injured tissues. The IR injury, as it relates to crush injuries in particular and all ischemic injuries in general, has the following components: endothelium and vascular dysfunction, adhesion molecules, reactive oxygen species (ROS), proinflammatory cytokines and signaling pathways, the complement system, and the ubiquitin-proteasome system.

Endothelium and Vascular Dysfunction

The crucial role of the endothelium in the IR injury is becoming better defined.[12,13] The endothelium is a multifunctional, dynamic structure that regulates blood flow, permeability, and cell trafficking functions in a biphasic manner, quiescent or activated.[14] Quiescent endothelial cells have an anticoagulant, antiadhesive, and vasodilatory phenotype. Activated endothelial cells express procoagulant, proadhesive, and vasoconstrictive properties.[15] The endothelium is normally bathed by flowing blood and surrounded by underlying parenchymal cells, and thereby is exposed to circulating blood cells, pH, pressure, oxygen content, and soluble plasma proteins. Physiologic and dysfunctional responses of the microcirculation endothelium vary with the level of the vasculature.[16,17]

Arterioles

Impaired endothelium-dependent vasodilation occurs secondary to the ischemic-hypoxic insult.[18,19] Vasospasm after reperfusion is thought to be caused by impairment of nitric oxide (·NO) production.[20] ROS are not likely to be

the cause of impaired endothelium-mediated vasodilation.[21]

Capillaries

Inadequate restitution of perfusion to ischemic muscles—the so called no-reflow phenomenon—arises from red blood cell sludging (rouleaux formation), leukocyte recruitment, and/or activated platelets.[22-25] The backup in flow disrupts the normal capillary filtration, tissue fluid resorption balance with the net effect of interstitial edema formation.[25] When the interstitial fluid pressure exceeds the capillary perfusion pressure, the microcirculation collapses. This defines the pathophysiology of the skeletal muscle-compartment syndrome.[25]

Postcapillary Venules

Release of ROS is mediated by interaction of neutrophils, platelets, and endothelial adhesion molecules.[26]

Adhesion Molecules

Cell adhesion molecules, predominantly selectins, integrins, and immunoglobulins, mediate leukocyte (and platelet)-endothelial cell interactions in the microvasculature and are relevant to the IR injury[27] (Table 20.4).

Selectins

After an ischemic insult, selectins interfere with leukocyte rolling.[26] Further activation results in firm adhesion and then transendothelial migration of the neutrophil with subsequent release of ROS.[28] This is mediated by the interaction of integrins and cell adhesion

Table 20.4 Adhesion Molecules Associated with Ischemia-Reperfusion Injury

FAMILIES	STRUCTURE	TYPES	LOCATION	LIGAND	FUNCTION
Immunoglobulins	Immunoglobulin-like	ICAM-1, ICAM-2, PECAM-1, and VCAM-1	Endothelium	CD11/CD18	Adherence, emigration
Integrins	Glycoproteins with two subunits (α, β)	CD11/CD18	Leukocytes	ICAM-1, ICAM-2	Adherence
Selectins	Lectin-like	E-, L-, and P-selectins	Endothelium, leukocytes and platelets	E-, L-, and P-selectins	Rolling

CD, cluster of differentiation; E, endothelial; ICAM, intercellular adhesion molecule; L, leukocyte; P, platelets; PECAM, platelet endothelial adhesion molecule; VCAM, vascular cell adhesion molecule.

molecule immunoglobulins.[27] Blockage of cell adhesion molecule in human trials using monoclonal antibodies, as opposed to animal models, has not been effective in trauma, stroke, myocardial infarction, and neonatal cardiopulmonary bypass.[29]

Reactive Oxygen Species

ROS are radicals, also known as oxygen free radicals, that are distinguished by having an unpaired electron in their outer orbit. This gives them the ability to oxidize many biologic molecules such as lipids, proteins, and ribonucleic acids.[30] They are also involved in many physiologic reactions in organisms.[31] Much has been learned about ROS since 1954 when they were found to be mediators of radiation injury.[32-38]

The superoxide anion ($\cdot O_2^-$) is the primary ROS. It interacts with other molecules to generate secondary ROS.[39] The secondary ROS are the singlet oxygen, superoxide, and hydroxyl radicals. Characteristics of ROS include[30-39]:

- High instability and reactivity
- Promotion of chain reactions (e.g., lipid peroxidation)
- Generation of more ROS
- Short half-life (microseconds to seconds)
- Poor diffusion through cell membranes

In addition to oxygen radicals, chlorine and nitrogen radicals are involved in many biochemical reactions including IR injury.[40] ·NO appears to be one of the most important molecules in this group. It is synthesized by a family of enzymes, nitric oxide synthases (NOSs), that convert L-arginine into ·NO and citrulline. ·NO is a vasodilator, and this effect protects the endothelium during reperfusion. At least two forms of the enzyme are present in endothelial cells: (1) endothelial NOS, which is constitutively expressed, and (2) an inducible form. The inducible form releases ·NO in larger quantities during inflammatory and/or immunologic defense reactions, and it is involved in host tissue damage.[41] It is upregulated by inflammatory stimuli such as endotoxins, cytokines, and lipid mediators.[42]

In endothelial cells, NOSs compete with arginase for L-arginine. Arginase activity increases after IR injury, potentially depleting the pool of L-arginine necessary for ·NO production.[43] This may explain why vasodilation is impaired after IR injury of skeletal muscle.[18,19] Paradoxically, inhibition of inducible NOS has been reported to exacerbate injury in certain situations, suggesting that this form of NOS is protective as well.[44]

Sources of ROS relevant to the skeletal muscle IR injury are the enzymes xanthine oxidase and neutrophil-derived nicotinamide adenine dinucleotide phosphate (NADPH) oxidase.[45] Xanthine oxidase usually exists in nonischemic, healthy cells predominantly as an oxidized nicotinamide adenine dinucleotide (NAD^+)–dependent dehydrogenase.[45] Ischemia promotes conversion of xanthine dehydrogenase to xanthine oxidase with concomitant adenosine triphosphate utilization, resulting in the accumulation of the breakdown products, xanthine and hypoxanthine.[45] These breakdown products act as substrates for xanthine oxidase, which produces ROS during reperfusion when molecular oxygen is introduced.[45] Xanthine oxidase is localized in the sarcolemma and mitochondria of aerobic muscle fibers, and also is found in large quantities in capillary endothelial cells of skeletal muscle.[46,47]

The other relevant source of ROS in IR injury is neutrophil-bound NADPH oxidase.[48] This enzyme oxidizes cytoplasmic NADPH to $NADP^+$. This reduces molecular oxygen to superoxide, which can dismutate to form hydrogen peroxide, with the reactions generating the "respiratory burst" of the neutrophil.[48] Activated neutrophils also contain a variety of granular enzymes, some of which are involved in ROS production such as myeloperoxidase, which is not released except under pathologic conditions.

The effects of ROS are counterbalanced and/or regulated by several antioxidant mechanisms. Enzymatic mechanisms occur via superoxide dismutase, catalase, and glutathione peroxidase. Nonenzyme agents include vitamin E, vitamin C, beta-carotene, and heme-binding proteins such as ceruloplasmin, transferrin, haptoglobin, and albumin.[49]

Proinflammatory Cytokines and Signaling Pathways

Most cytokines normally are not detectable in healthy individuals. During serious illnesses and after trauma, cytokine level increases are common.[50] Within minutes to hours after reperfusion, active transcription of proinflammatory molecules, for example, tumor necrosis factor (TNF)-α, interleukin (IL)-1, and IL-6, begins. IL-6, which is produced from most cells, is induced by TNF-α and IL-1.[50]

Neutrophils are activated by IL-6 during injury in direct proportion to the extent of tissue damage; hence, IL-6 may be a prognostic marker.[51,52] Macrophages and neutrophils are the main sources of TNF-α and IL-1. These cytokines are up-regulated by ischemia.[53,54] Intracytoplasmic events are triggered by receptors of TNF-α, including activation of a nuclear factor that leads to apoptosis.[55] This nuclear factor acts as a transcriptor for gene expression of many inflammatory mediators.[56]

Cellular damage induced by ROS and other inflammatory compounds activate a complex intracellular pathway mediated by caspases (intracellular cysteine proteases) that lead to apoptosis.[57] Caspase inhibition has been observed to increase tolerance to ischemia and reduce apoptotic cell death in laboratory studies.[58,59]

Complement System

The complement system is an innate host defense and its role in IR injury is well established.[60] Production of complement components is regulated by proinflammatory cytokines, primarily TNF-α and IL-6.

The complement system is activated by three pathways: (1) the classical antigen–antibody–dependent pathway; (2) the lectin pathway; and (3) the alternative pathway. All three pathways converge on complement component 3 (C3).[60,61] Its inhibition leads to complete blockade of complement activation.[61] During IR injury, several activated components of the complement system up-regulate cell adhesion molecule and recruit inflammatory cells.[60] Blockade of these activated components is a strategy that has been tried to ameliorate IR injury but has had mixed results.[62]

Ubiquitin-Proteasome System

The ubiquitin-proteasome system is a nonlysosomal, multicatalytic proteinase pathway that has a central role in degradation of intracellular proteins.[63] It is postulated that ubiquitin-proteasome system inhibition ablates the up-regulation of nuclear factors that lead to apoptosis, and it has been studied in the IR injury of the brain, heart, liver, and skeletal muscle.[64-68]

MECHANISMS OF HYPERBARIC OXYGEN THERAPY APPLICABLE TO CRUSH INJURIES

Hyperoxygenation

Primary and secondary mechanisms occur with the inhalation of pure oxygen at greater than 1 atmosphere absolute (ATA) of pressure—the definition of HBOT. The primary mechanisms are hyperoxygenation, a transient effect, and reduction of bubble size. Secondary mechanisms occur as a consequence of the tissues' responses to increased oxygen tensions in the plasma and tissue fluids that result from hyperoxygenation (Table 20.5). Whereas effects from the primary mechanisms usually occur immediately, the effects from the secondary mechanisms take time to occur, justify repetitive oxygen treatments, tend to be long lasting, and contribute significantly to the desired outcomes observed from HBOT. Regardless, when HBOT is used, hyperoxygenation is the mechanism that predominates the decision making for justifying the use of this therapeutic modality.

The effect of breathing increased pressures of oxygen has a physiologic basis. It results in increased oxygen in the plasma in direct proportion to the pressure of the inhaled oxygen. This supplements hemoglobin oxygen delivery to tissues and is no more flow dependent than transport of other physically dissolved substances in the bloodstream. In low-flow states, sludging and stasis of the cellular elements in the microcirculation, or severe anemia, the hyperbaric oxygen laden plasma continues to stream through the microcirculation and provide oxygen for diffusion from the capillary to the surrounding tissue fluids.[69] In the immediate period after the crush injury when oxygen demands of the tissues are likely to be the greatest and tissue viability is most at risk, oxygen availability is low due to compromised flow in the microcirculation. This is an important indication and provides the rationale for the immediate use of HBOT in crush injuries.

Effects of Hyperoxygenation

The hyperoxygenation effects of HBOT are threefold[69] (Fig. 20.3). At a typical treatment pressure of 2 ATA, the plasma and tissue fluid oxygen tensions increase 10-fold from about 100 and 30 mm Hg, respectively, to more than 1000 mm Hg in the plasma and more than 300 mm Hg in the tissue fluids.[70] Second, as a consequence of the hyperoxygenation of the plasma, the oxygen-carrying capacity of the

Table 20.5 Secondary Effects of Hyperoxygenation (see Fig. 20.3)

PERTINENT TO CRUSH INJURIES		OTHER SECONDARY EFFECTS	
EFFECT	**COMMENT**	**EFFECT**	**COMMENT**
1. Vasoconstriction	α-Adrenergic-like effect	5. Inert gas and carbon monoxide washout	A hyperoxygenation effect that rapidly cleanses the blood of these gases
2. Function of host cellular factors in wound healing	30–40 mm Hg O_2 tensions in the tissues fluids required	6. Microbiologic	HBOT has direct effects on bacteria killing (anaerobes) and cessation of toxin production (gas gangrene)
3. Perturbation of the IRI	The IRI is probably the final common pathway in tissue damage from crush injuries	7. Alteration of the blood–brain barrier	A possible mechanism to increase delivery of antibiotics and other drugs to the brain and spinal cord
4. Preservation of RBC deformability	The 7-μm-wide RBCs must elongate to pass through the 5-μm-wide capillary	8. Isobaric counterdiffusion	Gas exchange in bubbles (O_2 in; inert gas out)

HBOT, hyperbaric oxygen therapy; IRI, ischemia-reperfusion injury; RBC, red blood cell.

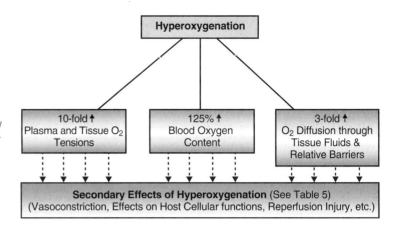

Figure 20.3 Hyperoxygenation effects of hyperbaric oxygen therapy. The three effects depicted above begin immediately on pressurization with hyperbaric oxygen. They lead to secondary effects. Whereas the hyperoxygenation effects are transient, the secondary effects tend to be long lasting and responsible ultimately for the salvage of tissue and healing of wounds.

blood is increased by 25% from approximately 20 volumes percent to about 25 volumes percent. The third effect of hyperoxygenation is a threefold increase in the diffusion distance of oxygen through tissue fluids and relative barriers such as edema, cicatrix, exudates, nonviable bone, cartilage, and the ischemic margins of a wound. These hyperoxygenation effects are transient, lasting during the HBOT period and continuing in the subcutaneous tissues for a 4-hour period and in the muscles for 1.5 hours.[70] Two important effects occur as a consequence of hyperoxygenation. First, during the period of transient hyperoxia using standard treatment pressures, almost enough oxygen is carried physically dissolved in the plasma to meet tissue oxygen requirements—even without red blood cells.[71] Second, the transient increases of oxygen in the tissues provide an oxygenated environment sufficient for the secondary mechanisms of HBOT to begin their actions.

Secondary Effects of Hyperoxygenation

Vasoconstriction

In the presence of hypoxia, tissue functions such as those necessary for wound healing and infection control are idle.[72] Hyperoxygenation has the potential to provide an oxygenated environment in the tissues sufficient for these functions to resume.[69,72] There are multiple secondary mechanisms of hyperoxygen-

ation; four have special pertinence to crush injuries. The first of these is vasoconstriction. This is a generalized effect in the vasoresponsive elements of the vascular system analogous to that seen with α-adrenergic agents. Vasoconstriction from hyperoxygenation reduces inflow by 20%, whereas oxygenation is maintained through hyperoxygenation.[73] With decreased inflow, yet maintenance of venous outflow, edema is reduced.[74,75] Benefits of edema reduction are twofold: First, oxygen availability is increased through reduction of the diffusion distance for oxygen through tissue fluids from the capillary to the cell; and second, reduced external pressure on the microcirculation improves flow.[75] For these effects to occur from HBOT, there still must be perfusion, even if only of the plasma, through the capillary bed. For example, in the fully manifested skeletal-muscle compartment syndrome, flow is obliterated in the microcirculation because the pressure of the edema fluid in the confined space of the injury exceeds that of the capillary perfusion pressure.[75]

Host Wound Healing Elements

Host factors such as fibroblast function, neutrophil oxidative killing, and osteogenesis are oxygen dependent.[72] If oxygen tensions in the wound environment are less than 30 mm Hg, as is anticipated in severe crush injuries, these wound healing and infection-controlling cells are unable to function.[72,76] As stated earlier, at the time the oxygen demands for the wound site are greatest, they are likely to be at the lowest of any time in the course of wound healing. This is the time when the host factors are mobilized to the wound site and initiate their wound healing and infection control functions.[72] It is a paradox that whereas measures to enhance blood oxygen saturations, monitored by pulse oximetry, are a standard of practice, the use of HBOT to improve oxygen availability to the crush injury site, and verifiable by juxtawound transcutaneous oxygen measurements, is not.

Role of Oxygen for Wound Healing

Oxygen is necessary for these wound healing factors to function. Without sufficient oxygen tensions in the wound margins, fibroblasts are unable to migrate to the wound site, multiply, and generate their matrix substances.[72] This latter function provides a substrate, that is, the matrix, for the amino acid precursors of wound healing such as lysine and hydroxylysine to initiate collage formation and heal the wound.[72] The other crucial function of the matrix is that it provides a scaffold for angiogenesis to restore the blood supply destroyed by the injury.[72] Without this activity the center of the wound will remain hypoxic and the wound will go on to a nonhealing state. Neutrophils likewise require tissue oxygen tensions at the 30- to 40-mm Hg range to generate the superoxides, peroxides, and halide species used to kill bacteria.[76] It is logical that the optimal time to complement the surgical and antibiotic measures to control the contamination introduced at the time of wounding is before the microorganisms begin multiplying at exponential rates. This is the time when the wound margins are most likely to be hypoxic and provide insufficient oxygen tensions for neutrophils to kill bacteria. Without functioning neutrophils, administration of antibiotics and surgical debridements often are inadequate to control infection The cells necessary for bone healing, especially the osteoclast, which is responsible for remodeling and resorbing dead bone, also require high oxygen tensions to function.[69]

Ischemia-Reperfusion Injury

Most in vitro and animal models utilizing HBOT for the IR injury in a variety of tissues demonstrate positive results.[77] Several studies have demonstrated decreased endothelial adhesion of neutrophils and improved survival of axial flaps, brain, muscle, and lung tissue with HBOT.[78-84] In a rat carbon monoxide model, the mechanism for the above observations appeared to be the down-regulation of cell adhesion molecules, specifically the B-integrin.[85-87] Other studies suggest that the perturbation for neutrophil adherence with HBOT is due to endothelial intercellular adhesion molecules.[88-90] Several studies have demonstrated the beneficial effects of HBOT in decreasing proinflammatory cytokines both in animals and humans.[91,92] In rat hemorrhagic shock and intestinal ischemic models, HBOT attenuated messenger RNA expression[91,92] and plasma levels of IL-6 and TNF-α. Although high concentrations of oxygen generate oxidative stresses, adaptive mechanisms to these have been identified including production of heme oxygenase-1, inducible heat shock proteins, catalase, and superoxide dismutase.[93-102] Reports on the effects of HBOT on apoptosis are mixed.[103-107]

Red Blood Cell Deformability

Because the erythrocyte diameter is 7.5 μm, it must deform (elongate) to pass through the 5-μm-wide capillary. As red blood cells age, they lose their ability to deform. When this occurs, they are removed by the reticuloendothelial system and their contents are recycled.[108] Rouleau formation, as is associated with hypoxia in the microcirculation, and sepsis are conditions that interfere with red blood cell deformability.[109,110] Red blood cells that are unable to deform will not pass through the capillary and off-load their oxygen to tissues. The consequences are tissue hypoxia and impaired ability to handle the bioburden introduced with the open fracture. HBOT may have a possible role because maintenance of red blood cell metabolism including membrane function is oxygen dependent and HBOT has been reported to improve red blood cell deformability.[111] This secondary mechanism of HBOT may have contributed to increased survival reported in an animal sepsis model.[112]

CLINICAL EXPERIENCES WITH HYPERBARIC OXYGEN IN THE MANAGEMENT OF CRUSH INJURIES

Introduction and Literature Review

Although there are reports of nearly a thousand case experiences using HBOT for crush injuries, almost all are retrospectively reported. The first report on the successful use of HBOT was published in 1961.[113] Subsequently, two literature reviews have been published. The first review, published in 1981, is a literature search of all published reports to that date (Table 20.6),[114] and second, published in 2005, is an evidentiary review (Table 20.7).[115] In the 1981 review, cases were tabulated as to being published in the English language literature (63 patients)[116-121] and the Soviet literature (634 patients).[122-126] The fact that the preponderance of patients (87%) was from Soviet reports reflects the strong interest of the then USSR (Union of Soviet Socialist Republics) in this subject and their direct application to crush, mangled extremity–type injuries as would stem from the battlefield. In the more recent review, Eastern Association for the Surgery of Trauma (EAST) recommendations to evaluate original articles were utilized.[127] Eight reports met the inclusion criteria for evidentiary information, but only one of the reports before 1981 (where outcomes were given primarily in subjective terms such as useful, improved, beneficial, effective, etc.) had sufficient statistical data to be included in the evidentiary review.[119] One noteworthy observation from the 1981 review was that the outcomes improved as the frequency of treatments increased (see Table 20.6).

The following is a summary of the studies included in the evidentiary review of crush injuries with associated problems. In 1973, Székely

and colleagues[119] reported on 19 crush-type injuries including those with severe injury to the upper and lower extremities, vascular trauma, extensive skin loss, and anaerobic infections associated with open fractures. Five cases included enough information to be included in the evidentiary review, although the authors acknowledged the difficulty they had in evaluating the role of HBOT in the overall outcomes. Measurement of skin temperatures in the injured limb and the intact limb were recorded and compared. It was a favorable prognostic sign if the skin temperature increased during HBOT and did not decrease significantly after the treatment was completed. The authors attributed this observation to increased metabolism of the injured tissues from the greater availability of oxygen as a consequence of HBOT. The authors concluded that HBOT has a role in some cases of severe limb damage. However, the assessment based on the five patients with complete information does not reveal an obvious benefit from HBOT.

Replantations: Chinese Experiences

A study from the Shanghai Sixth People's Hospital in 1975 included 21 traumatic amputations or near-amputations of the limbs and fingers.[128] Eighteen cases involved the upper extremities, two cases involved single fingers, and one the lower extremity. The average time of limb ischemia before replantation was 16 hours with a range of 6 to 36 hours. All patients received HBOT after surgery. Limb survival occurred in 10 of 15 detached limbs, including 2 fingers that were ischemic for less than 10 hours, and in 4 of 6 patients with ischemic times greater than 20 hours. This study is noteworthy for the high survival rates observed in those patients with prolonged ischemia times.

Vascular Injuries

In 1977, Monies-Chass and coauthors[129] reported outcomes on seven healthy young patients who suffered severe vascular trauma to their lower extremities and subsequently

Table 20.6 English and Soviet Union Citations Published on Crush Injuries—1981 Review[114]

FIRST AUTHOR (YEAR)	TYPE OF INJURY	NO. OF SUBJECTS	OUTCOMES, COMMENTS
SOVIET CITATIONS PUBLISHED ON CRUSH INJURIES (N = 71)			
Illingworth (1961)[116]	Limb ischemias	2	100% benefit, massive gangrene averted; no HBOT information
Maudsley (1963)[117]	Crush injuries, open fractures	1	Apparent benefit; possible compartment syndrome; no HBOT information
Slack (1966)[118]	Traumatic ischemias of lower extremities	22	HBOT at 2.5 ATA, 1-2 hours daily*; 59% "responded well ... HBOT worthwhile"
Székely (1973)[119]	Severe injuries of extremities	19	HBOT at 2-2.5 ATA, 2 hours; 10 treatments; HBOT "useful" in 68%; from past experiences amputations would have been needed
Schramek (1977)[120]	Arterial injuries from battle casualties	7	HBOT at 2.8 ATA, 2 hours, 6 treatments/day*; 100% salvage; HBOT reversed ischemia after arterial repair and prevented major amputations
Loder (1979)[121]	Crush injuries	20	HBOT at 2.5 ATA, 1 hour, 3 treatments/day*; 50% complete recovery; 30% partial recovery; 20% failure; HBOT speeded demarcation and improved survival in doubtful cases
SOVIET CITATIONS PUBLISHED ON CRUSH INJURIES (N = 634)			
Lukich (1976)[122]	Peripheral ischemias, acute arterial obstructions, gangrene, slow-healing postoperative wounds)	325	69% good results, 21% moderate effects, 10% no benefits of HBOT; average of 12 HBOT treatments per patient
Davidkin (1977)[123]	Acute traumatic ischemias including open fractures, severed limbs, frost bite, etc.	134	HBOT effective in treating generalized or local hypoxia as a result of trauma; enhances local repair processes
Gismondi (1978)[124]	Arteriopathies	22	HBOT effective in curbing or limiting tissue damage in more than half the cases
Isakov (1979)[125]	Open traumas of the extremities	91	Multiple benefits, both systemically and locally, including: (1) accelerated recovery of neutrophil phagocytic activity, (2) quicker diminution of edema, (3) healing of fractures, and (4) prevention of suppuration in stump wounds
Lukich (1979)[126]	Regional ischemias	62	HBOT resulted in variable, primarily favorable responses

*Note how outcomes improved as frequency of treatments per day increased: Schramek (100% salvage) with 6 treatments/day > Loder (80% complete or partial recovery) with 3 treatments/day > Slack (59% responded well) with 1 treatment/day.
ATA, atmospheres absolute; HBOT, hyperbaric oxygen therapy.

received HBOT. The average time interval from injury to vascular repair was 9 (range, 4-20) hours. All patients underwent standard vascular repair, but after surgery, the limbs remained severely ischemic with accompanying findings of cyanosis and swelling. HBOT was begun 1 to 2 days after the operations were completed, with 9.5 treatments being the average. Ischemia reversed in six patients, and progression of early gangrene of the toes was halted in one patient after HBOT. In this latter patient, amputations were limited to the toes. Functional outcomes of the nine cases were not mentioned in the report. Purported benefits from HBOT were the reversal of ischemic changes in the threatened limbs and acceleration of the demarcation process of the gangrenous toes.

Table 20.7 Evidentiary Review of Crush Injuries Managed with Adjunctive HBOT

AUTHOR	STUDY DESIGN/ DATA LEVEL*	TYPE OF INJURY	HBOT PROTOCOL	OUTCOMES†	HBOT BENEFICIAL
Székely and colleagues[119]	Case series; no control subjects; L-III	5 cases with severe injury to the limbs; 3 with associated fractures	2 ATA; variable durations	2 died; 3 had primary amputations; a serious complication noted from HBOT	Not clearly established
No author[128]	Case series; no control subjects; L-III	21 patients with traumatically amputated limbs/fingers	2-3 ATA; daily/twice daily ~1 week	14 (67%) successfully reimplanted	Yes
Monies-Chass and colleagues[129]	Case series; no control subjects; L-III	7 patients with severe vascular trauma and fractures to the lower extremities; all treated surgically; all had ischemia after surgery	2.8 ATA; 2-hour treatments; 4-20 hours after surgery; mean = 9.5 HBOT treatments	Ischemia resolved in 6 (86.7%) cases; dry gangrene of toes required amputation in one patient; no complications from HBOT	Yes
Shupak and colleagues[130]	Case series; no control subjects; L-III	13 patients with traumatic injuries to lower limbs; 10 had major arterial injuries with fractures	2.4 ATA; twice daily after surgery; mean = 5 treatments	Complete limb salvage in 8 (61.5%); in 4 (30.8%) patients, ischemia level was lowered distally; no O₂ toxicity	Yes
Strauss and Hart[131]	Case series; no control subjects; L-III	20 patients with compartment syndromes; 10 had HBOT before fasciotomy; HBOT for 10 after fasciotomy	2.0 ATA; three/two times a day; mean = 12 treatments; second group mean = 36 treatments	Progression arrested in 100% of first group—none went on to fasciotomies; In second group, preservation of threatened flaps, edema reduction, accelerated angiogensis, and restoration of function were observed	Yes
Radonic and colleagues[132]	Retrospective case series L-III	13 patients with crural artery injuries; 10 with fractures; all surgeries and HBOT; 17 patients for comparison	2.18 ATA; 7-21 treatments; 1-2 hours	Outcomes very good to fair in 12 (92%) with HBOT; in non-HBOT patients, 68.8% had comparable outcomes	Yes
Bouachour and colleagues[133]	PRCT/L-I with placebo for control group	36 patients with fracture-crush injuries; all surgeries within 6 hours of injury; half received HBOT	90 minutes daily at 2.5 ATA for 6 days	17/18 (94%) healed with HBOT vs. 10/18 (55.5%) in control subjects; no complications from HBOT	Yes
Kiyoshige[135]	Small series; no control subjects; L-III	6 patients; 10 amputated digits; all had replantation and HBOT	2.0 ATA; 1-hour treatments for 5 days	Survival in 7 (70%)	Yes
Matos and colleagues[137]	Case series; no control subjects; L-III	23 patients with Gustilo Type III fracture-crush injuries; all had surgeries within 24 hours and HBOT within 72 hours	2.36 ATA; twice daily for 90 minutes; mean = 12 treatments	20 (86.9%) threatened limbs survived and healed	Yes

*Evidence level based on the Eastern Association for the Surgery of Trauma.[127] Criteria for inclusion included: (1) a minimum of five human subjects, (2) publications from 1965 through 2003, and (3) evaluation by a minimum of two trauma experts from different level 1 trauma centers in the United States. Levels of evidence are as follows: level I = prospective, randomized, controlled trials; level II = prospective, noncomparative clinical studies or a retrospective analysis derived from reliable data; level III = retrospective case series or database review.

†Outcomes and benefits of hyperbaric oxygen therapy (HBOT) in these reports are discussed further in the text.

ATA, atmospheres absolute; L, level of evidence; PRCT, prospective, randomized, controlled trial.

Crush Injuries: Penetrating and Blunt Trauma

A 1987 report from the Israel Naval Hyperbaric Institute by Shupak and coworkers[130] describes their experiences using HBOT as an adjunct to managing crush injuries of the extremities. Penetrating trauma accounted for five injuries and blunt trauma for eight. All patients had extensive soft-tissue involvement and peripheral neurologic deficits. Ten of the 13 patients had associated major arterial injuries. All patients had surgery including fasciotomies before starting HBOT. The average time from surgery to starting HBOT was 11.5 (range, 0.5–36) hours. The indication for HBOT was worsening ischemia after surgery had been completed. The time delay from injury to starting HBOT was not given. Examination of the injured extremity including skin color, swelling, motor and sensory function, pulses, and skin temperatures at the line of demarcation between ischemic and healthy tissues was done before and after each HBOT treatment. HBOT was discontinued when no further improvement was noted after two successive treatments. Complete limb salvage was achieved in eight patients. Outcomes did not vary whether the injury was of the blunt or penetrating type. The authors conclude that HBOT is indicated after surgical treatment of crush injuries if doubt exists about the viability of the injured extremity.

Compartment Syndromes

A report on the experiences using HBOT as an adjunct for the management of skeletal muscle-compartment syndromes in 20 patients was published by Strauss and Hart in 1989.[131] The causes of the compartment syndromes were not specified. The patients were divided into two groups on the basis of whether HBOT treatments were initiated before or after fasciotomy surgery. Diagnoses were based on clinical findings, but supplemental information from an electronic manometer became available toward the latter part of the study. Compartment pressures ranged from 15 to 48 mm Hg in those patients for whom measurements were made. None of the 10 patients in whom HBOT was started before surgical decompression of their compartments went on to require fasciotomies. The authors conclude that initiation of HBOT during the lag phase (i.e., time from injury to the development of symptoms requiring fasciotomy) halted progression of the self-perpetuating ischemia-edema cycle and obviated the need for fasciotomy.

In the second group of patients, HBOT was started after fasciotomies had been done. The decisions for doing fasciotomies in this group were largely based on clinical findings at the time the patient was in the operating room for management of concomitant problems such as fractures, blood vessel injuries, and/or acute arterial occlusions. HBOT was started for this group because of anticipated tissue ischemia-related problems from preoperative or intraoperative observations. Objective benefits of HBOT for this group were difficult to quantify. Observations consistent with the mechanisms of HBOT included speeding of edema reduction, improved survivability of questionably viable tissues, more rapid demarcation of living and dead tissues, accelerated angiogenesis, and unexpected neurologic recovery (observed in two patients). The "soft" indications for starting HBOT were inversely related to the patient's host-function status; that is, the more compromised the patient, the more likely the authors were consulted for using HBOT as an adjunct to the management of the residuals of the patient's skeletal muscle-compartment syndromes. This inferred that when the surgeons anticipated poor outcomes in their postfasciotomy patients, HBOT was initiated to mitigate complications and speed coverage/closure of the fasciotomy wound.

Penetrating-Type Vascular Injuries

Radonic and colleagues[132] describe their experience using HBOT as an adjunct for managing 28 patients with combat-related crural (lower extremity) vascular injuries during the Croatian War. All injuries were of the penetrating type. All patients had injuries that required vascular, orthopedic, and plastic surgery management in addition to fasciotomies. Thirteen patients who had a combination of extensive bony and soft-tissue injuries coupled with an ischemic time of greater than 6 hours received HBOT as an adjunct to their management. Good prognostic signs associated with HBOT included increase in blood pressure, improved skin color, increase in temperature on the injured side, and maintenance of temperature. Outcomes were assessed at discharge from the hospital and were described as "very good," "good," or "fair." The authors conclude that HBOT helped decrease the amputation rate.

Crush Injuries and Fractures

A prospective, randomized, controlled study involving fractures associated with crush injuries of the legs was reported by Bouachour and colleagues[133] in 1996. Thirty-six patients were randomized into 2 groups of 18 each with usual orthopedic and surgical interventions in one arm and similar management plus adjunctive use of HBOT in the second. Patients with a history of peripheral vascular disease were excluded. Three findings confirmed the benefits of HBOT. The primary healing of fractures, the need for additional surgeries, and the healing of fractures in patients older than 40 years were all statistically significantly better in the HBOT arm. When a validity scale for prospective, randomized clinical trials was applied,[134] this study had design/methodology flaws, including failures to describe the randomization process, the severity of injury using a grading system, and mention of withdrawals or dropouts. Regardless, the data support the authors' conclusions that HBOT improved healing rates and reduced the need for repetitive surgeries in patients with severe leg fractures.

A second set of findings in Bouachour and colleagues' study[133] confirmed the importance of adequate oxygenation for healing. Transcutaneous oxygen measurements of the injured leg and of the contralateral leg were obtained to generate an index (i.e., $PtcO_2$

[injured leg]/$PtcO_2$ [contralateral leg]). In all fractures that healed, the indices were 0.9 or greater with the differences statistically significant. All patients who received HBOT had ratios greater than 0.9. This suggested that adequate tissue oxygenation made a difference in fracture healing, HBOT improved tissue oxygenation, and HBOT was the intervention that helped to achieve the differences in healing between the HBOT and control arms of the study.

Replantations: Japanese Experiences

Kiyoshige[135] has reported on replantation experiences of 10 digits in 6 patients who sustained crush, avulsion, and degloving amputations. Kiyoshige and coauthors[136] used a color monitoring system to assess postreplantation circulation before and after HBOT. Observations were divided into the following four groups: (1) uneventful, (2) congestion to survival, (3) congestion to necrosis, and (4) necrosis. Seven replants survived and three failed. The three failed digits demonstrated remarkable color changes during HBOT exposures. No color changes were observed in six of the seven surviving digits during the HBOT treatments. Kiyoshige concludes that the differences in color reactions to HBOT may be helpful in making early decisions to use salvage-directed interventions for threatened flaps.

Fracture-Crush Injuries

For completeness, an abstract by Matos and colleagues[137] is included in this review because it integrates evidentiary evidence pertaining to using HBOT for crush injuries and can be used to compare outcomes with those typically reported in the orthopedic literature. Twenty-three patients with Gustilo grade III open fracture-crush injuries were managed with usual orthopedic interventions plus adjunctive HBOT during a 2-year period (1997–1998). Subclassifications of the crush injuries included 7 (30.4%) Gustilo Type III-A (enough soft tissue to cover bone after debridement is completed),

13 (56.5%) Gustilo Type III-B (exposed bone after debridement), and 3 (13%) Gustilo Type III-C (concomitant vascular injury). Most patients received orthopedic and surgical treatment within 24 hours of injury and HBOT within 72 hours. Twenty patients (91.3%) had a successful outcome with preservation of the limb. Three patients (13%) required amputations. Outcomes based on subclassifications were not provided. For comparison purposes, an article published in the orthopedic literature of similar type fracture-crush injuries where HBOT was not used as an adjunct to management had an amputation rate of 22.6% (14 of 62 patients) and other unsatisfactory results in 21% (13 of 62 patients), giving an overall complication rate of 43.5%.[138]

Conclusions

Although the evidentiary evidence supporting the use of HBOT for crush injuries is scant, the conclusions are consistent; that is, HBOT is beneficial. Its effectiveness has been shown in a variety of crush injury types from blunt trauma to penetrating injuries, from compartment syndromes to open fractures, and from vascular trauma to replantations. The mechanisms of HBOT that are applicable to crush injuries and other traumatic ischemias mesh well with the understanding of the pathophysiology of these injuries. Consequently, when pairing the clinical experiences and laboratory data, justification for using HBOT as an adjunct for managing crush injuries is strong. However, in no situation should HBOT be used as a substitute for indicated surgical, orthopedic, and medical interventions.

With predictable complication rates from the most serious crush injury types, it is logical to attempt to improve outcomes with interventions that address the basic mechanisms that initiate the complications. This defines the role of HBOT for crush injuries. When the decision is made to use HBOT, current evidence suggests it should be started as soon after the injury as possible, preferably in the immediate postoperative period. If surgery is delayed, it is desirable to give HBOT while awaiting surgery. The side effects and complications of HBOT are so infrequent and/or minimal that contraindications for using this intervention as an adjunct in the management of crush injuries are almost nonexistent.[139]

Related Applications of Hyperbaric Oxygen for Traumatic Ischemias

The mechanisms of HBOT useful for crush injuries also have applications for related conditions where hypoxia is associated with trauma. These include skeletal muscle-compartment syndromes, thermal burns, cold injuries, threatened flaps and grafts, and compromised replantations. Throughout this chapter, the conditions have been referred to in various capacities including the evidentiary review. The strongest supporting information for using HBOT in skeletal-muscle compartment syndromes comes from methodologically sound laboratory studies.[75,140-144] These studies demonstrate that HBOT interrupts the self-perpetuating edema-ischemia cycle that accounts for the progression of compartment syndrome symptoms with time. Although clinical experiences with using HBOT for skeletal muscle-compartment syndromes are consistent with the expectations from the laboratory studies, a randomized, controlled trial, as is available for crush injuries, has yet to be conducted.[131,145-147]

REFERENCES

1. Gustilo RB, Williams DN: The use of antibiotics in the management of open fractures. Orthopedics 7:1617–1619, 1984.
2. Johansen K, Daines M, Howey T, et al: Objective criteria accurately predict amputation following lower extremity trauma. J Trauma 30:568–572, 1990.
3. Bondurant FJ, Cotler HB, Buckle R, et al: The medical and economic impact of severely injured lower extremities. J Trauma 28:1270–1273, 1988.
4. Gustilo RB, Mendoza RM, Williams DN: Problems in the management of type III (severe) open fractures: A new classification of type III open fractures. J Trauma 24:742–746, 1984.
5. Cierney G II, Mader JT, Penninck JJ: A clinical staging system for adult osteomyelitis. Contemp Orthop 10:17–37, 1985.

6. Christensen O: Mediation of cell volume regulation by Ca^{2+} influx through stretch-activated channels. Nature 330:66–68, 1987.

7. Malinoski DJ, Slater MS, Mullins RJ: Crush injury and rhabdomyolysis. Crit Care Clin 20:171–192, 2004.

8. Gonzalez D: Crush syndrome. Crit Care Med 33:S34–S41, 2005.

9. Gammie JS, Stukus DR, Pham SM, et al: Effect of ischemic time on survival in clinical lung transplantation. Ann Thorac Surg 68:2015–2019, 1999.

10. Pasupathy S, Homer-Vanniasinkam S: Surgical implications of ischemic preconditioning. Arch Surg 140:405–409, 2005.

11. Harris K, Walker PM, Mickel DA, et al: Metabolic response of skeletal muscle to ischemia. Am J Physiol 250:H213–H220, 1986.

12. Ward BJ, McCarthy A: Endothelial cell "swelling" in ischemia and reperfusion. J Mol Cell Cardiol 27:1293–1300, 1995.

13. Bychkov R, Pieper K, Ried C, et al: Hydrogen peroxide, potassium currents, and membrane potential in human endothelial cells. Circulation 99:1719–1725, 1999.

14. Cines DB, Pollak ES, Buck CA, et al: Endothelial cells in physiology and in the pathophysiology of vascular disorders. Blood 91:3527–3561, 1998.

15. Aird WC: Endothelial cell dynamics and complexity theory. Crit Care Med 30(suppl):S180–S185, 2002.

16. Rosenberg RD, Aird WC: Vascular-bed-specific hemostasis and hypercoagulable states. N Engl J Med 340:1555–1564, 1999.

17. Seal JB, Gewertz BL: Vascular dysfunction in ischemia-reperfusion injury. Ann Vasc Surg 19:572–584, 2005.

18. Meredith IT, Currie KE, Anderson TJ, et al: Postischemic vasodilation in human forearms is dependent on endothelium-derived nitric oxide. Am J Physiol Heart Circ Physiol 270:1435–1440, 1996.

19. Sternbergh WC, Makhoul RG, Adelman B: Nitric oxide mediated, endothelium-dependent vasodilation is selectively attenuated in the postischemic extremity. Surgery 114:960–967, 1993.

20. Seccombe JF, Pearson PJ, Schaff HV: Oxygen radical-mediated vascular injury selectively inhibits receptor-dependent release of nitric oxide from canine coronary arteries. J Thorac Cardiovasc Surg 107:505–509, 1994.

21. Shah KA, Samson SE, Grover AK, et al: Effects of peroxide on endothelial nitric oxide synthase in coronary arteries. Mol Cell Biochem 183:147–152, 1998.

22. Ames A, Wright RL, Kowada M, et al: Cerebral ischemia: The no-reflow phenomenon. Am J Pathol 52:437–453, 1968.

23. Jerome SN, Smith CW, Korthuis RJ: CD-18-dependent adherence reactions play an important role in the development of the no-reflow phenomenon. Am J Physiol 264:H479–H483, 1993.

24. Xu Y, Huo Y, Toufektsian MC, et al: Activated platelets contribute importantly to myocardial reperfusion injury. Am J Physiol Heart Circ Physiol 290:H692–H699, 2006.

25. Kurose I, Anderson DC, Miyasaka M, et al: Molecular determinants of reperfusion-induced leukocyte adhesion and vascular protein leakage. Circ Res 74:336–343, 1994.

26. Cooper D, Russell J, Chitman D, et al: Leukocyte dependence of platelet adhesion in postcapillary venules. Am J Physiol Heart Circ Physiol 286:H1895–H1900, 2004.

27. Krieglstein CF, Granger DN: Adhesion molecules and their role in vascular disease. Am J Hypertens 14:44–54, 2001.

28. Bulkley GB: The role of oxygen free radicals in human disease processes. Surgery 94:407–411, 1983.

29. Harlan JM, Winn RK: Leukocyte-endothelial interactions: Clinical trials of anti-adhesion therapy. Crit Care Med 30(suppl):214–219, 2002.

30. Southorn PA, Powis G: Free radicals in medicine. II. Involvement in human disease. Mayo Clin Proc 63:390–408, 1988.

31. Haddad JJ: Oxygen sensing and oxidant/redox-related pathways. Biochem Biophys Res Commun 316:969–977, 2004.

32. Gerschman R, Gilbert DL, Nye SW, et al: Oxygen poisoning and x-irradiation: A mechanism in common. Science 119:623–626, 1954.

33. McCord JM, Fridovich I: The utility of superoxide dismutase in studying free radical reactions. I. Radicals generated by the interaction of sulfite, dimethyl sulfoxide, and oxygen. J Biol Chem 244:6056–6063, 1969.

34. McCord JM, Fridovich I: The utility of superoxide dismutase in studying free radical reactions. II. The mechanism of the mediation of cytochrome c reduction by a variety of electron carriers. J Biol Chem 245:1374–1377, 1970.

35. Babior BM, Kipnes RS, Curnutte JT: Biological defense mechanisms. The production by leukocytes of superoxide, a potential bactericidal agent. J Clin Invest 52:741–744, 1973.

36. Granger DN, Sennett M, McElearney P, et al: Effect of local arterial hypotension on cat intestinal capillary permeability. Gastroenterology 79:474–480, 1980.

37. Granger DN, Rutili G, McCord JM: Superoxide radicals in feline intestinal ischemia. Gastroenterology 81:22–29, 1981.

38. Crimi E, Sica V, Williams-Ignarro S, et al: The role of oxidative stress in adult critical care. Free Radic Biol Med 40:398–406, 2006.

39. Bergamini CM, Gambetti S, Dondi A, et al: Oxygen, reactive oxygen species and tissue damage. Curr Pharm Design 10:1611–1626, 2004.

40. Kurose I, Wolf R, Grisham MB, et al: Modulation of ischemia/reperfusion-induced microvascular dysfunction by nitric oxide. Circ Res 74:376–382, 1994.

41. Tinker AC, Wallace AV: Selective inhibitors of inducible nitric oxide synthase: Potential agents for the treatment of inflammatory diseases? Curr Top Med Chem 6:77–92, 2006.

42. Laroux FS, Pavlick KP, Hines IN, et al: Role of nitric oxide in inflammation. Acta Physiol Scand 173:113–118, 2001.

43. Hein TW, Zhang C, Wang W, et al: Ischemia-reperfusion selectively impairs nitric oxide-mediated dilation in coronary arterioles: Counter-acting role of arginase. FASEB J 17:2328–2330, 2003.

44. Grisham MB, Jourd'Heuil D, Wink DA: Nitric oxide. I. Physiological chemistry of nitric oxide and its

metabolites: Implications in inflammation. Am J Physiol 276:G315-G321, 1999.

45. Gute DC, Ishida T, Yarimizu K, et al: Inflammatory responses to ischemia and reperfusion in skeletal muscle. Mol Cell Biochem 179:169-187, 1998.

46. Ibrahim B, Stoward PJ: The histochemical localization of xanthine oxidase. J Histochem 10:615-617, 1978.

47. Jarasch ED, Bruder G, Heid HW: Significance of xanthine oxidase in capillary endothelial cells. Acta Physiol Scand 548(suppl):39-46, 1986.

48. Weiss SJ: Tissue destruction by neutrophils. N Engl J Med 320:365-376, 1989.

49. Bast A, Haenen GR, Doelman CJ: Oxidants and antioxi- dants: State of the art. Am J Med 91(suppl):2-13, 1991.

50. Brown MJ, Nicholson ML, Bell P, et al: Cytokines and in- flammatory pathways in the pathogenesis of multiple organ failure following abdominal aortic aneurysm repair. Eur J Vasc Surg 22:485-495, 2001.

51. Roumen RM, Hendriks T, Van der Ven-Jongekrijg J, et al: Cytokine patterns in patients alter major vascular surgery, hemorrhagic shock, and severe blunt trauma. Relation with subsequent adult respiratory distress syndrome and multiple organ failure. Ann Surg 218:769-776, 1993.

52. Soda K, Kano Y, Kawakami M, et al: Excessive increase of serum interleukin 6 jeopardizes host defense against multi-bacterial infection. Cytokine 21:295-302, 2003.

53. Zhang F, Hu EC, Gerzenshtein J, et al: The expression of proinflammatory cytokines in the rat muscle flap with ischemia-reperfusion injury. Ann Plast Surg 54:313-317, 2005.

54. Germann G, Drucke D, Steinau HU: Adhesion receptors and cytokine profiles in controlled tourniquet isch- aemia in the upper extremity. J Hand Surg 22B:778- 782, 1997.

55. Chen G, Goeddel DV: TNF-R1 signaling: A beautiful pathway. Science 296:1634-1635, 2002.

56. Senftleben U, Karin M: The IKK/NF-kB pathway. Crit Care Med 30(suppl):18-26, 2002.

57. Fliss H, Gattinger D: Apoptosis in ischemic and reper- fused rat myocardium. Circ Res 79:949-956, 1996.

58. Sumer BD, Gastman BR, Gao F, et al: Caspase inhibition enhances ischemic tolerance of fasciocutaneous flaps. Laryngoscope 115:1358-1361, 2005.

59. Quadri SM, Segall L, de Perrot M, et al: Caspase inhibi- tion improves ischemia-reperfusion injury alter lung transplantation. Am J Transplant 5:292-299, 2005.

60. Kyriakides C, Austern W Jr, Wang Y, et al: Skeletal muscle reperfusion injury is mediated by neutrophils and the complement membrane attack complex. Am J Physiol 277:C1263-C1268, 1999.

61. Chan RK, Ibrahim SI, Verna N, et al: Ischaemia-reperfusion is an event triggered by immune complexes and comple- ment. Br J Surg 90:1470-1478, 2003.

62. Arumugam TV, Magnus T, Woodruff TM, et al: Comple- ment mediators in ischemia-reperfusion injury. Clin Chim Acta 374:33-45, 2006.

63. Ciechanover A: Intracellular protein degradation: From a vague idea thru the lysosome and the ubiquitin- proteasome system and onto human disease and drug targeting. Cell Death Differ 12:1178-1190, 2005.

64. Kukan M: Emerging roles of proteasomes in ischemia- reperfusion injury of organs. J Physiol Pharmacol 55:3-15, 2004.

65. Seiffert M, Gosenca D, Ponelies N, et al: Regulation of the ubiquitin proteasome system in mechanically injured human skeletal muscle. Physiol Res 56:227-233, 2007.

66. Pye J, Ardeshirpour F, McCain A, et al: Proteasome inhibition ablates activation of NF-κB in myocardial reperfusion and reduces reperfusion injury. Am J Physiol Heart Circ Physiol 284:H919-H926, 2003.

67. Elliot PJ, Zollner TM, Boehncke WH: Proteasome inhibition: A new anti-inflammatory strategy. J Mol Med 81:235-245, 2003.

68. Di Napoli M, McLaughlin B: The ubiquitin-proteasome system as a drug target in cerebrovascular disease: Therapeutic potential of proteasome inhibitors. Curr Opin Investig Drugs 6:686-699, 2005.

69. Strauss M: Crush injury, compartment syndrome and other acute traumatic peripheral ischemias. In: Kindwall EP (ed): Hyperbaric Medicine Practice, 2nd ed. rev. Flagstaff, Ariz, Best Publishing Company, 2004, pp 753-771.

70. Wells CH, Goodpasture JE, Horrigan DJ, et al: Tissue gas measurements during hyperbaric oxygen exposure. In: Smith G (ed): Proceed Sixth International Congress on Hyperbaric Medicine. Aberdeen, United Kingdom, Aberdeen University Press, 1977, pp 118-124.

71. Boerema I, Meijne NG, Brummelkamp WK, et al: Life without blood. A study of the influence of high atmo- spheric pressure and hypothermia on dilution of the blood. J Cardiovasc Surg 1:136-143, 1960.

72. Hunt TK, Linsey M, Grislis G, et al: The effect of differ- ing ambient oxygen tensions on wound infection. Ann Surg 181:35-39, 1975.

73. Bird AD, Telfer ABM: Effect of hyperbaric oxygen on limb circulation. Lancet 1:355-356, 1965.

74. Nylander G, Lewis D, Nordstrom H, et al: Reduction of postischemic edema with hyperbaric oxygen. Plast Reconstr Surg 76:596-603, 1985.

75. Strauss MB, Hargens AR, Gershuni DH, et al: Reduction of skeletal muscle necrosis using intermittent hyper- baric oxygen in a model compartment syndrome. J Bone Joint Surg 65A:656-662, 1983.

76. Hohn DC: Oxygen and leukocyte microbial killing. In: Davis JC, Hunt TK, eds. Hyperbaric oxygen therapy. Bethesda, Md, Undersea Medical Society, 1977, pp 101-110.

77. Buras J: Basic mechanisms of hyperbaric oxygen in the treatment of ischemia-reperfusion injury. Int Anesthesiol Clin 38:91-108, 2000.

78. Zamboni WA, Roth AC, Rusell RC, et al: The effect of acute hyperbaric oxygen therapy on axial pattern skin flap survival when administered during and after total ischemia. J Reconstr Microsurg 5:343-347, 1989.

79. Zamboni WA, Roth AC, Russell RC, et al: The effect of hyperbaric oxygen on reperfusion of ischemic axial skin flaps: A laser Doppler analysis. Ann Plast Surg 28:339-341, 1992.

80. Zamboni WA, Roth AC, Russell RC, et al: Morphologic analysis of the microcirculation during reperfusion of ischemic skeletal muscle and the effect of hyperbaric oxygen. Plast Reconstr Surg 91:1110-1123, 1993.

81. Atochin DN, Fisher D, Demchenko IT, et al: Neutrophil sequestration and the effect of hyperbaric oxygen in a rat model of temporary middle cerebral artery occlusion. Undersea Hyperb Med 27:185–190, 2000.

82. Steinberg H, Das DK, Cerreta JM, et al: Neutrophil kinetics in O2-exposed rabbits. J Appl Physiol 61:775–779, 1986.

83. Zamboni WA, Wong HP, Stephenson LL: Effect of hyperbaric oxygen on neutrophil concentration and pulmonary sequestration in reperfusion injury. Arch Surg 131:756–760, 1996.

84. Tjarnstrom J, Wikstrom T, Bagge U, et al: Effects of hyperbaric oxygen treatment on neutrophil activation and pulmonary sequestration in intestinal ischemia-reperfusion in rats. Eur Surg Res 31:147–154, 1999.

85. Thom SR: Functional inhibition of leukocyte B2 integrins by hyperbaric oxygen in carbon monoxide-mediated brain injury in rats. Toxicol Appl Pharmacol 123:248–256, 1993.

86. Thom S: Leukocytes in carbon monoxide-mediated brain oxidative injury. Toxicol Appl Pharmacol 123:234–247, 1993.

87. Thom SR: Effects of hyperoxia on neutrophil adhesion. Undersea Hyperb Med 31:123–131, 2004.

88. Larson JL, Stephenson LL, Zamboni WA: Effects of hyperbaric oxygen on neutrophil CD18 expression. Plast Reconstr Surg 105:1375–1381, 2000.

89. Hong JP, Kwon H, Chung YK, et al: The effect of hyperbaric oxygen on ischemia-reperfusion injury. An experimental study in a rat musculocutaneous flap. Ann Plast Surg 51:478–487, 2003.

90. Buras JA, Stahl GL, Svoboda K, et al: Hyperbaric oxygen downregulates ICAM-1 expression induced by hypoxia and hypoglycemia: The role of NOS. Am J Physiol Cell Physiol 278:C292–C302, 2000.

91. Yamashita M, Yamashita M: Hyperbaric oxygen treatment attenuates cytokine induction after massive hemorrhage. Am J Physiol Endocrinol Metab 278: E811–E816, 2000.

92. Yang Z, Bosco G, Montante A, et al: Hyperbaric O2 reduces intestinal ischemia-reperfusion-induced TNF-α production and lung neutrophil sequestration. Eur J Appl Physiol 85:96–103, 2001.

93. Mickel HS, Vaishnav YN, Kempski O, et al: Breathing 100% oxygen after global brain ischemia in Mongolian gerbils results in increased lipid peroxidation and increased mortality. Stroke 18:426–430, 1987.

94. Bernareggi M, Radice S, Rossoni G, et al: Hyperbaric oxygen increases plasma exudation in rat trachea: Involvement of nitric oxide. Br J Pharmacol 126:794–800, 1999.

95. Dennog C, Hartmann A, Frey G, et al: Detection of DNA damage after hyperbaric oxygen (HBO) therapy. Mutagenesis 11:605–609, 1996.

96. Speit G, Dennog C, Lampi L: Biological significance of DNA damage induced by hyperbaric oxygen. Mutagenesis 13:85–87, 1998.

97. Rothfuss A, Radermacher P, Speit G: Involvement of heme oxygenase-1 (HO-1) in the adaptive protection of human lymphocytes after hyperbaric oxygen (HBO) treatment. Carcinogenesis 22:1979–1985, 2001.

98. Speit G, Bonzheim I: Genotoxic and protective effects of hyperbaric oxygen in A549 lung cells. Mutagenesis 18:545–548, 2003.

99. Clark JE, Foresti R, Green CJ, et al: Dynamics of haem oxygenase-1 expression and bilirubin production in cellular protection against oxidative stress. Biochem J 34:615–619, 2000.

100. Dennog C, Radermacher P, Barnett YA, et al: Antioxidant status in humans after exposure to hyperbaric oxygen. Mutat Res 428:83–89, 1999.

101. Chang-Hyung K, Hong C, Yang-Sook C, et al: Hyperbaric oxygenation pretreatment induces catalase and reduces infarct size in ischemic rat myocardium. Eur J Physiol 442:519–525, 2001.

102. Gregorevic P, Lynch GS, Williams DA: Hyperbaric oxygen modulates antioxidant enzyme activity in rat skeletal muscles. Eur J Appl Physiol 86:24–27, 2001.

103. Vlodavsky E, Palzur E, Feinsod M, et al: Evaluation of the apoptosis-related proteins of the BCL-2 family in the traumatic penumbra area of the rat model of cerebral contusion, treated by hyperbaric oxygen: A quantitative immunohistochemical study. Acta Neuropathol 110:120–126, 2005.

104. Guimaraes FA, Taha MO, Simoes MJ, et al: Apoptosis and nuclear proliferation in rat small bowel submitted to hypothermic hyperbaric oxygenation for preservation.

105. Yuan LJ, Ueng S, Lin SS, et al: Attenuation of apoptosis and enhancement of proteoglycan synthesis in rabbit cartilage defects by hyperbaric oxygen treatment are related to the suppression of nitric oxide production. J Orthop Res 22:1126–1134, 2004.

106. Ganguly BJ, Tonomura N, Benson RM, et al: Hyperbaric oxygen enhances apoptosis in hematopoietic cells. Apoptosis 7:499–510, 2002.

107. Conconi MT, Baiguera S, Guidolin D, et al: Effects of hyperbaric oxygen on proliferative and apoptotic activities and reactive oxygen species generation in Mouse fibroblast 3T3/J2 cell line. J Investig Med 51:227–232, 2003.

108. Guyton AC, Hall JE: Medical Textbook of Physiology, 10th ed. Philadelphia, WB Saunders, 2000, p 389.

109. Hurd TC, Dasmhapatra KS, Rush BF, Machiedo GW: Red blood cell deformability in human and experimental sepsis. Arch Surg 123:217–220, 1988.

110. Powell RJ, Machiedo GW, Rush BF: Decreased red blood cell deformability and impaired oxygen utilization during human sepsis. Am Surg 59:65–68, 1993.

111. Mathieu D, Coget J, Vinkier L, et al: Red blood cell deformability and hyperbaric oxygen therapy [abstract]. HBO Review 6:280, 1985.

112. Thom SR, Lauermann MW, Hart GB: Intermittent hyperbaric oxygen therapy for reduction of mortality in experimental polymicrobial sepsis. J Infect Dis 154:504–510, 1986.

113. Smith G, Stevens J, Griffiths JC, et al: Near-avulsion of foot treated by replacement and subsequent prolonged exposure of patients to oxygen at two atmospheres pressure. Lancet 2:1122–1123, 1961.

114. Strauss MB: Role of hyperbaric oxygen in acute ischemias and crush injuries—an orthopedic perspective. HBO Rev 2:87–106, 1981.

115. Garcia-Covarrubias L, McSwain NE, Van Meter K, et al: Adjuvant hyperbaric oxygen therapy in the management of crush injury and traumatic ischemia: An evidenced-based approach. Am Surg 71:144–151, 2005.

116. Illingworth CFW, Smith G, Lawson DD, et al: Surgical and physiological observations in an experimental pressure chamber. Br J Surg 49:222-227, 1961.

117. Maudsley RH, Hopkinson WI, Williams KG: Vascular injury treated with high pressure oxygen in a mobile chamber. J Bone Joint Surg 2:346-350, 1963.

118. Slack WK, Thomas DA, De Jode LRJ: Hyperbaric oxygen in the treatment of trauma, ischemic disease of limbs and varicose ulceration. In: Brown IW, Cox BG (eds): Proceedings of the Third International Conference Hyperbaric Medicine. Washington, DC, National Academy of Science, National Research Council, Publication 1404, 1966. pp 621-624.

119. Székely O, Szánto G, Takats A: Hyperbaric oxygen therapy in injured subjects. Injury 4:294-300, 1973.

120. Schramek A, Hashmonai M: Vascular injuries in the extremities in battle casualties. Br J Surg 64:644-648, 1977.

121. Loder RE: Hyperbaric oxygen therapy in acute trauma. Ann R Coll Surg Engl 61:472-473, 1979.

122. Lukich VL, Fillimonova TS, Fokina LL, et al: Employment of hyperbaric oxygenation in out-patients. Khirurgiia 2:82-86, 1976.

123. Davidkin NF: Experience with clinical use of hyperbaric oxygenation in trauma and their complications. Ortop Traumatol Protez 9:33-35, 1977.

124. Gismondi AG, Colonna SS: Possible use of hyperbaric oxygen in the treatment of certain vascular diseases. Ann Med Nav 83:547-558, 1978.

125. Isakov YV, Atroschenko ZB, Bailik IF, et al: Hyperbaric oxygenation in the prophylaxis of wound infection in the open trauma of the locomotor system. Vestn Khir 123:117-121, 1979.

126. Lukich VL, Filimonova MV, Bazarova VS: Changes of the gaseous exchange in hyperbaric oxygenation in patients with regional ischemia. Vrach Delo 3:39-43, 1979.

127. EAST Ad Hoc Committee on Practice Management Guideline Development 2000. Utilizing Evidence Based Outcome Measures to Develop Practice Management Guidelines: A Primer. EAST Web site, 1998. Available at: http://www.east.org/tpg.html. Accessed April 12, 2003.

128. Hyperbaric oxygen therapy in replantation of severed limbs. A report of 21 cases. Chin Med J 1:197-204, 1975.

129. Monies-Chass I, Hashmonai M, Hoerer D, et al: Hyperbaric oxygen treatment as an adjuvant to reconstructive vascular surgery in trauma. Injury 8:274-277, 1977.

130. Shupak A, Gozal D, Ariel A, et al: Hyperbaric oxygenation in acute peripheral posttraumatic ischemia. J Hyperb Med 2:7-14, 1987.

131. Strauss MB, Hart GB: Hyperbaric oxygen and the skeletal muscle-compartment syndrome. Contemp Orthop 18:167-174, 1989.

132. Radonic V, Baric D, Petricevic A, et al: War injuries of the crural arteries. Br J Surg 82:777-783, 1995.

133. Bouachour G, Cronier P, Gouello JP, et al: Hyperbaric oxygen therapy in the management of crush injuries: A randomized double-blind placebo-controlled clinical trial. J Trauma 41:333-339, 1996.

134. Jadad AR, Moore RA, Carroll D, et al: Assessing the quality of reports of randomized clinical trials: Is blinding necessary? Controlled Clin Trials 17:1-12, 1996.

135. Kiyoshige Y: Effect of hyperbaric oxygen therapy as a monitoring technique for digital replantation survival. J Reconstr Microsurg 15:327-330, 1999.

136. Kiyoshige Y, Tsuchida H, Watanabe Y: Color monitoring after replantation. Plast Reconstr Surg 97:463-468, 1996.

137. Matos LA, Hutson JJ, Bonet H, et al: HBO as an adjunct treatment for limb salvage in crush injuries of the extremities [abstract]. Undersea Hyperb Med 26(suppl):66-67, 1999.

138. Caudle RJ, Stern PJ: Severe open fractures of the tibia. J Bone Joint Surg Am 69:801-807, 1987.

139. Kindwall EP: Contraindications and side effects to hyperbaric oxygen treatment. In: Kindwall EP, Whelan HT (eds): Hyperbaric Medicine Practice, 2nd ed. Flagstaff, Ariz, Best Publishing, 1999, pp 83-98.

140. Bartlett RL, Stroman RT, Nickels M, et al: Rabbit model of the use of fasciotomy and hyperbaric oxygen in the treatment of compartment syndrome. Undersea Hyperb Med 25(suppl):29, 1998.

141. Nylander G, Nordstr H, Granzen I, et al: Effects of hyperbaric oxygen in post-ischemic muscle. Scand J Plast Reconstr Surg 22:31-39, 1988.

142. Nylander, G, Otamiri DH, Larsson J: Lipid products in postischemic skeletal muscle and after treatment with hyperbaric oxygen. Sand J Plast Reconstr Surg 23:97-103, 1989.

143. Skyhar MJ, Hargens AR, Strauss MB, et al: Hyperbaric oxygen reduces edema and necrosis of skeletal muscle in compartment syndromes associate with hemorrhagic hypotension. J Bone Joint Surg 68A:1218-1224, 1986.

144. Strauss MB, Hargens AR, Gershuni DH, et al: Delayed use of hyperbaric oxygen for treatment of a model compartment syndrome. J Orthop Res 4:108-111, 1986.

145. Fitzpatrick DT, Murphy PT, Bryce M: Adjunctive treatment of compartment syndrome with hyperbaric oxygen. Mil Med 163:577-579, 1998.

146. Oriani G: Acute indications of HBO therapy-final report. In: Oriani G, Marroni A, Wattel F (eds): Handbook on Hyperbaric Medicine. New York, Springer, 1996, pp 93-103.

147. Strauss MB: Hyperbaric oxygen for crush injuries and compartment syndromes: Surgical considerations. In: Bakker DJ, Cramer FS (eds): Hyperbaric Surgery: Perioperative Care. Flagstaff, Ariz, Best Publishing, 2002, pp 341-359.

Evidence and Hyperbaric Oxygen Therapy

Summarizing the Literature and a Review of Some Unconventional Indications

21

Michael H. Bennett, MBBS, MD, MM(Clin Epi), FANZCA, Robert J. Turner, MBBS, FANZCA, DipDHM, Jan P. Lehm, MD, FANZCA, DipDHM, and Herbert B. Newton, MD, FAAN

The preceding chapters have detailed the physiology, medicine, and clinical evidence behind the commonly accepted indications for hyperbaric oxygen therapy (HBOT). This chapter introduces several indications that are not widely accepted, but where there is either a growing body of evidence in support of using HBOT, or where the application of HBOT as a routine is already advocated by some practitioners. For some of these indications, accumulating evidence may continue to support the effectiveness of HBOT, whereas for others, it appears more likely that any further evidence will confirm that HBOT does not improve important clinical outcomes.

To summarize the state of the clinical evidence for many of these indications, this chapter draws on recently published systematic reviews (SRs) of the use of HBOT. In particular, there has been a flurry of activity within the Cochrane Collaboration with the publication of 14 full reviews from 2002 to 2007. This chapter therefore begins with a discussion of the nature and purpose of an SR, as well as some details on how such reviews are generated. Then the case for and against 10 individual indications is discussed in detail.

SUMMARIZING THE CLINICAL EVIDENCE

Systematic Reviews

The growing acceptance of a formal, evidence-based approach to medicine has led to the development of explicit methodologies for summarizing the literature. An SR may be defined as a literature review that focuses on a specific question and that tries to identify, appraise, select, and synthesize all high-quality clinical research evidence relevant to that question.[1] Although increasing numbers of "independent" SRs are appearing in the medical literature, the Cochrane Collaboration, a global not-for-profit international organization involving thousands of academics and clinicians, has promulgated a particular methodology for SRs. There are currently more than 100,000 individual reviews on their database (www.thecochranelibrary.com). The cardinal feature that separates "systematic" reviews from the more general literature review is the systematic and explicit approach to each of the steps included in that definition. An SR will contain a clear articulation of the question the review is designed to address, clear inclusion and exclusion criteria, an explicit search strategy designed to be sensitive to appropriate literature, and an explicit methodology for the critical appraisal and synthesis of included information. These reviews should then present clear conclusions and recommendations consistent with the evidence located and appraised.

Although these reviews aim to include the evaluation of "all high-quality research evidence," they do not have to be confined to studies of a particular methodology. If there are no truly high-quality trials, then it is appropriate that a review examine in detail the highest quality evidence available. It is likely, however, that such reviews will be able to draw only weak recommendations for practice.

Meta-analysis

Meta-analysis is the quantitative analysis of the results included in an SR. In practice, this implies the combination of the results of several individual clinical trials using specialized statistical methodology. Such analyses are essentially observational, using trials as the unit of enrollment rather than individual patients. Although there is some room for dispute, most authorities agree that such analysis is likely to have high validity only if the individual trials are randomized controlled trials (RCTs). Although meta-analyses of cohort trials are not uncommon, the conclusions to be drawn from such reviews remain unclear.[2-4] If the included trials are subject to bias, then any meta-analysis is similarly subject to bias. The strength of meta-analysis lies in the ability to summarize a large volume of literature in a single publication and to produce clinically relevant conclusions. Meta-analysis can generate sufficient power from a series of smaller trials to answer important clinical questions. In the absence of meta-analysis, the combination of a series of small trials with low individual power can lead to confusion about appropriate therapeutic decisions.

Prior experience suggests that meta-analysis might not only make the evidence clear and unequivocal, but also avoid unnecessary and wasteful repetition of research performed in the belief that the "truth" is not yet evident. A good example is that described by Lau and colleagues[5] concerning trials of the use of streptokinase for the prevention of myocardial infarction. Lau found 33 such trials executed between 1959 and 1988. The authors performed a cumulative meta-analysis, repeating analysis with each study chronologically by publication date, and found a consistent and significant reduction in mortality with the use of streptokinase had already been found by 1973 (odds ratio [OR], 0.74; 95% confidence interval [CI], 0.59–0.92). At that time only eight trials involving 2432 subjects were available for analysis. The results of the 25 subsequent trials, enrolling an additional 34,542 patients, through 1988 had little or no effect on the OR. All those trial subjects had contributed limited information concerning the efficacy of streptokinase.

Reviews in This Chapter

This chapter reviews 10 conditions for which there is no general consensus that HBOT is indicated as a routine element of management. For some conditions, reasonable agreement exists that HBOT is *not* indicated; for others, it is probable that further work will define a place for HBOT.

Where possible, we have relied on published Cochrane SRs with meta-analysis. For a more detailed review of these indications, interested readers are referred to those reviews. Where no SR has been published, we have tried to present the available data in a systematic way.

SELECTED POTENTIAL INDICATIONS FOR HYPERBARIC OXYGEN THERAPY

Summary of the Literature

The Cochrane reviews referred to in these summaries are published in The Cochrane Library (Chichester, United Kingdom, John Wiley & Sons, Ltd.; www.thecochranelibrary.com). The relevant material is reproduced with permission. Cochrane reviews are updated regularly as new evidence emerges and in response to comments and criticisms. The Cochrane Library should be consulted for the most recent version of these reviews. Please note that the results of a Cochrane review can be interpreted differently, depending on people's perspectives and circumstances. The conclusions are the opinions of the authors and are not necessarily shared by The Cochrane Collaboration.

Acute Coronary Syndrome

Cardiovascular disease remains the leading cause of death in developed countries, and it is predicted to become the disease with the greatest global burden by 2020.[6] In the United Kingdom, coronary heart disease is the most common cause of premature death, causing 125,000 deaths from approximately 274,000 episodes in 2000, at a community cost of about £10 billion.[7,8] Because myocardial infarction (the presence of two of the following three conditions: chest pain, electrocardiographic changes, and increase of cardiac enzyme level) is not always diagnosable during an acute event, unstable and persisting ischemic heart pain (angina) with or without infarction are described together as acute coronary syndrome (ACS).

The main underlying problem in coronary heart disease is atherosclerosis, a degenerative process characterized by the formation of plaques composed of platelets, cells, matrix fibers, lipids, and tissue debris in the vessel lumen. Although such plaques are often complicated by ulceration of the vessel wall with obstruction to blood flow, such ulceration is not necessary for plaques to be problematic.[9] An unstable plaque (coronary atheroma vulnerable to rupture and fissure, and associated with thrombus formation) can lead to an ACS without the artery being totally occluded and infarction may follow.[10] A significant proportion of patients admitted with acute myocardial infarction will suffer a major morbidity or mortality, even when thrombolysis or angioplasty is used to relieve the obstruction.[11]

Therapy

The aim of acute therapy for ACS is to treat life-threatening arrhythmias (commonly ventricular fibrillation and bradycardia/asystole) and to prevent the development of heart failure by minimizing the extent of any myocardial infarction. Comprehensive and evidence-based guidelines for the early management of these conditions have been published in both Europe and the Unites States.[12,13] Acute measures include the administration of oxygen, glyccryl trinitrate, and morphine. The overall aim is to relieve pain, dilate the coronary arteries to improve oxygenation of the myocardium, and dilate venous capacitance vessels to relieve pulmonary congestion.

Additional measures shown to be of benefit include the administration of some combinations of aspirin, thrombolysis, heparin, antiplatelet agents (e.g., clopidogrel), and percutaneous stenting of the coronary vessels. Many of these interventions have been shown to be time critical; for example, thrombolysis is most effective within 3 hours of the onset of symptoms. Most recently, coronary angioplasty with or without stent placement has become the first-line treatment of myocardial infarction with S-T segment elevation when it can be delivered within 90 minutes of first contact. Preventative interventions should also be started early, and these include beta-blockers, statins, and angiotensin-converting enzyme inhibitors.

HBOT has been proposed as an adjunctive measure to improve outcome after ACS. The administration of HBOT is based on the arguments that the myocardium is hypoxic and that HBOT can reverse that hypoxia in areas that are marginally perfused. This effect is achieved by greatly increasing the diffusion gradient down which oxygen moves from the blood to the myocyte. Improved oxygen availability may also improve outcome through the effects of oxygen as a modulator of tissue repair. Oxygen has been shown to increase the expression of antioxidant enzymes in both tissues and plasma through an increase in glutathione levels,[14,15] to reduce the degree of lipid peroxidation[16] and to prevent the activation of neutrophils in response to endothelial damage, thus modifying ischemia-reperfusion injury.[17]

Evidence

First reported in a canine experimental model in 1958, hyperbaric oxygen (HBO) was associated with greatly improved survival in the short term (10% vs. 60% at 2 hours),[18] and generally positive findings were confirmed in a series of similar models over the next few years.[19-21] Some evidence also exists that HBOT may be further protective when used in combination with thrombolysis. In 1990, Thomas and colleagues[22] demonstrated a benefit in infarct size after the administration of both recombinant tissue plasminogen activator and HBOT at 2 ATA compared with either alone in a dog model. Not all trials have been supportive, however.[23,24] The relevance of all these animal models has been questioned because of interspecies differences in coronary anatomy, the absence of atherosclerotic disease, and the generally short delays to the institution of therapy.[25]

HBOT was first reported as a measure to treat acute myocardial infarction in a human subject in 1964.[26] Several uncontrolled human studies have been published since that time, generally with indications of benefit measured as a reduction in mortality or improvements in

hemodynamic or metabolic parameters.[27,28] These early clinical reports are summarized in Table 21.1.

Since 1973, there have been six RCTs reported where HBOT has been administered after ACS: Dekleva (2004)[31]; Sharifi (2004)[31a]; Stavitsky (1998)[31b]; Shandling (1997)[31c]; Swift (1992)[31d]; and Thurston (1973).[31e] All except Dekleva (2004) were appraised in a Cochrane SR.[32] The following summary incorporates the new data into the published review.

Cochrane Review

Search results identified seven reports of six clinical trials of HBOT for ACS; Shandling (1997) and Stavitsky (1998) are reports from the same Hyperbaric Oxygen Therapy for Myocardial Infarction (HOTMI) study, but they report different outcomes and were both included. Together, these trials include a total of 499 subjects, 247 subjects receiving HBOT and 252 control subjects (Table 21.2 provides a summary of the characteristics of these studies).

All studies involve the administration of 100% oxygen at 2 ATA for between 30 and 120 minutes; however, the total number of treatment sessions varies between studies. The lowest number administered is a single session (Stavitsky, 1998; Swift, 1992; Dekleva, 2004), whereas the highest is a maximum of 16 treatments within

Table 21.1 Summary of Nonrandom Clinical Reports on the Use of HBOT to Treat ACS

TRIAL	METHODOLOGY	THERAPY	OUTCOMES
Cameron and colleagues (1965)[27]	10 men with AMI within 24 hours	2 ATA 100% oxygen with 30-minute air break; 1 treatment only	Decreased cardiac output, increased SVR and SBP
Ashfield and colleagues (1969)[28]	40 patients with AMI within 24 hours and "seriously ill"	2 ATA 2 hours followed by 1 ATA on air; repeat for up to 4 days	15% mortality rate, improved pain and dyspnea
Veselka and colleagues (1999)[29]	17 patients with history of MI	Dobutamine stress echo followed by HBOT at 2 ATA for 90 minutes and TOE	HBO can detect viable myocardium with about the same performance as dobutamine
Moon and colleagues (1964)[26]	1 patient in cardiogenic shock	48 hours of HBOT	Successful outcome
Hood (1968)[30]	1 patient with refractory VT 3 weeks after anterolateral MI	3 ATA 100% oxygen for 15 minutes, then 2 ATA for 7 hours; 2 such sessions	Improvement in tachyarrhythmias; discharged day 25

Excludes Russian literature where no translation available.

AMI, acute myocardial infarction; ATA, atmospheres absolute; HBO, hyperbaric oxygen; HBOT, hyperbaric oxygen therapy; MI, myocardial infarction; SBP, systolic blood pressure; SVR, systemic vascular resistance; TOE, transesophageal echocardiogram; VT, ventricular tachycardia.

Table 21.2 Characteristics of Studies Included in the Review of HBOT for ACS

STUDY	METHODS	PARTICIPANTS	INTERVENTIONS	OUTCOMES
Stavitsky (1998)[31b]	Multicenter RCT; no blinding; 16 subjects excluded after randomization	138 subjects with AMI clinical diagnosis and who were eligible for thrombolysis were enrolled in emergency department	Control: thrombolysis, aspirin, heparin and IVI nitroglycerin. HBOT: same plus 2 ATA oxygen for 2 hours	Death, time to pain relief, enzyme change, LVEF
Shandling (1997)[31c]	As for Stavitsky, 1998	82 subjects (41 HBOT and 41 control)	As for Stavitsky, 1998	Length of stay
Sharifi (2004)[31a]	RCT; no blinding; 5 patients crossed allocation	69 subjects (33 HBOT, 36 control) with AMI or unstable angina; excluded if pain or S-T segments unresolved after 30 minutes	Control: stenting and aspirin, heparin, and clopidogrel HBOT: same, plus 2 ATA oxygen for 90 minutes at 1 and 18 hours	MACE, adverse events
Swift (1992)[31d]	RCT (2 active for each control); no loss to follow-up; subjects and assessors blind	34 subjects (24 HBOT, 10 control) with clinical diagnosis of AMI within the past week, plus abnormal wall motion on TOE	Control: echo, 2 ATA breathing air for 30 minutes and repeat HBOT: oxygen at 2 ATA between echoes	Improved left ventricular function on echocardiography
Thurston (1973)[31e]	RCT; no blinding after allocation to group	221 subjects (110 HBOT, 111 control) with strong clinical probability of AMI at admission; 13 later excluded	Control: "coronary care including oxygen by mask" HBOT: 48 hours of oxygen at 2 ATA for 2 hours, followed by 1 hour on air at 1 ATA	Death, significant dysrhythmias, adverse effects
Dekleva (2004)[31]	RCT using random number table; outcome assessor blind	74 subjects (37 each group) with AMI within 24 hours	Control: streptokinase 1.5 mU/L HBOT: plus 60 minutes oxygen at 2 ATA	Enzyme changes, LVEF

AMI, acute myocardial infarction; ATA, atmospheres absolute; HBOT, hyperbaric oxygen therapy; IVI, intravenous by infusion; LVEF, left ventricular ejection fraction; MACE, major adverse coronary event; RCT, randomized, controlled trial; TOE, transesophageal echo.

48 hours (Thurston, 1973). All trials include participants with acute myocardial infarction, and Sharifi (2004) also includes individuals presenting with unstable angina. Only Swift (1992) describes allocation concealment and blinded subjects to allocation with a sham HBOT session. The time from presentation to enrollment varied from within 1 week (Swift, 1992) to within 24 hours (Thurston, 1973; Dekleva, 2004) and within 6 hours (Stavitsky, 1998; Shandling, 1997). Sharifi (2004) does not state any time. The primary purpose of three of these reports is the treatment of acute myocardial infarction with HBOT, whereas for Swift (1992) it is the use of HBOT in acute myocardial infarction patients to identify myocardial segments capable of functional improvement, and for Sharifi (2004) the

effect of HBOT on restenosis after percutaneous coronary interventions.

Stavitsky (1998), Shandling (1997), and Dekleva (2004) exclude subjects who were not suitable for thrombolysis (e.g., recent stroke) and those in cardiogenic shock, whereas Swift (1992) and Dekleva (2004) exclude those with uncontrolled heart failure and/or significant ongoing angina. Comparator therapies also varied between trials, and the details were not always clearly stated. All trials used HBOT as an adjunctive procedure to "standard" care.

Three trials report the number of subjects who died at any time after enrollment (Sharifi 2004; Stavitsky 1998; Thurston 1973). Fewer subjects died after HBOT, but the difference is not statistically significant (9.7% vs. 14.1%; the relative risk [RR] of dying was 0.64; 95% CI, 0.38-1.06; $P = 0.08$), and there was no statistically significant reduction on subgroup analysis for those presenting in cardiogenic shock (cardiogenic shock: RR, 0.57; 95% CI, 0.3-1.09; $P = 0.09$; without cardiogenic shock: RR, 0.65; 95% CI, 0.35-1.2; $P = 0.17$) (Fig. 21.1).

The risk for suffering a major adverse coronary event (MACE) was reported by Sharifi (2004) at 8 months, with one subject (4.2%) suffering a MACE after HBOT versus eight subjects (35.1%) in the control group (RR, 0.12; 95% CI, 0.01-0.61; $P = 0.01$). The number needed to treat (NNT) to avoid one extra MACE was four (95% CI, 3-10).

Thurston (1973) reports the incidence of significant dysrhythmia (complete heart block, ventricular fibrillation, or asystole). Twenty-five such events were reported in the patients receiving HBOT versus 43 such events in the control group, and patients receiving HBOT were significantly less likely to suffer one of these dysrhythmias (RR, 0.59; 95% CI, 0.39-0.89, $P = 0.01$; NNT = 6; 95% CI, 3-24). Separate analyses for each of the three dysrhythmias suggested HBOT patients were significantly less likely to experience complete heart block (RR, 0.32; 95% CI, 0.12-0.84; $P = 0.02$) but not ventricular fibrillation (RR, 0.78; 95% CI, 0.36-1.71; $P = 0.54$) or asystole (RR, 0.73; 95% CI, 0.73-1.56; $P = 0.42$).

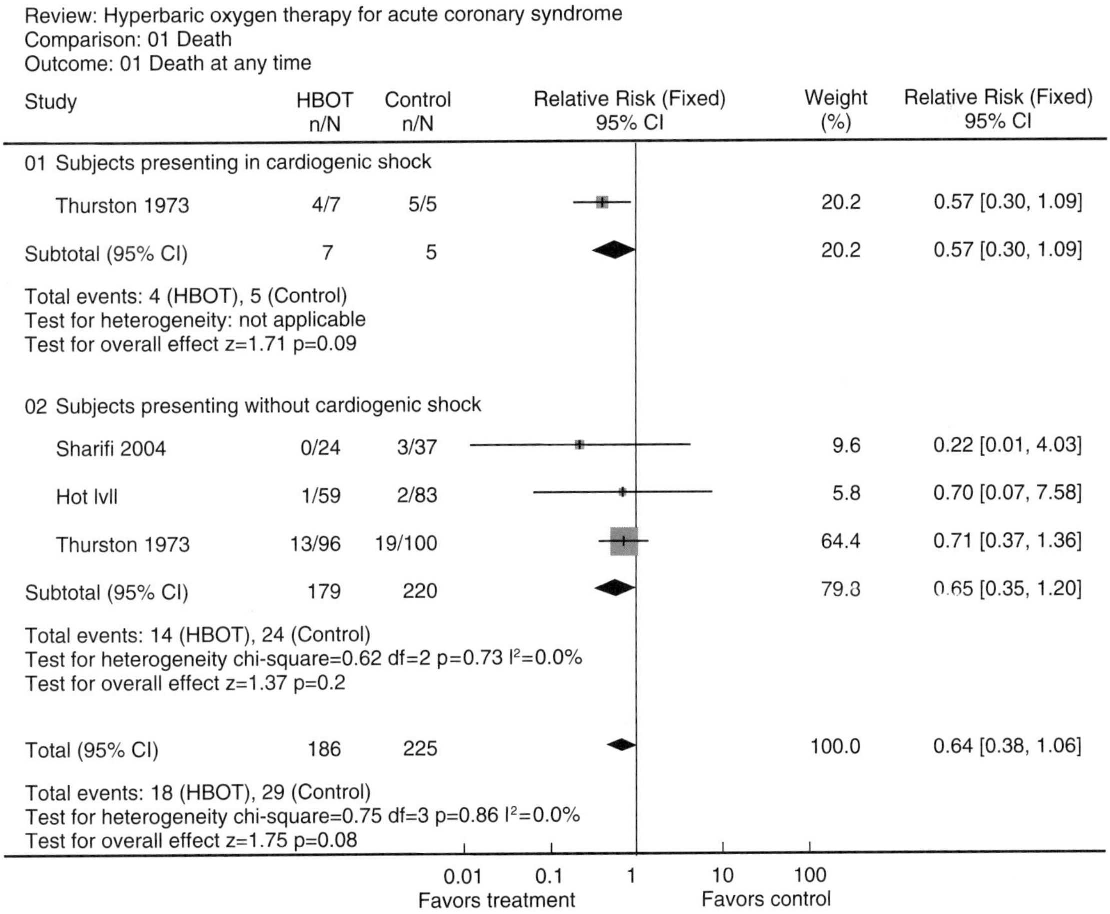

Review: Hyperbaric oxygen therapy for acute coronary syndrome
Comparison: 01 Death
Outcome: 01 Death at any time

Study	HBOT n/N	Control n/N	Relative Risk (Fixed) 95% CI	Weight (%)	Relative Risk (Fixed) 95% CI
01 Subjects presenting in cardiogenic shock					
Thurston 1973	4/7	5/5		20.2	0.57 [0.30, 1.09]
Subtotal (95% CI)	7	5		20.2	0.57 [0.30, 1.09]
Total events: 4 (HBOT), 5 (Control)					
Test for heterogeneity: not applicable					
Test for overall effect z=1.71 p=0.09					
02 Subjects presenting without cardiogenic shock					
Sharifi 2004	0/24	3/37		9.6	0.22 [0.01, 4.03]
Hot lvll	1/59	2/83		5.8	0.70 [0.07, 7.58]
Thurston 1973	13/96	19/100		64.4	0.71 [0.37, 1.36]
Subtotal (95% CI)	179	220		79.3	0.65 [0.35, 1.20]
Total events: 14 (HBOT), 24 (Control)					
Test for heterogeneity chi-square=0.62 df=2 p=0.73 I²=0.0%					
Test for overall effect z=1.37 p=0.2					
Total (95% CI)	186	225		100.0	0.64 [0.38, 1.06]
Total events: 18 (HBOT), 29 (Control)					
Test for heterogeneity chi-square=0.75 df=3 p=0.86 I²=0.0%					
Test for overall effect z=1.75 p=0.08					

0.01   0.1   1   10   100
Favors treatment   Favors control

Figure 21.1 Forest plot of the risk for death with hyperbaric oxygen therapy (HBOT). Subgroup analysis by presence or absence of cardiogenic shock. CI, confidence interval. *(From Bennett MH, Jepson N, Lehm JP: Hyperbaric oxygen therapy for acute coronary syndrome. Chichester, United Kingdom, John Wiley & Sons, Ltd. Cochrane Database Syst Rev (2):CD004818, 2005. Copyright Cochrane Collaboration, reproduced with permission.)*

Stavitsky (1998) reports statistically shorter mean time to pain relief in the HBOT group (261 vs. 614 minutes; 95% CI, 219-488, $P < 0.0001$), and both Stavitsky (1998) and Dekleva (2004) report lower peak creatine phosphokinase levels after HBOT, but not significantly so. Three trials report on improvements in left ventricular function. Swift (1992) reports the number of individuals where improved function could be demonstrated on echocardiography after HBOT (12 showed improved function in at least one segment after HBOT vs. zero with control; RR, 0.09; 95% CI, 0.01-1.4; $P = 0.09$), whereas Stavitsky (1998) and Dekleva (2004) both report nonsignificant improvements in left ventricular ejection fraction.

Shandling (1997) reported the length of stay in the first 63 subjects of their Hyperbaric Oxygen Therapy for Myocardial Infarction study. The mean days of hospital stay for the HBOT group was 7.4 versus 9.2 days for the control group. This difference was not statistically significant (weighted mean difference [MD], 1.8 days; 95% CI, 3.7 days to -0.1 days; $P = 0.06$).

Conclusions

The rationale for the use of HBOT for ACS is clear, and both the animal and uncontrolled human data suggest there may be a window of opportunity after both the primary event and revascularization where treatment may be beneficial. Limited evidence has been reported that HBOT reduces the incidence of both MACE and complete heart block and reduces the time to relief from angina when administered to patients with ACS. Although there is a trend toward favorable outcomes, no reliable data from these trials exist to confirm or refute any effect of HBOT on mortality, length of stay, or left ventricular contractility. A possibility of bias exists because of different anatomic locations and extent of myocardial damage on entry to these small trials, as well as from nonblinded management decisions in all except Swift (1992). Patient inclusion criteria are not standard and are reported poorly in some trials. Although all trials use some form of "standard" cardiac therapy in a dedicated unit designed to maximize outcome, these comparator therapies are generally poorly described.

Pooled data for clinical outcomes of interest could be performed only with respect to the risk for death and adverse effects. Although the risk for dying is not significantly improved after HBOT, there is some trend in that direction (RR, 0.64; $P = 0.08$) and the absolute risk difference of 3.2% suggests an NNT of around 31 patients to prevent 1 death by the addition of HBOT. Only one trial (Thurston, 1973) reports the fate of those presenting in cardiogenic shock, and although there is no statistically significant difference between groups in this small sample, it is worth noting that all survivors are from the HBOT group (three from seven subjects vs. none from five). The one small study that reports MACE rather than death alone (Sharifi, 2004) also suggests better outcome with the use of HBOT. This possible treatment effect would be of great clinical importance and deserves further investigation. Currently, given the small numbers and the sensitivity of the risk for both death and MACE to the allocation of withdrawals, this result should be interpreted with extreme caution. The routine adjunctive use of HBOT in these patients cannot yet be justified by the clinical evidence.

Given the indicative findings of improved outcomes with the use of HBOT in these patients, however, there is a case for large randomized trials of high methodologic rigor to define the true extent of benefit (if any) from the administration of HBOT. Specifically, more information is required on the subset of disease severity and timing of therapy most likely to result in benefit from this therapy. Given the activity of HBOT in modifying ischemia-reperfusion injury, attention should be given to combinations of HBOT and thrombolysis in the early treatment of acute coronary events and the prevention of restenosis after stent placement.

Acute Traumatic Brain Injury

Traumatic brain injury (TBI) is a significant cause of premature death and disability. Each year, there are at least 10 million new head injuries worldwide, and these account for a high proportion of deaths in young adults.[33,34] In the United States, there are more than 50,000 deaths due to TBI each year. The major causes are motor vehicle crashes, falls, and violence (including attempted suicide). Prevention strategies, including restraints for vehicle occupants, are now legally enforced in many countries. However, although road death rates are decreasing in most industrialized countries, they are increasing in many rapidly motorizing countries, particularly in Asia. For example, road death rates in China are already similar to those in the United States.[35] Head injuries are associated with long-term disability in many patients. In the United States, for example, 2% of the population (5.3 million citizens) is living with disability as a result of TBI,[33] and this places considerable medical, social, and financial burden on both families and health systems.[36]

Brain injury has a primary and secondary component. At the time of impact, there is a variable degree of irreversible damage to the neurologic tissue (primary injury). After this, a chain of events occurs in which there is ongoing injury to the brain through edema, hypoxia, and ischemia secondary to raised tissue or intracranial pressure (ICP), release of excitotoxic levels of excitatory neurotransmitters (e.g., glutamate), and impaired calcium homeostasis (secondary injury).[37,38]

Therapy

Therapy for TBI focuses on prevention or minimization, or both, of secondary injury by ensuring adequate oxygenation, hemodynamics, control of intracranial hypertension, and strategies to reduce cellular injury. A number of therapies, including barbiturates, calcium channel antagonists, steroids, hyperventilation, mannitol, hypothermia, and anticonvulsants, have been investigated, though none has shown unequivocal efficacy in reducing poor outcome.[39-43]

HBOT is a further adjunctive therapy that has been proposed to improve outcome in acute brain injury. Since the 1960s, there have been reports that HBOT improves the outcome after brain trauma.[44] Administration of HBOT is based on the observation that hypoxia after closed head trauma is an integral part of the secondary injury described earlier. Hypoxic neurons that perform anaerobic metabolism result in acidosis and an unsustainable reduction in cellular metabolic reserve.[45] As the hypoxic situation persists, neurons lose their ability to maintain ionic homeostasis, and free oxygen radicals accumulate and degrade cell membranes.[46,47] Eventually, irreversible changes result in unavoidable cell death. When ischemia is severe enough, these changes occur rapidly, but some evidence exists that these effects can occur over a period of days.[48] This gives some basis to the assertion that a therapy designed to increase oxygen availability in the early period after TBI may improve long-term outcome. HBOT may also reduce tissue edema by an osmotic effect,[49] and any agent that has a positive effect on brain swelling after trauma may also contribute to improved outcomes. On the other hand, oxygen in high doses is potentially toxic to normally perfused tissue, and the brain is particularly at risk.[50] For this reason, it is appropriate to postulate that, in some TBI patients, HBOT may do more harm through the action of increased free oxygen radical damage than good through the restoration of aerobic metabolism.

Evidence

Several animal models of head injury support the hypothesis that HBOT across a range of pressures may be beneficial through restoring oxygenation to damaged tissue or inflammatory modulation of ischemia-reperfusion injury. In a rat model of lateral fluid percussion injury, Daugherty and colleagues[51] administered HBOT at 1.5 ATA for 1 hour beginning 1 hour after injury and demonstrated improvements in brain Po_2 and mitochondrial redox potential suggesting there was more rapid recovery of aerobic metabolism in that group compared with animals exposed to 30% oxygen or 100% oxygen at 1 ATA. In a cold injury-induced lesion model in rabbits, Niklas and coauthors[52] confirm similar increases in Po_2, together with reductions in both the area of necrotic brain on microscopy and mortality (0% vs. 20%), after three sessions of HBOT at 2.5 ATA for 90 minutes beginning 1 hour after injury. Palzur and investigators[53] draw similar conclusions after exposure of rats to a brain contusion model and HBOT at 2.8 ATA. In an elegant experiment using a model similar to that of Daugherty and colleagues, Rogatsky and researchers[54] demonstrate a protective effect of HBOT at 1.5 ATA on the post-traumatic increase in ICP, both in rate and greatest values reached, and a reduction in mortality.

Most recently, Vlodavsky and colleagues[55] have implicated inflammatory modulation as a potentially important mechanism for benefit through the demonstration of reduced neutrophil infiltration into injured brain after exposure to HBOT at 2.8 ATA, together with a reduction in the expression of a family of enzymes associated with deleterious outcomes in TBI—the matrix metalloproteinases. The direct implication is that, at least at this high dose, HBOT decreases secondary injury and cell death and reduces reactive neuroinflammation after TBI.

The relevance of many of these encouraging findings for human brain injury is not yet clear. None of these animal models was intended to reproduce the time delays and potential adverse events after clinical trauma. The longest delay between insult and starting HBOT in these models is 3 hours, for example.[55] Unfortunately, despite these supportive findings and 40 years of interest in the delivery of HBOT in these patients, little clinical evidence of effectiveness exists.

HBOT has been shown to reduce both ICP and cerebrospinal fluid pressure in patients with brain injuries,[56,57] improve gray matter metabolic activity on single-photon emission computed tomography scan,[58] and improve glucose metabolism.[59] Some studies suggest that any effect of HBOT may not be uniform across all patients with brain injuries. For example, Hayakawa and coauthors[57] demonstrate that cerebrospinal fluid pressure rebounded to greater levels after HBOT than at pretreatment estimation in some patients, whereas others showed persistent reductions. It is possible that HBOT has a positive effect in a subgroup of patients with moderate injury, but not in those with extensive cerebral

injury. Furthermore, repeated exposure to HBOT may be required to attain consistent changes.[60] Clinical reports have attributed a wide range of improvements to HBOT including cognitive and motor skills, improved attention span, and increased verbalization.[56,58] These improvements are, however, difficult to ascribe to any single treatment modality because HBOT was most often applied in conjunction with intensive supportive and rehabilitative therapies.

For all these reasons, it is conceivable that the addition of HBOT might improve survival from serious brain injury without improving the proportion of those who survive with a useful functional level, whereas at the same time increasing overall costs of therapy. A Cochrane review has examined the randomized clinical evidence for any net benefit or harm.[61]

Cochrane Review

A Cochrane review identifies four randomized trials in which patients received HBOT for acute TBI: Ren (2001),[61a] Rockswold (1992),[61b] Artru (1976),[61c] and Holbach (1974).[61d] These trials include data on 382 participants: 199 in the HBOT group, and 183 in the control group. The largest trial (Rockswold, 1992) accounts for 44% of cases. Individual study characteristics are given in Table 21.3.

All four trials enrolled participants with closed head injury, but inclusion criteria varied. Rockswold (1992) accepted those with a Glasgow Coma Score of less than 10 for between 6 and 24 hours; Ren (2001) accepted subjects with a Glasgow Coma Score of less than 9 for up to 3 days after trauma. The other two older trials do not specify inclusion criteria, other than "closed head injury and comatose." Treatment pressures (1.5–2.5 ATA, or 152–253.3 kPa), time schedule (60–90 minutes), and number of sessions (10–40 sessions) of HBOT differ among studies. Similarly, some variation exists in comparator therapies and the time to final assessment. No study describes the method of randomization, clearly conceals allocation from the individual responsible for randomization, or uses a sham therapy.

Table 21.3 Characteristics of the Studies Included in the Cochrane Review of TBI

STUDY	METHODS	SUBJECTS	INTERVENTIONS	OUTCOMES
Artru (1976)[61c]	No blinding; 60 patients; inclusion depended on availability of hyperbaric chamber	Closed head injury and coma; stratified in 9 subgroups of severity and pathology	HBOT (n = 31): 2.5 ATA for 1 hour daily for 10 days, followed by 4 days rest and repeat if not responding Control (n = 29): standard care included hyperventilation and frusemide	Death, unfavorable outcome, adverse events
Holbach (1974)[61d]	Quasi-randomized, unblinded; 99 patients	Closed head injury and coma with "acute midbrain syndrome"	HBOT (n = 31): 1.5 ATA daily, regimen unknown Control (n = 29): "usual intensive care regimen"	Complete recovery, mortality
Ren (2001)[61a]	No blinding reported; 55 patients	Closed head injury, GCS score < 9; randomized on day 3 after stabilized	HBOT (n = 31): 2.5 ATA for a total of 400–600 minutes every 4 days, repeated 3 or 4 times Control (n = 20): dehydration, steroids, and antibiotics	Favorable GOS, change in GCS
Rockswold (1992)[61b]	Observers blinded, but not patients or caregivers	Closed head injury with GCS < 10 for >6 hours and <24 hours	HBOT: 1.5 ATA for 1 hour every 8 hours for 2 weeks or until death or waking (average number of treatments is 21) Control: "intensive neurosurgical care"	Favorable outcome (GOS, 1 or 2), mortality, intracranial pressure, adverse events

ATA, atmospheres absolute; GCS, Glasgow Coma Scale; GOS, Glasgow Outcome Scale; HBOT, hyperbaric oxygen therapy.

The primary combined outcome for the review is the attainment of a good functional outcome. This is defined in these studies as any one of the following: Glasgow Outcome Score less than 3, "return of consciousness," "complete recovery," or classified as "independent." At early outcome (0-4 weeks), 36% of patients had a good outcome in the HBOT group versus 14% in the control group. Pooled analysis suggests, however, that there is no significant difference between groups (RR with HBOT: 2.66; 95% CI, 0.73–9.69; $P = 0.06$). When combining all trials at final outcome, 109 subjects (51%) in the HBOT group had a good outcome versus 61 (34%) in the control group; however, this difference was not statistically significant (RR, 1.94; 95% CI, 0.92–4.08; $P = 0.08$). This result is likely to be subject to important heterogeneity between trials ($I^2 = 81\%$) and should be interpreted with caution (Fig. 21.2). This may well reflect differences in actual pathology of those included in different trials or the evolution of general therapy between the 1970s and 1990s.

Three of these trials report mortality at some time (Holbach at 12 days, Artru, and Rockswold at 12 months) involving 327 participants. There was significantly increased mortality with control therapy (RR, 1.46; 95% CI, 1.13–1.87; $P = 0.003$). Heterogeneity between studies was low ($I^2 = 0\%$). The NNT to avoid 1 death by applying HBOT was 7 (95% CI, 4–22) (Fig. 21.3).

Only Rockswold reports the effects of therapy on ICP. The effect of HBOT was complicated by a change in the experimental protocol during the period of recruitment. Although overall there was no difference in the mean maximum ICP between the two groups (MD, 3.1 mm Hg lower with HBOT; 95% CI, −9.6 to +3.4 mm Hg), the authors noted greater than expected ICP in the early HBOT participants. Because this was likely to represent pain from middle-ear barotrauma, the last 46 subjects recruited to HBOT had precompression myringotomy tubes inserted to allow free equalization of middle-ear

Review: Hyperbaric oxygen therapy for the adjunctive treatment of traumatic brain injury
Comparison: 01 Good functional outcome (GOS <3 or similar)
Outcome: 06 Good functional outcome at final follow-up

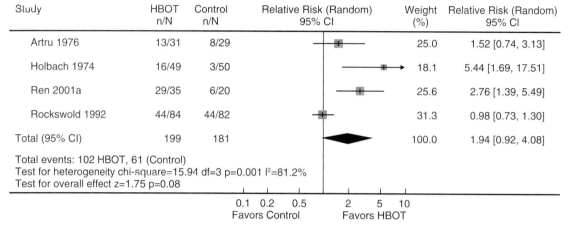

Study	HBOT n/N	Control n/N	Relative Risk (Random) 95% CI	Weight (%)	Relative Risk (Random) 95% CI
Artru 1976	13/31	8/29		25.0	1.52 [0.74, 3.13]
Holbach 1974	16/49	3/50		18.1	5.44 [1.69, 17.51]
Ren 2001a	29/35	6/20		25.6	2.76 [1.39, 5.49]
Rockswold 1992	44/84	44/82		31.3	0.98 [0.73, 1.30]
Total (95% CI)	199	181		100.0	1.94 [0.92, 4.08]

Total events: 102 HBOT, 61 (Control)
Test for heterogeneity chi-square=15.94 df=3 p=0.001 I²=81.2%
Test for overall effect z=1.75 p=0.08

0.1   0.2   0.5   2   5   10
    Favors Control   Favors HBOT

Figure 21.2 Forest plot for good functional outcome at final assessment. Considerable heterogeneity ($I^2 = 81\%$) exists, and this result should be interpreted with great caution. CI, confidence interval; GOS, Glasgow Outcome Scale; HBOT, hyperbaric oxygen therapy. *(From Bennett MH, Trytko BE, Jonker B: Hyperbaric oxygen therapy for the adjunctive treatment of traumatic brain injury [Cochrane review]. Cochrane Database Syst Rev (4):CD004609, 2004. Copyright Cochrane Collaboration, reproduced with permission.)*

pressures. Comparing the standard care group with the HBOT subjects with and without myringotomy, researchers found a significant decline in ICP with HBOT plus myringotomy, but no difference without myringotomy (MD with myringotomy: -8.2 mm Hg; 95% CI, -14.7 to -1.7 mm Hg; $P = 0.01$; MD without myringotomy: $+2.7$ mm Hg; 95% CI, -5.9 to $+11.3$ mm Hg; $P = 0.54$).

With regard to adverse events, Rockswold reports generalized seizures in two participants in the HBOT group versus none in the control group (RR, 0.2; $P = 0.3$) and a further two with hemotympanum from middle-ear barotrauma (RR, 0.2; $P = 0.03$). Two trials report participants with significant pulmonary effects. Rockswold reports 10 individuals with increasing oxygen requirements and infiltrates

Review: Hyperbaric oxygen therapy for the adjunctive treatment of traumatic brain injury
Comparison: 02 Death at final follow-up
Outcome: 01 Death at final follow-up

Study	Control n/N	HBOT n/N	Relative Risk (Fixed) 95% CI	Weight (%)	Relative Risk (Fixed) 95% CI
Artru 1976	16/29	15/31		26.6	1.14 [0.70, 1.86]
Holbach 1974	37/50	26/49		48.1	1.39 [1.02, 1.90]
Rockswold 1992	26/82	14/84		25.3	1.90 [1.07. 3.38]
Total (95% CI)	161	164		100.0	1.46 [1.13, 1.87]

Total events: 79 (Control), 55 (HBOT)
Test for heterogeneity chi-square=1.86 df=2 p=0.39 I²=0.0%
Test for overall effect z=2.95 p=0.003

0.1   0.2   0.5   1   2   5   10
    Favors Control   Favors HBOT

Figure 21.3 Forest plot for death at the final follow-up of each study. *(From Bennett MH, Trytko BE, Jonker B: Hyperbaric oxygen therapy for the adjunctive treatment of traumatic brain injury [Cochrane review]. Cochrane Database Syst Rev (4):CD004609, 2004. Copyright Cochrane Collaboration, reproduced with permission.)*

on chest radiograph, whereas Artru and colleagues[60] report 5 patients with respiratory symptoms including cyanosis and hyperpnea so severe as to imply "impending hyperoxic pneumonia." Overall, therefore, 15 patients (13% of those receiving HBOT) had severe pulmonary complications, whereas no such complications were reported in the standard therapy arm. This difference is statistically significant (RR, 0.06; 95% CI, 0.01-0.47; $P = 0.007$). There was no indication of heterogeneity between trials ($I^2 = 0\%$), and this analysis suggests we might expect to treat eight patients with HBOT to cause this adverse effect in one individual (number needed to harm, 8; 95% CI, 5-15).

Conclusions

Good biologic plausibility exists for the application of HBOT for TBI, and this position is generally supported by a number of small animal studies and some isolated case reports. However, although some evidence from RCTs that HBOT reduces mortality after closed head injury has been reported, there is less confidence that the addition of HBOT to standard therapy increases the chance of recovery to independence.

The single randomized trial that examines ICP as a proxy for beneficial effects did suggest that ICP was lower immediately after HBOT when patients had received middle-ear ventilation tubes. These tubes avoid middle-ear barotrauma on compression—a highly painful and stimulating condition that might be expected to increase ICP, regardless of the underlying brain injury. Any clinical benefit may come at the cost of significant pulmonary complications. These complications are rare in general hyperbaric practice[62] and may be related specifically to the head injuries suffered by these patients.

Although some experimental and anecdotal evidence suggests benefit, in an SR of the randomized evidence, only 382 participants were available for evaluation. The methodology was poor in some of these trials, and there was variability and poor reporting of entry criteria and the nature and timing of outcomes. In particular, a possibility of bias exists because of different times to entry in these small trials, as well as from nonblinded management decisions in all trials. The effect of age, oxygen dose, nature of comparative therapies, and severity of injury on the effectiveness of HBOT cannot be estimated given the data available.

In summary, limited evidence exists that HBOT reduces mortality in patients with acute TBI, but no clear evidence of improved functional outcome. The small number of studies, the modest numbers of patients, and the methodologic and reporting inadequacies of the primary studies included in this review demand a cautious interpretation. The routine use of HBOT for these patients is not yet justified on the basis of this clinical evidence.

The precise mechanisms whereby HBOT may exert a beneficial effect are still a matter of speculation. It is appropriate that laboratory investigations continue to elucidate the most promising timing and dose of HBOT after trauma. There is a case for large, randomized trials of high methodologic rigor to define the true extent of benefit (if any) from the administration of HBOT.

Neonatal Hypoxic Encephalopathy

Neonatal encephalopathy is a clinical syndrome of abnormal neurologic function detected within the first few days of life in the term or near-term neonate. Where an episode of peripartum hypoxia can be identified, neonatal encephalopathy is called *neonatal hypoxic encephalopathy* (NHE). It is important to make this differentiation because many cases of neonatal encephalopathy are not related to hypoxia.[63,64] NHE is characterized by abnormalities in cortical function (lethargy, coma, and/or seizures), brainstem function (cranial nerve abnormalities), tone (hypotonia), and/or reflexes (absent or hyporeflexic).[65] The relation among NHE, cerebral palsy (CP), and development delay is not always clear in the literature, perhaps because pathophysiology and diagnosis is not always clearly identifiable at the time of injury. Our understanding of the relation of NHE to CP is summarized in Figure 21.4, and this is the scheme used throughout this chapter. Whatever the exact mechanism, neonates

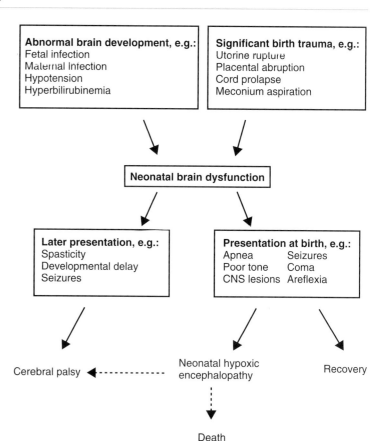

Figure 21.4 A simple scheme for defining the clinical relation between neonatal hypoxic encephalopathy and cerebral palsy.

identified as having NHE may in the long term experience developmental delay, CP, epilepsy, or any combination of these three. The standard treatment for NHE includes rapid resuscitation and cardiorespiratory support; however, many supplemental therapies have been proposed. HBOT is one such adjunctive therapy and has been adopted widely in China.

The prevalence of fetal and newborn asphyxia at delivery is approximately 25 per 1000 live births.[66] Most of these infants do not suffer any permanent injury, and the incidence of NHE is significantly lower, between 0.5 and 1 per 1000 births. Although not common, the permanent cerebral damage that results from NHE is a significant health burden with high medical and social costs.[67]

The cause of NHE is variable, but any event suggestive of fetal ischemia and occurring in the peripartum period may result in NHE. Recognized precipitating events include birth catastrophes such as cord prolapse, uterine

rupture, placental abruption, maternal cardiac arrest, and fetal exsanguination. In some cases, the cause remains undefined.[65] Perinatal observations such as fetal heart rate abnormalities and low Apgar scores (0–3 beyond 5 minutes) suggest an event that may result in NHE. Fetal cerebral hypoxia that is severe enough to lead to NHE is almost always associated with other hypoxic organ injuries that manifest in the days after delivery. The diagnosis of NHE is made on clinical findings and perinatal events, often supported by evidence of fetal hypoxia at birth, most commonly low scalp pH readings or a metabolic acidosis as measured by fetal umbilical blood gas measurement.[65,68]

Therapy

Prevention of NHE is of primary importance and focuses on rapid treatment of those conditions that may result in neonatal asphyxia.

Such therapies are aimed at maintaining optimal maternal hemodynamics and oxygenation to maximize delivery of oxygen to the fetus. Once identified, the treatment of NHE is rapid delivery where possible, followed by prompt resuscitation of the newborn. Although no interventions have been identified that clearly improve outcome with respect to death or disability,[67] a number of therapies have been proposed, including corticosteroids and magnesium.[69,70] In 2005, two clinical trials of therapeutic hypothermia were published, both of which suggest there may be some benefit in this modality of treatment.[71,72] More work is required to establish the place of hypothermia for routine treatment of these cases.

HBOT has also been advocated for the treatment of NHE. The technique was first described in a clinical study by Hutchison and coauthors[73] published in 1966. This non-blinded, randomized trial examined the mortality rate in 218 neonates with apnea or ineffective breathing at birth. The control group (111 neonates) received standard care with tracheal intubation and positive pressure ventilation, whereas the trial group received HBOT (up to a maximum of 4 ATA) for 30 minutes *and no other attempt at cardiopulmonary resuscitation* (107 neonates). No significant difference in mortality exists between the groups (13.5% control vs. 17.8% HBOT), suggesting that HBOT may be of similar benefit to intubation and ventilation for treating neonatal asphyxia. Although difficult to advocate, it would be interesting to know what the mortality rate with no active intervention might be compared with both these options.

The physiologic rationale for the use of HBOT in NHE is yet to be fully elucidated. Several possibilities have been postulated and include improved oxygenation to areas of marginal ischemia, down-regulation of cyclo-oxygenase-2, reduced striatal dopamine release, re-establishment of striatal metabolism, reductions in postischemic increases in vascular permeability, and reduction in secondary brain injury mediated by polymorphonuclear neutrophils.[74]

Evidence

Some evidence suggests that HBOT may be of benefit after ischemic brain injury in the adult animal. In several animal models, HBOT has been shown to reduce brain injury that occurs as a result of both focal and global ischemic insults.[75-82]

Since the initial trial report,[73] there has been little further data published in the Western literature, and certainly no further controlled clinical trials. Although the treatment of NHE with HBOT is not commonly reported in the West, a substantial number of reports has been published in the Chinese literature. These reports vary significantly in methodology, selection criteria, treatment protocols, and outcome measures. The results of these Chinese trials have been reviewed by Liu and colleagues.[83] In this article, the authors investigate the clinical effects of HBOT for NHE in an SR of the Chinese literature. In total, 126 citations were identified concerning HBOT for brain injury; however, only 20 trials met the selection criteria of "randomised or quasi-randomised controlled trials of treatment with HBO compared with 'usual care' in full term infants (more than 36 weeks gestation) with hypoxic ischemic encephalopathy and a history of perinatal asphyxia."[83] All of these trials were conducted in China.

Liu and colleagues[83] report that neonates treated with HBOT appeared to have more favorable outcomes when compared with the control groups in almost all of the trials. The combined odds of dying after HBOT compared with control were 0.26 (95% CI, 0.14-0.46) and for having neurologic sequelae were 0.41 (95% CI, 0.27-0.61). The conclusion of the review is that treatment with HBOT "possibly reduces mortality and neurological sequelae in term neonates with hypoxia-ischemic encephalopathy."[83] Unfortunately, the generally poor methodologic quality and reporting of these trials drew the authors to conclude they could not together constitute reliable proof of effect. They recommend a large RCT is required to generate reliable evidence.

Conclusions

NHE is a severe complication of birth as-phyxia. The mainstays of management include preventative measures, rapid resuscitation, and more recently, hypothermia. HBOT has been described for the treatment of NHE, but most of the recent reports are from Chinese studies of variable investigational rigor. There appears to be some indication that HBOT may be a useful treatment for NHE; however, there is further requirement for well-conducted RCTs before definitive recommendations can be made.

Cerebral Palsy

CP is not a specific diagnosis, but rather an "umbrella term" describing the clinical presentation of nonprogressive motor deficits in children during the first year of life and that can arise from a broad spectrum of causative factors.[84] Intellectual abnormalities may be present, but there are always physical abnormalities present for the term *CP* to be appropriate.[85] Children with CP present with developmental delay and static (i.e., nonprogressive) motor deficits (see Fig. 21.4).[84] The motor deficits are variable and can include weakness, incoordination, spasticity, clonus, rigidity, and muscle spasms. Spasticity can be quite debilitating and, if left untreated, can lead to muscle fibrosis, musculoskeletal deformities, and contractures. In addition, abnormal movements may be noted in some patients, including athetosis, chorea, and dystonia. Other clinical features that can be associated with CP include epilepsy, bowel and bladder dysfunction, hearing loss, visual impairment, and poor nutritional status caused by pseudobulbar palsy. Overall, approximately 36% of patients with CP experience development of epilepsy, with onset during the first year of life in more than two thirds of the cohort.[86]

CP is the most common severe physical disability of childhood with a prevalence of 2 to 3 per 1000 school-aged children, and it is most commonly seen in premature and low-birth-weight neonates.[87,88] Prevalence and incidence have been increasing in the recent past, possibly because of both better reporting and improvements in the survival of low-birth-weight neonates.[87,89] Approximately 85% of neonates born weighing less than 1500 grams now survive, and up to 15% of these survivors are likely to exhibit significant spastic motor deficits.[85,90] The estimated annual total cost of care for these patients in 2002 was $8.2 billion.[88]

In about 50% of cases, no definite cause for CP can be identified, whereas the remainder may be caused by a wide variety of factors including hypoxia-ischemia, stroke, trauma, infections, and chromosomal and genetic syndromes.[91-94] The neuropathology is also variable but usually includes one or more of the following conditions: periventricular leukomalacia, germinal matrix hemorrhage (often associated with periventricular leukomalacia), cerebral artery distribution infarcts, and gray matter ischemic lesions of the thalamus and basal ganglia.[95] Immature oligodendrocytes of the developing white matter appear to be susceptible to injury from free radicals, excitotoxic overstimulation, and proinflammatory cytokines,[95] any or all of which may be associated with hypoxic-ischemic events.[96-98] Immature cells are susceptible to free radical damage because they have lower concentrations of the antioxidant superoxide dismutase,[96] whereas excitotoxic injury can occur more easily because developing oligodendrocytes overexpress AMPA-kainate receptors, which are stimulated by kainate released during hypoxic-ischemic events.[97] Proinflammatory cytokines, including interferon-γ, tumor necrosis factor-α, and interleukin-2 and -6, are generated during hypoxia and ischemia, and have been demonstrated in regions of periventricular leukomalacia.[95] Both interferon-γ and tumor necrosis factor-α have toxic effects on developing oligodendrocytes.[99]

The clinical diagnosis of CP requires an extensive workup, including neuroimaging with magnetic resonance imaging (MRI).[96] MRI is sensitive to damage in the fetal and infant brain that could result in CP (e.g., periventricular leukomalacia). In neonates, there is typically a short period between a clinical hypoxic insult and the development of clinical manifestations. This suggests there may be a short window of therapeutic opportunity available to ameliorate or even reverse the cerebral damage.[85,100] Early diagnosis is therefore highly desirable.

Unfortunately, diagnosis may be difficult in the neonate. Clinical suspicion will be raised by the identification of specific events during gestation and delivery, but such events are often unrecognized, and diagnosis then relies on clinical examination, neurophysiologic monitoring, and neurologic imaging. Seizures are nonspecific and may manifest only through autonomic changes, apneas, and heart rate changes rather than overt movements. They may be missed.[101]

Surprisingly, little has been written concerning how HBOT might produce benefit. Most justification for therapy has been based on clinical results of both controlled and uncontrolled studies, rather than the development of a clear scientific rationale. Neubauer[102] has reported changes on single-photon emission computed tomography images before and after therapy that demonstrate improved blood flow. These findings imply improved function and, therefore, clinical status, and Neubauer associates these changes in particular with improvements noted by parents. The "idling neuron" hypothesis has been suggested to explain clinical findings, with the assumption that HBOT can improve blood flow to inactive but viable neurons.[103]

Some of the authors of an RCT published in 2001[103a] have suggested that pressure might have a therapeutic benefit unrelated to hyperoxia.[104] Little evidence is available to support this suggestion. Marois and Vanasse cite a rat model of acute cerebrovascular injury and a case series of 11 patients treated for "chronic toxic encephalopathy" with 10 exposures to 24% oxygen at 1.3 ATA.[105] At this time, neither the presence of an ischemic penumbra in CP nor benefit from the administration of low-pressure air have been widely accepted.

Therapy

Therapy for CP may be directed to prevent or ameliorate the injury in the acute phase, or to improve function in a established case. In neonates, there is typically a latent period of 6 to 48 hours between a hypoxic insult and

development of clinical manifestations, suggesting there may be a short window of therapeutic opportunity available to ameliorate or even reverse the cerebral damage.[85,100] Although HBOT has been advocated in both situations, clinical reports have almost exclusively involved HBOT for children between the ages of 3 and 12 years.

Conventional treatment options include physical and occupational therapy; drug therapy for spasticity; orthopedic procedures (e.g., orthotic devices, tendon lengthening); and neurosurgical intervention in selected cases (e.g., dorsal rhizotomy, peripheral neurotomy).[84,106,107] Spasticity should be treated (i.e., tone reduction) when there is unequivocal evidence for interference with function, positioning, care, or comfort level. Drug therapy includes baclofen (most commonly used), diazepam, dantrolene, and tizanidine. Children that are intolerant of or refractory to oral medications can be considered for intrathecal baclofen therapy.

Steroids have been a traditional therapeutic approach to prevention. Experimental evidence suggests these agents must be administered at least 24 hours before any hypoxic insult to improve neurologic outcome.

HBOT has been advocated for the improvement of both functional and cognitive ability. The use of HBOT acutely at the time of delivery is discussed elsewhere in this chapter (see Neonatal Hypoxic Encephalopathy section earlier in this chapter). HBOT is most often advocated at "mild" doses, typically between 1.3 and 1.75 ATA, on the basis that higher doses are more likely to produce toxic effects in the brain.[102,104,108] Children are usually compressed once or twice daily for 60 minutes, with a course of therapy ranging from 20 to 70 sessions over weeks to months.

Evidence

The first substantial account of the use of HBOT for CP was given at the 1989 Undersea and Hyperbaric Medical Society Annual Scientific Meeting, when Machado[109] reported his experience over 10 years treating 230 children in Sao Paulo. Using a regimen of 20 sessions at 1.5 ATA daily or twice daily, Machado reported a "clear reduction" in spasticity in 218 (94.8%) of his cohorts that persisted in about 75% of those who could be followed for 6 months. He also reported an improvement in general health and attention in most of the group.

Subsequent reports including three RCTs bring the total numbers to approximately 710 children,[102,103a,108,111-114] yet controversy continues unabated about the role of hyperbaric therapy, with each subsequent publication followed by a flurry of correspondence (Table 21.4).

In general, these reports suggest clinically important improvements in the gross motor function measure. This comprehensive measure, designed and validated for CP, consists of 88 items (recently available in a shortened version with 66 items) designed to document changes in motor function including lying, rolling, jumping, walking, and so forth.[117] For example, in the first peer-reviewed report of a case series of 25 children, the gross motor function measure improved an average of 5.3%, which is both clinically important and comparable with

Table 21.4 Summary of Clinical Evidence for the Use of HBOT for CP

STUDY	METHODS	SUBJECTS	INTERVENTIONS	OUTCOMES
Machado (1989)[109]*	Case series	230 children with CP (all types)	100% O_2 at 1.5 ATA for 1 hour, once or twice daily to 20 total	Reduced spasticity, improved attention, reduced convulsions
Montgomery and colleagues (1999)[108]	Case series	25 children 3–8 years old with spastic diplegia	95% O_2 at 1.75 ATA for 1 hour once or twice daily to 20 total	GMFM improved 5.3%, better walking; parents noted improved alertness and communication
Nuthall and colleagues (2000)[111]	2 cases	Children with CP	Required admission to ICU after HBOT	1 regurgitated feed, 1 experienced development of acute respiratory failure and seizures
Packard (2000)[113]*	RCT—no blinding or sham	26 children 1–5 years old with moderate-to-severe CP	100% O_2 at 1.5 ATA for 1 hour twice daily to 40 sessions; immediate treatment vs. delayed treatment at 6 months	Parents noted improved mobility, attention, and speech; no change on blinded assessment of Peabody score
Collet and colleagues (2001)[103a]†	RCT with blinding and sham	111 children 3–12 years old	100% O_2 at 1.75 ATA vs. 1.3 ATA air, both for 1 hour daily to 40 sessions	GFMF improved about 3% in both groups; no differences in neuropsychologic outcomes
Neubauer (2001)[102]*	Case series	About 250 children 6 weeks to 14 years old	Up to 1.5 ATA 100% O_2 for 1 hour; example cited had 77 treatments	90% have improved SPECT and parental ratings of function
Chavdarov (2002)[114]*	Case series	50 children, various types	1.5–1.7 ATA for 30 minutes daily to 20 total	4 withdrawn with adverse effects; improved motor function in 13%, mental function 6%
Mathai and colleagues (2005)[112]*	RCT with blinding and sham	20 children 1–10 years old, all types	3 cycles of 100% O_2 at 1.5 ATA for 1 hour daily to 30, then 1-month intervals (90 total); sham breathing air	Improved GMFM with HBOT; no differences in SPECT or spasticity; some improvement in speech

*Not published in peer-reviewed literature.
†Also includes separate reports of neuropsychological outcomes (Hardy and colleagues, 2002[115]) and adverse effects of therapy (Muller-Bolla and colleagues, 2006[116]).
ATA, atmospheres absolute; CP, cerebral palsy; GMFM, gross motor function measure; RCT, randomized, controlled trial; SPECT, single-photon emission computed tomography.

other accepted therapeutic measures.[108] Many of these reports also suggest improvements in both motor and cognitive skills on parental evaluation, and these promising results were used as the basis for a well-conducted randomized study in Quebec, which began recruiting patients in 2000.[103a]

The three published reports of randomized studies have also been generally positive. Unfortunately, two of these have not been published in peer-reviewed literature, and it is difficult to make a full appraisal.[112,113] Dr. Maurine Packard presented the "Cornell Study" at a meeting in Graz, Austria, in 2000. Her account has been reproduced on a national parent-to-parent Web site devoted to the care of children with disabilities, but it does not appear to have been published elsewhere. This study enrolled 26 children aged 15 months to 5 years who were randomly assigned to immediate HBOT (40 treatments at 1.5 ATA for 1 hour) or delayed HBOT on the same schedule 6 months later. No attempt was made to blind any participants or provide a sham therapy. Six of those recruited were later withdrawn for a variety of reasons, leaving 20 children to participate in the analysis. Most parents reported improvements in mobility (83%), attention (78%), and language (87%) over the treatment period (combined results of both groups after treatment). There were, however, no statistically significant differences between the groups on any of the observer blinded assessments for cognitive function or motor skills on testing after the immediate group had completed therapy or 2 months later. Dr. Packard concludes that for some children, HBOT can improve motor skills, attention, language, and play, and that the changes observed may be caused by either increased oxygen or intensive contact between child and parent, or a combination of factors.

In a study presented in the proceedings of the combined European Underwater and Biomedical Society and International Congress on Hyperbaric Medicine meeting in Barcelona in 2005, Mathai and coauthors[112] report the results of 20 children randomized to 90 treatments with 100% oxygen or air at 1.5 ATA.

This small trial of an intensive treatment regimen demonstrated statistically significant improvements in gross motor function measure in the oxygen group (4.9%) compared with sham, but no such changes in language, single-photon emission computed tomography scans, or spasticity scores. The authors conclude that HBOT appears to be associated with some benefit.

The most methodologically sound trial yet published is that by Collet and coworkers in *The Lancet*.[103a] These authors randomized 111 children to receive 40 sessions of either 100% oxygen at 1.75 ATA or a sham therapy with air at 1.3 ATA. Both arms of this study show improvements with gross motor function measure (3.4% with oxygen, 3.1% with air at 3 months), but there are no significant differences between groups on any motor or cognitive outcome reported in any of the three accounts of this trial. The 1.75 ATA oxygen schedule is associated with mild barotrauma on examination of the tympanic membrane.[103a,115,116] The authors conclude that either both treatment schedules were equally effective, there was a learning effect, or a participation effect of some kind was present. They find the latter to be the most plausible of these possibilities.

Controversy surrounded the Quebec RCT even before publication. A Scientific Advisory Committee was asked to evaluate the scientific validity of the study and to examine critically the hypotheses developed to explain the results.[118] The committee concluded they had no reservations about the scientific validity of the results, but questioned the mechanism of action for HBOT and recommended that no further clinical trials in children should be undertaken *"unless there is more basic science data to guide the design of future trials."*[119]

The committee examined each of the potential mechanisms in detail. They found no scientific support for a therapeutic effect of oxygen while breathing air at 1.3 ATA. This dose is equivalent to breathing 28% oxygen at 1 ATA and has not been shown previously to have profound effects outside the context of poor cardiorespiratory function. They believe a therapeutic effect of pressure even less likely given the inhibition of healing with a hyperbaric control in a model of burn injury.[119] They also conclude that a learning effect was possible but unlikely given the methodology of the investigators, and that although the improvements could have been the result of a normal evolution over time in this young group, insufficient data were available with which to compare the findings.

The committee therefore believed the most plausible explanation for these findings was a participation effect where a highly motivated group of parents and researchers have positively influenced both function and cognitive ability equally in both blinded arms of the trial. The same effect might operate in any unblinded clinical trial in this area,[120] and there is evidence for the association between participation in clinical trials and improved outcome across a broad range of patients, including children.[121,122] A positive influence may arise from a selection effect (the most motivated group is entered into trials), a placebo effect, an increased compliance with therapy, or a combination of all three. The inclusion of a highly motivated group in an intensive protocol involving repeated compression over several weeks and sustained contact with other motivated families appears a likely scenario for positive reinforcement of any perceived improvement.

Conclusions

We cannot be certain of the real explanation for these results until we have more data. It does appear more likely that a participation effect is operating than a putative pressure effect or one related to the administration of 28% oxygen at 1 ATA equivalent. Even if the latter were true, the proper interpretation of the data would seem to be the administration of the safer and cheaper alternative of 1.3 ATA air than 100% oxygen at 1.75 ATA. As far as we are aware, no one has adopted the practice of administering 28% oxygen outside the chamber environment.

Where do we go from here? All concede the need for further research, but the most productive directions are difficult. Although there is little more to be gained from continu-

ing open series, there are two potentially productive avenues. First, it is important for all patients with chronic brain injury that work continues at the basic science level to elucidate a proven mechanism of action for HBOT (or indeed pressure alone). This is critically important in children because of the potential for greater gain in the young and developing brain. Animal models continue to be generally supportive for acute hypoxic-ischemic brain injury in the adult, but little work has been conducted for chronic or pediatric injury. Furthermore, the concept of the ischemic penumbra remains contentious, and the correct interpretation of single-photon emission computed tomography scans in this context is unclear.

Second, clinical studies of the highest possible methodologic rigor are necessary. The experiences after the publication of the Quebec study illustrate the intensity with which any future trials will be examined. We believe the most pertinent trial would compare the efficacy of HBOT (1.3–2.0 ATA, 1 hour daily for 4–6 weeks) to a sham air therapy and a sham using 100% oxygen therapy (both with transitory trivial compression). Any future trials would need to consider appropriate, effective randomization and blinding of all participants and investigators; appropriate sample sizes with power to detect clinically important differences; careful definition and selection of target patients, with stratification for different CP types; appropriate and carefully defined comparator therapy; appropriate outcome measures, including those previously reported; careful elucidation of any adverse effects; and the cost-utility of the therapy.

This is a considerable challenge for any research group, particularly for clinical hyperbaric facilities, and cannot be mounted in the absence of support from the pediatric neurology community. The onus is on enthusiasts who are already convinced of the efficacy of HBOT for CP to encourage and prosecute these trials if they wish to persuade the skeptical. The skeptics should be keen to help in the interests of rational and cost-effective use of scarce resources but cannot be expected to drive an agenda for which they have little expectation of success.

Multiple Sclerosis

Multiple sclerosis (MS) is a chronic neurologic disease in which there is patchy inflammation, demyelination, and gliosis in the central nervous system (CNS). Although there is marked racial and geographic variability in prevalence, MS occurs most widely in races of Northern European ancestry (30–150/100,000)[123] and is the commonest cause of chronic neurologic disability in such countries. The disease frequently affects young adults, with a mean age at onset in the late 20s.[124,125]

Considerable variability exists in both presenting clinical features and the progression of disability across the spectrum of MS. Definitive diagnosis has proved to be a difficult problem, but one of great importance to the individual. A diagnosis of MS requires the elimination of alternative conditions that may mimic the disease, and clinical considerations remain paramount in making the diagnosis. Traditionally, diagnosis has been dependent on a patient experiencing two "attacks" of neurologic dysfunction (e.g., optic neuritis, transverse myelitis, double vision, or numbness and tingling of the legs). These attacks may be years apart, and not all patients who have had a single attack will go on to experience development of MS. An overview of the current status of diagnosis and classification of MS has been given by Murray.[126] About 85% of patients present with the "relapsing-remitting" form of MS, characterized by discrete, episodic relapses followed by partial or complete recovery. The remaining 15% present with a slowly progressing set of neurologic problems—the "primary progressive" form of MS. Over time patients with the relapsing-remitting form may become progressive (secondary progressive) or have a mild course with little progress (benign), and patients with primary progress MS may develop discrete relapses (progressive-relapsing). In practice, much overlap exists between these categories.

A further problem is that the development of MRI technology has shown that typical MS lesions are present long before the development of clinical symptoms and are more widespread than previously thought.[127] Evidence suggests there is a correlation between the number and size of early white matter lesions and the degree of subsequent disability over at least 15 years.[128] Although the early identification of individuals at risk leaves a window during which therapy can be delivered, it is not yet clear whether aggressive immunomodulatory therapy should be commenced at this stage or left until a second attack confirms the diagnosis.

Despite many recent advances in immunology, genetics, molecular biology, and related fields, the cause of MS remains uncertain.[129] The view that MS is an inflammatory, autoimmune demyelinating disease in genetically susceptible individuals has been challenged for some years but remains the generally accepted model.[129,130] The current prevailing hypothesis is that exposure to unknown environmental antigens in genetically susceptible individuals results in activation of certain T-cell populations toward myelin protein and proteolipid complexes. This triggers a massive inflammatory process that results in tissue destruction within the CNS.

The histologic changes described in MS are remarkably constant.[131] Discrete areas of inflammation appear and evolve within the CNS, showing a marked perivenular distribution. The lesions are mainly in the white matter but extend into the gray matter and may occur in the cerebral hemispheres, cerebellum, spinal cord, and optic nerves. Perivascular cuffing with lymphocytes, breakdown of the blood–brain barrier (BBB), and egress of inflammatory cells from the intravascular compartment are followed by cascading inflammatory activation. The area in which these series of events occurs is known as a plaque. Damage to myelin sheaths and oligodendrocytes and degeneration of axons cause the neurologic deficits by which the disease becomes apparent. The presence of thinly myelinated sheaths in some chronic lesions suggests that partial remyelination may occur. MRI data have also indicated that breakdown of the BBB is an extremely early event in the evolution of an inflammatory lesion in MS.[127]

It is widely held that this process, and subsequent development of a plaque, is immunologically mediated. The case has been summarized by Frohman and coworkers.[132] The most obvious feature of the acute lesion is a vigorous inflammatory response with abundant lymphocytes and macrophages, together with some plasma cells and eosinophils. The proinflammatory cytokines tumor necrosis factor-α, interferon-γ, and interleukin-2 can be shown on cells within the lesion. Many of the features of MS in humans can be reproduced using various experimental models of allergic encephalitis using animals where myelin and myelin peptides are injected into genetically susceptible individuals. Despite the current wide adoption and success of immunosuppressive therapy in MS, however (corticosteroids, β-interferons, glatiramer acetate), the evidence for an immunologic process remains circumstantial and the relevance of these experimental models has been questioned.

Some authors have noted that inflammation is a feature of neurodegenerative diseases of the CNS, and they go on to suggest that the inflammatory changes summarized earlier are reactive rather than causative. As an example, Chaudhuri points out that immune cells are a feature of a number of neurologic disorders including stroke, where a sevenfold increase in circulating and cerebrospinal fluid myelin-antigen–reactive T cells is accepted as a response to acute brain injury rather than its cause.[133-135] Furthermore, several features of MS are highly suggestive of a disorder of metabolic regulation including the protective effect of sunlight and sex steroids during pregnancy. After histopathologic analysis of a series of early lesions, Barnett and Prineas[136] have also proposed that all MS lesions may start with apoptosis of oligodendrocytes secondary to an ischemic or metabolic insult yet to be identified, rather than inflammation being the primary event. The possibility that MS is caused by an infectious agent remains; however, no putative organism has ever been isolated despite an extensive search.

With regard to the possible effectiveness of HBOT, it has been proposed that MS is, in fact, a vascular-ischemic event.[130] The similarity noted between the diffuse neurologic abnormalities associated with gas embolism and decompression sickness on the one hand, and MS on the other, suggest there may be a vascular association. Relevant features include the observation of perivenular lesions,[137] abnormal permeability of vessels in MS,[138] and abnormal vessel reactivity.[139] The close anatomic relation between MS plaques and venules in the CNS was first remarked on in 1863.[140] Acute lesions often extend along the vessels in a sleevelike manner, and both thrombosis and perivascular hemorrhages have been described.[137]

In a 1982 review, James[141] suggests that the sudden onset of neurologic symptoms in the absence of generalized illness could be explained as an embolic phenomenon. Based partly on data produced by Dow and Berglund in 1942,[142] James postulated that a subacute form of fat embolization similar to that after trauma, and associated with damage to the BBB, may be responsible. Such emboli could be triggered by a number of stimuli and, in theory at least, might lead to downstream hypoxia, endothelial damage, and leakage of reactive oxygen species and hydrolyzed fats into the interstitium. Damage to myelin could then produce the typical plaque over time. The reduced vascularity of the cortex in comparison with the white matter was postulated to explain the anatomic distribution of lesions. This mechanism is summarized in Figure 21.5.

Gottlieb and Neubauer[130] developed this "vascular-ischemic model" further, suggesting that MS may be viewed as a wound in the CNS resulting from vascular dysfunction and an ischemia-reperfusion event. They suggest that the described immunologic changes are a result of this dysfunction, rather than the primary cause of the clinical syndrome.

A modified vascular hypothesis has again been proposed, with attempts to include both immunologic and vascular processes in the general pathogenesis of MS.[143] Minagar and coauthors[143] suggest that breaching of the BBB is a consequence of endothelial dysfunction, in turn mediated by leukocyte-endothelial interactions. Either leucocytes or cerebral vascular endothelial cells may act as the primary

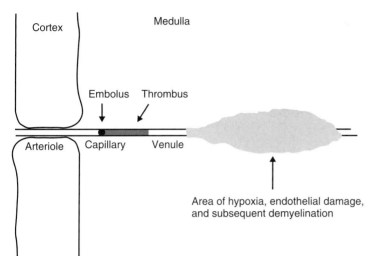

Figure 21.5 Theoretical pathology of plaque formation from James (1982)[141] and based on data from Dow and Berglund (1942).[142] Fat embolus causes downstream hypoxia, thrombus formation, and endothelial damage. Leakage of reactive species into the interstitium damages myelin and promotes plaque formation.

antigen-presenting cells in this process, but the result is chemotaxis between them, opening of the endothelial tight junctions that characterize the BBB, and entry of activated T cells and macrophages to the cerebral interstitium. The resulting cascade of inflammatory response damages both cellular elements and myelin. Pharmacologic agents designed to specifically target adhesion molecules along the BBB have already been introduced into clinical practice, although the first, natalizumab, has been withdrawn because of reports of progressive multifocal leukoencephalopathy in patients while taking the drug.[144,145]

Clinical Evaluation of Multiple Sclerosis

Although MRI findings are now widely accepted as surrogate outcomes for disease extent and progression, clinical outcomes were the standard measure by which the success or failure of therapeutic interventions were judged at least until the early 1990s. This covers the period of intense interest in the use of HBOT for MS. Although there are several proposed clinical assessment schemes, by far the most popular are those developed by Kurtzke.[146,147] The Kurtzke Extended Disability Status Scale (EDSS) and the Kurtzke Functional Status Scale (FSS) were intended to be used together to reproducibly describe the degree of functional impairment across seven systems (FSS) and a score for overall disability (EDSS).[146,147] The

scales are summarized in Table 21.5. Most of the clinical literature examining the effectiveness of HBOT for MS used one or both of these scales to compare functional and global impairment at enrollment and each outcome period in order to determine the benefit or otherwise of therapy. The implications are discussed later in this chapter.

Therapy

MS is currently an incurable disease. In general, there are three approaches to treatment: the prevention of disease progression and reduction of relapse rate, the treatment of acute exacerbations, and the treatment of chronic symptoms. HBOT has been postulated to modify disease progression and to reduce relapse rate, but it is not advanced for the control of acute exacerbations or chronic symptoms.

For the most part, measures aimed at altering disease progression and relapse are immunosuppressive or immunomodulatory, or both. Drugs used in MS include interferon-β, glatiramer acetate, intravenous immunoglobulin, mitoxantrone, methotrexate, and corticosteroids. The most commonly used options have been evaluated by the American Academy of Neurology and the MS Council for Clinical Practice Guidelines.[148] Current therapy consists of the administration of one or more of these partially effective, disease-modifying treatments to appropriate patients. The identification of nonresponders is

Table 21.5 Summary of Descriptors for Each Score of the Kurtzke Expanded Disability Status Score and the Kurtzke Functional Status Score[146,147]

EDSS	FSS
0 = Normal neurologic examination	Pyramidal: 0 = normal; 1 = signs without disability; 2 = mild disability; ... 6 = quadriplegia; ... 9 = unknown
1.0 = No disability; minimal signs on 1 FS	Cerebellar: 0 = normal; 1 = signs without disability; 2 = mild ataxia; ... 5 = unable to perform coordinated movements because of ataxia; ... 9 = unknown
1.5 = No disability; minimal signs on >1 FS.	Brainstem: 0 = normal; 1 = signs only; 2 = moderate nystagmus; ... 5 = inability to swallow or speak; ... 9 = unknown
2.0 = Minimal disability in 1 FS	Sensory: 0 = normal; 1 = vibration or figure writing decreased in one or two limbs; 2 = mild decrease in touch, pain, or position sense; ... 6 = sensation lost below head; ... 9 = unknown
2.5 = Minimal disability in 2 FSs	Visual: 0 = normal; 1 = scotoma with corrected acuity >20/30; 2 = scotoma with worse eye corrected acuity 20/30 to 20/59; ... 6 = worse eye corrected acuity <20/200 and better eye <20/60; ... 9 = normal
3.0 = Moderate disability in 1 FS, or mild disability in 3–4 FSs; fully ambulatory	Mental: 0 = normal; 1 = mood alteration; 2 = mild decrease in mentation; ... 5 = dementia severe or incompetent; 9 = unknown
3.5 = fully ambulatory; moderate disability in 3–4 FSs	Bladder/bowel: 0 = normal; 1 = mild urinary hesitance, urgency, or retention; 2 = moderate same or occasional incontinence; ... 6 = loss of bladder and bowel function; ... 9 = unknown
4.0 = fully ambulatory, walk without aid 500 m; up and about 12 hr/day despite relatively severe disability	Other
4.5 = Fully ambulatory, walk 300 m without aid; up and about much of day, able to work a full day but may have some limitation of full activity or require minimal assistance	
5.0 = Ambulatory without aid for 200 m; disability impairs full daily activities	
5.5 = Ambulatory for about 100 m; disability precludes full daily activity	
6.0 = Intermittent or unilateral constant assistance required to walk 100 m with or without resting	
6.5 = Constant bilateral support required to walk 20 m without resting	
7.0 = Unable to walk beyond 5 m with aid; essentially restricted to wheelchair; wheels self, transfers alone	
7.5 = A few steps only; restricted to wheelchair, needs aid to transfer; wheels self but may need motorized chair for full day's activities	
8.0 = Essentially restricted to bed, chair, or wheeled; may be out of bed much of the day; retains self-care functions; generally effective use of arms	
8.5 = Essentially restricted to bed much of the day; some effective use of arms, some self-care functions	
9.0 = Helpless bed patient; can communicate and eat	
9.5 = Unable to communicate effectively, eat, or swallow	
10 = Dead	

EDSS, Expanded Disability Status Score; FS, functional score; FSS, Functional Status Score.

problematic, and no absolute criteria exist by which to plan the timing of new or additional therapy.

Interferon-β is the agent for which there is the best evidence of efficacy, and several large, placebo-controlled RCTs have been published between 1998 and 2006.[149-157] These trials suggest a limited benefit in relapsing-remitting and secondary progressive MS, although all the trials have methodologic limitations. Benefits, in terms of reduced relapse rate and se-

verity, are achieved at high annual cost per patient (U.K. estimate between £10,000 and £20,000).[158] Adverse side effects are common, particularly flu-like symptoms and injection site reactions.

Some randomized evidence for the efficacy of glatiramer acetate, acetate azathioprine, cyclosporin, intravenous immunoglobulin, methotrexone, and mitoxantrone also exists in some clinical situations; however, the place of these agents remains less certain.

In his 1982 article suggesting MS was a vascular-ischemic event, James[141] proposes the use of HBOT administration as a treatment on the basis of the demonstrated ability of HBOT to produce vasoconstriction with increased oxygen delivery and some anecdotal evidence of efficacy.[159-161] In the subsequent 10 years a flurry of activity produced a number of RCTs in the United Kingdom, United States, Australia, and Europe despite widespread skepticism concerning the postulated pathophysiology. These trials have been summarized in a review paper by Bennett and Heard in 2001.[162] The nonrandomized clinical evidence is summarized in Table 21.6.

Evidence

The early reports had for the most part supported a role for HBOT in preventing progression of MS and indeed reducing disability across a wide range of patients. Both neurologists and hyperbaricists tended to divide into enthusiasts or staunch opponents of this approach, and the place of HBOT remained controversial. In the late 1980s, Kindwall and coauthors[163] initiated a national data register for MS patients undergoing HBOT. A total of 170 neurologists across 22 institutions in the United States contributed to this 2-year longitudinal study, and a total of 312 patients were enrolled. Kindwall and coauthors[163] describe a high dropout rate (only 76% finished the initial course of 20 treatments), and at completion of the 2-year study period, only 28 of the original 312 patients

remained in treatment (9%). The mean deterioration on the Kurtzke EDSS score was 0.93 or almost a full step from the beginning of treatment until the last evaluation. These disappointing results led the Undersea and Hyperbaric Medical Society to confirm that MS should not be an approved indication.

Many neurologists practicing in this area continue to believe such treatment is unlikely to be helpful, and HBOT is not widely available for this indication in many countries. An informal longitudinal case series published only on the Internet suggests significant benefit from the application of HBOT to patients with a variety of MS presentations.[164] This group claims significant benefit with HBOT for the prevention of long-term deterioration by regular maintenance therapy. The Multiple Sclerosis National Therapy Centres data derive from in excess of 1,000,000 treatment occasions and suggest widespread improvements in both symptomatology and mobility. Some of the claims are summarized in Table 21.7. These data are likely to be significantly biased in favor of apparent effectiveness because the only patients for whom we have late assessments are those who continue treatment over several years. As was the case with Kindwall and coauthors' study,[163] those dropping out are likely to be those who found little or no benefit from HBOT.

The evidence from comparative trials has been far less positive than that suggested by this U.K. experience. Worthington, in a nonrandomized crossover trial involving 51 patients with

Table 21.6 Selected Clinical Evidence for the Treatment of MS with HBOT

METHODOLOGY	AUTHOR	SUBJECTS (N)	CONCLUSION
Comparative trial with non-random crossover design	Worthington and colleagues (1987)[165]	51	Minor benefit from hyperbaric oxygen therapy
Comparative, nonrandom	Pallotta (1982)[166a]	22	Reduced relapse
Case series	Boschetty and Cernoch (1970)[159]	26	Transient symptomatic improvement (15/26)
Case series: no peer review*	No authors (2006)[164]	703	Improved disability scores and symptomatology
Qualitative review	Gottlieb and Neubauer (1988)[130]	14 trials	Suggest poor trials and data misinterpreted

*Internet publication only. No authors formally recognized but advice of James and Perrin acknowledged.

Table 21.7 Longitudinal Data from Multiple Sclerosis National Therapy Centres Data[164]

SYMPTOM	IMPROVED (%)	NO CHANGE (%)	WORSE (%)
Fatigue	70	22	8
Speech	64	34	1
Balance	59	37	4
Bladder control	68	30	0
Walking	77	19	4

chronic-progressive and relapsing-remitting disease, found some minor benefits after 20 HBOT sessions (peak flow and finger tapping improved), although walking and mobility were improved after the placebo sessions. Self-care activities decreased during the course of the trial for each group.[165]

In a qualitative review of the literature, Gottlieb and Neubauer[130] suggest many of the RCTs conducted were methodologically flawed, and that the authors may have misinterpreted the trial data. Of particular concern to these authors was the possibility that the dose of oxygen was too high and that few trials included ongoing "top-up" treatments after the original course of HBOT. Neubauer[166] recommends a starting pressure of 1.5 ATA with graduated introduction of greater pressures titrated to the patient response. It is of note, however, that the original positive RCT used 2 ATA oxygen and showed positive results at 1-year follow-up despite not including "top-up" treatments.[167] Neubauer and Gottlieb contend that the effective dose was lower in this trial because of inefficient oxygen delivery by the masks used in this trial, and they conclude that, despite generally poor results, these trials justify the use of HBOT when interpreted in the light of their own vascular-ischemic pathophysiologic model. After the publication of further randomized trials, Kleijnen and Knipschild[168] conducted a semiquantitative analysis and concluded "the majority of controlled trials could not show positive effects." They considered 8 of 14 trials to be of reasonable to high quality, and of these, only one trial (Fischer and colleagues[167]) showed a result in favor of HBOT. In 2004, Bennett and Heard[169] published a formal Cochrane SR with meta-analysis.

Cochrane Review

The Cochrane review on MS identifies 10 reports of 9 RCTs, all published between 1983 and 1990: Fischer and colleagues (1983),[167] Barnes (1985),[169a] Neiman (1985),[169b] Wood (1985),[169c] Confavreux (1986),[169d] L'Hermitte (1986),[169e] Harpur (1986),[169f] Wiles (1986),[169g] Barnes (1987),[169h] and Oriani (1990).[169i] In total, these trials include data on 504 participants, 260 receiving HBOT and 244 control or sham therapy. The details are summarized in Table 21.8.

The dose of oxygen per treatment session varied between studies from 1.75 ATA for 90 minutes (Harpur, 1986) to 2.5 ATA for 90 minutes (Confavreux, 1986; Oriani, 1990). All others used 2.0 ATA for 90 minutes. Whereas all trials used an initial course of 20 treatment sessions over 4 weeks, two (Harpur, 1986; Oriani, 1990) continued to administer "top-up" treatments. Similarly, there were differences in sham therapies, inclusion criteria, and exclusion criteria (see Table 21.8). The mildest cases on admission were those in Oriani (1990), where the entry criteria were EDSS score less than 5 and the mean scores were 3.39 (standard deviation, 1.16) in the active group and 2.97 (standard deviation, 0.84) in the control group, whereas the most severely affected were the participants enrolled by Confavreux (1986) (active group: mean EDSS score, 6.2; standard deviation, 0.7; control group: mean EDSS score, 6.9, standard deviation, 1.4). The majority of studies enrolled participants with scores between 3 and 8.

The participants and outcome assessors were blinded in all studies, although only Harpur (1986) attempted to test the success

Table 21.8 Characteristics of the Studies Included in the Cochrane Review of HBOT for MS

STUDY	METHODS	PARTICIPANTS	INTERVENTIONS	OUTCOMES
Barnes (1985)[169a]	Participants and observers blinded; 6/12 outcome	120 patients with EDSS score < 8: 60 sham, 60 HBOT	Active: HBOT 20 daily sessions at 2.0 ATA for 90 minutes Control: air at 1.1 ATA	EDSS, sphincter, pyramidal function, relapse, adverse effects
Barnes (1987)[169h]	1-year outcome	As above	As above	EDSS, sphincter, pyramidal function, relapse
Confavreux (1986)[169d]	Participants and observers blinded; steroids for some	17 MS patients with EDSS score of 3-8: 9 sham, 8 HBOT	Active: HBOT 20 daily sessions at 2.5 ATA for 90 minutes Control: air at 1.1 or 1.2 ATA	EDSS, sphincter, pyramidal function, adverse effects
Fischer (1983)[167]	Participants and observers blinded	40 MS patients with EDSS score < 6: 20 sham, 20 HBOT	Active: HBOT 20 daily sessions at 2.0 ATA for 90 minutes Control: 10% oxygen at 2.0 ATA	EDSS, sphincter, pyramidal function, relapse, adverse effects
Harpur (1986)[169f]	Participants and observers blinded	82 MS patients with EDSS score of 3-7.5: 41 sham, 41 HBOT	Active: HBOT 20 daily sessions at 1.75 ATA for 90 minutes; 7 "booster" sessions over 6 months Control: 12.5% oxygen at 1.75 ATA plus 7 "booster" sessions	EDSS, sphincter function, relapse, FSS
L'Hermitte (1986)[169e]	Participants and observers blinded; two active vs. one control group	49 MS patients with group EDSS score mean approximately 5.25: 15 sham, 34 HBOT	Active: (1) HBOT 20 daily sessions at 2.3 ATA plus diazepam 5 mg for 90 minutes; (2) HBOT at 2.0ATA Control: 10.5% oxygen at 2.0 or 2.3 ATA	EDSS, relapse, FSS, adverse effects during therapy
Neiman (1985)[169b]	Participants and observers blinded	24 MS patients with mean EDSS scores 6 (active) and 6.1 (control): 12 sham, 12 HBOT	Active: HBOT 20 daily sessions at 2.0 ATA for 90 minutes Control: Air at 1.2 ATA for 5 minutes	EDSS, bladder sphincter function, FSS
Oriani (1990)[169i]	Participants and observers blinded	44 MS patients with EDSS score < 5; mean EDSS scores 3.39 (active) and 2.97 (control): 22 sham, 22 HBOT	Active: HBOT 20 daily sessions at 2.5 ATA for 90 minutes. 5 "booster" sessions each month to 1 year Control: air at 2.5 ATA, plus 5 "booster" sessions	EDSS, sphincter, pyramidal function, FSS
Wiles (1986)[169g]	Participants and observers blinded	84 MS patients with mean EDSS scores of 5.4 (active) and 5.9 (control): 42 sham, 42 HBOT	Active: HBOT 20 daily sessions at 2.0 ATA for 90 minutes Control: air at 1.1 ATA	Bladder sphincter function, adverse effects during therapy
Wood (1985)[169c]	Participants and observers blinded	44 MS patients with EDSS score <3 to 8: 23 sham, 21 HBOT	Active: HBOT 20 daily sessions at 2.0 ATA for 90 minutes Control: 10% oxygen at 2.0 ATA	EDSS, sphincter, pyramidal function, adverse effects during therapy

ATA, atmospheres absolute; EDSS, Extended Disability Status Scale; FSS, Functional Status Score; HBOT, hyperbaric oxygen therapy; MS, multiple sclerosis.

of patient blinding by questionnaire (no numeric result reported). Overall, 31 (7.7%) of the patients enrolled in these trials were lost to follow-up, and sensitivity analysis was made using best- and worst-case outcome analyses to examine any potentially important effects when appropriate.

Most of these trials reported on improvements in disability using the EDSS. There were no benefits in mean EDSS at the completion of 20 treatments (mean change in active group compared with sham, -0.07; 95% CI, -0.23 to 0.09; $P = 0.4$) or at 6 months (-0.22; 95% CI, -0.54 to 0.09; $P = 0.17$); however, there was a statistically significant benefit at 1 year after completion of initial course (-0.85; 95% CI, -1.28 to -0.42; $P = 0.0001$). The only two out

of the nine trials that reported mean EDSS at 1 year were also the only two generally positive trials (Figs. 21.6 and 21.7). Similarly, the proportion of participants improved by at least one point on the EDSS did not differ at completion of 20 treatments (not improving with HBOT OR, 0.33; 95% CI, 0.09-1.18; $P = 0.09$) or at 6 months (OR, 0.42; 95% CI, 0.16-1.08; $P = 0.07$), but again, a statistically significant benefit from HBOT did exist at 1 year (OR, 0.2; 95% CI, 0.06-0.72; $P = 0.01$). Thirteen subjects (14.3%) in the HBOT group improved, and four subjects (4.5%) in the sham group improved. This analysis largely reflects the Oriani (1990) study, to which it contributes 84.7% of the weight. The result was sensitive to the allocation of dropouts with a loss of any significant

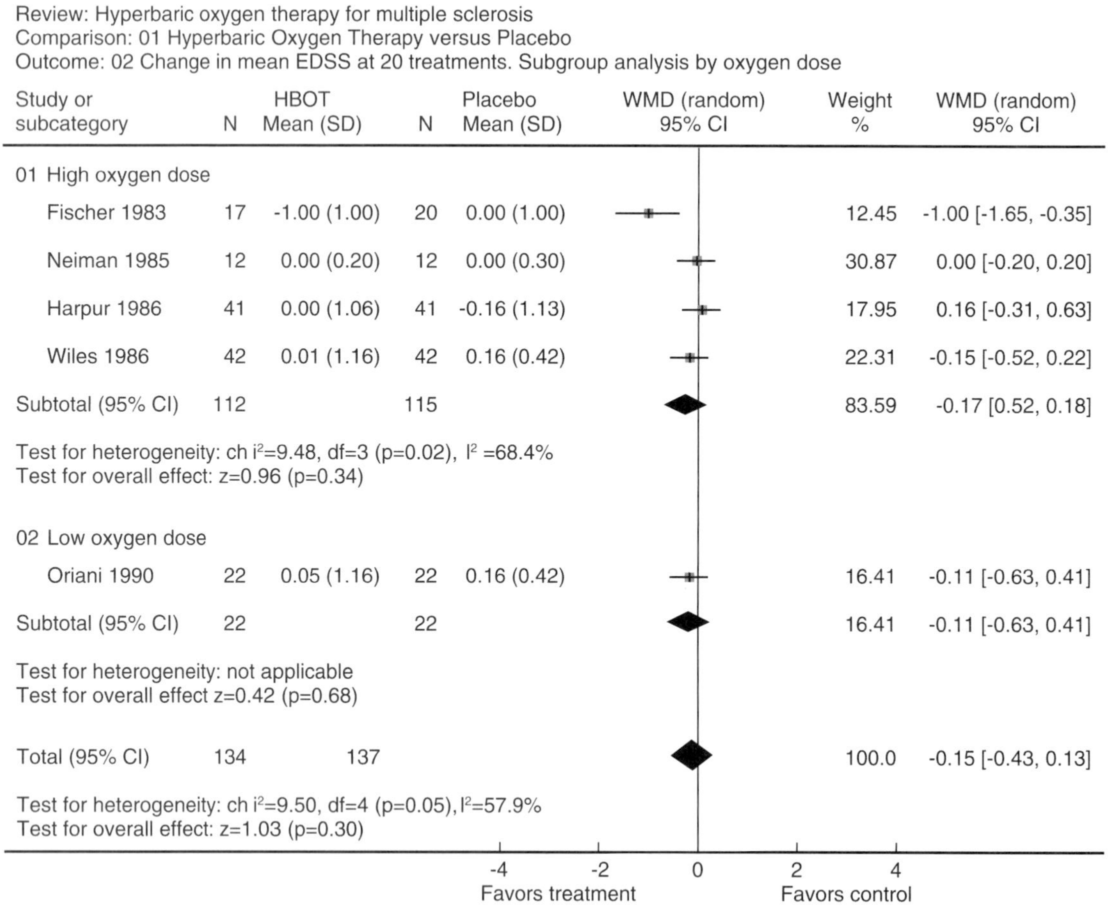

Review: Hyperbaric oxygen therapy for multiple sclerosis
Comparison: 01 Hyperbaric Oxygen Therapy versus Placebo
Outcome: 02 Change in mean EDSS at 20 treatments. Subgroup analysis by oxygen dose

Study or subcategory	N	HBOT Mean (SD)	N	Placebo Mean (SD)	WMD (random) 95% CI	Weight %	WMD (random) 95% CI
01 High oxygen dose							
Fischer 1983	17	-1.00 (1.00)	20	0.00 (1.00)		12.45	-1.00 [-1.65, -0.35]
Neiman 1985	12	0.00 (0.20)	12	0.00 (0.30)		30.87	0.00 [-0.20, 0.20]
Harpur 1986	41	0.00 (1.06)	41	-0.16 (1.13)		17.95	0.16 [-0.31, 0.63]
Wiles 1986	42	0.01 (1.16)	42	0.16 (0.42)		22.31	-0.15 [-0.52, 0.22]
Subtotal (95% CI)	112		115			83.59	-0.17 [0.52, 0.18]

Test for heterogeneity: ch i²=9.48, df=3 (p=0.02), I² =68.4%
Test for overall effect: z=0.96 (p=0.34)

02 Low oxygen dose							
Oriani 1990	22	0.05 (1.16)	22	0.16 (0.42)		16.41	-0.11 [-0.63, 0.41]
Subtotal (95% CI)	22		22			16.41	-0.11 [-0.63, 0.41]

Test for heterogeneity: not applicable
Test for overall effect z=0.42 (p=0.68)

Total (95% CI)	134		137			100.0	-0.15 [-0.43, 0.13]

Test for heterogeneity: ch i²=9.50, df=4 (p=0.05), I²=57.9%
Test for overall effect: z=1.03 (p=0.30)

```
        -4      -2       0       2       4
          Favors treatment    Favors control
```

Figure 21.6 Forest plot for improvement in Extended Disability Status Scale (EDSS) score after 20 treatments; subgroup analysis by oxygen dose. CI, confidence interval; HBOT, hyperbaric oxygen therapy; SD, standard deviation; WMD, weighted mean difference. *(From Bennett M, Heard R: Hyperbaric oxygen therapy for multiple sclerosis. Chichester, United Kingdom, John Wiley & Sons, Ltd. Cochrane Database Syst Rev (1):CD003057, 2004. Copyright Cochrane Collaboration, reproduced with permission.)*

Review: Hyperbaric oxygen therapy for multiple sclerosis
Comparison: 01 Hyperbaric Oxygen Therapy versus Placebo
Outcome: 02 Change in mean EDSS at 12 months

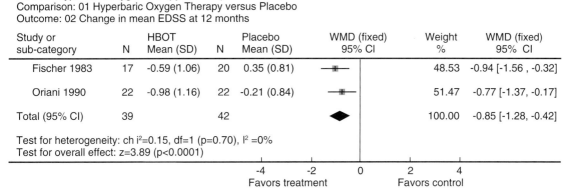

Study or sub-category	N	HBOT Mean (SD)	N	Placebo Mean (SD)	WMD (fixed) 95% CI	Weight %	WMD (fixed) 95% CI
Fischer 1983	17	-0.59 (1.06)	20	0.35 (0.81)		48.53	-0.94 [-1.56 , -0.32]
Oriani 1990	22	-0.98 (1.16)	22	-0.21 (0.84)		51.47	-0.77 [-1.37, -0.17]
Total (95% CI)	39		42			100.00	-0.85 [-1.28, -0.42]

Test for heterogeneity: ch i^2=0.15, df=1 (p=0.70), I^2 =0%
Test for overall effect: z=3.89 (p<0.0001)

$$-4 \quad -2 \quad 0 \quad 2 \quad 4$$
Favors treatment   Favors control

Figure 21.7 Forest plot for improvement in Extended Disability Status Scale (EDSS) score after 12 months. CI, confidence interval; HBOT, hyperbaric oxygen therapy; SD, standard deviation; WMD, weighted mean difference. *(From Bennett M, Heard R: Hyperbaric oxygen therapy for multiple sclerosis. Chichester, United Kingdom, John Wiley & Sons, Ltd. Cochrane Database Syst Rev (1):CD003057, 2004. Copyright Cochrane Collaboration, reproduced with permission.)*

advantage from the administration of HBOT with worst-case assumptions (OR, 1.34; 95% CI, 0.08-21.75; P = 0.21). The analysis suggests that 10 individuals would need to be treated with HBOT to achieve 1 extra patient with an improvement in EDSS score of 1 point at 1 year, but as many as 71 individuals may need to be treated (NNT = 10; 95% CI, 5-71).

On the basis that HBOT may prevent deterioration rather than improve disability, several trials recorded the proportion of patients experiencing deterioration. There was, however, no significant reduction in the odds of experiencing an exacerbation at completion of initial course of HBOT (OR, 0.31; 95% CI, 0.01-7.80; P = 0.5), 6 months (OR, 0.74; 95% CI, 0.25-2.22; P = 0.6), or at 1 year (OR, 0.38; 95% CI, 0.04-3.22; P = 0.4). At the final follow-up, 25.9% of patients in the HBOT group had suffered an exacerbation versus 36.9% in the sham group.

Many trials also recorded information on functional outcomes using the FSS. There were no significantly increased odds of improving in global FSS scores after HBOT at completion of therapy (OR, 1.17; 95% CI, 0.59-2.33; P = 0.65) or at 6 months (OR, 1.09; 95% CI, 0.55-2.18; P = 0.8). Only Oriani (1990) reports this outcome at 1 year, and 41% of patients in both arms had improved FSS scores. Similarly, there were no significant benefits from HBOT for maintaining bladder and bowel sphincter function (e.g., odds of not improving with HBOT at 6 months is 0.50; 95% CI, 0.08-2.94; P = 0.4).

At 1 year, 17.2% of participants had improved in the HBOT group and 5.7% in the sham group (P = 0.09).

In contrast, although there was no evidence of benefit for pyramidal function immediately after therapy, there was statistically significant benefit at both 6-month and 1-year assessments (e.g., at 1 year, the odds of not improving with HBOT were 0.13; 95% CI, 0.03-0.58; P = 0.007). At that time, 13.2% of patients improved in the HBOT group compared with 4.5% in the sham group. These results largely reflect the outcome in a single trial (Oriani, 1990) and suggest that at least 6 patients would need to be treated with HBOT to improve 1 extra individual, but perhaps as many as 197 patients would need to be treated (NNT = 11; 95% CI, 6-197).

These trials suggest that there were significantly increased odds of deteriorating vision after the administration of HBOT (OR, 24.87; 95% CI, 1.44-428.50; P = 0.03). The analysis suggests the NNT with HBOT to get one further complaint of visual disturbance is low (NNT = 1; 95% CI, 1-2). Approximately 55% of patients suffered deterioration in the HBOT group, and three participants (2.3%) experienced this in the sham group. No statistically significant increase occurred in the odds of aural barotrauma after the administration of HBOT (OR, 2.94; 95% CI, 0.62-13.91; P = 0.17), although no data were recorded on any other adverse effects of therapy.

Conclusions

The pathophysiology of MS remains uncertain and is an area of active research. Immune mechanisms appear likely to remain central to the development of the clinical syndrome, and given the known immunologic effects of hyperoxia, it remains possible that HBOT could have a role in disease modification. Animal models of MS are problematic and not universally accepted; therefore, preclinical evidence of HBOT remains thin. In contrast, a considerable body of clinical evidence exists on which to base treatment recommendations.

Despite encouraging reports in the literature, Bennett and Heard[169] conclude there was little evidence of a significant effect for the administration of HBOT in a formal SR with meta-analysis of the randomized evidence. There were no clear and clinically important benefits evident from HBOT administration with respect to important clinical outcomes. Although a modest benefit was demonstrated in mean EDSS score at 12 months, this result is uncertain given that only two trials reported on this outcome at this time (16% of the total participants in the review), and they were the only trials of the nine to suggest benefit at earlier assessment times. Similarly, the modest benefit suggested at 12 months in the proportion of participants with improved EDSS scores reflected a single trial (Oriani, 1990), which contributed 84.7% of the weight to that analysis and was sensitive to the allocation of dropouts. All other trials reporting this outcome at 6 months suggested no clinically useful benefit, and it appears biologically implausible that a benefit be absent at 6 months after treatment and present at 12 months. Furthermore, the reduction in mean EDSS in the HBOT group at 12 months was only 0.84 points, a barely detectable difference on clinical examination.

Of the 20 separate outcome factors where meta-analysis was possible, significant benefit was suggested in only 3. None of the subgroup analyses undertaken (oxygen course, nature of sham and oxygen treatment pressure) could explain the heterogeneity between the results of Fischer (1983) and Oriani (1990) (benefit suggested) and the other seven trials (no evidence of benefit).

Proponents of HBOT suggest that a long course of treatment may be required to demonstrate benefit,[170] and that those trials giving only 20 treatments are flawed in this regard. Others also maintain that treatments greater than 2 ATA are toxic and unhelpful.[130,166] Both these assertions are difficult to sustain, however, in that of the two trials contributing to this significant result, one gave a short course at only 2 ATA (Fischer, 1983), whereas the other continued with top-up treatments to 12 months and used 2.5 ATA (Oriani, 1990), and both showed benefits after 20 treatments and 6 months. Furthermore, the only other trial to administer a longer course of treatments (Harpur, 1986) failed to suggest any benefit in EDSS at 20 treatments or 6 months (no data at 12 months). There is no reason to extrapolate that data from other trials, including Harpur (1986), would have confirmed a benefit after 12 months after having failed to do so at earlier analyses.

In summary, no consistent evidence confirms a beneficial effect of HBOT for the treatment of MS, and routine use does not appear to be justified on the basis of the available evidence. The small number of analyses suggestive of benefit in the Cochrane meta-analysis were isolated, difficult to ascribe with biological plausibility, and would need to be confirmed in future well-designed trials. The cost to achieve any benefit is likely to be high.

The published clinical evidence is dated and difficult to interpret compared with contemporary investigations. Although there is a case for further research, there is little indication that strong and clinically useful treatment effects are likely. It is possible, however, that modest treatment benefits may be present in a subset of disease severity or classification. One of the two trials indicating some benefits (Oriani, 1990), for example, enrolled patients with relatively mild disabilities, and it may be that HBOT has a role in mild disease. Any future trials will need to be planned carefully and will need to include MRI data and validated quality-of-life instruments. Finally, any future trials should assess both the safety and cost of therapy. It is likely that only staunch advocates would be willing to pursue such investigations.

Acute Ischemic Stroke

Stroke may be defined as a sudden neurologic deficit that is of presumed vascular origin.[171] It is both a leading cause of mortality worldwide, accounting for an estimated 5.4 million deaths in 2001 (9.6% of all deaths), and a leading cause of disability, accounting for 6% of all disability-adjusted life-years in developed countries.[172] About one third of survivors require significant assistance in daily life at 1 year after an event.[171,173]

Stroke is divided into two broad subgroups: ischemic and hemorrhagic, with the former accounting for 73% to 86% of all cases.[174] On average, ischemic stroke has a lower case fatality rate than hemorrhagic stroke (23% vs. 62% at 1 year). Accepted treatment for ischemic stroke includes anticoagulation and thrombolysis, whereas in hemorrhagic stroke, such measures are likely to promote further bleeding.[171,173] Therefore, an early and accurate diagnosis is desirable.[171] Because clinical assessment is unreliable in determining the stroke type, neuroimaging (preferably using computerized tomography [CT] scan) is required for optimal management.[175]

During a cerebral ischemic event, neurologic tissue suffers hypoxia. When hypoxia is prolonged, neurons lose their ability to maintain ionic homeostasis. Free oxygen radicals accumulate and degrade the cell membranes,[46,47] leading to irreversible changes resulting in unavoidable cell death. These changes may occur rapidly and before therapy can be instituted, but in some patients, the symptoms worsen gradually or in a stepwise fashion over a matter of hours or days.[48] This latter observation suggests that the close management of hemodynamic, respiratory, and metabolic factors designed to maintain oxygenation might be beneficial.

Therapy

Great emphasis is placed on the prevention of cerebral ischemic events through lifestyle change and pharmacology aimed at reducing general cardiovascular risk. The recognition and modification of risk factors is a continuing challenge beyond the scope of this chapter, but evidence emerging from MRI using diffusion-weighted techniques suggests that silent ischemic events are common both before and after clinically apparent episodes of ischemia, and this technique may be useful to monitor the effect of any intervention.[176,177]

Intensive stroke management protocols, thrombolysis, and antiplatelet therapy have been shown to positively influence the outcome after acute events.[178-180] Within these protocols, accepted adjunctive measures designed to assist recovery from acute stroke include nutritional supplementation using enteral nutrition via nasogastric tube,[181] tight control of blood glucose,[182] and measures to control arterial blood pressure.[183] The most important therapeutic decision is whether to administer thrombolysis, and this decision is based on timing and exclusion of hemorrhagic stroke by brain imaging techniques.

HBOT has been proposed for the adjunctive treatment of ischemic stroke since the 1960s.[184,185] The potential benefits of HBOT include the reversal of hypoxia through increased oxygen delivery and reduction of cerebral edema.[49,56] Several specific and potentially beneficial effects of hyperoxia include decreased lipid peroxidation, inhibition of leukocyte activation, and restoration of the functional BBB.[76,77,186] It has been proposed that HBOT protects marginally viable brain (often termed "the ischemic penumbra") from further damage on reperfusion through these mechanisms that act to regulate abnormal cellular metabolites.[187,188] Conversely, oxygen in high doses may increase oxidative stress through the production of oxygen free radical species and is potentially toxic.[189] Indeed, the brain is particularly at risk.[50] Furthermore, HBOT has effects on cerebral blood flow that may promote further neuronal damage, including both reductions in CBF secondary to hyperoxic vasospasm and through an inverse steal phenomenon.[190] For these reasons, it is appropriate to postulate that, in some stroke patients, HBOT may do more harm than good.

Evidence

The majority of animal studies support the use of HBOT and these were thoroughly examined by Helms and colleagues in 2005.[191] The models used involve the permanent or temporary occlusion of cerebral arteries using ties or intravascular filaments, whereas the time to institution of HBOT in these animals varies from a few minutes to 24 hours (Table 21.9). In general, outcomes were improved with HBOT in both ischemia-reperfusion models and permanent occlusion models, with infarct size reductions being the most common outcome estimated. Although there was a greater variability in results after permanent occlusion, the beneficial effect of HBOT after temporary occlusions seemed to hold for delays to treatment of up to several hours in most of these studies. Nevertheless, some evidence exists of reduced benefit with increasing delays to treatment[192,193] and (disturbingly) worse outcomes with HBOT at 12-hour delay.[193]

Despite this generally encouraging animal evidence and 40 years of interest in the delivery of HBOT in stroke patients, little comparative evidence of effectiveness existed before the 1990s. Most reports were of single or multiple cases, with the largest study being a series of 122 cases reported in 1980.[194] A review of these studies calculated that more than half of the patients improved clinically or electrophysiologically with HBOT and concluded there was a case for setting up controlled studies.[190] Since 1991, three such RCTs have been reported in the literature, and these were recently included in a Cochrane review.[195]

Cochrane Review

The Cochrane review on acute ischemic stroke includes randomized trials enrolling patients with confirmed acute ischemic stroke and using HBO as an adjunct to standard care.

Outcomes on 106 patients, 52 in the HBOT group and 54 in the control group, are reported. Individual study characteristics are summarized in Table 21.10.

Significant variations exist in the methodology across these trials. Rusyniak (2003) and Nighoghossian (1995) enrolled patients within 24 hours of stroke onset, whereas Anderson (1991) accepted patients up to 2 weeks later. Rusyniak delivered a single therapy session at 2.5 ATA for 60 minutes, whereas both Nighoghossian and Anderson gave multiple treatments at 1.5 ATA.

All these trials were small and had low power to detect useful clinical differences between groups. The extent and severity of deficit on enrollment was poorly described and difficult to compare across trials given that all three used different neurologic and health status scales to establish baseline status.

All trials did, however, report death at between 3 and 6 months (Fig. 21.8). At that time, there were no significant differences in mortality (three deaths [6%] in those receiving HBOT vs. five [10%] with sham therapy), and the RR of dying after receiving HBOT was 0.61 (95% CI, 0.17–2.2; $P = 0.45$). No indication of significant heterogeneity between trials ($I^2 = 0\%$) was present.

Each of the three trials used functional scale scores, and a summary of these outcomes at final follow-up is presented in Table 21.11. Anderson (1991) also reports that mean infarct volume was smaller in the control group at 4 months (29.0 vs. 49.2 cm^3), but not significantly so (MD, 20.2 cm^3; 95% CI, −13.4 to 53.8; $P = 0.24$).

Claustrophobia was a significant problem in the monoplace vessels used in all trials for both arms. In the intensive therapy protocol used by Anderson (1991), for example, 39% of participants could not complete scheduled therapy.

Conclusions

The ischemic nature of the event, plus the majority of animal evidence, mean that a rational case can be made for the use of HBOT for stroke. The animal and uncontrolled human data suggest early treatment is more likely to

Table 21.9 Summary of Animal Studies of Focal Cerebral Ischemia Where HBOT Was Compared with Normobaric Air or Oxygen

TRIAL, ANIMAL, AND VESSEL OCCLUDED	TIME TO HBOT	OXYGEN DOSE	OUTCOME
Weinstein (1986),[192] gerbil, 20-minute bilateral CCA	0	1.5 ATA for 15 minutes once	Improved survival
Yang (2002),[192a] rat, 1-hour MCA	0	2.8 ATA for 15 minutes once	Neuroprotection implied by reduced extracellular dopamine
Miljkovic-Lolic and colleagues (2003),[74] rat, 1-hour MCA	0	3 ATA for 1 hour once	Reduced infarct volume, leukocyte infiltrate, and myeloperoxidase
Sunami (2000),[192b] rat, permanent right MCA and right CCA	10 minutes	3 ATA for 2 hours once	Reduced infarct volume
Hjelde (2002),[192c] rat, permanent MCA*	10 minutes	2 ATA for 3 hours 50 minutes once	No difference in ischemic volume or myeloperoxidase
Veltkamp and colleagues (2000),[81] rat, 1-hour 15-minute MCA	15 minutes	1.5 ATA for 1 hour or 2.0 ATA for 1 hour	Reduced infarct volume and better behaviorally with 2.5 ATA HBO
Burt (1987),[192d] gerbil, permanent CCA	<30 minutes	1.5 ATA for 36 or 18 hours with long air breaks† once	Reduced chance of infarct with intermittent, shorter HBO
Reitan (1990),[78] gerbil, permanent CCA	40 minutes	2.5 ATA for 2 or 4 hours†	Improved survival
Veltkamp (2005),[192e] rat, 2-hour MCA	40 minutes	3.0 ATA for 1 hour once	Reduced BBB permeability, smaller infarcts
Veltkamp and colleagues (2006),[82] rat, 2-hour MCA	45 minutes	3.0 ATA for 1 hour once	Reduced evidence of ischemic biochemical degradation
Corkill (1985),[192f] gerbil, permanent CCA	1 hour	1 or 1.5 ATA for up to 1 hour† once	More HBO reduced color density differences between sides
Gunther (2005),[192g] rat, permanent MCA	15 minutes to 6 hours*	2.5 ATA for 90 minutes once or 4 times on day 1*	Early HBO reduced infarct size, late at 6 hours and repeated HBO did not*
Roos (1998),[192h] rat, 3–90-minute MCA*	Not stated. Probably immediately after occlusion	2 ATA for 30 minutes once or daily for 4 days	No benefit
Schäbitz (2004),[79] rat, permanent MCA	2 hours	2 ATA for 1 hour once	Reduced infarct volume and deficit
Calvert (2006),[192i] rat, permanent CCA*	2 hours	2.5 ATA for 2 hours once vs. NBO control	No difference in the reduction of hypoxia inducible factor
Kawamura (1990),[192j] rat, 4-hour MCA	3 hours	2 ATA for 30 minutes once	Reduced infarct volume and edema
Lou (2006),[192k] rat, 90-minute MCA	3 hours	3 ATA for 1 hour once	Reduced infarct area and improved deficit
Lou and colleagues (2004),[193] rat, 90-minute MCA and permanent MCA*	3, 6, and 12 hours	3 ATA for 1 hour once	Transient: improved outcome early, worse outcome late* Permanent: worse outcome*
Weinstein and colleagues (1987),[193a] cat, 6- and 24-hour* MCA	Variable up to 6 hours	1.5 ATA 40 minutes once at 6 or 24 hours†	Function improved and reduced infarct size with HBO up to 3rd hour of 6-hour occlusion, but not 4th of 12-hour occlusion*
Badr and colleagues (2001),[187] rat, 2-hour MCA	6 hours	3 ATA for 1 hour once	Reduced biochemical evidence of ischemia
Yin (2005),[193b] rat, 2-hour MCA	6 or 24 hours	2.5 ATA 2 hours daily for 6 days	Improved outcome at both times
Yin (2002),[193c] rat, 2-hour MCA	8 hours	3 ATA for 1 hour once	Reduced infarct area
Yin (2003),[193d] rat, 2-hour MCA occlusion	8 hours	2.5 ATA for 2 hours once	Reduced infarct area, neurologic scores and apoptosis

Ranked by interval from occlusion to institution of hyperbaric oxygen therapy (HBOT).
  *No benefit from HBOT found.
  †Complex treatment schedules (see citation for details).
  BBB, blood–brain barrier; CCA, common carotid artery; HBO, hyperbaric oxygen; MCA, middle cerebral artery; NBO, normobaric oxygen.

Table 21.10 Characteristics of the Included Studies of HBOT for Acute Ischemic Stroke

STUDY	METHODS	SUBJECTS	INTERVENTIONS	OUTCOMES
Anderson (1991)[195a]	RCT stratified for disease severity and blinded; powered to find a 30% relative improvement in HBOT group with 45 subjects in each group (stopped early)	39 adults with ischemic stroke within 2 weeks, greater than 20 severity score out of 100; internal carotid territory	Neurologic intensive care Control: sham at 1.5 ATA for 60 m within 6 hours and then every 8 hours to a total of 15 over 5 days HBOT: 100% oxygen as above	Neurologic examination at day 5, week 6, year 1; infarct volume on CT scan at 4 months
Nighoghossian (1995)[195b]	RCT with sham therapy; 17 allocated to each arm; 7 subjects withdrawn	34 adults with stroke confirmed with CT within 24 hours suggestive of middle cerebral artery occlusion and scoring less than 80 on the Orgogozo scale (100 is normal)	Low-dose heparin and supportive care Control: sham at 1.2 ATA daily for 40 minutes for 10 days HBOT: 100% oxygen at 1.5 ATA on the same schedule	Neurologic examination on three scales: Orgogozo (100 to 0), Trouillas (0 to 10), and Rankin Disability scales; adverse effects of HBOT
Rusyniak (2003)[195c]	RCT stratified by time to 24 hours with allocation concealment and blinding of subjects and investigators	33 adults with ischemic stroke presenting within 24 hours of onset of neurologic deficit; all subjects scored less than 23 points on the NIHSS	Control: sham at 1.14 ATA for 60 minutes HBOT: 100% oxygen at 2.5 ATA on the same schedule as above	NIHSS at 24 hours and 90 days; Barthel Index, Rankin Scale, and Glasgow Outcome Scale at 90 days; mortality; adverse effects

ATA, atmospheres absolute; CT, computed tomography; HBOT, hyperbaric oxygen therapy; NIHSS, National Institutes of Health Status Scale; RCT, randomized, controlled trial.

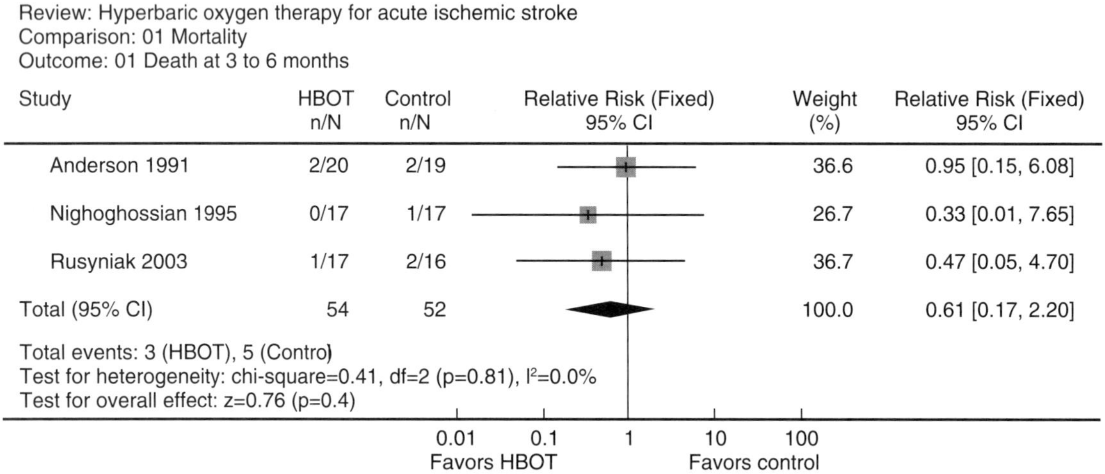

Review: Hyperbaric oxygen therapy for acute ischemic stroke
Comparison: 01 Mortality
Outcome: 01 Death at 3 to 6 months

Study	HBOT n/N	Control n/N	Relative Risk (Fixed) 95% CI	Weight (%)	Relative Risk (Fixed) 95% CI
Anderson 1991	2/20	2/19		36.6	0.95 [0.15, 6.08]
Nighoghossian 1995	0/17	1/17		26.7	0.33 [0.01, 7.65]
Rusyniak 2003	1/17	2/16		36.7	0.47 [0.05, 4.70]
Total (95% CI)	54	52		100.0	0.61 [0.17, 2.20]

Total events: 3 (HBOT), 5 (Contro)
Test for heterogeneity: chi-square=0.41, df=2 (p=0.81), I²=0.0%
Test for overall effect: z=0.76 (p=0.4)

```
0.01    0.1      1      10     100
  Favors HBOT        Favors control
```

Figure 21.8 Forest plot of mortality at 3 to 6 months after ischemic stroke. CI, confidence interval; SD, standard deviation. *(From Bennett MH, Wasiak J, Schnabel A, et al: Hyperbaric oxygen therapy for acute ischaemic stroke. Chichester, United Kingdom, John Wiley & Sons, Ltd. Cochrane Database Syst Rev (3):CD004954, 2005. Copyright Cochrane Collaboration, reproduced with permission.)*

Table 21.11 Summary of Functional and Activities of Daily Living Scales Used as Outcomes in the Randomized Controlled Trials of HBOT for Ischemic Stroke

FUNCTIONAL SCALE	TRIALS	CONTROL	HBOT	DIFFERENCE (95% CI)	P
Mean neurologic score* (lower score = better outcome)	Anderson (1991): 1 year	25.8	31.4	5.6 (−15.1 to 26.2)	0.59
Mean Orgogozo Scale (higher score = better outcome)	Nighoghossian (1995): 1 year	78.2	50.3	27.9 (4.0–51.8)†	0.02
Mean Trouillas Disability Scale (lower score = better outcome)	Nighoghossian (1995): 1 year	4.1	6.3	2.2 (0.15–4.3)†	0.04
Mean Modified Rankin Functional Assessment Scale (lower score = better outcome)	Nighoghossian (1995): 1 year	2.4	3.0	0.6 (−0.18 to 1.4)	0.13
Number of participants to achieve a good outcome‡	Rusyniak (2003): 90 days	10.0	6.0	RR 1.8 (0.8–3.7)	0.13
Barthel Index: 95 or 100 (good outcome)	Rusyniak (2003): 90 days	9.0	8.0	RR 0.8 (0.43–1.6)	0.6

*Score designed specifically for Anderson (1991).[195a]
†Significant differences.
‡Either National Institute of Health Stroke Scale < 2, Rankin Scale score < 2, or Glasgow Outcome Scale score = 5.
CI, confidence interval; HBOT, hyperbaric oxygen therapy; RR, relative risk.

produce benefit, and that late treatment (around 24 hours) may be harmful. There is, however, no convincing evidence from RCTs that HBOT improves outcome. Pooled data do not suggest any significant benefit in mortality in the 6 months after presentation. Although there was some indication from one trial (Nighoghossian, 1995) for improvement in one disability scale (Trouillas) and one clinical descriptive scale (Orgogozo), these improvements were not reflected in other trials or functional scales and were present at 1 year but not 6 months after therapy was completed. There does not appear to be a plausible explanation for this apparent late effect. Furthermore, the analysis of these ordinal scales to produce mean scores for group comparisons may not be appropriate.[196] One review concludes that of nine stroke scales tested, the National Institutes of Health Stroke Scale was one of the three most reliable, whereas the Barthel Index was the most reliable disability scale.[197]

Little clinical data exist on which to base treatment recommendations. The routine use of HBOT in stroke patients cannot be justified from the results of randomized trials at this time. However, given the small numbers of subjects in the trials included, we cannot be certain that a benefit from HBOT has been excluded. Any further trials should be planned carefully to provide information on the effect of disease severity, the appropriate oxygen dose, and the timing of therapy.

Idiopathic Sudden Sensorineural Hearing Loss and Tinnitus

Idiopathic sudden sensorineural hearing loss (ISSHL) is an acute hearing impairment with an incidence of about 8 to 15 per 100,000 of the population per year.[198] Although the cause and pathophysiology remain unclear,[199] ISSHL is most commonly defined as a greater than 30-dB sensorineural hearing loss occurring in at least three contiguous audiometric frequencies over 72 hours or less.[200] Tinnitus may be defined as the perception of sound in the absence of external acoustic stimulation. The incidence rate is probably about 10% to 20% of adults in the developed countries.[201-202] Brief episodes of tinnitus are probably normal, and clinically significant tinnitus is usually defined by applying one of several classification systems proposed.[204,205]

Because of the abrupt onset in many patients, a vascular cause for ISSHL has been suggested,[206] but other possibilities include viral infection, autoimmune disease, and inner-ear membrane rupture.[201,207] Histologically, postmortem samples have shown atrophy of the cochlear and a loss of neurons, but findings are quite variable.[207] The cause of tinnitus is equally obscure, although it is often associated with ISSHL—up to 90% of patients with ISSHL also complain of tinnitus.[208] The most widely discussed theories include excessive or abnormal spontaneous activity in the auditory system and related cerebral areas[209] and abnormal signal processing with "feedback."[210,211]

Therapy

Treatments for ISSHL are often aimed at improving the oxygenation of the inner ear and include vasodilators, plasma expanders, steroids, anticoagulants, diuretics, and antivirals. None has been proved of benefit in large, randomized trials or meta-analyses. A Cochrane review concerning the use of steroids was inconclusive,[212] whereas another concerning the use of vasodilators has been withdrawn.[213] Assessment of the effectiveness of therapy is complicated by a high rate of spontaneous recovery, as much as 65% in some studies,[214] and the variable periods for which hearing loss has been present before the institution of therapy. Specific therapies for tinnitus have tended to focus on the impact of the noise on quality of life and mood and include antidepressants anticonvulsants, and benzodiazepines or focus on trying to mask the noise itself with white noise generators. A variety of psychotherapeutic and "habituation" programs is also advocated to help the sufferer deal with the problem.[215] A Cochrane review of the use of Ginkgo biloba found no reliable evidence either way,[216] whereas a review of antidepressants is under way.[217]

HBOT has been proposed since the late 1960s to improve both ISSHL and tinnitus, based on the arguments that both hearing loss and tinnitus may result from a hypoxic event in the cochlear apparatus and that HBOT may be able to reverse that oxygen deficit.[218] The

great increase in plasma P_{O_2} during HBOT promotes oxygen diffusion into the perilymph, where the sensory apparatus (hair cells) is dependent on diffusion for oxygenation. High tensions of oxygen may persist for some time after each treatment; perilymph P_{O_2} has been reported at 58% greater than normal at 1 hour after removal from the hyperoxic environment.[218]

Evidence

Since the early 1970s, many patients have been reported in cohort studies comparing a wide range of both medical and hyperbaric treatment regimens. In his 1998 review, Lamm[218] documents 50 clinical studies involving more than 4000 patients who received HBOT after unsuccessful medical therapy. Many reports have been available only in German or Japanese.[219] Those appearing in English are summarized in Table 21.12, together with several more recent studies examining the use of HBOT early after hearing loss, generally in conjunction with pharmacologic agents. Typically, these trials suggest that after HBOT, a greater proportion of patients will have a significant return of hearing, and that mean hearing gains are also greater in the HBOT groups. Furthermore, it is strongly suggested that earlier therapy is more likely to succeed, although there is a likely bias from the high level of spontaneous improvement observed in these patients no matter which therapy is administered.

Much less work has been reported specifically for the treatment of tinnitus. Gul and co-workers[220] treated patients with acute-onset tinnitus and found a combined approach with intravenous polypharmacy and HBOT was less successful than pharmacology alone (80% vs. 66% reported improvements). Tan and colleagues[221] report mixed results using HBOT for the treatment of chronic tinnitus. Twenty percent could not tolerate compression, whereas 10% complained of worse tinnitus and 30% reported an improvement.

Since 1999 there have been six randomized clinical trials published in this area. Five have been included in a Cochrane review,[222] whereas

Table 21.12 Summary of Nonrandom Clinical Trials of the Use of HBOT for the Treatment of Acute Sudden Sensorineural Hearing Loss

TRIAL	METHODOLOGY	THERAPY	OUTCOMES
Goto (1979)[223a]	91 patients with ISSHL	Group 1 (21 patients): vasodilators, steroids, vitamin B Group 2 (49): 2.4 ATA HBO for 90 minutes on 20 occasions and stellate ganglion block Group 3 (20): all of the above	Greater improvement with combined therapy within 2 weeks of onset
Nakashima and colleagues (1998)[219]	Cohort of 692 patients with SSHL; 149 had HBOT added when not responding (within 14 days of onset)	All patients: vitamin B complex, vasodilator and "metabolic activators" HBOT: 2 ATA for 60 minutes, 14-20 treatments	Some recovery after HBOT
Aslan (2002)[223b]	50 patients with sudden deafness	25 patients treated with betahistine, prednisone, and stellate ganglion block for 5 days 25 patients as above plus HBOT 2.4 ATA for 90 minutes twice daily for 7 days, then daily for 6 days (20 treatments total)	Thresholds better with addition of HBOT
Sparacia (2003)[223c]	24 patients with SSHL	16 patients within 2 weeks compared with 8 patients 15-30 days; HBOT at 2.2 ATA 120 minutes for 20-40 days	75% good recovery in first group vs. no patient with good result in the second
Racic (2003)[223d]	115 patients with ISSHL with onset within 7 days	64 treated with intravenous pentoxifyl-line 50-300 mg/day; 51 treated with HBOT 2.8 ATA for 60 minutes, twice daily for a maximum of 30 sessions	Greater mean gain in hearing with HBOT; differences persist for 9 months
Horn (2005)[223e]	9 patients with ISSHL after failure of 2 weeks of medical therapy	HBOT at 2 ATA for 90 minutes daily for 10 days	3 patients responded with "dramatic improvements"
Satar (2006)[223f]	54 consecutive patients with ISSHL	17 medical therapy: complex, including anti-inflammatory drugs, vitamin B complex, nicotinamide, steroid, vitamin C, etc., twice daily for 7 days (within 15 days of onset) 37 as above plus HBOT 2.5 ATA for 90 minutes twice daily for 3 days and then 75 minutes daily for 2 weeks (within 5 days of onset)	No differences in recovery between groups

ATA, atmospheres absolute; HBO, hyperbaric oxygen; HBOT, hyperbaric oxygen therapy; ISSHL, idiopathic sudden sensorineural hearing loss; SSHL, sudden sensorineural hearing loss.

the sixth is also included in a later summary of that review.[223] The results and conclusions are summarized in the following section.

Cochrane Review

A comprehensive search of the literature for trials of HBOT for the treatment of either ISSHL or tinnitus produced 16 articles of interest, of which 6 were accepted for inclusion into the formal review as relevant RCTs: Cavallazzi (1996),[223g] Fattori (2001),[223h] Schwab (1998),[223i] Hoffmann (1995; two studies),[223j,223k] and Topuz (2004).[223l] Five of these included patients with acute presentation of ISSHL with or without tinnitus, whereas one enrolled subjects with at least a 6-month history of ISSHL, tinnitus, or both (Hoffmann [1995 chronic] provided two trial reports, one on acute and one on chronic hearing loss). The total number of patients enrolled was 304, with 163 in the HBOT group and 141 in the control group. The characteristics of these trials are summarized in Table 21.13.

Table 21.13 Characteristics of Studies Included in the Cochrane Review of HBOT for the Treatment of ISSHL or Tinnitus

STUDY	METHODS	PARTICIPANTS	INTERVENTIONS	OUTCOMES
Cavallazzi (1996)[223g]	Method of allocation not clear, no blinding	64 subjects with ISSHL, time course unknown; stratified into mild, moderate, severe, and "deep"	Control: multidrug therapy: heparin, betamethasone, nicotinic acid, flunarizine, antivirals, citidinephospho-coline, dextran, and vitamins HBOT: as above plus oxygen at 2.5 ATA for 60 minutes daily for 15 sessions over 3 weeks	PTA recovery (%)
Fattori (2001)[223h]	Method of randomization not clear, no blinding	50 subjects with ISSHL referred within 48 hours; stratified into mild, moderate, and severe.	Control: vasodilator therapy: 10-day course intravenous 200 mg/day buflomedil HBOT: oxygen at 2.2 ATA for 90 minutes daily for 10 days	PTA recovery (%) Mean PTA recovery (%)
Hoffmann (1995)[223k]	Method of randomization not clear, patients and assessors blinded	44 subjects with ISSHL for >6 months	Control: Air breathing at 1.5 ATA for 45 minutes daily, 5 days each week for 3 weeks HBOT: 100% oxygen on the same schedule as control subjects	Improved hearing (%) Tinnitus (%)
Hoffmann (1995)[223j]	Method of randomization not clear, no blinding	20 subjects with ISSHL not improved after 14 days of drug treatment with hydroxyethyl starch, pentoxifylline, and cortisone	Control: no treatment HBOT: oxygen at 1.5 ATA for 45 minutes daily, 5 days each week for 2-4 weeks (10-20 sessions)	Mean PTA recovery (dB) Tinnitus (%)
Schwab (1998)[223i]	Method of randomization not clear, no blinding	75 subjects with ISSHL seen within 2 weeks and without any prior therapy	Control: no treatment HBOT: oxygen at 1.5 ATA for 45 minutes daily, for 2-4 weeks (10-20 sessions)	Mean PTA recovery (dB) Tinnitus (0-10)
Topuz (2004)[223l]	Method of randomization not clear, no blinding	51 subjects with ISSHL seen within 2 weeks and without any prior therapy	Control: prednisone, Rheomacrodex, diazepam, and pentoxifylline HBOT: as above plus oxygen at 2.5 ATA for 90 minutes to 25 treatments in 3 weeks	Mean PTA recovery (dB)

ATA, atmospheres absolute; HBOT, hyperbaric oxygen therapy; ISSHL, idiopathic sudden sensorineural hearing loss; PTA, pure-tone average.

Inclusion criteria varied among the five studies dealing with acute presentation. Hoffmann (1995 acute) accepted only patients who had not improved after 2 weeks of pharmacologic therapy, Fattori (2001) accepted patients untreated within 48 hours of hearing loss, whereas Schwab (1998) and Topuz (2004) accepted patients up to 2 weeks after hearing loss. Cavallazzi (1996) did not define entry criteria. Treatment pressure (1.5-2.5 ATA), time schedule (45-90 minutes), and number of sessions (10-25 sessions) of HBOT differed some-

what among studies. Similarly, some variation existed in comparator therapies.

Statistical pooling was not possible for the majority of preplanned outcome measures because of lack of suitable data (Table 21.14). Cavallazzi (1996) and Fattori (2001) report on the proportion of subjects with better than 50% improvement in hearing immediately after the course of therapy. Fifty-five percent improved in the HBOT group versus 36% in the control group, but this difference is not statistically significant (RR with HBOT: 1.53;

Table 21.14 Summary of Pooled Outcomes from RCTs of HBOT for ISSHL and Tinnitus

OUTCOME	STUDIES	EFFICACY DATA		
		RR OR WMD (95% CI)	P	NNT
ACUTE PRESENTATION				
>50% return in hearing (proportion by PTA)	Cavallazzi (1996)[223] Fattori (2001)[223g]	RR: 1.53 (0.85-2.78)	0.16	
>25% return in hearing (proportion by PTA)	Cavallazzi (1996)[223] Fattori (2001)[223g]	RR: 1.39 (1.05-1.84)*	0.02	5 (3-20)
Mean improvement in PTA (%)	Fattori (2001)[223g]	WMD: 37.3 (21.75-52.85)*	<0.0001	
Mean hearing improvement (dB)	Hoffmann (1995)[223i] Schwab (1998)[223h] Topuz (2004)[223k]	WMD (severe loss): 37.7 (22.9-52.5)* WMD (moderate): 19.3 (5.2-33.4)* WMD (mild): 0.2 (−10.0 to 10.4)	<0.0001 (severe) 0.007 (moderate) 0.97 (severe)	
Mean improvement in tinnitus score (0-10)	Schwab (1998)[223h] Hoffmann (1995)[223i]	Improved 3.1 and 4.0 units more in HBOT, respectively		
CHRONIC PRESENTATION				
Some improvement in hearing (proportion)	Hoffmann (1995)[223j]	RR: 0.64 (0.30-1.33)	0.23	
Some improvement in tinnitus (proportion)	Hoffmann (1995)[223j]	RR: 0.44 (0.16-1.23)	0.12	

*Significant outcomes (statistical difference is assumed if the 95% confidence interval [CI] does not include the value 1.0).

  HBOT, hyperbaric oxygen therapy; ISSHL, idiopathic sudden sensorineural hearing loss; NNT, number needed to treat; PTA, pure-tone average; RCT, randomized, controlled trial; RR, relative risk; WMD, weighted mean difference.

95% CI, 0.85-2.78; $P = 0.16$). The same two trials reported the proportion of subjects with better than 25% improvement. In the HBOT group, 78% showed improvement compared with 56% in the control group (RR, 1.39; 95% CI, 1.05-1.84; $P = 0.02$). Subgroup analysis did not suggest a different response for different grades of severity on enrollment. The absolute risk difference of 22% represents an NNT to achieve 1 extra good outcome of 5 (95% CI, 3-20) (Fig. 21.9).

A statistically significant improvement existed in pure-tone average thresholds with HBOT expressed as percentage improvement (Fattori, 2001; weighted MD, 37% in favor of HBOT; 95% CI, 22-53%; $P < 0.001$) and as mean improvement in hearing expressed as decibels (dB) (Hoffmann, 1995; Topuz, 2004; Schwab, 1998).

Only Schwab (1998) and Hoffmann (1995 acute) (53 subjects) report on improvements in acute tinnitus. Although these trials report a greater mean improvement in tinnitus (using a visual analog scale between 0 and 10) in the HBOT arm than the control arm (3.1 and 0.4 units, respectively), neither trial reports standard deviation around those means, making further analysis impossible. The single trial that enrolled patients with a chronic presentation did not suggest any statistically significant differences in recovery of hearing or tinnitus.

Conclusions

Despite the promising results of many of the uncontrolled trials and cohort studies, analysis of the randomized evidence found limited evidence that HBOT improves hearing when applied as an early treatment in ISSHL. Only 6 trials with 304 participants were available for evaluation, and meta-analysis was not appropriate or possible for a number of important clinical outcomes. The trials are generally of moderate methodologic quality only, and both outcomes and methodology are poorly reported. Of particular concern is the high

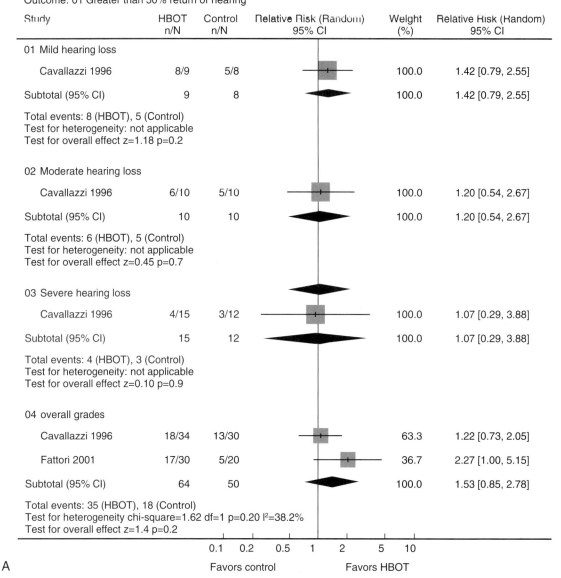

Review: Hyperbaric oxygen idiopathic sudden sensorineural hearing loss and tinnitus
Comparison: 01 Acute presentation. Recovery of hearing as measured by audiometry
Outcome: 01 Greater than 50% return of hearing

Study	HBOT n/N	Control n/N	Relative Risk (Random) 95% CI	Weight (%)	Relative Risk (Random) 95% CI
01 Mild hearing loss					
Cavallazzi 1996	8/9	5/8		100.0	1.42 [0.79, 2.55]
Subtotal (95% CI)	9	8		100.0	1.42 [0.79, 2.55]
Total events: 8 (HBOT), 5 (Control) Test for heterogeneity: not applicable Test for overall effect z=1.18 p=0.2					
02 Moderate hearing loss					
Cavallazzi 1996	6/10	5/10		100.0	1.20 [0.54, 2.67]
Subtotal (95% CI)	10	10		100.0	1.20 [0.54, 2.67]
Total events: 6 (HBOT), 5 (Control) Test for heterogeneity: not applicable Test for overall effect z=0.45 p=0.7					
03 Severe hearing loss					
Cavallazzi 1996	4/15	3/12		100.0	1.07 [0.29, 3.88]
Subtotal (95% CI)	15	12		100.0	1.07 [0.29, 3.88]
Total events: 4 (HBOT), 3 (Control) Test for heterogeneity: not applicable Test for overall effect z=0.10 p=0.9					
04 overall grades					
Cavallazzi 1996	18/34	13/30		63.3	1.22 [0.73, 2.05]
Fattori 2001	17/30	5/20		36.7	2.27 [1.00, 5.15]
Subtotal (95% CI)	64	50		100.0	1.53 [0.85, 2.78]
Total events: 35 (HBOT), 18 (Control) Test for heterogeneity chi-square=1.62 df=1 p=0.20 I^2=38.2% Test for overall effect z=1.4 p=0.2					

0.1 0.2   0.5   1   2   5   10
A   Favors control   Favors HBOT

Figure 21.9 Forest plot of treatment effect for acute presentation of idiopathic sudden sensorineural hearing loss (ISSHL). Proportion of subjects attaining 50% *(A)* and 25% *(B)* improvement in pure-tone average (PTA) hearing loss at the completion of therapy with subgroup analysis by severity grade on enrollment. CI, confidence interval; HBOT, hyperbaric oxygen therapy. *(From Bennett MH, Kertesz T, Yeung P: Hyperbaric oxygen for idiopathic sudden sensorineural hearing loss and tinnitus. Chichester, United Kingdom, John Wiley & Sons, Ltd. Cochrane Database Syst Rev (1):CD004739, 2007. Copyright Cochrane Collaboration, reproduced with permission.)*

rate of spontaneous recovery from ISSHL that may bias the results because of different entry times, as well as the nonblinded management decisions in all trials.

Given the available evidence, it is hard to justify the routine use of HBOT in these patients. There is certainly a case for large, randomized trials of high methodologic rigor to define the true extent of benefit (if any) from the administration of HBOT. Specifically, more information is required on the subset of disease severity and time of presentation most likely to be associated with a benefit from this therapy, the effect of differing oxygen dosage, and the effect of other therapies administered simultaneously. Attention should

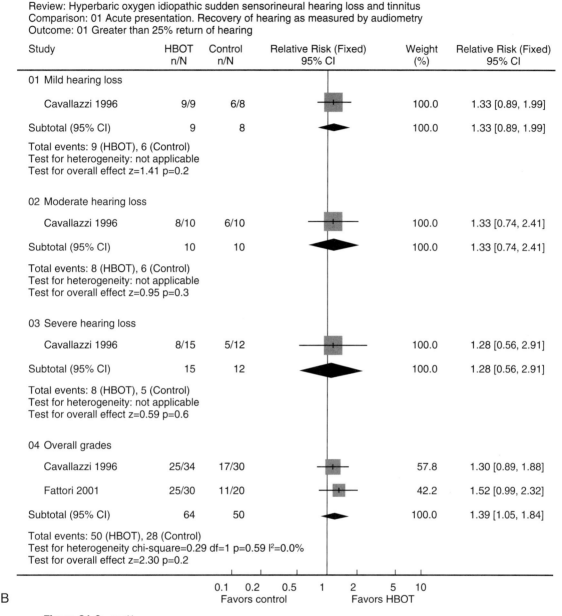

Review: Hyperbaric oxygen idiopathic sudden sensorineural hearing loss and tinnitus
Comparison: 01 Acute presentation. Recovery of hearing as measured by audiometry
Outcome: 01 Greater than 25% return of hearing

Figure 21.9, cont'd

Athletic Soft-Tissue Injuries and Delayed-Onset Muscle Soreness

Soft-tissue injuries are common and range from minor abrasions and bruising to major disruption of tendons, ligaments, and muscles. Although it is difficult to obtain accurate estimates of the impact of soft-tissue injuries in isolation, injuries in general result in tens of millions of emergency department visits and cost hundreds of billions of health-care dollars per annum in the United States alone.[224] In a recent examination of high-school athletic injuries in Ohio, the Centers for Disease Control and Prevention estimate the rate of injuries at 2.4 per 1000 athletes each year.[225] Soft-tissue injuries are commonly associated with athletic activity, and they occur in both elite and recreational athletes. In both these groups, soft-tissue injuries may be associated with considerable loss of work and health costs.[226] The causes of soft-tissue injuries are diverse and may involve acute traumatic impact, repetitive strain and overuse, or muscle injury induced by unaccustomed exercise.[226a,227]

Of particular interest to researchers is the phenomenon of delayed-onset muscle soreness (DOMS). Familiar to most individuals at some time, this is the name given to the syndrome of pain, swelling, and stiffness in muscles in the days after a bout of unaccustomed activity. One review confirms that the mechanisms, treatment strategies, and impact on athletic performance remain uncertain.[228] Putative mechanisms include lactic acid accumulation, muscle spasms, connective tissue damage, inflammation, and enzyme efflux secondary to muscle cell damage. DOMS is frequently used as an experimental soft-tissue injury in human research because it is both self-limiting and reliably reproduced in individuals unaccustomed to exercise.

Therapy

Accepted treatments for athletic soft-tissue injuries may be classified broadly as rest; local measures to reduce edema (e.g., massage, cryotherapy, elevation); drug therapy (typically nonsteroidal anti-inflammatory agents); stretching or further exercise (particularly for DOMS); surgical; and rehabilitative.[228-230] The ultimate aim of treatment is to restore pain-free function and enable the return to activity in the shortest time compatible with a low risk for reinjury. None of these interventions has been shown to clearly achieve these aims in the context of clinical trials, and some of the most commonly applied treatments have been thrown into question through SRs of the evidence.[231-233]

It has been suggested since 1982 that HBOT may accelerate injury recovery.[234] HBOT has been shown in a number of injury models to reduce edema and preserve microcirculation through vasoconstriction with enhanced oxygen delivery, a direct osmotic effect, and the inactivation of white cell adhesion.[49,235-237]

Evidence

The first clinical report of athletic injury treated with HBOT was published in 1993; it describes a 55% reduction in days lost to injury when Scottish soccer players suffering from a variety of injuries were treated with HBOT.[238] Since then, a number of anecdotal reports in the nonmedical media suggest that the use of HBOT has become commonplace in some elite sporting clubs. An SR of the randomized evidence has been published and the findings of that review are summarized in the following section.[239]

Cochrane Review

Nine trials published in eight reports between 1996 and 2003 were included in this review: Soolsma (1996),[239a] Borromeo (1997),[239b] Staples (1999),[239c] Mekjavic (2000),[239d] Harrison (2001),[239e] Webster (2002),[239f] Babul (2003),[239g] and Germain (2003).[239h] In total, these trials present results for 197 participants, and details are presented in Table 21.15.

Two trials evaluate HBOT for treating acute soft-tissue injury. Borromeo (1997) enrolled individuals with acute ankle sprains presenting within 72 hours to an orthopedic surgeon, whereas Soolsma (1996) enrolled individuals with grade II medial collateral ligament injuries in one knee who similarly presented within 72 hours. The other seven trials include young adult unconditioned volunteers who underwent exercise designed to produce DOMS under controlled conditions.

All authors administered HBOT between 2.0 and 2.5 ATA, and the total number of individual treatment sessions varied from 3 to 10. The mean time between injury and compression was 33 hours in Borromeo (1997) and 74 hours in Soolsma (1996), whereas most DOMS trials administered oxygen or sham therapy within 4 hours of exercise.

The trials were generally of fair to high quality and reported data on the time to full functional recovery, the proportion returning to full function and three secondary outcomes of interest (functional assessments, pain and swelling, and muscle strength).

Table 21.15 Characteristics of Randomized Trials Included in the Cochrane Review of HBOT for the Treatment of Soft-Tissue Injuries

STUDY	METHODS	SUBJECTS	INTERVENTIONS	OUTCOMES
Babul (2003)[239g]	Randomized and blinded; complex design	16 female healthy volunteers; provocative exercise of quadriceps muscle	HBOT: 2.0 ATA for 60 minutes at 4, 24, 48, and 72 hours after injury Control: sham at 1.2 ATA on air on the same schedule	Pain score, strength, swelling
Borromeo (1997)[239b]	Randomized and blinded; intention-to-treat analysis[239g]	32 adults with lateral ankle sprain within 72 hours	Splint, crutches, NSAID, active ROM HBOT: 2.0 ATA for 90 minutes, 3 sessions over 7 days Control: sham at 1.1 ATA on air for 90 minutes, same schedule	Healed, time to healing, pain score, swelling
Germain (2003)[239h]	Randomized, not blinded; numbers in each arm assumed equal	16 healthy volunteers; provocative exercise of quadriceps muscle	HBOT: 95% oxygen at 2.5 ATA for 100 minutes at 1 and 6 hours, then 1 treatment the next day and 2 treatments on the next day separated by 6 hours Control: no specific therapy	Pain score, strength, swelling
Harrison (2001)[239e]	Randomized, partial blinding; complex experimental design; SD calculated from SEM	21 male healthy volunteers; provocative exercise of elbow flexors	HBOT (2 groups): (1) Immediate: 2.5 ATA for 100 minutes; treatments immediately after injury and after 24, 48, 72, and 96 hours (2) Delayed: immediate sham (on air at minimal pressure), then the same HBOT schedule as group 1. Control: no specific therapy	Pain, strength, swelling
Mekjavic (2000)[239d]	Randomized, patient and statistician blind; intention-to-treat analysis; results from graphs	24 male healthy volunteers; provocative exercise of elbow flexors	HBOT: 60 minutes daily at 2.5 ATA Control: 2.5 ATA, 8% oxygen for 60 minutes), once daily	Pain, strength, swelling
Soolsma (1996)[239a]	Randomized and blinded; long delay to therapy; significant losses to follow-up	19 adults with grade II injury to the medial collateral ligament of the knee	Regular icing, stretching, and strengthening exercise rehabilitation program. Within 96 hours: HBOT: 2.0 ATA for 60 minutes, 10 sessions over 2 weeks Control: sham 1.2 ATA on air	Recovery index, pain, ROM, strength, swelling
Staples (1999a)[239c*]	Randomized and blinded; SD calculated from SEM; significant losses to follow-up.	49 male healthy volunteers; provocative exercise of quadriceps muscle	Phase 1 HBOT: (1) 2.0 ATA for 1 hour at 0, 24, and 48 hours after exercise, followed by 2 sham treatments at 72 and 96 hours; (2) sham at 0 and 24 hours, followed by HBOT at 48, 72, and 96 hours Control: (1) no specific intervention; (2) sham at 1.2 ATA breathing air at 0, 24, 48, 72, and 96 hours	Pain score, strength
Staples (1999b)[239c*]	As Staples 1999a	30 male healthy volunteers; as Staples 1999a	Phase 2 HBOT: (1) as Staples 1999a; (2) same HBOT on 5 occasions at 0, 24, 48, 72, and 96 hours Control: Sham as Staples 1999a	Pain score, strength
Webster (2002)[239f]	Randomized and blinded; results taken from graphs	12 male healthy volunteers; provocative exercise of gastrocnemius	HBOT: 2.5 ATA for 60 minutes at 3, 24, and 48 hours after injury Control: sham at 1.3 ATA on air on the same schedule.	Pain score, strength, swelling

*Two trials reported in a single publication.
ATA, atmospheres absolute; NSAID, nonsteroidal anti-inflammatory drug; ROM, range of motion; SD, standard deviation; SEM, standard error of the mean.

Participants entered into all the DOMS trials were young healthy volunteers who were not conditioned athletes and who had not exercised vigorously before entry into the studies. All trials except Germain (2003) used blinding with sham therapy.

For acute ligament injury, Borromeo (1997) reports that all subjects with ankle sprain returned to preinjury activity, and that there was no significant difference in the time taken to reach full recovery between treatment groups (MD, 0.30 day in favor of HBOT; 95% CI, −3.08 to 3.68 days). Neither Borromeo (1997) nor Soolsma (1996) found any significant differences between groups in the functional scores attained after therapy, although Borromeo (1997) did report a significantly greater improvement in scores in the HBOT group compared with those in the control group (MD, 1.40; 95% CI, 0.15-2.65; $P = 0.03$). Because all participants recovered completely, the clinical significance of this finding is unlikely to be great. Soolsma (1996) reports a reduction in pain for the HBOT group compared with control after 10 treatments, but not after 5 treatments or at 4 weeks of follow-up. There were no other reported differences in pain or swelling for either study of ligament injury.

For DOMS, most of the included trials assessed pain scores, swelling, and strength, although not all trials contributed data to all outcomes. In those trials that applied immediate HBOT after exercise, no significant differences in pain scores existed between the two groups at 24 hours or at end of treatment, but statistically significant differences were in favor of the control group at 48 (MD, 0.88; 95% CI, 0.09-1.67) and 72 hours (MD, 0.72; 95% CI, 0.06-1.37). These analyses are summarized in Figure 21.10. Similarly, there were no significant differences between groups in favor of HBOT at any time when HBOT was delayed for 24 hours, but at 72 hours, there were lower pain scores in the control group (MD, 0.85; 95% CI, 0.06-1.64). No statistically significant differences were present between the HBOT and control groups for any trial in regard to swelling or muscle strength.

Conclusions

In summary, despite some physiologic rationale and promising early reports, little good evidence for benefit from the use of HBOT for soft-tissue injuries or DOMS has been reported. The nine randomized trials in general report a uniform lack of benefit for HBOT. Only two of these trials included actual injuries, so the data in this area are sparse. The concentration of these studies on a short-term, self-limiting injury with a 100% recovery rate (DOMS) demands a cautious interpretation of the results.

The routine use of HBOT in athletic injuries cannot be justified on the evidence available. Indeed, there seems little case for further examination of the use of HBOT in DOMS. Although more information may be useful on a range of real clinical injuries, subsets of injury severity, and time of presentation, any further investigations would need to be carefully justified and any future trials would need to be carefully planned.

Thermal Burns

Thermal burns remain an important source of morbidity and mortality. In the United States, approximately 2 million people are burned each year, with about 155 individuals per million requiring hospital admission in the United States and 6500 dying.[240,241] Globally, there were 238,000 fire-related deaths in 2000, with low- and middle-income countries bearing 95% of the global burden. Annual mortality per 100,000 people is 1.3 in North America but 5.5 in Africa.[242]

Burns are a complex and evolving injury, with both local and systemic consequences—the latter manifesting once the burn area is greater than about 20% of the body surface area.[243] Locally, the burn wound tends to extend in the acute phase of the injury secondary to microvascular changes, profound activation of white cells and platelets, and the development of edema. Many small vessels are directly coagulated by the application of heat, whereas others will thrombose later.[244] The systemic response to burning is characterized

Review: Hyperbaric oxygen therapy for delayed-onset muscle soreness and closed soft-tissue injury
Comparison: 02 Induced DOMS: HBOT versus control
Outcome: 01 Pain score (10=worst pain) after exercise (immediate treatment)

Study	HBOT		Control		WMD (fixed) 95% CI	Weight (%)	WMD (fixed) 95% CI
	N	Mean (SD)	N	Mean (SD)			
01 24 hours							
Harrison 2001	5	5.96 (2.37)	6	5.19 (1.79)		9.9	0.77 [-1.75, 3.29]
Mekjavic 2000	12	4.42 (2.24)	12	3.51 (3.20)		12.9	0.91 [-1.30, 3.12]
Staples 1999a	9	4.84 (1.25)	18	4.62 (1.33)		60.4	0.22 [-0.80, 1.24]
Staples 1999b	20	3.81 (2.52)	10	3.78 (2.58)		16.7	0.03 [-1.91, 1.97]
Subtotal (95% CI)	46		46			100.0	0.33 [-0.46, 1.13]

Test for heterogeneity chi-squared=0.52 df=3 p=0.92 I^2=0.0%
Test for overall effect z=0.82 p=0.4

02 48 hours							
Harrison 2001	5	6.63 (2.58)	6	6.83 (2.36)		7.1	-0.20 [-3.15, 2.75]
Mekjavic 2000	12	6.77 (1.85)	12	5.56 (2.40)		21.0	1.21 [-0.50, 2.92]
Staples 1999a	9	4.84 (1.28)	18	3.86 (1.33)		57.3	0.98 [-0.06, 2.02]
Staples 1999b	20	3.50 (2.63)	10	2.96 (2.74)		14.6	0.54 [-1.51, 2.59]
Subtotal (95% CI)	46		46			100.0	0.88 [0.09, 1.67]

Test for heterogeneity chi-square=0.80 df=3 p=0.85 I^2=0.0%
Test for overall effect z=2.20 p=0.03

03 72 hours							
Harrison 2001	5	6.92 (2.15)	6	6.15 (2.12)		6.7	0.77 [-1.77, 3.31]
Mekjavic 2000	12	5.12 (2.38)	12	4.60 (2.24)		12.5	0.52 [-1.33, 2.37]
Staples 1999a	9	3.19 (1.09)	18	2.16 (1.13)		55.0	1.03 [0.15, 1.91]
Staples 1999b	20	1.56 (1.61)	10	1.42 (1.74)		25.8	0.14 [-1.15, 1.43]
Subtotal (95% CI)	46		46			100.0	0.72 [0.06, 1.37]

Test for heterogeneity chi-square=1.30 df=3 p=0.73 I^2=0.0%
Test for overall effect z=2.15 p=0.03

04 Days 4 to 7							
Harrison 2001	5	1.31 (0.65)	6	1.89 (0.85)		7.6	-0.58 [-1.47, 0.31]
Mekjavic 2000	12	0.60 (0.49)	12	0.51 (0.35)		51.6	0.09 [-0.25, 0.43]
Staples 1999a	9	1.36 (0.56)	18	1.29 (0.56)		29.8	0.07 [-0.38, 0.52]
Staples 1999b	20	0.62 (0.97)	10	0.71 (0.97)		11.0	-0.09 [-0.83, 0.65]
Subtotal (95% CI)	46		46			100.0	0.01 [-0.23, -0.26]

Test for heterogeneity chi-square=2.05 df=3 p=0.56 I^2=0.0%
Test for overall effect z=0.11 p=0.0

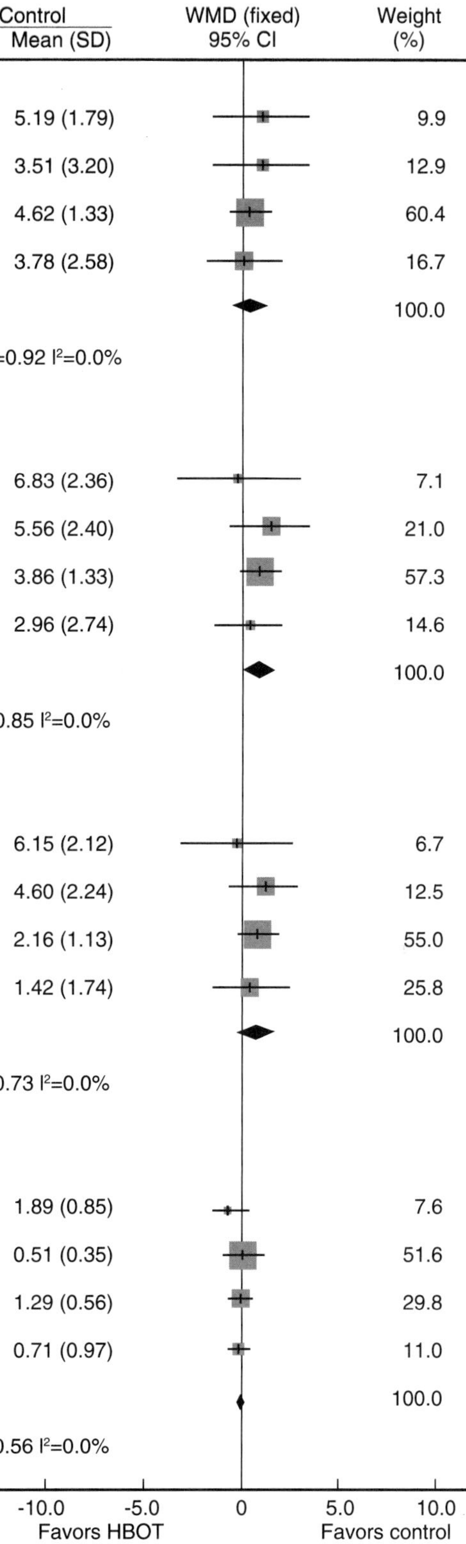

-10.0   -5.0   0   5.0   10.0
Favors HBOT   Favors control

Figure 21.10 Forest plot for pain scores at all times after immediate application of hyperbaric oxygen therapy (HBOT) after exercise. There is no indication of a benefit from HBOT at any time. CI, confidence interval; DOMS, delayed-onset muscle soreness; SD, standard deviation. *(From Bennett MH, Best TM, Babul S, et al: Hyperbaric oxygen therapy for delayed onset muscle soreness and closed soft tissue injury. Chichester, United Kingdom, John Wiley & Sons, Ltd. Cochrane Database Syst Rev (4):CD004713, 2005. Copyright Cochrane Collaboration, reproduced with permission.)*

by interstitial edema in distant organs, secondary to a combination of wound-released mediators and hypoproteinaemia.[245,246]

Therapy

Burns are a difficult treatment challenge and ideally the province of specialized units with high-volume workloads. Early treatment can positively influence mortality rate and involves appropriate fluid resuscitation, usually involving attainment of resuscitation targets using consensus formulas for initial fluid administration,[243] together with topical agents to control pain, limit direct fluid losses, and slow bacterial growth. Over the past two decades, early closure of full-thickness wounds has improved the outcome from extensive burns through the prevention of wound colonization and infection.[243] Temporary skin substitutes are used widely on a similar rationale when formal closure is not an option.

It has been suggested since 1965 that HBOT may improve outcome after thermal burns when Wada[247] serendipitously observed more rapid healing of second-degree burns in a group of coal miners who were being treated with HBOT for carbon monoxide poisoning. In 1970, Gruber and colleagues[248] demonstrated that the area subadjacent to a full-thickness injury was hypoxic and could be raised to normal or supranormal levels through the administration of oxygen under pressure. Since then, HBOT has been shown to reduce edema and preserve microcirculation in a number of injury models, including burns, through vasoconstriction with enhanced oxygen delivery, a direct osmotic effect, and the inactivation of white cell adhesion.[49,235,237] The preservation of microcirculation persists for some hours at least after hyperbaric oxygen exposure[249,250] and further exerts beneficial effects on infections in hypoxic tissues through a variety of mechanisms.[251]

Evidence

A significant body of experimental evidence exists using a variety of animal burn models. Although many of these are reported only in abstracts or proceedings and are difficult to locate, most have been summarized by Cianci and Sato.[252] A short list with a summary of the findings is presented in Table 21.16. In general, these models have suggested that early institution of HBOT after thermal burns may result in reduced edema and fluid resuscitation requirements, improved preservation of dermal architecture, improved vascularity, and improved immune response. Some models did, however, suggest no benefit or even poorer healing with the application of HBOT, and it is not clear which factors are important to ensure a positive outcome.

There have been relatively few clinical reports of effectiveness for HBOT, however. An experimental model of burn injury suggested some reduction in hyperemia, exudate, and wound size, but no overall improvement in healing,[119] whereas small, nonrandom, comparative trials have reported lower mortality and shorter hospital stays after HBOT in patients with significant burns.[253-255] In contrast, a comparative study of 72 matched patients suggests more renal failure and sepsis (although fewer grafts) in the HBOT group.[256]

Cochrane Review

In 2004, Villanueva and colleagues published a Cochrane review on the treatment of thermal burns with HBOT.[256a] Their initial search produced 22 possible relevant articles, but examination of the full text of these articles identified only 2 RCTs with relevant clinical outcomes: Brannen (1997)[256b] and Hart (1974).[256c] The characteristics of these trials are summarized in Table 21.17.

Both studies were considered to be of modest methodologic quality. Hart (1974) uses a double-blind method and describes the randomization method used ("sealed envelopes"), but enrolled only a small number of participants (low power). Brannen (1997) gives few details of the methodology used. Neither trial reports any losses to follow-up or withdrawals from treatment. Because of significant heterogeneity in the patients enrolled in these two studies, as well as the incompatibility of the outcome measures used, data from the two

Table 21.16 Summary of Animal Experimental Models of HBOT for Burn Injury

STUDY	MODEL	OUTCOME
Ketchum (1967)[257a]	Rats	Reduced healing time and infection with HBO
Bornside (1968)[257b]	Rats: examining HBO combined with antibiotics vs. antibiotics alone	Unknown
Ikeda (1968)[257c]	Rabbits	Reduced edema with HBO
Ketchum (1970)[257d]	Rats	Increased microvascularity
Perrins (1970)[257e]	Scalded pig	No benefit
Hartwig (1974)[257f]	Unknown	Increased microvascularity and reduced healing time, inflammation with HBO
Wells (1977)[257g]	Dogs with flame injury	Reduced fluid extravasation with HBO
Korn (1977)[257h]	Guinea pig	Improved epithelialization
Niccole (1977)[257i]	Rats	No advantage of HBO over SSD
Nylander (1984)[257j]	Mice	Reduction of edema with HBO
Saunders (1989)[257k]	Unclear	Improved microcirculation, dermal elements, and collagen quality
Stewart (1994)[257l]	Unclear	Improved dermal elements
Tenenhaus (1994)[257m]	Mice with 32% TBSA burns	Reduction in bacterial colonies but increased mortality with HBO
Germonpre (1996)[257n]	Rats with 5% TBSA burn	Improved preservation of basement membrane and reduced leucocyte infiltration with HBO
Shoshani (1998)[257o]	Guinea pigs given deep burn	Worse re-epithelialization with HBO
Akin (2002)[257p]	Rats	Reduced bacterial counts and translocation through intestinal wall with HBO
Bilic (2005)[257q]	Rats given 20% TBSA deep burn	Improved edema, neoangiogenesis, preserved dermal follicles, and epithelialization

HBO, hyperbaric oxygen; TBSA, total body surface area.

studies could not be pooled and are described individually.

Brannen (1997) reports no difference in mortality (seven patients [11%] in each group), whereas Hart (1974) does not report any mortality in his group. Neither study reports the rate of major morbidities such as wound infection. Brannen (1997) reports no differences in the length of stay or the number of surgeries performed.

Hart (1974) reports that mean healing times were significantly shorter in patients exposed to HBOT (mean: 19.7 vs. 43.8 days; $P < 0.001$), and that fluid requirements were also smaller in the HBOT group (mean: 2.2 mL/kg vs. 3.4 mL/kg; no statistical analysis reported). One of two grafts required in the sham group did not succeed, whereas all three required in the HBOT group succeeded (RR for failed graft without HBOT, 2.0; 95% CI, 0.5–8.0).

In summary, the review could include only data from two trials, and no meta-analysis could

be performed for any outcome. The two trials included a modest total of only 141 patients, of which 125 were in Brannen's trial (1997). Furthermore, the two trials were published 23 years apart, and the comparator therapy is likely to have been significantly different. The Hart (1974) trial was particularly constrained by a lack of power to detect useful clinical differences, and the finding that HBOT was no more effective than placebo in regard to length of stay, mortality, or number of surgeries may have been erroneous for this reason alone.

Mean healing times were reported by Hart (1974) and showed promising results, with times being shorter in patients exposed to HBOT. However, no definition of "healing" was given, and no description was given as to the extent of wound size and depth at presentation. Acute fluid requirements and other outcomes such as successful skin grafting were reported "better" in those receiving HBOT, but no formal

Table 21.17   Characteristics of Randomized Trials Included in the Cochrane Review of HBOT for the Treatment of Burns

STUDY	METHODS	SUBJECTS	INTERVENTIONS	OUTCOMES
Hart (1974)[256c]	Randomized and blinded	16 (14 male) acutely burned patients with 10–50% BSA; admitted within 24 hours	Control: routine burn management with crystalloid titrated to CVP and urine output; colloids after 24 hours if required; dressing with SSD; sham therapy breathing air at a trivial pressure. HBOT: 2 ATA for 90 minutes every 8 hours on day 1, then twice daily until healed	Mortality, acute fluid requirement, mean healing time and number of grafts
Brannen (1997)[256b]	Randomized, no blinding	125 (94 male) acutely burned patients; area not given; admitted within 24 hours	Control: routine burn management HBOT: as above plus 2 ATA for 90 minutes twice daily for a minimum of 5 days, maximum 1 treatment per 1% BSA burnt.	Mortality, acute fluid requirement, length of stay, number of operations

ATA, atmospheres absolute; BSA, body surface area; CVP, central venous pressure; HBOT, hyperbaric oxygen therapy; SSD, siver sulfadiazine.

analysis was made. Neither trial measured long-term outcomes. In an accompanying analysis of a series of 191 patients treated at the author's facility (138 with HBOT), Hart (1974) reports that the overall mortality rate for those treated with HBOT was 9% (less than predicted on the basis of a national series rate), and that 92 of 138 patients also survived to undergo autografting, with an average of 1.35 grafts per patient.

Conclusions

Although there are some promising results from nonrandom clinical reports and one small RCT, insufficient evidence is available to support the routine use of HBOT for patients with thermal burns. Given that some centers use HBOT routinely, there is a case for further randomized trials of high methodologic rigor to define the true extent of benefit from the administration of HBOT to patients with thermal burns. Specifically, more information is required on the subset of burn severity or size most likely to benefit from this therapy and the oxygen dose most appropriate. Any future trials would need to consider appropriate sample sizes with power to detect expected differences and careful definition and selection of target patients.

Dysfertility

Infertility is a major health issue throughout the world. It is estimated that every sixth couple has a problem conceiving and needs assistance to achieve pregnancy.[257] Many factors affect fertility and often no single causative factor can be identified. Known prognostic indicators in the female include age, ovarian reserve, and past reproductive history, while the important factors in the male are the spermatozoa count and motility. Fertilization and successful endometrial implantation are only the first of many steps required for a normal pregnancy and delivery. Congenital malformations, placental hypoxia, fetal hypoxia and other pregnancy disorders can result in threatened miscarriage. Spontaneous abortion occurs in around 15% of pregnancies in the first trimester.

In vitro fertilization (IVF) techniques in various forms are used to help infertile couples conceive their own biologic children. Despite many technologic advances in IVF, results are variable, and effective measures to promote fertilization, implantation, and gestation remain an active area of research. HBOT has been suggested as a possible means to improve the success rate of both "natural" and IVF pregnancies—particularly in Russia, where a number of pregnancy-related conditions are regarded as established indications for HBOT.[258] In the Western sphere to date, there has been much less enthusiasm for HBOT in this area.

Pathophysiology

Angiogenesis, blood flow, and oxygen play an important role in many fertility processes. The evidence comes mainly from recent improvements in ultrasound and Doppler techniques, particularly the development of transvaginal ultrasound probes.

Ovarian blood flow is known to increase in the preovulatory phase compared with the early follicular phase.[259] Huey and coworkers[260] demonstrate that perifollicular blood flow can predict oocyte development competence in IVF, but they have also suggested that follicular Po_2, Pco_2, and pH were not predictive of embryonic development. Van Blerkom and colleagues[261] demonstrate the importance of oxygen in oocyte meiosis by associating reduced oxygen content in ovarian follicular fluid with an increased rate of abnormalities in the organization of chromosomes on the metaphase spindle. Such abnormalities may result in segregation disorders and mosaicisms in the early embryo. Sufficient oxygen therefore appears necessary for appropriate development of the early embryo.

Despite many advances in IVF techniques, a large number of embryos do not implant for reasons that remain uncertain.[257] One important factor appears to be the quality of the endometrium. Good endometrial quality relies on the anatomy of the cavum and uterus as a whole, optimal hormonal status, absence of endometrial waves, and good vascularization and oxygenation. Many pharmacologic agents have been used in an attempt to improve blood supply to the uterus and subendometrium, but there have been no convincingly favorable results. One of the most important factors used to estimate endometrial quality is the endometrial thickness. If the endometrium is less than 7 mm thick at the time of ovulation, pregnancy is unlikely. However, if the thickness is more than 14 mm,

implantation rates are reduced and miscarriage rates increased.[262] Apart from simple thickness, it appears that the quality of texture and reflectivity of the endometrium are important. A trilaminar rather than a bilaminar endometrium on ultrasound has been correlated with increased pregnancy rates, whereas the absence of adequate capillary network in the subendometrium at the time of ovulation is incompatible with pregnancy.[257,263]

Evidence

Several Russian reports (only abstracts are available in English) associate benefits from HBOT for the treatment of dysfertility.[264-266] Zadoev and coauthors[264] report that HBOT was able to improve spermatic morphology and functional characteristics in male individuals with chronic prostatitis associated with infertility. Asribekova and researchers[265] have analyzed hormone receptors in women with late habitual abortions. Reception of both progesterone and estrogen in the nuclei and estrogen binding in the endometrial cytosol was significantly raised in a group of women with frequent miscarriages compared with healthy women. The hormone receptor ratio in the cytosol in the secretory phase was also increased in the women with habitual late abortions. Giving HBOT (no details of treatments given) to this group resulted in complete normalization of sex hormone reception.

Evidence to support the use of HBOT in the Western literature is sparse. A pilot study by Van Voorhis[259] focuses on a group of women with a poor prognosis for pregnancy through IVF techniques. Ten women older than 39 years, or aged 35 to 39 years with a history of a previous unsuccessful IVF attempt, were treated with daily HBOT (100% oxygen at 2.4 ATA for 90 minutes) Monday to Friday from day 3 of the menstrual cycle until the day before oocyte retrieval (median number of treatments, 9.5). All patients received the usual protocol and medications for IVF procedures at that institution. The study group was compared with another eligible group of women unwilling to undergo HBOT, and final outcomes were also compared with results from historical control subjects. Cycle cancellation rates for a poor ovarian response were high in all groups. In completed cycles, comparison with historical but not concurrent control subjects suggested improved estrogen response, implantation, and pregnancy rates after HBOT. Comparison with concurrent control subjects showed a greater number of embryos from the IVF cycle and a greater level of vascular endothelial growth factor in follicular fluid. The authors speculate that HBOT causes an increase in the level of vascular endothelial growth factor in follicular fluid similar to the increase seen in hypoxic wounds treated with HBOT. Two women receiving HBOT and IVF became pregnant and delivered healthy infants (40%) compared with 3 of 13 women in the concurrent control group (43%). The conclusion of this small pilot study is that there was no evidence of benefit for HBOT on the chance of delivering a healthy infant.

A 2006 study by Mitrovic and coworkers[257] aimed to evaluate the effect of HBOT on the endometrium using transvaginal color Doppler. Thirty-two women with unexplained infertility were entered into the study over a 3-year period. It is referred to as a randomized study; however, no details of randomization are provided. HBOT was given for 7 consecutive days beginning with day 5 of the menstrual cycle. Each treatment lasted 70 minutes at 2.3 ATA. Transvaginal Doppler sonography was conducted from day 8 until ovulation from 1 month before to 1 month after HBOT. A control group of patients received 100% oxygen at 1 ATA on the same schedule. All patients used only moderate stimulants of ovulation and had never before used IVF techniques. Thickness of the endometrium measured at the time of ovulation was, on average, 11.1 mm in the cycle where HBOT was administered compared with 7.7 mm in the cycle before HBOT. The endometrial thickness was similar to non-HBOT cycles in the control group. In HBOT cycles, the desired sonographic quality was obtained in 84% of patients in the preovulatory phase compared with only 9% in cycles where HBOT was not given. Mapping of subendothelial blood vessels in HBOT cycles demonstrated a low resistance compared with non-HBOT cycles. This was interpreted as a sign of the evolution of an intensive capillary network with low resistance as a result of angiogenesis.

It is interesting to reflect that studies in wounds have indicated angiogenesis increases in a linear fashion through 20 HBOT sessions before a plateau is reached.[267] The seven hyperbaric exposures in Mitrovic and coworkers'[257] study might have been too few to expect significant angiogenesis; nevertheless, significant changes on transvaginal Doppler were noted. Mitrovic concluded that the application of HBOT results in both optimization of endometrial quality and adequate subendometrial vascularization and oxygenation.

No randomized, controlled clinical studies of HBOT and IVF procedures have been reported, but two case reports of successful pregnancies after IVF in association with HBOT have been published in English.[263,268] Leverment and colleagues[263] report a case of secondary infertility in a 32-year-old woman who experienced development of endometrial scarring after a postpartum hemorrhage and uterine packing. She had five unsuccessful IVF cycles and ultrasound had demonstrated an endometrial thickness of only 4 mm. The patient's husband (a medical practitioner) proposed using HBOT to assist endometrial development. The patient received HBOT in the form of 10 daily treatments at 2.0 ATA for 90 minutes from day 1 to 10 of the menstrual cycle. The usual estrogen-progesterone protocol was followed, and this time the patient received sildenafil (a vasodilator) vaginally from days 3 to 15. Sildenafil had been given orally for previous IVF attempts. Ultrasound on day 10 measured endometrial thickness as 6 mm. Embryo transfer took place on day 20 and a single pregnancy followed. A healthy infant was born by caesarean section.

Mitrovic and coworkers[257] report a case of primary infertility in a 36-year-old woman who had previously received two unsuccessful embryo transfers before undergoing HBOT. She received HBOT at 2.3 ATA for 70 minutes from day 5 of the cycle to day 13. Endometrial thickness was measured at 11 mm during the hyperbaric cycle with no mention of previous estimates. She had hormone therapy and received two embryos, resulting in two implanted gestational sacs. She delivered two healthy infants at 38 weeks' gestation.

Conclusions

Some physiologic evidence exists that HBOT may be beneficial for oocyte development in the follicular stage, as well as evidence that HBOT may benefit endometrial proliferation and development for implantation. A small pilot series found no improvement in the pregnancy rate by combining IVF and HBOT in a cohort of patients with a poor prognosis for pregnancy. Two case reports suggest HBOT was associated with successful pregnancy when used in combination with IVF. More work in this area is required before HBOT could be regarded as an established therapy in this area. A need exists for further elucidation of the basic science behind HBOT effects on the ovary and endometrium, as well as careful clinical investigation of effectiveness, including further information on the optimal timing and dosage of HBOT. This is an exciting area for future researchers.

REFERENCES

1. Phillips B, Ball C, Sackett D, et al: Oxford Centre for Evidence-based Medicine Levels of Evidence. Oxford Centre for Evidence-based Medicine. Available at: http://www.cebm.net/index.aspx?0=1025. Accessed January 2008.
2. Tolley EA, Headley AS: Meta-analyses: What they can and cannot tell us about clinical research. Curr Opin Nutrit Metab Care 8:181, 2005.
3. Freemantle N, Mason J, Eccles M: Deriving treatment recommendations from evidence within randomized trials. Int J Technol Assess Health Care 15:304-315, 1999.
4. Pogue J, Yusuf S: Overcoming the limitations of current meta-analysis of randomised controlled trials. Lancet 351:47-52, 1998.
5. Lau J, Antman EM, Kulpenick B, et al: Cumulative meta-analysis of therapeutic trials for myocardial infarction. N Engl J Med 327:248-254, 1992.
6. Tunstall-Pedoe H, Kuulasmaa K, Tolonen H, et al: The WHO MONICA Project. MONICA Monograph and Multimedia Sourcebook. Geneva, World Health Organization, 2003, pp 170-183.
7. British Heart Foundation: Coronary heart disease statistics. Available at: www.dphpc.ox.ac.uk/bhfhprg/stats/2000/2002/keyfacts/index html. Accessed January 2008.
8. Poulter N: Global risk of cardiovascular disease. Heart 89:ii2-ii5, 2003.
9. Naghavi M, Libby P, Falk E, et al: From vulnerable plaque to vulnerable patient: A call for new definitions and risk assessment strategies: Part I. Circulation 108:1664-1672, 2003.
10. Heistad D: Unstable coronary-artery plaques. N Engl J Med 349:2285-2287, 2003.
11. Weaver WD, Simes RJ, Betriu A, et al: Comparison of primary coronary angioplasty and intravenous thrombolytic therapy for acute myocardial infarction: A quantitative review. JAMA 278:2093-2098, 1997.
12. Antman EM, Anbe DT, Armstrong PW, et al: ACC/AHA guidelines for the management of patients with ST-elevation myocardial infarction—executive summary. Circulation 110:588-636, 2004.
13. Arntz H-R, Bossaert L, Filippatos GS: European Resuscitation Council guidelines for resuscitation 2005. Section 5. Initial management of acute coronary syndromes. Resuscitation 67:S87-S96, 2005.
14. Speit G, Dennog C, Eichorn U, et al: Induction of heme oxygenase-1 and adaptive protection against the induction of DNA damage after hyperbaric oxygen treatment. Cardiogenesis 21:1795-1799, 2000.
15. Harabin AL, Braisted JC, Flynn ET: Response of antioxidant enzymes to intermittent and continuous hyperbaric oxygen. J Appl Physiol 69:328-335, 1990.
16. Thom SR, Elbuken M: Oxygen-dependent antagonism of lipid peroxidation in the rat. Free Radic Biol Med 10:413-426, 1991.
17. Tjarnstrom J, Wikstrom T, Bagge U: Effects of hyperbaric oxygen treatment on neutrophil activation and pulmonary sequestration in intestinal ischemia-reperfusion in rats. Eur Surg Res 31:147-154, 1999.
18. Smith G, Lawson DA: Experimental coronary arterial occlusion: Effects of the administration of oxygen under pressure. Scot Med J 3:346-350, 1958.
19. Smith GD, Lawson D: The protective effect of inhalation of oxygen at two atmospheres absolute pressure in coronary arterial occlusion. Surg Gynecol Obstet 112:320-322, 1962.
20. Trapp WG, Creighton R: Experimental studies of increased atmospheric pressure on myocardial ischemia after coronary ligation. J Thorac Cardiovasc Surg 47:687-692, 1964.
21. Meijne NG, Bulterijs A, Eloff SJ: An experimental investigation into the influence of administration of oxygen under increased atmospheric pressure upon coronary perfusion. J Cardiovasc Surg 4:521-525, 1963.
22. Thomas MP, Brown LA, Sponseller DR, et al: Myocardial infarct size reduction by the synergistic effect of hyperbaric oxygen and recombinant tissue plasminogen activator. Am Heart J 120:791-800, 1990.
23. Robertson HF: The effect of hyperbaric oxygenation on myocardial infarction in dogs. Can J Surg 9:81-90, 1966.
24. Holloway DH Jr, Whalen RE, Saltzman HA, et al: Hyperbaric oxygenation in the treatment of acute coronary artery embolization in dogs. J Lab Clin Med 66:596-603, 1965.
25. Whalen RE, Saltzman HA: Hyperbaric oxygenation in the treatment of acute myocardial infarction. Prog Cardiovasc Dis 10:575-583, 1968.

26. Moon AJ, Williams KG, Hopkinson WI: A patient with coronary thrombosis treated with hyperbaric oxygen. Lancet 1:18-20, 1964.

27. Cameron AJ, Gibb BH, Ledingham I. A controlled clinical trial of hyperbaric oxygen in the treatment of acute myocardial infarction. In: Hyperbaric Oxygenation: Proceedings of the Second International Congress. London, ES Livingstone, 1965.

28. Ashfield R, Drew CE, Gavey CJ: Severe acute myocardial infarction treated with hyperbaric oxygen. Postgrad Med J 45:648-653, 1969.

29. Veselka J, Mates M, Dolezal V: Detection of viable myocardium: Comparison of dobutamine echocardiography and echocardiography after hyperbaric oxygenation. Undersea Hyperb Med 26:9-13, 1999.

30. Hood WB, Yenikomshian S, Norman JC, et al: Treatment of refractory ventricular tachysystole with hyperbaric oxygenation. Am J Cardiol 22(5):738-741, 1968.

31. Dekleva M, Nesovic A, Vlahovic A, et al: Adjunctive effect of hyperbaric oxygen treatment after thrombolysis on left ventricular function in patients with acute myocardial infarction. Am Heart J 148:1-7, 2004.

31a. Sharifi M, Fares W, Abdel-Karim I, et al: Usefulness of hyperbaric oxygen therapy to inhibit restenosis after percutaneous coronary intervention for acute myocardial infarction or unstable angina pectoris. Am J Cardiol 93:1533-1535, 2004.

31b. Stavitsky Y, Shandling AH, Ellestad MH, et al: Hyperbaric oxygen and thrombolysis in myocardial infarction: The "HOT MI" randomised multicenter study. Cardiol 90:131-136, 1998.

31c. Shandling AH, Ellestad MH, Hart GB, et al: Hyperbaric oxygen and thrombolysis in myocardial infarction: The "HOT MI" pilot study. Am Heart J 134:544-550, 1997.

31d. Swift PC, Turner JH, Oxer HF, et al: Myocardial hibernation identified by hyperbaric oxygen treatment and echocardiography in postinfarction patients: Comparison with exercise thallium scintigraphy. American Heart Journal 124:1151-1158, 1992.

31e. Thurston GJ, Greenwood TW, Bending MR, et al: A controlled investigation into the effects of hyperbaric oxygen on mortality following acute myocardial infarction. Quarterly Journal of Medicine XLII:751-770, 1973.

32. Bennett MH, Jepson N, Lehm JP: Hyperbaric oxygen therapy for acute coronary syndrome. Chichester, United Kingdom, John Wiley & Sons, Ltd. Cochrane Database Syst Rev (2):CD004818, 2005.

33. Thurman DJ, Alverson C, Browne DD: Traumatic brain injury in the United States: A report to Congress. Bethesda, MD, U.S. Department of Health and Human Services, National Center for Injury Prevention and Control, 1999.

34. Alexander E: Global Spine and Head Injury Prevention Project (SHIP). Surg Neurol 38:478-479, 1992.

35. Roberts I: Letter from Chengdu: China takes to the roads. BMJ 310:1311-1313, 1995.

36. Fearnside MR, Gurka JA: The challenge of traumatic brain injury. Med J Aust 167:293-294, 1997.

37. Fiskum G: Mitochondrial participation in ischemic and traumatic neural cell death. J Neurotrauma 17:843-855, 2000.

38. Tymianski M, Tator CH: Normal and abnormal calcium homeostasis in neurons: A basis for the pathophysiology of traumatic and ischemic central nervous system injury. Neurosurgery 38:1176-1195, 1996.

39. Schierhout G, Roberts I: Anti-epileptic drugs for preventing seizures following acute traumatic brain injury (Cochrane review). Cochrane Database Syst Rev (4):CD000173, 2001.

40. Roberts I: Barbiturates for acute traumatic brain injury (Cochrane review). Chichester, United Kingdom, John Wiley & Sons, Ltd. Cochrane Database Syst Rev (2): CD000033, 2000.

41. Langham J, Goldfrad C, Teasdale G, et al: Calcium channel blockers for acute traumatic brain injury (Cochrane review). Chichester, United Kingdom, John Wiley & Sons, Ltd. Cochrane Database Syst Rev (4):CD000565, 2003.

42. Alderson P, Roberts I: Corticosteroids for acute traumatic brain injury (Cochrane review). Chichester, United Kingdom, John Wiley & Sons, Ltd. Cochrane Database Syst Rev (1):CD000196, 2005.

43. Roberts I, Schierhout G: Hyperventilation therapy for acute traumatic brain injury (Cochrane review). Chichester, United Kingdom, John Wiley & Sons, Ltd. Cochrane Database Syst Rev (2):CD000566, 2000.

44. Fasano VA, Nunno T De, Urciolo R, et al: First observation on the use of oxygen under high pressure for the treatment of traumatic coma. In: Boerema I, Brummelkamp WH, Meijne NG (eds): Clinical Application of Hyperbaric Oxygen. Amsterdam, Elsevier, 1964, pp 168-173.

45. Muizelaar JP: Cerebral blood flow, cerebral blood volume and cerebral metabolism after severe head injury. Textbook of Head Injury. London, WB Saunders, 1989, pp 221-240.

46. Ikeda Y, Long DM: The molecular basis of brain injury and brain edema: The role of oxygen free radicals. Neurosurgery 27:1-11, 1990.

47. Siesjo BK, Agardh CD, Bengtsson F: Free radicals and brain damage. Cerebrovasc Brain Metab Rev 1:165-211, 1989.

48. Robertson CS, Narayan RK, Gokaslan ZL, et al: Cerebral arteriovenous oxygen difference as an estimate of cerebral blood flow in comatose patients. J Neurosurg 70:222-230, 1989.

49. Hills BA: A role for oxygen-induced osmosis in hyperbaric oxygen therapy. Med Hypotheses 52:259-263, 1999.

50. Clark JM: Oxygen toxicity. The Physiology and Medicine of Diving, 3rd ed. New York, Saunders, 1982, pp 200-238.

51. Daugherty WP, Levasseur JE, Sun D, et al: Effects of hyperbaric oxygen therapy on cerebral oxygenation and mitochondrial function following moderate lateral fluid-percussion injury in rats. J Neurosurg 101:499-504, 2004.

52. Niklas A, Brock D, Schober R, et al: Continuous measurements of cerebral tissue oxygen pressure during hyperbaric oxygenation—HBO effects on brain edema and necrosis after severe brain trauma in rabbits. J Neurol Sci 219:77-82, 2004.

53. Palzur E, Vlodavsky E, Mulla H, et al: Hyperbaric oxygen therapy for reduction of secondary brain damage in head injury: An animal model of brain contusion. J Neurotrauma 21:41-48, 2004.

54. Rogatsky GG, Kamenir Y, Mayevski A: Effect of hyperbaric oxygenation on intracranial pressure elevation rate in rats during the early phase of severe traumatic brain injury. Brain Res 1047:131-136, 2005.

55. Vlodavsky E, Palzur E, Soustiel JF: Hyperbaric oxygen therapy reduces neuroinflammation and expression of matrix metalloproteinase-9 in the rat model of traumatic brain injury. Neuropathol Appl Neurobiol 32:40-50, 2006.

56. Sukoff MH, Ragatz RE: Hyperbaric oxygenation for the treatment of acute cerebral edema. Neurosurgery 10:29-38, 1982.

57. Hayakawa T, Kanai N, Kuroda R: Response of cerebrospinal fluid pressure to hyperbaric oxygenation. J Neurol Neurosurg Psychiatry 34:580-586, 1971.

58. Neubauer RA, Gottlieb SF, Pevsner NH: Hyperbaric oxygen for treatment of closed head injury. South Med J 87:933-936, 1994.

59. Holbach KH, Caroli A, Wassmann H: Cerebral energy metabolism in patients with brain lesions of normo- and hyperbaric oxygen pressures. J Neurol 217:17-30, 1977.

60. Artru F, Philippon B, Gau F, et al: Cerebral blood flow, cerebral metabolism and cerebrospinal fluid biochemistry in brain-injured patients after exposure to hyperbaric oxygen. Eur Neurol 14:351-364, 1976.

61. Bennett MH, Trytko BE, Jonker B: Hyperbaric oxygen therapy for the adjunctive treatment of traumatic brain injury (Cochrane review). Cochrane Database Sys Rev (4):CD004609, 2004.

61a. Ren H, Wang W, Ge Z: Glasgow coma scale, brain electrical activity mapping and Glasgow outcome score after hyperbaric oxygen treatment of severe brain injury. Chin J Traumatol 4(4):239-241, 2001.

61b. Rockswold GL, Ford SE, Anderson DC, et al: Results of a prospective randomized trial for treatment of severely brain-injured patients with hyperbaric oxygen. J Neurosurg 76(6):929-934, 1992.

61c. Artru F, Chacornac R, Deleuze R: Hyperbaric oxygenation for severe head injuries. Preliminary results of a controlled study. Eur Neurol 14(4):310-318, 1976.

61d. Holbach KH, Wassmann H, Kolberg T: Improved reversibility of the traumatic midbrain syndrome using hyperbaric oxygen. Acta Neurochirurgica 30(3-4):247-256, 1974.

62. Leach RM, Lees PJ, Wilmshurst P: ABC of oxygen: Hyperbaric oxygen therapy. BMJ 317:1140-1143, 1998.

63. Adamson SJ, Alessandri LM, Badawi N, et al: Predictors of neonatal encephalopathy in full-term infants. BMJ 311:598-602, 1995.

64. Nelson KB, Liviton A: How much of neonatal encephalopathy is due to birth asphyxia? Am J Dis Child 145:1325-1331, 1991.

65. Hankins GDV, Speer M: Defining the pathogenesis and pathophysiology of neonatal encephalopathy and cerebral palsy. Obstet Gynecol 102:628-636, 2006.

66. Low JA: Determining the contribution of asphyxia to brain damage in the neonate. J Obstet Gynaecol Res 30:276-286, 2004.

67. Higgins R: Hypoxic ischemic encephalopathy and hypothermia: A critical look. Obstet Gynecol 106:1385-1387, 2005.

68. Perlman JM, Tack ED, Martin T, et al: Acute systemic organ injury in term infants after asphyxia. Am J Dis Child 143:617-620, 1989.

69. Whitelaw A: A systematic review of therapy after hypoxia-ischaemic brain injury in the perinatal period. Semin Neonatol 5:33-40, 2000.

70. Kent A, Kecskes Z: Magnesium sulfate for term infants following perinatal asphyxia (protocol). John Wiley & Sons, Ltd. Cochrane Database Sys Rev 2, 2003.

71. Gluckman PD, Wyatt JS, Azzopardi D, et al: Selective head cooling with mild systemic hypothermia after neonatal encephalopathy: Multicenter randomized trial. Lancet 365:663-670, 2005.

72. Shankaran S, Laptook AR, Ehrenkranz RA, et al: Whole body hypothermia for neonates with hypoxic-ischemic encephalopathy. N Engl J Med 353:1574-1584, 2005.

73. Hutchison JH, Kerr MM, Inall JA, et al: Controlled trials of hyperbaric oxygen and tracheal intubation in asphyxia neonatorum. Lancet 7444:935-939, 1966.

74. Miljovic-Lolic M, Silbergleit R, Fiskum G, et al: Neuroprotective effects of hyperbaric oxygen treatment in experimental focal cerebral ischemia are associated with reduced brain leukocyte myeloperoxidase activity. Brain Res 971:90-94, 2003.

75. Iwatsuki N, Takahashi M, Ono K, et al: Hyperbaric oxygen combined with nicardipine administration accelerates neurologic recovery after cerebral ischemia in a canine model. Crit Care Med 22:858-863, 1994.

76. Mink RB, Dutka AJ: Hyperbaric oxygen after global cerebral ischemia in rabbits does not promote brain lipid peroxidation. Crit Care Med 23:1398-1404, 1995.

77. Mink RB, Dutka AJ: Hyperbaric oxygen after global cerebral ischemia in rabbits reduces brain vascular permeability and blood flow. Stroke 26:2307-2312, 1995.

78. Reitan JA, Kien ND, Thorup S, et al: Hyperbaric oxygen increases survival following carotid ligation in gerbils. Stroke 21:119-123, 1990.

79. Schabitz WR, Schade H, Heiland S, et al: Neuroprotection by hyperbaric oxygenation after experimental focal cerebral ischemia monitored by MRI. Stroke 35:1175-1179, 2004.

80. Takahashi M, Iwatsuki N, Ono K, et al: Hyperbaric oxygen therapy accelerates neurologic recovery after 15-minute complete global cerebral ischemia in dogs. Crit Care Med 20:1588-1594, 1992.

81. Veltkamp R, Warner DS, Domoki F, et al: Hyperbaric oxygen decreases infarct size and behavioral deficit after transient focal cerebral ischemia in rats. Brain Res 853:68-73, 2000.

82. Veltkamp M, Bieber K, Wagner S, et al: Hyperbaric oxygen reduces basal lamina degradation after transient focal cerebral ischemia in rats. Brain Res 1076:231-237, 2006.

83. Liu Z, Xiong T, Meads C: Clinical effectiveness of treatment with hyperbaric oxygen for neonatal hypoxic-ischaemic encephalopathy: Systematic review of Chinese literature. BMJ 333:374, 2006.

84. Jan MM: Cerebral palsy: Comprehensive review and update. Ann Saudi Med 26:123-132, 2006.

85. Amato M, Donati F: Update on perinatal hypoxic insult: Mechanism, diagnosis and interventions. Eur J Paed Neurol 4:203-209, 2000.

86. Zafeiriou DI, Kontopoulos EE, Tsikoulas I: Characteristics and prognosis of epilepsy in children with cerebral palsy. J Child Neurol 14:289-294, 1999.

87. Paneth N, Hong T, Korzeniewski S: The descriptive epidemiology of cerebral palsy. Clin Perinatol 33:251-267, 2006.

88. Koman LA, Smith BP, Shilt JS: Cerebral palsy. Lancet 363:1619-1631, 2004.

89. O'Shea TM, Preisser JS, Klinepeter KL, et al: Trends in mortality and cerebral palsy in a geographically based cohort of very low birth weight neonates born between 1982 to 1994. Pediatrics 101:642-647, 1998.

90. Hack M, Freidman H, Fanaroff A: Outcomes of extremely low birth weight infants. Pediatrics 98:913-937, 1996.

91. Kirton A, deVeber G: Cerebral palsy secondary to perinatal ischemic stroke. Clin Perinatol 33:367-386, 2006.

92. Noetzel MJ: Perinatal trauma and cerebral palsy. Clin Perinatol 33:355-366, 2006.

93. Hermansen MC, Hermansen MG: Perinatal infections and cerebral palsy. Clin Perinatol 33:315-333, 2006.

94. Menkes JH, Flores-Sarnat L: Cerebral palsy due to chromosomal anomalies and continuous gene syndromes. Clin Perinatol 33:481-501, 2006.

95. Folkerth RD: Neuropathologic substrate of cerebral palsy. J Child Neurol 20:940-949, 2005.

96. Baud O, Haynes RF, Wang H: Developmental up-regulation of MnSOD in rat oligodendrocytes confers protection against oxidative injury. Eur J Neurosci 20:29-40, 2004.

97. Deng W, Rosenberg PA, Volpe JJ, et al: Calcium-permeable AMPA/kainite receptors mediate toxicity and preconditioning by oxygen-glucose deprivation in oligodendrocyte precursors. Proc Nat Acad Sci U S A 100:6801-6806, 2003.

98. Liu HN, Giasson BI, Mushynski WE, et al: AMPA receptor-mediated toxicity in oligodendrocyte progenitors involves free radical generation and activation of JNK, calpain, and caspase 3. J Neurochem 82:398-409, 2002.

99. Agresti C, Bernardo A, Del Russo N: Synergistic stimulation of MHC class I and IRF-1 gene expression by IFN-gamma and TNF-alpha in oligodendrocytes. Eur J Neurosci 10:2975-2983, 1998.

100. Perlman JM: Intervention strategies for neonatal hypoxic-ischaemic cerebral injury. Clin Ther 28:1353-1365, 2006.

101. Mizrahi EM, Kellaway P: Characterization and classification of neonatal seizures. Neurology 37:1837-1844, 1987.

102. Neubauer RA: Hyperbaric oxygenation for cerebral palsy. Lancet 357:2052, 2001.

103. Neubauer RA, Gottlieb SF, Kagan RL: Enhancing 'idling' neurons. Lancet 335:542, 1990.

103a. Collet JP, Vanasse M, Marois P, et al: Hyperbaric oxygen for children with cerebral palsy: A randomised multicentre trial. HBO-CP Research Group. Lancet 357(9256):582-586, 2001.

104. Marois P, Vanasse M: Hyperbaric oxygen therapy and cerebral palsy. Dev Med Child Neurol 45:646-647, 2003.

105. Heuser G, Heuser SA, Rodelander D, et al: Treatment of neurologically impaired adults and children with 'mild' hyperbaric oxygenation (1.3 ATA and 24% oxygen). In:

Joiner JT (ed): Proceedings of the 2nd International Symposium on Hyperbaric Oxygenation for Cerebral Palsy and the Brain-Injured Child. Flagstaff, Ariz, Best Publishing, 2002, pp 109-115.

106. Patel DR: Therapeutic interventions in cerebral palsy. Indian J Pediatr 72:979-983, 2005.

107. Steinbok P: Selection of treatment modalities in children with spastic cerebral palsy. Neurosurg Focus 21:1-8, 2006.

108. Montgomery D, Goldberg J, Amar M, et al: Effects of hyperbaric oxygen therapy on children with spastic diplegic cerebral palsy: A pilot project. Undersea Hyperb Med 26:235-242, 1999.

109. Machado JJ: Clinically observed reduction of spasticity in patients with neurological diseases and in children with cerebral palsy from hyperbaric oxygen therapy: 1989. Available at: http://www.hbotoday.com/treatment/clinical/researchstudies/hbobrazil.shtml. Accessed January 2008.

110. Reference deleted in proofs.

111. Nuthall G, Seear M, Lepawsky M, et al: Hyperbaric oxygen therapy for cerebral palsy: Two complications of treatment. Pediatrics 106:E80, 2000.

112. Mathai SS, Bansali P, Singh Gill B, et al: Effects of hyperbaric oxygen therapy in children with cerebral palsy. In: Desola J (ed): Proceedings of the International Conference on Diving and Hyperbaric Medicine, Barcelona 7-10 September 2005. Barcelona, Spain, European Underwater and Biomedical Society, 2005, pp 193-197.

113. Packard M: The Cornell Study. 2000. Available at: http://www.netnet.net/mums/Cornell.htm. Accessed January 2008.

114. Chavdarov I: The effects of hyperbaric oxygenation on psycho-motor functions by children with cerebral palsy. In: Joiner JT (ed): Proceedings of the 2nd International Symposium on Hyperbaric Oxygenation for Cerebral Palsy and the Brain-Injured Child. Flagstaff, Ariz, Best Publishing, 2002, pp 91-96.

115. Hardy P, Collet JP, Goldberg J, et al: Neuropsychological effects of hyperbaric oxygen therapy in cerebral palsy. Dev Med Child Neurol 44:436-446, 2002.

116. Muller-Bolla M, Collet JP, Ducruet T, et al: Side effects of hyperbaric oxygen therapy in children with cerebral palsy. Undersea Hyperb Med 33:237-244, 2006.

117. Russell D, Rosenbaum P, Avery L, et al: The Gross Motor Function Measure (GMFM-66 & GMFM-88) User's Manual. Cambridge, Cambridge University Press, 2002.

118. Scientific Advisory Committee: Hyperbaric oxygen therapy for children with cerebral palsy: A multicenter randomised clinical trial. Quebec, Canada, Fonds dela recherche en sante du Quebec, 2000.

119. Niezgoda JA, Cianci P, Folden BW, et al: The effect of hyperbaric oxygen therapy on a burn wound model in human volunteers. Plast Reconstr Surg 99:1620-1625, 1997.

120. Essex C: Hyperbaric oxygen and cerebral palsy: No proven benefit and potentially harmful. Dev Med Child Neurol 45:213-215, 2003.

121. Edwards SJ, Lilford RJ, Braunholtz DA, et al: Ethical issues in the design and conduct of randomised controlled trials: A review. Health Technol Assess 2:1-132, 1998.

122. Lantos JD: The "inclusion benefit" in clinical trials. J Pediatr 134:130-131, 1999.

123. Compston D: The genetic epidemiology of multiple sclerosis. In: Compston A, McDonald I, Noseworthy J (eds): McAlpine's Multiple Sclerosis, 4 ed. Amsterdam, Elsevier, 1998, pp 45-142.

124. Weinschenker BG, Bass B, Rice GP: The natural history of multiple sclerosis: A geographically based study. 1. Clinical course and disability. Brain 112:133-146, 1989.

125. Pittock SJ, Mayr WT, McClelland RL: Disability profile of MS didn't change over 10 years in a population-based prevalence cohort. Neurology 62:601-606, 2004.

126. Murray TJ. Diagnosis and treatment of multiple sclerosis. BMJ 332:525-527, 2004.

127. Silver N, Lai M, Symms M, et al: Serial magnetisation transfer imaging to characterize the early evolution of new MS lesions. Neurology 51:758-764, 1998.

128. Brex PA, Ciccarelli O, O'Riordan JI, et al: A longitudinal study of abnormalities on MRI and disability from multiple sclerosis. N Engl J Med 346:158-164, 2002.

129. Ludwin SK: The pathogenesis of multiple sclerosis: Relating human pathology to experimental studies. J Neuropathol Exp Neurol 65:305-318, 2006.

130. Gottlieb SF, Neubauer RA: Multiple sclerosis: Its etiology, pathogenesis and therapeutics with emphasis on the controversial use of HBO. J Hyperb Med 3:143-164, 1988.

131. Prineas J, Barnard R, Revesz T, et al: Multiple sclerosis. Pathology of recurrent lesions. Brain 116:681-693, 1993.

132. Frohman EM, Racke MK, Raine CS: Multiple sclerosis—the plaque and its pathogenesis. N Engl J Med 354:942-955, 2006.

133. Hemmer B, Archelos JJ, Hartung HP: New concepts in the immunopathogenesis of multiple sclerosis. Nat Rev Neurosci 3:291-301, 2002.

134. Chaudhuri A, Behan PO: Multiple sclerosis is not an autoimmune disease. Arch Neurol 61:1610-1612, 2004.

135. Wang WZ, Olsson T, Kostulas V: Myelin antigen reactive T-cells in cerebrovascular diseases. Clin Exp Neurol 88:157-162, 1992.

136. Barnett MH, Prineas J: Relapsing and remitting multiple sclerosis: Pathology of the newly forming lesion. Ann Neurol 55:458-468, 2004.

137. Scheinker M: Histogenesis of the early lesions of multiple sclerosis. Arch Neurol 49:178-185, 1943.

138. Aita JF, Bennett DR, Anderson RE, et al: Cranial CT appearance of acute multiple sclerosis. Neurology 28:251-255, 1978.

139. Brickner RM: The significance of localized vasoconstrictions in multiple sclerosis; transient sudden miniature attacks of multiple sclerosis. Res Publ Assoc Res Nerv Ment Dis 28:236-244, 1950.

140. Rindfleisch E: Histologische detail zu der degeneration von gehirn und ruckenmark. Virchows Arch (Pathol Anat) 26:478-483, 1863.

141. James PB: Evidence for subacute fat embolism as the cause of multiple sclerosis. Lancet 1:380-386, 1982.

142. Dow RS, Berglund G: Vascular pattern of lesions of multiple sclerosis. Arch Neurol 47:1-18, 1942.

143. Minagar A, Wenche J, Jiminez JJ, et al: Multiple sclerosis as a vascular disease. Neurol Res 28:230-235, 2006.

144. Miller D, Khan OA, Sheremata WA: A controlled trial of natalizumab for relapsing multiple sclerosis. N Engl J Med 348:15-23, 2003.

145. Chaudhuri A: Lessons for clinical trials from natalizumab in multiple sclerosis. BMJ 332:416-419, 2006.

146. Kurtzke JF: Further notes on disability evaluation in multiple sclerosis with scale modifications. Neurology (Minneapolis) 15:654-661, 1965.

147. Kurtzke JF: Rating neurological impairment in multiple sclerosis: An expanded disability status scale (EDSS). Neurology 33:1444-1452, 1983.

148. Goodin DS, Frohman EM, Garmany GP, et al: Disease modifying therapies in multiple sclerosis. Neurology 58:169-178, 2002.

149. Barbero P, Bergui M, Versino E, et al: Every-other-day interferon beta-1b versus once-weekly interferon beta-1a for multiple sclerosis (INCOMIN Trial) II: Analysis of MRI responses to treatment and correlation with NAb. Mult Scler 12:72-76, 2006.

150. Li DKB, Zhao GJ, Paty D: Randomised controlled trial of interferon-beta-1a in secondary progresssive MS: MRI results. Neurology 56:1505-1513, 2001.

151. PRISMS (Prevention of Relapses and Disability by Interferon beta-1a Subcutaneously in Multiple Sclerosis) Study Group: Randomised double-blind placebo-controlled study of interferon beta-1a in relapsing/remitting multiple sclerosis. Lancet 352:1498-1504, 1998.

152. Simon JH, Lull J, Jacobs LD, et al: A longitudinal study of T1 hypointense lesions in relapsing MS. MSCRG trial of interferon beta-1a. Multiple Sclerosis Collaborative Research Group. Neurology 55:185-192, 2000.

153. The Once Weekly Interferon for MS Study Group: Evidence of interferon beta-1a dose response in relapsing-remitting MS: The OWIMS Study. Neurology 54:679-686, 1999.

154. Patti F, L'Episcopo MR, Cataldi ML, et al: Natural interferon-beta treatment of relapsing-remitting and secondary-progressive multiple sclerosis patients. A two-year study. Acta Neurol Scand 100:283-289, 1999.

155. European Study Group: The European Study Group on interferon beta-1b in secondary progressive MS: Placebo-controlled multicentre randomised trial of interferon beta-1b in treatment of secondary progressive multiple sclerosis. Lancet 352:1491-1497, 1998.

156. SPECTRIMS Study Group: Randomised controlled trial of interferon-beta-1a in secondary progressive MS: Clinical results. Neurology 56:1496-1504, 2001.

157. Johnson KP, Brooks BR, Ford CC, et al: Sustained clinical benefits of glatiramer acetate in relapsing multiple sclerosis patients observed for 6 years. Mult Scler 6:255-266, 2000.

158. Clegg A, Bryant J, Milne R: Disease-modifying drugs for multiple sclerosis: A rapid and systematic review. Health Technol Assess 4:i-iv, 1-101, 2000.

159. Boschetty V, Cernoch J: Use of hyperbaric oxygen in various neurologic diseases (preliminary report). Bratisl Lek Listy 53:298-302, 1970.

160. Neubauer RA: Treatment of multiple sclerosis with monoplace hyperbaric oxygenation. J Fla Med Assoc 65:101, 1978.

161. Neubauer RA: Exposure of multiple sclerosis patients to hyperbaric oxygen at 1.5-2 ATA. A preliminary report. J Fla Med Assoc 67:498-504, 1980.

162. Bennett M, Heard R: Treatment of multiple sclerosis with hyperbaric oxygen therapy. Undersea Hyperb Med 28:117-122, 2001.

163. Kindwall EP, McQuillen MP, Khatri BO, et al: Treatment of multiple sclerosis with hyperbaric oxygen. Results of a national registry. Arch Neurol 48:195-199, 1991.

164. Multiple Sclerosis National Therapy Centres. The experience of MS National Therapy Centres in treating MS with prolonged courses of high dosage oxygenation. Available at: http://www.ms-selfhelp.org/html/oxygen_3.html. Accessed January 2008.

165. Worthington J, DeSouza L, Forti A, et al: A double-blind controlled crossover trial investigating the efficacy of hyperbaric oxygen in patients with multiple sclerosis. In: Rose FC, Jones R (eds): Multiple Sclerosis: Immunological, Diagnostic and Therapeutic Aspects. London, John Libbey, 1987, pp 229-240.

166. Neubauer RA: Hyperbaric oxygen therapy of multiple sclerosis. A multi-centre survey. Lauderdale-By-The-Sea, Fla, RA Neubauer, 1983.

166a. Pallotta R: Hyperbaric therapy for multiple sclerosis. Minerva-Medica 73(42):2947-2954, 1982.

167. Fischer BH, Marks M, Reich T: Hyperbaric-oxygen treatment of multiple sclerosis. A randomized, placebo-controlled, double-blind study. N Engl J Med 308:181-186, 1983.

168. Kleijnen J, Knipschild P: Hyperbaric oxygen for multiple sclerosis. Review of controlled trials. Acta Neurol Scand 91:330-334, 1995.

169. Bennett M, Heard R: Hyperbaric oxygen therapy for multiple sclerosis. Chichester, United Kingdom, John Wiley & Sons, Ltd. Cochrane Database Syst Rev (1):CD003057, 2004.

169a. Barnes MP, Bates D, Cartlidge NE, et al: Hyperbaric oxygen and multiple sclerosis: Short-term results of a placebo-controlled, double-blind trial. Lancet 1:297-300, 1985.

169b. Neiman J, Nilsson BY, Barr PO, et al: Hyperbaric oxygen in chronic progressive multiple sclerosis: Visual evoked potentials and clinical effects. J Neurol Neurosurg Psychiatry 48:497-500, 1985.

169c. Wood J, Stell R, Unsworth I, et al: A double-blind trial of hyperbaric oxygen in the treatment of multiple sclerosis. Med J Aust 143:238-240, 1985.

169d. Confavreux C, Mathieu C, Chacornac R, et al: Ineffectiveness of hyperbaric oxygen therapy in multiple sclerosis: A randomized placebo-controlled double-blind study. Presse Med 15:1319-1322, 1986.

169e. L'Hermitte F, Roullet E, Lyon-Caen O: Hyperbaric oxygen treatment of chronic multiple sclerosis: Results of a placebo-controlled double-blind study in 49 patients. Revue Neurologique (Paris) 142:201-206, 1986.

169f. Harpur GD, Suke R, Bass BH, et al: Hyperbaric oxygen therapy in chronic stable multiple sclerosis: Double-blind study. Neurology 136:988-991, 1986.

169g. Wiles CM, Clarke CR, Irwin HP, et al: Hyperbaric oxygen in multiple sclerosis: A double blind trial. Br Med J (Clin Res Ed) 292:367-371, 1986.

169h. Barnes MP, Bates D, Cartlidge NE, et al: Hyperbaric oxygen and multiple sclerosis: Final results of a placebo-controlled, double-blind trial. J Neurol Neurosurg Psychiatry 50:1402-1406, 1987.

169i. Oriani G, Barbieri S, Cislaghi G, et al: Long-term hyperbaric oxygen in multiple sclerosis: A placebo-controlled, double-blind trial with evoked potentials studies. Journal of Hyperbaric Medicine 5:237-245, 1990.

170. James PB: Hyperbaric oxygen and multiple sclerosis. Lancet 1:572, 1985.

171. Bath PM, Lees KR: ABC of arterial and venous disease. Acute stroke. BMJ 320:920-923, 2000.

172. Lopez AD, Mathers CD, Ezzati M, et al: Global and regional burden of disease and risk factors, 2001. Systematic analysis of population health data. Lancet 367:1747-1757, 2006.

173. Bamford J, Sandercock P, Dennis M, et al: Classification and natural history of clinically identifiable subtypes of cerebral infarction. Lancet 337:1521-1526, 1991.

174. Sudlow CL, Warlow CP: Comparable studies of the incidence of stroke and its pathological types: Results from an international collaboration. International Stroke Incidence Collaboration. Stroke 28:491-499, 1997.

175. Wardlaw JM, Keir SL, Seymour J, et al: What is the best imaging strategy for acute stroke? Health Technol Assess 8:1-180, 2004.

176. Kang D-W, Latour LL, Chalela JA, et al: Early and late recurrence of ischemic lesion on MRI. Neurology 63:2261-2265, 2004.

177. Chalela JA, Merino JG, Warach S: Update on stroke. Curr Opin Neurol 17:447-451, 2004.

178. Chinese Acute Stroke Trial Collaborative Group: CAST: Randomised placebo-controlled trial of early aspirin use in 20,000 patients with acute ischaemic stroke. Lancet 349:1641-1649, 1997.

179. The International Stroke Trial Collaborative Group: The International Stroke Trial (IST): A randomised trial of aspirin, subcutaneous heparin, both, or neither among 19435 patients with acute ischaemic stroke. International Stroke Trial Collaborative Group. Lancet 349:1569-1581, 1997.

180. Stroke Unit Trialists' Collaboration: Organised inpatient (stroke unit) care for stroke (Cochrane review). Chichester, United Kingdom, John Wiley & Sons, Ltd. Cochrane Database Syst Rev (4):CD000197, 2007.

181. Prosser-Loose EJ, Paterson PG: The FOOD Trial Collaboration: Nutritional supplementation strategies and acute stroke outcome. Nutr Rev 64:289-294, 2006.

182. Baird TA, Parsons MW, Phan T, et al: Persistent post-stroke hyperglycaemia is independently associated with infarct expansion and worse clinical outcome. Stroke 34:2208-2214, 2003.

183. Aslanyan S, Fazekas F, Weir CJ, et al: Effect of blood pressure during the acute period of ischemic stroke on stroke outcome: A tertiary analysis of the GAIN International Trial. Stroke 34:2420-2425, 2003.

184. Hart GB, Thompson RE: The treatment of cerebral ischemia with hyperbaric oxygen (OHP). Stroke 2:247-250, 1971.

185. Ingvar DH, Lassen NA: Treatment of focal cerebral ischaemia with hyperbaric oxygen. Report of 4 cases. Acta Neurol Scand 41:92-95, 1965.

186. Thom SR: Functional inhibition of leukocyte B2 integrins by hyperbaric oxygen in carbon monoxide-mediated brain injury in rats. Toxicol Appl Pharmacol 123:248-256, 1993.

187. Badr AE, Yin W, Mychaskiw G, et al: Effect of hyperbaric oxygen on striatal metabolites: A microdialysis study in awake freely moving rats after MCA occlusion. Brain Res 916:85-90, 2001.

188. Selman WR, Lust WD, Pundik S, et al: Compromised metabolic recovery following spontaneous spreading depression in the penumbra. Brain Res 999:167-174, 2004.

189. Yusa T, Beckman JS, Crapo JD, et al: Hyperoxia increases H2O2 production by brain in vivo. J Appl Physiol 63:353-358, 1987.

190. Nighoghossian N, Trouillas P: Hyperbaric oxygen in the treatment of acute ischemic stroke: An unsettled issue. J Neurol Sci 150:27-31, 1997.

191. Helms AK, Whelan HT, Torbey MT: Hyperbaric oxygen therapy of cerebral ischemia. Cerebrovasc Dis 20:417-426, 2005.

192. Weinstein PR, Anderson GG, Telles DA: Results of hyperbaric oxygen therapy during temporary middle cerebral artery occlusion in unanesthetized cats. Neurosurgery 20:518-524, 1987.

192a. Yang ZJ, Camporesi C, Yang X, et al: Hyperbaric oxygenation mitigates focal cerebral injury and reduces striatal dopamine release in a rat model of transient middle cerebral artery occlusion. Eur J Appl Physiol 87(2):101-107, 2002.

192b. Sunami K, Takeda Y, Hashimoto M, et al: Hyperbaric oxygen reduces infarct volume in rats by increasing oxygen supply to the ischemic periphery. Crit Care Med 28(8):2831-2836, 2000.

192c. Hjelde A, Hjelstuen M, Haraldseth O, et al: Hyperbaric oxygen and neutrophil accumulation/tissue damage during permanent focal cerebral ischaemia in rats. Eur J Appl Physiol 86(5):401-405, 2002.

192d. Burt JT, Kapp JP, Smith RR: Hyperbaric oxygen and cerebral infarction in the gerbil. Surg Neurol 28(4):265-268, 1987.

192e. Veltkamp R, Siebing DA, Sun L, et al: Hyperbaric oxygen reduces blood-brain barrier damage and edema after transient focal cerebral ischemia. Stroke 36(8):1679-1683, 2005.

192f. Corkill G, Van Housen K, Hein L, et al: Videodensitometric estimation of the protective effect of hyperbaric oxygen in the ischemic gerbil brain. Surg Neurol 24(2):206-210, 1985.

192g. Günther A, Küppers-Tiedt L, Schneider PM, et al: Reduced infarct volume and differential effects on glial cell activation after hyperbaric oxygen treatment in rat permanent focal cerebral ischaemia. Eur J Neurosci 21(11):3189-3194, 2005.

192h. Roos JA, Jackson-Friedman C, Lyden P: Effects of hyperbaric oxygen on neurologic outcome for cerebral ischemia in rats. Acad Emerg Med 5(1):18-24, 1998.

192i. Calvert JW, Yin W, Patel M, et al: Hyperbaric oxygenation prevented brain injury induced by hypoxia-ischemia in a neonatal rat model. Brain Res 951(1):1-8, 2002.

192j. Kawamura S, Yasui N, Shirasawa M, et al: Therapeutic effects of hyperbaric oxygenation on acute focal cerebral ischemia in rats. Surg Neurol 34(2):101-106, 1990.

192k. Lou M, Chen Y, Ding M, et al: Involvement of the mitochondrial ATP-sensitive potassium channel in the neuroprotective effect of hyperbaric oxygenation after cerebral ischemia. Brain Res Bull 69(2):109-116, 2006.

193. Lou M, Eschenfelder CC, Herdegen T, et al: Therapeutic window for use of hyperbaric oxygenation in focal transient ischemia in rats. Stroke 35:578-583, 2004.

193a. Weinstein PR, Anderson GG, Telles DA: Results of hyperbaric oxygen therapy during temporary middle cerebral artery occlusion in unanesthetized cats. Neurosurgery 20(4):518-524, 1987.

193b. Yin D, Zhang JH: Delayed and multiple hyperbaric oxygen treatments expand therapeutic window in rat focal cerebral ischemic model. Neurocrit Care 2(2):206-211, 2005.

193c. Yin W, Badr AE, Mychaskiw G, et al: Down regulation of COX-2 is involved in hyperbaric oxygen treatment in a rat transient focal cerebral ischemia model. Brain Res 926(1-2):165-171, 2002.

193d. Yin D, Zhou C, Kusaka I, et al: Inhibition of apoptosis by hyperbaric oxygen in a rat focal cerebral ischemic model. J Cereb Blood Flow Metab 23(7):855-864, 2003.

194. Neubauer RA, End E: Hyperbaric oxygenation as an adjunct therapy in strokes due to thrombosis. A review of 122 patients. Stroke 11:297-300, 1980.

195. Bennett MH, Wasiak J, Schnabel A, et al: Hyperbaric oxygen therapy for acute ischaemic stroke. Chichester, United Kingdom, John Wiley & Sons, Ltd. Cochrane Database Syst Rev (3):CD004954, 2005.

195a. Anderson DC, Bottini AG, Jagiella WM, et al: A pilot study of hyperbaric oxygen in the treatment of human stroke. Stroke 22(9):1137-1142, 1991.

195b. Nighoghossian N, Trouillas M, Adeleine P, et al: Hyperbaric oxygen in the treatment of acute ischaemic stroke: A double-blind pilot study. Stroke 26:1369-1372, 1995.

195c. Rusyniak DE, Kirk MA, May JD, et al: Hyperbaric oxygen therapy in acute ischemic stroke: Results of the Hyperbaric Oxygen in Acute Ischemic Stroke Trial Pilot Study. Stroke 34(2):571-574, 2003.

196. Van Gijn J: Measurement of outcome in stroke prevention trials. Cerebrovasc Dis 2(suppl 2):23-34, 1992.

197. D'Olhaberriague L, Mitsias P: A reappraisal of reliability and validity studies in stroke. Stroke 27:2331-2336, 1998.

198. Stokroos RJ, Albers FW, Van Cauwenberge P: Diagnosis and treatment of idiopathic sudden sensorineural hearing loss (ISSHL): A survey in the Netherlands and Flanders. Acta Otorhinolaryngol Belg 50:237-245, 1996.

199. Haberkamp TJ, Tanyeri HM: The management of idiopathic sudden sensorineural hearing loss. Am J Otolaryngol 20:587-592, 1999.

200. Hughes GB, Freedman MA, Haberkamp TJ, et al: Sudden sensorineural hearing loss. Otolaryngol Clin North Am 29:393-405, 1996.

201. Thurmond M, Amedee RG: Sudden sensorineural hearing loss: Etiologies and treatments. J Louisiana State Med Soc 150:200-203, 1998.

202. Coles DA, Davis AC: Tinnitus: Its epidemiology and management. Copenhagen, 14th Danavox Jubilee Foundation, 1990.

203. Reference deleted in proofs.

204. Dauman R, Tyler RS: Some considerations on the classification of tinnitus. Proceedings of the Fourth International Tinnitus Seminar. Bordeaux, France. Amsterdam, Kugler, 1992, pp 225-229.

205. Stephens D, Hetu R: Impairment, disability and handicap in Audiology: Towards a consensus. Audiology 30:185-200, 1991.

206. Belal A: Pathology of vascular sensorineural hearing impairment. Laryngoscope 90:1831-1839, 1980.

207. Yoon TH, Paparella MM, Schachern PA, et al: Histopathology of sudden hearing loss. Laryngoscope 100:707-715, 1990.

208. Parnes SM: Current concepts in the clinical management of patients with tinnitus. Eur Arch Otorhinolaryngol 254:406-409, 1997.

209. Kaltenbach JA: Neurophysiologic mechanisms of tinnitus. J Am Acad Audiol 11:125-137, 2000.

210. Cacace AT: Expanding the biological basis of tinnitus: Crossmodal origins and the role of neuroplasticity. Hearing Res 175:112-132, 2003.

211. Jastreboff PJ: Phantom auditory perception (Tinnitus): Mechanisms of generation and perception. Neurosci Res 8:221-254, 1990.

212. Wei BPC, Mubiru S, O'Leary S: Steroids for idiopathic sudden sensorineural hearing loss. Chichester, United Kingdom, John Wiley & Sons, Ltd. Cochrane Database Syst Rev (2):CD003998, 2006.

213. Liang CY, Gong Y, Li J, et al: Vasodilator agents for sudden sensorineural hearing loss. Chichester, United Kingdom, John Wiley & Sons, Ltd. Cochrane Database Syst Rev (1):CD003422, 2002.

214. Mattox DE, Simmons FB: Natural history of sudden sensorineural hearing loss. Ann Otolaryngol Rhinolaryngol Laryngol 86:463-480, 1977.

215. Noell CA, Meyerhoff WL: Tinnitus. Diagnosis and treatment of this elusive symptom. Geriatrics 58:28-34, 2003.

216. Hilton M, Stuart E: Ginkgo biloba for tinnitus. Chichester, United Kingdom, John Wiley & Sons, Ltd. Cochrane Database Syst Rev (2):CD003852, 2004.

217. Baldo P, Cook JA, Dooley L, et al: Antidepressants for tinnitus. Chichester, United Kingdom, John Wiley & Sons, Ltd. Cochrane Database Syst Rev (4): CD003853, 2001.

218. Lamm K, Lamm H, Arnold W: Effect of hyperbaric oxygen therapy in comparison to conventional or placebo therapy or no treatment in idiopathic sudden hearing loss, acoustic trauma, noise-induced hearing loss and tinnitus. A literature survey. Adv Otorhinolaryngol 54:86-99, 1998.

219. Nakashima T, Fukuta S, Yanagita N: Hyperbaric oxygen therapy for sudden deafness. Adv Otorhinolaryngol 54:100-109, 1998.

220. Gul H, Nowak R, Buchner F-A, et al: Different treatment modalities of tinnitus at the EuromedClinic. Int Tinnitus J 6:50-53, 2000.

221. Tan J, Tange RA, Dreschler WA, et al: Long-term effect of hyperbaric oxygenation treatment on chronic distressing tinnitus. Scand Audiol 28:91-96, 1999.

222. Bennett MH, Kertesz T, Yeung P: Hyperbaric oxygen for idiopathic sudden sensorineural hearing loss and tinnitus. Chichester, United Kingdom, John Wiley & Sons, Ltd. Cochrane Database Syst Rev (1):CD004739, 2007.

223. Bennett MH, Kertesz T, Yeung P: Hyperbaric oxygen therapy for idiopathic sudden sensorineural hearing loss and tinnitus: A systematic review of randomized controlled trials. J Laryngol Otol 119:791-798, 2005.

223a. Goto F, Fujita T, Kitani Y, et al: Hyperbaric oxygen and stellate ganglion blocks for idiopathic sudden hearing loss. Acta Otolaryngol 88(5-6):335-342, 1979.

223b. Aslan I, Oysu C, Veyseller B, et al: Does the addition of hyperbaric oxygen therapy to the conventional treatment modalities influence the outcome of sudden deafness? Otolaryngol Head Neck Surg 126(2):121-126, 2002.

223c. Sparacia B, Sparacia, G: Hyperbaric oxygen therapy in treatment of sudden deafness. Acta Medica Mediterranea 19(2):95-102, 2003.

223d. Racic G, Maslovara S, Roje Z, et al: Hyperbaric oxygen in the treatment of sudden hearing loss. ORL J Otorhinolaryngol Relat Spec 65(6):317-320, 2003.

223e. Horn CE, Himel HN, Selesnick SH: Hyperbaric oxygen therapy for sudden sensorineural hearing loss: A prospective trial of patients failing steroid and antiviral treatment. Otol Neurotol 26(5):882-889, 2005.

223f. Satar B, Hidir Y, Yetiser S: Effectiveness of hyperbaric oxygen therapy in idiopathic sudden hearing loss. J Laryngol Otol 120(8):665-669, 2006.

223g. Cavallazzi G, Pignataro L, Capaccio P: Italian experience in hyperbaric oxygen therapy for idiopathic sudden sensorineural hearing loss. Proceedings of the International Joint Meeting on Hyperbaric and Underwater Medicine. European Undersea and Baromedical Society, 1996, pp 647-649.

223h. Fattori B, Berrettini S, Casani A, et al: Sudden hypoacusis treated with hyperbaric oxygen therapy. Ear Nose and Throat Journal 80:655-660, 2001.

223i. Schwab B, Flunkert C, Heermann R, et al: HBO in the therapy of cochlear dysfunctions—first results of a randomized study. EUBS Diving and Hyperbaric Medicine, Collected manuscripts of XXIV Annual Scientific Meeting of the European Underwater and Baromedical Society, 1998, pp 40-42.

223j. Hoffmann G, Bohmer D, Desloovere C: Hyperbaric oxygenation as a treatment for sudden deafness and acute tinnitus. Proceedings of the Eleventh International Congress on Hyperbaric Medicine, 1995, pp 146-151.

223k. Hoffmann G, Bohmer D, Desloovere C: Hyperbaric oxygenation as a treatment of chronic forms of inner ear hearing loss and tinnitus. Proceedings of the Eleventh International Congress on Hyperbaric Medicine, 1995, pp 141-145.

223l. Topuz E, Yigit O, Cinar U, et al: Should hyperbaric oxygen be added to treatment in idiopathic sudden sensorineural hearing loss? Eur Arch Otorhinolaryngol 261:393-396, 2004.

224. Finnegan M: Injury prevention: Editorial comment. Clin Orthop Relat Res (409):2, 2003.

225. Centers for Disease Control and Prevention (CDC): Sports-related injuries among high school athletes— United States, 2005-06 school year. Morb Mortal Wkly Rep 55:1037-1040, 2006.

226. Van Mechelen W: The severity of sports injuries. Sports Med 24:176-180, 1997.

226a. Leach RE: Hyperbaric oxygen therapy in sports. Am J Sports Med 26(4)489-490, 1998.

227. Babul S, Rhodes EC: The role of hyperbaric oxygen therapy in sports medicine. Sports Med 30:395-403, 2000.

228. Cheung K, Hume P, Maxwell L: Delayed onset muscle soreness: Treatment strategies and performance factors. Sports Med 33:145-164, 2003.

229. Kader D, Saxena A, Movin T, et al: Achilles tendinopathy: Some aspects of basic science and clinical management. Br J Sports Med 36:239-249, 2002.

230. Perryman JR, Hershman EB: The acute management of soft tissue injuries of the knee. Orthoped Clin North Am 33:575-585, 2002.

231. Bleakley C, McDonough S, MacAuley D: The use of ice in the treatment of acute soft-tissue injury. A systematic review of randomised controlled trials. Am J Sports Med 32:251-261, 2004.

232. Amendola A, Williams G, Foster D: Evidence-based approach to treatment of acute traumatic syndesmosis (high ankle) sprains. Sports Med Arthrosc 14:232-236, 2006.

233. Nassab PF, Schickendantz MS: Evaluation and treatment of medial ulnar collateral ligament injuries in the throwing athlete. Sports Med Arthrosc 14:221-231, 2006.

234. Oriani G, Barnini C, Marroni G: Hyperbaric oxygen therapy in the treatment of various orthopedic disorders. Minerva Med 73:2983-2988, 1982.

235. Nylander G, Lewis D, Nordstrom H, et al: Reduction of postischemic edema with hyperbaric oxygen. Plast Reconstr Surg 76:596-603, 1985.

236. Staples JR, Clement DB, McKenzie DC: The effects of intermittent hyperbaric oxygen on biochemical muscle metabolites of eccentrically exercised rats [abstract]. Can J Appl Physiol 20(suppl):49, 1995.

237. Thom SR, Mendiguren H, Nebolon M, et al: Temporary inhibition of human neutrophil B2 integrin function by hyperbaric oxygen. Clin Res 42:130A, 1994.

238. James PB, Scott B, Allen MW: Hyperbaric oxygen therapy in sports injuries. Physiotherapy 79:571-572, 1993.

239. Bennett MH, Best TM, Babul S, et al: Hyperbaric oxygen therapy for delayed onset muscle soreness and closed soft tissue injury. Chichester, United Kingdom, John Wiley & Sons, Ltd. Cochrane Database Syst Rev (4): CD004713, 2005.

239a. Soolsma SJ: The effect of intermittent hyperbaric oxygen on short term recovery from grade II medial collateral ligament injuries [thesis]. Vancouver, Calif, University of British Columbia, 1996.

239b. Borromeo CN, Ryan JL, Marchetto PA, et al: Hyperbaric oxygen therapy for acute ankle sprains. Am J Sports Med 25(5):619-625, 1997.

239c. Staples JR, Clement DB, Taunton JE, et al: Effects of hyperbaric oxygen on a human model of injury. Am J Sports Med 27(5):600-605, 1999.

239d. Mekjavic IB, Exner JA, Tesch PA, et al: Hyperbaric oxygen therapy does not affect recovery from delayed onset muscle soreness. Med Sci Sports Exerc 32(3):558-563, 2000.

239e. Harrison BC, Robinson D, Davison BJ, et al: Treatment of exercise-induced muscle injury via hyperbaric oxygen therapy. Med Sci Sports Exerc 33(1):36-42, 2001.

239f. Webster AL, Syrotuik DG, Bell GJ, et al: Effects of hyperbaric oxygen on recovery from exercise-induced muscle damage in humans. Clin J Sport Med 12(3):139-150, 2002.

239g. Babul S, Rhodes EC, Taunton JE, et al: Effects of intermittent exposure to hyperbaric oxygen for the treatment of an acute soft tissue injury. Clin J Sport Med 13:138-147, 2003.

239h. Germain G, Delaney J, Moore G, et al: Effect of hyperbaric oxygen therapy on exercise-induced muscle soreness. Undersea Hyperb Med 30(2):135-145, 2003.

240. Bessey PQ, Arons RR, DiMaggio CJ, et al: The vulnerabilities of age: Burns in children and older adults. Surgery 140:705-717, 2006.

241. Brigham PA, McLoughlin E: Burn incidence and medical care use in the United States: Estimates, trends, and data sources. J Burn Care Rehab 17:95-107, 1996.

242. WHO: The injury chartbook: A graphic overview of the global burden of injuries. Geneva, World Health Organization, 2002.

243. Sheridan RL: Burns. Crit Care Med 30:S500-S514, 2002.

244. Boykin JV, Eriksson E, Pittman RN: In vivo microcirculation of a scald burn and the progression of postburn dermal ischemia. Plast Reconstr Surg 66:191-198, 1980.

245. Demling RH, Niehaus G, Perea A: Effect of burn-induced hypoproteinemia on pulmonary transvascular fluid filtration rate. Surgery 85:339-343, 1979.

246. Youn YK, LaLonde C, Demling R: The role of mediators in the response to thermal injury. World J Surg 16:30-36, 1992.

247. Wada J, Ikeda T, Kamata K: Oxygen hyperbaric treatment for carbon monoxide poisoning and severe burns in coal mine gas explosion. Igakunoayumi (Japan) 54:68, 1965.

248. Gruber RP, Brinkley B, Amato JJ: Hyperbaric oxygen and pedicle flaps, skin grafts, and burns. Plast Reconstr Surg 45:24-30, 1970.

249. Ueno S, Tanabe G, Kihara K: Early post-operative hyperbaric oxygen therapy modifies neutrophile activation. Hepatogastroenterology 46:1798-1799, 1999.

250. Reference deleted in proofs.

251. Knighton DR, Halliday B, Hunt TK: Oxygen as an antibiotic: The effect of inspired oxygen on infection. Arch Surg 119:199-204, 1984.

252. Cianci P, Sato R: Adjunctive hyperbaric oxygen therapy in the treatment of thermal burns: A review. Burns 20:5-14, 1994.

253. Grossman A: Hyperbaric oxygen in the treatment of burns. Ann Plast Surg 1:163-171, 1978.

254. Niu A, Yang C, Lee H, et al: Burns treated with adjunctive hyperbaric oxygen therapy: A comparative study in humans. J Hyperb Med 2:75-85, 1987.

255. Cianci P, Lueders H, Lee H, et al: Adjunctive hyperbaric oxygen reduces the need for surgery in 40-80% burns. J Hyperb Med 3:97-101, 1988.

256. Waisbren B, Schutz D, Colletine G, et al: Hyperbaric oxygen in severe burns. Burns Incl Therm Inj 8:176-179, 1982.

256a. Villanueva E, Bennett MH, Wasiak J, et al: Hyperbaric oxygen therapy for thermal burns. Cochrane Database Syst Rev (2):CD004727, 2004.

256b. Brannen AL, Still J, Haynes M: A randomized prospective trial of hyperbaric oxygen in a referral burn center population. Am Surg 63:205-208, 1997.

256c. Hart G, O'Reilly R, Broussard N, et al: Treatment of burns with hyperbaric oxygen. Surgery, Gynecology and Obstetrics 139(5):693-696, 1974.

257. Mitrovic A, Nikolic B, Dragojevic S, et al: Hyperbaric oxygenation as a possible therapy of choice for infertility treatment. Bosnian J Basic Med Sci 6:21-24, 2006.

257a. Ketchum SA, Thomas AN, Hall AD: Effect of hyperbaric oxygen on small first, second, and third degree burns. Surgical Forums 18:65-67, 1967.

257b. Bornside GH, Nance FC: High-pressure oxygen combined with antibiotics in the therapy of experimental burn wounds. Antimicrob Agents Chemother 8:497-500, 1968.

257c. Ikeda K, Ajiki H, Nagao H, et al: Hyperbaric oxygen therapy of burns. Geka Chiryo 18(6):689-693, 1968.

257d. Ketchum F, Thomas A, Hall AD: Angiographic studies of the effect of hyperbaric oxygen on burn wound revascularisation. In: Wada J, Iwa T (eds): Proceedings of the Fourth International Congress on Hyperbaric Medicine. London, Balliere, 1970, pp 383-394.

257e. Perrins D: Failed attempt to limit tissue destruction in scalds of pig skin with HBO. In: Wada J, Iwa T (eds): Proceedings of the Fourth International Congress on Hyperbaric Medicine. London, Balliere, 1970, p 381.

257f. Härtwig J, Kirste G: Experimental studies on revascularization of burns during hyperbaric oxygen therapy. Zentralbl Chir 99(35):1112-1117, 1974.

257g. Wells CH, Hilton JG: Effects of hyperbaric oxygen on postburn plasma extravasation. In: Davis JC, Hunt TK (eds): Hyperbaric Oxygen Therapy. Bethesda, Md, Undersea Medical Society, 1977, pp 259-265.

257h. Korn HN, Wheeler ES, Miller TA: Effect of hyperbaric oxygen on second-degree burn wound healing. Arch Surg 112(6):732-737, 1977.

257i. Niccole MW, Thornton JW, Danet RT, et al: Hyperbaric oxygen in burn management: A controlled study. Surgery 82(5):727-733, 1977.

257j. Nylander G, Nordström H, Eriksson E: Effects of hyperbaric oxygen on oedema formation after a scald burn. Burns Incl Therm Inj 10(3):193-196, 1984.

257k. Saunders J, Fritz E, Ko F, et al: The effects of hyperbaric oxygen on dermal ischemia following thermal injury. 21st Annual meeting of the American Burn Association, New Orleans, Louisiana, March 1989.

257l. Stewart RJ, Mason SW, Taira MT, et al: Effect of radical scavengers and hyperbaric oxygen on smoke-induced pulmonary edema. Undersea Hyperb Med 21(1):21-30, 1994.

257m. Tenenhaus M, Hansbrough JF, Zapata-Sirvent R, et al: Treatment of burned mice with hyperbaric oxygen reduces mesenteric bacteria but not pulmonary neutrophil deposition. Arch Surg 129(12):1338-1342, 1994.

257n. Germonpre P, Reper P, Vanderkelen A: Hyperbaric oxygen therapy and piracetam decreases the early extension of deep partial thickness burns. Burns 22(6):468-473, 1996.

257o. Shoshani O, Shupak A, Barak A, et al: Hyperbaric oxygen therapy for deep second degree burns: An experimental study in the guinea pig. Br J Plast Surg 51(1):67-73, 1998.

257p. Akin ML, Gulluoglu BM, Erenoglu C, et al: Hyperbaric oxygen prevents bacterial translocation in thermally injured rats. Journal of Investigative Surgery 15(6):303-310, 2002.

257q. Bilic I, Petri NM, Bezic J, et al: Effects of hyperbaric oxygen therapy on experimental burn wound healing in rats: A randomized controlled study. Undersca Hyperb Med 32(1):1-9, 2005.

258. Jain KK: Textbook of hyperbaric medicine. Seattle, Hogrefe and Huber, 1999.

259. Van Voorhis BJ, Greensmith JE, Dokras A, et al: Hyperbaric oxygen and ovarian follicular stimulation for in vitro fertilization: A pilot study. Fertil Steril 83:226-228, 2005.

260. Huey S, Abuhamad A, Barroso G, et al: Perifollicular blood flow Doppler indices, but not follicular pO2, pCO2, or pH, predict oocyte developmental competence in in vitro fertilization. Fertil Steril 72:707-712, 1999.

261. Van Blerkom J, Antczak M, Schrader R: The developmental potential of the human oocyte is related to the dissolved oxygen content of follicular fluid: Association with vascular endothelial growth factor levels and perifollicular blood flow characteristics. Hum Reprod 12:1047-1055, 1997.

262. Gonen Y, Casper RF: Prediction of implantation by the sonographic appearance of the endometrium during controlled ovarian stimulation for in vitro fertilization (IVF). J In Vitro Fert Embryo Transf 7:146-152, 1990.

263. Leverment J, Turner R, Bowman M, et al: Report of the use of hyperbaric oxygen therapy (HBO2) in an unusual case of secondary infertility. Undersea Hyperb Med 31:245-250, 2004.

264. Zadoev SA, Evdokimov VV, Rumiantsev VB, et al: [Hyperbaric oxygenation in the treatment of patients with chronic congestive prostatitis and lower fertility]. Urologiia 1:27-30, 2001.

265. Asribekova MK, Karpova SK, Murashko LE, et al: [State of the sex hormone receptor in the endometrium of women with late habitual abortion]. Probl Endokrinol (Mosk) 37:26-28, 1991.

266. Chaika VK, Kvashenko VP, Akimova IK: Hyperbaric oxygenation in the prevention of uterine dysfunctions in toxemia of pregnancy. Akusherstvo i Ginekologiya (7):15-17, 1990.

267. Marx RE, Johnson RP: Problem wounds in oral and maxillo-facial surgery: The role of hyperbaric oxygen. In: Hunt TK (ed): Problem Wounds: The Role of Oxygen. Flagstaff, Ariz, Best Publishing Company, 1988, pp 65-123.

268. Mitrovic A, Brkic P, Nikolic B, et al: Hyperbaric oxygen and in vitro fertilisation. Aust N Z J Obstet Gynaecol 46:456-457, 2006.

Side V

Effects and Complications

Effects 22
of Pressure

Avi Shupak, MD, and Peter Gilbey, MD

MIDDLE EAR BAROTRAUMA

Middle ear barotrauma is the most common complication of hyperbaric oxygen therapy (HBOT) with reported incidence rates of 2% to 82%.[1-9] This large variability might be explained by differences in the criteria used for diagnosis (complaints of pain vs. otoscopic findings); the characteristics of the treated population (young military personnel with scuba diving experience vs. patients with high risk for middle ear barotrauma); the level of the patient's instruction and training in middle ear clearing maneuvers; chamber compression rate; and the patient's posture in the chamber (sitting vs. lying down).

PATHOGENESIS OF EAR BAROTRAUMA

The structures of importance in the pathogenesis of ear barotrauma are the tympanic membrane, eustachian tube (ET), middle ear cavity, and oval and round windows (Fig. 22.1).

Normally, the pressure in the middle ear is near ambient, which ensures free vibration of the tympanic membrane and efficient transduction of sound energy to the middle and inner ears. Barotrauma is the damage to tissues caused by an inability to maintain near equivalence between middle ear and ambient pressures.

Because the middle ear is a closed, relatively noncollapsible, temperature-stable, mucosa-lined bony cavity, its pressure is a direct function of the contained gas volume, changing only with gas transfer to or from the middle ear. Small fluctuations in middle ear pressure gradients can be buffered by the limited mobility of the tympanic membrane. However, tympanic membrane displacement can fully compensate only for volume changes of up to 0.2 to 0.3 mL, and buffers negative pressures of up to about 23 mm Hg in a middle ear having an average

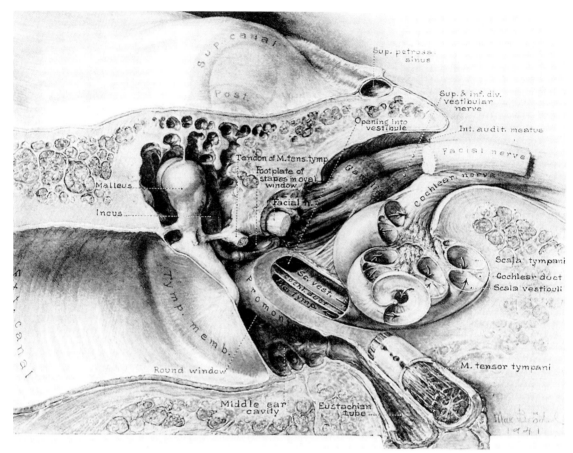

Figure 22.1 Coronal illustration of the ear. *(From Brodel M: Three Unpublished Drawings of the Anatomy of the Human Ear. Philadelphia, WB Saunders, 1946, by permission.)*

volume of 10 mL.[10] The main physiologic pathways for gas exchange between the middle ear and the external environment are gas diffusion through the mucosa and pressure equilibration via the ET (see Fig. 22.1). Gas exchange between the middle ear and mixed venous blood depends mainly on the slow diffusion of nitrogen at a rate of 0.0008 mm Hg/min.[11] Although this mechanism is of importance under stable ambient pressure conditions, the slow rate of transmucosal gas exchange makes it irrelevant when large and rapid changes in ambient pressure are encountered. In contrast, gas flow across the ET is a brisk, gradient-dependent, bolus exchange of gases between the nasopharynx and the tympanic cavity, and it is the main mechanism for middle ear pressure equilibration during HBOT. The ET lumen is collapsed under resting conditions and has to be forced open for middle ear pressure equal-

ization to occur. According to Boyle's Law, the volume of the tympanic cavity will increase during decompression, exerting increasing force on the ET. Passive opening of the tube will occur at middle ear-to-ambient overpressures of 23 to 38 mm Hg.[12] In contrast, when the ambient pressure increases during compression, the increased nasopharyngeal pressure and the mucosal surface tension keep the ET closed. Ear clearing would require voluntary contraction of the tensor veli palatine muscle or active maneuvers aiming to forcefully introduce air via the ET.[13] Active, pressure-driven ET opening occurs when the nasopharyngeal pressure is increased by Valsalva or Toynbee maneuvers or ET pressure can be reduced for some individuals by yawning or mandibular repositioning.

Patients with limited ability for active ET opening such as infants, children, sedated, comatose, and ventilated patients or those with concurrent nasopharyngeal inflammation, caused by viral infection, allergy, or gastroesophageal reflux, might not achieve efficient middle ear pressure equilibration when the ambient pressure increases and thus suffer from ear barotrauma. It should be emphasized that active ET opening under terrestrial conditions, as evident from tympanic membrane movement during the Valsalva maneuver, does not assure good ET ventilatory function during chamber compression.[14,15]

Several factors explain the high vulnerability of the middle ear to barotrauma under hyperbaric conditions. The rapid increase in ambient pressure during compression can overburden the middle ear pressure–regulating ability if frequent active pressure equalization is not practiced. When the tissue pressure surrounding the ET lumen exceeds the maximal force exerted by active contraction of the tensor veli palatini muscle, "locking" of the tube takes place.[16] This phenomenon occurs around unequalized pressure gradients of 90 mm Hg. Then, equalization can be accomplished only by introduction of air to the ET by a forceful Valsalva maneuver, which is associated with increased risk for inner ear barotrauma. Hyperbaric chamber tests have shown that higher pressures are required for active equalization with increasing rates of pressure change.[17] Increasing the ambient pressure leads to an increase in tympanic cavity mucosal volume, resulting in reduced patency of the ET.[18] In the monoplace chamber, patients lie down throughout treatment, and acute cases in the multiplace chamber are usually treated while recumbent. The supine position results in increased central venous pressure and leads to venous congestion and greater difficulty in ear clearing.[14] Increased middle ear and systemic oxygen partial pressures, such as those encountered during HBOT, cause negative middle ear pressure and serous fluid transudation.[19,20] This reflects down-regulation of ET ventilatory function[21,22] and is not secondary merely to middle ear oxygen absorption.[23] Failure of the middle ear pressure regulation mechanism is explained by the vulnerability of the middle ear chemoreceptor tissue to hyperoxia,[24]

similar to that described for the carotid body.[25] This tissue is an essential sensory component of the neural feedback circuits that control the ET function.[26]

Inner ear barotrauma is also related to middle ear pressure equalization difficulties. Increased intracranial pressure resulting from forceful efforts to equalize pressure might be transmitted to the inner ear mainly through the cochlear aqueduct.[27,28] Alternatively, successful opening of the ET when a significant underpressure exists in the middle ear might cause a brisk lateral displacement of the ossicular chain, resulting in inward movement of the round window membrane with a perilymphatic fluid wave directed toward the scala vestibuli.[29] These forces may cause rupture of Reissner's membrane, the basilar membrane, and a labyrinthine window fistula with consequent impairment of inner ear function.[30,31] Further damage might be caused by gas bubbles introduced through a perilymph fistula to the scala tympani and scala vestibuli that expand during decompression.[32,33] Whereas middle ear barotrauma is frequent among divers and patients undergoing HBOT, inner ear barotrauma seldom follows[27,34,35] and has never been described in a clinical hyperbaric patient, although it might be underreported.[36] Detachment of the tectorial membrane of the organ of Corti, outer hair cell edema and broken stereocilia, and perilymphatic hemorrhage have been reported in the guinea pig after repeated hyperbaric exposures to 3 to 5 atmospheres absolute (ATA) in a protocol that did not produce any signs of decompression sickness in the animals.[37] However, this hyperbaric-induced cochlear degeneration has not been substantiated to date by any human study.[15]

CLINICAL PRESENTATION OF MIDDLE EAR BAROTRAUMA

If pressure equalization fails during compression, the developing pressure gradient causes maximal extension of the tympanic membrane with stretching and tearing of its structural elements. Tympanic membrane retraction is followed by focal hemorrhages, middle ear mucosal swelling, capillary dilatation, transudate leakage, hemotympanum, and finally, inward rupture of the tympanic membrane.[38] When tympanic membrane perforation takes place, it mostly occurs in the anterior part of the pars tensa area where mobility is maximal and the proportion of elastic fibers is minimal.[39,40] Larger ruptures are associated with lower tensile strength of the tympanic membrane. The median pressure gradient resulting in tympanic membrane perforation is 1.2 ATA for subjects 50 to 90 years old[39] and 1.6 to 1.7 ATA for the younger population.[16] The critical pressure gradient for tympanic membrane rupture to occur is inversely correlated with the patient's age and might reach 0.5 ATA in older adults.[39] This is due to decreased vascularity and cellularity of the tympanic membrane decreasing its elasticity.[40] Also, atrophic scars or myringosclerosis foci that reduce the drum tensile strength are associated with increased risk for perforation at pressure gradients of only 0.3 to 0.8 ATA.[39]

When the pressure gradient across the tympanic membrane exceeds 60 mm Hg, most patients will experience various degrees of pain, a pressure sensation, and possibly a hearing loss.[41] Although symptoms can vary among patients, the diagnosis and severity classification of middle ear barotrauma are based on otoscopy findings. Middle ear barotrauma was first classified by Teed,[42] then later modified by MacFie[43] and also Edmonds and colleagues.[38] The modified Teed's scale includes six severity categories from normal examination in the face of subjective reports of ear pain or fullness (grade 0) to the presence of tympanic membrane rupture (grade 5) (Table 22.1). Although the use of middle ear barotrauma severity classification may standardize medical communication, it does not have any advantage over the detailed description of otoscopic findings.

PREVENTION OF MIDDLE EAR BAROTRAUMA

Meticulous teaching and training of the patient in various pressure equalization techniques and emphasizing the importance of frequent autoinflation, particularly during the early stages of chamber compression when maximal volume changes occur, can prevent middle ear barotrauma. It is no less important to establish good communication and agreed-on signs between the chamber attendant and patients so that compression can be halted immediately on the appearance of the first symptoms of evolving ear barotrauma.

The Frenzel maneuver is aimed at the active contraction of the tensor veli palatini muscle and accessory pharyngeal muscles, which open the ET. It is performed by pinching the nose, closing the glottis, and keeping the mouth closed while moving the jaw forward and down and pushing the tongue against the soft palate to force air through the ET. Valsalva maneuver is used when active contraction of the pharyngeal muscles fails to clear the ears. Air is introduced to the ET by forceful expiration while keeping the glottis and mouth closed and pinching the nose.

A slower chamber compression rate is related to a lower incidence of middle ear barotrauma.[5,7] In general, the compression rate should be matched to the patient's ability to achieve efficient middle ear pressure equalization on the one hand and the medical need to reach the treatment pressure in a timely fashion on the other hand.

Patients at high risk for ET failure should be identified so that preventive measures can be taken before the commencement of HBOT. Active ET opening is a voluntary process that requires collaboration, anatomic ability to build a positive nasopharyngeal pressure gradient, and

Table 22.1 Modified Teed's Classification of Middle Ear Barotrauma

GRADE	FINDINGS ON OTOSCOPY
0	Normal examination
1	Tympanic membrane injection or retraction
2	Slightly hemorrhagic tympanic membrane
3	Grossly hemorrhagic tympanic membrane
4	Hemotympanum
5	Tympanic membrane perforation

skill in the performance of the required maneuver. These prerequisites are compromised in the sedated, comatose, ventilated patients, and those having a tracheotomy.[36,44] The pediatric and elderly patient might not cooperate or have the ability to perform autoinflation. Greater risk for ear barotrauma was also reported for patients suffering from radionecrosis of the head and neck region in whom ET dysfunction is probably related to radiation effects.[4,45] Whereas inability to perform middle ear autoinflation before the commencement of HBOT marks high risk for the evolution of middle ear barotrauma during treatment,[15,44] successful bedside autoinflation does not assure successful ET ventilatory function under hyperbaric condition.[14] About 37% of patients demonstrating autoinflation before HBOT as evidenced by lateral movement of the tympanic membrane during otoscopy still sustained middle ear barotrauma.[15] Moreover, the results of laboratory ET function tests are inconsistent when it comes to predicting hyperbaric-related barotrauma. Tympanometry reflects middle ear compliance at a specific instant, and normal results do not assure uneventful middle ear clearing during compression.[14,46] Findings on the pretreatment nine-step inflation/deflation test showed no correlation to future occurrence of middle ear barotrauma,[9] and the swallow test was of no practical value.[47] Yet abnormal sonotubometry (sound transmission via the ET as detected by microphone placed in the external auditory canal) and tubotympano-aerodynamography (the wave pattern of tympanic membrane impedance in response to changes in nasopharyngeal pressure) values were suggested to predict the occurrence of middle ear barotrauma among patients given HBOT.[48] Mastoid pneumatization has previously been suggested as an important factor in middle ear pressure regulation. The findings of two studies that reported significant correlation between middle ear barotrauma and mastoid area were contradictory. Less mastoid pneumatization was found among sport divers who were prone to middle ear barotrauma.[49] In contrast, significantly larger areas of the mastoids were documented among commercial airline passengers who had experienced middle ear barotrauma.[50] Two further studies related to hyperbaric chamber operation found no correlation between mastoid pneumatization and the occurrence of middle ear barotrauma.[6,51]

Concurrent inflammation caused by viral infection, allergy, or gastroesophageal reflux might compromise ET ventilatory function because of nasopharyngeal congestion at the ET orifice.[8] The value of decongestants in preventing middle ear barotrauma has not yet been definitively established. The topical decongestant oxymetazoline taken 15 minutes before chamber compression did not alter subjective or objective barotrauma during HBOT.[52] Yet 60 to 120 mg oral pseudoephedrine predive and preflight taken 30 minutes before the exposure to changing ambient pressure significantly decreased the incidence and severity of middle ear barotrauma.[53,54] Also, several clinical series have suggested topical and systemic decongestants as a measure to lower middle ear complications associated with HBOT.[9,55,56] When middle ear clearing cannot be achieved by the various pressure-equalizing techniques, autoinflation by a nasal balloon (Otovent; Abigo Medical AB, Askim, Sweden) has been reported to be effective in preventing barotrauma during flights.[57] The balloon is held airtight to one nostril, the opposite nostril compressed, and the mouth closed, and at the same time the subject inflates the balloon through the nose. This method was recommended for the prevention of flight-associated middle ear barotrauma but has not yet been studied under hyperbaric chamber conditions. Pressure equalizing earplugs have recently been advertised to prevent middle ear barotrauma during flying (EarPlanes, JetEars, FliteMates, QuietEars, among others)[58,59] and diving (Doc's ProPlugs).[58] The theoretical rationale of this device is that delayed air movement into the external ear canal will allow more time for pressure equalization in the middle ear via the ET. The application of pressure-equalizing earplugs during a simulated flight did not prevent middle ear barotrauma among the study subjects, and higher grades of barotrauma by Teed's classification were found in the study group.[59] Although no study currently has been conducted to investigate the potential advantage of these earplugs during HBOT, it is unlikely that any benefit would be found because of the significantly larger and faster ambient pressure changes during compression in the hyperbaric chamber when compared with a commercial flight.

The middle ear and ET are rich in surfactant serving as a surface tension–lowering and antiadhesive agent. Lowering the surface tension by rinsing the ET with synthetic surfactant or using nebulized or aerosolized surfactant has led to reduced opening pressure of the tube and better aeration of the middle ear in several animal models of secretory and purulent otitis media.[60] A single study that has evaluated the role of natural and artificial ET surfactant in the treatment of altitude-induced barotrauma in the guinea pig found rapid resolution of barotrauma while treating the animals with both kinds of surfactant.[61] Although of theoretical value, no current evidence proves that surfactant might prevent middle ear barotrauma in humans under hyperbaric conditions.

Vitamins C and E applied as free radical scavengers in divers breathing 100% oxygen did not prevent the hyperoxia-induced ET ventilatory function impairment[62] and are probably of no value in preventing middle ear barotrauma in the chamber.

TREATMENT OF MIDDLE EAR BAROTRAUMA

Most cases of middle ear barotrauma occur only once and resolve spontaneously if the patient is not further exposed to hyperbaric conditions for several days.[3] If HBOT must be resumed earlier, myringotomy or insertion of ventilation tubes will assure middle ear clearing and prevent additional barotrauma. In the case of tympanic membrane perforation, the patient should avoid water from entering the middle ear because this will predispose to infection and may delay healing. In more than 90% of noninfected ears, spontaneous healing of the rupture will occur within 3 months.[32] Surgical intervention is recommended only if spontaneous

closure of the perforation has not occurred within 6 months or in the uncommon case of cholesteatoma associated with a large, unhealed perforation or that developing behind a closed tympanic membrane secondary to seeding of the tympanic cavity with squamous epithelium from the ruptured ear drum.[63]

MYRINGOTOMY AND MYRINGOSTOMY

The need for myringotomy (incising the tympanic membrane) or myringostomy (incising the tympanic membrane and insertion of ventilation tubes) was reported in various clinical series in 2.2% to 48% of the patients treated with HBOT.[4,7,9,46,57,58,65,66] The greatest intervention rate of 61% was reported among patients with an artificial airway.[44]

Myringotomy or myringostomy tube placement should be considered in two groups of patients: (1) patients definitely unable to auto-inflate because of lack of cooperation or possibly the presence of a tracheostomy or endotracheal tube (in these cases, bilateral intervention may be required), and (2) patients who suffer increasing pain and have otoscopic evidence of barotrauma that does not improve after receiving decongestants. If HBOT cannot be deferred for several days until middle ear barotrauma resolves, myringotomy or ventilation tube insertion is indicated in the involved side (Figs. 22.2 and 22.3).

The decision whether to perform knife, thermal, or laser myringotomy or to place ventilation tubes is dependent on the specific circumstances. If barotrauma is encountered during HBOT for a life-threatening condition, urgent in-chamber knife myringotomy may be indicated. For elective intervention, the method for middle ear ventilation is chosen according to the anticipated length of HBOT, available equipment, and surgical expertise. Knife myringotomy is the simplest procedure and is performed by widely available instruments. However, the tympanic membrane incision heals in several days and revision may be required.

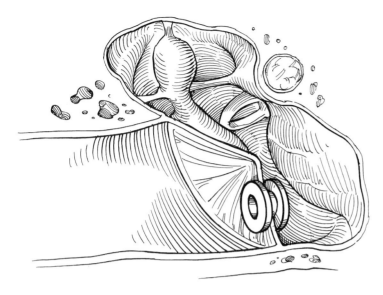

Figure 22.2 Coronal section illustration of the right ear with myringotomy tube in place. *(From Coker NJ, Jenkins HA [eds]: Myringotomy and Tympanostomy Tube Placement. Atlas of Otologic Surgery. Philadelphia, WB Saunders, 2001, p 103, by permission.)*

Myringotomy tube placement requires a surgical microscope, whereas thermal and laser myringotomy necessitate additional specific equipment.[65-68] Placement of myringostomy tubes is generally well tolerated. Complications include otorrhea in 5% to 20% of cases and persistent tympanic membrane perforations in less than 5%.[69,70] Higher complication rates after tube placement were reported among patients given HBOT, with otorrhea developing in 29% and persistent perforation in 26%.[56] The high-risk characteristics of the patient population, such as impaired tympanic perforation healing and tendency to acquire infections in patients with diabetes, ET dysfunction, and increased rate of chronic otitis media with effusion in patients undergoing head and neck irradiation, might explain this observation. The greatest complication rate was observed when the tubes were left for spontaneous extrusion to take place after the termination of HBOT; therefore, active removal of the tubes was recommended at the end of HBOT.[56,67] Advocates of electrocautery (thermal) and laser myringotomy report lesser complication rates when compared with insertion of ventilation tubes with satisfactory middle ear aeration for several weeks and no need for an additional surgical procedure for tube removal at the end of HBOT.[65-68] Thermal myringotomy was associated with an otorrhea rate of 4%. Most perforations were patent at the fifth postoperative week, but 15% failed to close by 6 months.[68] CO_2 laser myringotomy was less painful and had significantly lower incidence of otorrhea (6%) compared with ventilation tube placement (38%).[67] Laser myringotomy is probably suitable for patients receiving HBOT for several weeks only because the tympanic membranes are usually closed within 3 weeks,[65,66] and recurrence of middle ear barotrauma because of tympanic membrane healing was reported in 25% of patients receiving HBOT for an average of 4 weeks.[67]

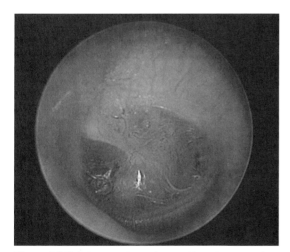

Figure 22.3 Left tympanic membrane with myringotomy tube in the anteroinferior quadrant. **(See Color Plate 29.)**

MYRINGOTOMY TECHNIQUE

When an urgent myringotomy is required and any delay in the commencement of chamber compression, even for minutes, might result in a life-threatening situation, a myringotomy can be performed with no anesthesia by the HBOT practitioner. Under this circumstance, intravenous sedation is a valid option depending on the patient's general condition and need for in-chamber neurologic evaluation to monitor the response to HBOT.

Myringotomy Incision

Sterilization of the tympanic membrane and external auditory canal before the procedure is not required. An angled myringotomy knife should be used to make the incision. If a myringotomy knife is not available, a simple substitute is a 25- or 22-gauge disposable spinal needle, which may be angled as needed.

The tympanic membrane is divided into virtual quadrants. A vertical axis, determined by the malleus handle, designates the 12- and 6-o'clock positions on the tympanic ring and divides the tympanic membrane into anterior and posterior halves. A horizontal line through the umbo divides it into superior and inferior halves (Fig. 22.4).

Myringotomy is preferably performed in the anterior-inferior quadrant of the tympanic membrane to avoid the middle ear ossicles, ligaments, horizontal segment of the facial nerve, and round window. However, in cases with an obstructing bulge in the anterior bony external ear canal, it may also be performed inferiorly or in the posteroinferior quadrant. The myringotomy should always be placed in healthy areas of the tympanic membrane because incisions in atrophic areas or through tympanosclerotic plaques may not heal, leaving permanent perforations.[71]

Either a radial or a circumferential incision may be used.[73] If urgent in-chamber myringotomy is indicated, a simple full-thickness puncture of the tympanic membrane will suffice for immediate middle ear pressure

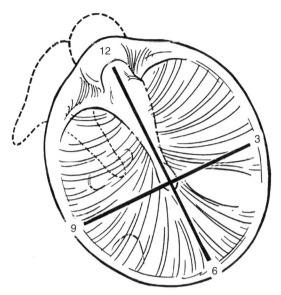

Figure 22.4 The tympanic membrane is divided into quadrants. A vertical axis, determined by the malleus handle, designates the 12- and 6-o'clock positions on the tympanic ring; the 90-degree horizontal axis delineates the 3- and 9-o'clock sites. The incus and stapes are located underneath the posterosuperior quadrant, and the round window is beneath the posteroinferior quadrant. *(From Coker NJ, Jenkins HA [eds]: Myringotomy and Tympanostomy Tube Placement. Atlas of Otologic Surgery. Philadelphia, WB Saunders, 2001, p 100, by permission.)*

equalization. Because the tympanic membrane is often retracted, it is advisable to keep the incision peripheral, a few millimeters from the tympanic membrane annulus, to avoid the knife from impinging the medial bony wall of the tympanic cavity.

Ototopical antibiotic drops can be considered in the immediate postoperative period in an effort to reduce the risk for otorrhea, particularly when there is a mucoid effusion present during myringotomy.[73] The patient should be instructed to avoid water from entering the ear for as long as the myringotomy is patent because water entering the ear would increase the risk for middle ear infection and resulting otorrhea.

PARANASAL SINUS BAROTRAUMA

The paranasal sinuses consist of bony cavities lined by mucosa. Sinus aeration is achieved via ostia openings to the nasal cavity at the middle and upper meatuses. The mucosa-coated bony canals that communicate the sinuses with the nasal cavity are permanently patent and pressure equalization is completely passive during both compression and decompression (Fig. 22.5). If the free passage of air in and out of the sinuses is compromised by anatomic variations such as deviation of the nasal septum, concha bullosa or other narrowing of the sinus openings, the presence of polyps, and acute or chronic inflammation of the nasal or sinus mucosa, sinus barotrauma may occur. When the sinus orifice is blocked during chamber compression, mucosal edema, fluid transudation, capillary tears, submucosal hemorrhage, and eventually hemorrhage into the sinus cavity may occur. During decompression, the increased air volume may exert high enough pressure to overcome the obstruction of the sinus duct and blood may flow out of the sinus cavity to the nose. Occasionally, sinus barotrauma will occur during decompression when inflamed tissue or viscous secretion blocks the sinus cavity in a ball-valve mechanism.

The reported incidence of sinus barotrauma is much lower than that of middle ear barotrauma.[3] Most sinus barotrauma occurs during compression and involves the frontal sinus. This is explained by the long and tortuous route of the nasofrontal duct through the anterior ethmoidal labyrinth, which makes it highly vulnerable to inflammatory reactions that often affect this area. The cardinal symptoms are headache, facial and malar pain localized to the frontal or maxillary sinuses, and bleeding from the nose after decompression.[74,75] Neurologic symptoms may affect the adjacent fifth cranial nerve, especially the infraorbital nerve.[76-78]

Rare sequelae of sinus barotrauma were reported in diving and air travel including orbital emphysema, cerebral empyema, pneumocephalus, and blindness.[79-82] Abnormal radiologic signs are found most commonly when imaging the maxillary sinuses. These include mucosal thickening and occasional fluid–air levels.

Symptoms are usually resolved by the use of topical decongestants and secretolytic agents. Antibiotics are indicated only if the barotrauma

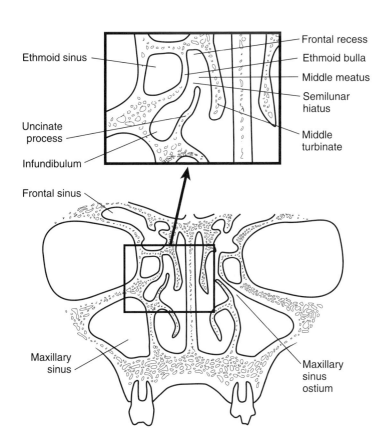

Ethmoid sinus

Uncinate process

Infundibulum

Frontal sinus

Maxillary sinus

Frontal recess

Ethmoid bulla

Middle meatus

Semilunar hiatus

Middle turbinate

Maxillary sinus ostium

Figure 22.5 Coronal scheme of the paranasal sinuses demonstrating the natural aeration/drainage passages. *(Based on Gustafson RO, Kern EB: Office endoscopy—when, why, what and how. Otolaryngol Clin North Am 22:683–689, 1989, by permission.)*

is complicated by secondary acute sinusitis, and they are not indicated prophylactically.[75] If recurrent sinus barotrauma is encountered, nasal endoscopy and high-resolution axial computed tomography of the sinuses are indicated for the diagnosis of possible surgically treatable anatomic abnormalities.[83,84] Minimal surgical intervention applying functional endoscopic techniques[85] aiming at the improvement of sinus drainage at the ethmoidal infundibulum and the frontal recess (see Fig. 22.5) has proved to be successful in several case series of recurrent sinus barotrauma in aviators.[84,86,87]

BARODONTALGIA AND ODONTOCREXIS

Barodontalgia refers to dental pain resulting from environmental pressure changes, and odontocrexis is the physical disruption of teeth during compression or decompression.[88,89] It may occur after expansion of gas within or near a defective tooth. Defects include cavities, incomplete root fillings, devitalized pulp, and periapical cysts. Restored teeth are more likely to be involved.[88] Pain usually involves the posterior maxillary teeth and results from compromised blood supply to the tooth, direct pressure on exposed nerve endings, and microleakage of tooth restoration materials.[88,90] Barodontalgia and odontocrexis have been reported in aircrew and divers[82,88] but not among patients who received HBOT.

SPECIAL CONSIDERATIONS

Cochlear Implants

The benefits of cochlear implant use have been well documented, with continuing evidence that implantation at an earlier age increases performance in regard to speech development. As more people of all age groups receive cochlear implants, potential hyperbaric exposure of the device will become more common. Cochlear implant systems consist of a subcutaneous receiver/stimulator unit, an electrode array implanted into the

cochlea, and an external antenna and speech processor. Although the external hardware can be removed, the effects of the rapidly changing ambient pressure on the implanted components are unavoidable. Commercially available cochlear implants have a housing made of either medical-grade ceramics or titanium that is hermetically sealed to prevent device failure from exposure of internal components to the corrosive effects of body fluids. In a recent study, the functioning of the receiver/stimulator, housing, and hermetic seals of the Clarion 1.2 (Advanced Bionics Corp., Sylmar, Calif), MED-EL Combi-40+ (MED-EL Corp., Innsbruck, Austria), and Nucleus-22 and Nucleus-24 (Cochlear Corp., Lane Cove, New South Wales, Australia) cochlear implants were not affected by repeated hyperbaric exposures from 2.4 to 6 ATA with compression rates of 10 to 82.5 feet/min and decompression rates of 5 to 20 feet/min.[91] Additional anecdotal case studies have reported proper functioning of cochlear implants after HBOT and diving.[92,93] Despite the above-mentioned reports, it is recommended that the cochlear implant manufacturer be consulted before the commencement of HBOT to acquire specific instructions for the cochlear implant system in question to ensure patient safety, avoid device malfunction, and maintain the manufacturer's warranty.

Stapedectomy

Since Shea[94] successfully replaced an otosclerotic stapes with a polyethylene tube for the first time in 1956, stapedectomy has been frequently performed using a variety of surgical techniques and different designs of prosthesis as an effective procedure for improving conductive hearing loss caused by otosclerosis.

Poststapedectomy patients have two potential problems when exposed to the hyperbaric environment. The first problem is lateral dislodgment of the stapes prosthesis with return of conductive hearing loss on the one hand, or inward movement with damage to the underlying labyrinthine membranes causing vertigo and sensorineural hearing loss on the other hand. The placement of a stapedial prosthesis eliminates the resistance of the stapes annular ligament, and changes in the ambient pressure, which induce displacement of the tympanic membrane, can now freely move the prosthesis as a piston in and out of the vestibule. It has been suggested that if the patient can tolerate external ear canal pressure changes of ± 400 mm H_2O, which can be applied by a clinical tympanometer, without vertigo, he or she may be safely exposed to hyperbaric conditions.[95]

The second problem is increased rate of inner ear barotrauma because of the inherent risk for perilymph fistula after stapedectomy with incidence rates of 3.2% to 10%,[96-98] and the reported association between ear barotrauma and perilymph fistula.[27,29-31,35] A survey of practicing otologic surgeons in the United States showed lack of consensus regarding poststapedectomy restrictions of diving and air travel and revealed no significant differences in the rate of inner ear barotrauma regardless of the surgical technique used and postoperative restrictions imposed.[99] In a recent survey of 2222 patients who had stapedectomy, 22 reported recreational scuba activities and 9 were engaged in skydiving. No significant diving-related long-term effects indicative of labyrinthine injury were seen in any of the patients.[100] Other studies reported no occurrence of inner ear barotrauma in poststapedectomy military aircrew members who have returned to active flight duty[101,102] and subjects who resumed diving activity after stapedectomy.[58] The results of these studies are supported by animal models that found no increased risk for inner ear insults in guinea pigs, cats, and monkeys exposed to hyperbaric pressure after stapedectomy.[103-105]

Practicing otologists' recommendations regarding the period after stapedectomy in which the patient should avoid large changes in ambient pressure ranged from 2 days to 6 months.[99] A balanced recommendation would be to avoid exposure to hyperbaric conditions 4 weeks after stapes surgery. This time interval would allow the safe adherence and maturation of the connective tissue pieces that are often placed under and around the stapes prosthesis in the oval window as a seal to prevent a perilymphatic leak and to attenuate extreme vertical movements of the prosthesis. During HBOT, the poststapedectomy patient should be followed carefully and treated for the earliest sign of ET dysfunction. The presence of a stapes prosthesis is not a contraindication for placement of myringotomy tubes.[106]

Tympanoplasty and Ossicular Prostheses

Patients having tympanoplasty because of a previous tympanic membrane perforation present increased risk for recurrent ear drum rupture during HBOT because of reduced thickness and elasticity of the tympanic membrane. Tympanic membranes that have been reconstructed with cartilage pieces and not merely by fascia were reported to better resist extreme barometric changes.[107]

Special caution should be practiced in a patient with total ossicular replacement prostheses. Penetration of the stapes footplate by the prosthesis and consequent inner ear damage have been reported secondary to changes in ambient pressure.[108]

REFERENCES

1. Stone JA, Loar H, Rudge FW: An eleven-year review of hyperbaric oxygenation in a military clinical setting. Undersea Biomed Res 18(suppl):80, 1991.
2. Younberg JT, Myers RM: Complications from hyperbaric oxygen therapy? Ann Emerg Med 19:1356, 1990.
3. Plafki C, Peters P, Almeling M, et al: Complications and side-effects of hyperbaric oxygen therapy. Aviat Space Environ Med 71:119-124, 2000.
4. Blanshard J, Toma A, Bryson P, et al: Middle ear barotrauma in patients undergoing hyperbaric oxygen therapy. Clin Otolaryngol 21:400-403, 1996.
5. Fitzpatrick DT, Franck BA, Mason KT, et al: Risk factors for symptomatic otic and sinus barotrauma in a multiplace hyperbaric chamber. Undersea Hyperb Med 26:243-247, 1999.
6. Ueda H, Shien CW, Miyazawa T, et al: Otological complications of hyperbaric oxygen therapy. Adv Otorhinolaryngol 54:119-126, 1998.
7. Vahidova D, Sen P, Papaesch M, et al: Does the slow compression technique decrease the incidence of middle-ear barotrauma? J Laryngol Otol 120:446-449, 2006.
8. Igarashi Y, Watanabe Y, Mizukoshi K: Middle ear barotrauma associated with hyperbaric oxygenation

treatment. Acta Otolaryngol (Stockh) 504(suppl):-143-145, 1993.

9. Fernau JL, Hirsch BE, Derkay C, et al: Hyperbaric oxygen therapy: Effect on middle ear and Eustachian tube function. Laryngoscope 102:48-52, 1992.

10. Sade J, Ar A: Middle ear and auditory tube: Middle ear clearance, gas exchange, and pressure regulation. Otolaryngol Head Neck Surg 116:499-524, 1997.

11. Doyle WJ, Alper CM, Seroky JT, et al: Exchange rates of gases across the tympanic membrane in rhesus monkeys. Acta Otolaryngol (Stockh) 118:567-573, 1998.

12. Cantekin EI, Saez CA, Bluestone CD, et al: Airflow through the Eustachian tube. Ann Otol Rhinol Laryngol 88:603-612, 1979.

13. Bluestone CD, Doyle WJ: Anatomy and physiology of the Eustachian tube and middle ear related to otitis media. J Allergy Clin Immunol 81:997-1003, 1998.

14. Shupak A, Sharoni Z, Ostfeld E, et al: Pressure chamber tympanometry in diving candidates. Ann Otol Rhinol Laryngol 100:658-660, 1991.

15. Beuerlein M, Nelson RN, Welling DB: Inner and middle ear hyperbaric oxygen-induced barotrauma. Laryngoscope 107:1350-1356, 1997.

16. Keller AP Jr: A study of the relationship of air pressure to myringorupture. Laryngoscope 68:2015-2029, 1958.

17. Groth P, Ivarsson A, Tjernstrom O, et al: The effect of pressure change rate on the Eustachian tube function in pressure chamber tests. Acta Otolaryngol (Stockh) 99:67-73, 1985.

18. Andreasson L, Ingelstedt S, Ivarsson A, et al: Pressure-dependent variation in volume of mucosal lining of the middle ear. Acta Otolaryngol (Stockh) 81:442-449, 1976.

19. Shupak A, Attias J, Aviv J, et al: Oxygen diving-induced middle ear under-aeration. Acta Otolaryngol (Stockh) 115:422-426, 1995.

20. Strauss MB, Lee WS, Cantrell RW: Serous otitis media in divers breathing 100 percent oxygen. Aerospace Med 45:434-437, 1974.

21. Shupak A, Tabari R, Swarts JD, et al: Effects of middle ear oxygen and carbon dioxide tensions on Eustachian tube ventilatory function. Laryngoscope 106:221-224, 1996.

22. Shupak A, Tabari R, Swarts JD, et al: Effects of systemic hyperoxia on Eustachian tube ventilatory function. Laryngoscope 107:1409-1413, 1997.

23. Buckingham RA, Stuart DR, Geick MR, et al: Experimental evidence against middle ear gas absorption. Laryngoscope 95:437-442, 1985.

24. Ylikoski J, Panula P: Neuropeptides in the middle ear mucosa. ORL J Otorhinolaryngol Relat Spec 50:176-182, 1988.

25. Lahiri S, Mulligan E, Andronikou S, et al: Carotid body chemosensory function in prolonged normobaric hypoxia in the cat. J App Physiol 62:1924-1931, 1987.

26. Eden AR, Gannon PJ: Neural control of middle ear aeration. Arch Otolaryngol Head Neck Surg 113:133-137, 1987.

27. Shupak A: Recurrent Diving-Related Inner Ear Barotrauma. Otol Neurotol 2006;27:1193-1196.

28. Thalen OE, Wit HP, Segenhout JM, et al: Dynamics of inner ear pressure change caused by intracranial pressure manipulation in the guinea pig. Acta Otolaryngol (Stockh) 121:470-476, 2001.

29. Goodhill V: Leaking Labyrinth lesions, deafness, tinnitus and dizziness. Ann Otol Rhinol Laryngol 90:99-106, 1981.

30. Kobayashi T, Gyo K, Yanagihara N: Combined rupture of Reissner's membrane and round window: An experimental study in guinea pigs. Am J Otol 20:179-182, 1999.

31. Nakashima T, Itoh M, Watanabe Y, et al: Auditory and vestibular disorders due to barotrauma. Ann Otol Rhinol Laryngol 97:145-152, 1988.

32. Molvaer OI: Otorhinolaryngological aspects of diving. In: Brubakk AO, Neuman TS (eds): Bennett and Elliott's Physiology and Medicine of Diving, 5 ed. St. Louis, Saunders, 2003, pp 227-264.

33. Axelsson A, Miller J, Silverman M: Anatomical effects of sudden middle ear pressure changes. Ann Otol Rhinol Laryngol 88:368-376, 1979.

34. Shupak A, Doweck I, Greenberg E, et al: Diving-related inner ear injuries. Laryngoscope 101:173-179, 1991.

35. Shupak A, Gil A, Nachum Z, Miller S, et al: Inner ear decompression sickness and inner ear barotrauma in recreational divers: A long-term follow-up. Laryngoscope 113:2141-2147, 2003.

36. Capes JP, Tomaszewski C: Prophylaxis against middle ear barotrauma in US hyperbaric oxygen therapy centers. Am J Emerg Med 14:645-648, 1996.

37. Zheng XY, Gong JH: Cochlear degeneration in guinea pigs after repeated hyperbaric exposures. Aviat Space Environ Med 63:360-363, 1992.

38. Edmonds C, Lowry C, Pennefather J: Diving and Subaquatic Medicine, 3rd ed. Oxford, Butterworth-Heinemann, 1992, pp 115-139.

39. Jensen JH, Bonding P: Experimental pressure induced rupture of the tympanic membrane in man. Acta Otolaryngol (Stockh) 113:62-67, 1993.

40. Ruah CB, Schachern PA, Zeltermann D, et al: Age-related morphologic changes in the human tympanic membrane. A light and electron microscopic study. Arch Otolaryngol Head Neck Surg 117:627-634, 1991.

41. Neblett LM: Otolaryngology and sport scuba diving. Ann Otol Rhinol Laryngol 115(suppl):1-12, 1985.

42. Teed RW: Factors producing obstruction of the auditory tube in submarine personnel. US Naval Med Bull 42:293-306, 1944.

43. MacFie DD: ENT problems of diving. Med Serv J Canada 20:845-861, 1964.

44. Presswood G, Zamboni WA, Stephenson LL, et al: Effect of artificial airway on ear complications from hyperbaric oxygen. Laryngoscope 104:1383-1384, 1994.

45. Young YH, Lin KL, Ko JY: Otitis media with effusion in patients with nasopharyngeal carcinoma postirradiation. Arch Otolaryngol Head Neck Surg 121:765-768, 1995.

46. Ashton DH, Watson LA: The use of tympanometry in predicting otitic barotrauma. Aviat Space Environ Med 61:56-61, 1990.

47. Schuchman G, Joachims HZ: Tympanometric assessment of Eustachian tube function of divers. Ear Hear 6:325-328, 1985.

48. Miyazawa T, Ueda H, Yanagita N: Eustachian tube function and middle ear barotrauma associated with extremes in atmospheric pressure. Ann Otol Rhinol Laryngol 105:887-892, 1996.

49. Uzun C, Adali MK, Koten M, et al: Relationship between mastoid pneumatization and middle ear barotrauma in divers. Laryngoscope 112:287-291, 2002.

50. Sade J, Ar A, Fuchs C: Barotrauma vis-à-vis the "chronic otitis media syndrome": two conditions with middle ear gas deficiency. Is secretory otitis media a contraindication to air travel? Ann Otol Rhinol Laryngol 112:230-235, 2003.

51. Toklu AS, Shupak A, Yildiz S, et al: Aural barotrauma in submarine escape: Is mastoid pneumatization of significance? Laryngoscope 115:1305-1309, 2005.

52. Carlson B, Jones J, Brown M, et al: Prevention of hyperbaric-associated middle ear barotraumas. Ann Emerg Med 21:70-73, 1992.

53. Brown M, Jones J, Krohner J: Pseudoephedrine for the prevention of barotitis media: A controlled clinical trial in underwater divers. Ann Emerg Med 21:849-852, 1992.

54. Csortan E, Jones J, Haan M, et al: Efficacy of pseudoephedrine for the prevention of barotrauma during air travel. Ann Emerg Med 23:1324-1327, 1994.

55. Giebfried JW, Lawson W, Biller HF: Complications of hyperbaric oxygen in the treatment of head and neck disease. Otolaryngol Head Neck Surg 94:508-512, 1986.

56. Clements KS, Vrabec JT, Mader JT: Complications of myringostomy tubes inserted for facilitation of hyperbaric oxygen therapy. Arch Otolaryngol Head Neck Surg 124:278-280, 1998.

57. Stangerup SE, Klokker M, Vesterhauge S, et al: Point prevalence of barotitis and its prevention and treatment with nasal balloon inflation: A prospective, controlled study. Otol Neurotol 25:89-94, 2004.

58. Becker GD, Parell JC: Barotrauma of the ears and sinuses after scuba diving. Eur Arch Otorhinolaryngol 258:159-163, 2001.

59. Klokker M, Vesterhauge S, Jansen EC: Pressure-equalizing earplugs do not prevent barotrauma on descent from 8000 ft cabin attitude. Aviat Space Environ Med 76:1079-1082, 2005.

60. McGuire JF: Surfactant in the middle ear and Eustachian tube: A review. Int J Pediatr Otorhinolaryngol 66:1-15, 2002.

61. Feng LN, Chen WX, Cong R, et al: Therapeutic effects of Eustachian tube surfactant in barotitis media in guinea pigs. Aviat Space Environ Med 74:707-710, 2003.

62. Mutzbauer TS, Neubauer B, Mueller PHJ, et al: Can Eustachian tube ventilatory function impairment after oxygen diving be influenced by application of free radical scavenger vitamin C and E? Laryngoscope 111:861-866, 2001.

63. Kronenberg J, Ben-Shoshan J, Modan M, et al: Blast injury and cholesteatoma. Am J Otol 9:127-130, 1988.

64. Reference deleted in proofs.

65. Bent JP, April MM, Ward RF: Atypical indications for OtoScan laser-assisted myringotomy. Laryngoscope 111:87-89, 2001.

66. Bent JP, April MM, Ward RF, et al: Role of OtoScan-assisted laser myringotomy in hyperbaric oxygen therapy. Undersea Hyper Med 27:159-161, 2000.

67. Vrabec JT, Clements KS, Mader JT: Short-term tympanostomy in conjunction with hyperbaric oxygen therapy. Laryngoscope 108:1124-1128, 1998.

68. Potocki SE, Hoffman DS: Thermal myringotomy for Eustachian tube dysfunction in hyperbaric oxygen therapy. Otolaryngol Head Neck Surg 121:185-189, 1999.

69. Luxford WM, Sheehy JL: Myringotomy and ventilation tubes: A report of 1568 ears. Laryngoscope 92:1293-1297, 1982.

70. McLelland CA: Incidence of complications from use of tympanostomy tubes. Arch Otolaryngol 106:97-99, 1980.

71. Coker NJ, Jenkins HA (eds): Atlas of Otologic Surgery. Philadelphia, WB Saunders, 2001, pp 100-103.

72. Reference deleted in proofs.

73. Inglis GA, Gates GA: Acute otitis media and otitis media with effusion. In: Cummings CW, Flint PW, Harker LA (eds): Cummings Otolaryngology-Head & Neck Surgery. Philadelphia, Elsevier Mosby, 2005, pp 4456-4464.

74. Fagan P, McKenzie B, Edmonds C: Sinus barotrauma in divers. Ann Otol Rhinol Laryngol 85:61-64, 1976.

75. Edmonds C: Sinus barotrauma: A bigger picture. SPUMS J 24:13-19, 1994.

76. Murrison AW, Smith DJ, Francis TJ, et al: Maxillary sinus barotrauma with fifth cranial nerve involvement. J Laryngol Otol 105:217-219, 1991.

77. Butler FK, Bove AA: Infraorbital hypoesthesia after maxillary sinus barotrauma. Undersea Hyperb Med 26:257-259, 1999.

78. Neuman TS, Settle H, Beaver G, Linaweaver P: Maxillary sinus barotrauma with cranial nerve involvement. Aviat Space Environ Med 46:314-315, 1975.

79. Zimmer-Galler IE, Bartley GB: Orbital emphysema: Case reports and review of the literature. Mayo Clin Proc 69:115-121, 1994.

80. Parell GJ, Becker GD: Neurological consequences of scuba diving with chronic sinusitis. Laryngoscope 110:1358-1360, 2000.

81. Mahabir RC, Szymczak A, Sutherland GR: Intracerebral pneumatocele presenting after air travel. J Neurosurg 101:340-342, 2004.

82. Brandt MT: Oral and maxillofacial aspects of diving medicine. Mil Med 169:137-141, 2004.

83. Zinreich SJ, Kennedy DW, Rosenbaum AE, et al: Paranasal sinuses: CT imaging requirements for endoscopic surgery. Radiology 163:769-775, 1987.

84. O'Reilly BJ, McRae A, Lupa H: The role of functional endoscopic sinus surgery in the management of recurrent sinus barotrauma. Aviat Space Environ Med 66:876-879, 1995.

85. Stammberger H, Hawke M (eds): Essentials of Endoscopic Sinus Surgery. St. Louis, Mosby, 1993, pp 1-12.

86. Larsen AS, Buchwald C, Vesterhauge S: Sinus barotrauma—late diagnosis and treatment with computer-aided endoscopic surgery. Aviat Space Environ Med 74:180-183, 2003.

87. Parsons DS, Chambers DW, Boyd EM: Long term follow-up of aviators after functional endoscopic sinus surgery for sinus barotrauma. Aviat Space Environ Med 68:1029-1034, 1997.

88. Lyons KM, Rodda JC, Hood JA: Barodontalgia: A review, and the influence of simulated diving on microleak-

age and on the retention of full cast crowns. Mil Med 164:221-227, 1999.

89. Calder IM, Ramsey JD: Odontocrexis: The effects of rapid decompression on restored teeth. J Dent 11:318-323, 1983.

90. Parris C, Frenkiel S: Effects and management of barometric change on cavities in the head and neck. J Otolaryngol 24:46-50, 1995.

91. Backous DD, Dunford RG, Segel P, et al: Effects of hyperbaric exposure on the integrity of the internal components of commercially available cochlear implants systems. Otol Neurotol 23:463-467, 2002.

92. Schweitzer VG, Burtka MJ: Cochlear implant flap necrosis: Adjunct hyperbaric oxygen therapy for prevention of explantation. Am J Otol 12:71-75, 1991.

93. Kompis M, Vibert D, Senn P, et al: Scuba diving with cochlear implants. Ann Otol Rhinol Laryngol 112:425-427, 2003.

94. Shea JJ: A personal history of stapedectomy. Am J Otol 19:2-12, 1998.

95. Huttenbrink K-B: Biomechanics of stapesplasty: A review. Otol Neurotol 24:548-559, 2003.

96. Sheehy JL, Nelson RA, House HP: Revision stapedectomy: A review of 258 cases. Laryngoscope 91:43-51, 1981.

97. Seltzer S, McCabe BF: Perilymph fistula: The Iowa experience. Laryngoscope 96:37-49, 1986.

98. Glasscock ME, Stopper IS, Haynes S, et al: Twenty-five years of experience with stapedectomy. Laryngoscope 105:899-904, 1995.

99. Harrill WC, Jenkins HA, Coker NJ: Barotrauma after stapes surgery: A survey of recommended restrictions and clinical experience. Am J Otol 17:835-845, 1996.

100. House JW, Toh EH, Perez A: Diving after stapedectomy: Clinical experience and recommendations. Otolaryngol Head Neck Surg 125:356-360, 2001.

101. Thiringer K, Ariaga MA: Stapedectomy in military aircrew. Otolaryngol Head Neck Surg 118:9-15, 1998.

102. Katzav J, Lippy WH, Shamiss A: Stapedectomy in combat pilots. Am J Otol 17:847-849, 1996.

103. Antonelli PJ, Adamczyk M, Appelton CM, et al: Inner ear barotrauma after stapedectomy in the guinea pig. Laryngoscope 109:1991-1995, 1999.

104. Garlington JC, Singleton GT: Rapid decompression and compression in the stapedectomized cat. Aerosp Med 40:475-478, 1969.

105. Fletcher JL, Robertson CD, Loeb EM: Effects of high intensity impulse noise and rapid changes in pressure upon stapedectomized monkeys. Acta Otolaryngol (Stockh) 68:6-13, 1969.

106. Farmer JC: Comment on: Barotrauma after stapes surgery: A survey of recommended restrictions and clinical experience. Am J Otol 17:845-846, 1996.

107. Velepic M, Bonifacic M, Manestar D, et al: Cartilage palisade tympanoplasty and diving. Otol Neurotol 22:430-432, 2001.

108. Pau HW: Inner ear damage in TORP-operated ears: Experimental study on danger from environmental air pressure changes. Ann Otol Rhinol Laryngol 108:745-749, 1999.

Oxygen Toxicity

James M. Clark, MD, PhD

Therapeutic applications of hyperbaric oxygenation, as is true for many therapeutic agents and procedures, have an intrinsic potential for producing mild-to-severe adverse effects. When hyperbaric oxygen therapy (HBOT) is used appropriately, however, serious adverse effects are rare,[1] and those that do occur are nearly always reversible.[2] The existence of potent antioxidant defense mechanisms and repair processes provide a favorable risk-to-benefit ratio by slowing the development of oxygen poisoning and hastening recovery from its subclinical effects.[3,4] Studies designed to determine human limits of oxygen tolerance for therapeutic applications of hyperoxia must necessarily use exposure conditions that produce measurable toxic effects in human volunteers. It is important to recognize that therapeutic exposures seldom, if ever, approach these limits.

During exposure to any level of hyperoxia, the sequence and severity of adverse effects in different organs and tissues are determined by interactions between the relative susceptibilities of the tissues and the local oxygen partial pressures to which they are exposed. At each local site, the oxygen tension is, in turn, dependent on the balance that exists among factors such as the arterial partial pressure of oxygen (Pa_{O_2}), capillary density, blood flow, and tissue metabolic rate. Because these factors are diverse throughout the body, specific organs and tissues are exposed to a range of oxygen tensions during oxygen breathing at any ambient pressure (Fig. 23.1).[5,6] Although Pa_{O_2} levels are expected to be uniform in all circulatory beds, capillary and venous levels can vary widely, especially at oxygen pressures that are high enough to provide metabolic needs from physically dissolved oxygen with little or no reduction of oxyhemoglobin.

PATHOLOGIC EFFECTS OF OXYGEN TOXICITY

The diversity and progression of toxic effects caused by extreme to lethal degrees of oxygen exposure are summarized in Figure 23.2.[5,7] The severity of oxygen poisoning increases progressively with increase of the inspired partial pressure of oxygen (Po_2) and with greater duration of exposure. In rats exposed to lethal degrees of pulmonary oxygen poisoning, pathologic effects include destruction of capillary endothelium and alveolar epithelium, alveolar cell hyperplasia, edema, hemorrhage, arteriolar thickening and hyalinization, fibrin formation, atelectasis, consolidation, severe impairment of gas exchange, hypoxemia, and death.[8,9] Manifestations of central nervous system (CNS) oxygen poisoning include effects ranging from localized muscle twitching to tonic-clonic generalized seizures. With continued exposure past the onset of these signs, progressive neural destruction, paralysis, and death may occur.[5,10] Effects of lethal exposures on the eye include retinal separation, destruction of visual cells, and blindness.[11,12] Other effects include erythrocyte hemolysis,[13,14] renal damage,[15,16] and myocardial pathology.[17] Effects on the liver[18,19] and endocrine organs[20,21] may also occur. Thet[22] has described in detail the nature and time courses of

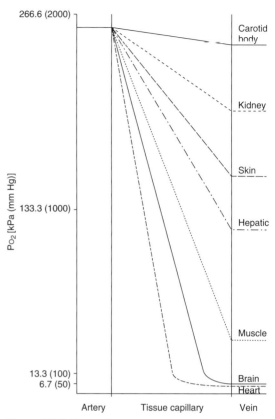

Figure 23.1 Range of oxygen pressure in different organs and tissues during oxygen breathing at 3.5 atmospheres absolute (ATA) (352 kPa). The curve for brain represents average measurements of arterial and internal jugular venous blood partial pressure of oxygen (Po_2) in 16 conscious men.[6] Venous values and capillary Po_2 changes for other organs and tissues are calculated from measured arterial values and tabulated values of tissue oxygen consumption and blood flow in humans. Even within an organ or tissue, inequalities of metabolic rate and blood flow should cause local differences in Po_2. Cells near the arterial end of a capillary are exposed to much greater Po_2 levels than other cells near the venous end. Pathologic states and drug effects on circulation or metabolism should be expected to alter the patterns shown here. (*From Lambertsen CJ: Effects of oxygen at high partial pressure. In: Fenn WO, Rahn H [eds]: Handbook of Physiology, Section 3: Respiration, Vol II. Washington, DC, American Physiological Society, 1965, pp 1027–1046; and Lambertsen CJ: Effects of hyperoxia on organs and their tissues. In: Robin ED [ed]: Extrapulmonary Manifestations of Respiratory Disease. Lung Biology in Health and Disease, Vol 8. New York, Marcel Dekker, 1978, pp 239–303, by permission.*)

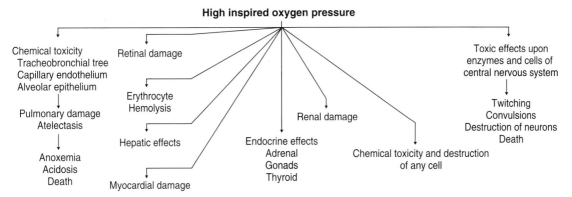

Figure 23.2 Diversity and progression of toxic effects produced by exposure to increased oxygen pressures. *(From Clark JM: The toxicity of oxygen. Am Rev Resp Dis 110:40–50, 1974, extending a concept used by Lambertsen CJ: Effects of oxygen at high partial pressure. In: Fenn WO, Rahn H [eds]: Handbook of Physiology, Section 3: Respiration, Vol II. Washington, DC, American Physiological Society, 1965, pp 1027–1046, by permission.)*

biochemical and morphologic changes that occur during recovery from pulmonary oxygen poisoning. Balentine[23] has written an excellent, comprehensive review of pathologic effects caused by oxygen poisoning in specific organs and tissues.

MECHANISMS OF OXIDANT DAMAGE AND ANTIOXIDANT DEFENSES

Detailed descriptions of potential biochemical mechanisms of oxidant damage and opposing antioxidant defenses, as provided previously,[2] are beyond the scope of this chapter. Available information and generally accepted interpretations are described briefly.

FREE RADICALS AND OTHER REACTIVE SPECIES

Gerschman and coworkers[24,25] first proposed that increased concentrations of free radical intermediates during exposure to hyperoxia provided a biochemical basis for oxygen toxicity. Adverse effects are initiated when oxygen is reduced by one electron to form superoxide and/or by two electrons to form hydrogen peroxide.[3,26] The superoxide anion is a by-product of cellular metabolism, and its rate of formation is accelerated by increased

oxygen pressures.[27] Superoxide is produced at both the ubiquinone and reduced nicotinamide adenine dinucleotide sites on the electron transport chain.[3,28,29] Additional sources are the endoplasmic reticulum and microsomes.[30] Other toxic species that may be generated by reactions with superoxide include hydroperoxy and hydroxyl radicals and singlet oxygen.[31] It is generally agreed that the secondary generation of more reactive intermediates, rather than direct interactions with superoxide and hydrogen peroxide, accounts for most of the oxidant damage to cellular components and membranes that occurs during exposure to hyperoxia.[29]

Sharing many biophysical characteristics with oxygen, nitric oxide (·NO) is another physiologic gas that provides an important source of free radicals. Both gases have paramagnetic properties, similar solubility in biological fluids, and an ability to diffuse freely across cell membranes. At a rate that is nearly diffusion limited, ·NO reacts with superoxide to produce the powerful oxidant peroxynitrite.[32] Much of the peroxynitrite formed in vivo reacts rapidly with carbon dioxide to produce a nitrocarbonate intermediate that is an efficient nitrating agent.[33] This reaction also produces intermediates that can affect other tissues in secondary reactions.[34]

Activated neutrophils can release into the extracellular environment a variety of reactive species including superoxide, hydrogen peroxide, hydroxyl radical, hypochlorous acid, and peroxynitrite.[29,35-37] The extracellular location of these species may make them less susceptible to opposition by intracellular antioxidant defenses.[29,37] In animals exposed to oxygen at 1.0 atmosphere absolute (ATA; 101 kPa), early observations in rats that neutrophil accumulation in the pulmonary vasculature and lung interstitium[37-40] was associated with rapid exacerbation of pulmonary damage[40] and, conversely, that pulmonary pathology in rabbits was decreased by prior systemic depletion of neutrophils[35] were interpreted as an indication that neutrophil activation was a primary causal factor in the pulmonary toxicity of oxygen.[41] However, subsequent studies have confirmed that, although neutrophil-derived oxygen radicals can increase the severity of pulmonary oxygen poisoning, they are not required for its development.[29,40]

FREE RADICAL INTERACTIONS WITH PLASMA MEMBRANES

Free radical interactions with plasma membranes can produce many types of damage with a variety of functional consequences (Fig. 23.3). The actions of membrane-bound enzymes can produce additional toxic radicals and other biologically active products.

Free radical damage to membranes can occur as lipid peroxidation, amino acid oxidation, protein strand scission, and various cross-linking reactions among lipids and proteins. Peroxidation of membrane unsaturated fatty acids, structural protein oxidation, and inactivation of membrane-bound enzymes can cause the loss of secretory and other important membrane functions by increasing membrane permeability and reducing transmembrane ion gradients.

Lipid Peroxidation

Cell membranes contain polyunsaturated fatty acids that can react with oxygen free radicals to generate lipid peroxides and peroxy radicals that, in turn, interact adversely with many of the same cellular constituents targeted by the initial free radicals.[3,4] These reactions, which are potentiated by the presence of metals, can become autocatalytic after initiation to exacerbate the damage by oxidizing many polyunsaturated fatty acid molecules for each initiation event. Because lipid radicals are hydrophobic and interact extensively with membrane-associated fatty acids, the resulting peroxidation may have adverse effects on membrane permeability and microviscosity. In addition, critical membrane functions such as deformability, ion

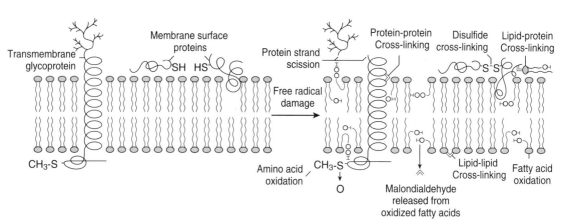

Figure 23.3 Potential sites of free radical damage to plasma membranes. Free radicals can initiate lipid peroxidation, which produces short-chain fatty acyl derivatives and the by-product malondialdehyde. Reactions with malondialdehyde can mediate a variety of cross-linking reactions. Free radicals can also catalyze amino acid oxidation, protein-protein cross-linking, and protein strand scission. *(From Freeman BA, Crapo JD: Biology of disease: Free radicals and tissue injury. Lab Invest 47:412–426, 1982, by permission.)*

transport, and enzyme activities can be altered by cross-linking and polymerization of membrane components caused by malondialdehyde, which is produced by peroxidation of fatty acids that contain three or more double bonds (see Fig. 23.3).

Lipid peroxidation occurs in rat and mouse cerebral cortical slices that are exposed to hyperoxia[42,43] and has been correlated in the rat with partial inactivation of NaK-ATPase.[44] Greater levels of lipid peroxidation in mouse as compared with rat brain slices were associated with an earlier onset of oxygen convulsions in the mice.[43] Both normal and tocopherol-deficient mice exposed to oxygen at 4.0 ATA (404 kPa) for 1 hour convulsed and had increased levels of brain lipid peroxides.[45] Tocopherol-supplemented mice exposed to the same conditions had neither convulsions nor brain lipid peroxidation. In contrast, brain lipid peroxide concentrations did not correlate with convulsions in rats breathing oxygen at 3.0 to 6.0 ATA (303–606 kPa).[46]

Hyperoxia-induced lipid peroxidation was exacerbated by the presence of Fe^{2+} in rat brain cortical slices,[44] and in homogenates from different brain regions, a linear relation existed between endogenous iron content and degree of lipid peroxidation.[47] An important role for iron as a potentiator of lipid peroxidation is supported by the observation that lipid peroxidation in rat brain homogenates exposed to hyperoxia was inhibited to a greater degree by addition of ceruloplasmin and deferoxamine than by superoxide dismutase (SOD) or catalase.[48]

Lipid peroxidation also occurs in the lungs and liver during exposure to hyperoxia.[29] In isolated perfused lungs from normal and tocopherol-deficient rats, rates of lipid peroxide formation increased, respectively, by about 50% and more than 500% during exposure to oxygen at 4.0 ATA (404 kPa).[49] The rate of lipid peroxidation increased in lung tissues exposed to O_2 at 0.8 to 1.0 ATA (81–101 kPa) for 2 to 7 days,[50-52] in liver tissue from rats exposed to 0.8 ATA (81 kPa) O_2 for 5 days,[52] and in isolated perfused liver exposed to O_2 at 4.0 ATA (404 kPa).[49]

Metabolism of Arachidonic Acid

There are indications that products of arachidonic acid metabolism are involved at least indirectly in the development of oxygen poisoning.[3] The membrane-associated enzymes cyclooxygenase and lipoxygenase react with arachidonic acid to initiate metabolic pathways that produce active radicals at several intermediate steps, as well as a variety of biologically active products including prostaglandins, thromboxanes, and leukotrienes.

Smith and colleagues[53,54] measured thromboxane and prostacyclin metabolite concentrations in bronchoalveolar lavage (BAL) fluid obtained from mice exposed to O_2 at 1.0 ATA (101 kPa) for up to 4 days. In an initial study,[53] the thromboxane metabolite concentration remained stable, whereas that of the prostacyclin metabolite increased threefold on exposure day 4. Inhibition of cyclo-oxygenase during exposure by giving indomethacin was associated with reduced concentration of prostacyclin metabolite, increased lung damage, and decreased survival time. Results were considered to be consistent with a protective role for prostacyclin and/or with diversion of arachidonic acid metabolism through the lipoxygenase pathway with detrimental effects.

Subsequently, a related study[54] using the same animal model demonstrated a positive correlation between severity of lung damage and BAL fluid concentration of sulfidopeptide leukotrienes. Observation of similar BAL fluid changes in neutropenic mice excluded neutrophils as a major source of the leukotrienes. Additional support for involvement of lipoxygenase products in the development of pulmonary oxygen poisoning is provided by the finding that rats exposed to O_2 at 1.0 ATA (101 kPa) for up to 72 hours had a progressive increase in BAL fluid leukotriene B_4 concentration concurrently with increased numbers of neutrophils in lavage fluid and reduced activity of nicotinamide adenine dinucleotide phosphate-cytochrome c reductase in lung microsomes.[55] Administration of low and high doses of a lipoxygenase inhibitor caused dose-dependent reductions in leukotriene B_4 concentration and neutrophil numbers in BAL fluid, as well as decreased mortality and prevention of the previously observed reduction in cytochrome c reductase activity. The authors conclude that the increased leukotriene B_4 concentration provided a chemoattractant for neutrophils that then exacerbated the damage caused by pulmonary oxygen toxicity.

Protein Damage by Free Radicals

Susceptibility of a protein to free radical attack and severity of the resulting damage are determined by several factors, including the nature of the free radical, cellular location and amino acid composition of the protein, the molecular location of susceptible amino acids, and their influences on protein conformation and activity.[3,56] In addition, the functional impact of a given degree of damage is influenced by the availability and efficacy of mechanisms for its reversal or repair. Because amino acids with sulfur atoms and/or unsaturated bonds are readily modified by free radicals, susceptible proteins include those that contain tryptophane, tyrosine, phenylalanine, histidine, methionine, or cysteine.[3,56] Peroxynitrite commonly modifies proteins by reacting with tyrosine residues to form S-nitrotyrosine. This selective process is influenced by both location of the tyrosine and its surrounding electrostatic characteristics.[56] Although cysteine can also be S-nitrosylated, this modification reverses more rapidly and has less biologic significance.

Using a system that generated hydroxyl and superoxide radicals by ^{60}Co radiation in the presence of oxygen, Davies[57-61] demonstrated a direct and quantitative relation between proteolytic susceptibility and protein damage induced by oxygen radicals. Protein degradation caused by oxygen radicals preceded the onset of lipid peroxidation and occurred independently of membrane damage by lipid peroxidation products.[61] Membrane transport proteins appear to be unusually susceptible to adverse interactions with oxygen radicals.[62]

ANTIOXIDANT DEFENSES

Survival in an aerobic environment required the evolutionary development of biochemical defenses against oxygen-derived free radicals.[3,4,63,64] Examples of potential oxidant-antioxidant interactions in the lung are summarized in Figure 23.4. Antioxidant defenses have been characterized as a multilayered system that evolved to counteract the adverse effects triggered by the univalent reduction of molecular oxygen.[4] A first line of defense in this system involves the action of enzymes, such as cytochrome oxidase, that can reduce molecular oxygen to water without producing reactive intermediates, thereby avoiding the univalent pathway and reducing the pool of active radicals that must be opposed by other means.

Metalloenzymes known as SODs constitute a second line of defense by catalyzing the dismutation of superoxide anion to form hydrogen peroxide.[3,4,27] A third line of antioxidant defense is provided by enzymes, such as catalase and glutathione peroxidase, that catalyze the removal of hydrogen peroxide produced either indirectly by superoxide anion dismutation or directly by reoxidation of reduced flavoenzymes.[4]

Biologic antioxidants such as vitamin E act as a fourth line of defense by reacting rapidly with chain propagating fatty acid radicals to form a stable α-tocopherol radical and terminate the chain reaction.[4] The hydrophobic properties of vitamin E cause it to partition within biologic membranes, thereby enhancing its effectiveness against fatty acid radicals.

Reversal of oxidant damage by reactivation of oxidized enzymes and reduction of oxidized tissue components constitutes a fifth line of defense[4] that appears to be provided mainly by interactions with reduced glutathione, producing oxidized glutathione as a by-product.[31] Concurrent activation of the pentose shunt pathway of glucose metabolism (see Fig. 23.4) supplies the nicotinamide adenine dinucleotide phosphate that is required to regenerate reduced glutathione.[31,65]

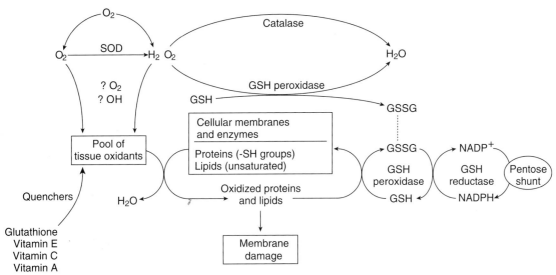

Figure 23.4 Oxidant-antioxidant interactions in the lung. Possible metabolic events induced by the increase of inspired partial pressure of oxygen (Po_2) are represented. The sequence is initiated by enhanced generation of superoxide anion, H_2O_2, and possibly other active species such as singlet oxygen and hydroxyl radicals to form a pool of tissue oxidants. These oxidants may damage cell membranes and intracellular enzymes by oxidizing tissue proteins and lipids. The tissue oxidant pool is diminished and free-radical chain reactions are stopped by interactions of quenchers with active species and oxidized tissue components. Superoxide anions can be removed specifically by superoxide dismutase (SOD). Damaged tissues may also be repaired by reduction of oxidized components by glutathione (GSH) to form oxidized glutathione (GSSG). Regeneration of GSH from GSSG may be accomplished by interaction with reduced nicotinamide adenine dinucleotide phosphate (NADPH), which is, in turn, restored by action of the pentose shunt pathway of glucose metabolism. The extent of lung damage may be determined by the net result of opposing radical-producing and -quenching actions with concurrent interactions between tissue-damaging and tissue-repairing processes. *(From Fisher AB, Bassett DJP, Forman HJ: Oxygen toxicity of the lung: Biochemical aspects. In: Fishman AP, Renkin EM [eds]: Pulmonary Edema. Bethesda, MD, American Physiological Society, 1979, pp 207–216, by permission.)*

Increasing evidence exists that the protective roles of classical antioxidant enzymes such as SOD, catalase, and glutathione peroxidase may be supplemented by other cellular and molecular responses to oxidative stress in mammalian cells.[66] Heme oxygenase-1, also known as heat shock protein 32, is highly induced by oxidant stress and has been proposed for a possible protective role against oxidant-induced lung injury.[67] Potential mechanisms for an antioxidant action include catalysis of the oxidative degradation of heme, which can function as a cellular pro-oxidant, and production of bilirubin as an end product that has antioxidant properties. Increased levels of heme oxygenase-1 were measured in lymphocytes obtained from healthy humans 24 hours after breathing O_2 at 2.5 ATA (252 kPa) for 60 minutes on a 20-minute O_2/5-minute air intermittent schedule.[68] Reversible breakage of

DNA strands found in lymphocytes after a single exposure to this profile did not occur after the second or subsequent exposures. In addition, lymphocytes isolated from blood obtained 24 hours after the initial exposure were resistant to DNA damage by hydrogen peroxide in vitro. In a related investigation,[69] synthesis of heat shock protein 70 was also induced in lymphocytes by a single 3 × 20-minute O_2 exposure at 2.5 ATA (252 kPa), whereas red blood cell concentrations of SOD, catalase, and glutathione peroxidase were not altered. The principle that heat shock proteins can provide cross-protection against oxidant injury is supported by the observation that hyperthermic preconditioning of cultured human umbilical vein endothelial cells significantly reduced the cellular damage caused by subsequent exposure to hydrogen peroxide.[70] In addition, heat acclimation of rats before O_2 exposure at

6.0 ATA (606 kPa) doubled the period of latency before the onset of electroencephalographic spikes in association with increased brain levels of heat shock protein 72.[71] During a 4-week period of deacclimation to heat, reversal of the gain in seizure latency correlated directly with decreasing levels of heat shock protein 72.

CLINICAL MANIFESTATIONS OF OXYGEN POISONING

Even at partial pressures that will ultimately produce severe oxidant damage, it is possible to breathe oxygen for a period with no overt manifestations of oxygen poisoning.[2,6] The duration of this "latent" period is inversely proportional to the level of inspired Po_2 such that there is a hyperbolic relation between inspired oxygen pressure and exposure duration required to produce a specific degree or type of oxygen poisoning (Fig. 23.5). Although it is now known that biochemical effects of oxygen toxicity are initiated rapidly at any level of hyperoxia with no actual latent period,[2,6,9,72] this early exposure interval provides an asymptomatic period of slowly developing oxidant injury from which complete recovery will occur promptly on return to normoxia.[6]

Similar hyperbolic relations have been demonstrated for the following effects of oxygen toxicity: inactivation of respiration in rat brain slices[73]; conduction block in isolated cat nerve[74]; erythrocyte hemolysis in mice[75]; death of Drosophila,[76] mice,[77] and rats[78,79]; pulmonary and neurologic symptoms in men[73,80]; and impairment of pulmonary function in men.[2] Because oxygen free radicals attack the basic cellular units of all life forms, it is reasonable to assume that hyperbolic oxygen pressure–exposure duration relations exist for all manifestations of oxygen poisoning.

NEUROLOGIC EFFECTS OF OXYGEN TOXICITY

In preparation for the initial use of closed circuit oxygen rebreathing systems in military covert operations during World War II, Donald[10,81] in the Royal Navy and Yarbrough and coworkers[82] in the U.S. Navy conducted extensive studies of CNS oxygen tolerance in large numbers of divers. These studies had as a primary focus the determination of onset times for symptoms and signs of CNS oxygen poisoning at oxygen pressures up to 4.0 ATA (404 kPa) in an attempt to identify a reliable early warning before the onset of convulsions. Observed effects include the diverse symptoms and signs summarized in Table 23.1. Unfortunately, minor symptoms did not occur consistently before the subject convulsed. In addition, any preconvulsive

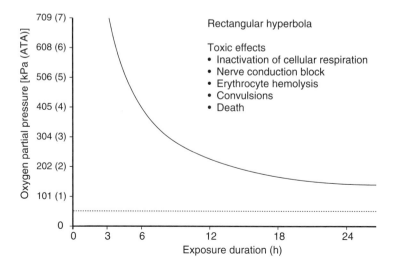

Figure 23.5 Inspired oxygen pressure–exposure duration relation for specific manifestations of oxygen poisoning. *(From Clark JM: The toxicity of oxygen. Am Rev Respir Dis 110:40–50, 1974, by permission.)*

Table 23.1 Effects of Central Nervous System Oxygen Poisoning in Healthy Humans

Facial pallor	Unpleasant olfactory sensations
Sweating	Unpleasant gustatory sensations
Bradycardia	Respiratory changes
Choking sensation	Panting
Sleepiness	Grunting
Depression	Hiccoughs
Euphoria	nspiratory predominance
Apprehension	Diaphragmatic spasms
Changes of behavior	Severe nausea
Fidgeting	Spasmodic vomiting
Disinterest	Vertigo
Clumsiness	Fibrillation of lips
Visual symptoms	Lip twitching
Loss of acuity	Twitching of cheek and nose
Dazzle	Palpitations
Lateral movement	Epigastric tensions
Decrease of intensity	Syncope
Constriction of visual field	Convulsions
Acoustic symptoms	
Music	
Bell ringing	
Knocking	

Adapted from Donald KW: Oxygen poisoning in man. I & II. Br Med J 1:667–672, 712–717, 1947; and Donald KW: Oxygen and the Diver. Harley Swan, United Kingdom, The SPA Ltd, 1992, by permission.

aura that did occur was sometimes followed by seizures so rapidly that it had little practical value as a warning.

Attempts by investigators in both navies to determine safe limits for breathing oxygen at increased pressures were further hindered by the consistent observation of wide variation in CNS oxygen tolerance among different individuals breathing oxygen at the same pressure (Fig. 23.6). Even in the same diver, onset times for neurologic effects of oxygen toxicity varied widely on different days (Fig. 23.7) such that his overall variability over a period of 90 days (Fig. 23.8) resembled that for single exposures of 36 different divers (see Fig. 23.6). The basis for CNS oxygen tolerance variability in the same or different individuals remains unexplained after failed attempts at correlation with factors such as age, weight, physical fitness, smoking, alcohol ingestion, psychologic stability, or personality traits.[10,81]

The seizure caused by oxygen toxicity is a generalized tonic-clonic convulsion that may occur suddenly without warning or it may be preceded by an aura or sequence of premonitory sensations.[6] Onset of the convulsion consists of a rigid tonic phase, with abrupt loss of consciousness and powerful extension of the neck and all four extremities. An initial opening of the mouth permits insertion of a padded spacer between the teeth to prevent laceration of the tongue. The tonic phase is followed within about 30 seconds by a clonic phase involving repeated, powerful, generalized muscle contractions for about 1 minute before gradual cessation. An apneic period that persists throughout both the tonic and clonic phases is followed by vigorous hyperventilation stimulated by retained carbon dioxide and a metabolic acidosis.

Hyperoxic seizures usually stop spontaneously on resumption of air breathing without therapeutic intervention. Return of consciousness within a few minutes after the convulsion is usually followed by a 5 to 30-minute postictal period during which mental alertness returns gradually. Brain oxygenation is

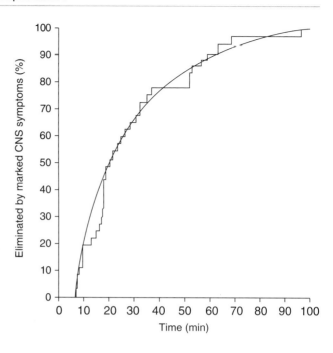

Figure 23.6 Incidence of neurologic effects in 36 divers breathing O_2 at 3.7 atmospheres absolute (ATA; 373 kPa) for intervals of 6 to 96 minutes. Each exposure was terminated when the diver experienced one of the neurologic effects listed in Table 23.1. *(From Donald KW: Oxygen and the Diver. Harley Swan, United Kingdom, The SPA Ltd., 1992; and Donald KW: Oxygen poisoning in man. I & II. Br Med J 1:667–672, 712–717, 1947, by permission.)*

maintained during the convulsion by the concurrent high alveolar Po_2, arterial hypercapnia, and increased cerebral blood flow (CBF). If the patient is not intubated, decompression should be delayed until regular breathing has resumed. Apart from the possibility of physical injury, a single oxygen convulsion does not produce residual effects.[6,81,82]

Carbon Dioxide Effects on Neurologic Oxygen Tolerance

An accelerated onset of neurologic oxygen poisoning at oxygen pressures of 3.0 ATA (303 kPa) or higher by mild-to-moderate increases of arterial partial pressure of carbon dioxide (Pa_{CO_2}) has been well documented.[9]

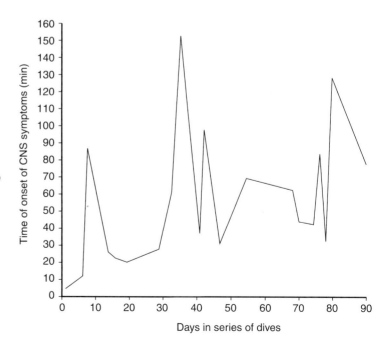

Figure 23.7 Oxygen tolerance variability within the same individual on different days. On 20 different days over a total period of 90 days, the same diver breathed O_2 at 70 feet (21 m) until he experienced neurologic symptoms or signs. Exposure durations are indicated. *(From Donald KW: Oxygen and the Diver. Harley Swan, United Kingdom, The SPA Ltd., 1992; and Donald KW: Oxygen poisoning in man. I & II. Br Med J 1:667–672, 712–717, 1947, by permission.)*

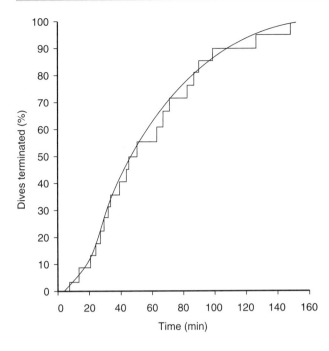

Figure 23.8 Oxygen tolerance variability within the same individual. Data shown in Figure 23.7 are replotted to indicate durations of individual exposures expressed as percentages of the total number of exposures. *(From Donald KW: Oxygen and the Diver. Harley Swan, United Kingdom, The SPA Ltd., 1992; and Donald KW: Oxygen poisoning in man. I & II. Br Med J 1:667–672, 712–717, 1947, by permission.)*

Arterial hypercapnia can also cause convulsions to occur at oxygen pressures at least as low as 2.0 ATA (202 kPa) where they do not normally occur at rest even in exposures as long as 12 hours.[83] Cerebral vasodilation with an associated increase in brain oxygen tension has been proposed as the basis for the detrimental effects of hypercapnia on CNS oxygen tolerance.[84] This conclusion is supported by the observation that internal jugular venous P_{O_2} in four resting men increased from an average value of 76 mm Hg (10.1 kPa) while breathing O_2 at 3.5 ATA (354 kPa) to 1000 mm Hg (133 kPa) when 2% CO_2 was added to the inspired gas. Average Pa_{CO_2} increased from 37 mm Hg (4.9 kPa) on O_2 alone to 58 mm Hg (7.7 kPa) on O_2/CO_2.[84] In rats breathing O_2 at 2.0 to 5.0 ATA (202–505 kPa), cerebral tissue P_{O_2} increased significantly when concentrations of 0.8% to 5.0% CO_2 in O_2 were inspired.[85,86]

It is widely accepted that the cerebral vasodilation caused by arterial hypercapnia is initiated by the increase in perivascular $[H^+]$ induced by freely diffusible CO_2.[87,88] However, more recent information indicates that ·NO may be involved in this process. Evidence for and against this hypothesis has been reviewed by Iadecola and coauthors.[89] Although a large majority of studies indicated that the cerebrovascular response to hypercapnia is reduced by inhibition of nitric oxide synthase (NOS), a few investigators found little or no effect. Some of the discrepancies may be explained by the observation in rats that, whereas NOS inhibition significantly reduced hypercapnic vasodilation over a Pa_{CO_2} range of 40 to 80 mm Hg (5.3–10.6 kPa), it had little or no effect at greater P_{CO_2} levels.[90] Iadecola and coauthors[89] concluded that, although ·NO synthesis appeared to be involved in hypercapnic vasodilation, ·NO may not be the final mediator acting on vascular smooth muscle and other vasodilator agents are likely participants.

Effects of Hyperoxia on Cerebral Blood Flow

Attempts to measure quantitatively the effects of hyperoxia on CBF have produced results that vary somewhat with different methods of measurement. Early studies in humans using the Kety–Schmidt N_2O uptake method indicated that CBF is reduced by 13% to 15% during O_2 breathing at 1.0 ATA (101 kPa)[91,92] and by 25% at 3.5 ATA (354 kPa).[92] Measurements of CBF responses to hyperoxia are complicated by the fact that the increase in Pa_{O_2} triggers a cascade of physiologic events that ultimately cause mild hyperventilation, arterial hypocapnia, and decreased CBF.[5,6] Intermediate steps include an increase in physically dissolved O_2, diminished reduction of venous oxyhemoglobin, altered CO_2 transport, and an increase in brain tissue Pco_2. The magnitude of Pa_{CO_2} reduction ranges from about 3 mm Hg (0.4 kPa) at 1.0 ATA (101 kPa) O_2 to a maximum of 7 to 8 mm Hg (0.9-1.1 kPa) at 2.0 to 2.5 ATA (202-252 kPa).[93]

Although the O_2 and related CO_2 effects on CBF are physiologically linked, they can be separated analytically by measuring CBF responses to a range of Pa_{CO_2} values in air and oxygen backgrounds.[94] The data in Figure 23.9, which were obtained with a noninvasive magnetic resonance imaging method over a total Pco_2 range of 40 to 52 mm Hg (5.3-6.9 kPa), reflect a 29% to 33% reduction in CBF during O_2 breathing at 1.0 ATA (101 kPa) with respect to CBF at equivalent Pa_{CO_2} levels during air breathing. The CBF, Pco_2 values for air breathing with no added CO_2 (see Fig. 23.9) are nearly identical to corresponding values for one of the subject groups that Kety and Schmidt[91] studied. However, the relative CBF decrement during O_2 breathing is about twice that found previously with the N_2O uptake

method.[91,92] In addition, the CBF, Pco_2 values for O_2 breathing with no added CO_2 (see Fig. 23.9) agree well with corresponding values obtained by using ^{133}Xe clearance to measure CBF.[95] The latter study[95] did not include air-breathing CBF measurements. Ohta[96] has used ^{133}Xe clearance to measure CBF at O_2 pressures of 0.5, 1.0, 1.5, 2.0, and 2.5 ATA (50, 101, 151, 202, and 252 kPa, respectively). With respect to air breathing at 1.0 ATA (101 kPa), CBF decreased by average values of 9%, 21%, 23%, 29%, and 19%, respectively. These results appear to be consistent with a near-maximal degree of vasoconstriction at an O_2 pressure of about 1.0 ATA (101 kPa). Although the data shown in Figure 23.9 clearly indicate an independent cerebral vasoconstrictive effect of hyperoxia, it is not currently possible to reconcile the varying magnitudes of this effect as determined by different methods of CBF measurement.

Hyperoxia-Nitric Oxide Interacting Effects on Cerebral Blood Flow

Demchenko and colleagues[97,98] proposed that the cerebral vasoconstriction induced by hyperoxia is mediated by reaction of superoxide with ·NO to decrease the availability of the vasodilator. In rats breathing O_2 at 5.0 ATA (505 kPa), CBF reduction did not

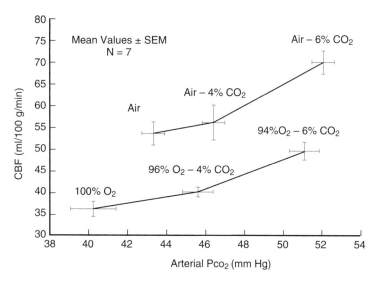

Figure 23.9 Relations of cerebral blood flow (CBF) to arterial partial pressure of carbon dioxide (Pco_2) in normal men breathing air or oxygen at 1.0 atmospheres absolute (101 kPa). SEM, standard error of the mean. *(From Floyd TF, Clark JM, Gelfand R, et al: Independent cerebral vasoconstrictive effects of hyperoxia and accompanying arterial hypocapnia at 1 ATA. J Appl Physiol 95:2453-2461, 2003, by permission.)*

occur when SOD was given before exposure.[97] Cerebral vasoconstriction also did not occur during O_2 breathing at either 3.0 or 5.0 ATA (303 or 505 kPa) in mice that were genetically altered to overexpress SOD.[98] In agreement with an absence of cerebral vasoconstriction and, therefore, delivery of a higher brain oxygen dose is the observation that SOD overexpression in mice exposed to O_2 at 6.0 ATA (606 kPa) was associated with a greater mortality rate than in nontransgenic mice.[99] In both transgenic and nontransgenic mice, mortality was reduced and seizure onset was delayed by inhibition of either SOD or NOS.

Several studies in rats exposed to O_2 pressures of 3.0 ATA (303 kPa) or greater have shown that an initial period of cerebral vasoconstriction is followed by delayed vasodilation before the onset of convulsions.[98,100-104] Although the biochemical basis for reversal of the initial vasoconstriction has not been fully explained, it is likely that interacting effects of hyperoxia and ·NO are involved (Fig. 23.10). In addition to the effect of superoxide on bioavailability of ·NO and modulation of this effect by SOD, results consistent with ·NO autooxidation were obtained in experiments designed to evaluate vascular ·NO bioavailability with an assay that used rat aortic rings exposed in vitro to O_2 at 2.8 ATA (283 kPa).[105] The same experiments indirectly demonstrated vascular ·NO production by a nonendothelial source. There were no indications of altered endothelial NOS activity after in vivo hyperoxia.

Concurrently with the hyperoxia-induced reduction of ·NO bioavailability, there are opposing effects that are also initiated by hyperoxia. In rats and genetically altered mice exposed to O_2 pressures of 0.2 to 2.8 ATA (20-283 kPa), there were rapid, dose-dependent increases of ·NO concentration in both the brain[106] and perivascular aortic area.[107] In both areas, activation of neuronal NOS was the dominant source of ·NO. Whereas neuronal NOS activation at 2.0 ATA (202 kPa) O_2 appeared to be related to an altered cellular redox state,[107] enzyme activation at 2.8 ATA (283 kPa) was considered to be mediated by an enhanced association of neuronal NOS with calmodulin that was facilitated by the molecular chaperone, heat shock protein 90.[106,107]

General agreement exists that brain ·NO production is increased in rats before the onset of seizures during exposure to O_2 pressures of 3.0 to 6.0 ATA (303-606 kPa).[102,108-112] Results obtained in genetic knockout mice are consistent with an early cerebral vasoconstriction related to superoxide-induced inactivation of endothelial NOS–derived ·NO, followed by delayed vasodilation that is dependent on both endothelial and neuronal NOS activation.[111,112] In addition to modulating an increased CBF and brain oxygen dose, ·NO production can have other toxic effects such as production of peroxynitrite[111] or amplification of an excitatory to inhibitory neurotransmitter imbalance by enhancing the release of glutamate and aspartate, and suppressing the release of γ-aminobutyric acid.[108,113,114]

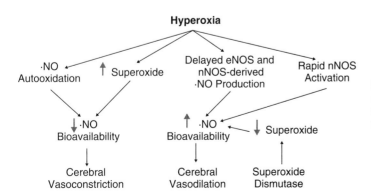

Figure 23.10 Interacting effects of hyperoxia and nitric oxide (·NO) on cerebral blood flow. eNOS, endothelial nitric oxide synthase; nNOS, neuronal nitric oxide synthase.

Rate of Development of Neurologic Oxygen Poisoning

As part of a multiyear, comprehensive investigation of human organ tolerance to continuous oxygen breathing at pressures of 3.0, 2.5, 2.0, and 1.5 ATA (303, 252, 202, and 151 kPa, respectively), referred to collectively as Predictive Studies V,[115] respiratory control parameters were measured as preconvulsive indices of neurologic oxygen poisoning.[93] Average changes in the timing component of ventilation, calculated as inspiratory time divided by total breath period (T_I/T_T), are shown in Figure 23.11. With the exception of the final measurement during O_2 breathing at 2.0 ATA (202 kPa), all of the remaining T_I/T_T values decrease progressively with increasing duration of O_2 breathing at each pressure. In contrast, average values obtained during air-breathing control periods scatter erratically about the control value. Linear regression lines and equations for each pressure are shown in Figure 23.11. The final data point at 2.0 ATA (202 kPa) was excluded from the regression because it was considered that the unique

inconsistency of this value was probably related to pulmonary symptoms experienced by some of the subjects at that time.[93,116] The increasing slope of the T_I/T_T changes at greater oxygen pressures is consistent with associated increments in the rate of development of neurologic oxygen poisoning.

Of the 13 subjects who breathed O_2 at 3.0 ATA (303 kPa) for up to 3.5 hours, 1 had a typical oxygen convulsion at 3.0 hours.[93,115] Ventilatory and end-tidal P_{CO_2} measurements for this subject are compared with averages for the other 12 subjects in Figure 23.12. Starting at about 2.5 hours of exposure, the subject who convulsed had an abrupt onset of an erratic breathing pattern with an associated 184% increase in expiratory time, 50% reduction in T_I/T_T, decreased respiratory rate and ventilation, and increase in end-tidal P_{CO_2} from 34 to 43 mm Hg (4.5–5.7 kPa).[93] Although not measured directly, concurrent increases in CBF and brain O_2 dose would be expected. Previously reported respiratory changes such as "inspiratory predominance" and "diaphragmatic spasms" (see Table 23.1) suggest that similar manifestations of neurologic oxygen poisoning occurred previously

Figure 23.11 Average changes in the timing component of ventilation in healthy men breathing oxygen at 3.0, 2.5, 2.0, and 1.5 atmospheres absolute (ATA) (303, 252, 202, and 151 kPa, respectively). The number of subjects in each group is 12, 8, 6, and 9, respectively. Control measurements during air breathing at 1.0 ATA (101 kPa) were performed in eight of the subjects exposed at 3.0 ATA (short air) and in five of the 1.5 ATA subjects (long air). *Dashed lines* are linear regressions through the average data connected by *solid lines*. Asterisks indicate statistically significant changes. T_I/T_T, inspiratory time divided by total breath period. *(From Gelfand R, Lambertsen CJ, Clark JM: Ventilatory effects of prolonged hyperoxia at pressures of 1.5-3.0 ATA. Aviat Space Environ Med 77:801–810, 2006.)*

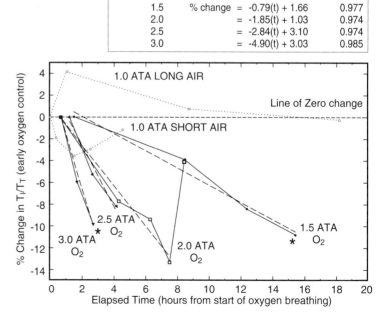

O_2 Pressure (ATA)	Linear Regression Equation	r^2
1.5	% change = -0.79(t) + 1.66	0.977
2.0	= -1.85(t) + 1.03	0.974
2.5	= -2.84(t) + 3.10	0.974
3.0	= -4.90(t) + 3.03	0.985

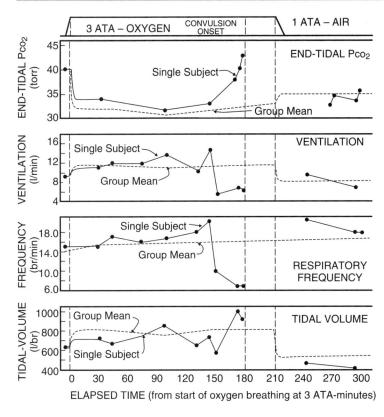

Figure 23.12 Changes in ventilation and end-tidal partial pressure of carbon dioxide (Pco_2) of a subject who convulsed compared with average changes in 12 other subjects who did not convulse during O_2 breathing at 3.0 atmospheres absolute (ATA; 303 kPa). *(From Lambertsen CJ, Clark JM, Gelfand R, et al: Definition of tolerance to continuous hyperoxia in man: An abstract report of Predictive Studies V. In: Bove AA, Bachrach AJ, Greenbaum LJ [eds]: Underwater and Hyperbaric Physiology IX. Bethesda, MD, Undersea and Hyperbaric Medical Society, 1987, pp 717–735, by permission.)*

in the absence of objective monitoring. Because only one subject convulsed in this series of experiments, the degree to which the observed respiratory changes can be generalized is unknown. Nevertheless, the toxic effects on respiratory control factors that caused the changes shown in Figure 23.12 may represent at least one mechanism for the preconvulsive CBF changes found repeatedly in rats.[98,100-104]

EFFECTS OF OXYGEN TOXICITY ON THE EYE

Ocular manifestations of oxygen poisoning are affected by many variables in addition to inspired Po_2 and exposure duration.[12] These include the age of the exposed individual, method of oxygen administration, and the presence of latent or overt conditions that may alter susceptibility to oxygen poisoning. Major influences of each of these conditions are described in the following sections.

Retinopathy of Prematurity

Retinopathy of prematurity is a unique condition caused by exposure of the premature infant to hyperoxia. Initially, there is constriction of the developing retinal vessels, followed by endothelial cell destruction and the arrest of retinal vascularization at an incomplete stage of development.[12,23] On removal from hyperoxia, there is a disorganized and profuse vascular proliferation by the remaining endothelial cells. This produces a fibrous mass of vascular tissue that ultimately causes irreversible retinal detachment and permanent blindness. Despite the fact that current management is generally aimed at maintaining conditions of stable and moderate oxygenation with Pa_{O_2} levels in the range of 60 to 80 mm Hg (8.0–10.6 kPa) and oxyhemoglobin saturations of 88% to 95%, retinopathy of prematurity remains prevalent among small premature infants.[117]

Effects on Peripheral Vision

Behnke and coworkers[118] first documented a progressive loss of peripheral vision to the point of near blindness (tunnel vision) in a man who breathed O_2 at 3.0 ATA (303 kPa) for 3.5 hours (Fig. 23.13). The visual loss was reversible and recovery was nearly complete within 50 minutes after resumption of air breathing. Similar visual changes were later reported by Donald[81] and Rosenberg and colleagues.[119] These early observations were confirmed and extended by Lambertsen and colleagues[115] in Predictive Studies V (Fig. 23.14). During O_2 breathing at 3.0 ATA (303 kPa), the visual field area remained near or above the pre-exposure control value for 2.5 to 3.0 hours, then decreased progressively until O_2 breathing was stopped at 3.5 hours. The average decrease in visual field area at 3.5 hours

was 50%, with individual decrements of 74% to 91% in the six subjects who had the largest changes. Complete recovery occurred within 45 minutes after return to air breathing. Visual acuity and visual-evoked cortical responses, both of which are determined primarily by central visual function, remained unchanged even in the subjects who had the largest visual field losses.

Extreme susceptibility to visual effects of oxygen toxicity was manifested in an individual who had recovered many years previously from retrobulbar neuritis in one eye.[120] During O_2 breathing at 2.0 ATA (202 kPa), the onset of progressive visual field contraction in the affected eye was noted at about 4 hours and was nearly complete by 6 hours. Although most of the visual field loss reversed within the first few hours of air breathing, complete recovery required more than 24 hours. This was considered to represent an exaggerated

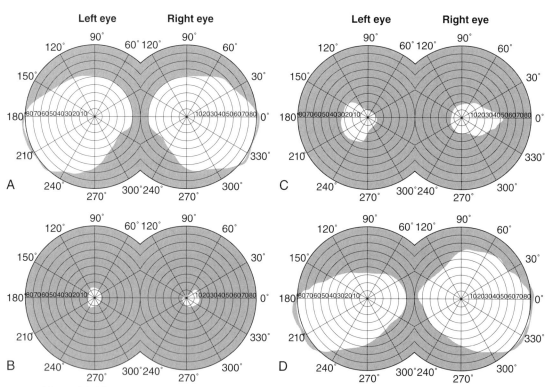

Figure 23.13 Perimetric measurements of visual fields in the same subject before and after 3.5 hours of oxygen breathing at 3.0 atmospheres absolute (ATA; 303 kPa). *A*, Normal pre-exposure visual fields. Visual fields were obtained 5 *(B)*, 25 *(C)*, and 50 *(D)* minutes after exposure. *(From Behnke AR, Forbes HS, Motley EP: Circulatory and visual effects of oxygen at 3 atmospheres pressure. Am J Physiol 114:436–442, 1936, by permission.)*

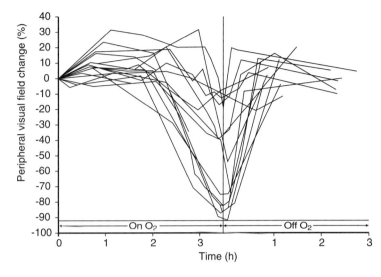

Figure 23.14 Peripheral visual field changes in healthy men during and after continuous O_2 exposure at 3.0 atmospheres absolute (ATA; 303 kPa) for 3.5 hours. Progressive decrements in peripheral vision developed after a delay and reversed rapidly after termination of oxygen breathing. Associated decrements in electroretinogram b-wave amplitude were less consistent and generally of smaller magnitude. Visual acuity and visual-evoked cortical responses were not changed. *(From Lambertsen CJ, Clark JM, Gelfand R, et al: Definition of tolerance to continuous hyperoxia in man: An abstract report of Predictive Studies V. In: Bove AA, Bachrach AJ, Greenbaum LJ [eds]: Underwater and Hyperbaric Physiology IX. Bethesda, MD, Undersea and Hyperbaric Medical Society, 1987, pp 717–735, by permission.)*

expression of oxygen effect related to the existence of an underlying neuronal and/or vascular defect.

Effects on Retinal Electrical Activity

Noell[121] and Bridges[122] studied in rabbits the effects of prolonged O_2 exposure on the electroretinogram (ERG), measured as the electrical response of the dark-adapted retina to a flash of light. Amplitude of the ERG was completely and reversibly suppressed by O_2 exposures ranging from nearly 2 days at 1.0 ATA (101 kPa) to less than 1 hour at 7.0 ATA (707 kPa). Recovery of the ERG did not occur if the O_2 exposure was continued sufficiently beyond the point of complete extinction, presumably to the point of visual cell damage or death.

Reversible decrements in ERG amplitude were also measured in healthy men during exposures to O_2 pressures of 3.0, 2.5, 2.0, and 1.5 ATA (303, 252, 202, and 151 kPa, respectively) for average durations of 3.4, 5.7, 8.8, and 17.7 hours, respectively.[2] Unexpectedly, the ERG changes did not correlate with concurrent reductions in visual field area. Whereas the largest visual field contractions were found during the relatively short exposures at 3.0 ATA (303 kPa), ERG amplitude decreased most consistently during the longer exposures at 2.0 ATA (202 kPa). The observed

lack of correlation for ERG and visual field effects of oxygen toxicity may reflect different sites of action or biochemical characteristics of the cells involved.

Oxygen Effects on the Lens of the Eye

Progressive myopia is an ocular effect of oxygen toxicity that occurs in some patients who receive daily 90- to 120-minute exposures to O_2 at 2.0-2.5 ATA (202–252 kPa) for chronic disease states.[123-127] Refractive changes occurred symmetrically in both eyes and appeared to progress throughout the duration of oxygen therapy. After completion of the therapy series, recovery was often rapid for the first few weeks and then continued more slowly for periods of several weeks to as long as a year (Fig. 23.15). Reversal was complete in most but not all patients.[123]

The cause of the progressive myopia induced by hyperoxia has been attributed to a reversible change in lens shape or metabolism.[123,124,128] Possible causes of myopia that have been excluded include changes in corneal curvature or intraocular tension[123] and change in the axial length of the eye.[128] Patients with diabetes and elderly patients appear to have a greater incidence of myopia.[124,128]

Evanger and colleagues[127] compared refractive changes in 20 patients using an oronasal

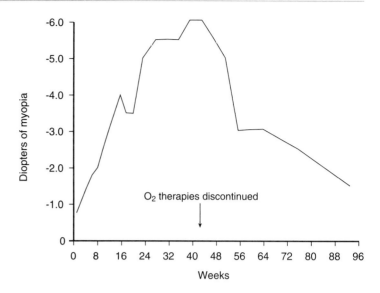

Figure 23.15 Onset and reversal of progressive myopia during and after a 44-week series of oxygen therapies. Each therapy consisted of 1 hour of oxygen breathing at 2.5 atmospheres absolute (ATA; 252 kPa) preceded and followed by 30-minute periods of compression and decompression. One treatment was given each day. *(From Lyne AJ: Ocular effects of hyperbaric oxygen. Trans Ophthalmol Soc U K 98:66–68, 1978, by permission.)*

mask with those in 12 other patients who received O_2 via a hood system. All patients received O_2 daily at 2.4 ATA (242 kPa) for 21 days. Each therapy consisted of three 30-minute O_2 cycles separated by 5-minute air breaks. Refraction was performed within 1 week before the start of the therapy series and then repeated within 2 to 4 days of completion and at regular intervals thereafter. Myopic shifts of at least 0.5 diopter occurred in 24 of 40 eyes (60%) in the mask group and in 20 of 24 eyes (83%) in the hood group. Maximal changes in spheric equivalents for all 20 patients given O_2 by mask had average values of −0.55 D and −0.53 D in right and left eyes, respectively, at 2 to 4 days after cessation of therapy. Refraction returned to baseline within 6 weeks. Corresponding average values of spherical equivalents for the 12 patients in the hood group were −1.06 D and −1.10 D. Maximal changes were found 12 to 16 days after cessation of therapy, and recovery occurred within 10 weeks. The investigators concluded that patients in the hood group received a more toxic dose to the lens because O_2 was delivered by diffusion across the cornea and by the arterial circulation. This conclusion is supported by the finding in rabbits that Po_2 of the aqueous humour was increased significantly by exposing the cornea to oxygen while the animal continued to breath air.[129]

Accelerated progression of pre-existing nuclear cataracts and formation of new cataracts were observed in a group of 25 patients who received extremely prolonged series of hyperbaric oxygen treatments.[130] Daily treatments consisting of 1 hour at 2.0 to 2.5 ATA (202–252 kPa) were given over 2 to 19 months for totals of 150 to 850 exposures. All of the patients developed myopia, and all but one had a refractive change of at least 1.0 D with an overall average maximal value of 3.0 D. On termination of therapy, the induced myopia reversed in most but not all patients, and myopia persisted in 11 patients for at least 6 months. Nuclear cataracts developed in 7 of 15 patients who started with clear lens nuclei and progressed in 8 of 10 patients who had pre-existing cataracts. Palmquist and colleagues[130] conclude that myopia appeared to be an early, reversible manifestation of lenticular oxygen toxicity, whereas cataract formation represented a more severe and less reversible toxic effect.

In what appears to be an exception to the general observation that newly formed cataracts occur only in therapy series that greatly exceed the 20 to 50 treatments used for most applications, early cataract development in a 49-year-old woman who had 48 treatments over a period of 11 weeks has been reported.[131] Each treatment consisted of O_2 breathing at 2.5 ATA (252 kPa) for three 30-minute periods separated by two 5-minute air breaks. Bilateral cataract formation was associated with a myopic shift that progressed over a period of 4 months after therapy to stabilize at 3.25 D. The cataracts and associated myopic shift were still present at 11 months after therapy. Although the patient did not have diabetes and was not taking steroids, the possibility of an undetected, predisposing condition should be considered.

Another unusual observation was documented in a 41-year-old woman who received 30 O_2 treatments at 2.4 ATA (242 kPa) for 90 minutes each treatment.[132] By the end of the therapy series, she noted subjective myopia that was not quantified. Ten days later, however, she described a rapid onset of an inability to read text. When she was evaluated on day 17, she had a 2-D hypermetropic shift that reversed over a period of about 10 weeks. Slit-lamp examination and ophthalmoscopy showed clear media and normal fundi. No underlying conditions were identified.

PULMONARY EFFECTS OF OXYGEN TOXICITY

Pulmonary effects of oxygen toxicity have been described extensively in previous reviews.[2,9] This presentation is necessarily more succinct. Most of the available information regarding toxic effects on the human lung has been obtained in healthy human volunteers who breathe oxygen until they experience early reversible degrees of pulmonary oxygen poisoning. Required exposure durations are well beyond those used in therapeutic applications with the possible exception of severe decompression sickness that requires saturation or multiple exposures.

The symptoms of pulmonary oxygen poisoning appear to be caused by a tracheobronchitis that starts in the substernal or carinal area and spreads throughout the tracheobronchial tree.[9,83] In subjects breathing O_2 at pressures of about 0.8, 1.0, and 2.0 ATA (81, 101, and 202 kPa, respectively), symptoms occur as early as 6, 4, and 3 hours, respectively. During O_2 breathing at 3.0 ATA (303 kPa), mild symptoms

may be experienced within 1 hour by sensitive individuals.[133] Beginning as a mild sensation that is accentuated by inspiration and occasionally induces a cough, the tracheal irritation becomes progressively more intense and widespread, in parallel with more frequent coughing. When extreme, the tracheal symptoms are characterized by a constant burning sensation that is exacerbated by inspiration and accompanied by uncontrollable coughing. The most severe symptoms are associated with dyspnea on exertion or even at rest. On cessation of O_2 breathing at 2.0 ATA (202 kPa), symptom intensity usually decreased rapidly within 2 to 4 hours.[83] Complete resolution of pulmonary symptoms occurred over about 1 to 3 days, although dyspnea on exertion sometimes persisted for several days.

Effects on Pulmonary Function

Effects of toxic oxygen exposures at 1.5, 2.0, 2.5, and 3.0 ATA (151, 202, 252, and 303 kPa, respectively) on selected indices of pulmonary function are summarized in Table 23.2.[116,133] The data indicate that patterns of pulmonary function deficits vary with different combinations of oxygen pressure and exposure duration. They also show that lung mechanical function is impaired earlier and more prominently than gas exchange function at each pressure. The functional deficits summarized in Table 23.2 probably represent the combined effects of direct oxidant injuries to pulmonary tissues and the exacerbation of those injuries by superimposed tissue reactions.

Additional variable patterns and degrees of effects on pulmonary function are illustrated by the changes in lung volumes and flow rates that are shown in Figure 23.16. At the end of the 1.5-ATA (151-kPa) O_2 exposures, changes in lung expiratory function ranged from essentially no change in maximal midexpiratory flow rate to a 25% decrement in peak expiratory flow rate, whereas all four indices of lung inspiratory function were uniformly decreased by 22% to 23%. In contrast, at the end of the O_2 exposures at 2.0 ATA (202 kPa), decrements in three of the four measures of lung inspiratory

Table 23.2 Effects of Continuous Oxygen Exposure at 151, 202, 252 and 303 kPa (1.5, 2.0, 2.5, and 3.0 ATA) on Selected Indices of Pulmonary Function in Humans

INDICES	151 KPA (1.5 ATA) (N)	202 KPA (2.0 ATA) (N)	252 KPA (2.5 ATA) (N)	303 KPA (3.0 ATA) (N)
Duration (hours)	17.7 ± 0.8	8.8 ± 1.7	5.7 ± 0.4	3.4 ± 0.3
Measurement time	End exposure	End exposure	After exposure	After exposure
FVC	$-20.4* \pm 11.6\%$ (9)	$-21.0* \pm 14.3\%$ (14)	$-11.9* \pm 15.6\%$ (8)	$-3.4 \pm 5.2\%$ (13)
FEV_1	$-14.0* \pm 16.2\%$ (9)	$-22.2* \pm 22.0\%$ (14)	$-21.7* \pm 29.2\%$ (8)	$-6.1* \pm 5.0\%$ (13)
FEF_{25-75}	$-1.0 \pm 27.0\%$ (9)	$-19.2* \pm 32.5\%$ (14)	$-30.8* \pm 34.3\%$ (8)	$-11.8* \pm 7.5\%$ (13)
$\%\Delta Vmax_{50}$†	$-19.9* \pm 22.9\%$ (9)	$-17.6* \pm 20.7\%$ (8)	$-20.4 \pm 46.9\%$ (8)	$-18.4* \pm 14.5\%$ (5)
D_{LCO}	$-10.8* \pm 8.5\%$ (9)	$-9.7* \pm 4.6\%$ (15)	$-7.7* \pm 4.4\%$ (8)	$-1.7 \pm 9.3\%$ (11)
$(A-a) \Delta Po_2$ (mm Hg)				
Before	12.3 ± 5.4 (6)	20.6 ± 6.9 (15)	16.1 ± 2.0 (8)	NM
After	$24.7* \pm 8.3$ (6)	18.6 ± 6.8 (15)	18.9 ± 4.1 (8)	NM

Measured at the end of exposure or during early postexposure period. Values shown are percentage changes from early exposure or pre-exposure control values with the one indicated exception. Values are presented as means ± standard deviation.
  $*P < 0.05$.
    †Values expressed as actual change rather than percentage change from early exposure or pre-exposure control.
    $(A-a) \Delta Po_2$, alveolar-arterial oxygen difference on air during exercise; ATA, atmospheres absolute; D_{LCO}, lung carbon monoxide diffusing capacity; FEF_{25-75}, maximal midexpiratory flow rate; FEV_1, 1 second forced expired volume; FVC, forced vital capacity; % $\Delta Vmax_{50}$, difference in maximal expiratory flow rates on helium/oxygen and air at 50% of forced expired volume expressed as percentage of the air flow rate; NM, not measured.
    From Clark JM, Jackson RM, Lambertsen CJ, et al: Pulmonary function in men after oxygen breathing at 3.0 ATA for 3.5 h. J Appl Physiol 71:878–885, 1991; and Clark JM, Lambertsen CJ, Gelfand R, et al: Effects of prolonged oxygen exposure at 1.5, 2.0, or 2.5 ATA on pulmonary function in men (Predictive Studies V). J Appl Physiol 86:243–259, 1999, by permission.

function were relatively greater than the corresponding measures of expiratory function. A third pattern of effects is represented by observations in two subjects who had unusually large changes in pulmonary function at 1.4 hours after cessation of O_2 breathing at 2.5 ATA (252 kPa). Although average reductions in expiratory and inspiratory forced vital capacity were nearly identical, decreases in the other three indices of lung expiratory function greatly exceeded the corresponding inspiratory changes. The observed different patterns of effects are also considered to represent varying combinations of direct and indirect effects of oxygen toxicity.

Rate of Development of Pulmonary Oxygen Poisoning

At regular intervals during continuous oxygen breathing at pressures of 1.5, 2.0, 2.5, and 3.0 ATA (151, 202, 252, and 303 kPa, respectively), each subject rated symptoms of chest pain, cough, chest tightness, and dyspnea as absent (0), mild (1+), moderate (2+), or severe (3+).[116,133] Average ratings of all four symptoms were combined for each subject

group to provide estimates of pulmonary symptom intensity with respect to exposure duration at each pressure (Fig. 23.17). Smooth curves drawn through the average symptom ratings indicate that rates of symptom development increased progressively at higher levels of inspired Po_2. The curves also show that pulmonary symptoms became moderately intense by the end of the longer oxygen exposures at 1.5 and 2.0 ATA (151 and 202 kPa) but remained generally mild during the exposures at 2.5 and 3.0 ATA (252 and 303 kPa).

Concurrently with the periodic subjective assessment of symptoms, the rates of development of pulmonary oxygen poisoning at 1.5, 2.0, and 2.5 ATA (151, 202, and 252 kPa, respectively) were monitored objectively by repeated performance of flow-volume maneuvers and spirometry.[116] Pulmonary function was evaluated quantitatively only before and after the 3.5-hour exposures at 3.0 ATA (303 kPa).[133] Vital capacity was selected for quantitative comparison of toxic effects at 1.5, 2.0, and 2.5 ATA (151, 202, and 252 kPa, respectively) because it decreased progressively and significantly at all three pressures (see Fig. 23.17) and because similar effects were observed in earlier studies at lower

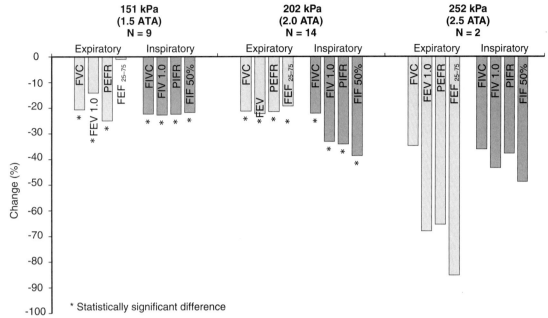

Figure 23.16 Average changes in expiratory and inspiratory lung volumes and flow rates after O_2 exposures at 1.5, 2.0, and 2.5 ATA (151, 202, and 252 kPa, respectively). Numbers of subjects at each pressure are indicated. FEF_{25-75}, maximal midexpiratory flow rate; $FEV_{1.0}$, 1 second forced expired volume; $FIF_{50\%}$, maximal inspiratory flow rate at 50% of inspired volume; $FIV_{1.0}$, 1 second forced inspired volume; FIVC, forced inspiratory vital capacity; FVC, forced vital capacity; PEFR, peak expiratory flow rate; PIFR, peak inspiratory flow rate. *$P, < 0.05$. *(From Clark JM, Lambertsen CJ, Gelfand R, et al: Effects of prolonged oxygen exposure at 1.5, 2.0, or 2.5 ATA on pulmonary function in men [Predictive Studies V]. J Appl Physiol 86:243–259, 1999, by permission.)*

pressures.[2,9] Average values of vital capacity declined more rapidly as inspired Po_2 increased from 1.5 to 2.5 ATA (151–252 kPa). Comparisons of pulmonary symptom and vital capacity curves for each pressure show that the initial decline in vital capacity consistently preceded the onset of symptoms, and that prominent decrements in vital capacity were sometimes associated with mild symptoms. As was found with neurologic manifestations of oxygen poisoning (see Fig. 23.6), the rate and magnitude of decline in vital capacity varied markedly among different individuals at the same oxygen pressure (Fig. 23.18).[83]

Rate of Recovery from Pulmonary Oxygen Poisoning

Recovery from pulmonary oxygen poisoning is a complex process that involves different rates of reversal of diverse toxic effects in different cells and tissues.[6,134] Complete recovery includes reversal of the intracellular bio-

chemical effects of oxygen toxicity together with recovery from tissue reactions to those effects. These components of reversal and recovery are expected to have different time courses, most of which cannot be measured directly. Recovery from functional deficit is likely to occur more rapidly than reversal or repair of structural damage.

Average rates of vital capacity recovery in groups of eight to nine subjects who were exposed to O_2 at 2.5, 2.0, or 1.5 ATA (252, 202, or 151 kPa, respectively) are shown in Figure 23.19.[116,135] In all three subject groups, vital capacity increased rapidly during the first 5 hours of recovery and returned to the pre-exposure control value within 15 to 30 hours. The slowest rate of recovery occurred after breathing O_2 at 1.5 ATA (151 kPa) for an average duration of 17.7 hours, but this may have been influenced by the performance of BAL in six of nine subjects at 8.5 to 10 hours of recovery.[116]

Individual variability in rates of vital capacity recovery for three subjects who breathed

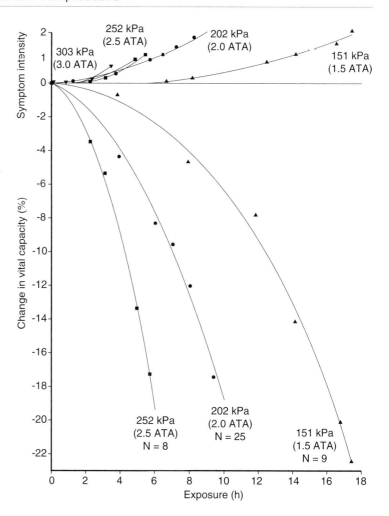

Figure 23.17 Rates of development of pulmonary symptoms and vital capacity decrements during continuous exposures to O₂ pressures of 3.0, 2.5, 2.0, and 1.5 atmospheres absolute (ATA; 303, 252, 202, and 151 kPa, respectively). Average symptom intensities were determined as described in the text. Vital capacity was not measured during O₂ exposure at 3.0 ATA (303 kPa) to allow more time for monitoring central nervous system functions.[115] Pulmonary function was evaluated 2 to 4 hours after the 3.0-ATA (303-kPa) exposures.[133] *(From Clark JM, Lambertsen CJ, Gelfand R, et al: Effects of prolonged oxygen exposure at 1.5, 2.0, or 2.5 ATA on pulmonary function in men [Predictive Studies V]. J Appl Physiol 86:243–259, 1999, by permission.)*

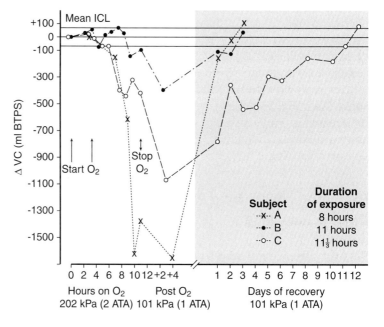

Figure 23.18 Individual variation in rates of development of, and recovery from, pulmonary oxygen poisoning. *Middle horizontal line* indicates the control value of vital capacity for each subject, and the *upper* and *lower lines* are 95% confidence limits for the subject with the widest limits. The start of O₂ breathing is adjusted on the graph to allow all three exposures to end at the same time. Note that rate of recovery is not necessarily proportional to magnitude of decrement in vital capacity. *(From Clark JM, Lambertsen CJ: Rate of development of pulmonary O₂ toxicity in man during O₂ breathing at 2.0 Ata. J Appl Physiol 30:739–752, 1971, by permission.)*

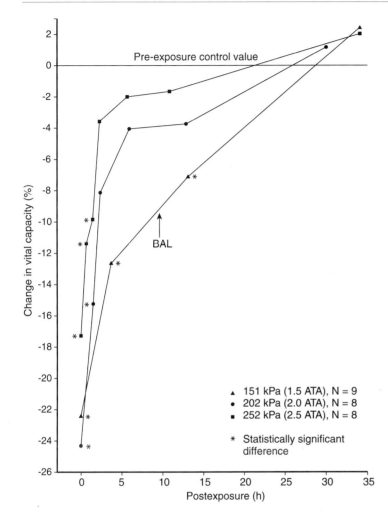

Figure 23.19 Rates of vital capacity recovery after O_2 exposure at 2.5, 2.0, and 1.5 ATA (252, 202, and 151 kPa, respectively). Average exposure durations were 5.7 hours at 2.5 ATA (252 kPa), 8.4 hours at 2.0 ATA (202 kPa), and 17.7 hours at 1.5 ATA (151 kPa). Lung volumes and flow rates were measured repeatedly during air breathing at 1.0 ATA (101 kPa) after termination of O_2 exposure. Pre-exposure control values were also measured at 1.0 ATA (101 kPa). Statistically significant decrements are indicated by an *asterisk. (From Clark JM, Lambertsen CJ, Gelfand R, et al: Effects of prolonged oxygen exposure at 1.5, 2.0, or 2.5 ATA on pulmonary function in men [Predictive Studies V]. J Appl Physiol 86:243–259, 1999, by permission.)*

O_2 at 2.0 ATA (202 kPa) for 8 to 11.3 hours is shown in Figure 23.18. The longest recovery period of 11 to 12 days occurred after an 11.3-hour exposure. A postexposure recovery period of several weeks was reported for one subject who breathed 0.98 ATA (99 kPa) O_2 for 74 hours.[136] The period of time required for complete recovery of vital capacity appears to be determined as much by the duration of the preceding exposure as by the magnitude of decrement. Oxygen exposures that are prolonged sufficiently to cause edema or other tissue reactions are likely to require longer recovery periods for complete resolution to occur.[134]

Of all the indices of pulmonary mechanical and gas exchange function that were measured after the prolonged oxygen exposures at 2.0 and 2.5 ATA (202 and 252 kPa), carbon monoxide diffusing capacity was the slowest to recover (Fig. 23.20).[116] Small but statistically significant decrements of about 6% to 11% persisted for at least 8 to 9 days. Extended follow-up measurements obtained from 2 weeks to 5 months after the oxygen exposures confirmed that average carbon monoxide diffusing capacity values had returned fully or to within 2% of the pre-exposure control values. Pulmonary diffusing capacity for carbon monoxide appears to be a sensitive index of complete recovery from pulmonary oxygen poisoning.

A single report claims that cumulative effects of pulmonary oxygen toxicity may be produced by a series of daily exposures that individually cause no measurable changes in pulmonary function.[137] In a group of 20 patients with no previous lung disease and no current smokers, each therapy consisted of three

Figure 23.20 Pulmonary diffusing capacity for carbon monoxide after O_2 exposure at 3.0, 2.5, 2.0, and 1.5 atmospheres absolute (ATA; 303, 252, 202, and 151 kPa, respectively). Average changes in carbon monoxide (CO) diffusing capacity relative to pre-exposure control values are shown, and statistically significant differences are indicated by an *asterisk*. Subsequent measurements of diffusing capacity in all subjects who were available for extended follow-up equaled or exceeded the pre-exposure control value. *(From Clark JM, Lambertsen CJ, Gelfand R, et al: Effects of prolonged oxygen exposure at 1.5, 2.0, or 2.5 ATA on pulmonary function in men [Predictive Studies V]. J Appl Physiol 86:243–259, 1999, by permission.)*

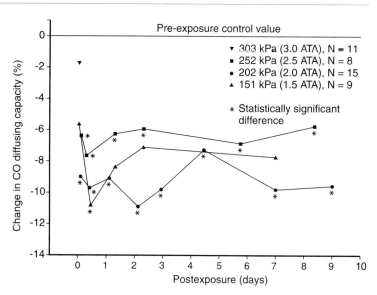

30-minute O_2 periods at 2.4 ATA (242 kPa) separated by two 5-minute air breaks. At the end of the therapy series given over 21 consecutive days, there were statistically significant, but quantitatively small, changes in lung expiratory function. Although the observed changes were clinically insignificant, they were still present 4 weeks later. Similar changes in lung expiratory function were not found in a different group of 18 patients that included smokers and had an average carbon monoxide diffusing capacity that was 81% of a normal reference population.[138] This group received 30 treatments over a period of 6 weeks. Each therapy consisted of 90 minutes of continuous O_2 breathing at 2.4 ATA (242 kPa). Additional measurements are needed to investigate the possibility of detectable cumulative effects from current therapy protocols.

Possible Interactions of Neurologic and Pulmonary Effects of Oxygen Toxicity

Two of eight subjects who breathed O_2 for 5 to 6 hours at 2.5 ATA (252 kPa) had unusually large changes in pulmonary mechanical function with abrupt decreases in lung volumes and midexpiratory flow rates during the last 2 hours of exposure, continued decline in lung expiratory function during the first post-

exposure hour, and nearly complete recovery over the next 3 to 4 hours (Fig. 23.21).[116] A similar pattern of changes in vital capacity was observed previously in one of the subjects studied during and after O_2 breathing at 2.0 ATA (202 kPa) (see Fig. 23.18).

The prominent magnitudes of the observed changes in lung volumes and flow rates, as well as their rapid rates of onset and reversal, are consistent with an exacerbation of localized manifestations of pulmonary oxygen poisoning by interaction with concurrent effects of neurologic oxygen toxicity. The observed large decreases in pulmonary mechanical function could have been caused by vagally induced bronchoconstriction, which is consistent with the sensation of chest tightness that was experienced by these subjects.[116] Results consistent with augmentation of vagal influences on cardiac function during O_2 breathing at 2.0, 2.5, or 3.0 ATA (202, 252, and 303 kPa, respectively) were also found in some individuals.[139]

DEFINITION OF OXYGEN TOLERANCE IN HUMANS

Human tolerance to oxygen toxicity must be defined over a range of useful pressures to derive maximal benefit from therapeutic applications of hyperoxia while avoiding concurrent adverse effects. Using decrease

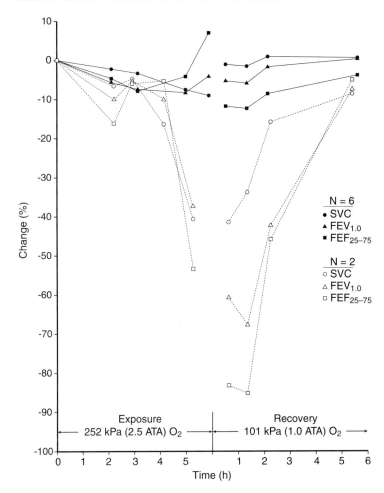

Figure 23.21 Pulmonary function changes during and after O_2 breathing at 2.5 atmospheres absolute (ATA; 252 kPa) for 5 to 6 hours. Average changes in slow vital capacity (SVC), 1-second forced expired volume ($FEV_{1.0}$), and maximal midexpiratory flow rate (FEF_{25-75}) for two subjects who had unusually large deficits are compared with corresponding values in six other subjects who had much smaller changes. Control measurements at 2.5 ATA (252 kPa) were obtained during early O_2 exposure. Pre-exposure control measurements at 1.0 ATA (101 kPa) were used for the postexposure data. *(From Clark JM, Lambertsen CJ, Gelfand R, et al: Effects of prolonged oxygen exposure at 1.5, 2.0, or 2.5 ATA on pulmonary function in men [Predictive Studies V]. J Appl Physiol 86:243–259, 1999, by permission.)*

in vital capacity as an index of pulmonary oxygen poisoning in conjunction with the empiric observation that the oxygen pressure-exposure duration relation for a specific manifestation of oxygen poisoning can be described by a rectangular hyperbola (see Fig. 23.5), investigators derived predictive curves to provide practical guidelines for applications of hyperoxia in therapy and diving.[2,9,140] The hyperbolic curves shown in Figure 23.22 describe oxygen pressure-exposure duration relations for average vital capacity decrements ranging from 2% to 20%. With vertical and horizontal asymptotes at zero time and 0.5 ATA (50 kPa) O_2, these initial pulmonary oxygen tolerance curves were derived from vital capacity data in 11 subjects exposed to O_2 at 2.0 ATA (202 kPa),[83] 4 subjects at 0.98 ATA (99 kPa),[136] and 6 subjects at 0.78 to 0.88 ATA (79–89 kPa).[141]

The vertical asymptote at zero time implies that onset and progression of pulmonary oxygen poisoning are immediate at an infinitely high oxygen pressure. Selection of 0.5 ATA (50 kPa) as the horizontal oxygen pressure asymptote was based on the absence of detectable changes in vital capacity during exposure to the oxygen pressure-exposure duration conditions summarized in Figure 23.23.

The data points on the curves in Figure 23.22 represent the maximum durations for the continuous oxygen exposures of Predictive Studies V.[116,133] Vital capacity data from 48-hour exposures to air at 5.0 ATA (505 kPa) (1.05 ATA or 106 kPa O_2) performed by Eckenhoff and colleagues[142] have also become available since the original tolerance curve derivation. Revision of the early pulmonary oxygen tolerance curves based on integration of an expanded dataset

PREDICTED PULMONARY OXYGEN TOLERANCE IN MAN

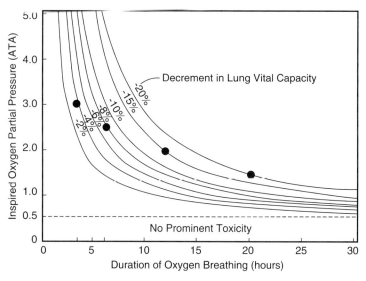

Figure 23.22 Predicted pulmonary oxygen tolerance in healthy men. *(From Clark JM: Pulmonary limits of oxygen tolerance in man. Exp Lung Res 14(suppl):897–910, 1988, by permission.)*

for open literature publication currently is in progress.

Unit Pulmonary Toxic Dose Concept

Many therapeutic applications of hyperoxia involve exposures to more than one oxygen pressure. Because oxygen poisoning occurs more rapidly at higher pressures, the same exposure duration does not cause equivalent degrees of intoxication at each pressure. Rather than calculating total oxygen dose as a sum of different oxygen pressures and exposure durations, this process has been facilitated by expressing exposures to different oxygen pressures in terms of an equivalent exposure to a standard reference level of hyperoxia. The "unit pulmonary toxic dose" concept was designed to express any toxic oxygen dose in terms of the number of minutes required to produce an equivalent degree of pulmonary effect during exposure to O_2 at 1.0 ATA (101 kPa).[143,144] Pending publication of the revised analysis of pulmonary oxygen tolerance, the numeric unit pulmonary toxic dose value for a given oxygen pressure–exposure duration condition may change, but the concept will remain the same.

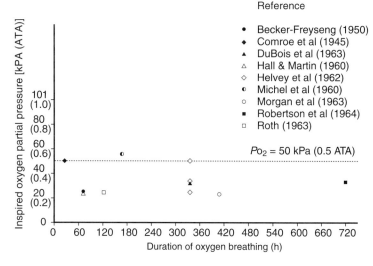

Figure 23.23 Pulmonary oxygen tolerance studies in healthy men that detected no objective evidence of pulmonary oxygen poisoning. Each symbol represents the average conditions of a separate study. Specific citations and numbers of subjects in each study are listed in a previous review.[2] *(From Clark JM, Thom SR: Oxygen under pressure. In: Brubakk AO, Neuman TS [eds]: Bennett and Elliott's Physiology and Medicine of Diving, 5th ed. Philadelphia, WB Saunders Company, 2003, pp 358–418, by permission.)*

Alternative mathematic descriptions of oxygen tolerance data have been proposed by Harabin and coworkers[145] using a nonlinear least-squares analysis with a simplified linear description of decrease in vital capacity, and by Arieli and colleagues[146] using a power expression to describe vital capacity changes. These alternatives have been discussed briefly in a previous review.[2]

Definition of Neurologic Oxygen Tolerance

The observed progressive decrements in the timing component of ventilation during O_2 breathing at 1.5, 2.0, 2.5, and 3.0 ATA (151, 202, 252, and 303 kPa, respectively) (see Fig. 23.11) provide an objective preconvulsive index of neurologic oxygen poisoning. Applying the same principles that were used to define pulmonary oxygen tolerance, the oxygen pressure–exposure duration relation for a specific neurologic effect of oxygen toxicity can be described by a rectangular hyperbola with vertical and horizontal asymptotes. Zero time is again selected as the vertical asymptote on the assumption that neurologic effects will occur immediately at an infinitely high oxygen pressure. The horizontal asymptote was determined analytically by plotting the slopes describing rates of decrease in T_I/T_T (see Fig. 23.11)

against the corresponding O_2 exposure pressures (Fig. 23.24) and extrapolating the resulting linear regression to a slope value of zero at 1.3 ATA (131 kPa), implying that T_I/T_T would remain stable at lower O_2 pressures.

Using a 5% decrease in T_I/T_T as a specific degree of toxic effect, the hyperbolic curve shown in Figure 23.25 predicts oxygen pressure–exposure duration relations that would produce this early preconvulsive manifestation of neurologic oxygen poisoning. With the selected asymptotes, location of the curve is determined by four data points obtained from the regression equations shown in Figure 23.11. For comparison with the neurologic curve, a pulmonary oxygen tolerance curve based on a 5% decrease in vital capacity is also shown in Figure 23.25. With asymptotes at zero time and 0.5 ATA (50 kPa), location of the pulmonary curve is determined by data points at 2.5, 2.0, and 1.5 ATA (252, 202, and 151 kPa, respectively) (see Fig. 23.17) and at 1.05 ATA (106 kPa) from Eckenhoff and colleagues.[142]

Limitations of Oxygen Tolerance Predictions

It is important to recognize that the curves in Figure 23.25 represent average responses to a toxic stress for which individual responses are

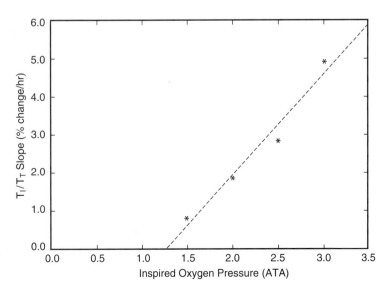

Figure 23.24 Derivation of a horizontal asymptote for neurologic oxygen tolerance curves. The inspiratory time divided by total breath period (T_I/T_T) slopes were obtained from the linear regressions shown in Figure 23.11. ATA, atmospheres absolute. *(From Gelfand R, Lambertsen CJ, Clark JM: Ventilatory effects of prolonged hyperoxia at pressures of 1.5-3.0 ATA. Aviat Space Environ Med 77:801–810, 2006.)*

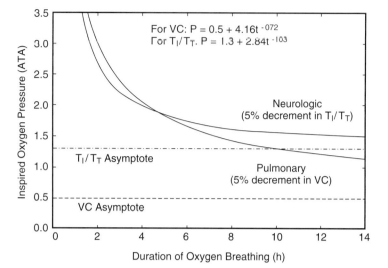

For VC: $P = 0.5 + 4.16t^{-.072}$
For T_I/T_T. $P = 1.3 + 2.84t^{-.103}$

Neurologic
(5% decrement in T_I/T_T)

T_I/T_T Asymptote

Pulmonary
(5% decrement in VC)

VC Asymptote

Inspired Oxygen Pressure (ATA)

Duration of Oxygen Breathing (h)

Figure 23.25 Comparison of neurologic and pulmonary oxygen tolerance in healthy men. ATA, atmospheres absolute; T_I/T_T, inspiratory time divided by total breath period; VC, vital capacity.

known to vary widely. Individual oxygen tolerance may also be affected by coexisting disease and drug influences. The curves are based on data obtained from single exposures of healthy subjects. Possible cumulative effects from repeated exposures have not been studied extensively. Even for single exposures, the curves represent conditions that produced measurable toxic effects. Although it would be justifiable to approach or even exceed the described limits for life-threatening conditions such as gas gangrene or severe decompression sickness, elective therapy protocols should stay as far to the left of the curves as possible while achieving desired therapeutic effects. Despite these reservations, HBOT has a high therapeutic index with a favorable risk-to-benefit ratio when it is used appropriately. In addition, the curves shown in Figure 23.25 were derived from data obtained during continuous oxygen exposures and, therefore, do not reflect the known amelioration of adverse effects by intermittent periods of breathing chamber air or a normoxic gas mixture (see later).

MODIFICATION OF OXYGEN TOLERANCE

Studies in animals have shown that the onset and rate of progression of oxygen poisoning can be influenced by a variety of conditions, procedures, and drugs.[9] Although few of these agents have been studied in humans exposed to hyperoxia, the animal data indicate that febrile patients or those with increased levels of catecholamines, adrenocortical hormones, or thyroid hormones may have an increased susceptibility to oxygen poisoning. The adverse effects of arterial hypercapnia on neurologic oxygen tolerance are well documented in humans and in animals.[9,84] Potential sources of CO_2 accumulation in a clinical setting include inadequate ventilation of an oxygen hood, excessive dead space in the oxygen delivery system, and narcotic respiratory depression in the patient. Patients who have chronic lung disease with hypercapnia may be at risk for development of seizures and pulmonary barotrauma.

Any patient who has a preexisting disorder or condition that can cause seizures may also have an increased susceptibility to oxygen-induced convulsions. In a group of 900 patients who received HBOT for carbon monoxide poisoning, the overall seizure incidence rate was 1.8%.[147] When the data were analyzed on the basis of maximum treatment pressure, the incidence rate ranged from 0.3% at 2.4 ATA (242 kPa) (N = 300) to 2.5% at 2.8 to 3.0 ATA (283–303 kPa) (N = 600). In patients who have no known predisposing conditions, the seizure incidence rate varies from an early estimate of 0.01% at treatment pressures of 2.0 to 3.0 ATA (202–303 kPa)[148,149] to more recent estimates of 0.015% (107,264 therapies), 0.030% (20,328 therapies), and 0.035%

(11,376 therapies) in three large surveys of patients treated at oxygen pressures of 2.4 to 2.6 ATA (242–263 kPa).[150] In a group of 998 patients who received a total of 2166 therapies for decompression sickness at peak pressures of 2.6 to 2.9 ATA (263–293 kPa), a seizure incidence rate of 0.6% was reported.[151]

Extension of Oxygen Tolerance

Several potential means for extension of oxygen tolerance[134] were discussed in a symposium[152] dedicated to that topic. To date, the only agent or procedure that has been demonstrated to be effective in humans is the interruption of oxygen breathing by periodic reduction of the inspired P_{O_2}. The practical value of this procedure was recognized in World War II field operations in which it was observed that a self-contained oxygen diver could reverse early signs of neurologic oxygen poisoning by ascending to a shallower depth for a period before returning to deeper water.[134] Subsequent studies in guinea pigs demonstrated that early manifestations of oxygen toxicity during O_2 breathing at 3.0 ATA (303 kPa) could be delayed significantly by alternating 30-minute periods of oxygen breathing with 10-minute

periods of normoxia (7% O_2).[153] In experiments designed to determine efficient methods for oxygen tolerance extension, Hall[154] evaluated many additional patterns of intermittent oxygen exposure in guinea pigs exposed to O_2 at 3.0 ATA (303 kPa). Selected results of the guinea pig experiments,[154] in conjunction with a study of human pulmonary tolerance to continuous O_2 breathing at 2.0 ATA (202 kPa),[83] were incorporated into the design of a related human study[155] that demonstrated that pulmonary tolerance to O_2 breathing at 2.0 ATA (202 kPa) could be more than doubled by alternating 20-minute O_2 exposure periods with 5-minute normoxic intervals (Fig. 23.26).

Harabin and coworkers[156] investigated the possibility that extension of oxygen tolerance by intermittent exposure may be related to increased activities of antioxidant enzymes. Guinea pigs and rats were exposed either continuously to O_2 at 2.8 ATA (283 kPa) or intermittently on a schedule that alternated 10-minute oxygen periods with 2.5-minute periods of air breathing (0.56 ATA or 56 kPa O_2). Activities of SOD, catalase, and glutathione peroxidase in the brain and lung of both species were measured at equivalent durations of continuous and intermittent oxygen exposure. Although the expected delay of

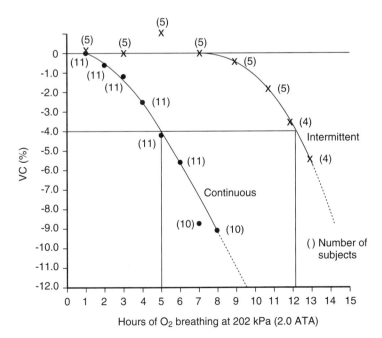

Figure 23.26 Extension of pulmonary oxygen tolerance at 2.0 atmospheres absolute (ATA; 202 kPa) in healthy men. The curve showing rate of decrease in vital capacity (VC) during continuous O_2 breathing was obtained from Clark and Lambertsen.[83] The curve for intermittent O_2 exposure was adapted from Hendricks and colleagues,[155] and the indicated duration of oxygen breathing represents a summation of all the intermittent, 20-minute O_2 periods. *(From Clark JM, Thom SR: Oxygen under pressure. In: Brubakk AO, Neuman TS [eds]: Bennett and Elliott's Physiology and Medicine of Diving, 5th ed. Philadelphia, WB Saunders Company, 2003, pp 358–418, by permission.)*

convulsions and lengthening of survival times were observed, concurrently with changes in antioxidant enzyme activities, the patterns of enzyme changes in both species were complex and did not correlate with the associated gains in oxygen tolerance.

Optimization of Oxygen Tolerance Extension by Intermittent Exposure

To identify effective intermittent exposure patterns for selective evaluation in human subjects, researchers exposed rats to systematically varied patterns of intermittent exposure at 4.0, 2.0, and 1.5 ATA (404, 202, and 151 kPa, respectively).[79] Oxygen exposure periods of 20, 60, or 120 minutes were each alternated with normoxic intervals whose durations were selected to provide oxygen/normoxia ratios of 4:1, 2:1, and 1:1 at each pressure. Hypothetically, it was expected that toxic effects of an excessively long oxygen period would not rapidly reverse during the subsequent normoxic interval. It was also anticipated that brief normoxic intervals would not allow adequate reversal of toxic effects from even relatively short oxygen periods.

Median survival times for all of the intermittent exposure patterns that were evaluated at 1.5, 2.0, and 4.0 ATA (151, 202, and 404 kPa, respectively) are plotted against durations of the corresponding normoxic intervals in Figure 23.27. In general, there was a nearly linear increase in survival time as the normoxic interval was lengthened, whereas the oxygen period remained constant at each pressure. One exception to the general rule occurred at 4.0 ATA (404 kPa) where survival time for the 120:30 oxygen/normoxia pattern was 12% shorter than the control survival time for continuous exposure. Typically, rats died during a 30-minute normoxic interval when the preceding 120-minute oxygen periods produced enough lung damage to cause lethal hypoxemia on return to a normoxic atmosphere. Additional exceptions occurred at both 4.0 and 2.0 ATA (404 and 202 kPa) where the 20:5 pattern was totally ineffective, presumably because the 5-minute normoxic interval did not allow adequate recovery.

During intermittent oxygen exposure at 1.5 ATA (151 kPa), however, none of the exceptions that occurred at higher pressures was observed (see Fig. 23.27). At this pressure, where oxygen poisoning would be

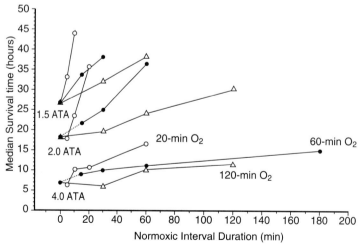

Figure 23.27 Relations of median survival times to normoxic interval durations for O_2 periods of 20 (open circles), 60 (solid circles), and 120 minutes (open triangles) at 1.5, 2.0, and 4.0 atmospheres absolute (ATA; 151, 202, and 404 kPa). Dashed lines in the curves for 60-minute O_2 periods at 2.0 and 4.0 ATA reflect that a 5-minute normoxic interval was not evaluated under those conditions. In general, there was a nearly linear increase in survival time as normoxic interval was lengthened, whereas the O_2 period remained constant. (From Clark JM, Lambertsen CJ, Gelfand R, Troxel AB: Optimization of oxygen tolerance extension in rats by intermittent exposure. J Appl Physiol 100:869–879, 2006, by permission.)

expected to develop more slowly, equivalent survival time extensions were obtained with the 120:30, 60:15, and 20:5 exposure patterns (Fig. 23.28). An exception that did occur at 1.5 ATA (151 kPa) was the observation that the 20:10 pattern was significantly more effective than either the 120:60 or 60:30 pattern. In addition, the combination of 120-minute oxygen periods with recovery intervals of equal duration produced no deaths in an exposure that was continued for 60 oxygen hours or 120 total hours. At the time of discontinuation, the rats did not appear to be in a preterminal state at an exposure duration that already represented a 126% increment in median survival time.

Berghage and Borkat[157] have proposed that the rate of development of oxygen poisoning during intermittent exposure is equivalent to that which occurs during continuous exposure to a constant oxygen pressure that is defined as a time-weighted average of the alternating oxygen and normoxic exposure periods. This hypothesis was examined by calculating time-weighted average oxygen pressures for each of the intermittent exposure patterns that were evaluated at 4.0, 2.0, and 1.5 ATA (404, 202, and 151 kPa), and then comparing the observed median survival time for each pattern to the predicted survival time for continuous exposure to the corresponding time-weighted average Po_2 (Fig. 23.29). Predicted survival times were determined by interpolation on the regression line fitted to observed survival times for continuous exposures at oxygen pressures of 4.0, 3.0, 2.0, 1.5, and 1.0 ATA (404, 303, 202, 151, and 101 kPa, respectively). Although many of the median survival times for intermittent exposure fall on or near the line for continuous exposure, many other intermittent exposure patterns, especially those performed at 4.0 ATA (404 kPa), produced survival time extensions that exceeded the predictions based on continuous exposures to the corresponding time-weighted average oxygen pressures.

Quantitative differences between observed and predicted survival times are summarized in Table 23.3 for all of the intermittent exposure patterns except for two in which no deaths occurred. The overall average deviation from the regression line in Figure 23.29 for

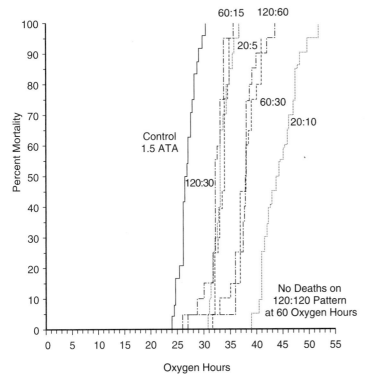

Figure 23.28 Survival time responses to intermittent exposure patterns at 1.5 atmospheres absolute (ATA; 151 kPa). The *solid, continuous exposure curve* represents survival times in 24 rats. Each intermittent exposure contained 20 rats. Each step indicates the death of one or more rats, plotted against accumulated O_2 hours. Survival times for rats that died during a normoxic interval are plotted at the end of the previous O_2 period. All 20 rats remained alive when the 120:120 intermittent exposure pattern was stopped at 60 O_2 hours. *(From Clark JM, Lambertsen CJ, Gelfand R, Troxel AB: Optimization of oxygen tolerance extension in rats by intermittent exposure. J Appl Physiol 100:869–879, 2006, by permission.)*

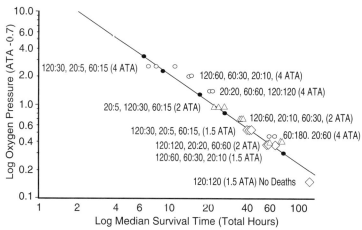

Figure 23.29 Log median survival times for continuous and intermittent exposures to O₂ pressures of 4.0, 3.0, 2.0, 1.5, and 1.0 atmospheres absolute (ATA; 404, 303, 202, 151, and 101 kPa, respectively), plotted against log O₂ pressure (ATA -0.7). The regression line is fitted to 5 points *(closed circles)* that represent survival times for continuous exposures to O₂ pressures of 4.0, 3.0, 2.0, 1.5, and 1.0 ATA. Inspired oxygen pressures for intermittent exposures are calculated as time-weighted averages.[157] Median survival times for intermittent exposures at 4.0, 2.0, and 1.5 ATA are represented, respectively, by *open circles, triangles,* and *diamonds. (From Clark JM, Lambertsen CJ, Gelfand R, Troxel AB: Optimization of oxygen tolerance extension in rats by intermittent exposure. J Appl Physiol 100:869–879, 2006, by permission.)*

the six patterns at 1.5 ATA (151 kPa) in which deaths occurred was −2%. The average deviation at 2.0 ATA (202 kPa) for the nine patterns in which deaths occurred was 12%, whereas the same patterns at 4.0 ATA (404 kPa) had an average deviation of 28%. Exclusion of the differences obtained for the 20:5 and 120:30 patterns at 2.0 and 4.0 ATA (202 and 404 kPa) results in average deviations of 16% and 38%, respectively, for the remaining seven patterns at each pressure. These results are consistent with the conclusion that some protective

Table 23.3 Percentage Change in Median Survival Time during Intermittent Oxygen Exposure at 4.0, 2.0, and 1.5 ATA (404, 202, and 151 kPa, Respectively) (with Respect to Interpolated Value on Regression Line for Continuous Exposure)

OXYGEN PERIOD		NORMOXIC INTERVAL (MIN)							
ATA	**MINUTES**	**5**	**10**	**15**	**20**	**30**	**60**	**120**	**180**
4.0	20	−4*	42		36		35		
	60			34		40	37		20
	120					−16	39	40	
2.0	20	−4	11		26				
	60			15		17	28		†
	120					3	10	5	
1.5	20	0	7						
	60			2		−7			
	120					−4	−9		†

*Percentage change in median survival time (total hours). Time-weighted average oxygen pressure calculated for each intermittent exposure pattern (see Fig. 23.29).
  †No deaths.
  ATA, atmospheres absolute.
  From Clark JM, Lambertsen CJ, Gelfand R, Troxel AB: Optimization of oxygen tolerance extension in rats by intermittent exposure. J Appl Physiol 100:869–879, 2006, by permission.

influence is activated more effectively by intermittent exposures to greater oxygen pressures. The observed differences in response to intermittent oxygen exposure at pressures of 1.5, 2.0, and 4.0 ATA (151, 202, and 404 kPa) also resemble the development of thermotolerance in which induction of a protective response requires a threshold level of stress and the magnitude of protection is proportional to the severity of the inducing stress.[158]

No direct evidence currently exists that heat shock or oxidation-specific stress proteins are involved in oxygen tolerance extension by intermittent exposure. However, the previously reviewed examples of cross-protection against oxidant stress provided by hyperthermic preconditioning of cultured human umbilical vein endothelial cells[70] or intact rats,[71] as well as the failure to find evidence for involvement of classical antioxidant enzymes,[156] indicate that this may be a fruitful area for future studies. Although intermittent exposure to 4.0 ATA (404 kPa) O_2 is not practical for therapeutic purposes, investigation of the biochemical basis for the increased oxygen tolerance associated with brief exposures to this Po_2 may ultimately provide more effective methods than those currently available for optimization of oxygen tolerance extension by intermittent exposure.

REFERENCES

1. Plafki C, Peters P, Almeling M, et al: Complications and side effects of hyperbaric oxygen therapy. Aviat Space Environ Med 71:119-124, 2000.
2. Clark JM, Thom SR: Oxygen under pressure. In: Brubakk AO, Neuman TS (eds): Bennett and Elliott's Physiology and Medicine of Diving, 5th ed. Philadelphia, WB Saunders Company, 2003, pp 358-418.
3. Freeman BA, Crapo JD: Biology of disease: Free radicals and tissue injury. Lab Invest 47:412-426, 1982.
4. Fridovich I, Freeman B: Antioxidant defenses in the lung. Annu Rev Physiol 48:693-702, 1986.
5. Lambertsen CJ: Effects of oxygen at high partial pressure. In: Fenn WO, Rahn H (eds): Handbook of Physiology, Section 3: Respiration, Vol II. Washington, DC, American Physiological Society, 1965, pp 1027-1046.
6. Lambertsen CJ: Effects of hyperoxia on organs and their tissues. In: Robin ED (ed): Extrapulmonary Manifestations of Respiratory Disease. Lung Biology in Health and Disease, Vol 8. New York, Marcel Dekker, 1978, pp 239-303.
7. Clark JM: The toxicity of oxygen. Am Rev Resp Dis 110:40-50, 1974.
8. Bean JW: Effects of oxygen at high pressure. Physiol Rev 25:1-147, 1945.
9. Clark JM, Lambertsen CJ: Pulmonary oxygen toxicity: A review. Pharmacol Rev 23:37-133, 1971.
10. Donald KW: Oxygen and the Diver. Harley Swan, United Kingdom, The SPA Ltd, 1992.
11. Beehler CC: Oxygen and the eye. Surv Ophthalmol 9:549-560, 1964.
12. Nichols CW, Lambertsen CJ: Effects of high oxygen pressures on the eye. N Engl J Med 281:25-30, 1969.
13. Mengel CE, Kann HE Jr, Lewis AM, Horton B: Mechanisms of in vivo hemolysis induced by hyperoxia. Aerosp Med 35:857-860, 1964.
14. Larkin EC, Adams JD, Williams WT, Duncan DM: Hematologic responses to hypobaric hyperoxia. Am J Physiol 223:431-437, 1972.
15. Hess RT, Menzel DB: Effect of dietary antioxidant level and oxygen exposure on the fine structure of the proximal convoluted tubules. Aerosp Med 42:646-649, 1971.
16. Resnick JS, Brown DM, Vernier RL: Oxygen toxicity in fetal organ culture. I. The developing kidney. Lab Invest 28:437-445, 1973.
17. Caulfield JB, Shelton RW, Burke JF: Cytotoxic effects of oxygen on striated muscle. Arch Pathol 94:127-132, 1972.
18. Schaffner F, Felig P: Changes in hepatic structure in rats produced by breathing pure oxygen. J Cell Biol 27:505-517, 1965.
19. Schaffner F, Roberts DK, Ginn FL, Ulvedal F: Electron microscopy of monkey liver after exposure of animals to pure oxygen atmosphere. Proc Soc Exp Biol Med 121:1200-1203, 1966.
20. Bean JW, Johnson PC: Adrenocortical response to single and repeated exposure to oxygen at high pressure. Am J Physiol 179:410-414, 1954.
21. Edstrom JE, Rockert H: The effect of oxygen at high pressure on the histology of the central nervous system and sympathetic and endocrine cells. Acta Physiol Scand 55:255-263, 1962.
22. Thet LA: Repair of oxygen-induced lung injury. In: Taylor AE, Matalon S, Ward P (eds): Physiology of Oxygen Radicals. Bethesda, MD, American Physiological Society, 1986, pp 87-108.
23. Balentine JD: Pathology of Oxygen Toxicity. New York, Academic Press, 1982.
24. Gerschman R, Gilbert DL, Nye SW, et al: Oxygen poisoning and x-irradiation: A mechanism in common. Science 119:623-626, 1954.
25. Gerschman R: Biological effects of oxygen. In: Dickens F, Neil E (eds): Oxygen in the Animal Organism. New York, Macmillan, 1964, pp 475-494.
26. Fridovich I: Superoxide anion radical ($O_2^{-}\cdot$), superoxide dismutases, and related matters. J Biol Chem 272:18515-18517, 1997.
27. McCord JM, Fridovich I: The biology and pathology of oxygen radicals. Ann Intern Med 89:122-127, 1978.
28. Fisher AB: Intracellular production of oxygen-derived free radicals. In: Halliwell B (ed): Oxygen Radicals and Tissue Injury. Bethesda, MD, Federation of American Societies for Experimental Biology, 1988, pp 34-39.

29. Jamieson D: Oxygen toxicity and reactive oxygen metabolites in mammals. Free Radic Biol Med 7:87-108, 1989.

30. Fisher AB, Forman HJ: Oxygen utilization and toxicity in the lungs. In: Fishman AP, Fisher AB (eds): Handbook of Physiology: The Respiratory System. Washington, DC, American Physiological Society, 1983, pp 231-251.

31. Fisher AB, Bassett DJP, Forman HJ: Oxygen toxicity of the lung: Biochemical aspects. In: Fishman AP, Renkin EM (eds): Pulmonary Edema. Bethesda, MD, American Physiological Society, 1979, pp 207-216.

32. Beckman JS, Koppenol WH: Nitric oxide, superoxide, and peroxynitrite: The good, the bad, and the ugly. Am J Physiol 271:C1424-C1437, 1996.

33. Gow A, Duran D, Thom SR, Ischiropoulos H: Carbon dioxide enhancement of peroxynitrite-mediated protein tyrosine nitration. Arch Biochem Biophys 333:42-48, 1996.

34. Squadrito GL, Pryor WA: Oxidative chemistry of nitric oxide: The roles of superoxide, peroxynitrite, and carbon dioxide. Free Radic Biol Med 25:392-403, 1998.

35. Shasby DM, Fox RB, Harada RN, Repine JE: Reduction of the edema of acute hyperoxic lung injury by granulocyte depletion. J Appl Physiol 52:1237-1244, 1982.

36. Weiss SJ, LoBuglio AF: Phagocyte-generated oxygen metabolites and cellular injury. Lab Invest 47:5-18, 1982.

37. Barry BE, Crapo JD: Patterns of accumulation of platelets and neutrophils in rat lungs during exposure to 100% and 85% oxygen. Am Rev Respir Dis 132:548-555, 1985.

38. Crapo JD, Barry BE, Foscue HA, Shelburne J: Structural and biochemical changes in rat lungs occurring during exposures to lethal and adaptive doses of oxygen. Am Rev Respir Dis 122:123-143, 1980.

39. Fox RB, Hoidal JR, Brown DM, Repine JE: Pulmonary inflammation due to oxygen toxicity: Involvement of chemotactic factors and polymorphonuclear leukocytes. Am Rev Respir Dis 123:521-523, 1981.

40. Crapo JD: Morphologic changes in pulmonary oxygen toxicity. Annu Rev Physiol 48:721-731, 1986.

41. Repine JE, Cheronis JC, Rodell TC, et al: Pulmonary oxygen toxicity and ischemia-reperfusion injury. A mechanism in common involving xanthine oxidase and neutrophils. Am Rev Respir Dis 136:483-485, 1987.

42. Kovachich GB, Mishra OP: Lipid peroxidation in rat brain cortical slices as measured by the thiobarbituric acid test. J Neurochem 35:1449-1452, 1980.

43. Dirks RC, Faiman MD: Free radical formation and lipid peroxidation in rat and mouse cerebral cortex slices exposed to high oxygen pressure. Brain Res 248:355-360, 1982.

44. Kovachich GB, Mishra OP: Partial inactivation of Na, K-ATPase in cortical brain slices incubated in normal Krebs-Ringer phosphate medium at 1 and at 10 atm oxygen pressures. J Neurochem 36:333-335, 1981.

45. Jerrett SA, Jefferson D, Mengel CE: Seizures, H_2O_2 formation and lipid peroxides in brain during exposure to oxygen under high pressure. Aerosp Med 44:40-44, 1973.

46. Becker NH, Galvin JF: Effect of oxygen-rich atmospheres on cerebral lipid peroxides. Aeromed Acta 33:985-987, 1962.

47. Zaleska MM, Floyd RA: Regional lipid peroxidation in rat brain in vitro: Possible role of endogenous iron. Neurochem Res 10:397-410, 1985.

48. Arai H, Kogure K, Sugioka K, Nakano M: Importance of two iron-reducing systems in lipid peroxidation of rat brain: Implications for oxygen toxicity in the central nervous system. Biochem Int 14:741-749, 1987.

49. Nishiki K, Jamieson D, Oshino N, Chance B: Oxygen toxicity in the perfused rat liver and lung under hyperbaric conditions. Biochem J 160:343-355, 1976.

50. Freeman BA, Topolosky MK, Crapo JD: Hyperoxia increases oxygen radical production in rat lung homogenates. Arch Biochem Biophys 216:477-484, 1982.

51. Januszkiewicz AJ, Faiman MD: The effect of in vivo hyperoxic exposure on the release of endogenous histamine from the rat isolated perfused lung. Toxicol Appl Pharmacol 72:134-141, 1984.

52. Webster NR, Toothill C, Cowen PN: Tissue responses to hyperoxia. Biochem Pathol Br J Anaesth 59:760-771, 1987.

53. Smith LJ, Sommers E, Hunt CE, Pachman L: Hyperoxic lung injury in mice: A possible protective role for prostacyclin. J Lab Clin Med 108:479-488, 1986.

54. Smith LJ, Shamsuddin M, Anderson J, Hsueh W: Hyperoxic lung damage in mice: Appearance and bioconversion of peptide leukotrienes. J Appl Physiol 64:944-951, 1988.

55. Taniguchi H, Taki F, Takagi K, et al: The role of leukotriene B4 in the genesis of oxygen toxicity in the lung. Am Rev Respir Dis 133:805-808, 1986.

56. Ara J, Przedborski S, Naini AB, et al: Inactivation of tyrosine hydroxylase by nitration following exposure to peroxynitrite and 1-methyl-4-phenyl-1,2,3,6-tetrahydropyridine (MPTP). Proc Natl Acad Sci U S A 95:7659-7663, 1998.

57. Davies KJ: Protein damage and degradation by oxygen radicals. I. General aspects. J Biol Chem 262:9895-9901, 1987.

58. Davies KJ, Delsignore ME, Lin SW: Protein damage and degradation by oxygen radicals. II. Modification of amino acids. J Biol Chem 262:9902-9907, 1987.

59. Davies KJ, Delsignore ME: Protein damage and degradation by oxygen radicals. III. Modification of secondary and tertiary structure. J Biol Chem 262:9908-9913, 1987.

60. Davies KJ, Lin SW, Pacifici RE: Protein damage and degradation by oxygen radicals. IV. Degradation of denatured protein. J Biol Chem 262:9914-9920, 1987.

61. Davies KJ, Goldberg AL: Oxygen radicals stimulate intracellular proteolysis and lipid peroxidation by independent mechanisms in erythrocytes. J Biol Chem 262:8220-8226, 1987.

62. Wolff S, Garner A, Dean R: Free radicals, lipids and protein degradation. Trends Biochem Sci 11:27-31, 1986.

63. Chance B, Sies H, Boveris A: Hydroperoxide metabolism in mammalian organs. Physiol Rev 59:527-605, 1979.

64. Forman HJ, Fisher AB: Antioxidant defenses. In: Gilbert DL (ed): Oxygen and Living Processes: An Interdisciplinary Approach. New York, Springer, 1981, pp 235-249.

65. Tierney D, Ayers L, Herzog S, Yang J: Pentose pathway and production of reduced nicotinamide adenine dinucleotide phosphate. A mechanism that may protect lungs from oxidants. Am Rev Respir Dis 108:1348-1351, 1973.

66. Camhi SL, Lee P, Choi AM: The oxidative stress response. New Horiz 3:170-182, 1995.

67. Choi AM, Alam J: Heme oxygenase-1: Function, regulation, and implication of a novel stress-inducible protein in oxidant-induced lung injury. Am J Respir Cell Mol Biol 15:9-19, 1996.

68. Speit G, Dennog C, Eichhorn U, et al: Induction of heme oxygenase-1 and adaptive protection against the induction of DNA damage after hyperbaric oxygen treatment. Carcinogenesis 21:1795-1799, 2000.

69. Dennog C, Radermacher P, Barnett YA, Speit G: Antioxidant status in humans after exposure to hyperbaric oxygen. Mutat Res 428:83-89, 1999.

70. Gill RR, Gbur CJ, Jr., Fisher BJ, et al: Heat shock provides delayed protection against oxidative injury in cultured human umbilical vein endothelial cells. J Mol Cell Cardiol 30:2739-2749, 1998.

71. Arieli Y, Eynan M, Gancz H, et al: Heat acclimation prolongs the time to central nervous system oxygen toxicity in the rat. Possible involvement of HSP72. Brain Res 962:15-20, 2003.

72. Haugaard N: Cellular mechanisms of oxygen toxicity. Physiol Rev 48:311-373, 1968.

73. Dickens F: The toxic effect of oxygen on nervous tissue. In: Elliott KAC, Page IH, Quastel JH (eds): Neurochemistry. Springfield, Ill, Thomas, 1962, pp 851-869.

74. Perot PL Jr, Stein SN: Conduction block in mammalian nerve produced by O_2 at high pressure. Am J Physiol 197:1243-1246, 1959.

75. Goldstein JR, Mengel CE: Hemolysis in mice exposed to varying levels of hyperoxia. Aerosp Med 40:12-13, 1969.

76. Fenn WO, Henning M, Philpott M: Oxygen poisoning in Drosophila. J Gen Physiol 50:1693-1707, 1967.

77. Gerschman R, Gilbert DL, Caccamise D: Effect of various substances on survival times of mice exposed to different high oxygen tensions. Am J Physiol 192:563-571, 1958.

78. Clark JM: Interacting effects of hypoxia adaptation and acute hypercapnia on oxygen tolerance in rats. J Appl Physiol 56:1191-1198, 1984.

79. Clark JM, Lambertsen CJ, Gelfand R, Troxel AB: Optimization of oxygen tolerance extension in rats by intermittent exposure. J Appl Physiol 100:869-879, 2006.

80. Welch BE, Morgan TE Jr, Clamann HG: Time-concentration effects in relation to oxygen toxicity in man. Fed Proc 22:1053-1056, 1963.

81. Donald KW: Oxygen poisoning in man. I & II. Br Med J 1:667-672, 712-717, 1947.

82. Yarbrough OD, Welham W, Brinton ES, Behnke AR: Symptoms of oxygen poisoning and limits of tolerance at rest and at work [Report No.: 01-47]. Washington, DC, Naval Experimental Diving Unit, 1947.

83. Clark JM, Lambertsen CJ: Rate of development of pulmonary O_2 toxicity in man during O_2 breathing at 2.0 Ata. J Appl Physiol 30:739-752, 1971.

84. Lambertsen CJ, Ewing JH, Kough RH, et al: Oxygen toxicity; arterial and internal jugular blood gas composition in man during inhalation of air, 100% O_2 and 2% CO_2 in O_2 at 3.5 atmospheres ambient pressure. J Appl Physiol 8:255-263, 1955.

85. Jamieson D, Vandenbrenk HA: Measurement of oxygen tensions in cerebral tissues of rats exposed to high pressures of oxygen. J Appl Physiol 18:869-876, 1963.

86. Bean JW: Cerebral O_2 in exposures to O_2 at atmospheric and higher pressure, and influence of CO_2. Am J Physiol 201:1192-1198, 1961.

87. Lassen NA: Brain extracellular pH: The main factor controlling cerebral blood flow. Scand J Clin Lab Invest 22:247-251, 1968.

88. Heistad D, Kontos H: Cerebral circulation. In: Abboud F, Shephard J (eds): Handbook of Physiology: The Cardiovascular System. Bethesda, MD, American Physiological Society, 1983, pp 137-182.

89. Iadecola C, Pelligrino DA, Moskowitz MA, Lassen NA: Nitric oxide synthase inhibition and cerebrovascular regulation. J Cereb Blood Flow Metab 14:175-192, 1994.

90. Iadecola C, Zhang F: Nitric oxide-dependent and -independent components of cerebrovasodilation elicited by hypercapnia. Am J Physiol 266:R546-R552, 1994.

91. Kety SS, Schmidt CF: The effects of altered arterial tensions of carbon dioxide and oxygen on cerebral blood flow and cerebral oxygen consumption of normal young men. J Clin Invest 27:484-492, 1948.

92. Lambertsen CJ, Dough RH, Cooper DY, et al: Oxygen toxicity; effects in man of oxygen inhalation at 1 and 3.5 atmospheres upon blood gas transport, cerebral circulation and cerebral metabolism. J Appl Physiol 5:471-486, 1953.

93. Gelfand R, Lambertsen CJ, Clark JM: Ventilatory effects of prolonged hyperoxia at pressures of 1.5-3.0 ATA. Aviat Space Environ Med 77:801-810, 2006.

94. Floyd TF, Clark JM, Gelfand R, et al: Independent cerebral vasoconstrictive effects of hyperoxia and accompanying arterial hypocapnia at 1 ATA. J Appl Physiol 95:2453-2461, 2003.

95. Clark JM, Skolnick BE, Gelfand R, et al: Relationship of ^{133}Xe cerebral blood flow to middle cerebral arterial flow velocity in men at rest. J Cereb Blood Flow Metab 16:1255-1262, 1996.

96. Ohta H: [The effect of hyperoxemia on cerebral blood flow in normal humans]. No To Shinkei 38:949-959, 1986.

97. Demchenko IT, Boso AE, Bennett PB, et al: Hyperbaric oxygen reduces cerebral blood flow by inactivating nitric oxide. Nitric Oxide 4:597-608, 2000.

98. Demchenko IT, Boso AE, O'Neill TJ, et al: Nitric oxide and cerebral blood flow responses to hyperbaric oxygen. J Appl Physiol 88:1381-1389, 2000.

99. Oury TD, Ho YS, Piantadosi CA, Crapo JD: Extracellular superoxide dismutase, nitric oxide, and central nervous system O_2 toxicity. Proc Natl Acad Sci U S A 89:9715-9719, 1992.

100. Bean JW, Lignell J, Coulson J: Regional cerebral blood flow, O_2, and EEG in exposures to O_2 at high pressure. J Appl Physiol 31:235-242, 1971.

101. Chavko M, Braisted JC, Outsa NJ, Harabin AL: Role of cerebral blood flow in seizures from hyperbaric oxygen exposure. Brain Res 791:75-82, 1998.

102. Demchenko IT, Boso AE, Whorton AR, Piantadosi CA: Nitric oxide production is enhanced in rat brain before oxygen-induced convulsions. Brain Res 917:253-261, 2001.

103. Demchenko IT, Oury TD, Crapo JD, Piantadosi CA: Regulation of the brain's vascular responses to oxygen. Circ Res 91:1031-1037, 2002.

104. Kurasako T, Takeda Y, Hirakawa M: Increase in cerebral blood flow as a predictor of hyperbaric oxygen-induced convulsion in artificially ventilated rats. Acta Med Okayama 54:15-20, 2000.

105. Hink J, Thom SR, Simonsen U, et al: Vascular reactivity and endothelial NOS activity in rat thoracic aorta during and after hyperbaric oxygen exposure. Am J Physiol Heart Circ Physiol 291:H1988-H1998, 2006.

106. Thom SR, Bhopale V, Fisher D, et al: Stimulation of nitric oxide synthase in cerebral cortex due to elevated partial pressures of oxygen: An oxidative stress response. J Neurobiol 51:85-100, 2002.

107. Thom SR, Fisher D, Zhang J, et al: Stimulation of perivascular nitric oxide synthesis by oxygen. Am J Physiol Heart Circ Physiol 284:H1230-H1239, 2003.

108. Elayan IM, Axley MJ, Prasad PV, et al: Effect of hyperbaric oxygen treatment on nitric oxide and oxygen free radicals in rat brain. J Neurophysiol 83:2022-2029, 2000.

109. Sato T, Takeda Y, Hagioka S, et al: Changes in nitric oxide production and cerebral blood flow before development of hyperbaric oxygen-induced seizures in rats. Brain Res 918:131-140, 2001.

110. Hagioka S, Takeda Y, Zhang S, et al: Effects of 7-nitroindazole and N-nitro-l-arginine methyl ester on changes in cerebral blood flow and nitric oxide production preceding development of hyperbaric oxygen-induced seizures in rats. Neurosci Lett 382:206-210, 2005.

111. Demchenko IT, Atochin DN, Boso AE, et al: Oxygen seizure latency and peroxynitrite formation in mice lacking neuronal or endothelial nitric oxide synthases. Neurosci Lett 344:53-56, 2003.

112. Atochin DN, Demchenko IT, Astern J, et al: Contributions of endothelial and neuronal nitric oxide synthases to cerebrovascular responses to hyperoxia. J Cereb Blood Flow Metab 23:1219-1226, 2003.

113. Bitterman N, Bitterman H: L-arginine-NO pathway and CNS oxygen toxicity. J Appl Physiol 84:1633-1638, 1998.

114. Demchenko IT, Piantadosi CA: Nitric oxide amplifies the excitatory to inhibitory neurotransmitter imbalance accelerating oxygen seizures. Undersea Hyperb Med 33:169-174, 2006.

115. Lambertsen CJ, Clark JM, Gelfand R, et al: Definition of tolerance to continuous hyperoxia in man: An abstract report of Predictive Studies V. In: Bove AA, Bachrach AJ, Greenbaum LJ (eds): Underwater and Hyperbaric Physiology IX. Bethesda, MD, Undersea and Hyperbaric Medical Society, 1987, pp 717-735.

116. Clark JM, Lambertsen CJ, Gelfand R, et al: Effects of prolonged oxygen exposure at 1.5, 2.0, or 2.5 ATA on pulmonary function in men (Predictive Studies V). J Appl Physiol 86:243-259, 1999.

117. Weinberger B, Laskin DL, Heck DE, Laskin JD: Oxygen toxicity in premature infants. Toxicol Appl Pharmacol 181:60-67, 2002.

118. Behnke AR, Forbes HS, Motley EP: Circulatory and visual effects of oxygen at 3 atmospheres pressure. Am J Physiol 114:436-442, 1936.

119. Rosenberg E, Shibata HR, MacLean LD: Blood gas and neurological responses to inhalation of oxygen at 3 atmospheres. Proc Soc Exp Biol Med 122:313-317, 1966.

120. Nichols CW, Lambertsen CJ, Clark JM: Transient unilateral loss of vision associated with oxygen at high pressure. Arch Ophthalmol 81:548-552, 1969.

121. Noell WK: Metabolic injuries of the visual cell. Am J Ophthalmol 40:60-70, 1955.

122. Bridges WZ: Electroretinographic manifestations of hyperbaric oxygen. Arch Ophthalmol 75:812-817, 1966.

123. Anderson B Jr, Farmer JC Jr: Hyperoxic myopia. Trans Am Ophthalmol Soc 76:116-124, 1978.

124. Lyne AJ: Ocular effects of hyperbaric oxygen. Trans Ophthalmol Soc U K 98:66-68, 1978.

125. Ross ME, Yolton DP, Yolton RL, Hyde KD: Myopia associated with hyperbaric oxygen therapy. Optom Vis Sci 73:487-494, 1996.

126. Fledelius HC, Jansen EC, Thorn J: Refractive change during hyperbaric oxygen therapy. A clinical trial including ultrasound oculometry. Acta Ophthalmol Scand 80:188-190, 2002.

127. Evanger K, Haugen OH, Irgens A, et al: Ocular refractive changes in patients receiving hyperbaric oxygen administered by oronasal mask or hood. Acta Ophthalmol Scand 82:449-453, 2004.

128. Anderson B, Shelton DL: Axial length in hyperoxic myopia. In: Bove AA, Bachrach AJ, Greenbaum LJ (eds): Underwater and Hyperbaric Physiology IX. Bethesda, MD, Undersea and Hyperbaric Medical Society, 1987, pp 607-611.

129. Heald K, Langham ME: Permeability of the cornea and the blood-aqueous barrier to oxygen. Br J Ophthalmol 40:705-720, 1956.

130. Palmquist BM, Philipson B, Barr PO: Nuclear cataract and myopia during hyperbaric oxygen therapy. Br J Ophthalmol 68:113-117, 1984.

131. Gesell LB, Trott A: De novo cataract development following a standard course of hyperbaric oxygen therapy. Undersea Hyperb Med 34:389-392, 2007.

132. Fledelius HC, Jansen E: Hypermetropic refractive change after hyperbaric oxygen therapy. Acta Ophthalmol Scand 82:313-314, 2004.

133. Clark JM, Jackson RM, Lambertsen CJ, et al: Pulmonary function in men after oxygen breathing at 3.0 ATA for 3.5 h. J Appl Physiol 71:878-885, 1991.

134. Lambertsen CJ: Extension of oxygen tolerance in man: Philosophy and significance. Exp Lung Res 14(suppl):1035-1058, 1988.

135. Clark JM: Pulmonary limits of oxygen tolerance in man. Exp Lung Res 14(suppl):897-910, 1988.

136. Caldwell PR, Lee WL Jr, Schildkraut HS, Archibald ER: Changes in lung volume, diffusing capacity, and blood gases in men breathing oxygen. J Appl Physiol 21:1477-1483, 1966.

137. Thorsen E, Aanderud L, Aasen TB: Effects of a standard hyperbaric oxygen treatment protocol on pulmonary function. Eur Respir J 12:1442-1445, 1998.

138. Pott F, Westergaard P, Mortensen J, Jansen EC: Hyperbaric oxygen treatment and pulmonary function. Undersea Hyperb Med 26:225-228, 1999.

139. Pisarello JB, Clark JM, Lambertsen CJ, Gelfand R: Human circulatory responses to prolonged hyperbaric hyperoxia in Predictive Studies V. In: Bove AA, Bachrach AJ, Greenbaum LJ (eds): Underwater and Hyperbaric Physiology IX. Bethesda, MD, Undersea and Hyperbaric Medical Society, 1987, pp 763-772.

140. Clark JM, Lambertsen CJ: Pulmonary oxygen tolerance and the rate of development of pulmonary oxygen toxicity in man at two atmospheres inspired oxygen tension. In: Lambertsen CJ (ed): Underwater Physiology. Baltimore, MD, Williams & Wilkins, 1967, pp 439-451.

141. Ohlsson WTL: A study on oxygen toxicity at atmospheric pressure. Acta Med Scand 128(suppl 190):1-93, 1947.

142. Eckenhoff RG, Dougherty JH Jr, Messier AA, et al: Progression of and recovery from pulmonary oxygen toxicity in humans exposed to 5 ATA air. Aviat Space Environ Med 58:658-667, 1987.

143. Bardin H, Lambertsen CJ: A quantitative method for calculating cumulative pulmonary oxygen toxicity: Use of the unit pulmonary toxicity dose (UPTD). Philadelphia, University of Pennsylvania, Institute for Environmental Medicine Report, 1970.

144. Wright WB: Use of the University of Pennsylvania Institute for Environmental Medicine procedure for calculation of cumulative pulmonary oxygen toxicity: US Navy Experimental Diving Unit Report 2-72. Washington, D.C., 1972.

145. Harabin AL, Homer LD, Weathersby PK, Flynn ET: An analysis of decrements in vital capacity as an index of pulmonary oxygen toxicity. J Appl Physiol 63:1130-1135, 1987.

146. Arieli R, Yalov A, Goldenshluger A: Modeling pulmonary and CNS O$_2$ toxicity and estimation of parameters for humans. J Appl Physiol 92:248-256, 2002.

147. Hampson NB, Simonson SG, Kramer CC, Piantadosi CA: Central nervous system oxygen toxicity during hyperbaric treatment of patients with carbon monoxide poisoning. Undersea Hyperb Med 23:215-219, 1996.

148. Davis JC, Dunn JM, Heimbach RD: Hyperbaric medicine: Patient selection, treatment procedures, and side effects. In: Davis JC, Hunt TK (eds): Problem Wounds: The Role of Oxygen. New York, Elsevier, 1988, pp 225-235.

149. Hart GB, Strauss MB: Central nervous system oxygen toxicity in a clinical setting. In: Bove AA, Bachrach AJ, Greenbaum LJ (eds): Undersea and Hyperbaric Physiology IX. Bethesda, MD, Undersea and Hyperbaric Medical Society, 1987, pp 695-699.

150. Hampson N, Atik D: Central nervous system oxygen toxicity during routine hyperbaric oxygen therapy. Undersea Hyperb Med 30:147-153, 2003.

151. Smerz RW: Incidence of oxygen toxicity during the treatment of dysbarism. Undersea Hyperb Med 31:199-202, 2004.

152. Clark JM (ed): Symposium on extension of oxygen tolerance. Exp Lung Res 14:865-1058, 1988.

153. Lambertsen CJ: Respiratory and circulatory actions of high oxygen pressure. In: Goff LG, (ed): Proceedings of the Underwater Physiology Symposium [Publication No 377]. Washington, DC, National Academy of Sciences–National Research Council, 1955, pp 25-38.

154. Hall DA: The influence of the systematic fluctuation of PO$_2$ upon the nature and rate of development of oxygen toxicity in guinea pigs [master's thesis]. Philadelphia, University of Pennsylvania, 1967.

155. Hendricks PL, Hall DA, Hunter WL Jr, Haley PJ: Extension of pulmonary O$_2$ tolerance in man at 2 ATA by intermittent O$_2$ exposure. J Appl Physiol 42:593-599, 1977.

156. Harabin AL, Braisted JC, Flynn ET: Response of antioxidant enzymes to intermittent and continuous hyperbaric oxygen. J Appl Physiol 69:328-335, 1990.

157. Berghage TE, Borkat FR: An oxygen toxicity computer [Report No.: 80-28]. Washington, D.C., Naval Health Research Center, Naval Medical Research and Development Command, 1980.

158. Perdrizet GA: Heat shock response and organ preservation: Models of stress conditioning. New York, Springer, Landes, 1997.

Ocular 24

Complications

in Hyperbaric

Oxygen Therapy

Frank K. Butler, Jr., MD, and Catherine Hagan, MD

The eye is a complex sensory organ that may be adversely affected as a side effect of hyperbaric oxygen therapy (HBOT). Aspects of anatomy and physiology of the eye affect HBOT. In addition, ocular contraindications to HBOT exist. Finally, the hyperbaric physician should be aware of the timing and conduct of pretreatment and post-treatment eye examinations, as well as examinations of ocular status appropriate for use in the hyperbaric chamber.

REVIEW OF PERTINENT ANATOMY AND PHYSIOLOGY OF THE EYE

To understand how the eye may be affected by environmental stressors, including HBOT, one must appreciate its unique anatomic and physiologic properties.[1] In the process of producing the sensory experience that we perceive as vision, incident light passes through the cornea of the eye, the anterior chamber, the pupil, the posterior chamber, the crystalline lens, and the vitreous body before reaching the retina (Fig. 24.1). The cornea provides approximately two thirds of the refracting power needed to focus light on the retina, with the lens providing the other third. The anterior chamber, posterior chamber, and vitreous body are filled with noncompressible fluid, which means that the eye should not be adversely affected by changes in pressure (barotrauma) unless a gas space exists adjacent to the eye (as with a face mask) or gas is iatrogenically or traumatically placed inside the eye. Light reaching the retina stimulates the photoreceptor cells, which then stimulate the ganglion cells. The confluence of the afferent portions of the ganglion cells is seen as the optic disc. These cells then exit the eye as the optic nerve to carry visual stimuli back to the occipital cortex of the brain via the optic nerve, chiasm, and tract. At the middle and posterior aspects of the eye, the globe is composed of three main layers: the whitish sclera, the vascular uveal tract, and the sensory retina. The uveal tract is fur-

ther divided into the posterior choroid, the iris visible in the anterior portion of the eye, and the intermediate ciliary body. The retina is likewise further divided into nine distinct layers.

Vision may be adversely affected by any factor that prevents light from reaching the retina or being sharply focused in the retinal plane. Vision may also be affected by environmental injury to the photoreceptor cells, injury to the occipital cortex, or any afferent structure carrying visual stimuli between these two areas.

The arterial supply to the eye is provided by the ophthalmic artery, a branch of the internal carotid artery that passes through the cavernous sinus. Some of the branches of the ophthalmic artery (lacrimal, supraorbital, ethmoidal, medial palpebral, frontal, dorsal nasal) supply orbital structures, whereas others (central artery of the retina, short and long posterior ciliaries, anterior ciliaries) supply the tissues of the globe.[1] The central retinal artery enters the globe within the substance of the optic nerve and supplies the inner layers of the retina. The long posterior ciliary arteries provide blood to the choroid and the outer layers of the retina. About 20 short posterior ciliary arteries and usually

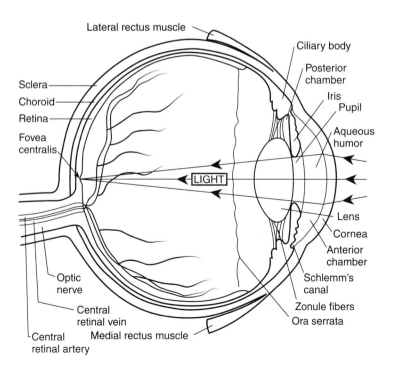

Figure 24.1 The eye.

2 long posterior ciliary arteries are present. The posterior ciliary vessels originate from the ophthalmic artery and supply the entire uveal tract, cilioretinal arteries, the sclera, the margin of the cornea, and the adjacent conjunctiva. The anterior ciliary arteries also arise from the ophthalmic artery, supply the extraocular muscles, and anastomose with the posterior ciliary vessels to form the major arterial circle of the iris, which supplies the iris and ciliary body. In approximately 15% to 30% of people, a cilioretinal artery is present. This artery is part of the ciliary arterial supply but supplies the area of the retina around the macula (central vision area).

The cornea and lens are avascular structures. The cornea receives its oxygen supply both from the precorneal tear film and the anterior chamber of the eye, whereas the oxygen supply to the lens is provided by the posterior chamber and the vitreous.[1]

OCULAR COMPLICATIONS OF HYPERBARIC OXYGEN THERAPY

Oxygen at high partial pressures may be toxic to multiple body tissues, including both the central nervous system (CNS) and the eye. Even in normoxic conditions, oxygen metabolism produces superoxide radicals and other potentially harmful reactive species. These substances are removed by superoxide dismutase and other cellular defense mechanisms. In hyperoxic conditions, these defense systems may be overwhelmed by increased radical production and oxygen toxicity may ensue.[2]

Central Nervous System Oxygen Toxicity

Systemic Manifestations

CNS oxygen toxicity is a complex, nonlinear disorder. Common systemic symptoms of CNS oxygen toxicity include muscle twitching, tinnitus, dysphoria, nausea, and generalized convulsion.[3-5] In exercising divers, CNS oxygen toxicity is not seen at shallow depths, but it begins to be a factor as the partial pressure of oxygen (Po_2) in the diver's breathing mix exceeds about 1.3 atmospheres absolute (ATA) and increases exponentially thereafter as the Po_2 continues to increase. CNS oxygen toxicity is characterized by sudden onset and (usually) a rapid relief from symptoms once the Po_2 is reduced to nontoxic levels. The risk for CNS oxygen toxicity is modified substantially by factors such as exercise, immersion, water temperature, total pressure, individual susceptibility, and the Pco_2 in the breathing mix. The dry, resting conditions experienced during HBOT reduce, but do not eliminate, the risk for CNS oxygen toxicity.

Ophthalmic Manifestations

Visual symptoms are a well-recognized manifestation of CNS oxygen toxicity.[3-6] The most commonly described ocular symptoms of CNS oxygen toxicity are eyelid twitching, blurred vision, and visual field constriction, although the latter symptom may represent retinal oxygen toxicity, as described later.[2] Visual hallucinations[4] and transient unilateral loss of vision[6] have also been reported. The single patient who experienced the unilateral visual loss had a previous history of retrobulbar optic neuritis in the index eye.[6] Loss of the peripheral visual field may be severe but is reversible on discontinuation of the hyperoxic exposure.

Treatment

When CNS oxygen toxicity is encountered, oxygen breathing should be discontinued immediately.[7] In most cases, symptoms resolve within several minutes, although some episodes progress to generalized convulsions despite a reduction in the Po_2. CNS oxygen toxicity typically is without residua, unless secondary trauma or other complications ensue from a convulsion. Oxygen breathing may be resumed 15 minutes after the symptoms of CNS oxygen toxicity subside. Should symptoms recur, consider reducing the P_{O_2} in the breathing mix.

Retinal Oxygen Toxicity

Oxygen can also be directly toxic to the tissues of the eye. As early as 1935, Behnke and colleagues[8] reported a reversible decrease in peripheral vision after oxygen breathing at 3.0 ATA. Lambertsen and Clark and their colleagues also observed a progressive decrease in peripheral vision associated with hyperoxic exposures that probably represents a form of retinal oxygen toxicity.[9,10] A decrease in peripheral vision was noted after approximately 2.5 hours of oxygen breathing at 3.0 ATA in a dry chamber. This decrease was progressive until oxygen breathing was stopped at 3.5 hours. The average decrement in visual field area was 50%. Recovery was complete in all subjects after 45 minutes of air breathing.[10] A decrease in electroretinographic amplitude was noted as well but did not correlate directly with the size of the visual field defect and returned to normal more slowly after the termination of the hyperoxic exposure.[10] Visual acuity and visual cortical-evoked responses remained normal in all subjects.

Retinal oxygen toxicity is not commonly reported as a complication of HBOT, but the incidence may be under-reported because visual fields are not typically monitored during the course of HBOT and the disorder is reversible after a return to normoxia.

Lenticular Oxygen Toxicity

Hyperoxic Myopia

The differential diagnosis of an acute myopic shift includes osmotic changes in the lens of the eye caused by the hyperosmolar state found in untreated diabetes mellitus, systemic medications (especially diuretics), miotic eye medications, and ciliary spasm. In the setting of repeated exposures to hyperoxia, however, the condition known as hyperoxic myopia must be included in the differential.[2]

Progressive myopic changes are a known complication of repetitive treatments with HBOT.[11-15] The rate of myopic change has been reported to be approximately 0.25 diopter/week with the change being progressive throughout the course of HBOT.[12] Hyperoxic myopia is generally attributed to oxidative changes causing an increase in the refractive power of the lens, because Anderson and Shelton[13] have shown that axial length and keratometry readings did not reveal a corneal or axial length basis for the myopic shift. Reversal of the myopic shift after discontinuation of the HBOT usually occurs within 3 to 6 weeks but may take as long as 6 to 12 months.[15] The P_{O_2} in these exposures typically varies from 2.0 - 3.0 ATA depending on the treatment protocol used, but hyperoxic myopia has also been reported in a closed-circuit mixed-gas scuba diver at a P_{O_2} of 1.3 ATA, a lower partial pressure than typically encountered in HBOT.[16] The myopic shift in that individual resolved over a 1-month period after completion of the hyperoxic exposures.

Cataract Formation

Palmquist and coauthors[14] have also reported cataract formation in patients undergoing a prolonged course of daily HBOT at 2.0 to 2.5 ATA.[14] Seven of 15 patients with clear lenses at the start of therapy experienced development of cataracts during their course of treatment. Fourteen of these 15 patients received a total HBOT time of between 300 and 850 hours. The lens opacities noted were not completely reversible after HBOT was discontinued. Figure 24.2 shows a slit-lamp photograph of a nuclear sclerotic cataract. Hyperoxic myopia and subsequent cataract formation may therefore be considered to represent two levels of severity of lenticular oxygen toxicity. The high success rate of modern cataract surgery makes cataract formation an easily manageable complication of HBOT, and this side effect is not necessarily a reason to discontinue therapy if there is a strong clinical indication for HBOT.

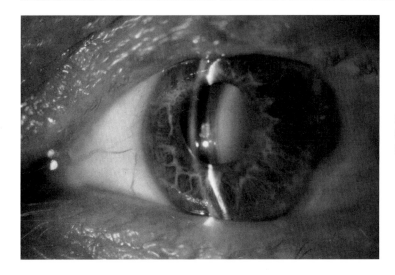

Figure 24.2 Slit-lamp image of a nuclear sclerotic cataract. **(See Color Plate 30.)** *(Courtesy Dr. David Harris.)*

Ocular Examination before Hyperbaric Oxygen Therapy

Documentation of ocular function before beginning HBOT allows the diving and hyperbaric medicine physician to have an objective measure of visual status. In this way, the benefit of therapy can be followed if HBOT is being performed for ocular indications, and any adverse effect of HBOT on visual status can be accurately quantified to guide therapeutic decisions. Any time that a patient is being considered for what is likely to be a prolonged course of HBOT, a more thorough pretreatment eye examination is indicated. The eye examination should include documentation of corrected and uncorrected visual acuity, refraction, color vision, status of the crystalline lens, and fundus examination. Automated visual perimetry should be included if clinically indicated. This examination should be repeated periodically when conducting long-term HBOT.

An exception to the above statement occurs when an individual is being recompressed on an emergent basis for disorders such as carbon monoxide poisoning, decompression sickness, or arterial gas embolism. Delays for eye examinations may theoretically result in worsening of patient's clinical condition and are not indicated especially because treatment regimens in these cases are typically short. If ocular signs or symptoms were part of the clinical presentation, as can occur with decompression sickness and arterial gas embolism, an abbreviated eye examination should be conducted periodically during treatment, and a complete eye examination as outlined in the previous paragraph should be conducted as soon as feasible after recompression. Automated visual perimetry should be included in these examinations if it is available.

OCULAR CONSIDERATIONS IN EVALUATIONS FOR HYPERBARIC OXYGEN THERAPY

Some ocular complications of HBOT can be avoided if candidates for HBOT are screened appropriately for ocular conditions that preclude safe compression in a hyperbaric chamber. From an ocular perspective, the HBOT evaluation for treatment is significantly different from those published for divers.[2] There is less concern about adequate visual acuity because the patient may be assisted as needed in the HBOT environment. Decompression issues are typically not a factor because the patient will be breathing 100% oxygen in most cases, except for short air breaks. The prescribed convalescent period before resumption of diving activity after ocular surgery should typically not be required because the potential for face-mask barotrauma and water intrusion into an ocular operative site will not be present in a recompression chamber. Recompression in a chamber after the various types of refractive surgery should likewise not pose a problem. Glaucoma is not a contraindication to HBOT, despite the presence of increased ambient (and intraocular) pressures. However, several ocular conditions do remain as contraindications to HBOT.

Enucleation (*only* if a hollow orbital prosthesis was used)

Some reports have described pressure-induced collapses of hollow silicone orbital implants at depths as shallow as 10 feet.[17] A hollow glass implant was also tested and did not implode at a maximum test depth of 115 feet, but diving with hollow glass implants cannot be recommended on the basis of this one test. Individuals with hollow orbital implants should not be subjected to increased ambient pressures. Most ocular implants currently in use, however, are not hollow and should not be considered a contraindication to diving or HBOT. The office of the ophthalmologist who performed the enucleation should be able to help in determining the nature of the orbital prosthesis that was implanted.

Presence of an Intraocular Gas Bubble

Intraocular gas is used by both vitreoretinal and anterior segment surgeons as an intraocular stent to maintain juxtaposition of the retina to the retinal pigment epithelium or the corneal endothelium to Descemet's membrane. Figure 24.3 shows a slit-lamp photograph of bubbles in the anterior chamber of the eye. Gas in the eye may cause intraocular barotrauma during compression or a central retinal artery occlusion during decompression and is an absolute contraindication to exposure to changes in ambient pressure.[18] Intraocular gas bubbles have been noted to expand even with the relatively small decrease in ambient pressure entailed in commercial air travel.[19,20] This expansion causes an increase in intraocular pressure[19,21] and may cause sudden blindness due to pressure-induced closure of the central retinal artery.[19,22] Should this occur, immediate recompression of the cabin to a lower altitude may be rapidly beneficial as the size of the gas bubble is reduced, the pressure in the eye is decreased, and blood flow in the central retinal artery is restored.[22] One important exception to the discussion about intraocular gas bubbles is the presence of gas bubbles in the eye that may occur as a manifestation of decompression sickness. Recompression and HBOT should be undertaken in this instance with the expectation that

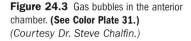

Figure 24.3 Gas bubbles in the anterior chamber. **(See Color Plate 31.)** *(Courtesy Dr. Steve Chalfin.)*

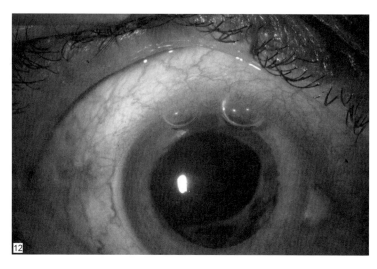

(1) the normal volume of the anterior chamber, posterior chamber, and vitreous before the formation of the gas bubble because of inert gas supersaturation will prevent compression barotraumas, and that (2) resolution of the intraocular bubbles because of HBOT will prevent an expanding gas phase on decompression with a resultant rise in intraocular pressure.

EVALUATING VISUAL FUNCTION DURING HYPERBARIC OXYGEN THERAPY

Individuals with decompression sickness or arterial gas embolism who present with ocular signs or symptoms will require evaluations of their visual status during treatment. Visual acuity should be measured with a near vision card (with refractive correction for age as appropriate). Color vision can be monitored with pseudo-isochromatic plates at depth, and central visual fields may be evaluated with repetitive Amsler grid testing. Large defects in peripheral vision may be detected with confrontation visual fields. These measures of visual function are easily accomplished in a multiplace chamber; some of them may also be feasible in a monoplace chamber.

MINIMIZING OCULAR COMPLICATIONS FROM HYPERBARIC OXYGEN THERAPY

Winkle and colleagues[23] demonstrate that exposing postradial keratotomy corneas to 100% nitrogen via goggles at 1 atmosphere for 2 hours caused a significant hyperopic shift of 1.24 diopters and corneal flattening of 1.19 diopters. Corneal thickness increased in both post-RK and control eyes but was not associated with a hyperopic shift in control eyes. This demonstrates that the Po_2 in the precorneal gas space is more important than inspired Po_2 in determining the physiologic effect of the gas mix on the cornea.[18] Jampol[24] demonstrates that 100% oxygen as the precorneal gas caused marked increases in the Po_2 in the

anterior chamber over those seen in animals breathing the same Po_2 but exposed to a precorneal oxygen fraction of 20%.

This research suggests that use of an oronasal mask as an oxygen delivery device instead of a hood should reduce the oxygen dose to the eye. In this way, the precorneal gas can be maintained nearer to a normal oxygen fraction. Evanger and coauthors[25] have studied this potential approach to reducing lenticular oxygen toxicity and demonstrate a reduction of the observed myopic shift by approximately 50% when HBOT patients were supplied with oxygen via mask instead of hood. Unfortunately, most patients find hoods more comfortable, but patients can be offered a choice when appropriate or possible.

REFERENCES

1. Lewis RA, Anderson RE, Friedlander MH, et al: Fundamentals and principles of ophthalmology. In: Basic and Clinical Science Course. San Francisco, American Academy of Ophthalmology, 1987, pp 24-102.
2. Butler FK: Diving and hyperbaric ophthalmology. Surv Ophthalmol 39:347-366, 1995.
3. Butler FK: Central nervous system oxygen toxicity in closed circuit SCUBA divers III. Panama City Beach, Fla, Navy Experimental Diving Unit [Report 5-86], 1986, pp 12-20.
4. Butler FK, Thalmann ED: Central nervous system oxygen toxicity in closed circuit SCUBA divers II. Undersea Biomed Res 13:193-223, 1986.
5. Butler FK, Thalmann ED: Central nervous system oxygen toxicity in closed circuit SCUBA divers. In: Bachrach AJ, Matzen MM (eds): Underwater Physiology VIII. Proceedings of the Eighth Symposium on Underwater Physiology. Bethesda, Md, Undersea Medical Society, 1984, pp 15-30.
6. Nichols CW, Lambertson CJ, Clark J: Transient unilateral loss of vision associated with oxygen at high pressure. Arch Ophthalmol 81:548-552, 1969.
7. U.S. Navy Diving Manual. Washington, D.C., Naval Sea Systems Command Publication SS521-AG-PRO-010 (0910-LP-103-8009). Rev. 5, August 15, 2005.
8. Behnke AR, Forbes HS, Motley EP: Circulatory and visual effects of oxygen at 3 atmospheres pressure. Am J Physiol 114:436-442, 1935.
9. Nichols GW, Lambertsen CJ: Effects of high oxygen pressures on the eye. N Engl J Med 281:25-30, 1969.
10. Lambertsen CJ, Clark JM, Gelfand R, et al: Definition of tolerance in continuous hyperoxia in man: An abstract report of Predictive Studies V. In: Bove AA, Bachrach AJ, Greenbaum LJ (eds): Proceedings of the Ninth International Symposium on Underwater and Hyperbaric Physiology. Bethesda, Md, Undersea and Hyperbaric Medical Society, 1987, pp 717-735.

11. Clark JM: Oxygen toxicity. In: Bennett PB, Elliott DH (eds): The Physiology and Medicine of Diving, 4th ed. London, WB Saunders, 1993, pp 121-169.

12. Anderson B, Farmer JC: Hyperoxic myopia. Trans Am Ophthalmol Soc LXXVI:116-124, 1978.

13. Anderson B, Shelton DL: Axial length in hyperoxic myopia. In: Bove AA, Bachrach AJ, Greenbaum LJ (eds): Ninth International Symposium on Underwater and Hyperbaric Physiology. Bethesda, Md, Undersea and Hyperbaric Medical Society, 1987, pp 607-611.

14. Palmquist BM, Philipson B, Barr PO: Nuclear cataract and myopia during hyperbaric oxygen therapy. Br J Ophthalmol 68:113-117, 1984.

15. Thom SR, Clark JM: The toxicity of oxygen, carbon monoxide, and carbon dioxide. In Bove AA, Davis JC (eds): Diving Medicine, 3rd ed. Philadelphia, WB Saunders, 1997, pp 131-145.

16. Butler FK, White E, Twa M: Hyperoxic myopia in a closed-circuit mixed-gas SCUBA diver. Undersea Hyperb Med 26:41-45, 1999.

17. Isenberg SJ, Diamant A: SCUBA diving after enucleation. Am J Ophthalmol 100:616-617, 1985.

18. Butler FK: The eye in the wilderness. In: Auerbach PS (ed): Wilderness Medicine, 5th ed. St Louis, Mosby, 2007, pp 604-624.

19. Kokame GT, Ing MR: Intraocular gas and low-altitude air flight. Retina 14:356-358, 1994.

20. Mills MD, Devenyi RG, Lam WC, et al: An assessment of intraocular pressure rise in patients with gas-filled eyes during simulated air flight. Ophthalmology 108:40, 2001.

21. Lincoff H, Weinburger D, Stergiu P: Air travel with intraocular gas II—clinical considerations. Arch Ophthalmol 107:907, 1989.

22. Polk JD, Rugaber C, Kohn G, et al: Central retinal artery occlusion by proxy: A cause for sudden blindness in an airline passenger. Aviat Space Environ Med 73:385, 2002.

23. Winkle KR, Mader TH, Parmley VC, et al: The etiology of refractive changes at high altitude after radial keratotomy. Ophthalmology 105:282-286, 1998.

24. Jampol LM: Oxygen therapy and intraocular oxygenation. Trans Am Ophthalmol Soc 85:407-437, 1987.

25. Evanger K, Haugen OH, Irgens A, et al: Ocular refractive changes in patients receiving hyperbaric oxygen administered by oronasal mask or hood. Acta Ophthalmol Scand 82:449-453, 2004.

Cardiovascular Aspects of Hyperbaric Oxygen Therapy

25

Alfred A. Bove, MD, PhD

All patients who receive hyperbaric oxygen therapy (HBOT) will experience development of some form of cardiovascular reaction to the hyperoxic environment either by expected regulatory modifications in cardiac and circulatory function, or possibly by unexpected reactions to HBOT caused by known or unknown comorbidities that are affected by the HBOT environment. When considering cardiovascular aspects of HBOT, it is worthwhile to examine the known effects of HBOT on circulatory regulation, cardiac function, and cardiovascular disease states, and to examine the value of HBOT in cardiovascular disorders.

OXYGEN EFFECTS ON CARDIOVASCULAR REGULATION

Exposure to partial pressures of oxygen (P_{O_2}) greater than 2 atmospheres absolute (ATA) is known to induce arteriolar vasoconstriction and increase systemic vascular resistance.[1] The mechanism for this change has been studied by a number of investigators. Abel and colleagues[1] have found that systemic vascular resistance was related to inspired P_{O_2} in a linear fashion until P_{O_2} reached 3 ATA. Systemic vascular resistance showed an increase of about 10% comparing air at 1 ATA with 100% oxygen at 3 ATA. Vasoconstriction mechanisms are thought to be related to reduction of nitric oxide ($\cdot$NO) production in endothelium that results for increased oxidation of the $\cdot$NO radical, and loss of the vasorelaxation effect of endothelial produced $\cdot$NO. Others suggest that alterations in other vasodilator compounds such as prostaglandins may play some role, and still others indicate that central vasoregulation is also affected by HBOT resulting in vasoconstriction. Figure 25.1 summarizes the hemodynamic effects of 1 and 3 ATA 100% oxygen.

VAGAL EFFECTS

Current evidence indicates that HBOT results in increased vagal activity with resultant sinus bradycardia. Some studies present evidence for a concomitant increase in sympathetic tone that results in systemic vasoconstriction and increased blood pressure. These changes are well tolerated in patients with normal cardiovascular function but can result in clinical deterioration in patients with compromised cardiac function. Shibata and coworkers[2] examined the heart rate response to 3 ATA P_{O_2}. Their data indicate

that parasympathetic activity and arterial-cardiac baroreflex function increased with hyperoxia in a dose-dependent manner. Their data support the parasympathetic stimulatory effects of increased P_{O_2} beyond 1 atmosphere. Sun and investigators[3] examined heart rate variability as a measure of autonomic integrity. They treated 23 patients with diabetic foot at 2 ATA for 90 minutes daily for 20 treatments. Compared with a control group, the patients who received HBOT showed an increase in RR-interval variability and high- and low-frequency power (indicators of parasympathetic or sympathetic activity) obtained by frequency analysis of the electrocardiogram. They interpreted these changes as indicating that HBOT increased vagal tone and improved cardiac neural regulation. Shibata and coworkers[2] evaluated neuroregulation in healthy subjects exposed to 21% to 100% oxygen at 1 ATA. They found a decreasing heart rate with increasing P_{O_2}, indicating that vagal tone was increased with increased P_{O_2}. In addition, frequency analysis of the electrocardiogram demonstrated that high-frequency variability changes indicated an increase in vagal tone. The low-frequency variability, however, was unchanged, suggesting that sympathetic activity was not changed by HBOT.

Lund and coauthors[4] examined the effects of HBOT and age on vagal activity. Their sub-

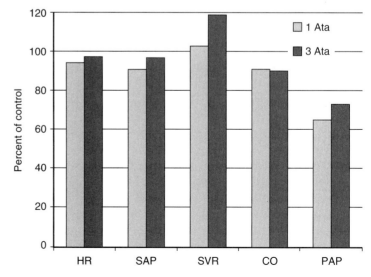

Figure 25.1 Changes in several hemodynamic measures comparing 100% oxygen at 1 and 3 atmospheres absolute (ATA). Values are percentage change from control (air at 1 ATA). CO, cardiac output; HR, heart rate; PAP, pulmonary arterial pressure; SAP, systolic arterial pressure; SVR, systemic vascular resistance. *(Data from Abel FL, McNamee JE, Cone DL, et al: Effects of hyperbaric oxygen on ventricular performance, pulmonary blood volume, and systemic and pulmonary vascular resistance. Undersea Hyperb Med 27:67–73, 2000.)*

jects were patients undergoing HBOT at 2.5 ATA for osteomyelitis and osteoradionecrosis. In patients older than 50 years, there were no effects of HBOT, but in younger patients, there was a positive vagal effect of HBOT. West and colleagues[5] examined the effect of HBOT at 2.8 ATA on vagal tone during exercise. Exposure did not show an effect on heart rate variability. This finding conflicts with the findings of Sun[3] noted earlier. Lund and coauthors[6] used heart rate variability and power analysis from the electrocardiogram to determine the effects of 2.5 ATA and confirmed the increased vagal tone associated with HBOT.

In addition to a reduced heart rate with HBOT exposure, changes in conduction and premature contractions can be found during HBOT. Eckenhoff and Knight[7] examined the cardiac rate and rhythm in 81 healthy subjects who were exposed to air saturation chamber experiments at depths of 2 to 132 feet sea water (fsw). They found heart rate reductions of 30% to 40% with prolongation of the $\dot{Q}T$ interval that was consistent with the reduced heart rate. Junctional escape rhythms or isolated premature beats were noted in 10% of their subjects. They found occasional ventricular premature beats during the exposures occurring at the same frequency as that found before exposure. These exposures were designed to simulate the diving environment, and the authors believe that the bradycardia noted in the exposures was related to both hyperoxia and increased pressure. Animal studies also confirm the HBOT effects observed in human studies. Doubt and Evans[8] examined the effects of Po_2 (2 ATA) and pressure (31 ATA by helium compression) on cardiac rhythm and conduction and cardiac contractility in anesthetized cats. Helium compression to 31.3 ATA decreased the heart rate and prolonged the PR and $\dot{Q}T$ intervals independently of changes in heart rate. They also note an increase in ventricular contractility. Increasing the Po_2 produced a further decrease in heart rate but a shortening of the $\dot{Q}T$ interval. Their data, and data from other studies noted earlier, indicate that separate pressure and oxygen effects result in increased

vagal tone. Shida and Lin[9] exposed awake rats to Po_2 up to 1590 torr using gas mixtures containing helium or nitrogen. In all cases, the bradycardia noted during hyperoxic exposure was related to the logarithm of Po_2, not to concentrations of nitrogen or helium. Pressure had small but measurable effects on the hyperoxic bradycardia. Lin and Shida[10] have reviewed the mechanisms for hyperbaric bradycardia. They identify two components of the bradycardia. They conclude that hyperoxia is the major factor responsible for initiating and maintaining hyperbaric bradycardia. They also have identified a nonoxygen-dependent bradycardia that is likely due to altered respiratory patterns that secondarily cause a reduction in heart rate. The above studies support a direct effect of HBOT on vagal tone, resulting in a bradycardia. The reduced heart rate appears to be the result of HBOT, increased pressure, and possibly to effects of hyperbaria (e.g., increased gas density or viscosity) on respiratory function.

HEMODYNAMICS

Changes in afterload resulting from oxygen-induced systemic vasoconstriction are noted earlier in this chapter. In the care of chronically ill patients undergoing HBOT for wound care, many patients will be susceptible to clinical deterioration because of cardiocirculatory instability induced by circulatory effects of HBOT. Molenat and investigators[11] have evaluated hemodynamic function using echocardiography at 1, 1.6, and 2.8 ATA in healthy subjects. Stroke volume, left atrial dimensions, and left ventricular (LV) dimensions were reduced under HBOT exposure, and indices of LV function showed a reduction in overall performance. Savitt and coworkers[12] studied 10 dogs with HBOT at 3 ATA and increasing arterial Po_2. LV stroke volume, cardiac output, coronary blood flow, and myocardial oxygen consumption were all significantly reduced. A reduction of cardiac dimensions, stroke volume, and cardiac output in the presence of an increased afterload would suggest that sympathetic tone is increased. The increased afterload also supports a sympathetic effect. Figure 25.1 shows typical changes in hemodynamics caused by oxygen breathing at 1 and 3 atmospheres.

MYOCARDIAL EFFECTS

In Wilson and colleagues' study,[13] 10 divers were subjected to saturation exposure to 50 to 60 fsw breathing nitrogen-oxygen mixtures. Bradycardia was noted in all divers, and it slowly reversed as the divers spent more time in the saturation exposure. By 8 days, the heart rate had returned to near control levels. Heart rate rapidly returned to baseline levels on decompression. In deeper exposures to 200 fsw, several divers demonstrated right-sided intraventricular conduction delay, suggesting that the right ventricle was under increased strain in these deeper exposures. As noted by other authors, the $\dot{Q}T$ interval increased in conjunction with the slower heart rate. Nelson and investigators[14] found no changes in cardiac metabolic enzymes after 4 weeks of HBOT at 2.4 ATA in rabbits. Doubt and Evans[15] studied anesthetized cats exposed to helium oxygen at 1000 fsw. They found a progressive delay between onset of electrical and mechanical contraction with depth. $\dot{Q}T$ interval increased with depth at all heart rates. Contractile indices were enhanced with depth. They suggested that excitation-contraction coupling was altered by the interaction between depth and heart rate. Although these effects were seen at high pressure, similar rate effects and $\dot{Q}T$ changes have been described at HBOT pressures.

PERIPHERAL VASCULAR EFFECTS

The vasoconstrictor effects of HBOT noted earlier are now thought to be caused in part by altered endothelial function resulting in reduction of endothelium-derived vasodilators. Hink and colleagues[16] found reduced endothelium-derived ·NO in isolated aortic rings from rats exposed to hyperbaric oxygen (HBO) at 2.8 ATA. The resultant increase in vascular tone supports the systemic vasoconstrictor effects of HBOT noted in several studies of human and animal exposures to HBO. They also found that extraendothelial ·NO was increased and attenuated the constrictor effects of norepinephrine. Further effects of HBOT on endothelium were proposed by Hong and coworkers,[17] who studied ischemia-reperfusion injury in a muscle flap preparation in the rat. Their data indicate that the cell adhesion molecule ICAM-1 (intercellular adhesion molecule-1) was reduced, thus allowing fewer neutrophils to adhere to endothelium in the HBOT animals. These data are relevant to ischemia-reperfusion in myocardium and suggest that HBOT might be beneficial in patients who undergo an ischemia-reperfusion event by revascularization during acute coronary syndrome (ACS). Tjärnström and colleagues[18] have examined endothelial cells in vitro after an 8-hour anoxic exposure followed by reperfusion with HBO at 1.5 ATA. Their data indicate that HBO stimulates the release of fibrinolytic factors that could prevent thromboses after ischemia-reperfusion. In a similar study of in vitro endothelial cell function, Buras and coworkers[19] also documented a reduction in ICAM-1 and resultant reduction in neutrophil adhesion to endothelial cells. They also found an HBO-induced increase in endothelial ·NO synthetase that may have contributed to the changes in ICAM-1 in this model. These findings were confirmed in humans by Ueno and researchers,[20] who examined 12 patients who underwent elective partial hepatectomy for liver cancer and were given 2 courses of HBOT at 2.0 ATM for 60 minutes at 3 hours and 24 hours after hepatectomy; these patients were compared with 12 hepatectomy patients who did not receive HBOT. In the HBOT group, peak levels of polymorphonuclear leukocyte elastase and thrombomodulin were diminished compared with the control group. The incidence of hyperbilirubinemia and hepatic failure was lower in the HBOT group compared with the control group. Thom and colleagues[21] report a reduction in β_2-integrin–dependent neutrophil adherence in healthy human subjects exposed to HBO at 3 ATA. Although these studies were undertaken in organs and tissue cultures not directly associated with cardiac tissue, the effects are similar in myocardium, and similar HBO effects on neutrophils, endothelium, and endothelial vasoactive mediators would be expected to occur in myocardial tissue subjected to an ischemia-reperfusion injury.

HYPERBARIC OXYGEN THERAPY IN CARDIAC DISEASES

Hypertension

Patients scheduled for HBOT for wound care are often patients with combined cardiovascular risks including hypertension. In these patients, therapy for hypertension should be maintained and blood pressure measures during therapy should be monitored because the known vasoconstrictive effects of HBOT may increase blood pressure during therapy. In general, the interaction of HBOT and hypertension is of minimal consequence and ordinary precautions will prevent any inordinate increase in blood pressure during HBOT. The vasoconstrictor effects of HBOT have been addressed in a number of studies. Hink and colleagues[16] suggest that a reduction in endothelial ·NO caused by oxidation of this vasodilator molecule results in reduced vasodilation and a subsequent increase in systemic vasoconstriction. Neubauer and investigators[22] have found a decrease in cardiac output, heart rate, and stroke volume when compared with 1-atmosphere data. Peripheral vascular tone increase may contribute to the reduced cardiac output. Abel and colleagues[1] have examined hemodynamic responses to HBOT at 3 ATA. They found a decrease in cardiac output, an increase in systemic vascular resistance, and no change in PVR. They suggest that HBOT acted by increased sympathetic activity and promote using caution in patients with heart failure. In patients with compromised LV function, an increased afterload caused by peripheral vasoconstriction may not be accompanied by an increase in blood pressure if the left ventricle cannot respond to the increased afterload with

increased energy output to maintain cardiac output constant.

Bergo and Tyssebotn[23] have examined the effects of CO_2 on HBOT effects on hemodynamics in rats exposed to 3 ATA. They confirm the HBOT-induced vasoconstriction described by other investigators. In their study, LV systolic pressure increased, cardiac output and heart rate decreased, and stroke volume remained constant. Increased P_{CO_2} did not alter the HBOT effects on cardiac function or peripheral resistance. However, HBOT-induced cerebral vasoconstriction was reversed by CO_2. Nakada and coauthors[24] found in rats exposed to 2 ATA HBOT increased levels of epinephrine and norepinephrine originating from the adrenal gland, again suggesting that sympathetic activity is part of the HBOT response. The above data suggest that critically ill patients and patients with hypertension should be monitored carefully while receiving HBOT to detect significant increases in blood pressure. This may require multiple measures of blood pressure while the patient is being treated with HBOT. Conventional treatment for increased blood pressure will be efficacious in the HBOT environment. Treatment should be directed toward peripheral vasodilation (e.g., calcium channel blockers, long-acting nitrates) if blood pressure requires management during HBOT.

Ischemic Heart Disease

The well-known relation of myocardial ischemia as the functional consequence of coronary artery disease would on first principles be amenable to HBOT. The development of an ACS is related to partial or total occlusion of a coronary artery with resultant reduction in coronary blood flow, inadequate oxygenation of myocardial tissue, and either dysfunction or death of segments of myocardium. The loss of myocardial function results in compromised pump function of the heart and often results in acute followed by chronic heart failure. Prevention of ischemic injury or death of myocardium is a continuously sought-after goal for patients with ACS, and many clinical trials have been devoted to the treatment of acute and chronic coronary disease. Important landmarks in therapy of ACS include surveillance and prevention of lethal arrhythmias, thrombolytic therapy to restore blood flow to myocardium distal to coronary arteries occluded by acute thrombus, and primary percutaneous coronary intervention to open occluded coronary arteries and restore blood flow. Current therapy of ACS includes thrombolytic therapy, acute percutaneous coronary intervention, and a number of drugs to improve cardiomyocyte recovery and prevent ventricular rcmodeling.[25] Hood and colleagues[26] describe a 37-year-old man with an acute myocardial infarction (AMI) who had refractory ventricular tachycardia that was successfully controlled with use of HBOT at 3 ATA for 7 hours. After HBOT, the patient was also weaned from vasopressors. Clinical trials have demonstrated that minimizing the time between onset of symptoms and intervention to restore flow through the infarct artery preserves myocardial function and reduces mortality from AMI.[27] A role for HBOT in management of ACS seems intuitive; however, the studies done to date have demonstrated either no effect or small contributions to overall outcome. Thomas and coworkers'[28] findings in experimental animals initiated some interest in HBOT in reducing infarct size, but the study was not repeated. In a randomized study of 112 AMI subjects, Stavitsky and investigators[29] randomized half of the patients to HBOT plus thrombolysis and half to thrombolysis without HBOT. They note small reductions in time to pain re-

lief and serum creatine kinase concentration, and a small increase in discharge ejection fraction (51.7%) compared with the usual care group (48.4%). None of the changes was statistically significant. There was some indication that HBOT might reduce pain symptoms in AMI, but no improvement in LV function or other objective measures were shown, and the trial was not designed to report mortality. Dekleva and researchers[30] randomized 74 patients with AMI to either thrombolysis with streptokinase alone or thrombolysis plus HBOT at 3 ATA. The HBOT group showed an improved ejection fraction 3 weeks after the infarction; LV end-diastolic and end-systolic volumes measured by echocardiography were smaller in the HBOT group. Bennett and colleagues[31] reviewed 4 clinical trials that included 462 patients with ACS who received HBOT. They found no change in mortality. Evidence existed of reductions in risk for subsequent major adverse coronary events and some dysrhythmias after HBOT, particularly complete heart block (Table 25.1). Time to pain relief was reduced by HBOT, but there was some evidence of claustrophobia in monoplace chambers. Ruiz and coauthors[32] describe improved survival in dogs with acute coronary ligation. Six of seven dogs provided HBOT at 2 ATA survived, whereas three of eight control animals survived ($P < 0.10$). All deaths were due to ventricular fibrillation.

Thomas and coworkers[28] have evaluated the effect of HBOT at 2 ATA combined with recombinant tissue plasminogen activator on infarct size in dogs when using triphenyltetra-

Table 25.1 Summary of Hyperbaric Oxygen Effects on 462 Patients with an Acute Myocardial Infarction

MEASURE	RR FOR HBOT	P
Survival	0.64	0.08
MACE	0.12	0.03
Dysrhythmia	0.59	0.01
Complete heart block	0.32	0.02
Monoplace claustrophobia	31.6	0.02
Time to pain relief	353 minutes	0.0001

HBOT, hyperbaric oxygen therapy; MACE, major adverse cardiovascular event; RR, risk ratio.
    Data from a meta-analysis of four clinical trials (Bennett M, Jepson N, Lehm J: Hyperbaric oxygen therapy for acute coronary syndrome. Cochrane Database Syst Rev 18:CD004818, 2005).

zolium staining where infarcted tissue does not show staining, and the demarcated infarct area can be quantitated to measure infarct size. They found a substantial improvement in infarct recovery with combined HBOT and recombinant tissue plasminogen activator. Their results have not been repeated since their initial experiment.

Mogelson and investigators[33] studied 23 dogs provided with HBOT immediately after occlusion of the left anterior descending coronary artery. Infarct size was not different from a control group, and creatine kinase release was also similar to the control group. They concluded that HBOT does not reduce infarct size in the conscious dog and does not affect creatine kinase release or disappearance. In a rat model, Kim and researchers[34] examined the effects of HBOT pretreatment on infarct size. Infarct size was reduced in their ischemic-reperfusion model. They believe that the reduced infarct size resulted from the induction of catalase in myocardium. Sterling and colleagues[35] have measured infarct size in an ischemia-reperfusion model in rabbits. Using triphenyltetrazolium staining, they were able to reduce infarct size when HBOT was provided at the time of reperfusion, but not when provided after the onset of reperfusion. Although their study involved a different experimental model, their results support Thomas and coworkers'[28] findings.

An interesting use of HBOT in chronic ischemic heart disease is described in the study by Swift and colleagues,[36] who evaluated 24 patients with single-photon emission computed tomography thallium-201 exercise scintigraphy. Improved contraction after HBOT was demonstrated in 20 of 62 damaged LV segments. Of 42 segments with fixed contraction abnormalities after HBOT, 8 had reversible thallium defects, 4 had normal thallium kinetics, and 30 had fixed thallium defects. The authors suggest that HBOT could be used to identify hibernating myocardium that would be amenable to revascularization.

Sharifi and coauthors[37] have found a reduced rate of clinical restenosis in patients who were given HBOT after percutaneous coronary intervention. Patients in the HBOT group underwent exposure at 2 ATA in a monoplace chamber 2 hours before or immediately after percutaneous coronary intervention and another 18 hours after the first exposure. With the administration of HBOT, appreciable changes were noted in the heart rate and blood pressure. The mean blood pressure increased by 20 mm Hg, and the mean heart rate decreased by 10 beats/min. The increase in blood pressure responded to the intravenous administration of nitroglycerin and enalapril. Their composite end point of death, myocardial infarction or target vessel revascularization, occurred in 1 of 24 patients in the HBOT group and 13 of 37 patients in the control group. The difference was significant ($P < 0.001$). As noted earlier, Hood and colleagues[26] treated a 37-year-old man with refractory ventricular tachycardia and AMI with two 7-hour exposures to HBOT. The authors found that HBOT was successful in reducing the ventricular rate and in abolishing the requirement for vasopressors. During the first exposure, when the patient was critically ill, the number of ventricular ectopic beats was reduced during hyperbaric oxygenation. In a subsequent study, Gilmour and investigators[38] pretreated eight dogs with HBOT at 3 ATA, then occluded the left anterior descending coronary artery and found the animals developed LV failure. HBOT was repeated 10 minutes after coronary occlusion and continued for 1 hour. No improvement in LV function was found compared with a control group that was provided room air. The authors conclude that the HBOT did not improve LV function after coronary occlusion. Although isolated cases of apparent success with HBOT in acute coronary occlusion have been presented, the majority of animal and human data suggest little or no benefit exists to treating patients with an AMI with HBOT.

PACEMAKERS AND IMPLANTABLE DEFIBRILLATORS

In general, most implantable pacemakers are designed to withstand pressures up to about 100 fsw to accommodate divers who might have an implanted device. Individual pacemaker characteristics, however, should be sought from the manufacturer to be certain that a patient with a pacemaker can be exposed to increased ambient pressure without harm. Kratz and co-workers[39] have found that hermetically sealed implantable pacemakers were tolerant of pressures used in HBOT, but external pacemakers failed under pressure, whereas the electrical characteristics of pacing leads did not change. They suggest that external pacing under hyperbaric conditions could be accomplished by attaching a permanent pacemaker to the patient's temporary external leads. Trigano and researchers[40] tested several implantable rate-responsive pacemakers in an experimental hyperbaric chamber. They found that all pacemakers paced properly under pressures to 60 meters sea water (197 fsw), even though case distortion was noted in several pacemakers. Accelerometers incorporated into pacemakers to detect physical activity also appeared to function properly at 30 and 60 meters sea water, although several devices showed pressure effects on accelerometer function. Pitkin[41] has reviewed current practices on use of defibrillation inside a hyperbaric chamber. He indicates that defibrillation can be accomplished safely and defines indications and contraindications to this procedure. Patients with implanted internal cardiac defibrillators can be exposed to treatment levels of increased pressure without harm to the device. Information from the manufacturer on pressure tolerance for a given device is important to have; however, to date, no case of an internal cardiac defibrillator firing in a patient undergoing HBOT has been reported. If risk for an arrhythmia is low, the device can be disabled during HBOT to avoid inappropriate shocks while in the chamber. This would be of particular importance in a monoplace chamber.

CONGENITAL HEART DISEASE

The cyanotic state that accompanies complex congenital heart disease with a right-to-left shunt has interested physiologists and clinicians for centuries. When the anatomic foundation of cyanotic heart disease became under-

stood, attempts to alleviate cyanosis were made by providing oxygen at 1 atmosphere with the initially surprising result that there was little change in cyanosis.[42] This is particularly true when the cyanosis is primarily due to venous admixture, not to pulmonary dysfunction. The cause for this finding was that the desaturated hemoglobin from the venous system was mixing with arterial blood with a hemoglobin saturation of nearly 100%, and addition of oxygen at 1 ATA did little to increase venous oxygen content; hence minimal improvement was found in arterial desaturation. However, the addition of oxygen at pressures greater than atmospheric pressure allows plasma to be saturated with oxygen, and delivery of oxygen to tissues does not require unloading of oxygen from hemoglobin. Under these conditions, hemoglobin remains fully saturated as it traverses the tissue beds to the venous system. Boerema[43] describes the value of HBOT in operating on infants with cyanotic heart disease. The first cases underwent surgery in Amsterdam in 1960. He states: "The babies immediately became pink and stayed so during the whole operation."[43] With HBOT at 3 ATA, the dissolved oxygen content of blood is 4 to 6 mL/dL and supplies all the oxygen requirements without need for hemoglobin. In the case of a cyanotic infant, venous blood becomes fully saturated, and the cyanosis caused by mixing of poorly oxygenated venous blood with arterial blood through a right-to-left shunt is eliminated. Infants that are then fully oxygenated have a greater rate of survival after surgery.

This fact started an era of cardiac surgery under hyperbaric conditions to allow surgery to be done in a fully oxygenated child or adult. Hitchcock and coauthors[44] reviewed the status of cardiac applications of HBOT in 1963. They identify use of HBOT in acute coronary occlusion, for cardiac surgery, and for arterial occlusion, particularly occlusion of the internal carotid artery causing stroke. Most of these applications had not been established in humans at that time, but animal studies showed promise for ultimate application to humans. Hitchcock and coauthors[44] describe the lack of efficacy in reducing serum transaminase levels after coronary ligation in dogs treated with oxygen at 2.5 ATA. They also note that, although total coronary occlusion would prohibit the beneficial effects of HBOT on the myocardium, the presence of collateral circulation would allow blood with high Po$_2$ to reach ischemic tissue. They performed cardiac surgery in a 19-foot diameter hyperbaric operating room (Fig. 25.2) that provided a working environment at 3 ATA.[45] Gross[46] has reviewed his experience on cardiac surgery in infants younger than 1 year. He has performed surgery in a hyperbaric chamber for cyanotic complex anomalies of the heart. He notes a substantial improvement in surgical mortality for infants who underwent surgery in a hyperbaric environment. Successful surgery on infants with tricuspid atresia, tetralogy of Fallot, and transposition of the great vessels in infants breathing oxygen at 3 ATA has been reported. Using HBOT, surgeons could achieve suspension of the circulation for 2 to 3 minutes, enough time to repair an intracardiac defect. More recently, application of extracorporeal circulation has been perfected for infants, and the need for surgery in hyperbaric operating rooms has disappeared. Gross[46] took advantage of the ability to fully oxygenate a cyanotic infant with a right-to-left shunt under hyperbaric

conditions to improve survival in these early attempts to repair complex congenital cardiac lesions. Levitsky and Hastreiter[47] discuss the need for an extracorporeal perfusion for infants to avoid the high costs of a hyperbaric surgical facility. Currently, hyperbaric operating suites have been abandoned in the United States.

HYPERBARIC OXYGEN THERAPY IN CARDIAC SURGERY

HBOT has been used for management of sternal wound healing after heart bypass surgery and for therapy of iatrogenic air embolism occurring in association with open-heart surgery. Recent studies have addressed the value of HBOT in minimizing neurocognitive changes known to occur after bypass surgery.

NEUROPROTECTION

More recently, HBOT has been tested for neuroprotection after heart bypass surgery. Alex and coworkers[48] have examined the effect of pretreatment with HBOT at 1.5 ATA on cognitive function. They found improvements in

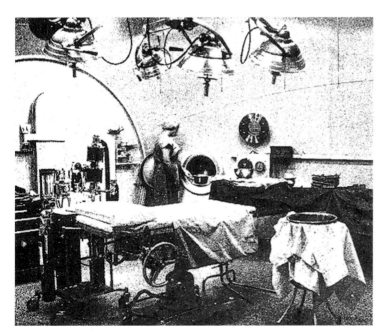

Figure 25.2 Photograph of Hitchcock's hyperbaric operating room ca. 1960. *(From Hitchcock CR, Haglin JJ: Hyperbaric oxygenation. Postgrad Med 38:157–169, 1965, by permission.)*

neuropsychometric function and reduction of inflammatory mediators produced by heart bypass surgery. Baumgartner and investigators[49] have found increased microemboli signals during HBOT at 2.5 ATA in patients with prosthetic heart valves. They interpreted these data to indicate that gaseous microemboli are produced by the prosthetic valves during HBOT exposure. The cause of neuropsychometric impairment after surgery is not well understood. In the case of evident air emboli, however, there is adequate knowledge to relate neuropsychometric impairment to either overt or occult gas embolism to the brain, and HBOT should be considered when air embolism is suspected (see Chapter 13).

IATROGENIC AIR EMBOLISM

Kol and others[50] used HBOT to manage air embolism complicating cardiac surgery. They found that a 17- to 20-hour delay resulted in significant residual neurologic impairment, whereas minimal delay to therapy resulted in full recovery. There is a case report of HBOT[51] for cerebral air embolism resulting from arterial air injection after cardiac surgery where the patient reported sudden onset of blindness after inadvertent injection of air into a radial artery. HBOT restored vision after one course of therapy at 60 fsw. Ziser and colleagues[52] describe 17 cases of accidental air embolism during cardiac surgery. All patients received HBOT. Approximately 47% (8 patients) achieved full recovery, 6 remained unconscious, and 3 died. Recovery was correlated with delay to HBOT. Patients treated within 5 hours of embolism demonstrated full or nearly full recovery, and long delays to therapy (9–20 hours) were characteristic of the patients with adverse outcomes. Toscano and coworkers[53] describe two cases of massive air embolism occurring during cardiac surgery that responded to HBOT. They recommend that all cases of accidental air embolism occurring during cardiac surgery be treated with HBOT. Takahashi and colleagues[54] reviewed their experience with iatrogenic arterial and pulmonary air embolism. Of their 34 reported cases, 16 arterial embolism

cases were related to cardiovascular procedures that included arteriography, ventriculography, and cardiac surgery. In many of the cases, the presence of air embolism to the brain was inferred by persistent neurologic impairment after expected recovery from anesthesia. HBOT was provided at 3 to 3.8 ATA of 100% oxygen for 90 minutes. In the 16 patients, 6 had a full recovery after 7 daily HBOT treatments, 5 had some residual neurologic defects but were not clinically impaired, and 5 died. Other causes of iatrogenic air embolism included hemodialysis and craniotomy. Their data suggest that a shorter time to treatment is an important predictor of outcome.

POSTBYPASS MEDIASTINITIS

Petzold and researchers[55] have used HBOT in conjunction with surgical debridement to treat a sternal wound infection in a patient who underwent orthotopic heart transplantation. HBOT had no adverse effects on the patient or the transplanted heart, and the authors believe that the added HBOT improved outcome in their immunosuppressed patient. Siondalski and others[56] have evaluated the combination of HBOT and aggressive surgical debridement to improve clinical outcomes in 55 patients with postoperative sternal wound infections or mediastinitis, or both, after sternotomy for cardiac surgery. Total hospital stay averaged 8 weeks; all patients were free of infection confirmed by culture before discharge. The authors did not use a control group but believe that the combined therapy improved outcome of these postoperative infections.

An interesting application of HBOT was studied by Todo and investigators,[57] who evaluated HBOT at 3 ATA for preserving explanted hearts in dogs in preparation for heart transplantation. This study would expand the heart donor pool in Japan to include donor hearts obtained after cardiac arrest with myocardial anoxia. The authors found that dog hearts could be preserved with a combination of hypothermia, HBOT, and a perfusate that included 2% magnesium sulfate in 2% glucose and 5% low-molecular-weight dextran. Hearts were transplanted up to 48 hours later and regained function.

In their review, Moon and Hart[58] describe methods for cardiac and other continuous monitoring techniques during HBOT. For critically ill patients, a multiplace chamber can be used as an extension of the intensive care unit; however, this application is accompanied by the increased operational complexity associated with chamber operation. As noted previously, patients with cardiac disorders can decompensate during HBOT, and measures should be prearranged to manage a cardiac patient whose condition deteriorates while receiving HBOT (see Chapter 7).

DRUG EFFECTS OF HYPERBARIC OXYGEN THERAPY

For most medications used by patients who might be candidates for HBOT, there are no known effects of HBOT on efficacy or dose effects of commonly used cardiovascular drugs. Specific instances of drug modification by HBOT are rare. Rump and coauthors[59] have examined the pharmacokinetics of lidocaine in human volunteers exposed to 2.5 ATA HBOT for 20 minutes alternating with 5-minute air breaks over a total of 75 minutes. Under HBOT, lidocaine injection caused dizziness and tinnitus, sweating, tre-mor, and coordination disturbances, even though maximum lidocaine concentrations were far less than therapeutic serum levels. The authors suggest that lidocaine side effects may result from interaction between lidocaine and HBOT. Davies and colleagues[60] demonstrate antagonistic effects of increased pressure to 12 ATA on anticonvulsant drugs. Their study includes diazepam, pentobarbital, and ethanol. However, similar effects have not been found at usual HBOT pressures. Rump and coauthors[61] have reviewed the literature on oxygen effects on a number of drug metabolic pathways. They conclude that "a single exposure to hyperbaric or hyperoxic conditions does not seem to affect single-dose pharmacokinetics of drugs eliminated by the kidney (gentamicin) or by the liver with a capacity-limited clearance (pentobarbital, the-ophylline, caffeine) or with a perfusion-limited clearance (pethidine, lidocaine)." Their conclusions were confirmed by Merritt and Slade's[62] study, which found no change in gentamicin pharmacokinetics under HBOT conditions. Whether Kramer and coworkers'[63] findings of an increased salicylate clearance in dogs exposed to 2.8 ATA of 100% oxygen can be extrapolated to humans is yet to be determined, although there appears to be no change in clinical efficacy of aspirin on platelet aggregation under HBOT conditions.

Seriakov and Feofanova[64] have evaluated the effects of HBOT on platelet aggregation and the effects of antiplatelet drugs. They found no changes in platelet aggregation and no changes in efficacy of aspirin or pentoxifylline in 65 coronary patients undergoing HBOT. Radcliff and Spencer describe changes in drug delivery rates[65] of a proprietary drug infusion system under hyperbaric conditions. In particular, infusion rates of propofol are slightly increased at 2 and 3 ATA.

Patients recommended for HBOT are likely to be taking one or more cardiovascular medications including antihypertensive medications. This class of medications that includes diuretics, calcium channel blockers, direct vasodilators, nitrates, beta-blockers, and aldosterone blockers is not known to change efficacy in HBOT environments. These medications can be continued during a course of HBOT, but usual care management dictates that they be reviewed in the context of the current medical condition. For example, a patient in shock from a clostridial infection would not be provided antihypertensive medications. Patients scheduled for HBOT should have blood pressure monitored before and after therapy. Patients who are undergoing HBOT and are critically ill should have blood pressure monitored during therapy. Therapy to maintain blood pressure during HBOT should be continued during therapy. No evidence is available to indicate an interaction between usual intravenous inotropic or pressor therapy and HBOT.

Weaver and Churchill[66] report on three cases of pulmonary edema that occurred during HBOT. One patient died. Two patients had diabetes, and one had severe aortic stenosis.

HBOT may contribute to pulmonary edema by increasing LV afterload, increasing LV filling pressures, increasing oxidative myocardial stress, decreasing LV compliance by oxygen radical-mediated reduction in ·NO antioxidant redox signal of right and left ventricles, inducing bradycardia with concomitant LV dysfunction, increasing pulmonary capillary permeability, or causing pulmonary oxygen toxicity. They indicate that patients with reduced LV function should be treated with caution.

REFERENCES

1. Abel FL, McNamee JE, Cone DL, et al: Effects of hyperbaric oxygen on ventricular performance, pulmonary blood volume, and systemic and pulmonary vascular resistance. Undersea Hyperb Med 27:67-73, 2000.
2. Shibata S, Iwasaki K, Ogawa Y, et al: Cardiovascular neuroregulation during acute exposure to 40, 70, and 100% oxygen at sea level. Aviat Space Environ Med 76:1105-1110, 2005.
3. Sun TB, Yang CC, Kuo TB: Effect of hyperbaric oxygen on cardiac neural regulation in diabetic individuals with foot complications. Diabet Med 23:360-366, 2006.
4. Lund VE, Kentala E, Scheinin H, et al: Effect of age and repeated hyperbaric oxygen treatments on vagal tone. Undersea Hyperb Med 32:111-119, 2005.
5. West BJ, Griffin LA, Frederick HJ, Moon RE: The independently fractal nature of respiration and heart rate during exercise under normobaric and hyperbaric conditions. Respir Physiol Neurobiol 145:219-233, 2005.
6. Lund V, Laine J, Laitio T, et al: Instantaneous beat-to-beat variability reflects vagal tone during hyperbaric hyperoxia. Undersea Hyperb Med 30:29-36, 2003.
7. Eckenhoff RG, Knight DR: Cardiac arrhythmias and heart rate changes in prolonged hyperbaric air exposures. Undersea Biomed Res 11:355-367, 1984.
8. Doubt TJ, Evans DE: Effects of hyperbaric oxygen exposure at 31.3 ATA on spontaneously beating cat hearts. J Appl Physiol 55:139-145, 1983.
9. Shida KK, Lin YC: Contribution of environmental factors in development of hyperbaric bradycardia. J Appl Physiol 50:731-735, 1981.
10. Lin YC, Shida KK: Mechanisms of hyperbaric bradycardia. Chin J Physiol 31:1-22, 1988.
11. Molenat F, Boussuges A, Grandfond A, et al: Haemodynamic effects of hyperbaric hyperoxia in healthy volunteers: an echocardiographic and Doppler study. Clin Sci (Lond) 106:389-395, 2004.
12. Savitt MA, Rankin JS, Elberry JR, et al: Influence of hyperbaric oxygen on left ventricular contractility, total coronary blood flow, and myocardial oxygen consumption in the conscious dog. Undersea Hyperb Med 21:169-183, 1994.
13. Wilson JM, Kligfield PD, Adams GM, et al: Human tecg changes during prolonged hyperbaric exposures breathing N2-O2 mixtures. J Appl Physiol 42:614-623, 1977.
14. Nelson AG, Wolf EG Jr, Hearon CM, Li B: Hyperbaric oxygenation treatments and metabolic enzymes in the heart and diaphragm. Undersea Hyperb Med 21:193-198, 1994.
15. Doubt TJ, Evans DE: Hyperbaric exposures alter cardiac excitation-contraction coupling. Undersea Biomed Res 9:131-145, 1982.
16. Hink J, Thom SR, Simonsen U, et al: Vascular reactivity and endothelial NOS activity in rat thoracic aorta during and after hyperbaric oxygen exposure. Am J Physiol Heart Circ Physiol 291:H1988-H1998, 2006.
17. Hong JP, Kwon H, Chung YK, Jung SH: The effect of hyperbaric oxygen on ischemia-reperfusion injury: An experimental study in a rat musculocutaneous flap. Ann Plast Surg 51:478-487, 2003.
18. Tjärnström J, Holmdahl L, Falk P, et al: Effects of hyperbaric oxygen on expression of fibrinolytic factors of human endothelium in a simulated ischaemia/reperfusion situation. Scand J Clin Lab Invest 61:539-545, 2001.
19. Buras JA, Stahl GL, Svoboda KK, Reenstra WR: Hyperbaric oxygen downregulates ICAM-1 expression induced by hypoxia and hypoglycemia: The role of NOS. Am J Physiol Cell Physiol 278:C292-C302, 2000.
20. Ueno S, Tanabe G, Kihara K, et al: Early post-operative hyperbaric oxygen therapy modifies neutrophile activation. Hepatogastroenterology 46:1798-1799, 1999.
21. Thom SR, Mendiguren I, Hardy K, et al: Inhibition of human neutrophil beta2-integrin-dependent adherence by hyperbaric O2. Am J Physiol 272:C770-C777, 1997.
22. Neubauer B, Tetzlaff K, Staschen CM, Bettinghausen E: Cardiac output changes during hyperbaric hyperoxia. Int Arch Occup Environ Health 74:119-122, 2001.
23. Bergo GW, Tyssebotn I: Cardiovascular effects of hyperbaric oxygen with and without addition of carbon dioxide. Eur J Appl Physiol Occup Physiol 80:264-275, 1999.
24. Nakada T, Koike H, Katayama T, et al: Increased adrenal epinephrine and norepinephrine in spontaneously hypertensive rats treated with hyperbaric oxygen. Hinyokika Kiyo 30:1357-1366, 1984.
25. Antman EM, Anbe DT, Armstrong PW, et al: ACC/AHA guidelines for the management of patients with ST-elevation myocardial infarction—executive summary: A report of the American College of Cardiology/American Heart Association Task Force on practice guidelines. J Am Coll Cardiol 44:671-719, 2004.
26. Hood WB, Yenikomshian S, Norman JC, Harold D: Levine HD treatment of refractory ventricular tachysystole with hyperbaric oxygenation. Am J Cardiol 22:738-741, 1968.
27. McNamara RL, Wang Y, Herrin J, et al, for the NRMI Investigators: Effect of door-to-balloon time on mortality in patients with ST-segment elevation myocardial infarction. J Am Coll Cardiol 47:2180-2186, 2006.
28. Thomas MP, Brown LA, Sponseller DR, et al: Myocardial infarct size reduction by the synergistic effect of hyperbaric oxygen and recombinant tissue plasminogen activator. Am Heart J 120:791-800, 1990.
29. Stavitsky Y, Shandling AH, Ellestad MH, et al: Hyperbaric Oxygen and Thrombolysis in Myocardial Infarction: The 'HOT MI' Randomized Multicenter Study. Cardiology 90:131-136, 1998.
30. Dekleva M, Neskovic AM, Vlahovic A, et al: Adjunctive effect of hyperbaric oxygen treatment after thrombolysis

on left ventricular function in patients with acute myocardial infarction. Am Heart J 148:589-566, 2004.

31. Bennett M, Jepson N, Lehm J: Hyperbaric oxygen therapy for acute coronary syndrome. Cochrane Database Syst Rev 18:CD004818, 2005.

32. Ruiz E, Haglin JJ, Hitchcock CR: Anemia and hyperbaric oxygenation in dogs subjected to coronary artery ligations. J Surg Res 13:339-348, 1972.

33. Mogelson S, Davidson J, Sobel BE, Roberts R: The effect of hyperbaric oxygen on infarct size in the conscious animal. Eur J Cardiol 12:135-146, 1981.

34. Kim CH, Choi H, Chun YS, et al: Hyperbaric oxygenation pretreatment induces catalase and reduces infarct size in ischemic rat myocardium. Pflugers Arch 442:519-525, 2001.

35. Sterling DL, Thornton JD, Swafford A, et al: Hyperbaric oxygen limits infarct size in ischemic rabbit myocardium in vivo. Circulation 88:1931-1936, 1993.

36. Swift PC, Turner JH, Oxer HF, et al: Myocardial hibernation identified by hyperbaric oxygen treatment and echocardiography in postinfarction patients: Comparison with exercise thallium scintigraphy. Am Heart J 124:1151-1158, 1992.

37. Sharifi M, Fares W, Abdel-Karim I, et al, Hyperbaric Oxygen Therapy in Percutaneous Coronary Interventions Investigators: Usefulness of hyperbaric oxygen therapy to inhibit restenosis after percutaneous coronary intervention for acute myocardial infarction or unstable angina pectoris. Am J Cardiol 93:1533-1535, 2004.

38. Gilmour DP, Hood WB Jr, Kumar R, et al: Experimental myocardial infarction. IX. Efficacy of hyperbaric oxygenation in ventricular failure after coronary occlusion in intact conscious dogs. Am J Cardiol 31:336-343, 1973.

39. Kratz JM, Blackburn JG, Leman RB, Crawford FA: Cardiac pacing under hyperbaric conditions. Ann Thorac Surg 36:66-68, 1983.

40. Trigano A, Lafay V, Blandeau O, et al: Activity-based rate-adaptive pacemakers under hyperbaric conditions. J Interv Card Electrophysiol 15:179-183, 2006.

41. Pitkin A: Defibrillation in hyperbaric chambers: A review. J R Nav Med Serv 85:150-157, 1999.

42. Friedman WF: Congenital heart disease in infancy and childhood. In: Braunwald E (ed): Heart Disease. Philadelphia, WB Saunders, 1980, pp 981-983.

43. Boerema I: The value of hyperbaric oxygen in thoracic surgery. Thorac Cardiovasc Surg 48:177-184, 1964.

44. Hitchcock CR, Harris RH, Haglin JJ: Hyperbaric oxygenation in cardiac and pulmonary disease. Dis Chest 44:622-632, 1963.

45. Hitchcock CR, Haglin JJ: Hyperbaric oxygenation. Postgrad Med 38:157-169, 1965.

46. Gross RE: Thoracic surgery for infants. J Thorac Cardiovasc Surg 48:152-176, 1964.

47. Levitsky S, Hastreiter AR: Cardiovascular surgical emergencies in the first year of life. Surg Clin North Am 52:61-75, 1972.

48. Alex J, Laden G, Cale AR, et al: Pretreatment with hyperbaric oxygen and its effect on neuropsychometric dysfunction and systemic inflammatory response after cardiopulmonary bypass: A prospective randomized double-blind trial. J Thorac Cardiovasc Surg 130:1623-1630, 2005.

49. Baumgartner RW, Frick A, Kremer C, et al: Microembolic signal counts increase during hyperbaric exposure in patients with prosthetic heart valves. J Thorac Cardiovasc Surg 122:1142-1146, 2001.

50. Kol S, Ammar R, Weisz G, Melamed Y: Hyperbaric oxygenation for arterial air embolism during cardiopulmonary bypass. Ann Thorac Surg 55:401-403, 1993.

51. Bove AA, Clark JM, Simon AJ, Lambertsen CJ: Successful therapy of cerebral air embolism with hyperbaric oxygen at 2.8 ATA. Undersea Biomed Res 9:76-80, 1982.

52. Ziser A, Adir Y, Lavon H, Shupak A: Hyperbaric oxygen therapy for massive arterial air embolism during cardiac operations. J Thorac Cardiovasc Surg 117:818-821, 1999.

53. Toscano M, Chiavarelli R, Tucci F, et al: Hyperbaric oxygenation in cerebral air embolism occurring during open-heart surgery. G Ital Cardiol 11:1301-1304, 1981.

54. Takahashi H, Kobayashi S, Hayase H, Sakakibara K: Iatrogenic air embolism: A review of 34 cases. In: 9th International Symposium on Underwater and Hyperbaric Physiology. Durham, NC, Undersea and Hyperbaric Medical Society, 1987, pp 931-948.

55. Petzold T, Feindt PR, Carl UM, Gams E: Hyperbaric oxygen therapy in deep sternal wound infection after heart transplantation. Chest 115:1455-1458, 1999.

56. Siondalski P, Keita L, Sicko Z, et al: Surgical treatment and adjunct hyperbaric therapy to improve healing of wound infection complications after sterno-mediastinitis. Pneumonol Alergol Pol 71:12-16, 2003.

57. Todo K, Nakae S, Wada J: Heart preservation with metabolic inhibitor, hypothermia, and hyperbaric oxygenation. Jpn J Surg 4:29-36, 1974.

58. Moon RE, Hart BB: Operational use and patient monitoring in a multiplace hyperbaric chamber. Respir Care Clin N Am 5:21-49, 1999.

59. Rump AF, Siekmann U, Fischer DC, Kalff G: Lidocaine pharmacokinetics during hyperbaric hyperoxia in humans. Aviat Space Environ Med 70:769-772, 1999.

60. Davies DL, Bolger MB, Brinton RD, et al: In vivo and in vitro hyperbaric studies in mice suggest novel sites of action for ethanol. Psychopharmacology (Berl) 141:339-350, 1999.

61. Rump AF, Siekmann U, Kalff G: Effects of hyperbaric and hyperoxic conditions on the disposition of drugs: Theoretical considerations and a review of the literature. Gen Pharmacol 32:127-133, 1999.

62. Merritt GJ, Slade JB: Influence of hyperbaric oxygen on the pharmacokinetics of single-dose gentamicin in healthy volunteers. Pharmacotherapy 13:382-385, 1993.

63. Kramer WG, Welch DW, Fife WP, et al: Salicylate pharmacokinetics in the dog at 6 ATA in air and at 2.8 ATA in 100% oxygen. Aviat Space Environ Med 54:682-684, 1983.

64. Seriakov VV, Feofanova ID: Hyperbaric oxygenation and antiaggregants: Effects on platelet function in patients with ischemic heart disease. Anesteziol Reanimatol (2):31-33, 1997.

65. Radcliffe JJ, Spencer I: Performance of the Baxter disposable patient-controlled analgesia infusor under hyperbaric conditions. Anaesthesia 49:796-797, 1994.

66. Weaver LK, Churchill S: Pulmonary edema associated with hyperbaric oxygen therapy. Chest 120:1407-409, 2001.

Contraindications to Hyperbaric Oxygen Therapy

26

D. Mathieu, MD, PhD

CONTRAINDICATIONS TO HYPERBARIC OXYGEN THERAPY

Hyperbaric oxygen therapy (HBOT) has been used in multiple clinical situations for more than 40 years. Some indications are now well established, and the level of evidence supporting its use is slowly increasing. However, no medical procedure is absolutely free of risk. The decision to use HBOT requires the assessment of the balance between the level of risk acceptable for the patient and his or her physician(s) and the expected benefit in the specific clinical situation. Thus, contraindications to HBOT may vary according to indication (absolute or relative), clinical setting (emergency or scheduled), patient condition (critical or ambulatory), and hyperbaric center capability (staff, equipment, location).

The first and major contraindication to treating a patient with HBOT is, of course, an inadequate hyperbaric facility. Examples include situations such as when the hyperbaric chamber is improper for medical use, the staff is not adequately trained, and there is a lack of equipment, procedures, or an emergency plan. These factors may seem self-evident, but accidents that have occurred in the past are sometimes still reported as adverse effects of HBOT. Widely accepted recommendations on hyperbaric facilities were issued by the European Committee for Hyperbaric Medicine in 1994[1]:

- The hyperbaric facility must have the adequate equipment, technical competence, staff and personal skill such that any potential accident, derangement, or problem will not be likely to interfere with the decision to accept a patient with an indication for HBOT.
- The hyperbaric facility must be located, equipped, and staffed in order to

guarantee the continuity of the treatment chain.

Currently, general agreement has been reached that patient management should be evidence based. However, that assertion may not apply well to patient safety for two main reasons: to expose a patient to highly predictable risk would be considered unethical even in the absence of any published evidence, and accidents and adverse effects are grossly under-reported in the medical literature.[2,3] In the industrial world, the control of risk uses the risk management method and is an essential component of the quality-control system.[4]

To better support the contraindications to HBOT, we follow that method and discuss first the potential hazards posed by HBOT, how to minimize patient complications by excluding those patients at special risk, and how to implement this process in clinical practice.

POTENTIAL HAZARDS POSED BY HYPERBARIC OXYGEN THERAPY

HBOT involves breathing oxygen at a pressure greater than atmospheric pressure. Although low, the incidence rate of adverse effects of HBOT is reported to be between 5 and 50 per 1000 hyperbaric exposures depending on the indication, clinical setting, and patient condition (Table 26.1). Injuries can occur because of changes in barometric pressure, high-pressure oxygen breathing, and the specific environment of the hyperbaric chamber.

Hazards Caused by Barometric Pressure Changes

Injuries caused by pressure changes are called *barotrauma*. They may be caused by a small change in pressure applied to intrapulmonary airways such as during artificial ventilation at ambient pressure, but the large changes in barometric pressure that occur during HBOT potentially put the patient at a special risk.[8,9]

Table 26.1 Incidence of Hyperbaric Oxygen Therapy Complications

AUTHORS	PLAFKI AND COLLEAGUES[5]	POISOT AND DELORT[6]	SHEFFIELD AND SMITH[7]	D. MATHIEU (UNPUBLISHED DATA)
Number of patients	782	1592	8078	6534
Number of exposures	11,376	17,420	166,701	61,259
Incidence per 1000 exposures				
All events	17	43	8.3	5.5
Middle ear barotrauma	3.8	1.2	4.4	1.5
Seizure	5	0.7	1.7	0.7

Barotrauma may affect any gas-containing cavity in the body: the ears, the sinuses, the lungs, the gut, or abnormal settings such as a dental abscess or pneumothorax.

Barotrauma during the compression phase occurs mainly in the ears and sinuses when entry of air into a cavity is impeded by obstruction, either anatomic or functional. Middle-ear barotrauma is the most frequent complication of HBOT and typically occurs in 0.1% to 0.5% of hyperbaric exposures, but it may arise in 1% to 9% of patients according to some series.[5,6] A few clinical series have reported astonishingly high rates of ear barotrauma such as 10% in Raphael and colleagues' study on CO poisoning[10] and 47% in Chavez and Adkinson's study on mandibular osteoradionecrosis.[11] These variations in incidence rates may be explained by differing clinical definitions, the clinical setting (emergency or chronic care), patient selection, patient education, compression protocol, and supervision.

Barotrauma may also occur during the decompression phase when gas that has entered a cavity during the compression is unable to escape. The resulting increase in intracavity gas pressure may lead to rupture and gas leakage to surrounding tissues and structures. If gas enters the circulation, it may embolize to the lungs and the systemic arteries with catastrophic consequences.

Lung barotrauma, although rare in the setting of HBOT, is the most threatening complication of HBOT. Decompression of 15 to 30 kPa (0.15–0.3 ATA) is sufficient to cause lung injury if the glottis is closed.[8] Lung barotrauma may cause hemoptysis, pneumothorax, pneumomediastinum, subcutaneous emphysema, or arterial gas embolism (see Chapter 13).

More insidious are injuries related to abnormal cavities that have become filled with air. A dental abscess may become exquisitely painful during pressure changes. A laryngocele or esophageal diverticula may overdistend during decompression and cause compression or even obstruction of the airways.[12] A simple pneumothorax may become a tension pneumothorax during decompression and cause respiratory distress, cardiovascular collapse, and cardiac arrest. Similarly, an airway obstruction such as that related to an asthma attack may theoretically cause an overexpansion injury during decompression. However, large case series suggesting this happens with any frequency do not exist. Similarly, the same mechanism may occur in patients with chronic obstructive pulmonary disease, although there is no published evidence that they are at a higher risk for pneumothorax. A rare but dramatic example of barotrauma is cerebral compression induced by the overexpansion of an intracranial pneumatocele during decompression.[13]

Hazards Caused by High-Pressure Oxygen Breathing

Oxygen toxicity occurs in three major forms: neurologic, pulmonary, and ocular.[14] Central nervous system oxygen toxicity is the most common manifestation of oxygen toxicity and manifests itself as a generalized tonic-clonic seizure ("grand mal" type). It may be heralded by facial twitching, nausea or vomiting, visual changes, and/or tachycardia. The incidence of oxygen convulsions during HBOT is reported to be between 0.1 and 30 per 1000 exposures.[15,16] This large range may be explained by variations in HBOT protocol, oxygen delivery systems, underlying pathology, and patient status.[17] Any patient with a low seizure threshold (epilepsy) or with a decreased seizure threshold (high fever, low glucose level, drugs such as corticosteroids) is at a high risk for an oxygen-induced seizure (see Chapter 23 for further description of central nervous system oxygen toxicity).

Pulmonary toxicity is rare and HBOT protocols have been designed to avoid its occurrence. However, exceptionally long treatment may induce respiratory symptoms.[18] Retinal oxygen toxicity is well known in premature newborns receiving oxygen therapy.[19] HBOT in newborns and young children requires special protocols and monitoring to prevent any risk[20,21] (see Chapter 6).

Prolonged series of HBOT may expose some patients to visual disturbances such as temporary myopia or difficulty with night vision.[14] Progressive cataract formation may occur in patients receiving more than 100 HBOT sessions[22] (see Chapter 24 for a discussion of the ophthalmologic issues associated with HBOT).

Hazards Caused by the Hyperbaric Chamber Environment

The hyperbaric chamber represents a special environment that may expose the patient to specific risks.[4] Only hazards that may be prevented by patient selection are discussed here.

Hazards Caused by Intensive Care Unit Patient Care

Many of the medical devices used to deliver care or to monitor patients have their function or their safety altered by the hyperbaric chamber environment. Regulation or Good Practice guidelines have been issued to guarantee a high level of safety, but they all require that any medical device has to be evaluated and approved for hyperbaric use before use in a hyperbaric chamber.[23-26]

This is of particular importance when a critically ill patient has to be treated with HBOT. Only hyperbaric centers equipped with medical devices allowing continuing intensive care unit monitoring and treatment and that are approved for hyperbaric use should treat such patients. Similarly, care for a critically ill patient requires specially trained personnel and specific organization and procedures.[27,28]

Hazards Caused by Oxygen Delivery Systems

Every oxygen delivery system has its own constraints. For example, demand valves require a specific breathing pattern, and because most patients are unfamiliar with this, they may experience an increase in work of breathing, leading to respiratory fatigue. The overboard dumping of expired gas increases the expiratory resistance and may cause an increased intrinsic positive end-expiratory pressure. Rebreathing may occur, leading to hypercapnia when ventilatory equipment has a large dead space and when minute ventilation is inadequate. A hood or an oversized mask is an example of such a situation.[28] Even in monoplace chambers where no special oxygen delivery system has to be used, the increased work of breathing because of the increased gas density and a decreased ventilatory drive in some patients may compromise respiratory status.[27]

Hazards Caused by Specific Patient Issues

Specific physiologic or pathologic conditions may expose a patient to a greater risk than usual or to a special risk.

Physiologic Conditions

Children: Infants and Young Children

Because of their usually normal respiratory capacity, children, especially infants and young children, may experience high tissue oxygen pressure and are therefore at greater risk for oxygen toxicity, in particular oxygen-induced seizures and retinal toxicity for newborns. Use of lower treatment pressures, short cycles of oxygen/air breaks, and constant monitoring of transcutaneous oxygen pressure are usually sufficient to assure safety. Antioxidant (vitamin C or E) supplementation has been proposed[20] but has not been fully evaluated in HBOT.

Older Adults

Older adults are also at special risk for problems during HBOT, not because of their age itself, but because they often have respiratory, cardiac, and/or vascular problems. Attention has to be paid to the respiratory and cardiac status during HBOT; a frequent pitfall is inadequate attention to the oxygen delivery system such as an unfitted mask or the demand valve set too high. Monitoring of transcutaneous pressure of oxygen and carbon dioxide may allow early detection of such problems.

Pregnant Women

The use of HBOT during pregnancy also raises some concerns because of the possible adverse effects on the fetus induced by high oxygen partial pressures, including teratogenicity, retinopathy, and cardiovascular effects, particularly alteration in placental blood flow and premature closure of the ductus arteriosus.[29-32] Experimental studies reporting increased fetal anomalies have used oxygen exposures far exceeding profiles of pressure and time that are used clinically.[29] Other experimental studies using typical protocols have not shown an increase in adverse fetal outcomes.[33-35] Clinical reports are also reassuring. The most extensive clinical experience has been reported from Russia, where more than 700 pregnant women have been treated with HBOT during all stage of gestation for hypoxemia of various origins.[36,37] According to these reports, HBOT significantly improves the condition of the mother and fetus and reduces perinatal complications and mortality. The lack of detrimental effects of HBOT on fetus and neonates has also been reported by some Western authors.[38-40]

A common indication for which a pregnant woman may require HBOT is carbon monoxide poisoning, and there is a moderate published experience with no adverse fetal consequence.[41,42]

Few reports have been published for other indications for HBOT; therefore, a careful assessment of benefit/risk balance is necessary, together with fetal monitoring.

Pathologic Conditions

Some patients may be exposed to special risk because of comorbidity, medications, or implanted medical devices. However, these situations should not be considered as contraindications to HBOT without an extensive evaluation and discussion.[43]

Patients with a History of Malignancy

The question whether HBOT may promote growth or recurrence of tumors has long been a matter of concern. Because cellular proliferation and angiogenesis promoted by HBOT are the rationale to use this treatment in delayed wound healing, it is understandable that those effects would be considered detrimental if they occurred in tumors.

Feldmeier and colleagues[44] evaluated this topic in 2003.[44] Careful review of cell culture and animal studies show that mechanisms of angiogenesis and cell proliferation are different between tumor growth and wound healing. Since the first article appeared in 1966 reporting that HBOT may have an enhancing effect of tumor growth,[45] published clinical studies suggest no more than a neutral effect of HBOT on tumor growth.[46-48] The authors conclude that the published literature provides little basis for HBOT to enhance malignant growth or metastases, and thus a history of malignancy should not be considered as a contraindication for HBOT (see Feldmeier and colleagues[44] for a complete discussion).

Patients with Diabetes Mellitus

It is a long-held belief that patients with diabetes experience a reduction in their insulin requirement and are therefore at increased risk for hypoglycemia when treated with HBOT. There are, however, no experimental studies and only a few, scant clinical reports on this problem. In clinical practice, hypoglycemia may occur in two different settings:

- *Patients with diabetes receiving adjunctive HBOT for an infection:* Infection can disturb diabetes management because of increases in insulin requirements. As the infection is treated, insulin doses will be reduced, and if this is not adequately addressed, hypoglycemia may occur during an HBOT session. These patients require close glycemic surveillance even inside the hyperbaric chamber.
- *Patients with "apparently" well-controlled diabetes receiving HBOT:* Several factors may contribute to the occurrence of a hypoglycemic episode during HBOT: fasting because of transportation and waiting time, maladjustment of antidiabetic drug regimen, and HBOT-induced changes in glycemic control. In particular, the decrease in catecholamine plasma level during hyperoxia may impair the hyperglycemic counter-reaction to a hypoglycemic episode and may explain its clinical expression.[49]

Patients with Implanted Medical Devices

Early pacemaker models were sensitive to pressure, but current models function normally in the hyperbaric environment. In case of doubt, it is wise to check with the manufacturer if a particular model may be exposed to high pressure[7] (see Chapter 25).

Patients with diabetes with implanted insulin pumps may also be referred for HBOT. A risk analysis does not demonstrate an increased risk.[25]

Patients Who Have Received Specific Medications

Bleomycin, a drug used in the treatment of various tumors, has long been recognized as an agent that may increase pulmonary oxygen toxicity. Experimental studies show that rats treated with bleomycin and oxygen exhibited an increase in the number of intra-alveolar cells and alveolar fibrin disposition at 24 and 48 hours.[50] Even though Rinaldo and investigators[51] have found a lesser degree of experimental lung injury when oxygen was administered 21 days after bleomycin, compared with 8 days, Goldiner and coauthors[52] have reported the occurrence of clinical lung toxicity with a mean period of 9.6 months between bleomycin administration and oxygen given during surgery. This study was challenged by Donat and Levy,[53] who reported no worsening of bleomycin lung toxicity by oxygen given perioperatively with a mean period of 6.4 months between bleomycin administration and oxygen therapy. Thus, the period when oxygen therapy appears to be safe after bleomycin administration has not been firmly established. A 1-year period is probably sufficient, so it appears that only recent treatment with bleomycin has to be considered a contraindication to HBOT.

Doxorubicin is another antitumor agent with which an increased mortality has been demonstrated in rats treated simultaneously with doxorubicin and HBOT.[54] No toxic effects have been reported in clinical use. It has been recommended that a 2- to 3-day interval between the last doxorubicin dose and administration of HBOT commences.[43]

Other drugs have also been considered as a concern when used concomitantly with HBOT. For example, cis-platinum (delay in fibroblast proliferation and collagen disposition), disulfiram (decrease in antioxidant production), and mafenide acetate (increase in local CO_2 production) have all been suggested to be contraindications to HBOT. Published evidence of clinically important side effects is weak, however, and these medications should not be considered as contraindications for HBOT.

Patients with Anxiety or Claustrophobia

Claustrophobia or confinement anxiety is a real concern and must not be underestimated because the incidence may be as high as 1% to 2% of the patients treated in a multiplace chamber[5-7] and 5% of patients treated in a monoplace chamber.[55] If not properly managed, claustrophobia leads to agitation and difficulty in oxygen administration, which may endanger the patient and others. Proper evaluation before treatment, sedation with a benzodiazepine, education, and reassurance by attendants inside and outside the chamber are usually sufficient to allow HBOT. A small number of patients (~1-2/1000) will not be able to control their anxiety and HBOT has to be interrupted or discontinued.[7]

GENERAL CONTRAINDICATIONS TO HYPERBARIC OXYGEN THERAPY

After the risk management methodology, contraindications to treatment are special situations that expose the patient to an unacceptable risk. Thus, defining contraindication cannot be done without taking into consideration the expected benefit of the treatment. For the purposes of this discussion, absolute contraindications to HBOT are conditions that pose a risk for death or major disability, and relative contraindications to HBOT are conditions where the potential risk is limited in intensity and duration[56] (Table 26.2).

Table 26.2 Contraindications to Hyperbaric Oxygen Therapy

ABSOLUTE

Unvented pneumothorax
Acute severe bronchospasm
Concomitant treatment with doxorubicin
Concomitant or recent treatment with bleomycin

RELATIVE

Upper airway infection
Allergic rhinitis
Chronic sinusitis and otitis
Chronic obstructive pulmonary disease with emphysema
History of pneumothorax or thoracic surgery
History of ear, nose, and throat surgery
Epilepsy
Optic neuritis
Arterial hypertension (uncontrolled)
Heart failure (uncontrolled)
Claustrophobia
Dangerous behavior

Absolute Contraindications

Major complications of HBOT include several pulmonary abnormalities and oxygen toxicity. Moreover, a patient should be treated with HBOT only if the medical and nursing staff and the chamber equipment are fit to care for the patient.

Absolute Contraindications Because of the Risk for Life-Threatening Barotrauma

Although there are only a few series reporting pulmonary barotrauma during HBOT,[57,58] the potential severity of this complication has always convinced hyperbaric physicians to carefully screen patients for conditions that may pose that risk.

Unvented Pneumothorax

Untreated pneumothorax is considered as an absolute contraindication because it can become a tension pneumothorax during decompression. A chest tube should be inserted before the patient begins HBOT. A chest radiograph is mandatory after tube insertion to confirm proper tube placement and venting. It is also an element of safe practice to obtain a chest radiograph before HBOT when a patient has been subjected to a procedure where there exists a risk for iatrogenic pneumothorax.

Venting is also required for other rare gas-filled structures if they might develop trapped gas during HBOT such as a lung pneumatocele, laryngocele, esophageal diverticulum, or intracranial pneumatocele.

Acute Severe Bronchospasm

Acute severe bronchospasm is an absolute contraindication because of the risk for intrapulmonary entrapped gas that will expand during decompression. Immediate treatment of bronchospasm with inhaled bronchodilators, steroids, and controlled ventilation should be available at the hyperbaric chamber for patients with asthma, patients with chronic obstructive pulmonary disease, and patients with smoke inhalation.

Absolute Contraindications Because of the Risk for Severely Disabling Oxygen Toxicity

Actual HBOT protocols have minimized the risk for severe oxygen toxicity. However, premature and young infants require special attention and protocols.

As reported earlier, some drugs enhance oxygen toxicity and are contraindications of HBOT, including:

- concomitant treatment with doxorubicin.
- concomitant or recent treatment with bleomycin.

Absolute Contraindications Because of an Unacceptable Risk for Endangering Patient Safety

A patient may be treated with HBOT only if the medical and nursing staff and the chamber equipment are fit to care for the patient. This especially applies to patients in critical condition (see Chapter 7 for an extended discussion of HBOT in critical care).

Relative Contraindications

Relative contraindications vary and have to be considered on a patient-by patient basis.[49] They may be classified according to the risk to be prevented.

Relative Contraindication Because of the Increased Risk for Barotrauma

Ear barotrauma is the most common side effect of HBOT. This complication is usually prevented by educating the patient about effective autoinsufflation techniques. For patients for whom the middle ear does not equilibrate, myringotomy and tympanostomy tube insertion may be required. Sinus barotrauma is the second most common side effect. Topical nasal decongestants are often used to prevent ear or sinus barotrauma, but they have not been proved effective.[59]

Upper airway infection, allergic rhinitis, and chronic sinusitis are relative contraindications to HBOT. Most frequently, these problems can be controlled, allowing HBOT to proceed.

Ear surgery for otosclerosis may also increase the risk for ear barotrauma, and transtympanic tube placement may be required before initiation of HBOT. Other forms of ear injury usually do not cause any problems.

Chronic obstructive pulmonary disease, especially emphysema, has been considered a contraindication for HBOT by some authors because of the expiratory obstruction and the risk for lung barotrauma. However, except during an acute severe bronchospastic attack, the degree of airway obstruction is never such that it causes substantial intrapulmonary gas retention assuming the decompression rate is slow as in usual HBOT protocols (1–2 m/min).

A history of pneumothorax or previous thoracic surgery has sometimes been reported as a contraindication to HBOT. These conditions do not usually pose a high risk unless an unvented space remains. However, physicians and attendants have to be aware of the patient's history and be prepared to manage a pneumothorax in the chamber.

Relative Contraindications Because of the Increased Risk for Oxygen Toxicity

To Reduce the Risk for Oxygen-Induced Convulsion

Various environmental and personal factors may modify the sensitivity to central nervous system oxygen toxicity, thus shortening the duration of the latent period and reducing the threshold pressure for the development of seizures.

Factors such as age, sex, circadian rhythm, temperature, and various drugs have been recognized to increase central nervous system oxygen toxicity, but the most potent factor is increased CO_2 concentrations. Thus, hypercapnia of any cause (hypoventilation, chronic obstructive pulmonary disease, effects of analgesics or narcotics, anesthesia, among others) should be avoided and patients with increased arterial CO_2 pressure closely monitored.[14]

Epilepsy has long been considered as a contraindication to HBOT. In fact, there is a lack of clinical evidence showing that patients with epilepsy have a greater risk for hyperoxic convulsions. Experimental studies suggest the mechanisms of epileptic and hyperoxic seizures are different.[60,61] In practice, patients with epilepsy who are medically well controlled may undergo HBOT without any major risk for seizure. Moreover, the consequences of oxygen-induced seizure in the HBOT environment are low. Close surveillance during HBOT, frequent air breaks, and adjustment of the anticonvulsant drug regimen (if needed) are usually sufficient to allow patients with a seizure disorder to be treated with HBOT.

To Reduce the Risk for Ocular Oxygen Toxicity

Premature and young infants are usually able to tolerate HBOT, but the risk for ocular toxicity must be considered. Lower oxygen pressure, frequent air breaks, and for some authors, antioxidant supplementation (vitamins C and E)[20] allow the treatment of these infants with a certain degree of safety. Optic neuritis has been reported as possibly implicated in a case of blindness occurring in a patient treated with HBOT. Although a causal relation was not clearly established, these patients should probably be followed with close ophthalmologic surveillance[43] (see Chapter 24).

Relative Contraindications Because of Increased Risks Related to the High Oxygen Pressure Environment

In healthy subjects, hyperoxia induces hemodynamic changes mainly because of hyperoxic vasoconstriction. There may be an increase in arterial pressure, bradycardia, and a decrease in cardiac output. The increase in ventricular afterload may be poorly tolerated and lead to ventricular failure, and the patient's cardiac function should be considered before HBOT if appropriate. Most patients with well-compensated heart failure experience few problems during HBOT.

Patients with chronic respiratory failure and hypercapnia may be at risk for acute hypoventilation because hyperoxic breathing suppresses the hypoxic respiratory drive. Although this risk is low in well-equilibrated patients, monitoring transcutaneous pressure of oxygen and carbon dioxide is important in these patients.

Relative Contraindications Because of Unacceptable Risks due to Psychologic and Behavioral Issues

Claustrophobia and anxiety should be controlled by psychological support or anxiolytic drugs, or both, to safely administer HBOT. Despite patient education and staff supervision, some patients may not comply with safety measures. Lack of compliance with safety measures despite staff efforts is a contraindication to HBOT.

CONSEQUENCES FOR CLINICAL PRACTICE

Once the potential hazards and contraindications to treatment are identified, there should be specific procedures to identify these issues to reduce patient risk. This is accomplished at the initial medical consultation and with a proper surveillance program.[15,28,56]

Initial Medical Consultation

During the initial medical consultation, the physician not only has to consider the indication for HBOT referral but also has to evaluate the patient for potential contraindications. A treatment-specific medical history and clinical examination should be performed. Otoscopy with observation of pressure equalization maneuvers is appropriate. A chest radiograph and, for adult patients, an electrocardiogram may be required. Pulmonary function tests with spirometry are useful to evaluate the respiratory condition of selected patients but are generally not needed.

The results of this initial medical consultation should be placed in the patient's record and there should be a specific plan for patient management during his or her stay at the hyperbaric facility that is available for review by all staff involved with the patient's hyperbaric treatment.

Patient Education

Except in the case of sedated patients or emergency patients, there should be an established program for patient education about the special requirements of the HBOT environment. Physiologic changes possibly experienced during HBOT have to be explained, and staff and equipment should be introduced. Ideally, the functioning of the equipment to be used should also be explained.

Ear pressure equalization maneuvers must be taught before the first HBOT session. Safety is also an important part of patient education: The need for cotton clothes, forbidden items, emergency measures in case of fire, or urgent decompression have to be explained. Patients should receive a document summarizing these items before initiating the treatment.

Chamber Attendance and Monitoring

The presence of a chamber attendant during the HBOT session is an important safety measure. Chamber attendants help patients to equalize ear pressure and they can monitor patients during the session. Their presence inside the multiplace chamber reassures patients and helps to avoid any unsuitable behavior.

CONCLUSION

As with any treatment, HBOT has its own side effects and contraindications. Even if the overall risk is low, contraindications have to be considered during the initial medical consultation to minimize the most severe risks: lung barotrauma and oxygen toxicity. Most medical conditions are only relative contraindications, and the balance between expected benefit from HBOT and anticipated risk has to be evaluated before a patient should undergo HBOT.[62]

REFERENCES

1. European Committee for Hyperbaric Medicine Recommendations of the jury of the first European Consensus Conference on Hyperbaric Medicine, Lille, 1994. In: Marroni A, Mathieu D, Wattel F (eds): The ECHM Collection, Vol. 1. Flagstaff, Ariz, Best Publishing Company, 2005, pp 133-142.
2. Sutton J, Standen P, Wallace A: Accidents to patients in hospital: A comparative study. Nurs Times 90:52-54, 1994.
3. Elnitsky C, Nichols B, Palmer K: Are hospital incidents being reported? J Nurs Adm 27:40-46, 1997.
4. Kot J, Houman R, Gough-Allen R: Safety in hyperbaric medicine. In: Mathieu D (ed): Handbook on Hyperbaric Medicine. Dordrecht, The Netherlands, Springer, 2006, pp 691-711.
5. Plafki C, Peters P, Almeling M, et al: Complications and side effects of hyperbaric oxygen therapy. Aviat Space Environ Med 71:119-124, 2000.
6. Poisot D, Delort G: Accidents survenus au cours de traitements hyperbares dans le service du centre hospitalier de Bordeaux. Med Sub Hyp 6:84-91, 1987.
7. Sheffield P, Smith A: Physiological and pharmacological bases of hyperbaric oxygen therapy. In: Bakker D, Cramer F (eds): Hyperbaric Surgery. Flagstaff, Ariz, Best Publishing Company, 1999, pp 63-109.
8. Hamilton-Farrell M, Bhattacharyya A: Barotrauma. Injury 35:359-370, 2004.
9. Roque F, Simao A: Barotraumatism. In: Mathieu D (ed): Handbook on Hyperbaric Medicine. Dordrecht, The Netherlands, Springer, 2006, pp 715-729.
10. Raphael JC, Elkharrat D, Jars-Guincestre MC, et al: Trials of normobaric and hyperbaric oxygen for acute carbon monoxide intoxication. Lancet 2:414-419, 1989.
11. Chavez J, Adkinson C: Adjunctive hyperbaric oxygen in irradiated patients requiring dental extractions: Outcome and complications. J Oral Maxillofac Surg 59:518-522, 2001.
12. Plante-Longchamp G: Une redoubtable contre-indication à la plongée sous marine: la laryngocele. Med Aeronaut Spat Med Subaqu Hyperbare 20:63-65, 1981.
13. Mahadir C, Szymczak A, Sutherland GR: Intracerebral pneumotocele presenting after air travel. J Neurosurg 101:340-342, 2004.
14. Bitterman N, Bitterman H: Oxygen toxicity. In: Mathieu D (ed): Handbook on Hyperbaric Medicine. Dordrecht, The Netherlands, Springer, 2006, pp 731-765.
15. Davis J, Dunn J, Heimbach R: Hyperbaric medicine: Patients selection, treatment procedures and side effects. In: Davis J, Hunt T (eds): Problem Wounds. The Role of Oxygen. New York, Elsevier, 1988, 225-235.
16. Hampson N, Simonson S, Kramer C, Piantadosi C: Central nervous system oxygen toxicity during hyperbaric treatment of patient with carbon monoxide poisoning. Undersea Hyperb Med 23:215-219, 1996.
17. Hampson N, Atik D: Central nervous system oxygen toxicity during routine hyperbaric oxygen therapy. Undersea Hyperb Med 30:147-153, 2003.
18. Louge P, Cantais E, Palmier B: Acute respiratory distress syndrome after prolonged hyperbaric oxygen therapy: A case of pulmonary oxygen toxicity? Ann Fr Anesth Reanim 20:559-562, 2001.

19. Palmer E, Flynn J, Hardy R, et al: Incidence and early course of retinopathy of prematurity. Ophthalmology 98:1628-1640, 1991.

20. Finer N, Schindler R, Grant G, et al: Effect of intramuscular vitamin E on frequency and severity of retrolental fibroplasia. A controlled trial. Lancet 1:1087-1091, 1982.

21. Torbati D, Peyman G, Wafapoar H, et al: Experimental retinopathy by hyperbaric oxygenation. Undersea Hyperb Med 22:31-39, 1995.

22. Palmquist B, Philipson B, Barr P: Nuclear cataract and myopia during hyperbaric oxygen therapy. Br J Ophthalmol 68:113-117, 1994.

23. Hyperbaric facilities. NFPA 99 standard for health care facilities chapter 19. In: Klein B (ed): Health Care Facilities Handbook, 5 ed. Quincy, Mass, National Fire Protection Association, 1996, pp 525-582.

24. EN 14 931: Pressure Vessels for Human Occupancy. Multiplace Pressure Chamber Systems for Hyperbaric Therapy. Performance, Safety Requirements and Testing. Brussels, Belgium, CEN, 2006.

25. COST Action B14. A European Code of Good Practice for hyperbaric oxygen therapy. Eur J Underwater Hyperb Med 5(suppl 1):43-61, 2004.

26. Chimiak J: Evaluating equipment and materials for use in a hyperbaric oxygen environment: The clinical hyperbaric evaluation and testing program. In: Workman N (ed): Hyperbaric Facility Safety. Flagstaff, Ariz, Best Publishing Company, 1999, pp 675-688.

27. Weaver L: Management of critically ill patients in the monoplace hyperbaric chamber. In: Kindwall E, Wheelan H (eds): Hyperbaric Medicine Practice, 2nd ed. Flagstaff, Ariz, Best Publishing Company, 1999, pp 245-322.

28. Kemmer A, Muth C, Mathieu D: Patient management. In: Mathieu D (ed): Handbook on Hyperbaric Medicine. Dorbrecht, The Netherlands, Springer, 2006, pp 651-669.

29. Ferm VH: Teratogenic effects of hyperbaric oxygen. Proc Soc Exp Biol Med 116:975-976, 1964.

30. Fujikura T: Retrolental fibroplasia and prematurity in newborn rabbits induced by maternal hyperoxia. Am J Obstet Gynecol 90:854-858, 1964.

31. Telford I, Miller P, Haas G: Hyperbaric oxygen causes fetal wastage in rats. Lancet 2:220-221, 1969.

32. Miller P, Telford I, Haas G: Effects of hyperbaric oxygen on cardiogenesis in the rat. Biol Neonate 17:44-52, 1971.

33. Cho S, Yun D: The experimental study on the effect oh hyperbaric oxygen on the pregnancy wastage of rats with acute carbon monoxide poisoning. Seoul J Med 23:67-75, 1982.

34. Gilman S, Greene K, Bradley M, Biersner R: Fetal development: Effects of simulated diving and hyperbaric oxygen treatment. Undersea Biomed Res 9:297-304, 1983.

35. Assali N, Kirschbaum THL, Dilts P: Effects of simulated diving and hyperbaric oxygen treatment on uteroplacental and fetal circulation. Circ Res 22:573-588, 1968.

36. Molzhaninov E, Chaika V, Domanova A: Experience and prospects of using hyperbaric oxygenation in obstetrics. In: Yefuni SN (ed): Proceeding of the Seventh International Congress on Hyperbaric Medicine, Moscow, 1981. Moscow, Russia, Nauka, 1983, pp 139-141.

37. Chaika V: The immediate and long term results to development of children born by mother with hyperbaric oxygenation. In: Yefuni SN (ed): Proceeding of the Seventh International Congress on Hyperbaric Medicine, Moscow, 1981. Moscow, Russia, Nauka, 1983, pp 364-367.

38. Ledingham I, McBride T, Jennett W: Fatal brain damage associated with cardiomypathy of pregnancy with notes on caesarean section in a hyperbaric chamber. Br Med J 4:285-287, 1968.

39. Sparacia B: HBO in the treatment of fetal growth deficiencies. In: Oriani G, Marroni A, Wattel F (eds): Handbook on hyperbaric medicine. Berlin, Springer, 1996, pp 791-797.

40. Barthelemy L, Michaud A: Traitement par l'oxygène hyperbare des insuffisances vasculaires foeto-placentaires. Med Sub Hyp Int 3:19-39, 1999.

41. Van Hoesen K, Camporesi E, Moon R, et al: Should hyperbaric oxygen be used to treat the pregnant patient for acute carbon monoxide poisoning? A case report and literature review. JAMA 261:1039-1043, 1989.

42. Elkharrat D, Raphaël JC, Korach JM, et al: Acute carbon monoxide intoxication and hyperbaric oxygen in pregnancy. Intensive Care Med 17:289-292, 1991.

43. Kindwall E: Contra-indications and side effects to hyperbaric oxygen therapy. In: Kindwall E, Weelan H (eds): Hyperbaric Medicine Practice, 2nd ed. Flagstaff, Ariz, Best Publishing Company, 1999, pp 83-97.

44. Feldmeier J, Carl U, Hartman K, Sminia P: Hyperbaric oxygen: Does it promote growth or recurrences of malignancy? Undersea Hyperb Med 30:1-18, 2003.

45. Johnson RJR, Lauchlan SC: Epidermoid carcinoma of the cervix treated by Co therapy and hyperbaric oxygen. In: Brown IW, Cox BG (eds): Proceedings of the Third International Congress on Hyperbaric Medicine. Washington, DC, National Academy of Sciences, 1966, pp 648-652.

46. Dische S: Hyperbaric oxygen. The medical research council trials and their clinical significance. Br J Radiol 51:888-894, 1979.

47. Denham W, Yeoh EK, Ward GG, et al: Radiation therapy in hyperbaric oxygen for head and neck cancer at Royal Adelaide Hospital 1964-1969. Int J Radiat Oncol Biol Phys 13:201-208, 1987.

48. Marx RE: Radiation injury to tissue. In: Kindwall E, Whelan H (eds): Hyperbaric Medicine Practice, 2nd ed. Flagstaff, Ariz, Best Publishing Company, 1999, pp 665-723.

49. Howley ET, Cox RH, Welch HG, Adams RP: Effect of hyperoxia on metabolic and cathecolamine responses to prolonged exercise. J Appl Physiol 54:59-63, 1983.

50. Berend N: The effect of bleomycin and oxygen on rat lung. Pathology 16:136-139, 1984.

51. Rinaldo J, Goldstein R, Snider G: Modification of oxygen toxicity after lung injury by bleomycin in hamsters. Am Rev Respir Dis 126:1030-1033, 1982.

52. Goldiner P, Carlon G, Cvitkovic E, et al: Factors influencing postoperative morbidity and mortality in patients treated with bleomycin. Br Med J 1:1664-1667, 1978.

53. Donat S, Levy D: Bleomycin associated pulmonary toxicity: Is perioperative oxygen restriction necessary? J Urol 160:1347-1352, 1998.

54. Upton PG, Yamaguchi KT, Myers S, et al: Effects of antioxidants and hyperbaric oxygen in ameliorating

experimental doxorubicin skin toxicity in the rat. Cancer Treat Rep 70:503-507, 1986.

55. Weaver L: Monoplace hyperbaric chamber use of US Navy Table 6: A 20 year experience. Undersea Hyperb Med 33:85-88, 2006.

56. Wattel F, Mathieu D, Bocquillon N, Linke JC: Pratique de l'oxygénothérapie hyperbare. Prise en charge des patients. In: Wattel F, Mathieu D (eds): Traité de Médecine Hyperbare. Paris, Ellipse, 2002, pp 544-561.

57. Unsworth IP: Pulmonary barotraumas in a hyperbaric chamber. Anesthesiology 28:675-678, 1973.

58. Murphy DG, Sloan EP, Hart RG, et al: Tension pneumothorax associated with hyperbaric oxygen therapy. Am J Emerg Med 9:176-179, 1991.

59. Carlson S, Jones J, Brown M, Hess C: Prevention of hyperbaric-associated middle ear barotrauma. Ann Emerg Med 21:1468-1471, 1992.

60. Vion-Dury J, LeGal La Salle G, Rougier I, Papy JJ: Effects of hyperbaric and hyperoxic conditions on amygdala-kindled seizures in rat. Exp Neurol 92:513-521, 1986.

61. Garcia-Cabrera I, Milgram NW, Berge OG: Electroencephalographic and behavioural correlates of seizure development in rats in response to hyperbaric exposure. Epilepsy Res 7:65-71, 1990.

62. European Committee for Hyperbaric Medicine: Recommendations of the jury of the 7th European Consensus Conference on Hyperbaric Medicine, Lille, 2004. Available at: http://www.echm.org. Accessed October 10, 2006.

Index

Page numbers followed by *f* indicate figures; those followed by *t* indicate tables.